RADIOLOGY
of
BONE DISEASES

THIRD EDITION

GEORGE B. GREENFIELD, M.D.

Chairman, Department of Radiology,
Mount Sinai Hospital Medical Center
Professor of Diagnostic Radiology,
Rush Medical College, Chicago, Illinois
Consultant Radiologist, Hines Veterans
Administration Hospital, Hines, Illinois

RADIOLOGY
of
BONE DISEASES

THIRD EDITION

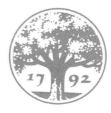

J. B. LIPPINCOTT COMPANY
Philadelphia and Toronto

Third Edition

Copyright © 1975 by J. B. Lippincott Company
Copyright © 1969 by J. B. Lippincott Company
Copyright © 1980 by George B. Greenfield, M.D. All rights reserved. No part of this book may be used or reproduced in any manner whatsoever without written permission except in the case of brief quotations embodied in critical articles and reviews. Printed in the United States of America. For information address J. B. Lippincott Company, East Washington Square, Philadelphia, Penna. 19105

ISBN-0-397-50432-2

Printed in the United States of America

3   5   6   4

Library of Congress Cataloging in Publication Data

Greenfield, George B
        Radiology of bone diseases.
        Includes bibliographies and index.
        1. Bones—Radiography. I. Title. [DNLM: 1. Bone and bones
—Radiography. WE200 G812r]
RC930.5.G73   1980   616.7'107572   80-12119
ISBN 0-397-50432-2

To
B. A. G., E. J. G., and S. A. G.

CONTENTS

1
THE ANALYTICAL APPROACH TO BONE RADIOLOGY

2
LOSS OF BONE DENSITY

3
ALTERATION OF BONE TEXTURE

6

THE CARDINAL ROENTGEN FEATURES 367

7

THE SOLITARY LESION

BENIGN TUMORS AND TUMORLIKE CONDITIONS OF BONE

DIFFERENTIAL DIAGNOSIS OF BENIGN CONDITIONS OF BONE

MISCELLANEOUS, RARE, AND NONDESCRIPT BONE LESIONS

8

THE SOFT TISSUES

9

THE JOINTS

PREFACE

Not only has there been clinical and scientific advancement in our knowledge of bone diseases over the past 5 years, but the role of the radiologist has become expanded.

It is no longer sufficient only to predict the histology of bone lesions. The radiologist must act in the capacity of a true consultant to guide the clinician through the maze of the newer imaging techniques, as well as standard techniques, in order to achieve maximum clinical and cost effectiveness.

The newer techniques, particularly that of CT Scanning, are introduced into this edition without obscuring the major emphasis on conventional radiologic examinations.

A suggested procedure for workup of a patient with suspect bone metastases is described.

The advances of the past 5 years in the radiographic diagnosis of bone diseases are interwoven in this new edition. The source material for this is 15 journals, including several foreign journals.

The recent advances in metabolic bone diseases and the subclassification of bone tumors are presented. Computer-generated tables of predilection sites of various primary bone tumors are also included, along with the reclassification of bone tumors according to the World Health Organization.

The three original objectives of this book, that is, the grouping of diseases by predominant roentgen features, the unification of scattered recent information in the literature, and the analytical approach, again are retained and emphasized.

George B. Greenfield, M.D.

PREFACE TO THE FIRST EDITION

The purpose of this book is threefold. The first is to present a well-illustrated volume of bone diseases in which the diseases are grouped according to roentgen features while maintaining an integral description of each entity. The second purpose is to unify the widely scattered information that has appeared in the radiological literature of the past decade. In addition, an analytical approach to the diagnosis of bone lesions is presented. This comprises basic understanding and objective analysis of specific roentgen features correlated with clinical and laboratory findings to determine a multidisciplinary "total information profile." This method can lead to a correct conclusion more often than can the method of pattern matching, and may permit reaching a diagnosis of entities that the observer has not previously seen.

The grouping of diseases by predominant roentgen features rather than by etiology renders the emergence of an illustrated section of differential diagnosis out of each segment of the book, and transforms the Table of Contents into a Table of Differential Diagnosis. It is also appropriate to include tables of diagnostic possibilities of many roentgen findings. The practical advantage of this arrangement to an observer who is trying to interpret a difficult radiograph is real.

This book also answers the need for a single volume that concisely unifies information that is widely scattered in the periodical literature.

The vast majority of illustrations are fresh and unpublished radiographs. It is hoped that they contribute a valuable addition to the literature and that these cases will be of help to people of all specialities who come into contact with bone disease.

George B. Greenfield, M.D.

ACKNOWLEDGMENTS

I wish to thank both the staff of the Radiology Department of Mount Sinai Hospital Medical Center for its support, and the physicians who contributed cases and are individually credited in the captions.

Also I would like to thank Mr. Z. Mandelstam again for his fine photography.

George B. Greenfield, M.D.

RADIOLOGY
of
BONE DISEASES

THIRD EDITION

1

THE ANALYTICAL APPROACH TO BONE RADIOLOGY

GENERAL CONSIDERATIONS

The diagnosis of bone lesions is a multidisciplinary task, involving the best efforts of the radiologist, the clinician, the clinical pathologist, and the anatomical pathologist. A widespread and erroneous belief among radiologists is that the pathologist, merely by looking down the barrel of the microscope, can confirm or negate the radiologist's intuitive diagnosis, which is often made by the "Aunt Minnie" method of instantaneous pattern recognition. Often, the clinical picture is not obtained or is completely ignored. Many radiologists never consider laboratory values because they are totally unfamiliar with them. The above factors contribute to an aura of pessimism surrounding radiographic diagnosis, based on a reputation of low accuracy and summarized by the sentiment: "All bone lesions look alike anyway." The similarities and differences among various bone lesions, however, are in the eye of the beholder, or more accurately, in the methodological organization of the mind of the beholder and his approach to the diagnosis of bone pathology.

The basic approach should be simple. The roentgen pattern should be accurately and objectively analyzed with respect to approximately 32 distinct, independent features. On the basis of this objective analysis, a list of differential diagnoses can be prepared. This list should be broad, so as not to exclude the correct diagnosis. The differential diagnoses are then applied to the particular case. The age of the patient is of prime importance, and the probabilities for the presence of many disease entities can be eliminated on this basis alone. The sex and the race of the patient are also important. These factors are correlated with the total clinical picture, and the biochemical values are determined. This effectively reduces the list to a few possibilities. A suitable biopsy site, if indicated, may then be determined from the roentgenogram, and adequate and representative biopsy material delivered to the pathologist. The objective analysis should be made before clinical influences prevail, so as not to prejudice an accurate description.

It is of fundamental importance to realize that the radiograph does not substitute for a biopsy, and that the possibilities for diagnosis on the basis of the radiograph alone are extremely limited in many instances, as is the possibility for establishing a diagnosis solely on the basis of a microscopic section, or solely on the clinical picture. It is the multidisciplinary, total information profile that should be the diagnostic procedural goal.

The clinical correlation of objective radiological patterns is an exercise in statistics. However, bone has a limited response to disease processes. There are many more diseases than avenues of bone response, so it should not be surprising that different lesions can have similar patterns. In addition, many lesions distinguished by a typical characteristic on roentgen films often present an atypical appearance. To these atypical lesions that may lack one or more distinctive features (*e.g.*, the "sunburst" appearance in osteosarcoma, or laminated periosteum in Ewing's sarcoma), an old adage seems applicable: "A three-legged dog is still a dog."

Only about one dozen primary bone tumors occur with appreciable frequency, of which most are readily diagnosable radiologically in their typical forms. A definitive diagnosis of certain asymptomatic benign entities, such as benign cortical defect or nonossifying fibroma, may be made on radiological grounds.

The statistical correlation for a solitary atypical lesion can be no better than a guess, which may be valid when applied on a percentage basis to a large population, but which is inadequate when applied to the individual patient. Thus, a definitive procedure such as amputation must never be performed on the basis of the roentgen picture alone, but only after adequate tissue sections have first been studied. The roentgen findings alone, isolated from clinical and pathologic reality, should be considered insufficient information in themselves for a definitive diagnosis.

The purpose of this book is to outline the many features of bone lesions to be evaluated radiologically and to present a differential diagnosis of roentgen signs. A brief sketch of physiology and pathology of the various disease entities is presented and arranged according to radiographic findings. This book does not delve deeply into the study of bone diseases; many excellent textbooks are available for such information. Physiology, particularly in the metabolic bone diseases, is stressed, because an understanding of biochemical processes is essential for diagnosis.

ANATOMY OF BONE

DEVELOPMENT

All connective tissues, including bone, are derived from pluripotential undifferentiated mesenchymal cells. These cells differentiate into chondroblasts and chondrocytes that form and maintain cartilage: osteoblasts that lay down osteoid matrix and form osteocytes; and osteoclasts that lyse bone in the continuous turnover processes.

The two physiological mechanisms of bone production and development in the embryo are enchondral and intramembranous ossification. The major portion of the bony structure is ossified in preformed cartilage with enchondral bone formation of the spongiosa. A periosteal collar forms, and the inner or cambium layer forms appositional bone by intramembranous ossification. The mechanism of growth in length is by enchondral ossification.

Several bones are not preformed in cartilage but through direct transition from mesenchyme; this is intramembranous ossification. These bones ossify slightly earlier than enchondral bones. They are listed below.

BONES OSSIFIED IN MEMBRANE

1. Parietal bone
2. Temporal bone (squama and tympanic parts)
3. Upper occipital squamosa
4. Frontal bone
5. Vomer
6. Medial plate of the pterygoid
7. Facial bones
8. Clavicles—develop secondary enchondral ossification centers
9. Mandible

The remainder of the long bones, cuboid bones, and flat bones are preformed in cartilage. These differences in bone production assume significance if generalized disease causes a disturbance of one mechanism but not the other.

The types of bones are the tubular bones, long and short, the flat bones, the cuboidal bones, and the mandible and clavicle.

OSSIFICATION

The tubular bones are composed of an epiphysis, epiphyseal cartilage plate or physis, zone of provisional calcification, metaphysis and diaphysis. The diaphysis is composed of the spongiosa and cortex and is covered by the periosteum. The periosteum is attached at the metaphysis and, in adults, along the shaft.

In addition to epiphyses, there are apophyses. An apophysis is an accessory ossification center that develops late and forms the protrusions from the shaft that serve as attachments for muscles and ligaments (*e.g.,* the greater trochanter). Apophyses do not contribute to a major growth in length of long bones. They have the same structure as epiphyses and fuse to the shaft in the same manner. Occasionally, epiphyseal and apophyseal centers may persist without fusion to become accessory ossicles (*e.g.,* os acromiale, os acetabuli). The number of epiphyseal and apophyseal centers of the long bones varies according to the bone, and these are summarized below.

SECONDARY OSSIFICATION CENTERS OF THE TUBULAR BONES

No epiphyses
  Middle phalanx of little toe
1 epiphysis
  Metacarpals
  Phalanges
2 epiphyses
  Radius
  Ulna
  Femur
  Tibia
  Fibula
3 epiphyses
  Humerus—Head, trochlea, and capitulum
1 apophysis
  Tibia—Tuberosity
  Radius—Tuberosity
2 apophyses
  Femur—Greater and lesser trochanters
4 apophyses
  Humerus —Greater and lesser tuberosities
             —Lateral and medial epicondyles

In addition to the usual centers, pseudoepiphyses or accessory epiphyses may be present as a normal variant or in disease states. These are most often observed in the metacarpals, metatarsals, and phalanges. Normally, in monoepiphyseal short bones, the cartilaginous end without an epiphysis ossifies from the shaft. Occasionally an ossification center appears at this end, converting it to an abnormal biepiphyseal bone. This accessory ossification center appears early, grows rapidly, and fuses precociously to the shaft. There may be a residual peripheral groove after fusion.

The clavicle is the first bone of the body to ossify. It ossifies from membrane, with cartilage growth at the ends. An epiphyseal ossification center appears at the medial end of the clavicle between the 16th and 20th years of life. The scapula ossifies in its body and from ossification centers in the coracoid process, followed by the acromion and inferior angle in later years. *The pelvis* develops from centers in the iliac, ischiac, and pubic bones, forming a Y-shaped synchondrosis at the acetabulum. A center in the os acetabuli appears in the 11th to 14th year. The epiphysis of the iliac crest appears about the 15th year.

A cartilaginous portion in the anterior segment of *the ribs* persists throughout life. Ossification centers on the heads and tubercles of ribs 1 to 10 appear at about the 11th year. At birth, the sternum has an ossification center in the manubrium and usually two unpaired and two paired centers in the body.

The tarsal and carpal bones ossify in cartilage, and the time and order of their appearance accurately indicates the age of the individual. Several bones such as the calcaneus and the talus have accessory ossification centers.

The vertebral bodies and the spinous processes ossify in the 6th fetal week to the 4th fetal month. The ring epiphyses appear around the superior and inferior margins of the vertebral bodies, except the atlas and coccygeal vertebrae, in the 8th to the 14th years. Apophyses at the posterior aspects of the spinous and transverse processes appear in the 16th to 20th years.

VASCULAR SUPPLY OF BONE

The vascular system of a bone consists of the nutrient vessels, periosteal vessels, metaphyseal vessels, and epiphyseal vessels (Fig. 1–1)

The nutrient vessels enter through the nutrient canal, branch upward and downward to supply the entire medullary cavity, then divide into radial branches that enter the cortex and anastomose with branches from the periosteal plexus in the haversian canals. The cortex thus has a double blood supply.

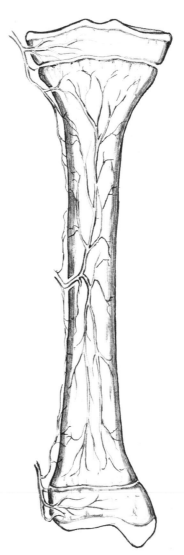

FIG. 1–1. Vascular supply of bone. The nutrient artery enters the medullary cavity by way of the nutrient foramen and branches proximally and distally. Radial branches to the cortex are given off, which anastomose with cortical branches from the periosteal plexus. Separate vessels to the epiphyseal ossification centers, which do not communicate with nutrient vessels until fusion of the physis has occurred, are present. The bone ends are supplied by the epiphyseal and metaphyseal vessels that branch into arterial arcades, which become progressively smaller and terminate in small capillary loops in the subchondral region. (Drawing courtesy of Dr. Carlos Escamilla, Associate Radiologist, Cook County Hospital. Data from Carey TJ: Anatomy, physiology, and pathology of the blood supply of bones. J Bone Joint Surg 50-A:766–783, 1968)

The nutrient canals appear as oblique grooves with sclerotic margins in the cortex, and are most prominent in infants. Their direction depends on the direction of enchondral bone growth, the vessels growing away from the end with the epiphysis of most rapid growth.

In the iliac bone there is a typical Y-shaped nutrient canal.

The periosteal vessels form a plexus of fine vessels that surround the shaft and penetrate to enter the haversian canals. When the periosteum is elevated, this blood supply is cut off. In the newborn, periosteal vessels contribute almost nothing to the blood supply of the cortex, owing to loose periosteal attachment. If the periosteum is elevated in early life, the cortex may be deprived of its potential collateral circulation.

Early in life the metaphyseal arteries are derived from the periarticular plexus. These vessels have very poor anastomoses and are virtually "end-arteries." As the bone grows, the periosteal plexus progressively supplies the peripheral parts of the metaphysis. The central four-fifths are supplied by the terminal branches of the nutrient artery. These vessels form arterial arcades.

The epiphyseal blood vessels do not communicate with those of the shaft until after fusion of the ossification center. The epiphysis is supplied by central vessels from the joint capsule, which enter through the nutrient foramina and ramify to form terminal capillary loops.

Veins exit from the long bones at three sites; accompanying the artery, at the articular ends, and as many small veins to the periosteum. Nerve fibers enter the bone with the blood vessels and extend into the haversian canals. The periosteum and bone are sensitive to pain. Sharpey's fibers extend from the bone to the periosteum.

The blood supply to the hip at an early age is of particular interest because of the frequency and severity of avascular disease. Retinacular branches of the medial and lateral circumflex femoral arteries supply the epiphysis, as well as vessels of the ligamentum teres. The latter vessels are usually insufficient to maintain viability of the head.

BONE MARROW

Bone marrow is of the same roentgen density as other soft tissues. It fills the medullary spaces of the tubular bones, the flat bones, the cuboidal bones, and the calvaria to the internal occipital protuberance. There is red marrow (blood-forming), fat marrow, fibrous marrow, and mixed marrow. In the child, all marrow spaces are filled with red marrow. In the adult, red marrow is normally found in the bones of the trunk and in the epiphyseal and metaphyseal segments of the long tubular bones. Compensatory mechanisms in certain disease states convert fat marrow into blood-forming marrow, and in more severe instances, extramedullary hematopoiesis results.

TYPES OF BONE DISEASES

The general etiological classification of diseases of bone is summarized below. In evaluating the differential diagnosis of a bone lesion, these entities should be considered.

DISEASES OF BONE

1. General metabolic
2. Inborn errors of metabolism
3. Endocrine
4. Hematologic
5. Inflammatory
6. Neoplastic
7. Congenital (including dysplasias and dysostoses)
8. Traumatic
9. Hamartomatous
10. Toxic
11. Trophic
12. Hypervitaminosis
13. Hypovitaminosis
14. Reticuloses
15. Lipoid storage disturbances
16. Cysts and other tumorlike conditions
17. Generalized bone disease of unknown etiology (*e.g.,* Paget's disease, fibrous dysplasia)
18. Muscular dystrophies
19. Bone changes associated with renal disease
20. Bone changes associated with cardiorespiratory disease
21. Bone changes associated with neurocutaneous diseases (phacomatoses)
22. Ischemic

THE ROENTGEN ANALYSIS OF BONE LESIONS

The features to observe in evaluating a radiograph of a bone are listed below.

The decision-making pattern in establishing a radiographic diagnosis should follow a logical order, based on the analysis of features and conforming to established criteria. As an example, if we were to evaluate a case of suspected bone tumor, we would follow this line of questioning:

Is it a *lesion* or is it *normal*?
Is it *solitary* or *multiple*?
Is it *malignant* or *benign*?
What is the *cell type*?

In many instances we cannot do more than decide on the malignancy or benignity of the lesion. The area of involvement or extent of the lesion must always be described.

It is important to understand the pathogenesis of the various observable features, for only then can their true significance in relation to the causal lesion be understood.

ROENTGEN FEATURES OF BONE LESIONS

 1. Loss of bone density
 2. Alteration of bone texture
 3. The epiphysis
 4. The physis or epiphyseal cartilage growth plate
 5. The zone of provisional calcification
 6. The metaphysis
 7. The medulla and spongiosa
 8. The cortex
 9. The endosteum
10. The periosteum
11. Shortening of bone
12. Lengthening of bone
13. Overconstriction or overtubulation of bone
14. Underconstriction or undertubulation of bone
15. Changes in contour or deformities of bone
16. Expansion of bone
17. Destruction of bone
18. Resorption of bone
19. Erosion of bone
20. Bone production or sclerosis
21. Calcification
22. Origin of the solitary lesion
23. Location of the lesion
24. Invasion or noninvasion
25. Size of the lesion
26. Shape of the lesion
27. Margination
28. Trabeculation
29. Bone maturation
30. Fracture
31. The soft tissues
32. The joint

DISCUSSION OF ROENTGEN FEATURES

Loss of bone density can occur generally as a result of osteoporosis, osteomalacia, hyperparathyroidism, and bone infiltrations, as well as spurious radiolucency due to radiographic technique. Osteoporosis is a decrease in bone mass; osteomalacia is a condition in which bone contains uncalcified osteoid; and hyperparathyroidism causes loss of bone density through increased osteoclastic activity. These three conditions can be differentiated readily by roentgen and biochemical means.

Alteration of bone texture. A coarsened trabecular pattern is due to resorption of bone trabeculae, allowing the remaining trabeculae to stand out in relief. Bone apposition of the remaining trabeculae causes true thickening. These changes commonly appear in infiltrative disease and in conditions having increased bone marrow activity.

The epiphysis is the end of a growing bone, or the section located at the growing end. Initially cartilaginous, it develops an ossification center that fuses to the shaft at maturity. The epiphysis protects the growth plate and produces articular cartilage. It is prone to dysplasia and ischemia. The time of appearance and fusion of the various ossification centers are indicators of skeletal maturity. The involvement of the ossification center in a disease process is an important differential point.

The physis or epiphyseal cartilage growth plate is the major area of growth in length of the long bones. It may be normal, narrowed, or widened in disease states. Abnormal spiculations or calcifications within the physis characterize several diseases.

The zone of provisional calcification is the layer of calcified cartilage of the physis adjacent to the metaphysis. It is normally only several cells thick and may be seen as a fine dense line. It may be absent, widened, interrupted, or intact, and constitutes an important differential feature of the rachitiform, trophic, and infectious diseases.

The metaphysis is the segment between the physis and the diaphysis. It consists of the primary and secondary spongiosa. Interference with formation or resorption of spongiosa originates in this region. A bone collar, or "ossification groove," composed of osteoclasts about the entire periphery of the metaphysis is istrumental in modeling of the shaft.

The medulla and spongiosa. The secondary spongiosa of the metaphysis becomes the spongy or cancellous bone of the medullary cavity, intimately associated with the bone marrow. In actuality, there is only one bone trabeculum with many ramifications that are all interconnected.

The cortex is composed of cancellous bone histologically similar to, but structurally different from, the spongiosa. The internal architecture—the haversian system—is continuously being remodeled. Cortical destruction can be caused by both malignant and benign processes. In general, a well-developed malignant process sweeps away the entire involved segment of cortex, but a benign process, such as osteomyelitis, destroys areas segmentally, leaving intact cortex in between. (An exception to this rule is Ewing's sarcoma.) Cortical thickening, absence, or thinning is also characteristic of various disease processes.

The endosteum is the membrane that covers the trabeculae and the inner margin of the cortex. It is composed only of a single layer, and has osteoblastic and osteoclastic properties. Endosteal scalloping of the inner margin of the cortex characterizes many disease processes. The endosteum is active in expanding lesions.

The periosteum is the membrane surrounding bone. It is composed of two layers; the outer or fibrous layer, and the inner or cambium layer. The cambium layer has osteoblastic and osteoclastic properties. The balance of activity between the endosteum and the periosteum determines bone mass in the constant turnover processes of bone.

Edema, hemorrhage, pus, or tumor cells can lift the periosteum from the shaft, after which reactive periosteal new bone formation takes place. The basic patterns of periosteal elevation are variations of solid or interrupted types. The latter may be spiculated or lamellated. A periosteal cuff called Codman's triangle may also be seen; this can be caused by both malignant and benign processes.

Shortening of bone can be a local phenomenon or part of a generalized dwarfing process. There are five patterns of generalized bone shortening, grouped according to segmental predominance:

a) Acromelic—distal, hands and feet
b) Rhizomelic—proximal humeri and femora
c) Mesomelic—middle, forearms and legs
d) Proportional
e) Deformed and asymmetrical

Lengthening of bone can be due to localized causes or to generalized disease, such as pituitary eosinophilic adenoma prior to epiphyseal fusion.

Overconstriction or overtubulation of bone results in long slender bones, or dolichostenomelia. There may be deformities and curvature or long bones.

Marked thinning and pseudarthroses may result. Various disease processes exhibit these findings.

Underconstriction or undertubulation of bone results from a failure of normal modeling processes. The normal proportion between shaft diameter and end diameter is lost, resulting in either a rectangular bone or an "Erlenmeyer flask" deformity.

Changes in contour or deformities of bone may be a significant diagnostic finding, as in exostoses. Not all exostoses are osteochondromas; the location and form differentiate the various types.

Expansion of bone is caused by endosteal resorption and periosteal apposition in a localized area. The rate of enlargement of the lesion must be slower than the ability of the periosteum to form new bone; otherwise destruction would result. At best, this feature indicates rate of growth of a lesion.

Destruction of bone is sometimes caused by osteoclastic activity stimulated by the lesion. An "osteoclastic front" precedes the lesional cells, and bone lysis involves a wider area histologically than lesional cells. Tumor cells also directly cause trabecular destruction, and osteoclasts may be difficult to find in these microscopic fields. Radiologically, approximately 30% to 50% of cancellous bone must be destroyed before changes are evident, but the exact figure depends upon the margination of the lesion and the radiographic technique. Radioisotope uptake scans can often show bone lesions when conventional films are negative. Three patterns of bone destruction can be differentiated radiologically which result from the degree of aggressiveness of the lesion:

a) Geographic—one or several well-defined holes
b) "Moth-eaten"—multiple moderate-sized holes, which may coalesce
c) Permeative—many tiny holes in cortical bone that become fewer in number away from the center of the lesion, thus causing lack of definition

Resorption of bone is loss of bone substance, either at the bone ends as in neurotrophic changes, or subperiosteally, which is the hallmark of hyperparathyroidism. The most common areas of bone resorption are the terminal tufts of the fingers and toes, and the distal clavicles. Neurotrophic disease may cause a pencil-like or a candlelike resorptive deformity.

Erosion of bone is evidenced by a smooth marginal or saucerlike cortical defect. It indicates the pressure effects of a process external to bone, such as an aneurysm or lymph node. It must be differentiated from invasion of bone by a neoplasm.

Bone production or sclerosis. Local lesional tissue or a generalized process may cause osteoblasts to form new bone. This reactive bone sclerosis must be differentiated from neoplastic new bone formation, which can be caused by the osteogenic or chondrogenic series of tumors. In addition, heterotopic new bone formation by metaplasia may occur in the soft tissues. Lack of absorption of primary spongiosa accounts for the increased bony density in osteopetrosis.

Calcification may be differentiated from ossification by its lack of organization into cortex and trabeculae. Calcification may be intra- or extraosseous. Calcification caused by a disturbance of calcium metabolism is called *metastatic.* If it occurs in devitalized tissues, it is called *dystrophic.* In bone, calcification is most likely to be seen in cartilaginous lesions and infarcts.

Origin of the solitary lesions. There are anatomical and histological reasons for the predilection for certain sites by many lesions. Bone tumors most often occur in the field of greatest activity of their analogous normal cells. Indeed, many tumors in atypical locations are not diagnosable radiographically. Hematogenous osteomyelitis has a predilection for the metaphyses because of the vascular anatomical structure. Origin is a prime fundamental consideration in the diagnosis of a solitary lesion.

Location of the lesion, as distinct from its origin, indicates the current status. For example, a giant-cell tumor is believed to originate from the metaphysis, but if the cartilage plate has closed, the tumor extends to the articular surface and is located at the bone end. If the tumor occurs prior to epiphyseal fusion, it does not appear at the bone end, but remains at its site of origin. The central or eccentric location of a lesion is also a fundamental consideration. We must evaluate location with respect to:

a) Which bone is involved
b) Epiphysis, physis, metaphysis, diaphysis
c) Cortical, medullary, or periosteal location
d) Articular surface
e) Soft tissue

Invasion or noninvasion is another consideration of prime diagnostic significance. A bone lesion of medullary or cortical origin invading soft tissue will have caused cortical destruction, but one of periosteal origin need not. Soft-tissue tumors can also invade bone.

The size of the lesion is an important consideration with respect to its rate of growth and growth potential. Various tumors are characterized by a typical size when first seen. Frequently, primary malignant bone tumors are not small when first seen.

The shape of the lesion is an indication of its nature. A rapidly growing lesion expands uniformly and has a circular shape. A unicameral bone cyst is a good example of an elongated lesion, the long axis being parallel to the bone shaft.

Margination, or *zone of transition,* is a result of the rate of growth of the lesion and the stimulation of osteoblasts. A sharply marginated lesion grows more slowly than a nonmarginated lesion. Faster growth results in aggressive destructive patterns.

Trabeculation results from uneven cortical expansion and erosion. The various apparent chambers usually communicate with each other. Lesions may be heavily trabeculated, or lightly trabeculated, as in giant-cell tumor. Some lesions may be truly compartmented.

Bone maturation refers to the time of appearance and fusion of the various epiphyseal and apophyseal ossification centers. This process is separate from that of bone growth. Maturation is controlled mainly by thyroid and gonadal hormones; growth is controlled by pituitary growth hormone as well as by the thyroid and gonadal hormones.

A fracture is an interruption of the continuity of bone. It may be traumatic or pathologic. When a fracture line is completely transverse, the bone should be suspected of being abnormal. Callus formation, particularly in march fractures, is not to be confused with bone tumor.

The soft tissues are not to be overlooked in the evaluation of generalized or localized bone lesions. One must consider invasion of soft tissue from bone lesions, soft-tissue edema, calcifications, ossifications, tumors, emphysema, and atrophy.

The joint is involved in the various arthritides, and may be an important clue in the diagnosis of a bone lesion. For example, if a destructive lesion of bone is present, and a joint picture of hemophilic arthropathy is noted, then hemophilic pseudotumor should be the prime consideration. Tuberculosis and rheumatoid arthritis may explain many bone changes.

IDENTIFICATION OF LESIONAL TISSUE

The roentgen image is the result of differential absorption of x-ray energy by various tissues and materials. The densities that can be discriminated are the following:

Air density. Air is the most radiolucent substance, as seen in the lungs or in subcutaneous emphysema.

Fat density. Fat is less radiolucent than air but more radiolucent than soft tissue. Retroperitoneal structures are visible because of the surrounding retroperitoneal fat. The muscle planes and joint capsules are outlined by fat. A lipoma may show increased radiolucency.

Water density (unit density or soft-tissue density). Because the major component of soft tissue is water, all soft tissues, organs, and blood pools normally cast the same density on the radiograph. Tumors, no matter how scirrhous, cannot be discerned on the roentgenogram by density changes if they are composed of ordinary soft tissue.

Intermediate density. An area of hemosiderosis, in the soft tissues or in the liver, will be slightly more radiopaque than normal soft tissue, but not nearly as dense as bone.

Calcific density. Calcification, if sufficient, and bone cast a dense, white shadow on the radiograph. Variations in bone density can be readily discerned in properly exposed radiographs.

Metallic density. Metals are more opaque than bones. A metallic foreign body can effectively block out all radiation from the underlying area of film.

The following tissues encountered in bone pathology may be identified on a physical and structural basis:

Fat is readily identifiable in an intra- or extraosseous lipoma by the radiolucent shadow that is cast. However, a low fat content may not be radiolucent. Necrotic fat may calcify.

Cartilage is characterized by amorphous spotty calcification, although this may be absent. Increased calcific density in a cartilage tumor may be due to:

a) Dystrophic calcification
b) Miniature foci of enchondral bone formation or
c) Marginal reactive bone sclerosis

Bone formation can be recognized by organization into cortex and trabeculae; this process should not be confused with calcification, although both are of the same order of density. A small amount of bone uniformly dispersed in a fibrous lesion gives a "ground glass" appearance.

Soft-tissue tumors or masses all cast the same unit or water density.

Soft-tissue emphysema, gas-forming abscess, or gas gangrene all cast a shadow of air density.

Hemosiderin deposits in the periarticular soft tissues, usually encountered about hemarthritic joints in hemophilia, can be recognized by slight increase in density.

Calcified vessels may be seen as thin linear or curvilinear streaks of calcification. Sometimes parallel lines appear.

Phleboliths are recognized as small round or ovoid calcifications, usually having a dense rim.

CORRELATION WITH CLINICAL AND LABORATORY FINDINGS

An objective list of differential diagnoses should be compiled without prejudice on the basis of the roentgen pattern. The probabilities of an entity considered in the differential diagnosis should then be compared to the probabilities derived from the clinical and laboratory picture.

The pertinent *clinical information,* when relevant, should include the following:

1. Age, sex, and race of patient
2. Duration of symptoms, severity, mode of relief
3. History of trauma, surgery, or radiation therapy
4. Type of onset (acute or insidious)
5. Pain or inflammatory signs (redness, heat, swelling)
6. Functional disturbance
7. Neurological signs or symptoms
8. History of systemic diseases
9. Visible deformity
10. Extent of involvement
11. Family history
12. Medications or treatment

Laboratory studies must include a CBC and

1. Serum calcium
2. Serum phosphorus
3. Serum alkaline phosphatase

The performance of these tests is the minimal requirement for the diagnosis of all significant bone lesions. In every giant-cell tumor, repeated determinations of the above three tests must be made in order to rule out hyperparathyroidism. Other laboratory studies, when applicable, include the following:

4. Serum uric acid
5. Urine studies for calcium, phosphorus, and abnormal components
6. Serum acid phosphatase
7. Calcium balance studies
8. Renal function studies
9. Hematological studies
10. Electrophoretic studies
11. Bioassays
12. Chromosome pattern

TABLE 1–1. NORMAL BIOCHEMICAL VALUES

Serum or Plasma Constituent	Normal Values (per 100 ml)
Calcium*	8.8–10.5 mg
Phosphorus*	2.7–4.5 mg
Alkaline phosphatase	2.0–4.5 units (Bodansky)
Acid phosphatase	0.5–2.0 units (Bodansky)
Uric acid	3.0–6.0 mg
Urea nitrogen	10.0–20.0 mg
Nonprotein Nitrogen	15.0–35.0 mg
Creatinine	1.0–2.0 mg
Hydroxyprolone	0.9–2.1 μg/ml

* The serum calcium and phosphorus levels are age- and sex-dependent.

Important normal biochemical values are summarized in Table 1–1.

RADIOGRAPHIC TECHNIQUES

Most bone lesions can be adequately demonstrated by conventional films of excellent quality. Tomography can often be useful to bring out occult features. Arteriography is useful to determine the extent of the lesion. The arteriographic pattern correlates well with the histological vascularity. It is claimed that arteriography can determine whether or not the mass is a neoplasm, if it is benign or malignant, what the blood supply is, and where the ideal spot is for a biopsy.[8,10] Radioisotope bone uptake scans can show increased bone activity much earlier than the lesion can be detected on films; however, the nature of the lesion cannot be ascertained. Lymphangiography may also be of value in specific cases. Magnification technique has also been used. Densitometric methods for the evaluation of bone mineral content have been described. In addition to radiodensitometry, radiogrammetry, or the measurement of the thickness of cortical bone, has gained acceptance. A method in common use is the photon absorption technique, utilizing the commercially available Norland Cameron Bone Mineral Analyzer. The source of gamma radiation is [125]I. The radius, or radius and ulna, are scanned and a direct readout system of bone mineral content is used. Changes in the appendicular skeleton are claimed to reflect axial skeletal changes. Methods using computed tomography for bone mineral analysis are claimed to be highly accurate.

Xeroradiography is a technique that has become widely used in mammography, but may find increasing applications in other soft-tissue work and in bone radiography. Among the advantages in superb resolution, up to 1,500 lines per inch. In addition, a long contrast scale makes possible the recording of detail of both soft tissue and bone on the same image. Small density differences become visible. Another important property is the edge enhancement effect, resulting in an accentuated border between densities.

Computed tomography is of proven value in the investigation of bone and soft-tissue lesions. An early lesion, at times, may be demonstrated in no other way. Soft-tissue extension of a bone lesion may accurately be determined by the unique cross-sectional view that this modality allows. The extent of a central skeletal tumor can be superbly demonstrated. Ultrasound is also useful to show the extent of an intra-abdominal or intrapelvic component of a bone tumor.

COMPUTER-AIDED DIAGNOSIS

Computer programs for diagnosis have been described in several areas.[20] Lodwick has developed a program for computer-aided diagnosis of primary bone tumors.[19] The various roentgen features, called *predictor variables*, are standardized and tabulated. They are systematically evaluated by the observer from the radiograph, and the information is transformed by suitable computer input for analysis using Bayes' theorem. The output is a differential diagnosis of probable predominant cell type, based on probabilities of association of each tumor with specific predictor variables. This is modified by the incidence of each tumor at large and by the frequency of association of each specific roentgen feature with a given tumor.

Tables of probabilities of association of each predictor variable with each tumor in the program have been developed. High accuracy is claimed for this system.

REFERENCES

1. Aegerter E, Kirkpatrick J A: Orthopedic Diseases, 4th ed. W B Saunders, 1975

2. Bauer C H: The use of radionuclides in orthopaedics, Part IV. Radionuclide scintimetry of the skeleton. J Bone Joint Surg 50–A:1681–1709, 1968

3. Caffey J, Silverman F N: Pediatric X-ray Diagnosis, 6th ed. Chicago, Year Book Publishers, 1972

4. Edeiken J, Hodes P J: Roentgen Diagnosis of Diseases of Bone, 2nd ed. Baltimore, Williams & Wilkins, 1973

5. Feist J H: The biologic basis of radiologic findings in bone disease: Recognition and interpretation of abnormal bone arthiteture. Radiol Clin N Amer 8:183–206, 1970

6. Goldsmith R S, Arnaud S B, Arnaud C D: Chemical determinants in the laboratory diagnosis of metabolic bone disease. In Clinical Aspects of Metabolic Bone Disease, pp 55–66. Excerpta Medica, Amsterdam, 1973

7. Greulich W W, Pyle S I: Radiographic Atlas of Skeletal Development of the Hand and Wrist, 2nd ed. Stanford C A, Stanford University Press; London, Oxford University Press, 1959

8. Halpern M, Freiberger R H: Arteriography as a diagnostic procedure in bone disease. Radiol Clin N Amer 8:277–288, 1970

9. Harper H A: Review of Physiological Chemistry, 14th ed. Los Altos, CA, Lange Medical Publications, 1973

10. Herzberg D L, Schreiber M H: Angiography in mass lesions of the extremities. Am J Roentgen 111:541–546, 1971

11. Hsia Y D: Inborn Errors in Metabolism. Part I: Clinical Aspects, 2nd ed. Chicago, Year Book Publishers, 1966

12. Jackson W P U: Calcium Metabolism and Bone Disease. London, Edward Arnold, 1967

13. Jaffe H L: Tumors and Tumorous Conditions of the Bones and Joints. Philadelphia, Lea & Febiger, 1958

14. Jaffe H L: Metabolic, Degenerative, and Inflammatory Diseases of Bones and Joints. Philadelphia, Lea & Febiger, 1972

15. Johnson L C: A general theory of bone tumors. Bull N Y Acad Med 29:164–171, 1953

16. Koehler A, Zimmer E A: Borderlands of the Normal and Early Pathologic in Skeletal Roentgenology, 10th ed. New York, Grune & Stratton, 1961

17. Lasser E C: Dynamic Factors in Roentgen Diagnosis. Baltimore, Williams & Wilkins, 1967

18. Lodwick G S: A Systemic Approach to the Roentgen Diagnosis of Bone Tumors. In Tumors of Bone and Soft Tissue. Chicago, Year Book Publishers, 1965

19. Lodwick G S: Solitary malignant tumors of bone: The application of predictor variables in diagnosis. Seminars Roentgen 1:293–313, 1966

20. Lusted L B: Introduction to Medical Decision Making. Springfield, Charles C Thomas, 1968

21. Maximow A A, Bloom W: A Textbook of Histology, 7th ed. Philadelphia, W B Saunders, 1957

22. Meschan I, Farrer–Meschan R M F: Roentgen Signs in Clinical Practice, Vol I. Philadelphia, W B Saunders, 1966

23. Murray R O, Jacobson H G: The Radiology of Skeleton Disorders. Exercises in Diagnosis, 2nd ed. Baltimore, William & Wilkins, 1977

24. Rubin P: Dynamic Classification of Bone Dysplasias. Chicago, Year Book Publishers, 1964

25. Sante L R: Principles of Roentgenological Interpretation, 9th ed, rev. Ann Arbor, Michigan, Edwards Brothers, 1952

26. Saville, P D: Biochemistry and radiologic diagnosis of bone disease. Radiol Clin N Amer 8:207–214, 1970

27. Sherman R S: The nature of radiologic diagnosis in disease of bone. Radiol Clin N Amer 8:227–240, 1970

28. Wertheimer L G, Lopes S L F: Arterial supply of the femoral head. J Bone Joint Surg 53–A:545–556, 1971

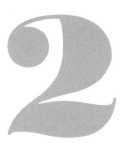

2

LOSS
OF
BONE
DENSITY

Normal bone structure and density depend upon the presence of a complex of multiple factors: normally functioning bone cells in adequate numbers, a sufficient nutritional state, normal endocrine balance, normal nerve and stress stimulations, and normal renal and gastrointestinal tract function (Fig. 2–1). The failure of any of these functions can lead to a radiographically detectable loss of bone density. The deficiency of a specific factor determines a definite clinicopathologic entity.

The three major metabolic diseases resulting in a generalized diffuse loss of bone density are osteoporosis, osteomalacia, and hyperparathyroidism. Infiltrative diseases, such as myeloma, leukemia, and storage diseases also cause diffuse loss of bone density.

Osteoporosis refers to a condition caused by diminution of bone mass. The bone substance is of normal quality. In osteomalacia there is abnormal bone with excess uncalcified osteoid. Hyperparathyroidism results in increased resorption of bone by osteoclasts. This is accompanied by proliferation of fibrous connective tissue. These three entities can be differentiated by roentgen and biochemical means.

OSTEOPOROSIS

Osteoporosis[115] is a skeletal condition, generalized or localized, in which the quantity of bone per unit volume is decreased in amount, but is normal in composition (Fig. 2–2).

Bone is in a constant state of remodeling. There are three functional types of bone cells: the osteoblast, the osteoclast, and the osteocyte.

The *osteoblast* is responsible for the deposition of bone matrix and its subsequent mineralization. This cell secretes soluble collagen, which aggregates into an extracellular array of fibrils. Nucleating points are established along the fibril in association with phosphate binding. The osteoblasts are said to form a continuous membrane over their working surface and may actively transport materials across

this membrane, initiating calcification. Further mineralization proceeds spontaneously if normal calcium and phosphorus concentrations are present. Osteoblasts secrete matrix at a rate of 1 micron per day. This unmineralized matrix constitutes an osteoid seam, which must "mature" 5 to 10 days in order to calcify. Deep in the osteoid seam is the "calcification front," an abrupt transition to mineralized matrix.

The *osteoclast* secretes enzymes which dissolve the mineral and lyse the matrix simultaneously. The osteoclast is usually a multinuclear giant cell, but functionally this need not be so. Resorption proceeds more rapidly than formation. An osteoclast, during its life span of a few days, resorbs up to eight times the amount of bone formed by an osteoblast during its life span of several weeks. Osteoclasts require a free surface, such as a vascular, trabecular, endosteal, or periosteal surface, from which to operate. They cannot resorb a surface that is covered with osteoid.

The *osteocyte* is contained in its lacuna, and has the capacity to resorb perilacunar bone. It probably is also able to redeposit bone. Ninety-nine percent of the anatomical surface of the skeleton is composed of the lacunar and canalicular sufaces. The osteocyte is thus in major relation to calcium homeostasis and the mechanical properties of bone.

Remodeling of bone is a process that continues from before birth until death. It continues beyond skeletal maturation. Adult metabolic disease usually is a result of bone remodeling activity. This process occurs on the periosteal, endosteal, and haversian surfaces. The rate of bone turnover, the amount of uncalcified osteoid, the net gain or loss of bony tissue, and the limitation of the amount of mineral that can be deposited are all determined directly by bone remodeling in the adult.

Remodeling does not occur at random, but, according to Frost,[47] in "packets" termed basic multicellular units (BMU). The BMU becomes activated by an unknown signal to a group of mesenchymal cells. Osteoclasts differentiate first and resorb approximately 0.05 mm³ of both organic and inorganic components of bone. Osteoclastic activity then

(Text continues on p. 18)

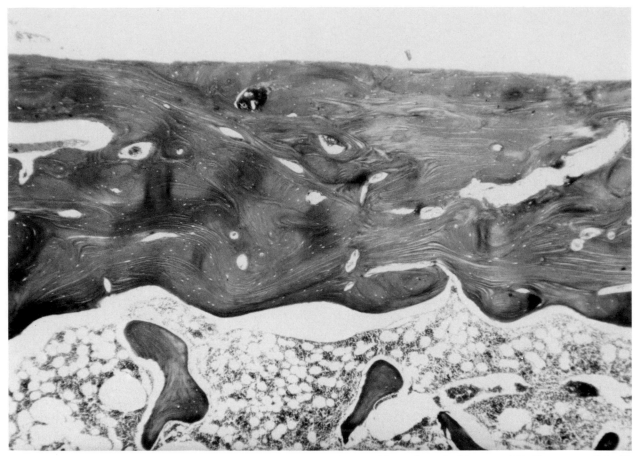

FIG. 2–1. Normal cortical bone. ×2.5. (Courtesy of Dr. R. Heredia, Dept. of Pathology, Mt. Sinai Hospital, Chicago, IL)

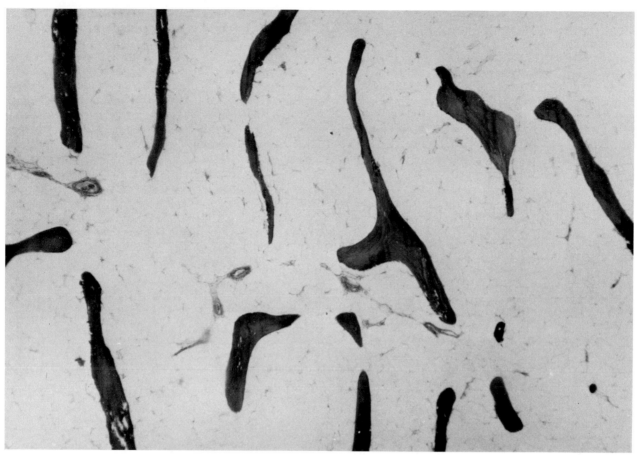

FIG. 2–2. Osteoporosis. Note the thin, sparse bone trabeculae. ×2.5. (Courtesy of Dr. R. Heredia, Dept. of Pathology, Mt. Sinai Hospital, Chicago, IL)

halts. Osteoblasts appear and form new bone matrix on the previously resorbed surfaces, and initiate mineralization. An almost equal amount of bone is formed. At the age of 30, the resorption phase of a typical BMU is 1 month, and the formation phase 3 months, for a total of 4 months. The BMU time gradually increases to approximately 5 months by age 65. Thus it is postulated that a predetermined sequence exists.

When the bone formation rate is less than the bone resorption rate, diminution of bone mass develops. These two processes are homeostatically linked. Other than a transient initial phase, both formation and resorption will change in the same direction. If both processes are accelerated there is a high remodeling rate, while if both are retarded there is a low remodeling rate. If bone formation lags behind bone resorption at either rate, osteoporosis will develop.

The osteoporoses are considered to be a heterogeneous group of disorders that may have remodeling rates from high to low. These diseases are of diverse etiologies, with only their end result in common.

Decreased bone mass leads to increased skeletal fragility, and results in fractures. In types of osteoporosis with a high remodeling rate (*e.g.,* thyrotoxicosis), the bone is less liable to fracture than in types of osteoporosis with a low remodeling rate (*e.g.,* osteogenesis imperfecta). The difference between the two conditions can be explained by the fact that in the high-remodeling-rate type of osteoporosis, microfractures caused by stress have a

FIG. 2–3. Osteoporosis—infant, age 1 month, with patent ductus arteriosus. **A.** There is loss of bone density of the spine, pelvis and upper femora. Subchondral demineralization leads to a "bone-within-a-bone" appearance of the lumbar spine. **B.** Same patient, 1 year later, showing the return to normal appearance of the spine.

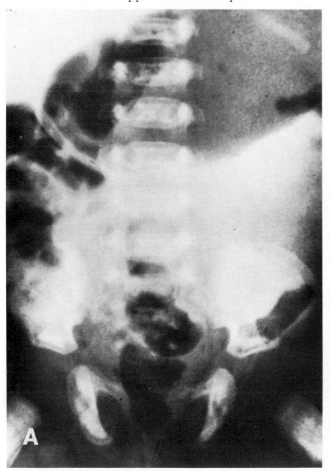

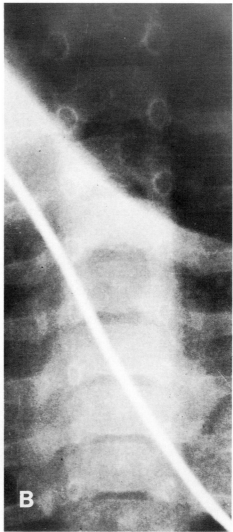

greater healing potential and progress less often to true fractures.

Bone mass increases steadily until adolescence, when the rate accelerates in both sexes. A difference in acceleration rate between the sexes appears at this time. Both sexes show an increase in bone mass until about the age of 35 years. Thereafter, bone mass decreases, beginning earlier and proceeding more rapidly in women, until 20% to 40% has been lost by the age of 65. Decrease in bone mass in women begins prior to the menopause, and is accelerated in the postmenopausal state. The rate of fractures therefore increases in aging persons, again particularly women. The incidence of hip fractures in women doubles every 5 years after the age of 60.

A universal age-related loss of skeletal mass occurs; this is part of the aging process rather than disease. It is not yet known whether the symptomatic manifestations of this process represent the superimposition of other osteopenogenic abnormalities, or exaggeration due to earlier initiation of bone loss with a lower initial bone mass.[43]

Biochemically, the serum concentrations of calcium, phosphorus, and alkaline phosphatase are normal in osteoporosis (except in osteogenesis imperfecta, in which the alkaline phosphatase may be elevated). The urinary calcium may be high in the active phase, but once the disease is established, the urinary calcium is normal or low. Negative calcium balance may also be present in the active state of the disease.

Osteoporosis is usually an irreversible process. Once bone loss has progressed beyond a certain point in adults, normal restitution cannot take place. There must be approximately a 50% loss of bone mass in order for the disease to be clinically significant, and 30% for it to be radiologically detectable.

Clinically, the disease is most manifest in the spine, with low back pain the most common symptom. In contrast to hyperparathyroidism and osteomalacia, and peripheral bones are neither painful nor tender. Vertebral collapse may cause loss of height. Fractures of the hip, wrist, and humerus are also common.

Bone mass results from the balance between periosteal and endosteal activity. If the endosteum resorbs bone, then the trabeculae are resorbed in a greater proportion than the cortex. Osteoporosis affects the spine more than other bones because the ratio of vertebral trabeculae to cortex is greater than that in peripheral bones. It is not limited, however, to the axial skeleton.

A widespread challenge has been made in recent years to Albright's concept that involutional osteo-

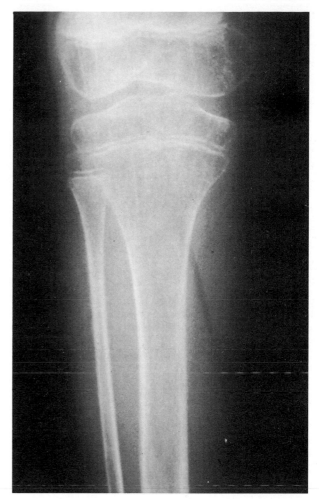

FIG. 2–4. Osteoporosis (leg) due to osteogenesis imperfecta. There is loss of bone density and thinning of the cortex. Note accentuation of the bone's trabecular pattern, with vertical striae of trabeculae in the epiphyses and in the proximal tibial metaphysis, and the relative increase in density of bone adjacent to the epiphyseal cartilage plate.

porosis is caused by diminished osteoblastic activity resulting from a deficiency of gonadal hormones. Most patients with postmenopausal osteoporosis have a normal rate of bone formation and an increased rate of bone resorption. Estrogens are believed to inhibit osteoclastic activity.

The normal progressive bone atrophy of advancing age may be modified by: (1) decrease in anabolic gonadal hormones, (2) excess of adrenal glucocorticoids, (3) diet, (4) exercise, and (5) heredity.

A lack of dietary calcium over a long period of time, inadequate calcium absorption, or chronic ex-

(*Text continues on p. 22*)

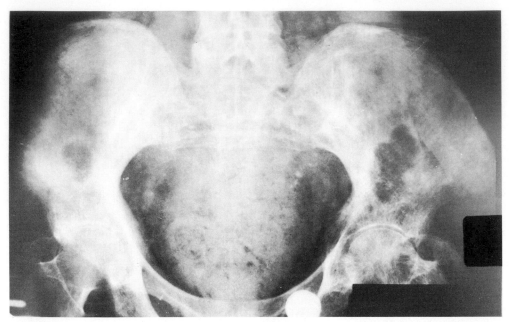

FIG. 2–5. Senile osteoporosis (pelvis) with accentuation of the trabecular pattern. Loss of the trabecular pattern in both iliac wings is noted, with accentuation of the trabecular pattern in the pelvic brim, and vertical trabeculae noted in the supra-acetabular region and the femoral head and neck.

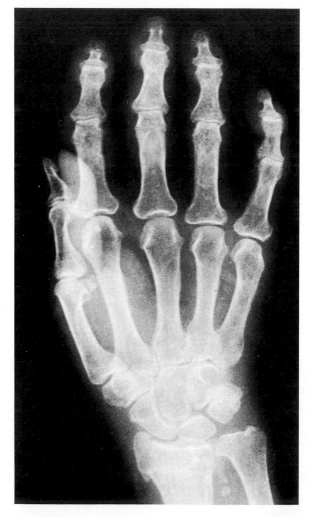

FIG. 2–6. Senile osteoporosis (hand). A uniform loss of bone density with a thin but sharply defined cortex is noted. A fracture of the distal radius is present. This represents a common site of fracture in osteoporosis, along with the hip and the vertebral bodies.

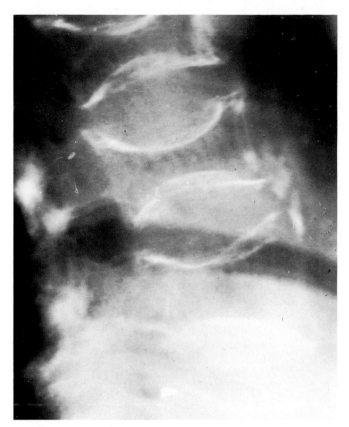

FIG. 2–7. Senile osteoporosis (dorsal spine). There is marked loss of bone density with thinning of the vertebral end-plates, which appear as a fine, dense line in contrast to the center of the vertebral bodies. Compressions, leading to a biconcave appearance and loss of height of several vertebral bodies, are seen.

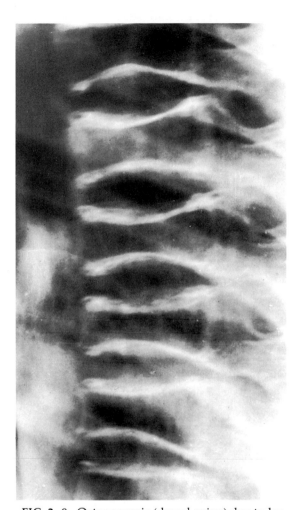

FIG. 2–8. Osteoporosis (dorsal spine) due to hypogonadism. There is marked loss of bone density of the vertebral bodies. The end-plates of the vertebrae appear dense in relation to the rest of the body. The vertebral epiphyseal rings are present and also appear dense. Note wedging of several vertebral bodies and biconcavity due to pressure from the nucleii pulposi. The intervertebral spaces are preserved.

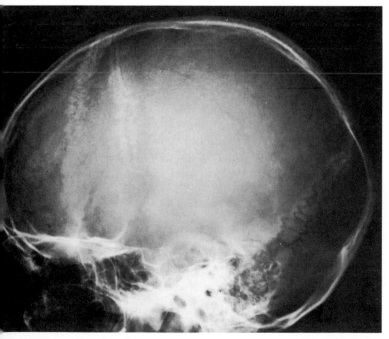

FIG. 2–9. Osteoporosis (skull) due to hypogonadism. Note loss of bone density of the calvarium and a relative increase in residual density in the areas immediately adjacent to the sutures. The thin and relatively dense inner and outer tables of the skull can be discerned in the frontal region. Deossification of the dorsum sellae, with a thin and relatively dense cortex, can also be seen.

21

cess urinary calcium loss have been shown to lead to osteoporosis.[105] Calcium is withdrawn from the skeletal reservoir, and there is a lysis of matrix. Continued resorption leads to osteoporosis. Humans have the ability of limited adaptation to low calcium intake by increasing intestinal absorption or decreasing urinary excretion.

Geographic and racial differences in the incidence and sex distribution of hip fractures as an indication of the severity of senile osteoporosis have been described in studies covering Britain, Sweden, Singapore, South Africa, and Hong Kong.[20] The highest reported incidence is in the Swedish, followed by the British, Hong Kong Chinese, Singapore Chinese, and South African Bantu, in that order. Fractures in women outnumber those in men in Sweden and Britain, while fractures in men exceed those in women in Singapore, and an equal sex incidence is found in Hong Kong. Age-related changes were found in all races and both sexes, with a progressive increase noted after the age of 45. Blacks have a larger average skeletal mass, and black women lose less bone at the endosteal surface than white women. The incidence of fractures is correspondingly less. White women over the age of 50 have the greatest risk of developing fractures secondary to osteoporosis.

About 5% of patients with osteoporosis have an associated disease in which an underlying disorder produces bone loss.[106]

GENERALIZED OSTEOPOROSIS

The causes of generalized osteoporosis are summarized below.

CLASSIFICATION OF GENERALIZED OSTEOPOROSIS

I. *Congenital*
1. Osteogenesis imperfecta
2. Neuromuscular diseases and dystrophies
3. Gonadal dysgenesis
4. Trisomy 18
5. Trisomy 13–15
6. Progeria
7. Ehlers–Danlos syndrome
II. *Acquired*
1. Osteoporosis of aging
2. Endocrine
    A. Hypogonadism
    (1) Ovaries
        (a) Turner's syndrome
        (b) Primary ovarian failure (menopause)
    (2) Testes
        (a) Hypogonadism
        (b) Eunuchoidism
        (c) Prepubertal castration syndrome
    B. Adrenal cortex
    (1) Cushing's syndrome due to adrenal cortical hyperplasia or neoplasm
    (2) Adrenal atrophy (adrenopause)
    (3) Addison's disease
    C. Pituitary
    (1) Cushing's syndrome due to basophilic adenoma
    (2) Acromegaly
    D. Thyroid
    (1) Hyperthyroidism
    E. Pancreas
    (1) Diabetes mellitus
    F. Nonendocrine tumors that secrete ACTH-like polypeptides
    (1) Oat-cell carcinoma
3. Disuse atrophy. Osteoporosis due to lack of stress stimulus
    A. Space flight osteoporosis[78]
4. Deficiency
    A. Vitamin C (scurvy)
    B. Protein deficiency
    C. Calcium deficiency
    D. Malnutrition
    E. Alcoholism
5. Liver disease, with or without jaundice
6. Hypoxemia
    A. Chronic pulmonary disease
    B. Congenital heart disease
7. Idiopathic. Osteoporosis in young people without demonstrable cause
8. Iatrogenic
    A. Excessive steroid therapy
    B. Heparin[58,113]
    C. Experimental hyperoxia
9. Inborn errors of metabolism
    A. Homocystinuria (defect in synthesis of protein)[129]

Idiopathic juvenile osteoporosis[28,31,56] is a rare condition that is not associated with the classic etiologies of osteoporosis. The age of onset is between 8 and 12 years. The patient complains of generalized or focal pain, and loss of height is observed.

The radiological findings are similar to those in other forms of osteoporosis: generalized loss of bone density, cortical thinning, vertebral body biconcavity and collapse, and long bone fractures. A familial history is lacking in these patients.

Negative calcium balance is present, but the other laboratory values are usually normal. The disease is usually self-limiting, with spontaneous radiological and clinical improvement.

Osteoporosis in children is usually secondary to liver disease, steroid therapy, Cushing's syndrome, thyrotoxicosis, Turner's syndrome, immobilization, or osteogenesis imperfecta.

Intestinal malabsorption of calcium, possibly associated with defective incorporation of calcium in bone, has been suggested as the basis for this condition.

Alcoholic bone disease may be a form of osteoporosis with a component of osteomalacia. The bone is of lower than normal density. Comparison in cases of sudden death in alcoholics under 40 years with nonalcoholics over 70 years showed an equal fat-free dry weight of iliac crest biopsies. A significant degree of intestinal malabsorption has been found in alcoholics with hypophosphatemia, hypokalemia, and elevated alkaline phosphatase.

A *"bone-within-a-bone" appearance of the infantile spine,*[14] owing to loss of bone density at the periphery of the vertebral body but with retention of a thin sharp cortical outline, is not uncommon. This is usually seen in infants 1 to 2 months of age. The bone subsequently returns to normal density. The evidence suggests that this appearance in a 1- to 2-month-old infant is a normal stage in the transformation of the architecture of the neonatal vertebra to that of later infancy (Fig. 2–3).

Rigg's syndrome[106] consists of osteoporosis, increased serum immunoreactive parathyroid hormone, and inappropriately low serum 1,25-dihydroxyvitamin D. Most patients with postmenopausal osteoporosis have normal or low values for serum immunoreactive parathyroid hormone (IPTH). A small subset are found to have increased values, up to two to three times higher than the normal means, and with low calcium levels. After surgical removal of hyperplastic parathyroid tissue in one of these patients, the serum IPTH decreased to normal. The researchers have suggested that the increased serum IPTH in these patients is caused by secondary hyperparathyroidism.

Radiologically, a definitive diagnosis of osteoporosis cannot be made on roentgen features alone. A generalized uniform loss of bone density can be seen in the following conditions: (1) osteoporosis, (2) osteomalacia, (3) hyperparathyroidism, and (4) infiltrations of marrow (*e.g.,* myeloma). Ca + Phos

The presence of characteristic radiographic findings of osteomalacia (Looser's lines), and hyperparathyroidism (subperiosteal resorption and brown tumor) distinguish these conditions. Biochemical findings distinguish among multiple myeloma, osteomalacia, and hyperparathyroidism. The

laboratory values in osteoporosis are characteristically normal. The roentgen diagnosis of generalized osteoporosis can only be made by the exclusion of other diseases, or in the presence of clinical evidence of this disease. In rapidly developing osteoporosis, endosteal resorption and widening of the haversian canals with a striated and spotty cortical appearance simulates a permeative destructive process.

The chief roentgen finding in established osteoporosis is a diminished density of bone. Cortical thinning with endosteal resorption and relative increase in density of the cortex and vertebral endplates may be seen (Fig. 2–4). The cortex is seen as a thin sharp line. There is preferential resorption of transverse trabeculae,[136] and accentuation of the remaining trabeculae along lines of stress (Fig. 2–5). Growth lines stand out in relief. The linea aspera of the femora become more apparent. The bones become brittle (Fig. 2–6) but do not bend, in contrast to hyperparathyroidism and osteomalacia. Osteogenesis imperfecta is the only form of osteoporosis in which the bones are frequently bowed,[117,136] These changes are most manifest in the spine and pelvis. The most common sites of fractures in postmenopausal and senile osteoporosis are the vertebral bodies, femoral necks, and wrists.

The vertebral changes consist of anterior wedging and biconcavity of the bodies owing to infractions of the vertebral end-plates from pressure of the nucleus pulposis (Fig. 2–7). Flattening of a vertebral body is only rarely seen and should suggest an infiltrative process. The intervertebral spaces are preserved (Fig. 2–8).

The more common causes of diminished bone density in the vertebrae are: (1) postmenopausal or senile osteoporosis, (2) steroid effect, Cushing's syndrome, or iatrogenic, (3) multiple myeloma, (4) hyperparathyroidism, (5) leukemia, (6) hemoglobinopathies, and (7) osteomalacia.

Vertebral spur formation caused by degenerative spinal changes is arrested or diminished in the presence of osteoporosis.

Initially, the skull shows a spotty loss of density of the calvarium. Later the bone adjacent to the sutures assumes a relatively sclerotic appearance (Fig. 2–9).

There can be thinning of the parietal bones owing to resorption of the external table. More commonly, the floor of the sella turcica and dorsum sellae become deossified. This finding must be differentiated from deossification caused by increased intracranial pressure or intrasellar tumor. Osteoporosis beginning early in life leads to excessive pneumatization of the paranasal sinuses and mastoids.

The caliber and size of the bone do not diminish in osteoporosis in the absence of fractures. Congenital or juvenile forms frequently lead to deficient development, with a bone smaller than normal.[136]

Striation of cortical bone, best seen in the metacarpals, has been described in over half of patients with moderate to severe thyrotoxicosis.[87] The radiological technique requires industrial film and 8× visual magnification. Similar changes are seen in acromegaly, and striation to a lesser extent in the endosteal zone is seen in involutional osteoporosis (Fig. 2–10).

Hypercallosis in the presence of osteoporosis may be present in osteogenesis imperfecta and in Cushing's syndrome from any cause. In Cushing's syndrome, aseptic necrosis of the femoral and humeral heads, as well as similar changes in the lateral femoral condyles and distal ends of the humeri in children, sometimes occur. Horizontal sclerotic bands adjacent to vertebral end-plates may be present (Figs. 2–11, 2–12). These bands are caused by hypercallus formation at multiple infractions. The vertebral end-plates in Cushing's syndrome may appear thick, with loss of sharp outline. Mottling of the calvarium is also seen in this condition. Partial resorption of the lamina dura has been reported. Osteoporosis of the spine in hypercortisonism will heal in children once the cause is removed, but not in adults. The differential diagnosis of loss of bone density in children is summarized below.

LOSS OF BONE DENSITY IN CHILDREN

> Leukemia
> Steroid therapy
> Cushing's syndrome
> Osteogenesis imperfecta tarda
> Idiopathic juvenile osteoporosis
> Still's disease
> Thyrotoxicosis
> Liver disease
> Turner's syndrome
> Paralysis

Quantitative radiography: The clinical determination of osteoporosis and its rational treatment depend upon reliable methods for assessment of bone density.

Radiologic estimation of bone mass utilizes four different approaches: densitometry,[144] radiogrammetry, photon-beam scanning, and computed tomography.[54]

The densitometric approach estimates bone mineral content by densitometric scans of radiographs compared to a standard aluminum wedge.

Radiogrammetry, by the method of Garn and Poznanski,[50] is based upon vernier caliper measurements of the total subperiosteal diameter and the medullary cavity width of the second metacarpal at its midshaft. These dimensions are compared with norms and standards according to age, sex, and race. This yields an estimate of the relative rates of subperiosteal surface apposition and endosteal surface resorption. Various diseases have been studied with respect to this resorption.

FIG. 2–10. Osteoporosis (proximal phalanges) with cortical striation, as may be seen in thyrotoxicosis and other conditions. Note fine ovoid radiolucencies with intracortical location, giving an appearance of striation of the cortex. Generalized loss of bone density with accentuation of the trabecular pattern in the distal metacarpals is present.

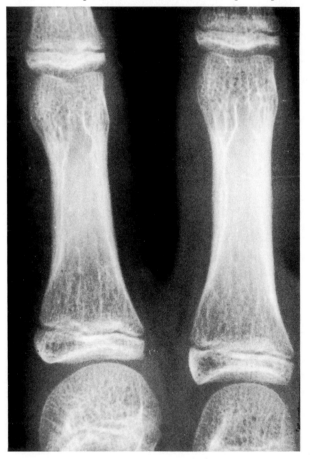

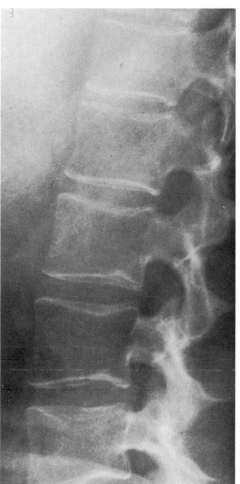

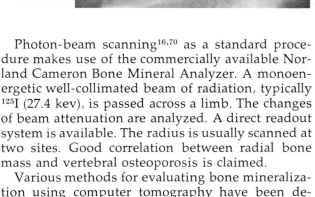

FIG. 2–11. Osteoporosis (lumbar spine) in a cirrhotic patient on steroid therapy—male, age 31 years. Note loss of bone density with thinning, and relative increase in density of the vertebral end-plates. Several areas of herniation of the nucleus pulposus into the vertebral end-plates may be noted in the lower lumbar region. (Courtesy of Dr. Morris Sokolov)

FIG. 2–12. Osteoporosis (lumbar spine)—follow-up film of patient in Fig. 2–11, after 6 weeks. Note multiple infractions at the vertebral end-plates, and increased density of the superior end-plates of several vertebrae owing to excess callus formation. Generalized loss of bone density persists with prominent callus formation, which is a typical steroid effect.

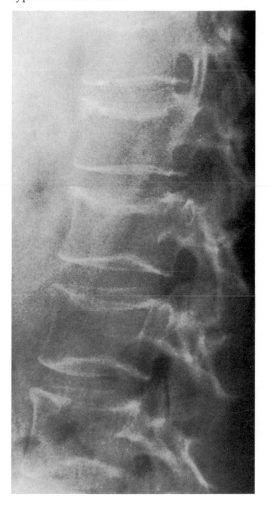

Photon-beam scanning[16,70] as a standard procedure makes use of the commercially available Norland Cameron Bone Mineral Analyzer. A monoenergetic well-collimated beam of radiation, typically [125]I (27.4 kev), is passed across a limb. The changes of beam attenuation are analyzed. A direct readout system is available. The radius is usually scanned at two sites. Good correlation between radial bone mass and vertebral osteoporosis is claimed.

Various methods for evaluating bone mineralization using computer tomography have been described.[91] Dual-energy and single-energy techniques have been developed, and high precision is claimed. The cost effectiveness of this procedure has not been determined as yet.

A different quantitative approach to the assessment of bone metabolism is the evaluation of cor-

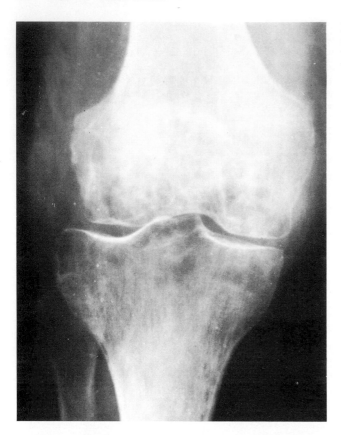

FIG. 2–13. Rapidly developing osteoporosis (knee) with spotty distribution. Note multiple areas of radiolucency in the distal femur and proximal tibia, some of which coalesce to give an almost destructive appearance.

FIG. 2–14. Localized osteoporosis (foot), early stage. Spotty and patchy areas of loss of bone density may be seen alternating with areas of normal bone density. The cortex in the major portion appears normal, although there is thinning in the involved spotty areas. This may be seen best at the inferior margin of the calcaneus.

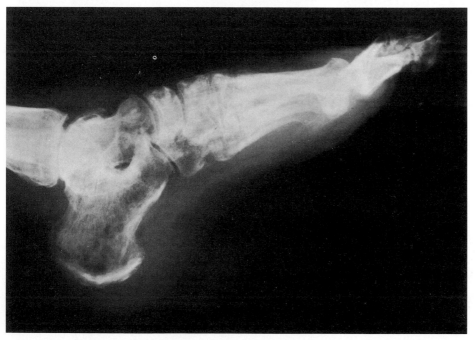

tical bone striations.[149] Fine-detail films are obtained of the first and second metacarpals. The striations seen are graded on a scale of 0–3+.

Hypermetabolic states of various etiologies, including growing children, high-remodeling-rate osteoporosis, osteomalacia, and hyperparathyroidism, show an increase in cortical striations.

The reader is referred to the Fourth International Conference on Bone Measurement for detailed descriptions of the various methods[80] (which are beyond the scope of this book).

These techniques permit studies of the effects of age, sex, race, genetics, and other variables on bone mass in the population. Epidemiologic studies of osteoporosis can be performed, and those individuals who risk developing a fracture can be identified.

LOCAL OSTEOPOROSIS

Wolff's law states: "Every change in the form and the function of a bone or of their function alone, is followed by certain definite changes in their internal architecture, and equally definite secondary alterations in their external conformation, in accordance with mathematical laws."

Local immobilization, in accord with Wolff's law, leads to osteoporosis. This has been shown to be a high-remodeling-rate type of osteoporosis.

In the event of a fracture, there is a greater loss of density distal to the fracture site, even though the degree of immobilization is the same for proximal and distal fragments. Impaired venous flow, neural changes, and withdrawal of tonic muscle pulls have been postulated to explain this finding.

The principal causes of local osteoporosis are summarized below.

CAUSES OF LOCAL OSTEOPOROSIS

1. Disuse atrophy (*e.g.*, fractures, casts) (Distal
2. Inflammatory
   A. Rheumatoid arthritis
   B. Osteomyelitis
   C. Tuberculosis
3. Tumors
   A. Malignant, primary, and metastatic
   B. Benign
4. Sudeck's atrophy
5. Muscular paralyses
6. Transitory demineralization of the femoral head
7. Denervation or tendon section

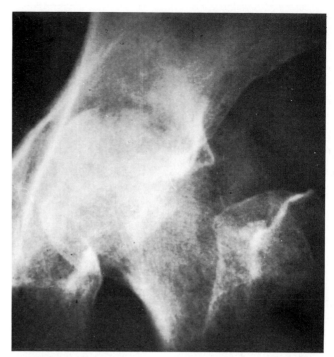

FIG. 2–15. Localized osteoporosis (right hip), secondary to septic arthritis. There is subchondral rarefaction of the upper portion of the femoral head and neck, with loss of distinctness of the cortical outline.

Radiologically, there is a spotty loss of density with mottled irregular rarefaction and endosteal resorption in early stages (Fig. 2–13, 2–14). Subchondral rarefaction accompanied by loss of sharp outline of the articular cortex occurs (Fig. 2–15), later progressing to a periarticular deossification (Fig. 2–16) owing to greater vascularity at this site. Finally a uniform loss of density occurs in the entire affected area with a thin smooth cortex (Fig. 2–17). There is often an associated reduction of muscle mass. In the event of a fracture, the greatest loss of density is in the distal fragment, and in the bones distal to the fracture in an adult patient. Return to normal density may occur in children and in men, but not in women.

In inflammatory conditions, pyogenic infections and tuberculosis can be differentiated by the ratio of destruction to osteoporosis. In pyogenic infections, destruction precedes osteoporosis. In tuberculosis the reverse is true. Localized severe osteoporosis in diabetes mellitus can mimic bone destruction. A surprising amount of restitution of

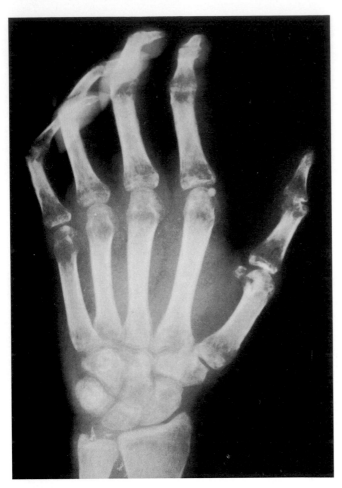

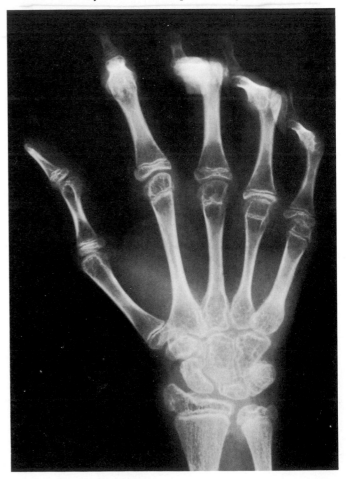

FIG. 2–16. Localized periarticular osteoporosis (hand) due to ulnar and median nerve paralysis. Note opaque sutures at the wrist. There is loss of bone density involving the periarticular regions of the phalanges and metacarpals, with preservation of normal density in the midshafts. The cortices in the involved areas are thinned. This will later progress to uniform osteoporosis. (From Greenfield GB, Escamilla CH, Schorsch HA: The hand as an indicator of generalized disease. Am J Roentgen 99:736–745, 1967)

FIG. 2–17. Localized osteoporosis (hand) secondary to juvenile rheumatoid arthritis. Note loss of bone density and thinning of the cortex. The diminished caliber of the shafts caused by lack of development may be seen.

bone may be witnessed following conservative therapy.[98]

Sudeck's atrophy is a rapid development of painful osteoporosis following trivial trauma, believed to have a neurovascular etiology. There is rapid appearance of spotty and periarticular osteoporosis (Fig. 2–18). Although the symptoms may subside, restitution of normal bone density usually never takes place. The soft tissue becomes swollen and tender, and then atrophic.

Partial transient osteoporosis,[75] a well-documented syndrome, includes transitory demineralization of the femoral head and migratory regional osteoporosis. Severe pain develops about a major joint, usually the hip, knee, or ankle in middle-aged or elderly adults. Initially the radiographs are normal. Osteoporosis is seen 1 to 2 months later. The symptoms subside in 4 to 10 months, and the osteoporotic areas subsequently remineralize. In about 30% of the cases the cause is unknown. In the remain-

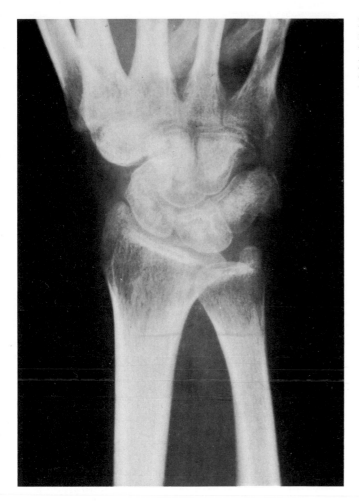

FIG. 2–18. Sudeck's atrophy (right wrist) 2 weeks following minor injury. There is severe periarticular osteoporosis with thin but intact cortices in the involved regions. The joint spaces are normal, thus differentiating this appearance from that of the arthritides. There was severe pain in this case.

osteoporosis and increased numbers of erythrocytes. Joint fluid studies are compatible with sterile synovitis.

Radiologically, severe loss of density of the femoral head with loss of outline of the articular cortical margin is characteristic. Mottling of the medullary bone may also be seen. Changes in the acetabulum and femoral neck may be similar but less marked. Complete healing is said to occur in 2 to 4 months, at times with a transient irregular increase in bone density.

Ischemic necrosis may develop following biopsy. The etiology is unknown. This condition appears similar to *migratory regional osteoporosis* (Duncan et al).[43] Sequential areas are involved, with a marked degree of localized osteoporosis, soft-tissue inflammatory reaction, and severe pain on weight-bearing. The hip may or may not be involved, along with the knee or foot. Each episode is similar to reflex sympathetic osteodystrophy. The duration of disability averages 3 to 4 months.

The repair of osteoporosis is slow; remaining trabeculae are increased in thickness, but those trabeculae that have been lost are not renewed.

der, trauma, surgery, neuralgia, herpes zoster, and vascular disturbances have been implicated.

Two types of distribution have been described; the radial form, which involves only one or two rays of the hand or foot, and the zonal form.

Transitory demineralization of the femoral head[92,112] is a self-limiting but disabling disorder of the hip. Other areas, such as the knee, ankle, and foot, may be episodically involved in some, but not all, patients. The sex ratio is 3:1, men to women. In the majority of women, the onset of symptoms is in the third trimester of pregnancy, and in all women observed there was involvement of the left hip. This finding suggests a mechanical compression of some type.

The main symptom is pain in the hip, which may radiate to the knee. Frequently there is inability to bear weight. Routine laboratory examinations are normal except for occasional elevation of the erythrocyte sedimentation rate. Bone biopsy reveals

OSTEOMALACIA

Osteomalacia[12,19,43] is a condition of the skeleton characterized by the accumulation of increased amounts of uncalcified osteoid. The appositional growth rate of bone is decreased, and the osteoid tissue fails to calcify, or does so extremely slowly. It is the end result of a defect in calcification which may arise from various causes.

The excess osteoid is present as an elevation in the percentage of total skeletal osteoid and bone surface covered by osteoid, with increased numbers and usually increased width of osteoid seams. There is a decreased rate of osteoid synthesis associated with a yet lower rate of mineralization. Normally, the delay between osteoid synthesis and mineralization is from 5 to 10 days. In osteomalacia, the time lag may become 3 months or longer. Furthermore, significant abnormalities are found in mineralized areas, including persistent large areas of decreased mineral density and low mineral content around many osteocytes.

Biochemically, reduction of the serum inorganic phosphorus level is frequently found in cases of osteomalacia. It is believed that hypophosphatemia is responsible for the metabolic bone disease that develops, particularly in association with rickets.[30] The serum calcium concentration is slightly low to normal, possibly due to absence of mobilizable bone calcium. Parathormone (parathyroid hormone) levels are usually elevated, presumably secondary to hypocalcemia. The alkaline phosphatase level is elevated except in cases of hypophosphatasia. Serum hydroxyproline levels are elevated.

There are three basic categories of osteomalacia:

1. Vitamin D deficiency
2. Hypophosphatemia with normal vitamin D intake
3. Defective nucleation without abnormalities of calcium, phosphorus, or vitamin D

VITAMIN D METABOLISM[7,135]

Functions of vitamin D.[30] The known functions of vitamin D result from its causing elevation of plasma calcium and phosphorus concentrations. The functions that are claimed by DeLuca are summarized below.

FUNCTIONS OF VITAMIN D[30]

1. Prevention of rickets and osteomalacia
2. Prevention of hypocalcemic tetany
3. A role in the prevention of osteoporosis
4. Prevention of muscle weakness

Ultraviolet radiation isomerizes vitamin D_3 by chemical photolysis from 7-dehydrocholesterol, which is present in the epidermal layer of the skin. The resulting vitamin D_3 is then absorbed and transported in the plasma bound to a specific globulin. Dietary vitamin D_2 (ergocalciferol) and vitamin D_3 (cholecalciferol) are absorbed from the duodenum and jejunum via lymphatic channels, bound to lipoproteins. The absorbed vitamin D admixes with endogenous vitamin D_3 and is either metabolized or stored in body tissues. The normal range of plasma vitamin D levels is 8 to 45 ng/ml.

Both vitamins D_3 and D_2 are metabolized by the liver, the former to 25-hydroxycholecalciferol (25-HCC), and the latter to 25-hydroxyergocalciferol (25-HEC). Both metabolites circulate bound to a plasma protein. It is considered that 25-HCC is the

first in a series of biologically active vitamin D_3 metabolites. This metabolite is transported to target organs (intestine, bone, and kidney) and to storage depots (muscle and fat). In the kidney, 25-HCC increases renal tubular resorption of inorganic phosphate. It is further metabolized in the proximal renal tubules to either 1,25-dihydroxycholecalciferol (1,25-DHCC), which has 13 times the biological activity of vitamin D_3, or 24,25-dihydroxycholecalciferol (24,25-DHCC), which may possibly be the initial event in the inactivation of the potent vitamin D molecule (Fig. 2-19).

The conversion of 25-HCC to 1,25-DHCC or 24,25-DHCC is thought to be strong feedback-regulated by the need for calcium or phosphorus. It is considered that 1,25-DHCC is the ultimate vitamin D_3 metabolite which governs the intestinal transport and absorption of calcium. Thus vitamin D_3 is the storage form, 25-HCC the major form, and 1,25-DHCC the ultimate active form regulating intestinal calcium absorption and bone remodeling.

Mechanism of calcium homeostasis.[30] Hypocalcemia results in PTH secretion (Fig. 2-20). PTH then acts on kidney and bone. In the kidney, PTH causes excretion of phosphorus and improves resorption of calcium. This process is said to require the presence of 1,25-DHCC and to stimulate its formation. Then 1,25-DHCC acts on the intestine to stimulate calcium transport. It acts upon bone, where, together with PTH, calcium is mobilized from the bone fluid compartment. Renal reabsorption of calcium is stimulated by 1,25-DHCC. The plasma calcium concentration then rises, which shuts down PTH secretion by the parathyroid. Thus, it can be seen that there is an interplay between the parathyroid gland and the vitamin D–endocrine system located within the kidney.

Clinically, muscular weakness and nonspecific pains that gradually increase in severity are present in osteomalacia. All bones may exhibit extreme tenderness. The patient walks with a waddling gait. Skeletal deformities eventually develop. The causes of osteomalacia and rickets are summarized below.

CAUSES OF OSTEOMALACIA AND RICKETS

1. Dietary calcium deficiency
2. Deficient absorption of calcium or phosphorus
   A. Vitamin D deficiency (or lack of exposure to sunshine)
   B. Malabsorption states
      (1) Celiac disease
      (2) Sprue
      (3) Idiopathic steatorrhea

(4) Pancreatic disease—exocrine
(5) Amyloidosis
(6) Postgastrectomy
(7) Regional ileitis
(8) Lymphoma of small bowel
(9) Small bowel fistula
(10) Chronic use of cathartics[42]
(11) Jejunoileal bypass[127]
  C. Obstructive jaundice
(1) Congenital (biliary atresia)
(2) Acquired (probable if jaundice is long-standing)
3. Enzyme abnormalities—hypophosphatasia
4. Excessive excretion of calcium or phosphorus by way of breast or placenta (puerperal osteomalacia)
5. Excessive utilization of calcium as fixed base
  A. Renal tubular acidosis
  B. Rickets following ureterosigmoidostomy[131] (hyperchloremia)
6. Renal
  A. Tubular (hypophosphatemic)
(1) Vitamin D-resistant rickets
(2) Fanconi syndrome
    (a) Primary
        i. Childhood type, with cystinosis
        ii. Adult type, without cystinosis
    (b) Acquired
        i. Multiple myeloma
        ii. Nephrotic syndrome
        iii. Neurofibromatosis
        iv. Heavy metal poisoning
        v. Beryllium poisoning
        vi. Ingestion of outdated tetracycline
        vii. Vitamin D intoxication in adults
(3) Secondary to inborn metabolic disturbances
    (a) Galactosemia
    (b) Tyrosinosis
    (c) Oxalosis
    (d) Wilson's disease[18]
  B. Glomerular (hyperphosphatemic)
(1) Renal osteodystrophy
7. Accelerated hepatic degradation of vitamin D_3 and 25-HCC
  A. Anticonvulsant medication
8. Pseudovitamin D-deficiency rickets or osteomalacia[10,32]
9. Tumor with ectopic humeral syndrome (sclerosing hemangioma or nonossifying fibroma)[99,114]
10. Antacid-induced osteomalacia and nephrolithiasis[148]
11. Liver cirrhosis[127]

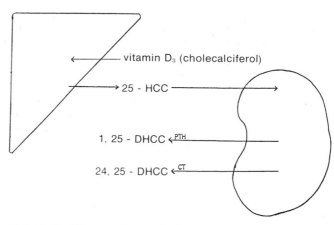

FIG. 2–19. Vitamin D metabolism.

FIG. 2–20. Calcium homeostasis.

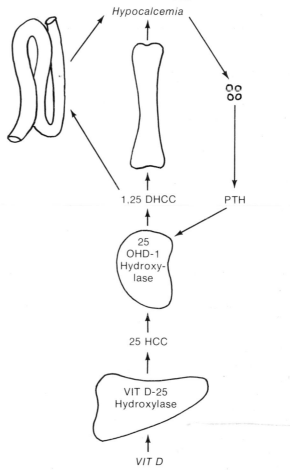

Renal disease can lead to bone changes from either tubular or glomerular causes. *Tubular disease* results in a low serum phosphorus level until renal failure supervenes. The three principal varieties of tubular disease usually associated with rickets are vitamin D-resistant rickets, renal tubular acidosis (hyperchloremic acidosis), and Fanconi syndrome.

In *vitamin D-resistant rickets or osteomalacia,* the proximal tubular resorption of phosphorus is diminished. Thirty-three types have been described. The most common is the X-linked dominant hypophosphatemic condition. This is characterized by low plasma phosphorus, normal calcium, low to normal plasma PTH levels, and phosphaturia without aminoaciduria. Another condition is known as vitamin D-dependency rickets. These patients have hypocalcemia, hypophosphatemia, elevated alkaline phosphatase, rickets, and aminoaciduria. The cause is thought to be a defect in 250HD-1 Hydroxylase. In very rare cases the first manifestation occurs in adult life.

One such family of 133 members has been reported. The hypophosphatemic children did not have rickets or bowing, the young adults had minimal bowing, and the involvement of adults over 40 years manifested progressive severe bowing. The condition is thought to be an X-linked dominant.

Renal tubular acidosis[25] is a state of tubular insufficiency with regard to renal excretion of hydrogen ions and/or resorption of bicarbonate ions out of proportion to, and in the absence of, glomerular insufficiency. The condition is classified into proximal and distal renal tubular acidoses. The distal defect represents the "classical" disease and is more severe. It can lead to cation wasting (calcium and potassium), rickets or osteomalacia, growth retardation, interstitial nephritis and uremia. Nephrocalcinosis occurs in 38% of patients, nephrolithiasis in 49% and osteomalacia in 29%. The combination of nephrocalcinosis and osteomalacia is most suggestive of renal tubular acidosis when hypervitaminosis D in the treatment of rickets is excluded.

Secondary renal tubular acidosis may be associated with hyperglobulinemic states, Fanconi syndrome, multiple myeloma, ulcerative colitis, collagen diseases, sarcoidosis, hydronephrosis, and medullary sponge kidney.

Fanconi syndrome results from multiple defects of renal tubular resorption. The condition may either be inherited as an autosomal recessive, or acquired from a variety of exogenous or endogenous nephrotoxic agents. There is generalized aminoaciduria together with excessive excretion of one or more of the following.

1. Phosphate, leading to hypophosphatemia, dwarfism, rickets, and osteomalacia
2. Glucose (renal glycosuria)
3. Potassium, leading to hypokalemia and muscle weakness
4. Calcium, with hypercalciuria but without nephrolithiasis and nephrocalcinosis
5. Water (polyuria)
6. Proteinuria and metabolic acidosis

The prognosis for primary Fanconi syndrome is poor and death may occur at puberty, usually from uremia. A decreased glomerular filtration rate may obscure the aminoaciduria.

Fanconi syndrome is not to be confused with limited aminoaciduria without other tubular defects, such as cystinuria, in which cystine, lysine, arginine, and ornithine are found in the urine. Renal tubular defects must be considered when the onset of rickets is over the age of 2 years, when rickets do not heal on ordinary doses of vitamin D, and when more than one member of a family is affected.

The roentgen findings of rickets are described under that heading in Chapter 4.

Glomerular disease results in renal osteodystrophy, discussed subsequently.

Prolonged use of *anticonvulsive medications*[152] has been found to result in rickets and osteomalacia. Up to 65% of institutionalized epileptics and 20% of outpatient epileptics (adult) are shown to have significant hypocalcemia, hypophosphatemia, and osteomalacia when bone biopsies are obtained. The condition responds to dietary vitamin D supplements. Plasma levels of 25-HCC and 25-HEC are decreased. The basis is thought to be drug-stimulated hepatic enzymatic activity, resulting in accelerated degradation of vitamin D_3 and 25-HCC to inactive metabolites.

Pseudovitamin D deficiency[10, 32] is an unusual hereditary bone disorder characterized by rickets or osteomalacia, very low serum calcium, and a normal or only slightly depressed serum phosphate. The disease is manifested by severe radiological changes of rickets or osteomalacia, pain, and myopathy. The diet is normal in vitamin D, malabsorption is not present, and renal function is normal. A very good response to large doses of vitamin D uniformly occurs. It has been proposed that this disease represents an abnormality of vitamin D metabolism associated with a resistance to parathormone-mediated renal phosphate excretion.

Tumor-induced osteomalacia and rickets, or ectopic humeral syndrome, refers to osteomalacia associated with a variety of bone and soft-tissue tumors.

It is a very rare condition. Surgical excision of the tumor results in remission of the osteomalacia. The mechanism is obscure. No hormones have been demonstrated to be secreted by the tumors.[77,104,151] The tumors that have been described as associated with osteomalacia are listed below.

BONE AND SOFT-TISSUE TUMORS THAT HAVE BEEN ASSOCIATED WITH OSTEOMALACIA

Sclerosing hemangioma
Nonossifying fibroma
Benign Osteoblastoma
Cavernous hemangioma of knee
Giant-cell tumor (malignant)
Giant-cell reparative granuloma
Hemangiopericytoma
Ossifying mesenchymal tumor

Atypical axial osteomalacia[41] is a rare condition of unknown etiology involving the central skeleton only radiologically. The condition occurs in elderly men, and the symptomatology is minimal. The cervical spine, lumbar spine, ribs and pelvis show coarsening of the trabecular pattern with thickening and disorganization. No pseudofractures are seen and the peripheral skeleton appears normal. Biopsy reveals an increased number of wide osteoid seams compatible with osteomalacia. The blood chemistries, however, are not suggestive of osteomalacia. The serum calcium and phosphorus values are normal.

Radiologically, in osteomalacia of all etiologies, there is a loss of bone density owing to the presence of nonmineralized osteoid (Fig. 2–21). Mottled radiolucent areas may appear, particularly in the skull. The bone trabecular pattern is coarsened, with loss of both longitudinal and transverse trabeculae. Thinning and lack of definition of the cortex may be seen. The endosteal edge of the cortex and the bony trabeculae are not as well defined as in osteoporosis. Fine-detail radiography of the hands shows intracortical striations in 60% of patients with osteomalacia.[84] The features distinguishing osteomalacia from osteoporosis are the presence of bone deformities and pseudofractures. Bowing deformities, chiefly of the pelvis, the vertebral column, the thorax, and the proximal extremities, are characteristic features. These result in kyphoscoliosis of the spine (Fig. 2–22), a "bell-shaped" thorax (Fig. 2–23), and deformities of the pelvis caused by weight-bearing, which give a triradiate shape to the pelvic lumen (Fig. 2–24). Bowing deformities of the long bones, particularly of the lower extremities, occur.

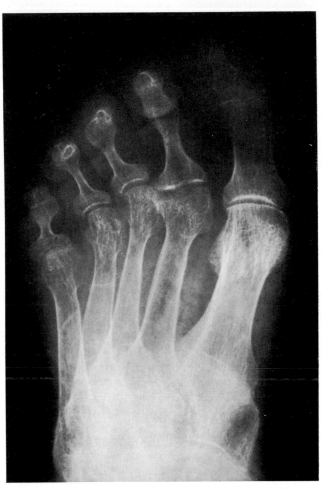

FIG. 2–21. Osteomalacia (foot) due to nontropical sprue —white female, age 56 years. Serum calcium 4.4 mg%, serum phosphorus 2.1 mg%, alkaline phosphatase 2.5 units. There is loss of bone density and thinning of the cortices. In the absence of other roentgen signs and of clinical and laboratory information, it would be impossible to distinguish this picture from one of osteoporosis.

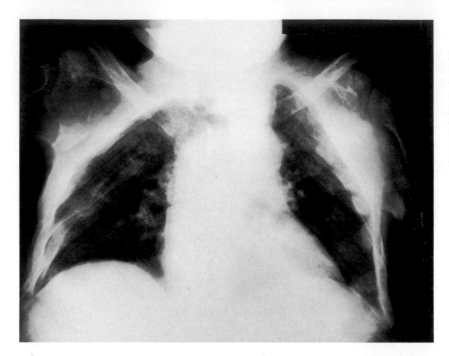

FIG. 2–22. Renal osteomalacia (dorsal spine, ribs, and scapulae)—female, age 49 years. Kyphoscoliosis of the dorsal spine, rib deformities, and fractures are present. Note loss of bone density with accentuation of the trabecular pattern in both scapulae. Pseudofractures may be seen bilaterally in the scapulae. The ribs appear mottled.

Pseudofractures (Looser's lines, or Milkman's syndrome) are usually present in the early stages of the disease. These are bilateral symmetrical bands of radiolucency located in:

1. Scapula (axillary margin as well as lateral and superior margins) (Fig. 2–25)
2. Femoral neck and femoral shafts (Fig. 2–26)
3. Pubic and ischeal rami
4. Ulna at the proximal third of the shaft
5. Radius at the distal third of the shaft
6. Ribs (Fig. 2–27)
7. Clavicle
8. Metacarpals, metatarsals, and phalanges (Fig. 2–28)

In later stages of the disease, sclerosis about the pseudofractures occurs and renders them more visible.[74] These zones are composed of osteoid and fibrous tissue and possibly represent healing reactions to infractions. No blood vessels have been consistently found at these sites. Pseudofractures are present in the following diseases:

1. Osteomalacia (sometimes prior to other visible changes)
2. Florid rickets (usually forearms are involved)
3. Paget's disease
4. Fibrous dysplasia
5. Hyperphosphatasia
6. Diseases in which osteomalacia is a secondary feature (*e.g.*, Wilson's disease).
7. Idiopathic[49]

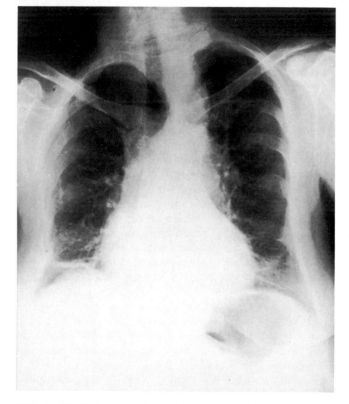

FIG. 2–23. Osteomalacia due to nontropical sprue; same patient as in Fig. 2–21. Note dorsal kyphosis and bell-shaped thorax, and generalized loss of bone density. There are pseudofractures at the axillary margins of both scapulae.

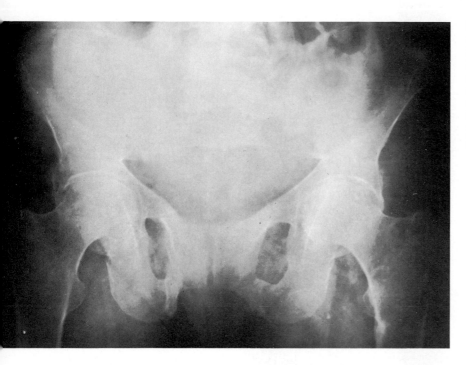

FIG. 2–24. Osteomalacia (pelvis) due to nontropical sprue. There is deformity of the pelvis with protrusio acetabuli. Bilateral and symmetrical pseudofractures of the pubis may be seen. Note bone deformity at the right ischiopubic junction, and generalized diminution of bone density. A pseudofracture of the proximal medial left femoral shaft is also present.

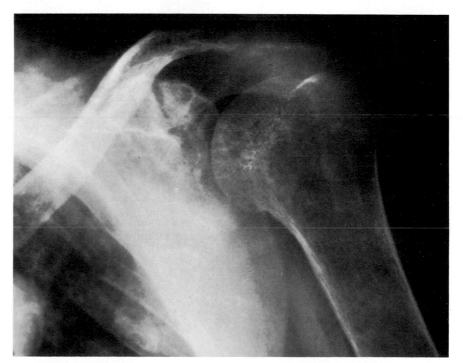

FIG. 2–25. Renal osteomalacia (left scapula); same patient as in Fig. 2–22. Note pseudofracture at the superior margin of the scapula, and marked deformity of the scapula. Definitive fractures of the left upper ribs may be seen.

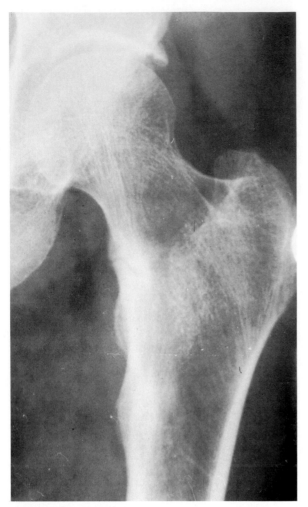

FIG. 2–26. Osteomalacia (hip) — pseudofracture of medial aspect of the base of the femoral neck. Note the area of linear radiolucency surrounded by a zone of sclerosis.

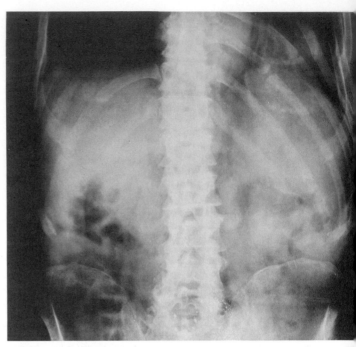

FIG. 2–27. Osteomalacia (ribs) — hypophosphatemic. Multiple fractures and pseudofractures in the lower ribs are seen. (Courtesy of Dr. Dharmashi V. Bhate, VA Hospital, Hines, IL)

FIG. 2–28. Renal osteomalacia (hands); same patient as in Fig. 2–25. Bilateral and symmetrical pseudofractures at the distal phalanges of both thumbs may be noted. A pseudofracture of the distal phalanx of the right fifth finger may also be seen. There is loss of bone density, accentuation of the trabecular pattern, and cortical thinning.

If the osteomalacic process continues. Looser's lines progress to complete fractures, often having considerable separation of fragments (Fig. 2–29). Pseudofractures are to be differentiated from pseudarthroses, which are commonly seen in neurofibromatosis. Osteomalacia and osteoporosis not infrequently coexist.

METABOLISM OF CALCIUM AND PHOSPHORUS

Calcium is absorbed chiefly in the proximal small bowel in the presence of vitamin D. The net absorption is about 15% of the intake, with the remainder egested in the feces. This figure takes into account approximately 400 mg per day of calcium secreted into the intestine in digestive juices. Interference with absorption, therefore, makes it possible to lose more calcium than was ingested because of these secretions. The factors that inhibit calcium absorption from the intestine are the following:

1. Lack of vitamin D
2. Presence of phosphate in the intestine. If excess phosphate is present, insoluble $Ca_3(PO_4)_2$ is formed. This occurs in uremia when phosphate is not cleared by the kidneys and secretion into the intestine occurs. This process partially explains the hypocalcemia occurring with uremia.
3. pH. Alkaline intestinal contents inhibit calcium absorption.
4. Presence of free fatty acids. In steatorrhea caused by primary intestinal malabsorption, free fatty acids combine with calcium to form insoluble soaps. Also, there is failure of vitamin D absorption. This explains the osteomalacia in these conditions.
5. Presence of phytic acid and oxalates

The normal serum calcium concentration is 8.8 to 10.5 mg %. The two main fractions are ionized calcium and protein-bound nonionized calcium; these are present in approximately equal amounts under

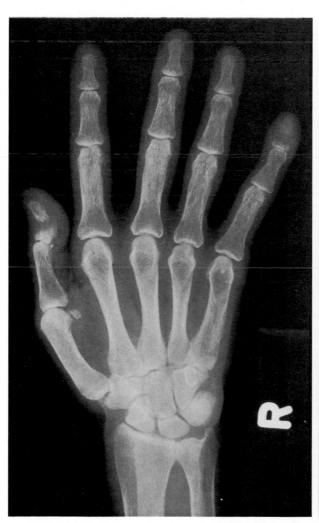
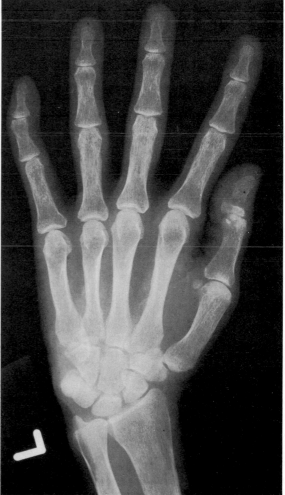

normal conditions. A small amount of citrate-linked calcium that is not ionized is also present. The ratio of ionized to nonionized calcium is increased in acidosis and decreased in alkalosis.

The calcium level is more labile in infants than in adults. Urinary calcium is derived from diffusible plasma calcium. Over 99% of glomerular filtered calcium is resorbed by the tubules. A small rise in plasma calcium may lead to a large rise in urinary calcium. The average urinary calcium excretion is about 100 to 200 mg per day. Vitamin D and parathormone are believed to exert some control over renal calcium excretion.

Phosphorus is present in the blood as inorganic phosphate chiefly in two ionic forms, $H_2PO_4^-$ and $HPO_4^=$, and in esters and phospholipids. The plasma phosphorus level, which refers to inorganic phosphates, is normally more variable than the calcium level. The normal adult range is 2.7 to 4.5 mg %. In the first few weeks of life, a level of 7 mg % is normal.

All plasma phosphate passes through the glomerular filter. Approximately 90% is resorbed by the proximal tubules. Parathormone exerts a major influence at this site, inhibiting net tubular resorption and thereby increasing urinary phosphate.

The relationship among plasma calcium, plasma phosphorus, CO_2, and pH is usually constant and may be expressed as follows[130]:

$$\frac{Ca^{++} \times (HCO_3)^- \times (HPO_4)^=}{pH} = K$$

Under normal circumstances the product of the calcium and phosphorus ion concentrations in mg % ranges from 30 to 40. The normal range values of serum calcium and phosphorus are age- and sex-dependent (Table 2-1).[43]

Many conditions can cause hyper- or hypocalcemia or hyper- or hypophosphatemia, and hyper- or hypocalciuria. Important causes are listed in Table 2-2.

TABLE 2–1. Normal Serum Values in Adults by Age and Sex (95% Confidence Limits)

Age (years)	Calcium (mg/100 ml)		Phosphorus (mg/100 ml)	
	M	**F**	**M**	**F**
20	9.1–10.2	8.8–10.0	2.5–4.5	2.8–4.7
30	9.0–10.1	8.8–10.0	2.4–4.3	2.5–4.2
50	8.9–10.0	8.8–10.0	2.2–4.1	2.7–4.4
70	8.8–9.9	8.8–10.0	2.0–3.9	2.9–4.8

(Modified from Goldsmith et al: In Clinical Aspects of Metabolic Bone Disease, Amsterdam, Excerpta Medica, 1973)

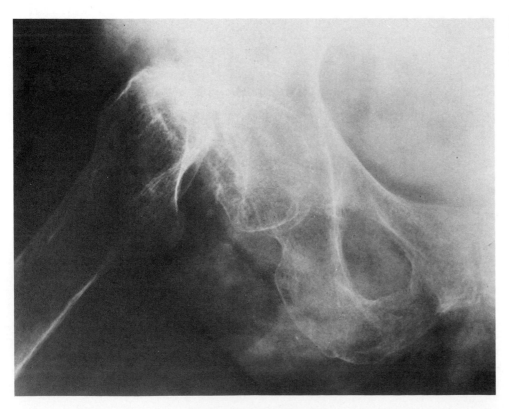

FIG. 2–29. Osteomalacia. Loss of bone density, as well as femoral neck fracture are noted.

TABLE 2–2. Causes of Altered Calcium and Phosphorus Concentrations

HYPERCALCEMIA

1. Hyperparathyroidism
2. Skeletal metastases
3. Hyperthyroidism or hypothyroidism
4. Rapid deossification of bone
5. Myelomatosis (sometimes accompanied by elevated serum protein)
6. Sarcoidosis
7. Reticuloses
8. Leukemias and lymphomas
9. Vitamin D intoxication
10. Idiopathic hypercalcemia
11. Adrenal insufficiency
12. Hypophosphatasia
13. Wermer's syndrome (familial multiple endocrine adenomas)
14. Secretion of parathormone-like substance from malignant tumors
15. Milk-alkali syndrome

HYPOCALCEMIA

1. Hypoparathyroidism
2. Vitamin D deficiency
3. Malabsorption states
4. Uremia
5. Uremic osteodystrophy
6. Hypoalbuminemic states
7. Pancreatitis
8. Neonates
9. Acidosis

HYPERPHOSPHATEMIA

1. Glomerular failure
2. Hypoparathyroidism
3. Hypervitaminosis D
4. Acromegaly
5. Skeletal metastases

HYPOPHOSPHATEMIA

1. Pregnancy
2. Hypovitaminosis D
   A. Vitamin D-deficient rickets
   B. Osteomalacia
2. Renal tubular dysfunction
   A. Fanconi syndrome
   B. Vitamin D-resistant rickets
4. Hyperparathyroidism
5. Malabsorption
6. Increased carbohydrate metabolism
7. Dietary deficiency
8. Skeletal metastases

HYPERCALCIURIA

1. Hypercalcemia
2. Widespread bone destruction
3. Active osteoporosis
4. Renal tubular disease
5. Primary hyperparathyroidism
6. Acidosis
7. Sarcoidosis
8. Vitamin D intoxication

HYPOCALCIURIA

1. Hypocalcemia
2. Active reconstruction of bone
3. Decreased glomerular filtration rate
4. Alkalosis
5. Vitamin D deficiency
6. Reduced amount of calcium absorbed from the intestine

HYPERPARATHYROIDISM

Parathyroid hormone[100] (PTH) is secreted from the parathyroid gland and from adenomas as an 84 amino acid peptide (molecular weight 9,500). Circulating immunoreactive PTH is smaller, with a molecular weight of about 7,000, and is immunologically dissimilar to extracted and secreted hormone. A precursor, proparathyroid hormone, has been demonstrated (molecular weight 11,500). At least two cleavages take place from biosynthesis to ultimate disappearance; pro PTH to PTH, and PTH to circulating PTH. These cleavage steps have been postulated as points of metabolic control to regulate the amount of biologically active hormone available for interaction with receptors in bone and kidney.

Fragments of PTH can be active, and it has been determined that the amino terminal portion of the molecule between residues 2 and 27 is necessary for activity. Radioimmunoassays with antibodies to permit selective measurement of limited regions of the hormone sequence have been developed. Immunoassays are clinically useful. The normal circulating PTH level is dependent on the serum calcium level, and shows a circadian rhythm with the highest value at 2:00 to 4:00 A.M. Assays of the 7,000 molecular weight form are thought to reflect the chronic state of parathyroid function, and are expected to be most useful in the routine clinical assessment of hyperparathyroidism (Arnaud et al).[43]

Parathyroid hormone exerts its major influences directly on the bone and the kidney, and secondary influences on the gastrointestinal tract and the mammary glands. In the kidney, PTH inhibits net tubular phosphate resorption, causing an increase in urinary phosphorus, and a decrease in serum inorganic phosphorus levels. It also increases calcium reabsorption.

In bone excess, PTH is associated with increased osteoclastic resorption and osteocytic osteolysis. Elevation of the serum calcium level correlates positively with immunoreactive PTH levels. The relationship is not linear, with inhibition of PTH efficacy at *higher serum calcium levels*. The initial calcium release from bone in response to PTH is believed to be due to osteocytic osteolysis. It is postulated that vitamin D has a permissive effect on PTH-induced osteoclastic proliferation, and that serum calcium regulation by PTH is vitamin D-dependent.

Control of the parathyroid glands is regulated by plasma calcium levels by a direct negative feedback mechanism. It has been conjectured that metabolites of vitamin D, such as 1,25-DHCC, act upon parathyroid cells, setting the point around which the serum calcium concentration controls the rate of PTH secretion (Rasmussen).[43]

Calcitonin (CT)[43,140] is a hormone produced by the parafollicular cells of the thyroid gland. Its administration causes reduction in serum calcium and phosphorus concentrations effected by reduction of bone resorption. It is a single chain polypeptide of 32 amino acids with a molecular weight of about 3,600. CT tends to negate the action of PTH on bone; however, it does not work at the same receptor site. It does not block PTH effects on the kidney. Its effect is greatest at high skeletal resorption rates, and it is almost without effect on serum calcium levels in the normal adult.

Hyperparathyroidism may be primary, secondary, or tertiary.

Hyperparathyroidism[5,43,53] refers to the condition of increased circulating PTH. Seventeen to 40% of patients with primary hyperparathyroidism exhibit demonstrable radiographic bone changes. Increased awareness of this condition, coupled with refinements in serum calcium determinations and revision of normal values, contributes to earlier diagnosis prior to the onset of roentgen abnormalities. The pathological designation of the skeletal effects of the hyperparathyroid state is "generalized osteitis fibrosa cystica," or osteitis fibrosa. In the radiological literature the condition is generally referred to as hyperparathyroidism. It should not be inferred, however, that in the absence of radiologically demonstrable skeletal changes, the patient is "negative for hyperparathyroidism."

The causes of primary hyperparathyroidism are: (1) parathyroid adenoma (may be associated with multiple endocrine adenomas), (2) parathyroid hyperplasia, (3) parathyroid carcinoma, (4) nonparathyroid tumors that secrete a parathormonelike substance, and (5) multiple endocrine neoplasia, type II (medullary carcinoma of thyroid, hyperparathyroidism, pheochromocytoma, Cushing's syndrome).

Secondary hyperparathyroidism is the response of the gland to chronic hypocalcemia, usually of renal glomerular disease, by means of the negative feedback regulatory mechanism.[101] Congenital hyperparathyroidism as a response of the fetal parathyroid gland to maternal hypoparathyroidism has been described[1] (Fig. 2–30).

Tertiary hyperparathyroidism refers to the condition of escape of the gland from the regulatory effects of serum calcium levels in patients following prolonged stimulation, such as renal hemodialysis. It is also known as autonomy of the parathyroid gland.

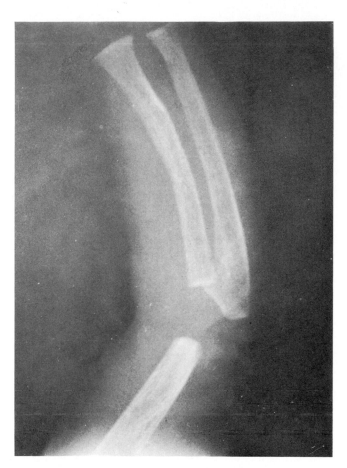

FIG. 2–30. Congenital hyperparathyroidism (forearm) due to reactive hyperplasia of the fetal parathyroid glands, secondary to absence of maternal parathyroid glands. Note loss of bone density, accentuation of the bony trabecular pattern, and deformity of the shaft of the radius from a healed intrauterine fracture.

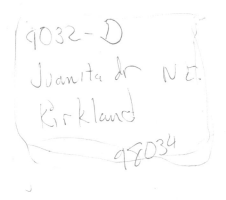

FIG. 2–31. Hyperparathyroidism. Note the large lacuna in bone with multinucleated giant cells. ×16. (Courtesy of Dr. R. Heredia, Dept. of Pathology, Mt. Sinai Hospital, Chicago, IL)

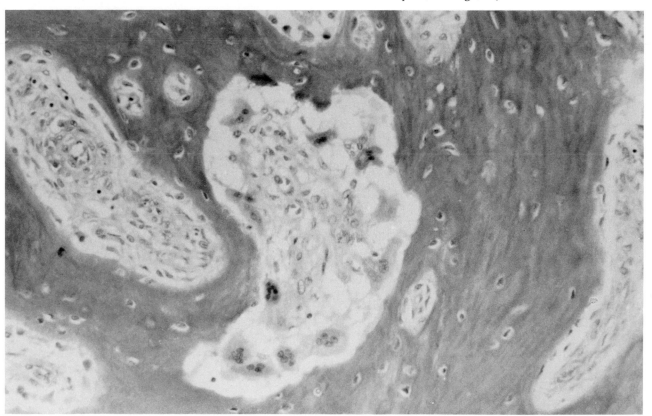

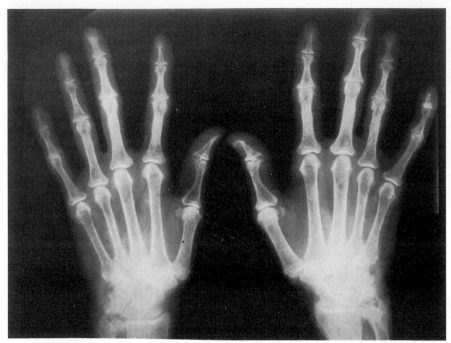

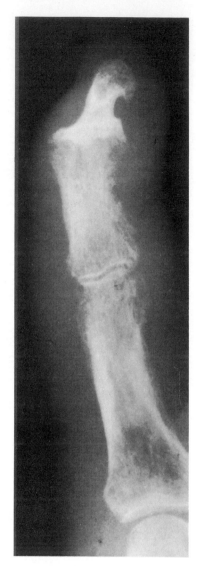

FIG. 2–32. Hyperparathyroidism (hands). Subperiosteal resorption of bone of the proximal and middle phalanges may be seen bilaterally on both the radial and the ulnar sides. Note loss of distinction and resorption of the terminal tufts of all the phalanges, and bony resorption around both ulnar styloid processes. There is a generalized loss of bone density, and cortical thinning.

FIG. 2–33. Hyperparathyroidism (fifth finger) showing subperiosteal bone resorption, most marked at the radial aspect of the middle phalanx. There is loss of cortical definition and a "lacelike" appearance at the resorbed site.

Histologically, the basic process is osteoclastic and osteocytic resorption and replacement of the resorbed bone by fibrous tissue (Fig. 2–31). Bone formed as a reaction to osteoclastic destruction shows alterations in quality and in the pattern of collagen fibrils. There is defective lamellar structure and failure of haversian system formation. Softening and deformity of the bone result. Cysts and brown tumors arise in the fibrous tissue overgrowth that replaces bone matrix, owing to focal hemorrhages. Numerous giant cells are present. Pathological changes precede roentgen changes.

Biochemically, the serum calcium concentration is raised only in primary hyperparathyroidism, and it may be only intermittently raised. In secondary hyperparathyroidism, the serum calcium level is normal or low. The serum phosphorus level is low until renal failure develops. The serum alkaline phosphatase is elevated if bone disease is present. In the presence of known primary hyperparathyroidism, subperiosteal bone resorption can be expected in all patients with an elevated serum alkaline phosphatase.[101] The urine calcium is elevated in primary disease, as well as the urine phosphorus, unless renal failure supervenes. Circulating PTH levels are elevated.

Clinically, the ratio of women to men with primary hyperparathyroidism is about 3 to 1, and the

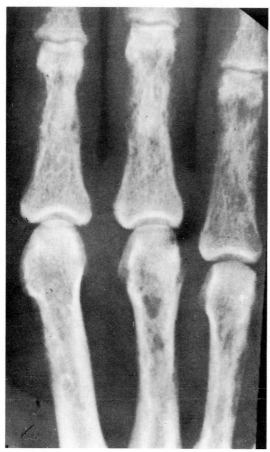

FIG. 2–34. Primary hyperparathyroidism (metacarpals and proximal phalanges). Note subperiosteal bone resportion, most marked on the radial sides of the proximal phalanges with a "scooped-out" appearance of the cortex, increased trabecular pattern, and medullary areas of radiolucency.

condition is most often encountered in the third to fifth decades of life. The symptoms are due to bone disease, hypercalcemia, and renal disease. Weakness, lethargy, polydypsia, and polyuria are frequent early complaints.

Patients with bone disease are in the minority. With skeletal involvement, bone pain and tenderness occur. Clubbing of the fingers may be present, as well as localized masses caused by brown tumors. Pathological fracture and, in later stages, deformities can be seen. Polyarthritis may also be present.

Hypercalcemia can lead to muscular weakness, gastrointestinal symptoms, including peptic ulcer and pancreatitis, and central nervous symptoms ranging from headaches to psychotic behavior. Calcium deposition in the kidneys may occur as nephrocalcinosis or nephrolithiasis. About 75% of

patients have renal involvement, with resulting renal colic and hypertension. Kidney damage may lead to terminal uremia. Primary hyperparathyroidism has been reported as being associated with benign monoclonal gammopathy.[118] It is also reported as presenting with acute paraplegia.[139]

Radiologically, the changes of primary and secondary hyperparathyroidism are similar, except that in the secondary form brown tumors are rare and osteosclerosis is more common.

Among the early changes are subperiosteal bone resorption, particularly along the radial margins of the middle phalanges, at the proximal metaphyseal-diaphyseal junction, distal clavicles (Figs. 2–32, 2–33, 2–34), and the medial aspect of the upper third of the tibia. This was first reported by Camp and Ochsner and described by Pugh as "a peculiar lacelike appearance of the bone beneath the periosteum."[101] The first sign is loss of normal cortical definition, followed by irregular lacy resorption. The endosteal margin initially remains intact. The process may progress to complete cortical resorption. This finding has only been observed in primary and secondary hyperparathyroidism. Subperiosteal bone resorption is thus the radiological hallmark of hyperparathyroidism; any area can be involved. The upper margins of the ribs, the pubis, the ischia, the calcaneus, and the proximal humeri are additional common sites for subperiosteal bone resorption, as well as the distal radius, ulna, the sternal ends of the clavicles,[142] and the dorsum sellae (Fig. 2–35).

Resorption of the cortex of the tooth socket or the lamina dura is a similar process (Figs. 2–36, 2–37). The periodontal membrane is not markedly thickened as is seen in scleroderma, and the teeth maintain their normal density. The alveolar anatomical landmarks are obscured. This finding is not specific and can be seen in the following:

1. Hyperparathyroidism
2. Paget's disease
3. Osteomalacia
4. Scleroderma
5. Hyperphosphatasia
6. Partial resorption reported in Cushing's syndrome
7. Burkitt's tumor
8. Pyorrhea
9. Dental caries

The calvarium shows granular deossification, and less often, cystlike areas. Both tables lose their sharp outlines and the calvarium is thickened (Figs. 2–38, 2–39).

(Text continues on p. 46)

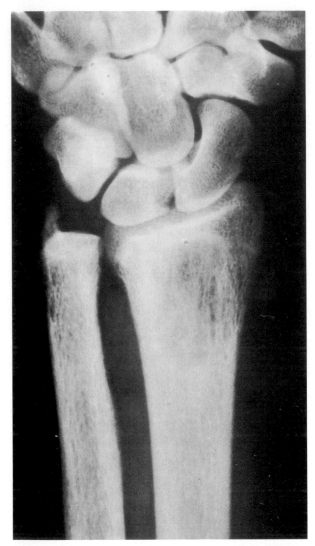

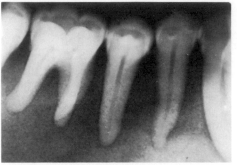

FIG. 2–36. Hyperparathyroidism (dental film). There is resorption of the lamina dura. The teeth are normal. The periodontal membrane, seen as a zone of radiolucency surrounding the teeth, is not widened. Bone texture shows a granular pattern.

FIG. 2–35. Secondary hyperparathyroidism (wrist) —subperiosteal resorption along the margins of the distal radius, ulna, and ulnar styloid process. Note increase in the trabecular pattern and loss of cortical definition. A localized loss of density at the radial metaphyses might be the beginning of an early brown tumor.

FIG. 2–37. Normal lamina dura (compare Fig. 2–36). There is a very fine marginal condensation of bone at the tooth socket, representing the intact lamina dura. This is normally separated from the tooth by the radiolucent periodontal membrane, which is 0.5 mm thick. The bony trabecular pattern appears normal.

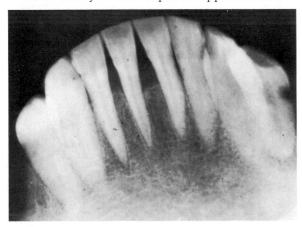

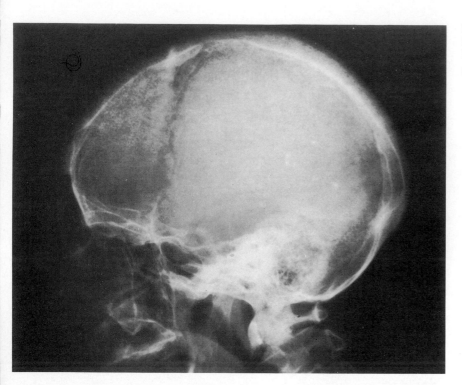

FIG. 2–38. Primary hyperparathyroidism (skull)—parathyroid adenoma. Note loss of bone density in the skull, with a granular pattern.

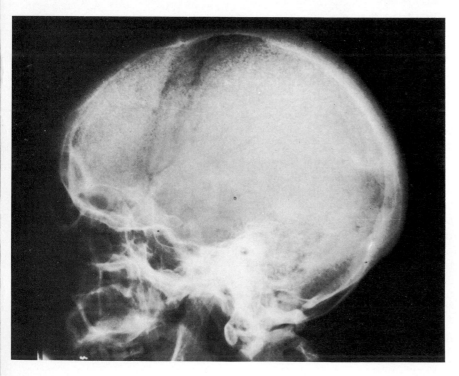

FIG. 2–39. Primary hyperparathyroidism (skull); same patient as in Fig. 2–38, 7 years after removal of parathyroid adenoma. Granular demineralized pattern of skull persists unchanged.

Generalized loss of bone density (Fig. 2–40) follows, with endosteal resorption. The trabecular pattern may be delicate, indistinct, or accentuated (Figs. 2–41, 2–42). A generalized "ground glass" appearance, with endosteal scalloping in the later stages of the disease, is occasionally seen (Fig. 2–43). Clubbing of the fingers with bone resorption of the terminal tufts of the phalanges appears, and may occur in the early stages of the disease prior to subperiosteal resorption. Resorption, particularly of the distal clavicles (Fig. 2–44), symphysis pubis, ischia (Fig. 2–45), sacroiliac joints, and tendinous insertions of the calcaneus, follows.

As the disease progresses, lightly trabeculated, expanding focal bone lesions, which can be quite destructive, appear. They are located chiefly in the mandible, pelvis (Fig. 2–46), ribs, and femora, but any bone may be involved at any site, even the orbit[66] (Figs. 2–47, 2–48, 2–49, 2–50). These lesions vary in size, and are brown tumors or true cysts resulting from intraosseous hemorrhages. True giant-cell tumors are also reported to be associated with these lesions, as well as skeletal metastases in the event of a parathyroid carcinoma. Periosteal reaction is sparse. Pathological fractures may occur. After removal of a parathyroid adenoma, a brown tumor often accumulates dense bone and persists for many years as a sclerotic focus (Figs. 2–51, 2–52, 2–53). It is important to differentiate a cellular brown tumor from a cyst, particularly in a weight-bearing bone. A cyst will not heal after parathyroidectomy, and the patient will remain at risk of a pathological fracture. The distinction on plain films is unreliable. The two may be differentiated by arteriography, or by demonstrating enhancement in the tumor area on post-infusion computed tomography.[35]

Further progression of the disease leads to bizarre deformities of bone. There may be basilar invagination of the skull, wedging, or biconcave deformities of the vertebral bodies and kyphoscoliosis. The pelvis may assume the same triradiate deformity as in osteomalacia (Figs. 2–54, 2–55). Pathological fractures occur (Fig. 2–56). Soft-tissue calcifications, calcified vessels (Fig. 2–57), articular cartilages (Fig. 2–58), menisci, joint capsules, and periarticular tissues occur, as well as nephrolithiasis and nephrocalcinosis. Soft-tissue calcification is more common in secondary hyperparathyroidism. Calcific deposits in the prostate, the salivary glands, and the pancreas are also sometimes present. Metastatic pulmonary calcification, more common in renal failure but also seen rarely in primary hyperparathyroidism, has been reported.[23]

(Text continues on p. 54)

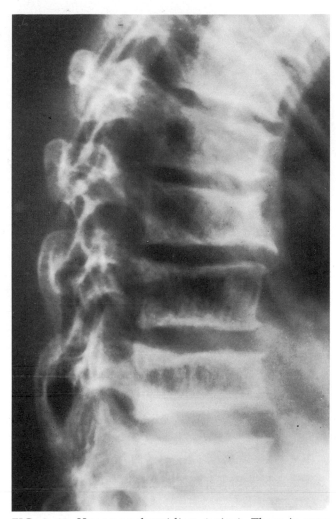

FIG. 2–40. Hyperparathyroidism (spine). There is very generalized loss of bone density, with relative increase in density of the vertebral end-plates and accentuation of trabeculae, which are vertically oriented. Note loss of height of several vertebral bodies.

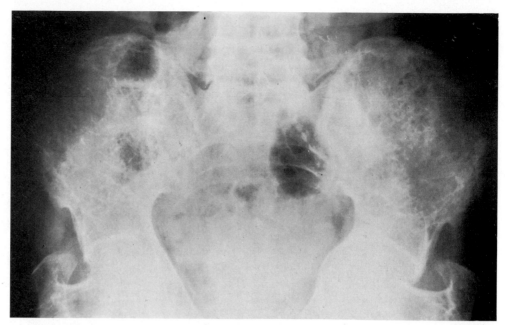

FIG. 2–41. Hyperparathyroidism (pelvis). There is marked alteration of the bone texture in the iliac wings, with resorption of the major portion of the bony trabeculae and accentuation of the few remaining trabeculae. Protrusion of the left acetabulum may also be noted.

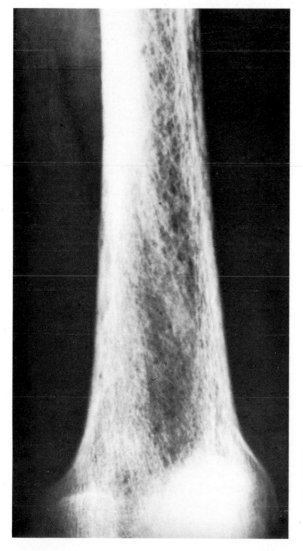

FIG. 2–42. Primary hyperparathyroidism (distal femur). Note the very marked accentuation of trabecular pattern. Cortical thickening at the upper medial aspect is also noted.

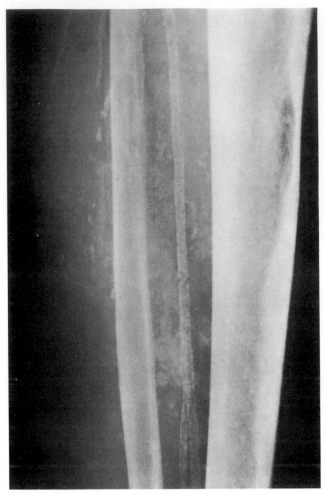

FIG. 2-43. Secondary hyperparathyroidism (tibia). Note uniform loss of bone density with a "ground glass" appearance and endosteal scalloping of the tibial cortex. Severe vascular calcification and subcutaneous ossifications are also present.

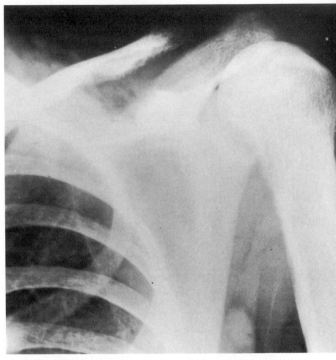

FIG. 2-44. Secondary hyperparathyroidism. Note marked bone resorption of the terminal clavicle, along the inferior aspect of the distal clavicle, and at the tip of the acromion. There is subperiosteal resorption along both the medial and the lateral margins of the proximal humerus, and resorption at the superior aspects of the third and fourth ribs, with loss of cortical definition. Accentuation of the trabecular pattern can also be seen.

FIG. 2-45. Hyperparathyroidism (pelvis). Note subperiosteal bone resorption along the ischia and the symphysis pubis, and loss of bone density and accentuated trabecular pattern in the femoral heads.

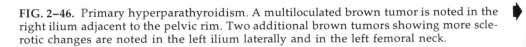

FIG. 2-46. Primary hyperparathyroidism. A multiloculated brown tumor is noted in the right ilium adjacent to the pelvic rim. Two additional brown tumors showing more sclerotic changes are noted in the left ilium laterally and in the left femoral neck.

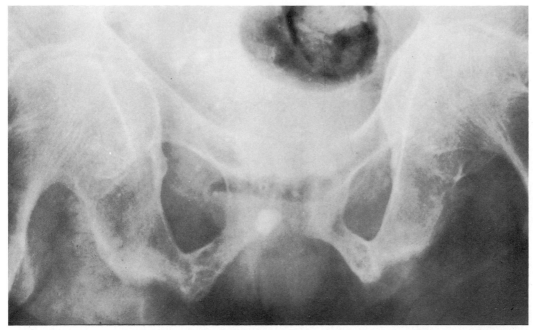

FIG. 2–45

FIG. 2–46

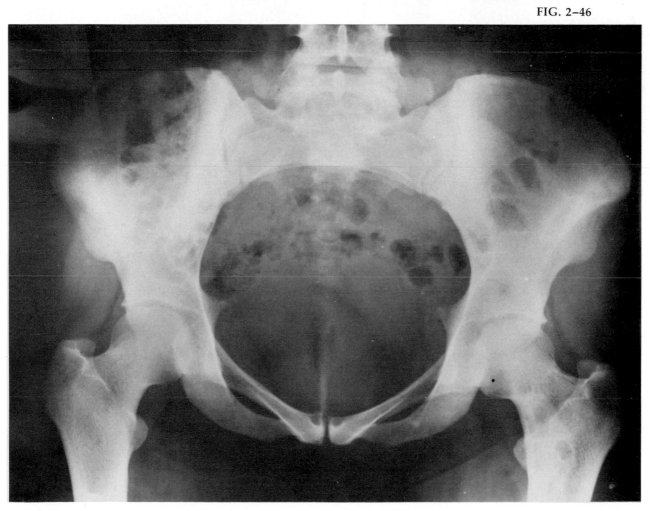

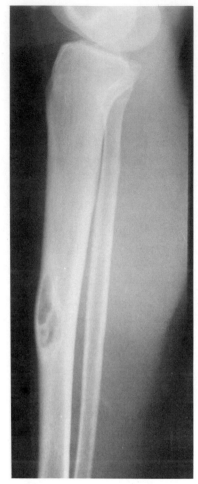

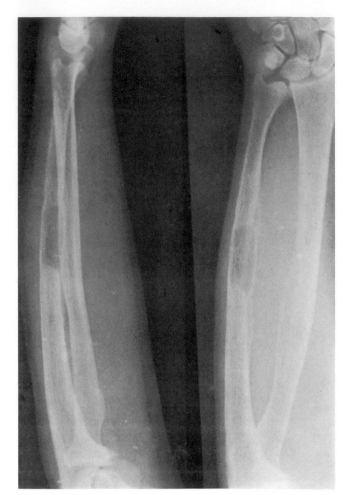

FIG. 2–47   FIG. 2–48

FIG. 2–47. Primary hyperparathyroidism. A slightly expansile loculated brown tumor is noted in the midtibial shaft.

FIG. 2–48. Hyperparathyroidism (forearm)—brown tumor. There is an expanding, lightly trabeculated, well-demarcated radiolucent lesion in the mid-diaphysis of the ulna.

FIG. 2–49. Primary hyperparathyroidism (forearm)—brown tumor. Note the expansile lightly trabeculated lesion at the distal ulna, not extending to the articular surface. Accentuation of the trabecular pattern of the radius is also seen.

FIG. 2–50. Primary hyperparathyroidism (skull)—brown tumor in the frontoparietal region. Note the multiple conglomerate radiolucent areas with some marginal sclerosis.

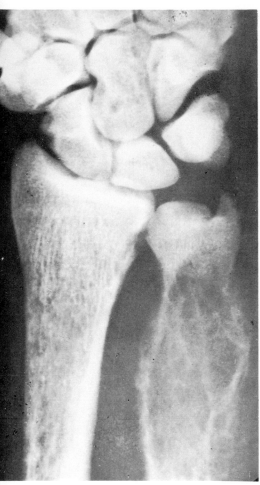

FIG. 2–49

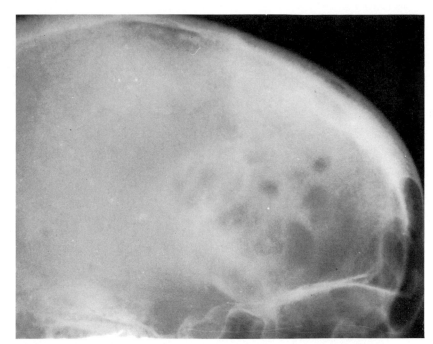

FIG. 2–50
FIG. 2–51

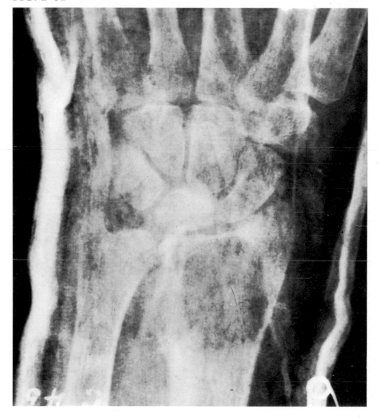

FIG. 2–51. Primary hyperparathyroidism (left wrist)—female, age 34 years. Picture is of left wrist in plaster cast, taken soon after biopsy; lesion was reported as a giant-cell tumor. Biochemical determinations revealed: serum calcium 15.4 mg%; serum phosphorus 2.9 mg%; alkaline phosphatase 4.7 u.

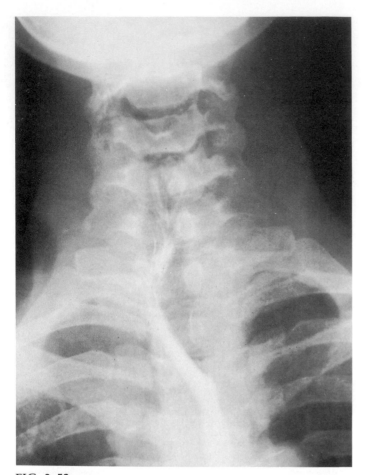

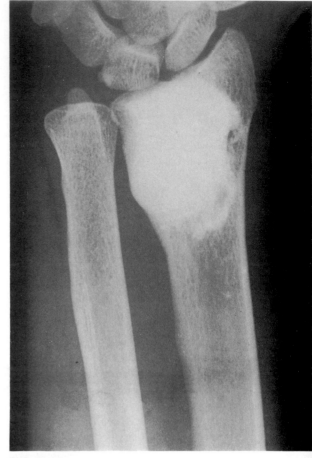

FIG. 2–52

FIG. 2–53

FIG. 2–54

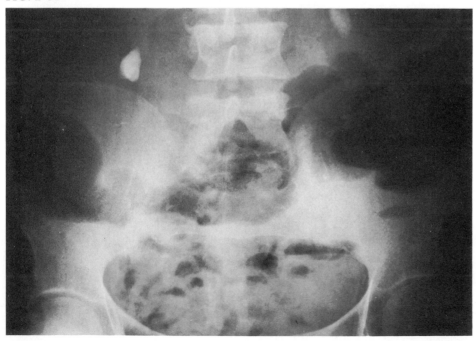

FIG. 2–52. Barium swallow of patient in Fig. 2–51. There is deviation of the cervical esophagus to the right. A 6.5 g parathyroid adenoma was removed surgically.

FIG. 2–53. Primary hyperparathyroidism (left wrist); same patient as in Figs. 2–51 and 2–52, 4 years after removal of parathyroid adenoma. Persistent residual sclerotic focus at site of previous brown tumor. The surrounding bone structure appears normal.

FIG. 2–54. Hyperparathyroidism (pelvis) — female, age 30 years. The bone structure appears normal. Bilateral renal calculi may be seen.

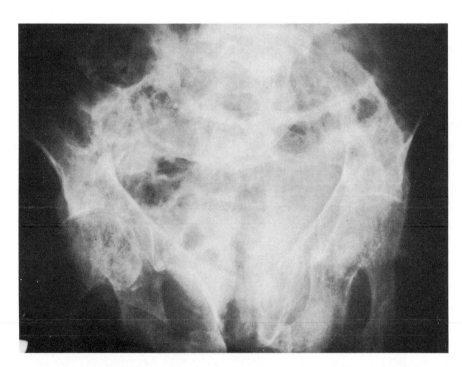

FIG. 2–55. Hyperparathyroidism (pelvis); same patient as in Fig. 2–54 after 4 years. There has been marked deossification of the pelvis with accentuation of the trabecular pattern. A triradiate deformity may be seen, similar to that which occurs in osteomalacia.

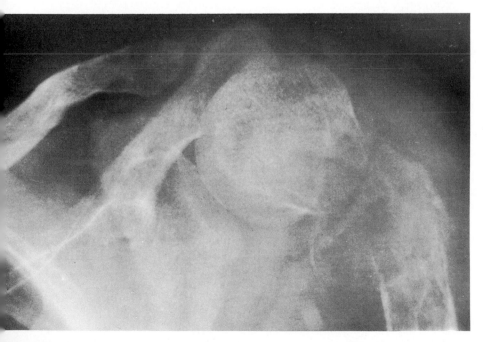

FIG. 2–56. Pathological fracture (proximal humerus) in patient with parathyroid carcinoma and hyperparathyroidism. Both bony metastases and brown tumors are present. The nature of this particular lesion was not determined. The two types of lesions may be radiologically indistinguishable, although the expanded shell of the lesion suggests that it is a brown tumor.

53

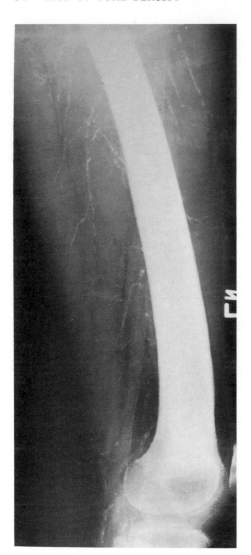

FIG. 2–57. Secondary hyperparathyroidism (thigh). Note extensive and severe calcification of the femoral artery and branches.

FIG. 2–58. Hyperparathyroidism (knees). Calcification of the articular cartilages of the knees may be noted bilaterally and symmetrically. For differential diagnosis see Chapter 8, pages 637–638.

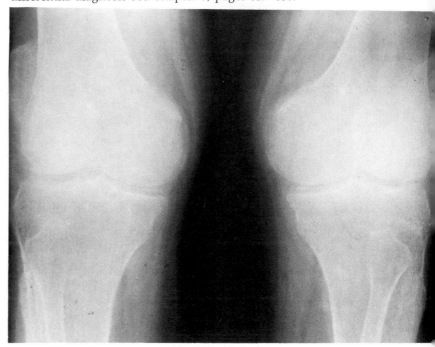

A solitary brown tumor may be the only bone manifestation of this disease. This is estimated to occur in 3% of cases. It is therefore important to determine the serum calcium and phosphorus levels when any solitary bone lesion that could conceivably represent a brown tumor is encountered.

If the disease occurs prior to epiphyseal closure, a radiographic picture similar to that of rickets occurs, owing to uncalcified metaphyseal osteoid.

Osteosclerosis occasionally is present, possibly caused by PTH or caused by the action of thyrocalcitonin. The spine is most commonly involved. This can take the form of a uniform increase in bone density, or the end-plates of vertebral bodies may become denser than the center giving a horizontal striped appearance, the "rugger jersey" (football sweater) spine (Figs. 2–59, 2–60). Other bones can also be involved (Fig. 2–61).

Osteosclerosis is usually encountered in renal osteodystrophy, but can also rarely appear in primary hyperparathyroidism. Peculiar cystic or erosive changes showing a predilection for the small joints of the hands and wrists have been described in this disease. The radiocarpal, radioulnar, and metacarpophalangeal joints are involved. Absence of joint space narrowing, as well as "whiskering" at the joint margins and associated cystic changes, may be present. The large joints may also be involved.[102]

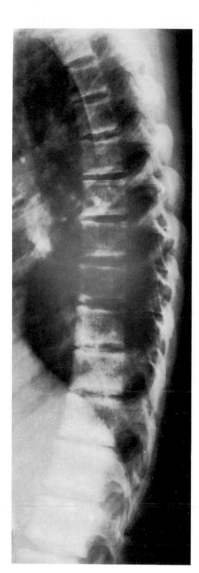

FIG. 2–59. Secondary hyperparathyroidism (spine)—"rugger jersey" spine. Osteosclerosis with greater density of the bone approaching the vertebral end-plates, giving a striped appearance.

FIG. 2–60. Secondary hyperparathyroidism (lumbar spine)—osteosclerosis with "rugger jersey" spine.

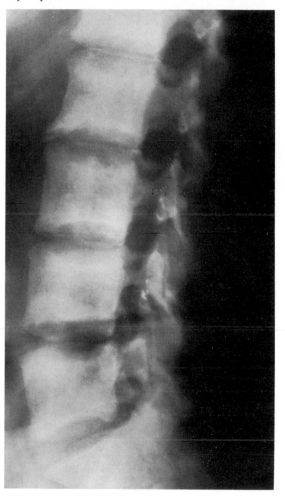

Chondrocalcinosis is common in primary hyperparathyroidism. Cartilage calcification in the wrists, knees, shoulders, hips, elbows, and symphysis pubis may be seen. Acute pseudogout may occur.

Restoration and bone density,[9] reconstruction of the cortex and lamina dura, and healing of pathological fractures take place following successful treatment of hyperparathyroidism. True bone cysts persist and brown tumors become sclerotic. The skull may have a residual pagetoid appearance and a residual increase in bone density. The resorbed terminal phalangeal tufts reform after treatment.

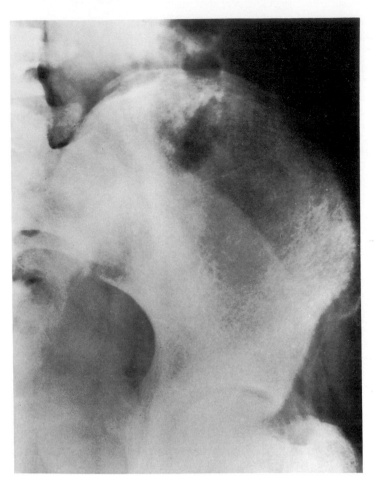

FIG. 2–61. Secondary hyperparathyroidism—osteosclerosis in female, age 17 years. There is accentuation of the trabecular pattern in the iliac wing. Note subperiosteal bone resorption along the iliac margin.

RENAL OSTEODYSTROPHY

Renal disease may be primarily tubular or glomerular. Tubular syndromes, such as vitamin D-resistant rickets, renal tubular acidosis, and Fanconi syndrome result in loss of phosphate and other metabolites in the urine. The resultant hypophosphatemia leads to rickets and osteomalacia. Although osteitis fibrosa is said sometimes to complicate these conditions as well as nutritional rickets, it is not predominantly a part of the roentgen spectrum of the above diseases.

Chronic glomerular renal disease, however, produces a wide spectrum of roentgenologically detectable changes in bone and soft tissue.

PATHOPHYSIOLOGY

Chronic glomerular renal disease with reduced renal mass and reduced glomerular filtration rate manifests itself in two basic forms: resistance to vitamin D and reduced renal clearance of phosphate[72] (Fig. 2–62).

Resistance to vitamin D can begin in the early phase of chronic renal failure and become increasingly severe as the disease progresses.[72] The resultant effect of this phenomenon is rickets in the immature skeleton and osteomalacia in the adult. The mechanism in renal hyperphosphatemic disease is not similar to that in vitamin D-deficient rickets or tubular disease with hypophosphatemia, where bone changes are associated with a low calcium-phosphate ion product. This product may be elevated in patients with chronic renal failure. There are several theories as to the manner in which bone matrix mineralization is blocked. Avioli and Slatopolsky,[111] cited by Robinson,[111] proposed that there is an abnormal metabolism of vitamin D_3 in patients with chronic renal failure. This is responsible for decreased intestinal absorption of calcium. Vitamin D is also implicated as having a direct effect on osteoid mineralization. The production of vitamin D antagonists, as well as failure of end-organ response, has also been speculated.

Reduced glomerular filtration rate results in reduced renal phosphate clearance. This plays the major pathogenetic role in the development of secondary hyperparathyroidism.[128] This causes a rise in the phosphate level in body fluids. A significant inverse correlation is present between free calcium ion concentration and diffusible inorganic phosphate concentration in severe renal failure.[72] Plasma calcium ion concentration decreases. This is not to imply a cause-and-effect relationship. By a direct negative feedback mechanism in response to hypocalcemia, the parathyroid glands may develop hyperplasia and hypertrophy, with an increased secretion of parathormone. There is a suggestion that the plasma magnesium concentration may also be implicated, with an increase causing inhibition, and a decrease causing stimulation of parathyroid secretion. This leads to increased circulating parathyroid hormone, which is the true state of secondary hyperparathyroidism. The high levels of circulating PTH are also maintained owing to decreased renal degradation of PTH.[128]

The bone may respond to parathormone in various degrees. If the bone is able to respond with an increased activity of osteoclasts and osteocytes, then the resultant effect is osteitis fibrosa. This leads to release of calcium. Parathormone also inhibits net tubular phosphate resorption, leading to an increase in urinary phosphate which, however, is limited by renal failure. A rise in the calcium-phosphate ion product leads to metastatic calcification. The increase in serum calcium concentration exerts an inhibitory effect on parathormone secretion.

The bone may respond poorly to parathormone. In 1948, Albright and Reifenstein suggested that patients with osteomalacia fail to show a response to parathormone because the bone is covered with osteoid tissue, which prevents resorption.[5] The coating of unmineralized osteoid tissue over all bony surfaces makes mineralized tissue unavailable to maintain normocalcemia. Another factor is the possibility that the parathormone in patients with chronic renal failure is altered, and that the observed skeletal resistance to parathormone is in part due to this alteration.[72] Low levels of 1,25-DHCC is thought to impair the response of the skeleton to the action of PTH.[128]

If there is lack of development of osteitis fibrosa, the predominant roentgen picture may be one of osteomalacia or osteoporosis.

Osteoporosis may be due to the general condition

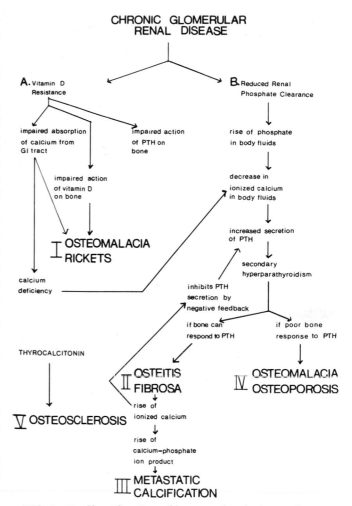

FIG. 2–62. Classification of bone and soft-tissue changes in chronic glomerular renal disease. (From Greenfield GB: Roentgen appearance of bone and soft-tissue changes in chronic renal disease. Am J Roentgen 116:749–757, 1972)

of the patient or local immobilization due to bone pain or fracture.

Some patients with renal disease have absolute overproduction of bone matrix, which may be mineralized sufficiently so that the bones appear excessively dense on roentgenograms.[111] In 1932, Selye gave mice small doses of parathormone for an extended period of time and observed osteosclerosis. This has also been more recently observed with parathyroid administration in thyroidectomized rats.[137] Thyrocalcitonin has been the subject of much recent investigation and has been shown to cause osteosclerosis.

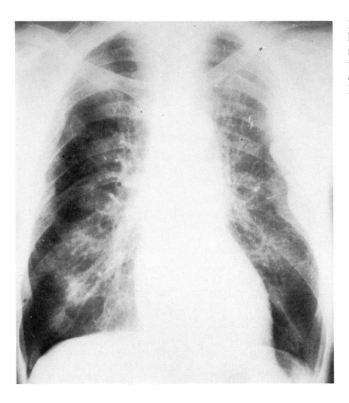

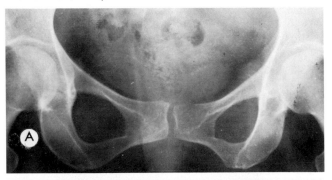

FIG. 2–63. Renal osteodystrophy (chest)—patient on renal hemodialysis. Osteomalacia of the chest is seen, demonstrating multiple healed rib fractures with deformity of the thorax. (From Greenfield GB: Roentgen appearance of bone and soft-tissue changes in chronic renal disease. Am J Roentgen 116:749–757, 1972)

FIG. 2–64. Renal osteodystrophy (pelvis)—patient on renal hemodialysis—osteomalacia. **A.** The pelvis is normal. **B.** Same patient 13 months later. There are symmetric pseudofractures at the ischia and pubic bones. (From Greenfield GB: Roentgen appearance of bone and soft-tissue changes in chronic renal disease. Am J Roentgen 116:749–757, 1972)

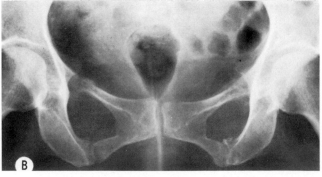

In severe renal failure of long duration, elevation of the serum calcium concentration may not exert an inhibitory effect on parathyroid secretion. This is referred to as autonomy of the parathyroid gland, or tertiary hyperparathyroidism.

The incidence of bone changes in chronic renal disease can approach 25% in untreated cases. In dialysis programs, bone changes become more severe as the dialysis progresses, and the incidence can approach 80% to 90%. Correlation between histological and radiological changes is high in estimating the severity of osteitis fibrosa, but is of no value in diagnosing the degree of osteomalacia.[29]

In successful renal transplantation, the visible changes tend to regress. A complication of renal transplantation, ischemic necrosis of bone involving several joints, has been reported in a high percentage of cases.[26]

ROENTGENOGRAPHIC FINDINGS

It can thus be seen that the spectrum of changes includes osteomalacia, osteitis fibrosa, osteoporosis, osteosclerosis, metastatic calcification, rickets (if in the immature skeleton), and possibly ischemic necrosis if renal transplantation has been performed.

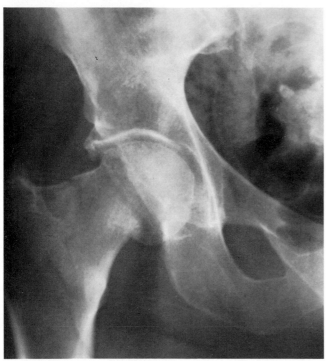

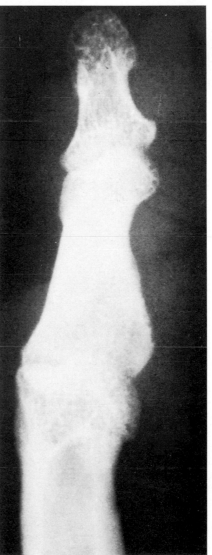

FIG. 2–65. Renal osteodystrophy (femur)—patient on renal hemodialysis—osteomalacia with fracture of the right femoral neck. (From Greenfield GB: Roentgen appearance of bone and soft-tissue changes in chronic renal disease. Am J Roentgen 116:749–757, 1972)

FIG. 2–66. Renal osteodystrophy (finger)—patient on renal hemodialysis—osteitis fibrosa, early change. There is minimal subperiosteal bone resorption of the radial side of the middle phalanx at the metaphyseal-diaphyseal junction. (From Greenfield GB: Roentgen appearance of bone and soft-tissue changes in chronic renal disease. Am J Roentgen 116:749–757, 1972)

Early in the course of renal failure, a picture of osteomalacia may predominate.

A common presentation is deformity of the chest with multiple fractures of the ribs (Fig. 2–63). Pseudofractures may also be seen in the scapulae, femora, pubes, and ischia (Figs. 2–64, 2–65). They sometimes have a symmetric distribution.

If bone can respond to parathormone, then the effects of secondary hyperparathyroidism will be predominant (Figs. 2–66, 2–67, 2–68). There may be an underlying osteoporosis due to general lack of mobility or to local factors of immobilization (Fig. 2–69). In the immature skeleton, osteomalacia manifests itself as rickets, with the typical widening of the epiphyseal cartilage plate and cupping and fraying of the metaphysis. This may be seen in combination with subperiosteal bone resorption and pseudofractures (Figs. 2–70, 2–71). Periosteal new bone formation has also been reported (Fig. 2–72).

Osteosclerosis can complicate the picture, as well as soft-tissue calcification (Fig. 2–74). The spine is the area most commonly involved (Figs. 2–59, 2–60) with sclerosis. The skull and long bones also may be involved with cortical thickening and sclerosis, giving an almost pagetoid appearance[109] (Fig. 2–73). Patients on renal dialysis have progressive changes of osteitis fibrosa. Following successful renal transplantation, the majority of patients become euparathyroid in 6 to 18 months, with regression of changes of osteitis fibrosa.[62]

(Text continues on p. 63)

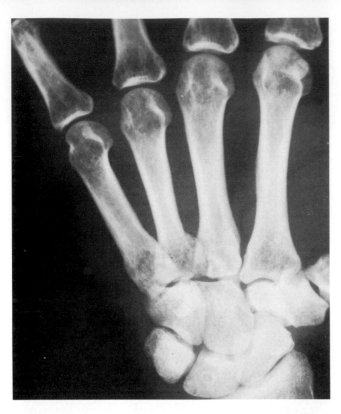

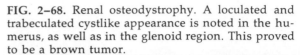

FIG. 2–67. Renal osteodystrophy (hand)—patient on renal hemodialysis—osteitis fibrosa. There is an expansile lesion at the base of the fourth metacarpal which is probably a cyst or brown tumor. The lesion was not biopsied. (From Greenfield GB: Roentgen appearance of bone and soft-tissue changes in chronic renal disease. Am J Roentgen 116:749–757, 1972)

FIG. 2–68. Renal osteodystrophy. A loculated and trabeculated cystlike appearance is noted in the humerus, as well as in the glenoid region. This proved to be a brown tumor.

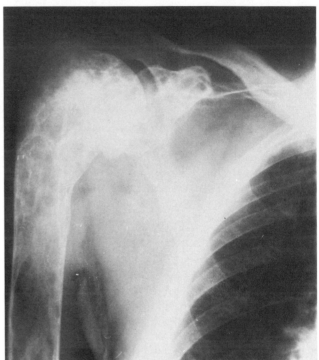

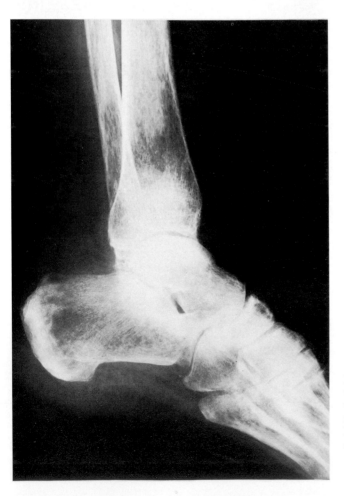

FIG. 2–69. Renal osteodystrophy (lower extremity)—patient on renal hemodialysis. There is permeative osteoporotic pattern in osteomalacia patient secondary to immobilization from hip fracture. (From Greenfield GB: Roentgen appearance of bone and soft-tissue changes in chronic renal disease. Am J Roentgen 116:749–757, 1972)

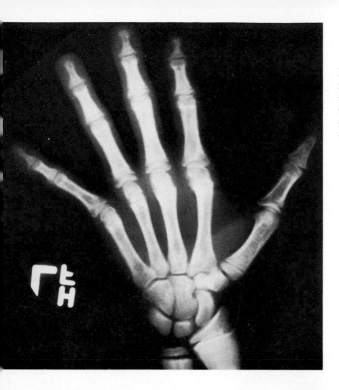

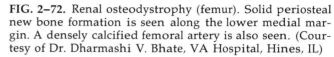

FIG. 2–70. Renal osteodystrophy (hand) — male, age 10 years, on renal hemodialysis. Subperiosteal bone resorption, resorption of the terminal phalanges, and rachitic changes manifested by widening of the epiphyseal cartilage plate, particularly at the distal ulna are noted. This indicates a combination of osteitis fibrosa with osteomalacia (rickets).

FIG. 2–72. Renal osteodystrophy (femur). Solid periosteal new bone formation is seen along the lower medial margin. A densely calcified femoral artery is also seen. (Courtesy of Dr. Dharmashi V. Bhate, VA Hospital, Hines, IL)

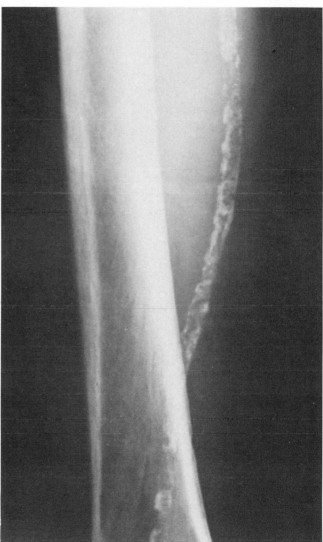

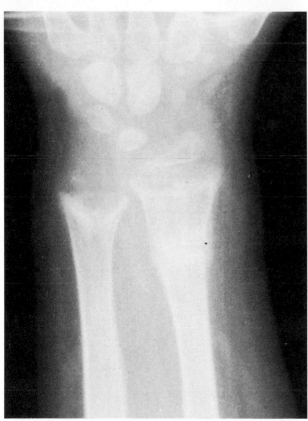

FIG. 2–71. Renal osteodystrophy (forearm) — patient on renal hemodialysis — renal rickets. There is widening of the epiphyseal cartilage plate with cupping and fraying of the metaphysis. A pseudofracture of the distal radius is present. (From Am J Roentgen 116:749–757, 1972)

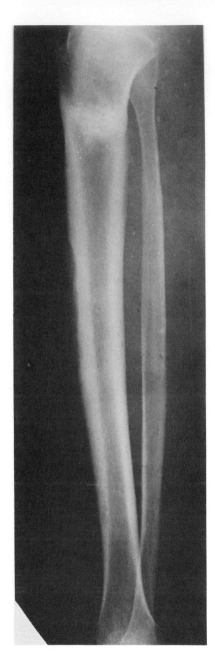

FIG. 2–73. Renal osteodystrophy (leg). Dense cortical thickening is seen with anterior irregularity, which is somewhat reminiscent of Paget's disease. A dense band at the junction of the metaphysis and diaphysis is also seen. (Courtesy of Dr. Dhasmashi V. Bhate, VA Hospital, Hines, IL)

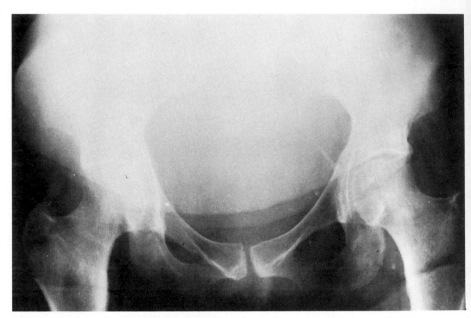

FIG. 2–74. Renal osteodystrophy (pelvis)—patient on renal hemodialysis. There is osteosclerosis of the pelvis associated with calcification of the left sacrospinous ligament in a patient with chronic renal disease. These findings were formerly thought to be characteristic of fluorosis. (From Greenfield GB: Roentgen appearance of bone and soft-tissue changes in chronic renal disease. Am J Roentgen 116:749–757, 1972)

FIG. 2–75. Renal failure. Patient is a 55-year-old diabetic on dialysis who developed gangrene of the penis. Multiple calcified vessels are noted. (Courtesy of Dr. Dharmashi V. Bhate, VA Hospital, Hines, IL)

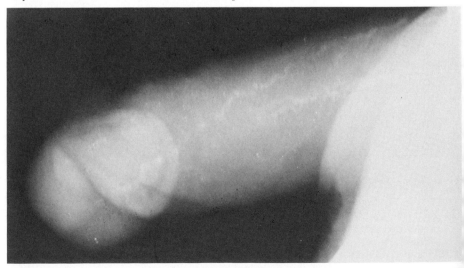

Subchondral resorption of bone may be seen, as well as widening and irregularity, owing predominantly to subchondral trabecular destruction, fibrosis, and new bone formation. This may involve the sternoclavicular joints, the sacroiliac joints, and the symphysis pubis.[103,116] The peripheral joints may show subchondral resorption, sclerosis, and collapse, as well as intraosseous cystic defects. Subchondral resorption under the vertebral end-plates may result in Schmorl's nodes.[103] Cases have been reported of renal osteodystrophy with central vertebral end-plate depressions resembling that seen in sickle-cell anemia.[154]

Cortical bone resorption may be seen in chronic renal failure by microradiographic techniques in up to 61% of patients. The findings include subperiosteal, intracortical, and endosteal bone resorption. Intracortical resorption indicates more extensive skeletal involvement than subperiosteal resorption alone.[85]

Ischemic necrosis has been reported following renal transplantation. This may be the result of immunosuppressive therapy. The roentgen appearance follows the usual course of subarticular fracture and bone collapse. The sites frequently involved are the hip, knee, and humeral head.

Demineralization, flattening, irregularity, and destruction of the head of the mandible with widening of the temporomandibular joint have been reported in patients on long-standing dialysis without transplant.[34] A medullary bone infarct has also been reported.

SOFT-TISSUE CALCIFICATION

Local and systematic factors interplay in the picture of soft-tissue calcification in chronic renal disease.[93] The most frequent sites of soft-tissue calcification are: arterial (Fig. 2–75), ocular, periarticular, cutaneous, subcutaneous, and visceral.

There are two types of arterial calcification that can be roentgenologically recognized: atheromatous and medial sclerosis. Arterial calcification seen in this condition is almost always medial sclerosis, usually resulting in the absence of ischemia. Several partients have been reported with long-standing chronic renal failure and secondary hyperparathyroidism who developed a syndrome of medial calcinosis of the small- and medium-sized arteries with subintimal thickening. These changes resulted in painful ischemic ulcers of the fingers, legs, or thighs, leading to gangrene. The patients required maintenance hemodialysis or had functioning renal homografts. These changes are similar to experimentally produced calciphylaxis, as de-

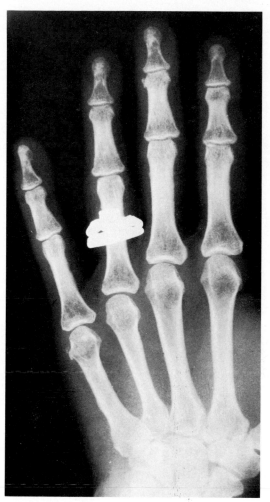

FIG. 2–76. Renal osteodystrophy (hand)—patient on renal hemodialysis. Periarticular soft-tissue calcifications of the distal interphalangeal joint of the middle finger and at the fifth metacarpophalangeal joint are noted. (From Greenfield GB: Roentgen appearance of bone and soft-tissue changes in chronic renal disease. Am J Roentgen 116:749–757, 1972)

scribed by Selye.[52] Corneal and conjunctival calcifications are common in patients on long-term dialysis.

Articular chondrocalcinosis occurs in primary hyperparathyroidism, but is rare in chronic renal disease with secondary hyperparathyroidism. Patients on long-term hemodialysis may rarely contract acute inflammatory joint involvement. Although rare, acute pseudogout has been reported in patients with chronic renal failure.[36] The patients may have atypical distributions. Some of the lesions may appear as gout. In other instances there is

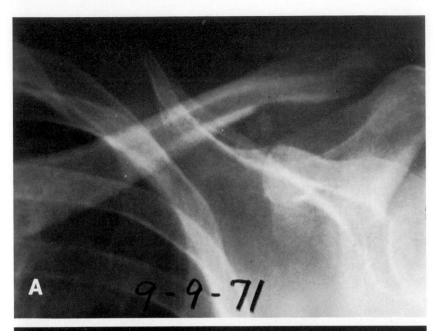

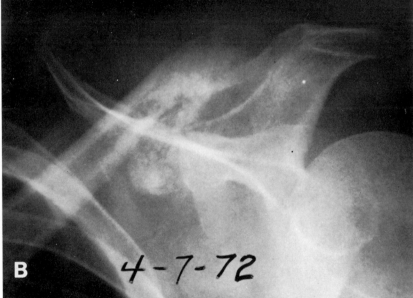

FIG. 2–77. Renal osteodystrophy (clavicle) — patient on renal hemodialysis. **A.** A small focus of soft-tissue calcification in the distal infraclavicular area, associated with slight erosion of the cortex, is noted. **B.** Same patient, 7 months later. There has been marked increase in size of the calcific density.

no evidence of gout or pseudogout. Olecranon bursitis, due to resting the elbow against a firm surface during dialysis for prolonged periods, has been reported.[27]

Periarticular calcification may appear following the inflammatory stage (Fig. 2–76), rarely associated with bone erosion, stimulating tumoral calcinosis (Fig. 2–77, 2–78). Severe pruritus may occur with subcutaneous and cutaneous calcifications. The lesions may be nodular, deposited in the periarticular regions, or may take the form of subcutaneous plaques with discoloration of the overlying skin.

Visceral calcification may occur in the lungs, kidneys, stomach, heart, and (rarely) liver. Calcifications in the lungs occur in the pulmonary alveolar septa and are usually not visible roentgenographically, but may produce a fine reticular, punctate, nodular, or segmental opacity. Severe myocardial calcification can be a major cause of death.

The term **renal osteodystrophy** is usually used to describe the bone changes in this condition.

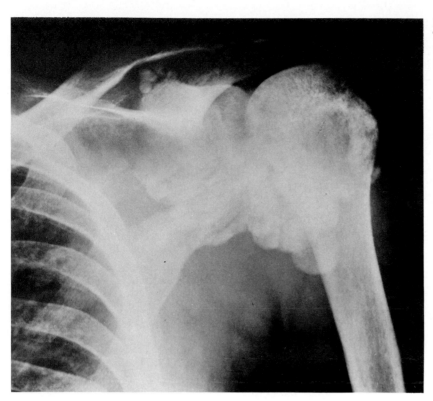

FIG. 2–78. Renal failure (shoulder). There are dense, large, calcific, lobulated areas about the shoulder region which give a tumoral calcinosis appearance.

REFERENCES

1. Aceto T et al: Intrauterine hyperparathyroidism: A complication of untreated maternal hypoparathyroidism. J Clin Endocr 26:487–492, May 1966

2. Adams R G, Harrison J F, Scott P: The development of cadmium-induced proteinurea, impaired renal function, and osteomalacia in alkaline battery workers. Quart J Med (new series) 38:425–443, 1969

3. Aegerter E, Kirkpatrick J A Jr: Orthopedic Diseases, 4th ed. Philadelphia, W B Saunders, 1975

4. Agus Z S, Goldberg M: Pathogenesis of uremic osteodystrophy. Radiol Clin N Amer 10:545–556, 1972

5. Albright F, Reifenstein, E C: The Parathyroid Glands and Metabolic Bone Disease: Selected Studies. Baltimore, Williams & Wilkins, 1948

6. Allen E H, Millard F J C, Nassim J R: Hypoparathyroidism. Arch Dis Child 43:295–301, 1968

7. Avioli L V: Vitamin D_3 metabolism in man and its relation to disorders of mineral metabolism. In Clinical Aspects of Metabolic Disease, Amsterdam, Excerpta Medica pp 355–366, 1973

8. Barnett E, Nordin B E C: The radiological diagnosis of osteoporosis: A new approach. Clin Radiol 11:166–174, 1960

9. Bartlett N L., Cochran D Q: Reparative processes in primary hyperparathyroidism. Radiol Clin N Amer 2:261–279, August 1964

10. Birtwell W M et al: An unusual hereditary osteomalacic disease. Pseudo-vitamin D deficiency. J Bone Joint Surg 52–A:1222–1228, 1970

11. Bishop M C, Boldero J L: Bone infarction not associated with caisson disease: A case report. Brit J. Radiol 46:139–142, 1973

12. Bonucci E, Denys–Martrajt H, Tun–Chot S, Hioco D J: Bone structure in osteomalacia, with special reference to ultrastructure. J Bone Joint Surg 51–B:511–528, 1969

13. Bradley J G, Huang H H, Ledley R S: Evaluation of calcium concentration in bones from CT scans. Radiol 128:103–107, 1978

14. Brill P W, Baker D H, Ewing M L: Bone-within-bone in the neonatal spine. Stress change or normal development. Radiology 108:363–366, 1973

15. Caffey J, Silverman F N: Pediatric X-ray Diagnosis, 6th ed. Chicago, Year Book Publishers, 1972

16. Cameron J R, Mazess R B, Sorenson J A: Precision and accuracy of bone mineral determination by direct photon absorptiometry. Invest Radiol 3:141–150, 1968

17. Campbell J E, Tam C S, Sheppard R H: "Brown tumor" of hyperparathyroidism induced with anticonvulsant medication. J Canad Assn Rad 28:73–78, 1977

18. Cavalino R, Grossman H: Wilson's disease presenting with rickets. Radiology 90:493–494, March, 1968

19. Chalmers J: Osteomalacia: Review of 93 cases. J Roy Coll Surg Edinb 13:255–275, 1968

20. Chalmers J, Ho K C: Geographical variations in senile osteoporosis. J Bone Joint Surg 52–B:667–675, 1970

21. Chiroff R T, Jowsey J: Effect of calcitonin on immobilization osteopenia. J Bone Joint Surg 52–A:1138–1146, 1970

22. Cochran M et al: Hypocalcemia and bone disease in renal failure. Nephron 10:113–140, 1973

23. Cohen A M et al: Metastatic pulmonary calcification in primary hyperparathyroidism. Arch Int Med 137:520–525, 1977

24. Cohen M E L, Cohen G F, Ahad V, Kaye M: Renal osteodystrophy in patients on chronic haemodialysis: A radiological study. Clin Radiol 21:124–134, 1970

25. Courey W R, Pfister R C: The radiographic findings in renal tubular acidosis. Analysis of 21 cases. Radiology 105:497–504, 1972

26. Cruess R L et al: Aseptic necrosis following renal transplantation. J Bone Joint Surg 50–A:1577–1590, 1968

27. Cruz C, Shah S V: Dialysis elbow. JAMA 238:243, 1977

28. Cumming W A: Idiopathic juvenile osteoporosis. J Canad Assn Radiol 21:19–26, 1970

29. Debnam J W et al: Radiological pathological correlations in uremic bone disease. Radiol 125:653–658, 1977

30. DeLuca H F: Vitamin D metabolism and function. Arch Intern Med 138:836–852, 1978

31. Dent C E, Friedman M: Idiopathic juvenile osteoporosis. Quart J Med 34:177–210, 1965

32. Dent C E, Friedman M, Watson L: Hereditary pseudovitamin D-deficiency rickets ("Heredetäre Pseudomangelrachitis"). J Bone Joint Surg 50–B:708–719, 1968

33. Dent C E, Hodson C J: Radiological changes associated with certain metabolic bone diseases. Brit J Radiol 27:605–618, 1954

34. Dick R, Jones D N: Temporo-mandibular joint changes in patients undergoing chronic haemodialysis. Clin Radiol 24:72–76, 1973

35. Doppman J K et al: Differential diagnosis of brown tumor vs cystic osteitis by arteriography and computed tomography. Radiol 131:339–340, 1979

36. Ellman M H, Brown N L, Katzenberg C A: Acute pseudogout in chronic renal failure. Arch Intern Med 139:795–796, 1979

37. Eugenidis N, Olah A J, Haas H G: Osteosclerosis in hyperparathyroidism. Radiology 105:265–276, 1972

38. Ferran J L, Luciani J C, Meunier P, Dumas R: Osteodystrophie rénale delénfant confrontations radiohistologiques. J Radiol Electrol 58:173–181, 1977

39. Fine R N, Isaacson A S, Payne V, Grushkin C M: Renal osteodystrophy in children: Effect of hemodialysis and renal homotransplantation. J Pediat 80:243–249, 1972

40. Fordham C C, Williams T F: Brown tumor and secondary hyperparathyroidism. New Eng J Med 269:129–131, 1963

41. Frame B, Frost H M, Ormond R S, Hunter R B: Atypical osteomalacia involving the axial skeleton. Ann Intern Med 55:632–639, 1961

42. Frame B, Guiang H L, Frost H M, Reynolds W A: Osteomalacia induced by laxative (phenolphthalein) ingestion. Arch Intern Med 128:794–796, 1971

43. Frame B, Parfitt A M, Duncan H: Clinical aspects of metabolic bone disease. Proceedings of an international symposium held at the Henry Ford Hospital, Detroit, Michigan, June 26–29, 1972. Amsterdam, Excerpta Medica, 1973

44. Frost H M: A new bone affection—feathering. J Bone Joint Surg 42–A:447–456, 1960

45. Frost H M: The Bone Dynamics in Osteoporosis and Osteomalacia. Springfield, IL, Charles C Thomas, 1966

46. Frost H M: Bone dynamics in metabolic bone disease. J Bone Joint Surg 48–A:1192–1203, 1966

47. Frost H M: The origin and nature of transients in human bone remodeling dynamics. In Clinical Aspects of Metabolic Bone Disease, pp 124–137. Amsterdam, Excerpta Medica, 1973

48. Frymoyer J W, Hodgkin W: Adult-onset vitamin D-resistant hypophosphatemic osteomalacia. J Bone Joint Surg 59–A:101–106, 1977

49. Fulkerson J P, Ozonoff M B: Multiple symmetrical fractures of bone of unresolved etiology. Am J Roentgen 129:313–316, 1977

50. Garn S M, Poznansky A K, Nagy J M: Bone measurement in the differential diagnosis of osteopenia and osteoporosis. Radiology 100:509–518, 1971

51. Genant H K, Kozin F, Bekerman C, McCarty D J, Sims J: The reflex sympathetic dystrophy syndrome. A comprehensive analysis using fine-detail radiography, photon absorptiometry, and bone and joint scintigraphy. Radiol 117:21–32, 1975

52. Gipstein R M et al: Calciphylaxis in man. Arch Intern Med 136:1273–1280, 1976

53. Gleason D C, Potchen E J: The diagnosis of hyperparathyroidism. Radiol Clin N Amer 5:277–287, 1967

54. Goldsmith N F et al: Bone-mineral determination in normal and osteoporotic women. J Bone Joint Surg 53–A:83–100, 1971

55. Goldsmith R S: Differential diagnosis of hypercalcemia. New Eng J Med 274:674–677, 1966

56. Gooding C A, Ball, J H: Idiopathic juvenile osteoporosis. Radiology 93:1249–1350, 1969

57. Greenfield G B: Roentgen appearance of bone and soft-tissue changes in chronic renal disease. Am J Roentgen 116:749–757, 1972

58. Griffith G C, Nichols G, Asher J D, Flanagan B: Heparin osteoporosis. JAMA 193:91–94, 1965

59. Griffiths H J, Ennis J T, Bailey G: Skeletal changes following renal transplantation. Radiol 113:621–626, 1974

60. Griffiths H J, Zimmerman R E: The clinical application of bone mineral analysis. Skel Rad 3:1–9, 1978

61. Hahn T J, Avioli L V: Anticonvulsant osteomalacia. Arch Intern Med 135:997–1000, 1975

62. Hampers C L, Katz A J, Wilson R E, Merrill J P: Calcium metabolism and osteodystrophy after renal transplantation. Arch Intern Med 124:282–291, 1969

63. Harper H A: Review of Physiological Chemistry, 14th ed. Los Altos, CA, Lange Medical Publications, 1973

64. Heath D A, Martin D J: Periosteal new bone formation in hyperparathyroidism associated with renal failure. Brit J Radiol 43:517–521, 1970

65. Hoffman R R, Campbell R E: Roentgenologic bone-island instability in hyperparathyroidism. Radiology 103:307–308, 1972

66. Holzer N J et al: Bone tumor of the orbit. JAMA 238:1758–1759, 1977

67. Houang M T W et al: Idiopathic juvenile osteoporosis. Skel Rad 3:17–23, 1978

68. Howell D S: Review article. Current concepts of calcification. J Bone Joint Surg 53–A:250–258, 1971

69. Jackson W P U: Calcium Metabolism and Bone Disease. London, Edward Arnold, 1967

70. Johnston C C, Smith D M, Nance W E, Bevan J: Evaluation of radial bone mass by the photon absorption technique. In Clinical Aspects of Metabolic Bone Disease, pp 28–36. Amsterdam, Excerpta Medica, 1973

71. Jowsey J, Massry S G, Coburn J W, Kleeman C R: Microradiographic studies of bone in renal osteodystrophy. Arch Intern Med 124:539–542, 1969

72. Kleeman C R: Divalent ion metabolism and osteodystrophy in chronic renal failure. Session I: Uremic osteodystrophy — basic concepts and clinical considerations. Arch Intern Med 124:261–321, 1969

73. Lalli A F, Lapides J: Osteosclerosis in renal disease. Am J Roentgen 93:924–926, 1965

74. LeMay M: The early radiological diagnosis of osteomalacia in adults. Radiology 70:373–378, 1958

75. Lequesne M et al: Partial transient osteoporosis. Skel Rad 2:1–9, 1977

76. Levin E J, Frand D F: Bone changes following ureteroileostomy. Am J Roentgen 118:347–355, 1973

77. Linovitz R J et al: Tumor-induced osteomalacia and rickets. A surgically curable syndrome. Report of 2 cases. J Bone Joint Surg 58–A:419–422, 1976

78. Mack P B, Vogt F B: Roentgenographic bone density changes in astronauts during representative Apollo space flight. Am J Roentgen 113:621–633, 1971

79. Massry S G et al: Secondary hyperparathyroidism in chronic renal failure: Clinical spectrum in uremia, during hemodialyses, and after renal transplantation. Arch Intern Med 124:431–441, 1969

80. Mazess R B: Fourth International Conference on Bone Measurement. Am J Roentgen 131:539–553, 1978 ·

81. McLean F C, Urist M R: Bone: An Introduction to the Physiology of Skeletal Tissue, 2nd ed. Chicago, University of Chicago Press, 1961

82. Meema H E et al: Arterial calcifications in severe chronic renal disease and their relationship to dialysis treatment, renal transplant, and parathyroidectomy. Radiology 121:315–321, 1976

83. Meema H E et al: Improved radiological diagnosis of azotemic osteodystrophy. Radiology 102:1–10, 1972

84. Meema H E, Meema S: Improved roentgenologic diagnosis of osteomalacia by microscopy of hand bones. Am J Roentgen 125:925–935, 1975

85. Meema H E, Oreopoulis D G, Meema S: A roentgenologic study of cortical bone resorption in chronic renal failure. Radiology 126:67–74, 1978

86. Meema H E, Oreopoulos D G, Rabmovich S, Husdan H, Rapoport A: Periosteal new bone formation (periosteal neostosis) in renal osteodystrophy: Relationship to osteosclerosis, osteitis fibrosa, and osteoid excess. Radiology 110:513–522, 1974

87. Meema H E, Schatz D L: Simple radiologic demonstration of cortical bone loss in thyrotoxicosis. Radiology 97:9–15, 1970

88. Meschan I, Farrer–Meschan R M R: Roentgen Signs in Clinical Practice, Vol I. Philadelphia, W B Saunders, 1966

89. Morgan D B: The metacarpal bone: A comparison of the various indices for the assessment of the amount of bone and for the detection of loss of bone. Clin Radiol 24:77–82, 1973

90. Nicholas J A, Saville P D, Brenner F: Osteoporosis, osteomalacia, and the skeletal system. J Bone Joint Surg 45–A:391–405, 1963

91. Orphanoudakis S C et al: Mineral analysis using single-energy computed tomography. Invest Rad 14:122–130, 1979

92. Pantazopoulos T, Exarchou E, Garofalidis G H: Idiopathic transient osteoporosis of the hip. J Bone Joint Surg 55–A:315–321, 1973

93. Parfitt A M: Soft-tissue calcification in uremia. Arch Intern Med 124:544–556, 1969

94. Parfitt A M: The quantitative approach to bone morphology. A critique of current methods, and their interpretation. In Clinical Aspects of Metabolic Bone Disease, pp 86–94. Amsterdam, Excerpta Medica, 1973

95. Parsons V: Divalent ion metabolism and the kidney. Nephron 10:157–173, 1973

96. Pitt M J, Haussler M R: Vitamin D: Biochemistry and clinical applications. Skel Rad 1:191–208, 1977

97. Platts M M, Grech P, McManners T, Cochran M: Skeletal changes in patients treated by regular haemodialysis in the Sheffield area. Brit J Radiol 46:585–593, 1973

98. Pogonowska M J, Collins L C, Dobson H L: Diabetic osteopathy. Radiology 89:265–271, 1967

99. Pollack J A, Shiller A L, Crawford J D: Rickets and myopathy cured by removal of a nonossifying fibroma of bone. Pediatrics 52:364–371, 1973

100. Potts J T et al: Parathyroid hormone: Chemical and immunochemical studies in relation to biosynthesis, secretion, and metabolism of the hormone. In Clinical Aspects of Metabolic Bone Disease, pp 208–214. Amsterdam, Excerpta Medica, 1973

101. Pugh D G: Subperiosteal resorption of bone. A roentgenologic manifestation of primary hyperparathyroidism and renal osteodystrophy. Am J Roentgen 66:577–586, 1951

102. Resnick D L: Erosive arthritis of the hand and wrist in hyperparathyroidism. Radiology 110:263–269, 1974

103. Resnick D, Niwayama G: Subchondral resorption of bone in renal osteodystrophy. Radiology 118:315–321, 1976

104. Reyton P, Shaw D G: Hypophosphatemic osteomalacia secondary to vascular tumors of bone and soft tissue. Skel Rad 1:21–24, 1976

105. Riggs L B et al: Calcium deficiency and osteoporosis. Observations in 166 patients and critical review of the literature. J Bone Joint Surg 49–A:915–924, 1967

106. Riggs L B et al: Osteoporosis, increased IPTH, and low serum 1,25-DH-vitamin D. Mayo Clin Proc 53:701–706, 1978

107. Ringe J D, Buurman R: The value of usual judgment of the calcium content of the skeleton. Fortschr Roentgenstr 128:546–550, 1978

108. Ritchie W G M, Winney R J, Davison A M, Robson J S: Periosteal new bone formation developing during hemodialysis for chronic renal failure. Brit J Radiol 48:656–661, 1975

109. Rittenberg G M, Meredith H C, Hungerford G D: The skull in renal osteodystrophy. Skel Rad 3:105–107, 1978

110. Ritz E et al: Skeletal complications of renal insufficiency and maintenance hemodialysis. Nephron 10:195–207, 1973

111. Robinson R A: Ultrastructural appearance of bone cells and matrix in renal osteodystrophy. Arch Intern Med 124:519–529, 1969

112. Rosen R A: Transitory demineralization of the femoral head. Radiology 94:509–512, 1970

113. Sackler J P, Liv L: Heparin-induced osteoporosis. Brit J Radiol 46:548–550, 1973

114. Salassa, R M, Jowsey J, Arnaud C D: Hypophosphatemic osteomalacia associated with "nonendocrine tumors." New Eng J Med 283:65–70, 1970

115. Saville P D: Osteoporosis: An overview. In Clinical Aspects of Metabolic Bone Disease, pp 293–302. Amsterdam, Excerpta Medica, 1973

116. Schabel S L, Burgener F A: Osteitis pubis in renal failure simulating chondrosarcoma. Brit J Radiol 48:1027–1028, 1975

117. Scherr D D: A severely deformed patient with osteogenesis imperfecta at the age of 54. J Bone Joint Surg 46–A:159–160, 1964

118. Schnur M J, Appel G B, Bilezikian J P: Primary hyperparathyroidism and benign monoclonal gammopathy. Arch Intern Med 137:1201–1203, 1977

119. Schwartz E E, Lantieri R, Tepuck J G: Erosion of the inferior aspect of the clavicle in secondary hyperparathyroidism. Am J Roentgen 129:291–295, 1978

120. Sellers A, Winfield A C, Massry S G: Resorption of condyloid process of mandible. An unusual manifestation of renal osteodystrophy. Arch Intern Med 131:727–728, 1973

121. Shapiro R: The biochemical basis of the skeletal changes in chronic uremia. Am J Roentgen 111:750–761, 1971

122. Shapiro R: Radiologic aspects of renal osteodystrophy. Radiol Clin N Amer 10:557–568, 1972

123. Sherlock S: Diseases of the Liver and Biliary System, 2nd ed. Oxford, Blackwell Scientific Publications, 1958

124. Simpson W, Ellis H A, Kerr D N S, McElroy M, McNay R A, Peart K N: Bone disease in long-term haemodialysis. Brit J Radiol 49:105–110, 1976

125. Simpson W, Kerr D N S, Hill A V L, Siddiqui J Y: Skeletal changes in patients on regular hemodialysis. Radiology 107:313–320, 1973

126. Simpson W, Young J R, Clark F: Pseudofractures resembling stress fractures in Punjabi immigrants with osteomalacia. Clin Radiol 24:83–89, 1973

127. Sitrin M, Meredith S, Rosenberg I H: Vitamin D deficiency and bone disease in gastrointestinal disorders. Arch Intern Med 138:886–888, 1978

128. Slatopolsky E et al: How important is phosphate in the pathogenesis of renal osteodystrophy? Arch Intern Med 138:848–852, 1978

129. Smith S W: Roentgen findings in homocystinuria. Am J Roentgen 100:147–154, 1967

130. Snapper I: Rare Manifestations of Metabolic Bone Disease. Their Practical Importance. Springfield, IL, Charles C Thomas, 1952

131. Specht E E: Rickets following ureterosigmoidostomy and chronic hyperchloremia. A case report. J Bone Joint Surg 49–A1422–1430, 1967

132. Spence A J, Lloyd–Roberts G C: Regional osteoporosis in osteoid osteoma. J Bone Joint Surg 43–B:501–507, 1961

133. Stanbury S W: Bone disease in uremia. Am J Med 44:714–724, 1968

134. Stanbury S W, Lumb G A, Mawer E R: Osteodystrophy developing spontaneously in course of chronic renal failure. Arch Intern Med 124:274–281, 1969

135. Stanbury S W et al: Vitamin D metabolism and renal bone disease. In Clinical Aspects of Metabolic Bone Disease, pp 562–573. Amsterdam, Excerpta Medica, 1973

136. Steinbach H T: The roentgen appearance of osteoporosis. Radiol Clin N Amer 2:191–207, 1964

137. Steiner R E: Physiological approach to radiology. Radiology 100:497–508, 1971

138. Strong C G: Hormonal influence on renal function. Med Clin N Amer 50:985–995, 1966

139. Sundaram M, Scholz C: Primary hyperparathyroidism presenting with acute paraplegia. Am J Roentgen 128:674–676, 1977

140. Symposium on thyrocalcitonin. J Bone Joint Surg 48–B:384–388, 1966

141. Tapia J, Stearns G, Ponseti I V: Vitamin D-resistant rickets. A long-term clinical study of 11 patients. J Bone Joint Surg 46–A:935–958, 1964

142. Teplick J G, Eftekhari F, Haskin M E: Erosion of the sternal ends of the clavicles. Radiology 113:323–326, 1974

143. Urist M R, Zaccalini P S, McDonald N S, Skoog W A: New approaches to the problem of osteoporosis. J Bone Joint Surg 44–B:464–484, 1962

144. Vose G P: Estimation of changes in bone calcium content by radiographic densitometry. Radiology 93:841–844, 1969

145. Vose G P: Review of roentgenographic bone demineraliza-

tion studies of the Gemini space flights. Am J Roentgen 121:1–4, 1974

146. Weber A L: Primary hyperoxaluria. Roentgenographic, clinical, and pathological findings. Am J Roentgen 100:155–161, 1967

147. Weller M, Edeiken J, Hodes P J: Renal osteodystrophy. Am J Roentgen 104:354–363, 1968

148. Wendenburgh H H, Baldauf G, Barwich D: Vitamin D-deficiency osteopathy after prolonged treatment with anticonvulsants. Fortschr Roentgenstr 124:7–10, 1976

149. Wilson J S, Genant H K: In vivo assessment of bone metabolism using the cortical striation index. Invest Rad 14:131–136, 1979

150. Yoshikawa S et al: Atypical vitamin D-resistant osteomalacia. Report of a case. J Bone Joint Surg 46–A:998–1007, 1964

151. Yoshikawa S et al: Benign osteoblastoma as a cause of osteomalacia. J Bone Joint Surg 59–B:279–286, 1977

152. Young L W, Forbes G B, Borgstedt A D, Bryson M F: Rickets and antiepileptic therapy. In Clinical Aspects of Metabolic Bone Disease, pp 394–396. Amsterdam, Excerpta Medica, 1973

153. Zimmerman H B: Osteosclerosis in chronic renal disease. Am J Roentgen 88:1152–1169, 1962

154. Ziter F M H: Central vertebral end-plate depression in chronic renal disease: Report of 2 cases. Am J Roentgen 132:809–811. 1979

3

ALTERATION
OF
BONE
TEXTURE

ARCHITECTURE OF BONE

A long bone can be seen radiologically as comprising a cortex and a medulla. The cortex is composed of a dense layer of bone called the *compacta.* The medulla has a loose structural meshwork of bone called the *spongiosa,* which extends into the marrow cavity.

The radiographic appearance of the bony trabecular pattern depends upon the amount, density, and orientation of the cancellous or spongy bone.

The compacta is composed of haversian canals with surrounding haversian lamellae. These are continuously being reformed. Interstitial lamellae between the haversian systems are present. An outer and inner circumferential layer of lamellae at the margins of the cortex encompass the compacta. The Volkmann's canals, which communicate between the haversian canals, are present, as well as Sharpey's fibers and elastic fibers running parallel to Volkmann's canals and perpendicular to the haversian system. These connect with the periosteum. The compacta becomes thinner at the metaphyseal end of a long bone, and the spongiosa increases near the metaphyses. The epiphyseal ossification center is surrounded by a thin layer of compacta with central spongiosa.

The calvarium is composed of an inner and outer layer of compacta and the diploë of spongiosa between them.

The cancellous bone or spongiosa extends into the marrow cavity in the central area of the tubular bones. These bone trabeculae orient along lines of stress, according to Wolff's law.

Resorptive and reconstructive mechanisms can bring about alteration of the trabecular architectural pattern. Processes that cause resorption of bone can diminish the trabecular pattern. Osteoporosis, osteomalacia, and hyperparathyroidism can all cause a diminished or coarsened trabecular pattern. Resorption of trabeculae accentuates the remaining trabeculae in relief. In addition, restorative activity of the endosteum can cause bone apposition of the remaining trabeculae, further accentuating the pattern. The trabeculae become oriented along new or old lines of stress, again reinforcing or accentuating the coarsened appearance. Selective resorption of horizontal trabeculae occurs in osteoporosis. Infiltrative processes, such as anemias caused by increased hematopoietic activity, storage diseases, and neoplastic diseases such as leukemia and multiple myeloma, can cause general alterations and coarsening of the trabecular pattern. The processes are basically similar. The bone pattern found in the diffuse type of multiple myeloma can have the same roentgenographic appearance as that shown by sickle-cell anemia, thalassemia or hyperparathyroidism.

GENERALIZED DISEASES THAT CAUSE ALTERATION OF BONE TEXTURE

THE ANEMIAS

The abnormal bone pattern of the anemias results from several factors. Marrow overactivity causes resorption of spongy bone, thus coarsening the bony trabecular pattern. Interruption of blood supply can lead to infarction, of which sickle-cell dactylitis in children and infants is a particular manifestation. Interruption of blood supply also leads to mature calcified infarcts in the tubular bones. In addition, ischemic necrosis occurs, particularly in the femoral head. Marrow overactivity in the skull can result in thickening of the calvarium and, in extreme cases, a "hair-on-end" appearance. In addition, localized loss of blood supply can cause retardation of growth, as occurs particularly in the centra of the vertebrae in sickle-cell anemia, giving rise to the typical biconcave or "fish" vertebrae. Generalized loss of stature is commonly present. Retardation of bone maturation and delayed puberty frequently occur, owing to chronic illness.

Sickle-cell anemia greatly predisposes the patient to salmonella osteomyelitis. Intestinal infarctions permit entry of the organisms. Salmonella osteomyelitis often occurs as a dactylitis or as a spondylitis. Soft-tissue masses from extramedullary hematopoiesis can be present, more often seen in thalassemia.

The hemoglobin molecule is composed of approximately 560 amino acids arranged in two pairs of wound polypeptide chains, with the heme groups situated between the loops of the chains. The normal adult hemoglobin (Hb A_1) has two pairs of polypeptide chains, an α chain with 141 amino acids and a β chain with 146 amino acids. The normal adult also has less than 0.4% of fetal hemoglobin (Hb F) present. The percentage of Hb F is markedly elevated in early infancy and in disease states, notably thalassemia. Hb F is composed of two α chains and two distinct chains termed γ chains. Normal adult hemoglobin also has present a minor hemoglobin component (Hb A_2) with two α chains and two distinct chains termed δ chains. These different hemoglobins can be identified by electrophoresis.

Abnormal hemoglobins that differ in their electrophoretic mobility have been assigned by convention a different letter of the alphabet in the order of their discovery. Exceptions to this classification are fetal hemoglobin (Hb F), sickle-cell hemoglobin (Hb S), and Hb M, which is associated with methemoglobinemia.

After the letters of the alphabet had been used up, it was agreed that newly discovered hemoglobins would be named after the geographic location in which the hemoglobin was found (*e.g.,* hemoglobin Mexico). If the characteristics of a lettered hemoglobin were present in a newly discovered one, the geographic designation was added as a subscript (*e.g.,* hemoglobin M$_{Saskatoon}$). If the structural abnormality was determined as to the amino acid substitution in the globin chain, this substitution was designated by a superscript to the globin chain involved (*e.g.,* hemoglobin S$\alpha_2\beta_2^{6\ glu\cdot val}$).

Over 170 inherited abnormalities of hemoglobin have been described. These are classified as: common α and β chain abnormalities (Hb's S, C, D, E); rare α and β chain abnormalities; methemoglobinemias; γ, δ and ϵ chain abnormalities; and, mixed heterozygous hemoglobinopathies.

SICKLE-CELL ANEMIA

Sickle-cell anemia[132] is a condition in which the red blood cells assume a reversible sickled or filamentous configuration at reduced oxygen tensions. This sickling phenomenon can be demonstrated with a drop of blood mixed with a 2% solution of sodium metabisulfite on a glass slide under a cover slip. Sickling appears within 15 minutes if the test is positive.

Sickling is caused by an abnormal hemoglobin, Hb S, which is genetically transmitted. Sickle-cell anemia affects those individuals who are homozygous for the sickle-cell gene (Hb SS). The entire abnormality is based on the substitution of valine for glutamic acid in the 6 position on the β-globin chain.[132] Several explanations for the molecular basis of sickling have been proposed, including valine-valine cyclization leading to monofilament formation. Several filaments may associate to form a hollow cable, seen on electron microscopy. During oxygenation, this coupling arrangement is lost and sickling ceases.

Several factors influence the severity of the disease. Oxygen tension is a prime factor, as sickling occurs when oxygen tension of the blood reaches 35 to 45 mm Hg. It must become still lower to induce sickling in individuals who are heterozygous for the sickle-cell gene. Another consideration is the percentage of hemoglobins S and F present. In homozygous sickle-cell anemia, the percentage of hemoglobin S may range from 70% to 99%. There is a rough inverse correlation between the percentage of fetal hemoglobin and the severity of clinical symptoms, those cells with the largest amount of hemoglobin F being less susceptible to sickling. Another factor is pH, with greater sickling occurring at lower pH, such as in the renal medulla. Increased blood viscosity, increased mechanical fragility of sickled cells, and extravascular hemolysis of sickled erythrocytes are phenomena that contribute to the course of events in this disease. There are two general types of sickle cells. One is a mildly sickled oat-shaped cell which reverts to normal shape upon oxygenation. The second is a filamentous form which seems to be irreversibly sickled.

The chain of events is that localized deoxygenation leads to erythrocyte sickling, increased blood viscosity, stasis, decrease in pH, and continued decrease in oxygen in the red cell to produce further and irreversible sickling. Protean symptoms are thus produced.

This disease is limited almost exclusively to blacks, except for a few white patients reported with inheritance of genes from parents with heterozygous sickle-thalassemia. It has also been reported in whites in Greece, Turkey, Italy, Sicily, and India.[41]

Sickle-cell trait (Hb SA) is found in 7% to 9% of black Americans. Sickle-cell anemia (Hb SS) occurs in approximately 1 of every 600 blacks. Hemoglobin SC disease is one-third as common as sickle-cell anemia.

The signs and symptoms of sickle-cell disease are due to anemia, which is caused by rapid destruction of abnormal erythrocytes. Jaundice is present. Increased bilirubin levels can lead to gallstones. Stasis and increased viscosity of the blood result from sickling, which causes thrombosis and infarction. Increased hematopoietic activity occurs in response to anemia. The spleen initially enlarges. Later in the disease there is splenic fibrosis, shrinkage, and calcification resulting from infarction. Severe abdominal symptoms, the so-called sickle-cell crises, result from mesenteric vascular thrombosis. Cardiomegaly and congestive heart failure due to anemia commonly occur. Renal papillary necrosis also results. A clinically benign form, termed *mild sickle-cell disease*,[120] exists, with no distinguishing hematological features.

One of the most common symptoms in infancy is swelling of the hands and feet, caused either by infarction or salmonella infection. Radiologically, this must be differentiated from benign cortical hyperostosis and vitamin A intoxication. Any black infant with dactylitis should be suspected of having sickle-cell anemia. Salmonella organisms gain entry from the intestine, and have a diaphyseal predilection for osteomyelitis peculiar to this disease.

The causative organism is most often *Salmonella paratyphosa,* although other gram-negative organisms such as *E. coli* and *Hemophilus influenzae* may rarely be responsible.

Salmonella paratyphosa is always pathogenic, and invades the intestinal lymphatics and regional lymph nodes as well as the reticuloendothelial system. The premise of intestinal microinfarctions need not be invoked to explain the mode of entry. The organisms then lodge in the bone marrow at sites of thromboses and infarcts, in accordance with the principle of *locus minoris resistentiae.* Unknown factors work either to increase the virulence of the salmonella organisms or to inhibit other bacteria which do not cause osteomyelitis in this disease, such as pneumococci or other gram-positive organisms. Salmonella osteomyelitis is not limited to sickle-cell anemia. It has been reported in other conditions[95] which are summarized below.

SALMONELLA OSTEOMYELITIS
MAY OCCUR IN:

Sickle-cell anemia
Other hemoglobinopathies
Typhoid fever
Cirrhosis of the liver
Systemic lupus
Leukemia
Lymphoma
Bartonellosis
Chronic osteomyelitis

Another important hemoglobinopathy involves hemoglobin C. The abnormality results from the substitution of glutamic acid for lysine in the 6th position from the N terminal of the β chain. It is found with greatest frequency in West Africa, where up to 28% of the population possess this hemoglobin. An incidence of 2% to 3% in the black population of the United States is reported, and sporadic cases have been reported in Italians.

Hemoglobin C trait, or Hb AC, is an asymptomatic condition without anemia.

Hemoglobin CC disease is characterized by mild clinical symptoms, moderate hemolytic anemia, and splenomegaly. The prognosis is good.

Hemoglobin SC disease is a heterozygous state in which the individual carries two abnormal alleles of the β chain, Hb S and Hb C. No hemoglobin A is present. The disease is similar to hemoglobin SS disease but is milder. Splenomegaly may be present.

Most patients with Hb SS disease do not live beyond the age of 30 to 40 years, but patients with Hb SC disease can live to an older age. Therefore, any patient over the age of 40 with changes of sickle-cell anemia demonstrated radiographically is most likely to have Hb SC disease. Sickle-cell disease and glucose-6-phosphate dehydrogenase deficiency coexist in Ghana and Saudi Arabia, with a reported favorable effect on sickle-cell anemia.

Sickle-cell trait, or heterozygous SA disease, ordinarily does not cause symptoms. The erythrocytes sickle under reduced oxygen tension. Splenic infarction during aerial flight has been reported, as well as recurrent hematuria and papillary necrosis. Ischemic necrosis of the femoral and humeral heads has also been reported.[103] These changes occur most often under conditions of stress. The patients have no anemia. Individuals with sickle-cell trait have a survival advantage in relationship to malaria, particularly young children with *Plasmodium falciparum* infection.

Hemoglobin S may be combined with thalassemia. If it occurs in the form of β thalassemia in which there is a complete suppression of β chain synthesis, the course is similar to that found in sickle-cell anemia.

Radiologically, the spine, the flat bones, and the long bones show loss of bone density and a coarsening of the trabecular pattern (Figs. 3–1, 3–2, 3–3). Loss of bone density of the spine is one of the important skeletal changes in sickle-cell disease. Very few other conditions cause radiolucency of the spine alone in young adults[85] (*e.g.,* Cushing's syndrome and steroid therapy). Sclerotic changes may also occur (Figs. 3–4, 3–5).

(*Text continues on p. 78*)

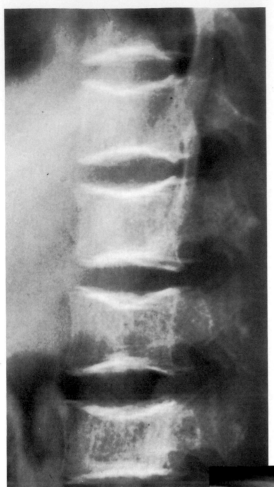

FIG. 3-1. Sickle-cell anemia—SS hemoglobin (lumbar spine). Loss of bone density is present with relative increase in density of the vertebral end-plates. There is a tendency toward biconcavity of the vertebral bodies. Note mild trabecular accentuation.

FIG. 3–2. Hemoglobin SC disease (chest). Coarsening of the trabecular pattern in all of the ribs is evident on this chest film.

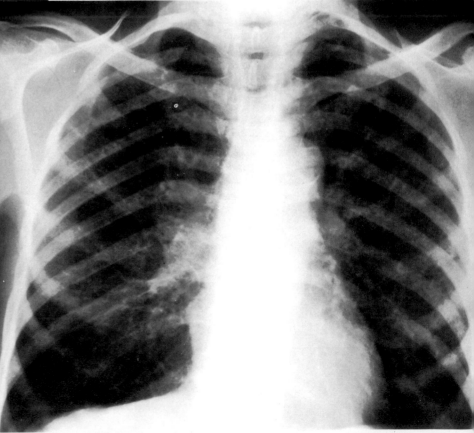

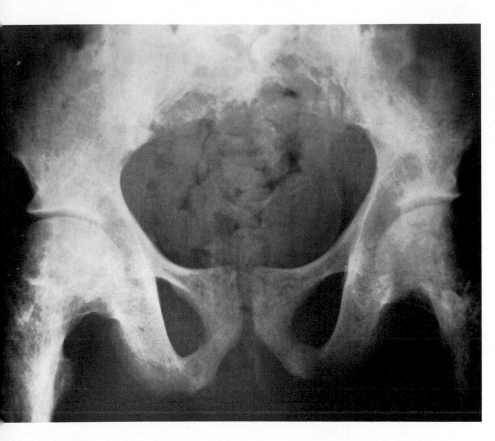

FIG. 3–3. Sickle-cell anemia (pelvis and hips). There is accentuation of the trabecular pattern in the pelvis, hips, and upper femora, and cortical thickening of the proximal femoral shafts. Small medullary bone infarcts in the femoral necks may also be seen.

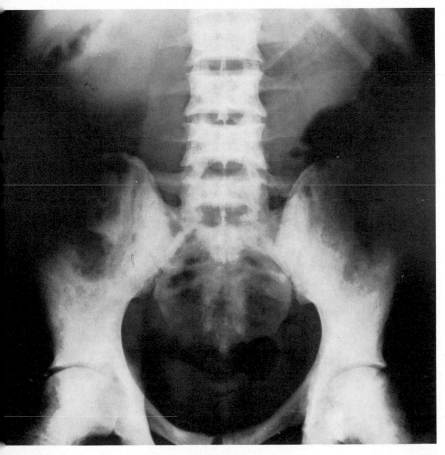

FIG. 3–4. Sickle-cell anemia. Note generalized sclerosis of the lumbar spine, pelvis, and hip joints, and coarsened bone trabecular pattern.

The spine also characteristically exhibits a uniform biconcave contour of all of the vertebral bodies (Fig. 3–6). This is referred to as "fish" vertebrae because of their similarity to vertebral bodies in certain species of fishes. Nonuniform involvement of the spine may also appear with a configuration similar to Schmorl's nodes (Figs. 3–7, 3–8). The etiology of this configuration is not usually caused by compression infractions as in osteoporosis, but is attributed to local inhibition of bone growth owing to ischemia at the centra, caused by interference with the blood supply from the nutrient artery.[105] The perforating metaphyseal arteries at the periphery of the vertebrae are not involved and allow growth at the periphery of the vertebral bodies. This condition is analogous to the cupping of the metaphyses from central ischemia also seen in this disease.

This deformity is uncommon before the age of 10 years. It becomes manifest before the end of the second decade.[106] In its typical appearance, a cuplike depression involving the central three-fifths of both upper and lower end-plates of several contiguous vertebral bodies is seen. Vertebral end-plate depression, although perhaps not in the typical sickle-cell form, may rarely be seen in other conditions. These are summarized as follows:[109,134,137]

CONDITIONS OTHER THAN SICKLE CELL IN WHICH VERTEBRAL BICONCAVITY HAS BEEN REPORTED

> Homocystinurea
> Hereditary spherocytosis
> Thalassemia major
> Gaucher's disease
> Renal osteodystrophy
> Osteopenia

The anterior vertebral notch in the middle of the anterior surface of the vertebral body may be exaggerated in children with sickle-cell disease, as well as in some other conditions.[79] These are summarized below.

EXAGGERATED ANTERIOR VERTEBRAL NOTCH IN CHILDREN[79]

> Sickle-cell disease
> Thalassemia major
> Gaucher's disease
> Metastatic neuroblastoma

In addition to loss of density, biconcavity of the bodies, and accentuation of the trabecular pattern, the spine is prone to salmonella osteomyelitis. This disease commonly involves the intervertebral disk spaces and contiguous vertebral bodies, causing deformity and gibbus formation. Infarction of the bodies leading to collapse may also occur.

FIG. 3–5. Sickle-cell anemia (legs) — sclerosis of the shafts of both tibiae and fibulae. The fibulae show cortical thickening and narrowing of the medullary canal. Coarsening of the trabecular pattern at the proximal ends of the bones is evident.

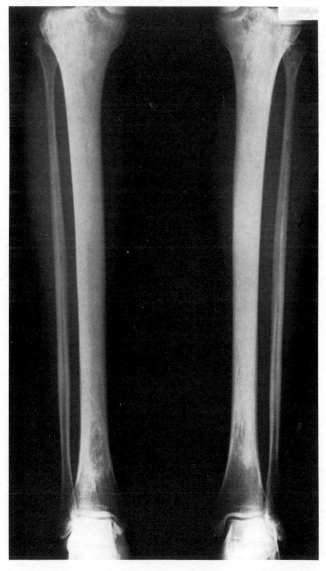

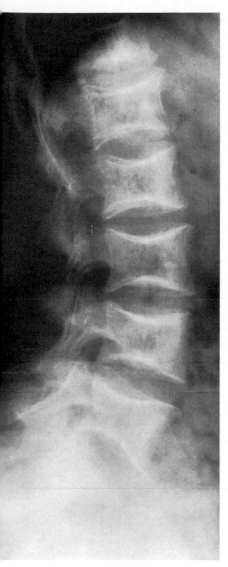

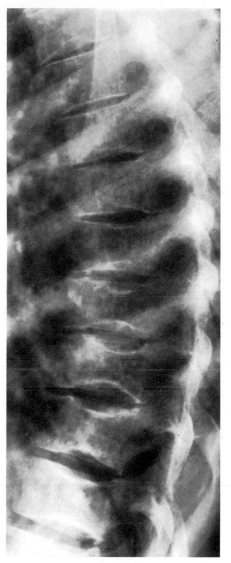

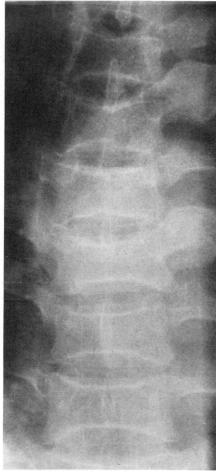

FIG. 3–6   FIG. 3–7   FIG. 3–8

FIG. 3–6. Sickle-cell anemia (lumbar spine). Note uniform biconcavity of all of the lumbar vertebral bodies. There is loss of bone density and coarsened trabecular pattern.

FIG. 3–7. Sickle-cell anemia (dorsal spine). Note nonuniform biconcavity of the dorsal vertebral bodies. Several bodies are not involved. In the upper and midregions, several Schmorl's nodes may be seen, and in the lower region the bodies assume the more typical "fish" vertebra. Also note coarsening of the trabecular pattern.

FIG. 3–8. Sickle-cell anemia (dorsal spine) — anteroposterior view. There is central cupping with small central depressions at the superior and inferior end-plates of several vertebral bodies.

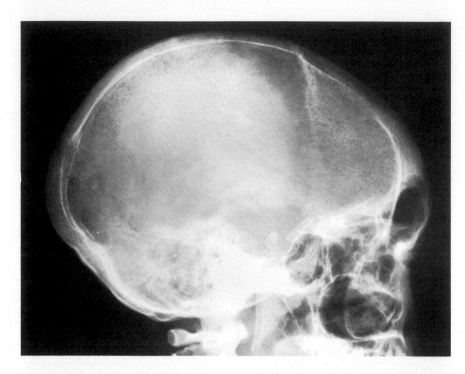

FIG. 3–9. Sickle-cell anemia (skull) —initial granular appearance with loss of bone density of the calvarium. On the basis of this picture alone, it would be difficult to differentiate this diagnosis from other causes of deossification, particularly hyperparathyroidism.

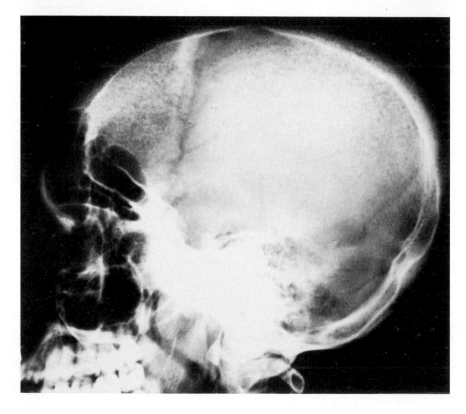

FIG. 3–10. Sickle-cell anemia (skull). A granular appearance of the frontal and parietal areas is noted, along with slight thickening of the calvarium and loss of bone density.

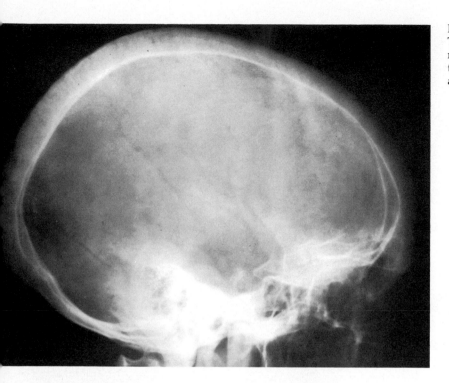

FIG. 3–11. Sickle-cell anemia (skull). There is thickening of the calvarium with no involvement below the internal occipital protuberance. Bone texture and density are normal.

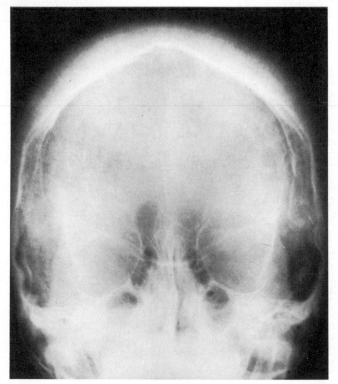

FIG. 3–12. Sickle-cell anemia (skull). Marked widening of the calvarium and parallel intraosseous striations may be seen. The paranasal sinuses are normally developed.

The skull initially shows a granular appearance (Figs. 3–9, 3–10), followed by marked widening of the diploic space (Figs. 3–11, 3–12) and thinning of the outer table. The areas involved are the frontal and the parieto-occipital regions. The calvarium is not involved below the internal occipital protuberance, because there is no marrow in this region; this is an important finding which serves to differentiate the anemias from other causes of calvarial thickening, such as fibrous dysplasia and Paget's disease. In extreme cases, perpendicular spiculated new bone formation appears, giving a "hair-on-end" appearance (Fig. 3–13). Radiolucent infarcts of the calvarium also may occur (Figs. 3–14, 3–15, 3–16). These lucencies, however, may represent focal marrow's hyperplasia. In a reported series of 194 patients, 25% of patients showed porous decrease in bone density, 22% showed widening of the diploë, and 5% showed "hair-on-end" striations.[116] This is a representative proportion.

In the hands and feet, early changes include periostitis at an early age, as well as destructive bone lesions. These result from either infarction (Figs. 3–17, 3–18), or salmonella infection (Fig. 3–19). In very young infants, these changes are more likely to be due to osteomyelitis, as Hb F has not as yet been replaced by Hb S; thus, infarction is not to

(Text continues on p. 85)

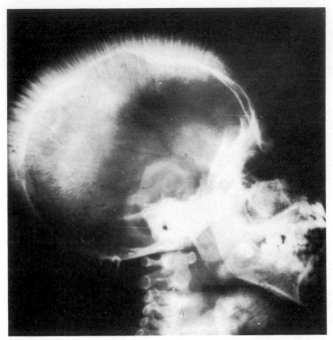

FIG. 3–13. Advanced sickle-cell anemia (skull). Note marked new bone formation perpendicular to the tables of the skull, causing so-called "hair-on-end" appearance. There is no involvement inferior to the internal occipital protuberance.

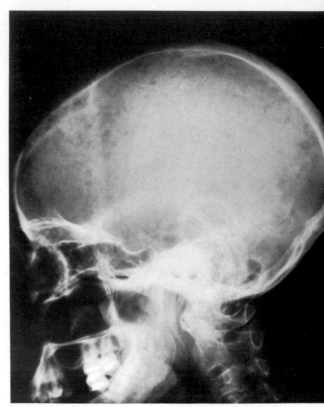

FIG. 3–14. Sickle-cell anemia (skull). Note multiple small, discrete radiolucencies that represent infarctions. Bone texture and density are otherwise normal.

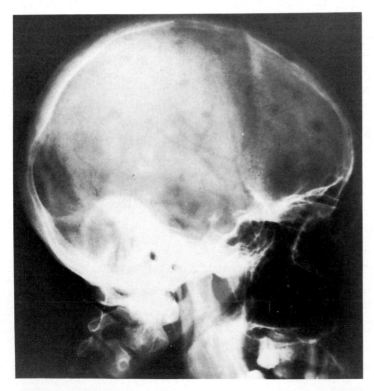

FIG. 3–15. Sickle-cell anemia (skull). Note several small radiolucencies in the calvarium, representing infarcts. The calvarium has a slightly granular texture. Calcification of the glomus of the choroid plexus may be noted incidentally.

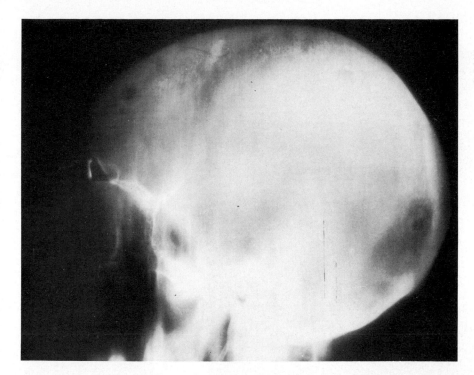

FIG. 3–16. Tomogram of skull in Fig. 3–15. Multiple well-defined radiolucencies represent the infarcts.

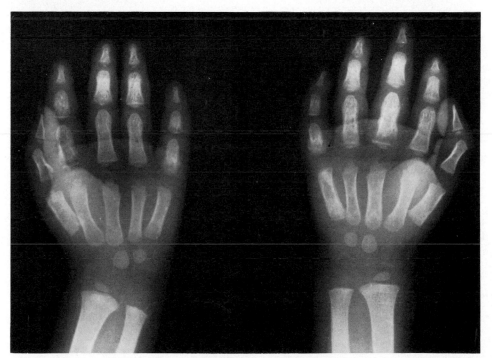

FIG. 3–17. Hemoglobin SC disease (hands)—young black female. Note destructive lesions in multiple phalanges bilaterally, and periosteal new bone formation. Also note that there is periosteal new bone formation of several metacarpals bilaterally without frank destructive changes. Blood culture was negative for salmonella organisms. This picture represents infarctions, the so-called hand-foot syndrome. It is impossible to distinguish radiologically between infection and infarction under these circumstances.

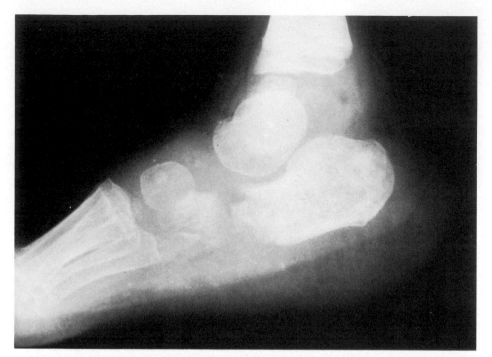

FIG. 3–18. Sickle-cell anemia (tarsal bones). Note destructive and mottled changes of the os calcis and cuboid bone, caused by infarction.

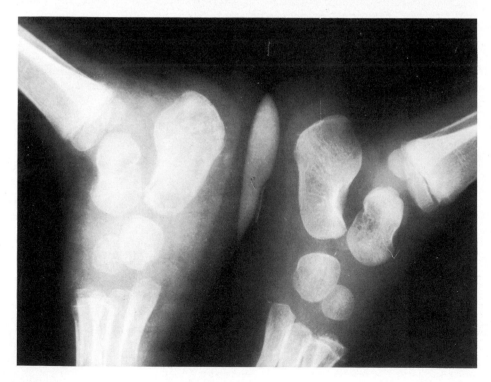

FIG. 3–19. Hemoglobin SC disease (tarsal bones). Mottled appearance of the right os calcis represents salmonella osteomyelitis. Compare Fig. 3–18, noting similarity in appearance to infarction.

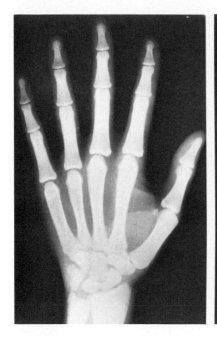
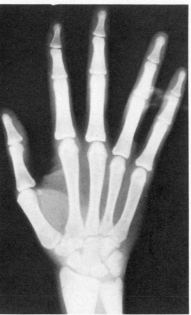

FIG. 3–20. Sickle-cell anemia (hands). Long, slender metacarpals and phalanges are noted.

be expected. The two cannot be readily differentiated by roentgen or clinical means. Infarction, or hand-foot syndrome, occurs at the average age of 18 months. Periosteal new bone formation and intramedullary densities appear 1 to 2 weeks after the onset of symptoms. The condition is self-limiting.[134] The hands may also show a long, slender form of metacarpals and phalanges, resembling those of Marfan's syndrome (Fig. 3–20). Later changes include cupping and conical epiphyses and shortening of the phalanges and metacarpals or metatarsals, leading to brachydactyly[31] (Figs. 3–21, 3–22, 3–23). The latter can have the same appearance as is found in pseudo- and pseudohypoparathyroidism, Turner's syndrome, idiopathic brachydactyly, or brachydactyly caused by local injury. The distribution is not, however, symmetrical, and the fourth metacarpals are not selectively involved. Widening of the medullary spaces may also occur (Figs. 3–24, 3–25).

The long bones may show changes caused by osteomyelitis or infarction, which are similar in appearance (Fig. 3–26). Periosteal elevation, destructive changes, endosteal resorption, and layering of new bone along the inner cortex of the medullary space, giving a "bone-within-a-bone" appearance, may be seen (Figs. 3–27, 3–28, 3–29, 3–30).

Infarctions of the long bones[16,17] may be cortical or medullary, the cortical type being far more common in sickle-cell disease. The majority of infarcts occur in the Hb SS genotype. Cortical infarcts may be complete, resulting in necrosis and rarefaction of the cortex, or incomplete, resulting in cortical thickening. The determining factor is the presence or absence of periosteal collateral circulation. In early infancy, the periosteum is loosely attached and contributes nothing to the vascular supply of the cortex. Therefore, in infancy and childhood, "active" infarcts develop with cortical rarefaction and destruction. The periosteum retains its osteogenic properties and forms new bone. In adults, cortical thickening results from recurring, small endocortical infarcts. In older patients "tramline" or "splitting" of the cortex occurs.

In children, "active" long bone infarcts occur most often in the intermediate segment between the central portion of the shaft and the metaphysis. This is thought to be the portion with the least oxygenation. The most common sites, in order, are the distal femur, proximal tibia, and distal humerus. In younger infants it is not uncommon for the central segments and both intermediate segments to be involved, resulting in infarction of virtually the entire diaphysis due to severe occlusion of the nutrient artery and no periosteal collateral. This is uncommon in the femur and tibia. Multiple infarctions occur more frequently than single ones. Symmetrical involvement is not uncommon, and occurs most frequently in the distal femora.

(Text continues on p. 89)

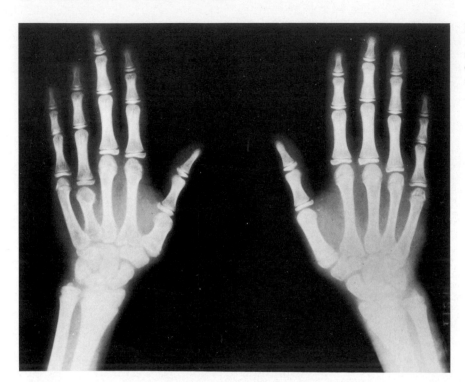

FIG. 3–21. Sickle-cell anemia (hands). The right hand shows shortening of first and fourth metacarpals. The hands are otherwise essentially normal.

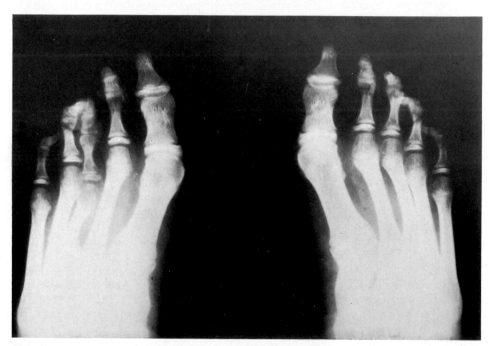

FIG. 3–22. Sickle-cell anemia (feet); same patient as in Fig. 3–21. There is shortening of the right third metatarsal.

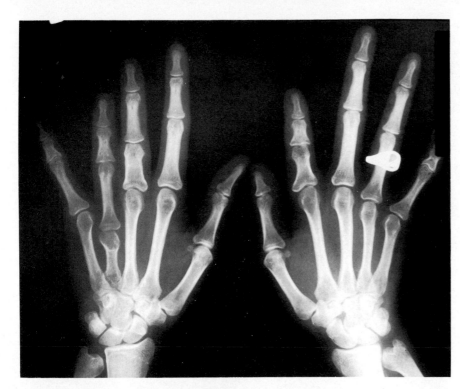

FIG. 3–23. Sickle-cell anemia (hands). Note shortening of the right proximal phalanx of the middle finger, with a cup-shaped proximal articular surface; of the right fourth metacarpal with flattening of the articular surface; of the right fourth middle phalanx, with normal-looking articular surfaces; of the right fifth middle phalanx, left first distal phalanx, left second proximal and middle phalanges, with cupping of the articular surface, and left fifth middle phalanx. (Courtesy of Dr. Antonio Pizarro, VA Hospital, Hines, IL)

FIG. 3–24. Sickle-cell anemia (hand). There is slight widening of the shafts and lack of tubulation in the metacarpals.

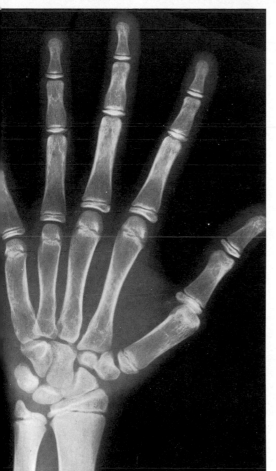

FIG. 3–25. Sickle-cell anemia (hands). Widening and lack of constriction of the shafts of the metacarpals and phalanges bilaterally, combined with loss of density and thinning of the cortices are noted. This finding is unusual in sickle-cell anemia.

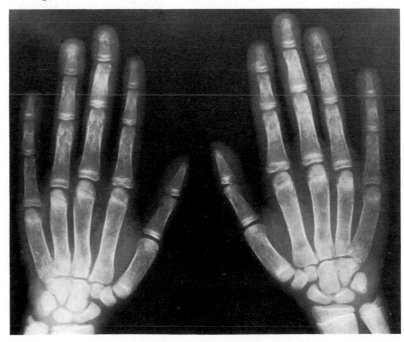

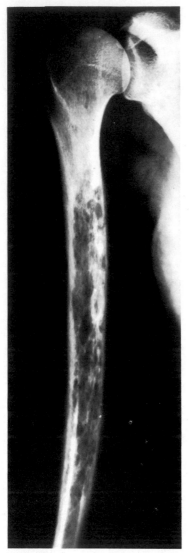

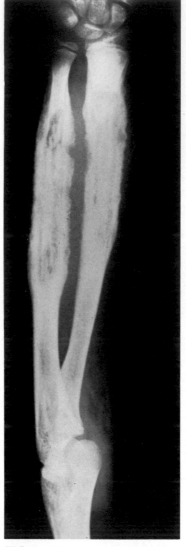

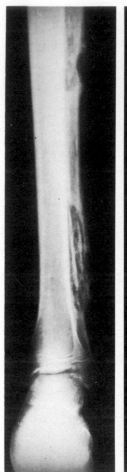

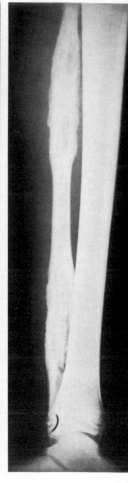

FIG. 3–26   FIG. 3–27   FIG. 3–28

FIG. 3–26. Hemoglobin SC disease (humerus)—osteomyelitis caused by infection with *E. coli.* There is extensive bony destruction of the shaft of the humerus. Note periosteal new bone formation and splitting of the cortex of the distal humerus. The osteomyelitis involves the diaphysis, rather than the metaphyses.

FIG. 3–27. Sickle-cell anemia (forearm)—black female, age 12 years—osteomyelitis. Note multiple draining sinuses. There is widening of the shafts of both radius and ulna, caused by involucrum formation, and dead cortex or sequestrum within an extensive destructive area, giving a "bone-within-a bone" appearance. The diaphyseal location of the osteomyelitis is apparent in both bones.

FIG. 3–28. Sickle-cell anemia (left leg)—osteomyelitis; same patient as in Fig. 3–27. Two separate areas of osteomyelitis—in the proximal shaft and in the distal shaft of the fibula—may be seen, with destructive changes and involucrum formation. Note the "bone-within-a-bone" appearance at the distal site.

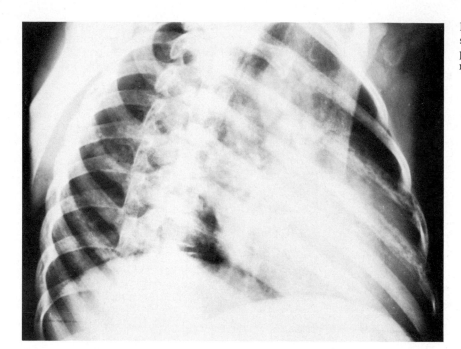

FIG. 3–29. Sickle-cell anemia (ribs)— salmonella osteomyelitis. Note the patchy destructive areas in several ribs.

In adults, the manifestation of cortical infarction is endocortical thickening due to periosteal collateral. In the event that edema elevates the periosteum cutting off collateral circulation, full cortical infarction may occur.

The complications of bone infarction are osteomyelitis and pathological fracture. The sequestra that form tend to resorb under medical management. Bone infarcts occur in many conditions, some of which are summarized below.

BONE INFARCTS

Sickle-cell disease
Idiopathic
Occlusive vascular disease
Osteomyelitis
Fibrosarcoma
Ewing's tumor
Gout
Gaucher's disease
Alcoholism
Pancreatitis
Polyarteritis nodosa
Caisson disease
Radiation

Osteomyelitis, rather than, or superimposed upon, infarction is suggested when massive longitudinal intracortical diaphyseal fissuring is present associated with overabundant involucrum formation. The involvement of multiple, often symmetrical sites with the above processes is highly consistent with infection. The most common sites involved are the diaphyses of the long bones, the humeri, femora, radii, ulnae, and fibulae.

Pathological fractures of the long and short bones may be due to thin cortices, owing to marrow hyperplasia, cortical infarcts, and osteomyelitis. Fractures due to minor trauma in sickle-cell disease at sites without infarction or infection are common.

Generalized "splitting" of the endosteal layer is very suggestive of sickle-cell disease (Fig. 3–31). In addition, areas of medullary infarction in the shafts of the bones may rarely be seen (Fig. 3–32). Bone infarcts, particularly in the femoral and humeral heads, occur, manifested as sporadic areas of necrosis (Fig. 3–33) or as areas of structural failure showing fragmentation, flattening of the heads and cyst formation (Figs. 3–34, 3–35, 3–36).

Ischemic necrosis of the femoral head is very common in sickle-cell disease.[30] It occurs in up to 60% of patients with hemoglobin SC disease, and in up to 12% of patients with homozygous sickle-cell anemia. It also occurs rarely in sickle-cell trait under stress conditions and in sickle-thalassemia. The radiographic development of ischemic changes follows the pattern common to other diseases in which this event occurs (see Chap. 4). Three basic patterns

(Text continues on p. 92)

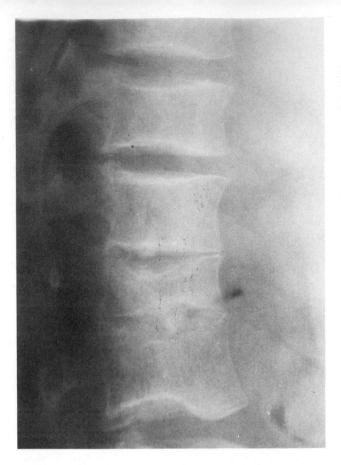

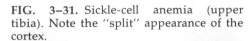

FIG. 3–30. Sickle-cell anemia (spine)—osteomyelitis. Notice destruction of the intervertebral space and a wedge shape of the adjacent vertebral body. Several biconcave vertebral bodies are noted.

FIG. 3–31. Sickle-cell anemia (upper tibia). Note the "split" appearance of the cortex.

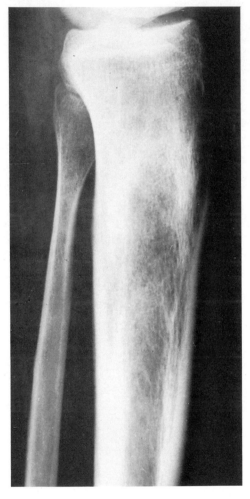

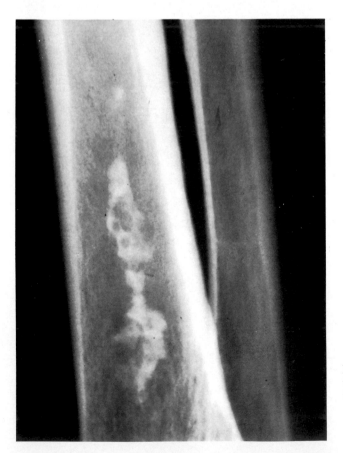

FIG. 3–32. Sickle-cell anemia (leg). Medullary infarction in the distal tibial shaft is seen as an intramedullary calcification with a serpiginous configuration.

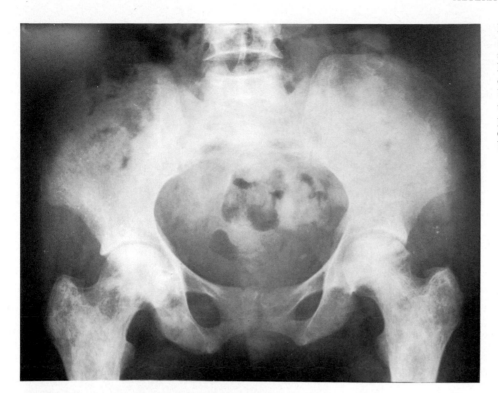

FIG. 3–33. Sickle-cell anemia (pelvis and hips). The hips show sclerosis of both femoral heads. There is a loss of bone density and accentuated trabecular pattern. "Splitting" of the cortex can be seen in the proximal femora. Biconcavity of the fourth lumbar vertebral body can also be seen.

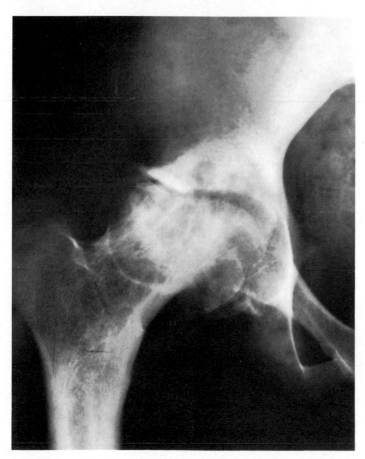

FIG. 3–34. Sickle-cell anemia—infarction and ischemic necrosis of the head of the femur following structural collapse. Note flattening of the head, secondary acetabular changes, increased density, and cyst formation.

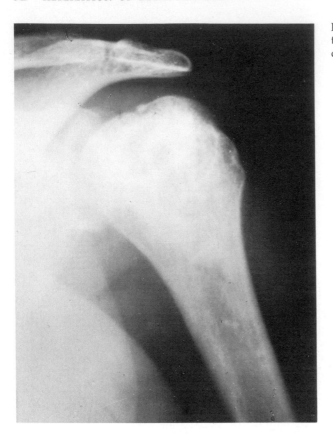

FIG. 3–35. Sickle-cell anemia. Note ischemic necrosis of the humeral head with sclerotic and radiolucent areas, and disruption of the articular cortex.

FIG. 3–36. Sickle-cell anemia (knees). Note residual deformity of the lateral aspect of the proximal left tibial epiphysis, which has resulted from epiphyseal infarction, causing unilateral genu valgum.

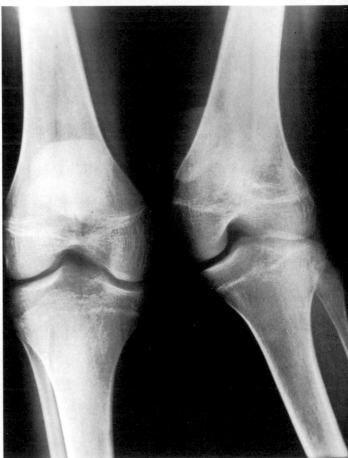

can be discerned. The first is a course similar to that of Legg–Perthes' disease, with ischemic necrosis of the femoral capital epiphysis, widening of the joint space, and thickening of the femoral neck. There is eventual replacement of the necrotic bone in the femoral head. In the second pattern, patients show a localized area of necrosis, with segmental flattening and destruction similar to osteochondrosis dissecans. In the third, they may show severe hip changes with flattening, secondary osteoarthritis, fragmentation, and destruction, with no spontaneous improvement expected.

An angled deformity of the ankle mortise, termed *tibiotalar slant*, has also been reported in sickle-cell anemia (Fig. 3–37). It is due to premature closure of the lateral tibial epiphysis owing to ischemia. It may be unilateral or bilateral, and is found in approximately 4% of patients. Tibiotalar slant may also be seen in juvenile rheumatoid arthritis, hemophilia, and multiple epiphyseal dysplasia.[72,117] Many sickle-cell patients are of short stature. Maturation of bone may be delayed (Figs. 3–38, 3–39).

Extramedullary hematopoiesis may be evident as a paraspinal soft-tissue shadow, although this condition more commonly occurs in thalassemia (Fig.

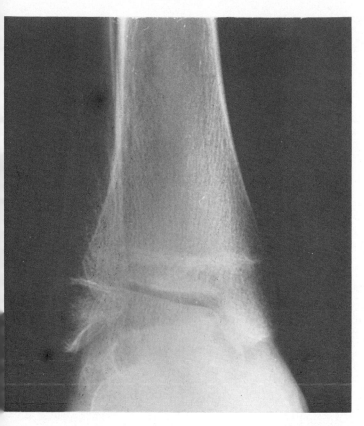

3–40). Hemarthrosis may rarely complicate sickle-cell disease (Fig. 3–41). Extramedullary hematopoiesis is a compensatory mechanism which occurs when the blood-forming organs are unable to supply body demand for red cells. It occurs most commonly in the congenital hemolytic anemias: hereditary spherocytosis; thalassemia, particularly the intermedia form; and, sickle-cell anemia. It has also been reported in myelofibrosis, polycythemia, erythroblastosis fetalis, leukemia, Hodgkin's disease, carcinomatosis, hyperparathyroidism, and rickets. It may occur idiopathically and may rarely cause neurologic symptoms due to spinal cord involvement.

The radiographic appearance of intrathoracic paraspinal extramedullary hematopoiesis is that of unilateral or bilateral well-demarcated masses in the posterior mediastinum at the level of the middle

FIG. 3–37. Sickle-cell anemia (ankle). Note the slope of the distal tibial articular surface with the lateral side more superior, giving the typical "tibiotalar slant."

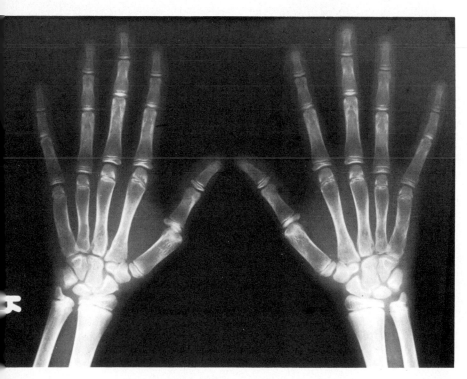

FIG. 3–38. Sickle-cell anemia (hands)— male, age 23 years. There is retarded growth and maturation, and lack of fusion of the secondary epiphyseal ossification centers. Note widening of the medullary cavity and lack of constriction of the first and the fifth metacarpals bilaterally.

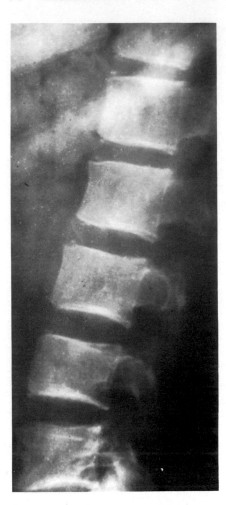

FIG. 3–39. Sickle-cell anemia (spine) — same patient as in Fig. 3–38; persistence of ring epiphyses of the vertebral bodies at age 23. Loss of bone density in the lumbar spine may be seen. Pituitary infarction was clinically suspected.

FIG. 3–40. Sickle-cell anemia. Note paraspinal soft-tissue mass bilaterally in the lower dorsal region, representing extramedullary hematopoiesis. This finding is more common in thalassemia major than in sickle-cell anemia. The bone changes of sickle-cell anemia are also present: biconcavity of the vertebral bodies and coarsened bony trabecular pattern.

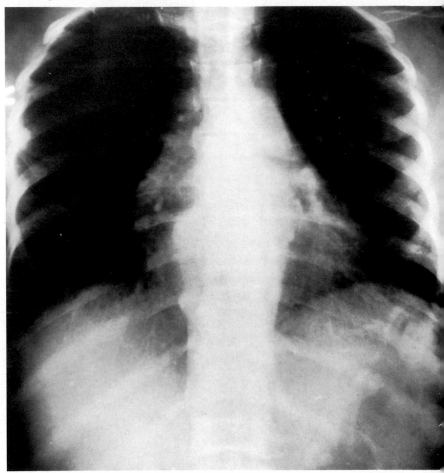

FIG. 3–41. Hemoglobin SC disease (knee) — lateral view. Note the cortical and medullary changes of the femur and tibia. Distention of the knee joint capsule is present. On aspiration this proved to be a hemarthrosis.

and lower thorax. The masses may be rounded or lobulated, or the lateral contour may form a single curve. No calcification is seen, and no erosion or reactive change of adjacent bone has been described.

Nonosseous changes of sickle-cell anemia include splenic infarction, cardiomegaly, cholelithiasis, pulmonary infections, vascular congestive changes, and renal papillary necrosis (Fig. 3–42).

THE THALASSEMIAS

Thalassemia comprises a group of heterogeneous disorders usually characterized by hereditary hypochromic microcytic anemia, based on a decreased rate of synthesis of one or more hemoglobin polypeptide chains.[132] The classification derives from the specific polypeptide chain involved; thus, there are α, β, δ, and $\delta\beta$ thalassemias. The hemoglobinopathies resulting from a single amino acid substitution are not considered to be thalassemias. However, an abnormal hemoglobin may be present in some forms of thalassemia, such as hemoglobin

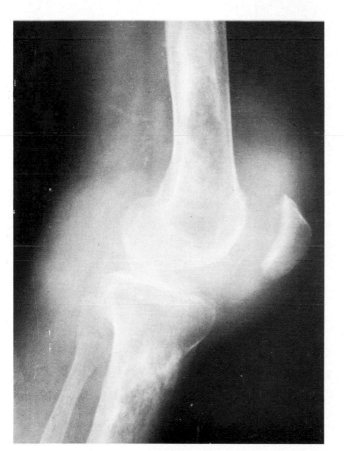

Barts (a tetramer of γ chains, or γ_4), hemoglobin H (a tetramer of β chains, or β_4), or the Lepore hemoglobins.

Heterozygotes are relatively mildly affected and are classed as thalassemia trait or thalassemia minor. Homozygotes, with two similar or identical genes for thalassemia, have a severe impairment of hemoglobin synthesis and are classed as thalassemia major. If a heterozygote is severely involved, the clinical picture may approach that of a mild thalassemia major and is classed as thalassemia intermedia.

A classification of the various types of thalassemia is as follows.[132]

1. β Thalassemia
   A. A_2 Thalassemia
   B. F Thalassemia
   C. A_2-F Thalassemia
2. δ Thalassemia
3. α Thalassemia
4. Thalessemia-like syndromes
   A. Lepore hemoglobins
   B. Hereditary persistence of fetal hemoglobin
5. Mixed heterozygotes (including sickle-thalessemia).

(Note: Hb A_1 = 2 $\alpha\beta$ chains; Hb A_2 = $2\alpha\gamma$ chains; Hb F = 2 $\alpha\delta$ chains.)

The "classical" type described by Cooley and Lee in 1925 is A_2 thalassemia, in which there is a decrease in the rate of synthesis of the β polypeptide chain of hemoglobin. This is the most common form and has also been termed Mediterranean anemia, or Cooley's anemia.

Thalessemia major is the homozygous form. It usually occurs in Mediterranean people, especially those of Italian, Sicilian, and Greek descent. The blood picture is of a severe microcytic, hypochromic anemia with elevated counts for reticulocytes, target cells, and stippled cells. There is anisocytosis. Normoblasts, erythroblasts, and leucocytosis may be present. In "classical" thalassemia, Hb A_2 is present in excess of 3%, in association with microcythemia. Hemoglobin F is usually present in amounts of 50% to 90%. Red-cell survival is decreased, serum bilirubin and fecal urobilinogen are increased, and the serum iron is elevated.

Clinically, severe anemia associated with jaundice usually appears in the latter half of the first year. A mongoloid facies, owing to swelling of the facial bones, is characteristic in early life. Splenomegaly and hepatomegaly are present, as well as cardiac enlargement beginning late in childhood. Marked skeletal dwarfism is evident after the age of 8 years,

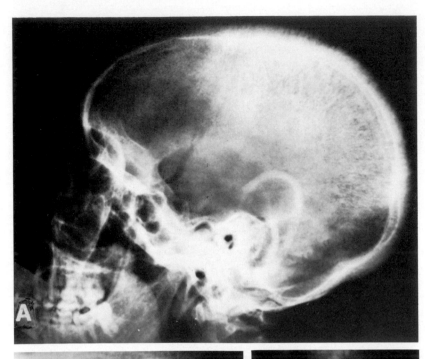

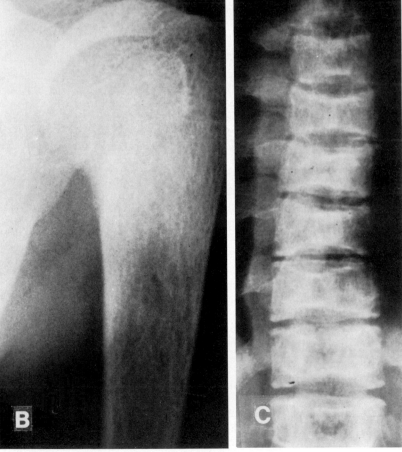

FIG. 3–42. Sickle-cell anemia with renal failure and changes of renal osteodystrophy, combined with bone changes of sickle-cell anemia. **A.** Skull. Note the "hair-on-end" appearance. **B.** Upper humerus. There is accentuation of the trabecular pattern and, in addition, subperiosteal resorption of the medial cortex. **C.** Spine (anteroposterior view). Shows bone sclerosis and biconcavity of several vertebral bodies.

and secondary sex characteristics are retarded. Later, maxillary hypertrophy with forward displacement of the incisors develops, giving the characteristic "rodent facies." Pathological fractures are common and are often multiple, usually involving the lower extremities. Compression fractures of the spine may also occur.[34] These patients rarely survive beyond adolescence.

Thalassemia minor represents the heterozygous state. It varies greatly in clinical severity and may be classified as follows:

1. Thalassemia minima or trait—Asymptomatic and without anemia
2. Typical thalassemia minor—Moderate anemia and splenomegaly, regularly increasing Hb A$_2$, and, at times, increasing Hb F
3. Thalassemia intermedia—Can approach in severity the milder forms of thalassemia major

Combinations of heterozygous states of thalassemia mixed with abnormal hemoglobins include: sickle-thalassemia (many cases in the United States reported in white patients); thalassemia-hemoglobin C disease (blacks and whites); and, thalassemia-hemoglobin E (southeast Asia). The clinical severity of these diseases varies.

Radiologically, bone changes result from erythroid hyperplasia of the marrow. Hyperplasia is more marked in thalassemia major than in any other anemia. All bones can be involved initially. If the patient survives to later life, the peripheral bone lesions may regress, and rarely sclerose, while the central skeletal lesions progress because of the conversion of red to yellow marrow in the peripheral skeleton.

The cortices are thinned. Resorption of the trabeculae gives a coarsened trabecular pattern (Fig. 3–43). There is underconstriction of bone, giving a square appearance of short tubular bones and an "Erlenmeyer flask" deformity of the long bones (Figs. 3–44, 3–45). These changes must be differentiated from those of Gaucher's disease in patients of an early age. The bone changes may appear at the second half of the first year of life.

In the skull the diploic space widens, with external displacement and thinning of the outer table (Fig. 3–46), which can assume a "hair-on-end" or perpendicularly striated appearance in extreme cases (Fig. 3–47). The earliest change takes place in the frontal bone. There is no involvement of the occipital bone inferior to the internal occipital protuberance owing to the lack of marrow in this area—an important point in differentiating thalassemia from nonhematological causes of widening of the calvarium (Figs. 3–48, 3–49).

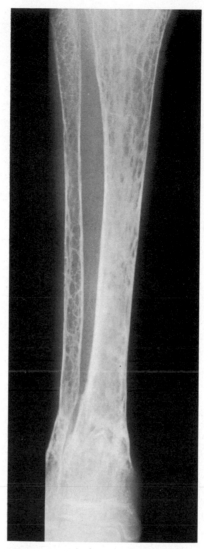

FIG. 3–43. Thalassemia major (leg). There is thinning of the cortices and marked accentuation of the bony trabecular pattern. Fractures at the lower leg have occurred. (Courtesy of Dr. Miguel Garces, Chicago, IL)

The facial bones are involved with marrow hyperplasia, causing lack of pneumatization of the frontal, maxillary, and sphenoid sinuses, as well as the mastoid air cells. The ethmoid sinuses alone are normally pneumatized, because of the lack of marrow in the ethmoid bone (Fig. 3–50). Hypertelorism may also occur. The facial bone changes are diagnostic of thalassemia and do not occur in sickle-cell anemia.

(Text continues on p. 100)

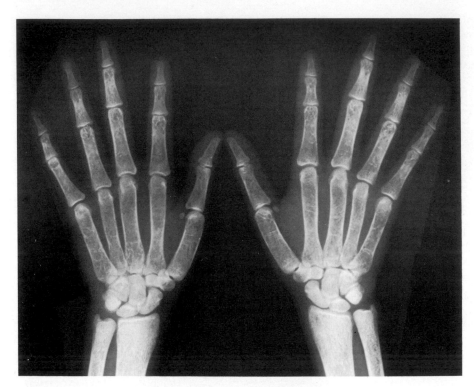

FIG. 3–44. Thalassemia major (hand)—female, age 24 years. There is loss of bone density, prominence of the bone trabecular pattern, underconstriction of the metacarpals and phalanges, giving them a rectangular appearance, and lack of tubulation of the distal radius and ulna. The changes in the hands did not regress on reaching adulthood, as sometimes happens.

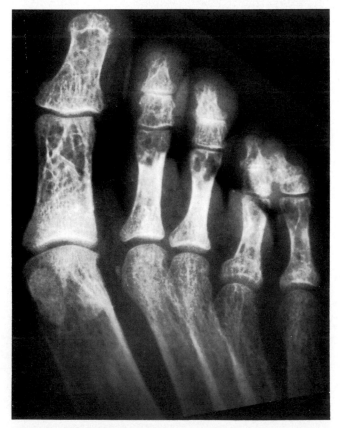

FIG. 3–45. Thalassemia major (foot); same patient as in Fig. 3–44. The rectangular, underconstricted shape of the first metatarsal is easily seen. Also note coarsening of the trabecular pattern.

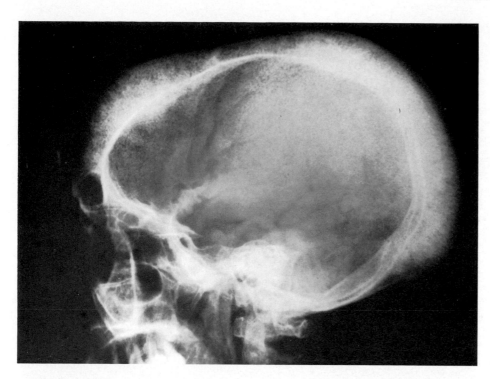

FIG. 3–46. Thalassemia major (skull). Note severe thickening of the calvarium in the frontal and parietal regions. This thickened area has a granular appearance, with a suggestion of striping perpendicular to the tables of the skull in the posterior parietal region. There is less thickening in the region of the coronal suture than in other areas, and there is no involvement below the occipital protuberance. The inner table is clearly defined, while the outer table lacks similar sharp definition. There is no encroachment into the cranial cavity.

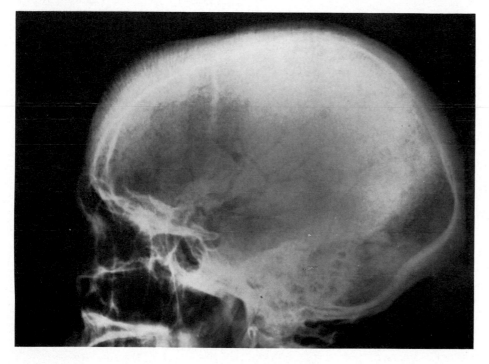

FIG. 3–47. Thalassemia major (skull). Note thickening of the calvarium, particularly in the frontal region, with striation perpendicular to the inner table of the skull. The inner margin of the calvarium is well defined, whereas the involved area of the outer margin lacks sharp definition.

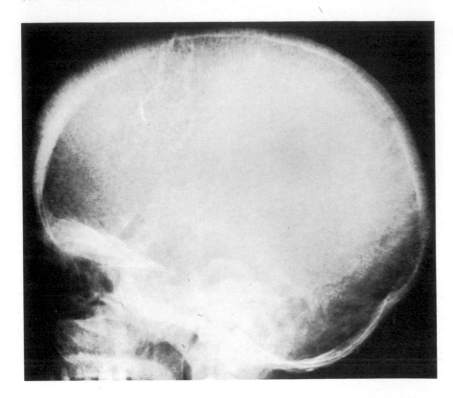

FIG. 3–48. Thalassemia major (skull). Note thickening of the calvarium, giving it a "hair-on-end" appearance, without involvement of the skull inferior to the internal occipital protuberance. Lack of development of all the paranasal sinuses except the ethmoids may also be seen. These features are characteristic of thalassemia.

FIG. 3–49. Thalassemia major (skull); same patient as in Fig. 3–48—posteroanterior view. Again, note thickening and "hair-on-end" pattern. There is lack of development of frontal and maxillary sinuses. Only ethmoid air cells are present. (Courtesy of Dr. Miguel Garces, Chicago, IL)

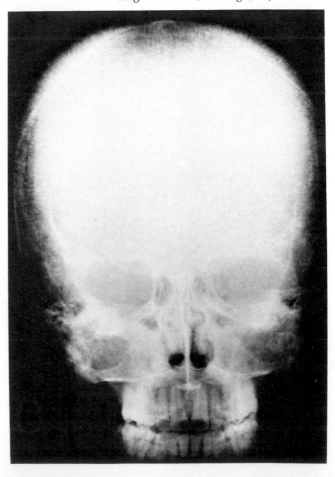

The ribs show a coarsened trabecular pattern, cortical thinning, loss of bone density, and widening. In particular, there is a central bulbous widening uniformly distributed in all ribs, which is characteristic (Fig. 3–51). An inferior "notch" may be present.

The spine also shows an altered trabecular pattern and loss of density. The biconcavity of the vertebral bodies so common in sickle-cell anemia is characteristically lacking in thalassemia (Fig. 3–52). A single case of spine changes "typical" of sickle-cell anemia in a patient with thalassemia major has been reported.[28] Exaggeration of the notch in the anterior vertebral bodies in infants may also be seen.[79] A large intrathoracic paraspinal soft-tissue mass of extramedullary hematopoiesis may also be present.[69] The pelvis shows deossification and alteration of the trabecular pattern (Figs. 3–53, 3–54).

The appearance of the secondary ossification centers is delayed, combined paradoxically with premature fusion to the shafts, causing stunted growth. Premature fusions are present in approximately one-quarter of patients over 10 years of age (Fig. 3–55). Transverse metaphyseal bands and pathological fractures may also occur. Bone infarcts, which are common in sickle-cell anemia, are rare. Secondary hemosiderosis[133] rarely results in opacification of the paravertebral lymph nodes and other

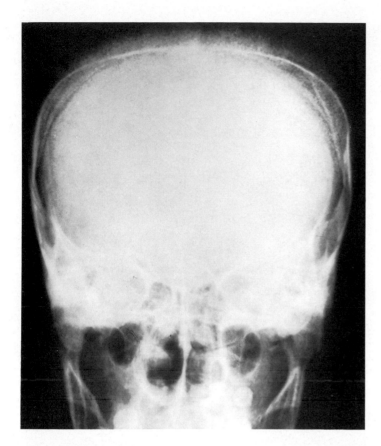

FIG. 3–50. Thalassemia major (skull). Note thickening of the calvarium and involvement of the frontal sinuses and hypoplasia of both maxillary antra. The mastoid processes may be seen, and there is lack of pneumatization. The ethmoid sinuses appear relatively clear.

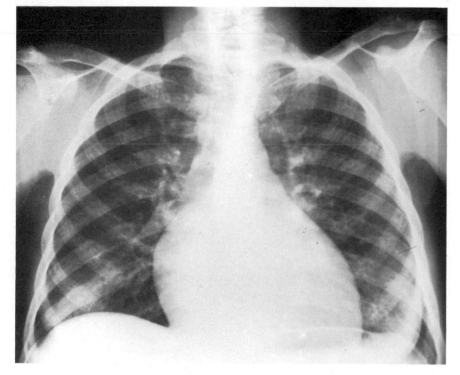

FIG. 3–51. Thalassemia major (chest). There is coarsening of the trabecular pattern of all the visualized bones. Note the central bulbous widening of all the ribs, a finding characteristic of thalassemia. The cortices of the ribs are thinned.

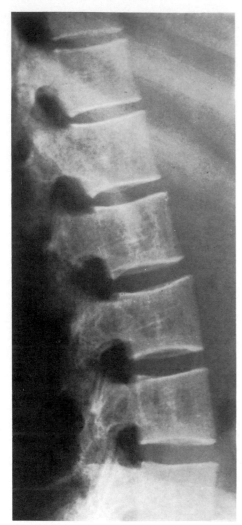

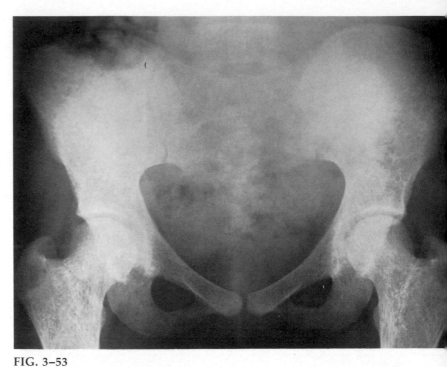

FIG. 3–53

FIG. 3–54

FIG. 3–52. Thalassemia major (lumbar spine). There is loss of bone density with a relative increase in the density of the vertebral end-plates, and coarsening of the trabecular pattern. The biconcavity so commonly seen in sickle-cell anemia is not present.

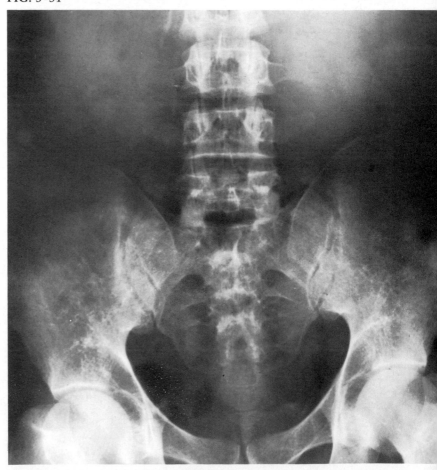

FIG. 3–53. Thalassemia major (pelvis). There is loss of bone density with coarsening and accentuation of the bony trabecular pattern. The density of the femoral heads is the same as that of the rest of the bone. There is no evidence of infarctions, as might be present in sickle-cell anemia.

FIG. 3–54. Thalassemia minor (spine and pelvis) — black male, age 50 years. Note coarsening of the bony trabecular pattern in the spine and pelvis, and loss of bone density. There is no evidence of biconcavity of the spine nor of infarction of the femoral heads.

FIG. 3–55. Thalassemia major (upper humerus). There is premature fusion of the humeral capital epiphysis, causing deformity. Cortical thinning, underconstriction of bone, and trabecular accentuation may also be noted.

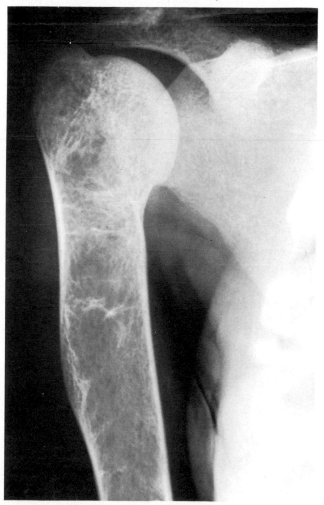

lymph nodes, as well as the liver, owing to massive iron deposition.

Thalassemia minor and heterozygous combinations can cause bone abnormalities of varying severity.

Sickle-cell β-*thalassemia disease*[107] is a doubly heterozygous disorder due to the inheritance of one gene for hemoglobin S and one gene for β-thalassemia. These mutant genes have an adverse effect on both the rate of hemoglobin synthesis, and the physicochemical properties of hemoglobin. The genes interact by suppressing the synthesis of normal β globin chains required for the formation of normal hemoglobin A. The abnormal β chain which forms hemoglobin S is suppressed to a lesser degree, resulting in an increased proportion of hemoglobin S within the red cell to the level at which sickling may occur. Laboratory diagnosis involves the quantitative determinations of hemoglobins S, A_2, and F. Hemoglobin S in this disease is usually present in concentrations of 60% to 85%. Proof of the presence of thalassemia depends upon the demonstration of increased concentrations of either hemoglobin A_2 or hemoglobin F, which are normally present in only trace amounts.

In one form, there is a twofold increase in hemoglobin A_2, and hemoglobin A is present at a concentration of 20% to 30%. In the other form, hemoglobin F reaches a level of 10% to 30%, and there is complete suppression of hemoglobin A synthesis.

The clinical and radiological severity of the disorder varies greatly. Blacks and Mediterranean people are most susceptible.

Radiologically, the abnormalities could be attributed to the effects of hemoglobin S, rather than thalassemia. Lesions produced by sickling and vascular occlusion are prominent. Two-thirds of patients are expected to show skeletal lesions, which are of the type seen in sickle-cell disease. "Splitting" of the cortex with thickening, ischemic necrosis of the femoral (Fig. 3–56) and humeral heads, biconcave and sclerotic vertebral bodies, and thickening of the calvarium in the frontal and parietal regions are all seen. The hand–foot syndrome may occur in infants.[67] Medullary bone infarcts may also occur (Figs. 3–56, 3–57). In addition, Salmonella osteomyelitis may occur in this condition, as in sickle-cell disease. Splenomegaly may be seen in adults, while it is not seen in sickle-cell anemia.

The stigmata of Cooley's anemia are not seen, because thalassemia serves only to permit the gene for hemoglobin S to gain expression.

The causes of a "hair-on-end" pattern in the skull[86] are summarized below.

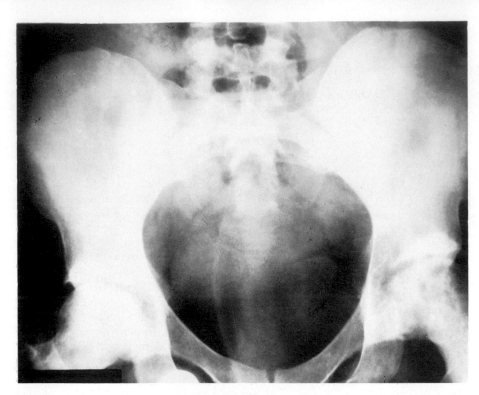

FIG. 3–56. Sickle-cell β-thalassemia disease (pelvis and hips). Bilateral ischemic necrosis of the femoral heads is noted.

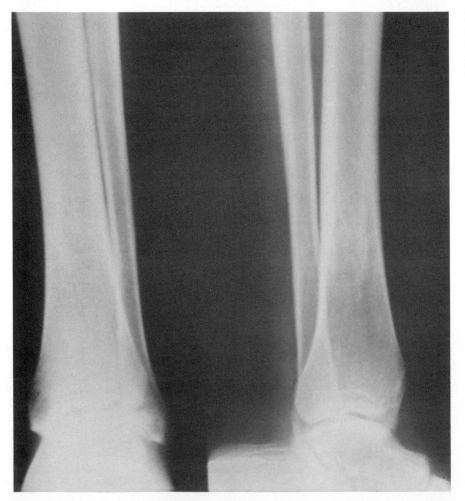

FIG. 3–57. Sickle thalassemia (distal leg). Note the amorphous calcification in the medulla of the distal tibia representing a medullary bone infarction.

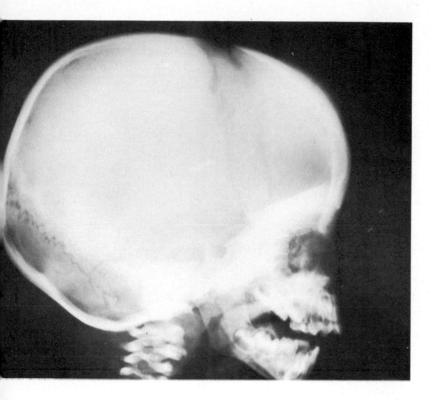

FIG. 3–58. Iron-deficiency anemia (skull)—white male, age 20 months, with diarrhea and failure to develop. Diagnosis of nutritional anemia was made and hemoglobin was found to be 4.3 g%. The skull shows thickening and widening in the frontal bone and, to a lesser extent, in the anterior parietal region. The bone texture and density appear otherwise normal.

DIFFERENTIAL DIAGNOSIS OF A "HAIR-ON-END" PATTERN IN THE SKULL

1. Congenital hemolytic anemias
   A. Thalassemias
   B. Sickle-cell disease
   C. Hereditary spherocytosis
   D. Hereditary elliptocytosis
   E. Hereditary nonspherocytic hemolytic anemia, pyruvate-kinase deficiency
2. Iron-deficiency anemia
3. Cyanotic congenital heart disease
4. Polycythemia vera in childhood
5. Metastases from neuroblastoma

BONE CHANGES IN OTHER ANEMIAS

Iron-deficiency anemia[2,97] in severe cases may show roentgenologic abnormalities, particularly in children. Mild to moderate osteoporosis with an associated atrophy of the outer table of the skull is reported to be the most common finding. The bones of the hands are commonly involved when osteoporosis is present, with findings of loss of density and thin cortices. Widening of the shaft and coarsening of the trabecular pattern are less often seen. Rarely, the skull may show widening of the diploic space (Fig. 3–58). In the long bones, changes suggestive of rickets have been reported in a low percentage of patients. Transverse metaphyseal striping may also be present (Fig. 3–59). The degree of osteoporosis does not correlate with the serum iron and hemoglobin levels, but may be related to the degree of protein caloric malnutrition. A smaller sella turcica has been reported in juveniles with severe iron deficiency.[104]

Hereditary spherocytosis also may cause calvarial thickening (Fig. 3–60), but long bone involvement is rare. The long bones may be involved if the disease is severe or if onset is in infancy. Vertebral end-plate depression has been reported (Fig. 3–60).[109]

Pyruvate-kinase-deficiency anemia[10] is an autosomal, recessive, nonspherocytic, hemolytic anemia in the homozygous state. Heterozygotes are normal. Second to glucose-6-phosphate dehydrogenase deficiency, it is the most common inherited enzyme deficiency in human erythrocytes. Hemolytic anemia, based on pyruvate-kinase deficiency, is probably the consequence of impaired glycolysis in the erythrocyte. The degree of clinical severity varies widely. Jaundice, splenomegaly, and cholelithiasis are found.

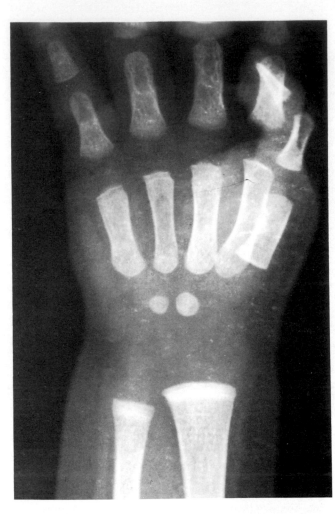

FIG. 3–59. Iron-deficiency anemia (wrist); same patient as in Fig. 3–58. Note horizontal metaphyseal striping, a nonspecific finding, at the distal radius and ulna.

FIG. 3–60. Hereditary spherocytosis (skull). Moderate thickening of the calvarium in the frontal and parietal regions is noted.

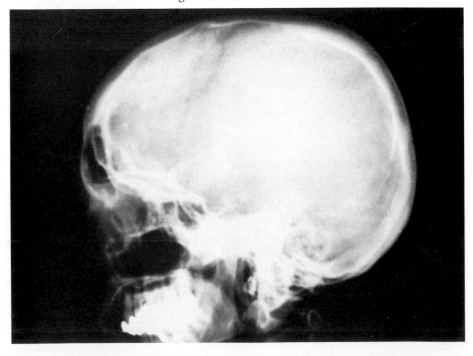

Radiologically, thickening of the diploic space leading to a "hair-on-end" appearance may be seen. Coarsening of the trabecular pattern of the long bones, with thinning of the cortices and failure of tubulation of the bone ends, has been reported in some patients. The paranasal sinuses remain aerated, in contrast to what happens in thalassemia.

HEMOGLOBINOPATHIES ASSOCIATED WITH UNSTABLE HEMOGLOBIN[132]

Unstable hemoglobins are thought to have arisen from mutations. They are structural variants of Hb A which undergo denaturation within the red cell, resulting in precipitation and formation of insoluble inclusions called Heinz bodies. This condition results in a disorder which has previously been referred to as congenital Heinz body anemia, and now is referred to as unstable hemoglobin hemolytic anemia. A large number of unstable hemoglobins are known. Their instability can arise from amino acid substitution, deletion, and replacement by proline. These factors alter the microgeometry of the hemoglobin molecule. The unstable hemoglobin variants are inherited as autosomal disorders. The clinical spectrum varies, and the severity of symptoms can be related to the degree of molecular instability. A compensated hemolytic anemia may be present or, in the event of a patient who carries a particularly unstable variant such as Hb–Hammersmith, a severe chronic hemolytic anemia may be present which is manifested in the first year of life. The diagnosis can be made in the laboratory. Deaths have been reported as resulting from these disorders. Thrombotic complications and gallstones occur, and bone changes are not well clarified.

CYANOTIC CONGENITAL HEART DISEASE[82]

Cyanotic congenital heart disease may produce skeletal abnormalities on the basis of erythroid hyperplasia secondary to chronic arterial unsaturation. The changes are similar to those seen in thalassemia.[122] In addition, changes of pulmonary hypertrophic osteoarthropathy, retarded bone maturation, and rib notching may be seen.

Extracardiac radiologic abnormalities have been summarized by Fellows and Rosenthal[39] as follows:

EXTRACARDIAC RADIOLOGIC ABNORMALITIES IN CYANOTIC CONGENITAL HEART DISEASE*

1. Skull
   A. Diploic thickening
   B. Macrocephaly
   C. Sinusitis
2. Skeleton (axial and peripheral)
   A. Bone marrow expansion
      (1) Generalized
      (2) Localized
   B. Periosteal new bone (pulmonary osteoarthropathy)
   C. Cortical sclerosis
   D. Rib notching
   E. Scoliosis
   F. Premature fusion of sternal ossification centers
   G. Retarded bone age
   H. Clubbing of fingers
3. Joints
   A. Effusion
   B. Gout
4. Abdomen
   A. Gallbladder
      (1) Calculi
   B. Kidneys
      (1) Enlargement (nonobstructive)
   C. Spleen
      (1) Enlargement

* Modified from Fellows KE, Rosenthal A. Am J Roentgen 114:371–379, 1972

The skull usually shows thickening in the supraorbital region or the posterior parietal area, where a "hair-on-end" appearance may be seen. A diffuse process may lead to macrocephaly in infants and young children. The incidence of sinusitis may be increased. Bone marrow hyperplasia results in medullary expansion and loss of normal diaphyseal constriction. The trabecular pattern is coarsened and the cortex is thinned. The changes are most prominent in the long bones, pelvis, spine, and sternum. Bone infarcts, such as those seen in sickle-cell disease, are absent. Localized expansion due to focal marrow hyperplasia may rarely be seen. Pulmonary hypertrophic osteoarthropathy, with diaphyseal periosteal new bone formation and clubbing of the fingers, may appear. Retardation of bone age may be present. Premature closure of sternal ossification centers is a frequent finding. Sclerosis is also expected to be present in some cases, as well as rib notching.

PAGET'S DISEASE (OSTEITIS DEFORMANS)

Paget's disease is a disease of unknown etiology in which there is initially a destruction of bone followed by a reparative process.

Geographic variations[110] in the prevalence of this disease have been reported. It is more frequent in the northern portions of the United States than in the southern, and is frequent in England and western Europe.

Histologically, the lesions are characterized by fibrosis and marked vascularity. There is marked enlargement of the haversian canals, making differentiation between the compacta and spongiosa difficult. A reparative process is concurrently present—osteoblastic and osteoclastic activity occur simultaneously. The result is distortion of architecture and a patternless arrangement, called the "mosaic structure," of haversian systems with their limiting cement lines. Intranuclear inclusions in osteoclasts are seen in electron micrographs.

Clinically, the disease occurs most commonly in middle life, although an occasional case in the third decade may be seen, and precocious onset[52] of Paget's disease has been reported. Three percent of all persons over 40 years of age (in prevalent areas) are affected with some form of the disease; this is usually monostotic and asymptomatic, occurring in the vertebra or pelvis. Men are affected twice as often as women. The lesions are seldom painful.

Deformities, particularly basilar invagination of the skull, can lead to severe neurological disturbances. The skull enlarges, and the patient complains of having to buy larger and larger sized hats.

The disease can be monostotic or polyostotic. The end result is a weakened, deformed, and thickened skeleton. Cardiovascular effects due to increased shunting of blood are common. Malignant degeneration occurs in a significant number of cases. This occurs most frequently in the seventh to eighth decade of life. An associated increase in incidence of hypertension and arteriosclerosis also occurs.

The serum calcium and phosphorus levels are normal. There is, however, a marked elevation of the serum alkaline phosphatase, which may be up to 20 times higher than normal. A sudden rise in an already elevated serum alkaline phosphatase level may herald the onset of an osteosarcoma.

Radiologically, four stages of Paget's disease may be discerned: Stage 1, the destructive phase; Stage 2, the combined phase; Stage 3, the sclerotic phase; and Stage 4, malignant change.

The combined phase is most commonly encountered and the roentgen findings in this phase are pathognomonic. The sclerotic phase occurs less frequently and is seen as a uniform area of bone sclerosis.

In the *skull,* the disease begins as a rarefied area called osteoporosis circumscripta, representing the destructive phase (Fig. 3–61). The area is well de-

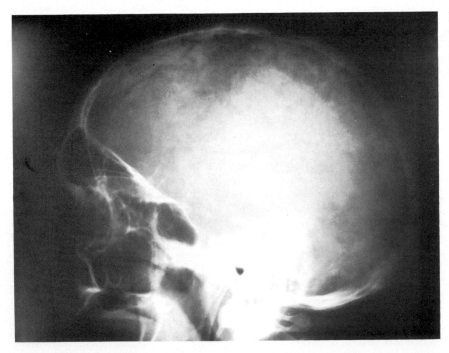

FIG. 3–61. Paget's disease (skull)—destructive phase in relatively early stage. Note loss of bone density in the parietal region, without a definitive circumscript margin.

marcated and involves the major portion of the calvarium. The outer table is destroyed, but characteristically the inner table is spared (Figs. 3–62, 3–63, 3–64, 3–65). Reparative processes begin as sclerosis of the inner table. Thickening of the diploë, and later of the outer table, follow. Irregular areas of sclerosis in the thickened diploë, the "cotton wool" appearance, are characteristic (Fig. 3–66). Basilar invagination results from bone softening. In the sclerotic phase, diffuse sclerosis of the skull may be seen with loss of differentiation between the tables and the diploë (Fig. 3–67). Dental changes include loss of lamina dura, resorption of bone near the apices of the teeth, and hypercementosis. The paranasal sinuses may be obliterated. The petrous pyramids are frequently involved. Tomograms of the petrous pyramids reveal demineralization regardless of their sclerotic appearance on conventional radiographs.[93]

In the *spine*, the most common finding is monostotic vertebral involvement in the combined phase. The vertebral body is enlarged. There is a rim of thickened cortex, giving a "picture frame" appearance. The trabecular pattern is coarsened and may be arranged in a vertically striated orientation (Fig. 3–68). This striated appearance of the body can be differentiated from hemangioma by the thickened cortex and increased size, which are not present in vertebral hemangioma. The neural arch may be thickened (Fig. 3–69). Monostotic Paget's disease of the vertebra may also be seen in the sclerotic phase. Enlargement of the body and "squaring" of the anterior margin, when present, help to differentiate this condition from osteoblastic metastases. In Hodgkin's disease there may be erosion of the anterior margin of a sclerotic vertebral body owing to pressure from contiguous enlarged lymph nodes, differentiating it from this condition.

The spine may be generally involved in polyostotic Paget's disease. The destructive phase, pathologic fractures, and the combined stage may coexist (Fig. 3–70, 3–71). In addition, uncalcified osteoid may give rise to a paraspinal soft-tissue mass.

The cervical spine is rarely involved, but when it is, it shows peculiarities in appearance and serious neurological sequelae, owing to spinal stenosis.[38] The latter is due to encroachment on the spinal canal by vertebral collapse, dislocation, or fracture. Bony overgrowth may encroach upon the intervertebral foramina, interfere with the blood supply to the spinal cord (resulting in myelomalacia), or lead to narrowing of the spinal canal (resulting in cord compression).

The destructive phase may lead to vertebral body collapse with intact intervertebral spaces. The neural arches are also likely to be involved, differentiating this process from metastases. In the combined phase, degenerative changes may obscure the diagnostic features of Paget's disease. The intervertebral disk of contiguously involved vertebral bodies may be replaced by bone, with resultant fusion. The sclerotic phase presents as a homogeneous dense vertebra. Again, involvement of the neural arch and spinous process helps in differentiating Paget's disease from carcinoma metastases. The atlas and axis may be involved,[23] with anterior subluxation of the atlas or bone hypertrophy, resulting in narrowing of the canal.

(Text continues on p. 115)

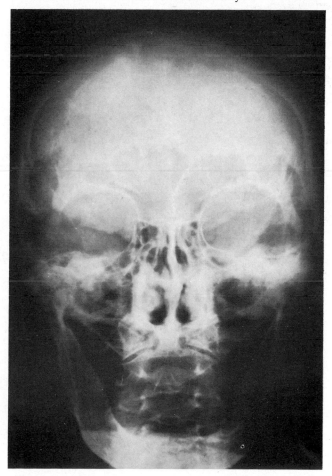

FIG. 3–62. Paget's disease (skull) — anteroposterior view — osteoporosis circumscripta. There is a sharply demarcated loss of bone density bilaterally of the occipital and temporal regions extending to the frontal area. The rest of the skull is normal in texture and density.

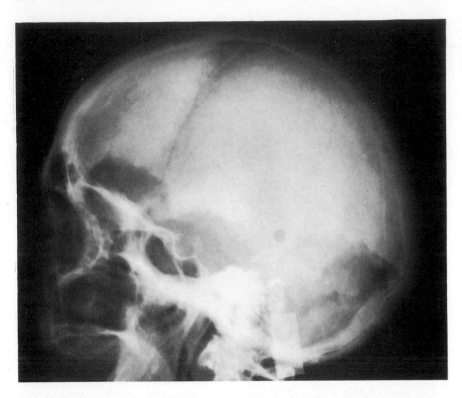

FIG. 3–63. Paget's disease—lateral view of the skull in Fig. 3–62—osteoporosis circumscripta. A sharply demarcated region of loss of bone density involving the occipital, temporal, and frontal areas may be seen. Also note that the inner table in the occipital area is preserved, while there is loss of definition of the outer table.

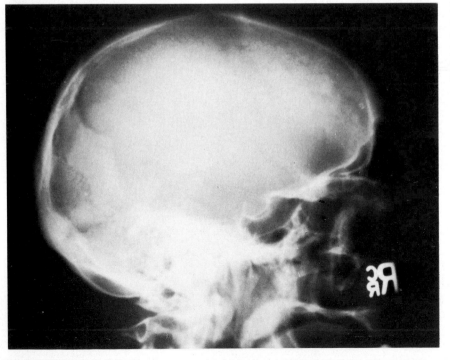

FIG. 3–64. Paget's disease (skull)—destructive phase—osteoporosis circumscripta. Loss of density in the parietal bone is noted, with a sharply marginated contour of normal bone in the occipital region.

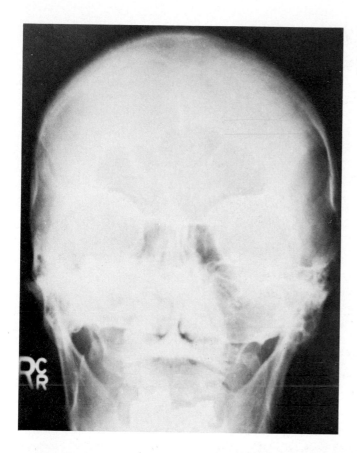

FIG. 3–65. Paget's disease (skull)—anteroposterior view—osteoporosis circumscripta. A sharply demarcated loss of bone density is seen in the parietal region on the left and to a lesser extent on the right.

FIG. 3–66. Paget's disease (skull)—conbined phase. Note marked thickening of the entire calvarium, with good definition of thickened inner and outer margins. Bony sclerotic patches give the characteristic "cotton wool" appearance.

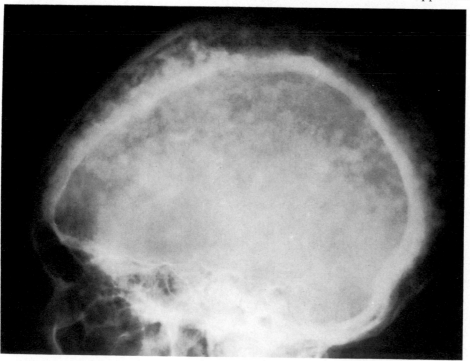

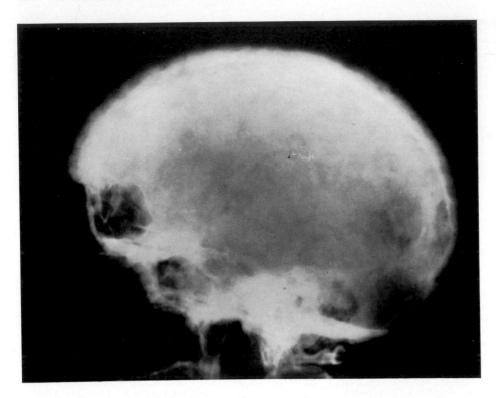

FIG. 3–67. Paget's disease (skull)—dense sclerotic phase. The calvarium shows a uniform marked increase in density, with scattered, relatively radiolucent patches.

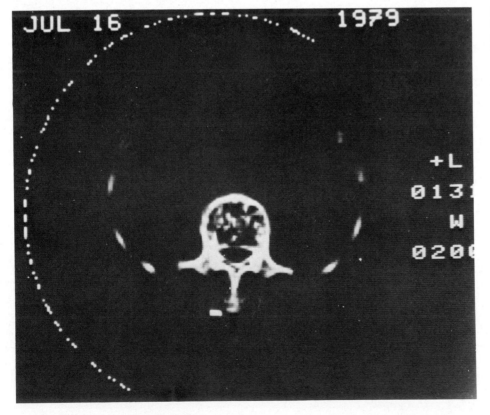

FIG. 3–68. Paget's disease—CT scan. Note the coarsened trabeculae within the vertebral body, seen on end.

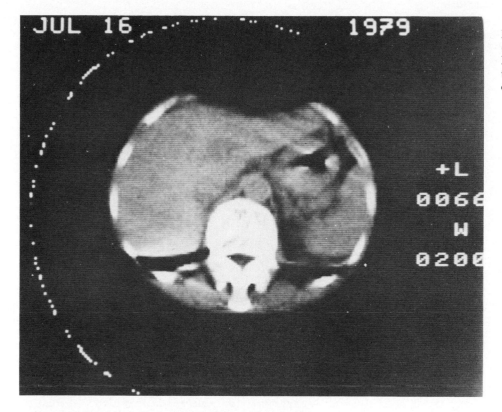

FIG. 3–69. Paget's disease (lumbar vertebrae) — CT scan. Note the marked thickening of the neural arch and increased density of the vertebral body.

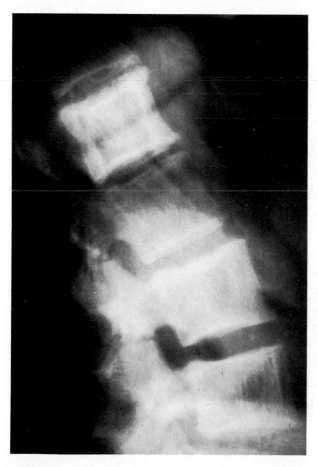

FIG. 3–70. Paget's disease — view of the spine showing the 12th dorsal vertebral body and the upper four lumbar vertebral bodies. There is mixed involvement of the spine. The 12th dorsal body is normal. The first lumbar vertebral body shows involvement in the combined phase of the disease, in which thickening of the anterior and posterior margins and of the vertebral end-plates gives it a "picture frame" appearance. The second lumbar vertebral body is normal. The third lumbar vertebral body is involved in the sclerotic phase, characterized by a uniform increase in density of the body and squaring of the anterior margin with lack of normal convexity (compare with anterior margin of L–1). The fourth lumbar vertebral body is involved in a transition between the combined phase and the sclerotic phase. It shows increased density of the vertebral body, with several prominent vertical trabeculae at the anterior aspect and squaring of its anterior margin.

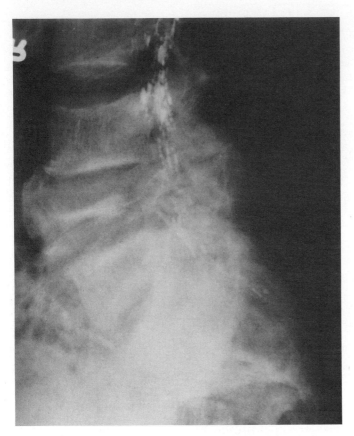

FIG. 3–71. Paget's disease—combined phase. Note the collapse of the fourth lumbar vertebral body. (Courtesy of Dr. Dharmashi V. Bhate, VA Hospital, Hines, IL)

FIG. 3–72. Paget's disease (pelvis)—combined phase. Cortical thickening and trabecular accentuation may be seen throughout the pelvis and right femur. There is widening of the bone contour caused by the thickened cortex. Note sclerosis of the right pubis as compared to the left pubis, and sclerotic changes in the left ilium. A transverse pathological fracture of the right proximal femoral shaft is also visible. Considerable vascular calcification is present. Compare with Fig. 3–74.

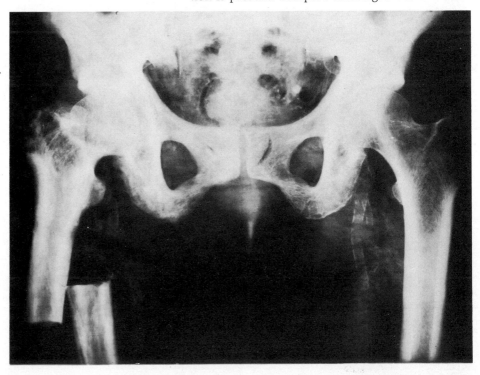

The *pelvis* is usually involved in approximately two-thirds of patients with Paget's disease, and usually with the combined stage of the disease.[47] It is rarely, if ever, observed in the radiolucent stage. There may be a small area of involvement, involvement of only one-half of the pelvis, or general involvement. The characteristic cortical thickening, enlargement of the pubis and ischium, and coarsened trabecular pattern are present, as well as thickening of the pelvic rim (Rim sign) (Fig. 3–72). Small irregular patches of bone sclerosis sometimes occur. In a reported series, 3 patients below the age of 40 years showed purely sclerotic lesions, which mimicked osteitis condensans ilii or sclerosing osteomyelitis, and then progressed with time to the combined stage of Paget's disease.[25] There may be deformity and protrusion of the acetabulum. Uniform narrowing of the hip joint space with medial migration of the femoral head is a common finding. Only minimal hypertrophic changes may be present.[47] The etiology of this Paget's arthritis is not known. Degenerative arthritis may be associated[48] (Fig. 3–73). When the pelvis is diffusely involved in the sclerotic phase, roentgen differentiation from osteoblastic metastases is difficult (Fig. 3–74). Widening of the bone, thickening of the cortex, and lack of soft-tissue mass serve as differential points.

The *ribs* are uncommonly involved. Single or multiple ribs can be affected (Fig. 3–75). There is widening and thickening of the bone. The *clavicles* and *scapula* may be involved in the combined or sclerotic phases (Figs. 3–76, 3–77).

Rarely, the sternum, calceneus, talus, patella (Fig. 3–78), a phalanx, or a metatarsal is involved. The hand may be involved, with the phalanges and metacarpals, and even less frequently the carpals, showing changes[54] (Fig. 3–80). Even the sesamoids may be involved (Fig. 3–79).

The long bones are commonly involved in the combined phase and rarely in the destructive phase.

The destructive phase typically begins at the end of a bone or at an apophysis such as the greater trochanter or tibial tubercle. The lesion extends along the shaft for a variable distance and ends in a typical, sharply demarcated, angular configuration,

(Text continues on p. 119)

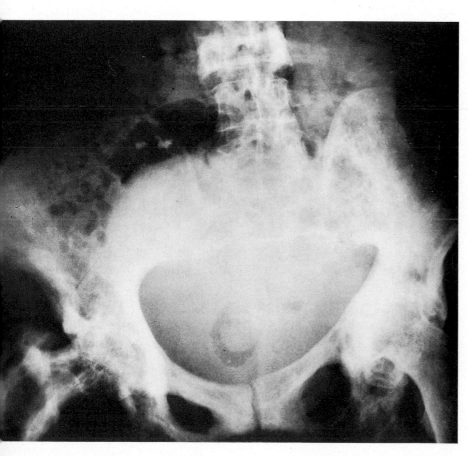

FIG. 3–73. Paget's disease (pelvis). Changes of advanced disease are present with cortical thickening and accentuation of the trabecular pattern, as well as enlargement of the caliber of bone. Bilateral arthritic changes are seen with narrowing of the joint spaces and medial migration of the femoral heads, particularly on the left, where slight protrusion is present. This entity represents a distinct Paget's arthritis.

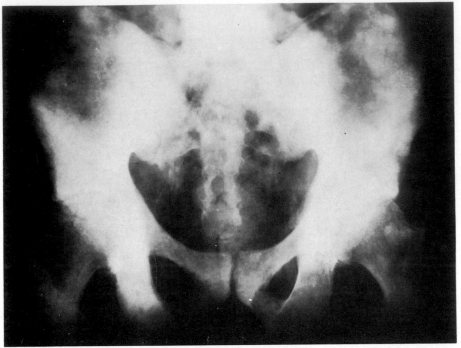

FIG. 3–74. Osteoblastic metastases (pelvis) from carcinoma of the prostate. (Compare with Paget's disease in Fig. 3–72.) There is no evidence of cortical thickening or trabecular accentuation. Sclerosis involving the right ilium and ischium, and patchy sclerotic changes in the left ilium and proximal femur, may be noted. The characteristic changes—cortical thickening and trabecular accentuation—are absent, rendering differentiation from the combined stage of Paget's disease readily possible.

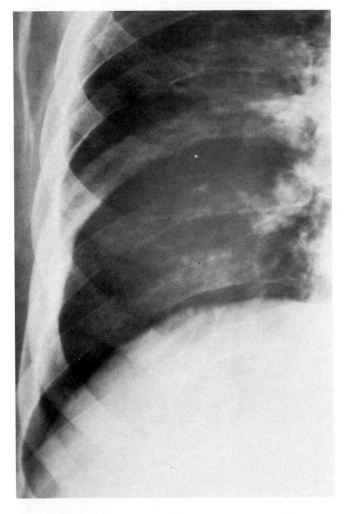

FIG. 3–75. Paget's disease—solitary rib involvement. Note cortical thickening and widening of the bone, similar to changes in other bones in Paget's disease. Increased density of the anterior aspect of the involved rib may also be seen.

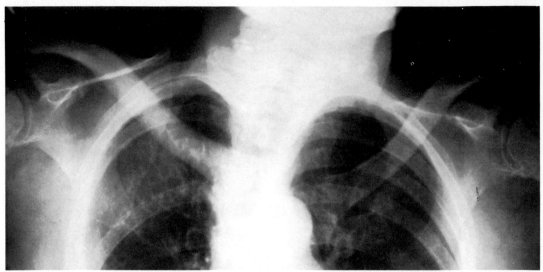

FIG. 3–76. Paget's disease of the right clavicle — sclerotic phase. There is uniform increase in density of the clavicle. (Incidental finding: postsurgical right rib resection.) Left clavicle appears normal by comparison.

FIG. 3–77. Paget's disease (left shoulder) — sclerotic phase. Note uniform increase in density of the scapula and clavicle.

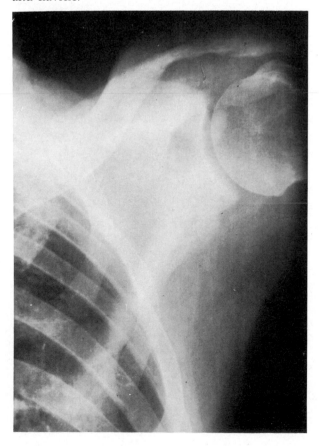

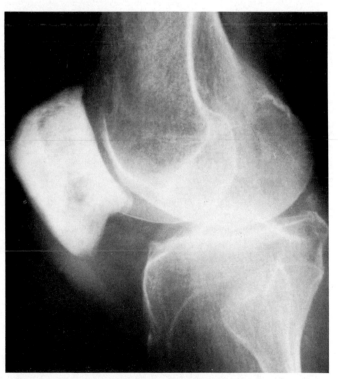

FIG. 3–78. Paget's disease (patella). Marked sclerosis, cortical thickening, and accentuation of the trabecular pattern, as well as enlargement of the patella, are noted.

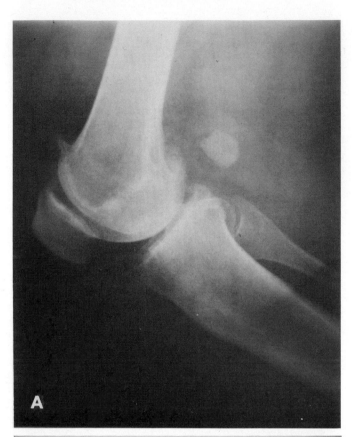

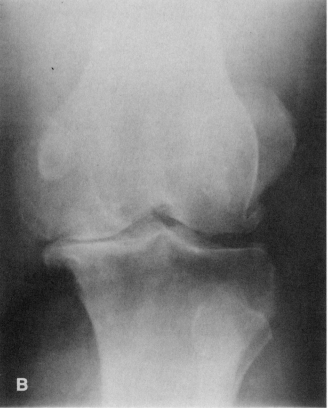

FIG. 3–79. Knee—anteroposterior (**A**) and lateral (**B**) views. Thickening and enlargement of the cyamella, with a sclerotic cortex indicating involvement with Paget's disease.

FIG. 3–80. Paget's disease (hand). Sclerosis, accentuation of the trabecular pattern, and enlargement of the caliber of the proximal phalanx of the middle finger are noted.

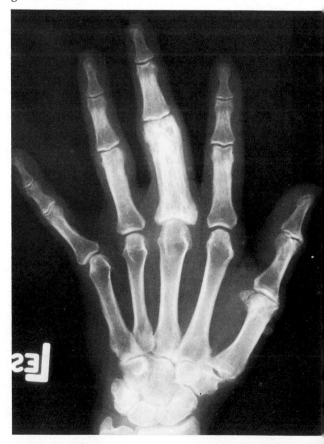

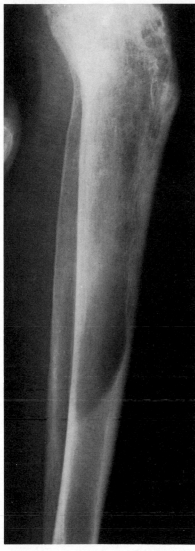

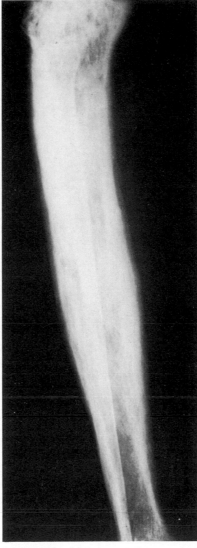

FIG. 3–81

FIG. 3–82

FIG. 3–81. Paget's disease (tibia)—destructive phase. There is an area of radiolucency extending from the proximal tibia and involving two-thirds of the shaft, ending in a sharply demarcated angular configuration (the so-called "blade of grass" appearance). Accentuation of the trabecular pattern at the proximal aspect of the tibia may also be seen.

FIG. 3–82. Paget's disease (tibia and fibula)—combined phase. Marked cortical thickening and widening of the bones, and accentuation of the trabecular pattern in the proximal and midportions, may be noted.

giving a "blade of grass" appearance (Fig. 3–81). An ovoid, cystlike,[115] expansile radiolucency in the anterior tibial cortex may also be present. One case has been reported which showed progression of a small, lucent, midanterior, tibial lesion to involvement of the entire tibia, with the combined stage of Paget's disease within the 12 years.[135]

In the combined stage, widening of the bone and thickening of the cortex are present, owing to resorptive and appositional processes. There is thickening of the trabeculae with disruption of the architectural pattern (Fig. 3–82), which may give a reticulated, lacelike, "soap bubble," or disorganized appearance. Incomplete fractures resembling pseudofractures of osteomalacia (Fig. 3–83) and pathological fractures (Fig. 3–85) of the transverse type occur in up to 8% of cases. These most com-

monly involve the femur. The incomplete fractures are stress fractures of the cortex that tend to heal at the periosteal and endosteal surfaces, leaving only a midcortical residual (Fig. 3–84). Softening of the bone leads to deformities (Fig. 3–86), particularly the "shepherd's crook" deformity of the upper femur (Fig. 3–87), and anterior bowing of the tibia (Fig. 3–88). The fibula is least likely to be involved.

Malignant degeneration, particularly in the form of osteogenic sarcoma, but also as other forms of sarcoma, may occur in widespread Paget's disease, with an incidence of about 10% (Figs. 3–89, 7–23). Osteosarcoma accounts for half of all secondary neoplasma, fibrosarcoma for an additional quarter, and the remainder are accounted for by chondrosarcoma, reticulosarcoma, pleomorphic, and unspecified types.[101] Giant-cell tumor has also been de-

(Text continues on p. 123)

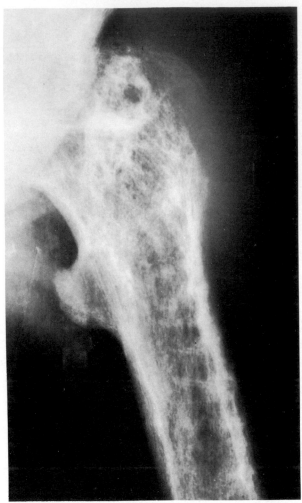

FIG. 3-83. Paget's disease (proximal femur) — combined phase. Note multiple incomplete or pseudo-fractures at the outer aspect of the femoral cortex, and cortical thickening and accentuated trabecular patterns characteristic of the combined phase of Paget's disease. No surgical procedure had ever been performed.

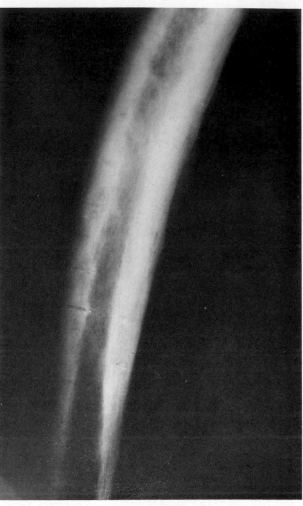

FIG. 3-84. Paget's disease (femur). Note the bowing of the femur. The thickening of the cortex and the small linear radiolucencies contained within the cortex represent incomplete or stress fractures.

FIG. 3-85. Paget's disease (femur) — combined phase. Transverse pathological fracture of the proximal third femoral shaft, the changes characteristic of Paget's disease — cortical thickening, trabecular accentuation, and sclerosis in the proximal femur and pelvis — may be noted.

FIG. 3-86. Paget's disease (radius and ulna). Note cortical thickening and trabecular accentuation, characteristic of the combined phase of Paget's disease, in both bones, and a curved deformity of the radius.

FIG. 3-87. Paget's disease (upper femur) — changes of the combined phase of the disease with cortical thickening and accentuated trabeculation. Note the "shepherd's crook" deformity of the proximal femur.

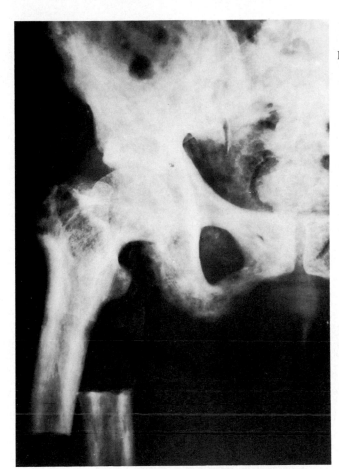

FIG. 3–85

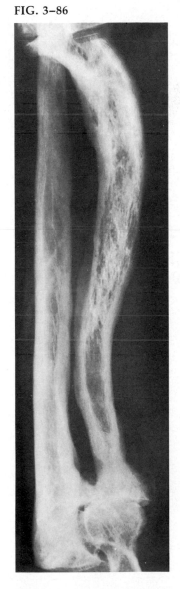

FIG. 3–86

FIG. 3–87

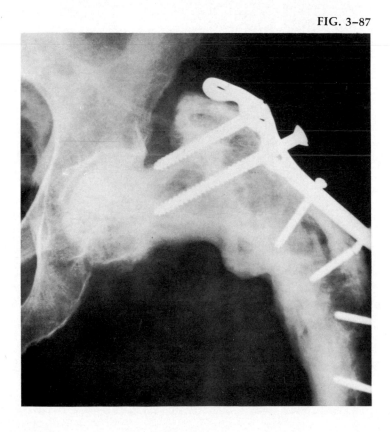

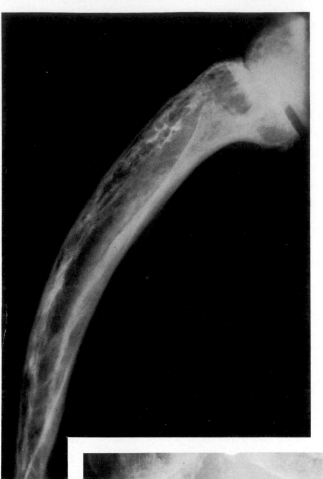

FIG. 3–88. Paget's disease (tibia). Characteristic changes of the combined phase of the disease—cortical thickening, trabecular accentuation, and several sclerotic patches—may be seen. There is also characteristic anterior bowing deformity of the tibia.

FIG. 3–89. Paget's disease (tibia)—malignant degeneration to osteosarcoma. Note characteristics of combined phase—cortical thickening and trabecular accentuation. There is also a destructive process involving the proximal tibia, and the mid- and lateral aspects of the articular surface have been destroyed. There is an ill-defined margin at the distal aspect. This represents osteosarcoma. The destructive tumor is seen to be situated anterior at the proximal tibia. The margins of the tumor are poorly defined.

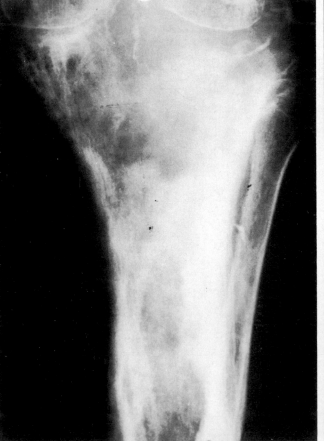

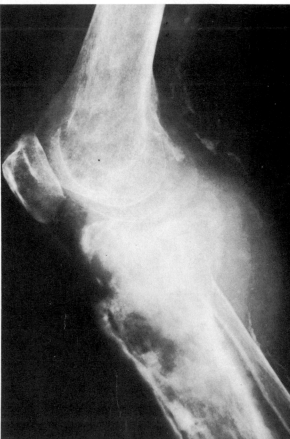

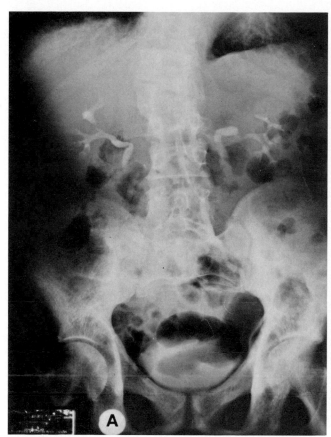

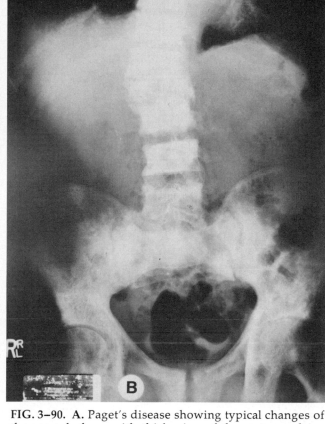

FIG. 3–90. **A.** Paget's disease showing typical changes of the second phase with thickening of the cortex and increased trabecular pattern. An old fracture of the second lumbar vertebra is noted. **B.** The same patient approximately 2 years later. The patient had developed a carcinoma of the prostate, and extensive osteoblastic metastases are superimposed upon Paget's disease in the spine, sacrum, and pelvis. A destructive lesion at the site of the previous fracture at L-2 is seen, illustrating the concept of locus minoris resistenciae.

scribed in association with Paget's disease.[62,113] Giant-cell tumors complicating Paget's disease have a predilection for the skull and facial bones. Benign giant-cell tumors have shown extreme bone resorption at their periphery. Malignant giant-cell tumors often follow a rapidly fatal course. Osteomyelitis superimposed upon Paget's disease may present a bizarre roentgen picture (Fig. 3–91).

Osteolytic areas occurring in Paget's disease may be based on various etiologies, summarized as follows:

DIFFERENTIAL DIAGNOSIS OF RADIOLUCENT AREAS IN PAGET'S DISEASE[5,13]

First stage of Paget's
Cystic degenerative changes
Radiolucency following fracture
Sarcomatous change
Giant-cell tumor
Coincidental lesions
    Metastases
    Myeloma[100]
    Brown tumor
Pseudomalignant manifestations[20]

An osteosarcoma developing in Paget's disease is most often osteolytic; however, a sclerotic lesion can occur. Osteoblastic metastases may be superimposed upon Paget's disease (Fig. 3–90).

Extramedullary hematopoiesis in Paget's disease has been reported in the dorsal paraspinal region and in the pelvis.[66] While this condition usually arises as a compensatory phenomenon in anemia, no anemia was present in the reported cases. It is thought that pathological fractures led to extrusion of marrow and resultant tumorous extramedullary hematopoiesis.

FIBROUS DYSPLASIA (FIBRO-OSSEOUS DYSPLASIA)

Fibrous dysplasia[43] is a developmental disturbance caused by a germ plasm defect involving proliferation and maturation of fibroblasts. Spicules of bone and islands of cartilage are interspaced in a matrix of collagenous tissue. The variable amount of the bone present accounts for the range of roentgen density, from a radiolucent to a "ground glass" appearance. The disease may be monostotic, monomelic, or polyostotic. When polyostotic, it is often unilateral.

Clinically, the disease begins in younger individuals and occasionally is seen in infants. Males and females have an approximately equal incidence. In polyostotic disease, localized pigmentations, or "café-au-lait" spots, are present in about one-third of patients. These have an irregular outline ("coast-of-Maine") as opposed to the smoothly marginated ("coast-of-California") "café-au-lait" spots seen in neurofibromatosis. Pigmentations do not occur in monostotic disease.

The following associated endocrine manifestations have been reported:[129]

1. Sexual precocity
2. Hyperthyroidism and goiter
3. Acromegaly
4. Cushing's syndrome
5. Acceleration of skeletal growth and maturation
6. Gynecomastia
7. Parathyroid enlargement

Sexual precocity, referred to as the McCune-Albright syndrome, occurs in up to 30% of females with polyostotic disease. It also occurs in males, but is very rare, with only 6 cases reported to date in the literature. This is true sexual precocity with acceleration of the normal process of release of gonadotropins by the anterior pituitary. Thyroid disorders

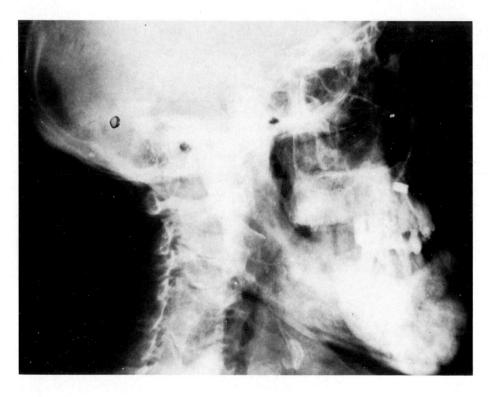

FIG. 3–91. Paget's disease (mandible) complicated by chronic draining osteomyelitis. Marked enlargement and patchy sclerosis of the mandible are noted.

are common, and hyperthyroidism is said to occur in 5% of cases. Acromegaly is a rare complication, with 5 cases reported to date. Cushing's syndrome has also been reported as a very rare associated condition. Acceleration of skeletal growth and maturation is very common even in the absence of sexual precocity.

Premature fusion of the epiphyses may result in reduced stature in spite of rapid early growth. Gynecomastia in males and parathyroid enlargement are reported as rare associations. One theory that has been proposed to explain endocrine changes in this disease is that a congenital abnormality of the hypothalamus causes overproduction of one or more releasing hormones, stimulating production by the anterior pituitary of gonadotropins, thyroid-stimulating hormone, growth hormone, and ACTH.[129]

Pain, bone deformities, and pathological fractures commonly occur. The serum calcium and phosphorus levels are normal. The alkaline phosphatase level may be elevated in some cases.

Radiologically, the monostotic form chiefly involves the long bones, with the majority of lesions in the femur and tibia.[59] The ribs and facial bones[32] are also frequently involved. The polyostotic form involves chiefly the femur, ilium, tibia, pubis, humerus, vibula, radius, scapula, and clavicle, in that order. Pathological fractures, chiefly at the femoral neck or intertrochanteric region, frequently occur.

There is usually more extensive involvement of bone at any given site in polyostotic disease. The majority of cases involve only one or a few bones. There is a high correlation between iliac and femoral involvement; if the ilium is involved, the femur is also likely to be involved, but the reverse is not true. In the long bones an expanding lesion may be seen, usually at the metaphysis. This can occur at any location, including the epiphysis before and after fusion,[88] and can involve a small portion or all of the bone (Figs. 3–92, 3–93, 3–94, 3–95). The cortex is intact, and may be thickened (Fig. 3–96). There is usually no periosteal elevated new bone formation. The lesion may be trabeculated (Fig. 3–97) or may vary from a radiolucent or cystlike area (Figs. 3–98, 3–99) to a uniform "ground glass" appearance (Fig. 3–100). Accentuation of the trabecular pattern also occurs (Fig. 3–101). The inner cortical margin may show scalloping or undulated thickening (Fig. 3–102). The entire bone may be widened (Figs. 3–103, 3–104). Marked deformities, particularly the "shepherd's crook" deformity of the proximal femur, occur in polyostotic disease. The tibia is commonly involved (Fig. 3–105). Patho-

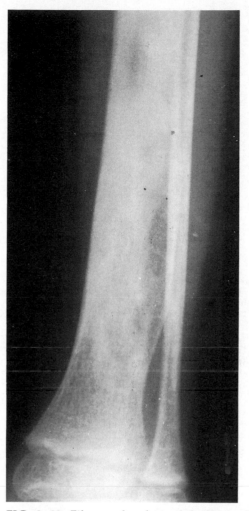

FIG. 3–92. Fibrous dysplasia (left tibia)—female, age 5 years. Note expansile lesion along the lateral margin of the tibia, cortical thickening and sclerotic changes. (Picture taken in 1951)

logical fractures sometimes occur (Fig. 3–106), and then there may be associated periosteal reaction. Pseudarthroses occur. Incomplete or pseudofractures may also be present (Figs. 3–107, 3–108, 3–109). Lesions which have been present for many years may show dense spotty or linear calcification similar to medullary bone infarction (Fig. 3–110). Sequestrum formation, or a sclerotic zone in the medullary cavity surrounded by a radiolucent area within a larger sclerotic zone, has been reported in 2 cases.

(Text continues on p. 133)

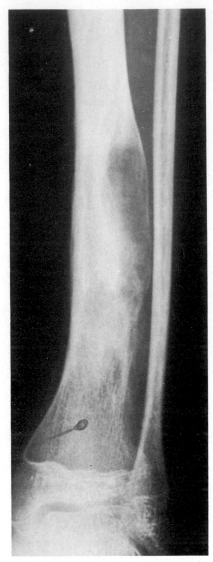

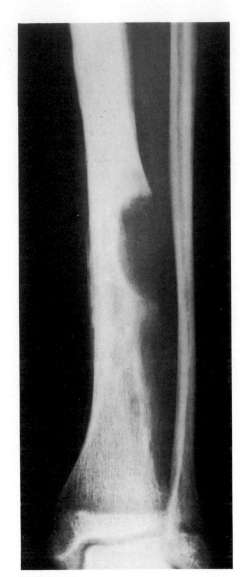

FIG. 3–93   FIG. 3–94

FIG. 3–93. Fibrous dysplasis (left tibia) — same patient as in Fig. 3–92, age 11 years. Normal growth of the left tibia has occurred, and the expansile lesion at the outer aspect of the distal tibia is again visible. There is now thinning of the cortex. Sclerosis at the proximal aspect, osteoporosis at the distal aspect, and over-constriction of the fibula may also be seen. (Picture taken in 1957)

FIG. 3–94. Fibrous dysplasia (left tibia) — same patient as in Figs. 3–92 and 3–93, age 12 years. The thinned cortical shell at the outer margin of the tibia has become so thin that it is invisible. There is now apparent scalloping of the outer margin of the lesion. Proximal sclerosis, cortical thickening and distal osteoporosis may again be noted, and a minimal amount of periosteal reaction at the medial aspect of the lesion, an unusual finding, is apparent. (Picture taken in 1958)

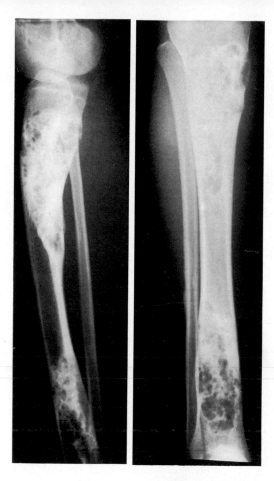

FIG. 3–95. Fibrous dysplasia (tibia). Note expansile, extensive multi-locular lesions at the proximal and distal metaphyseal areas, extending toward the diaphysis. Cortical thickening of the posterior tibial cortex is also present, and a similar lesion in the distal femur is partially visible.

FIG. 3–96. Fibrous dysplasia (proximal femur). Note cortical thickening, particularly of the medial cortex, with a localized area of greater thickening in the subtrochanteric region.

FIG. 3–97. Fibrous dysplasia (humerus). There is extensive involvement of the humerus with heavy trabeculation, cortical thickening, and expansion of the shaft of the bone in the distal humerus.

FIG. 3–97

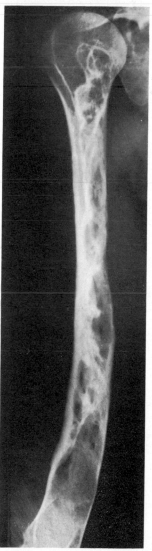

FIG. 3–96

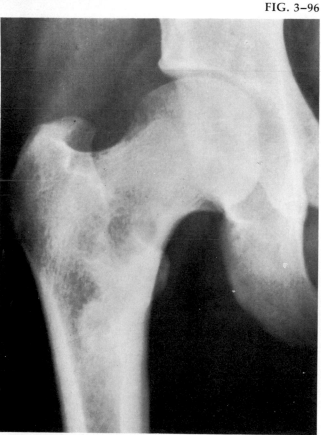

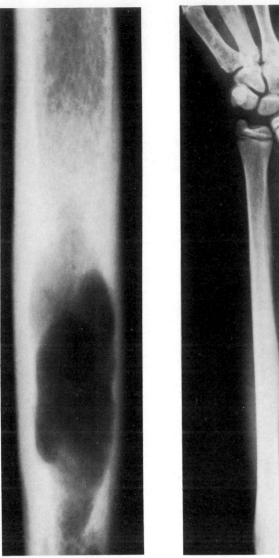

FIG. 3–99 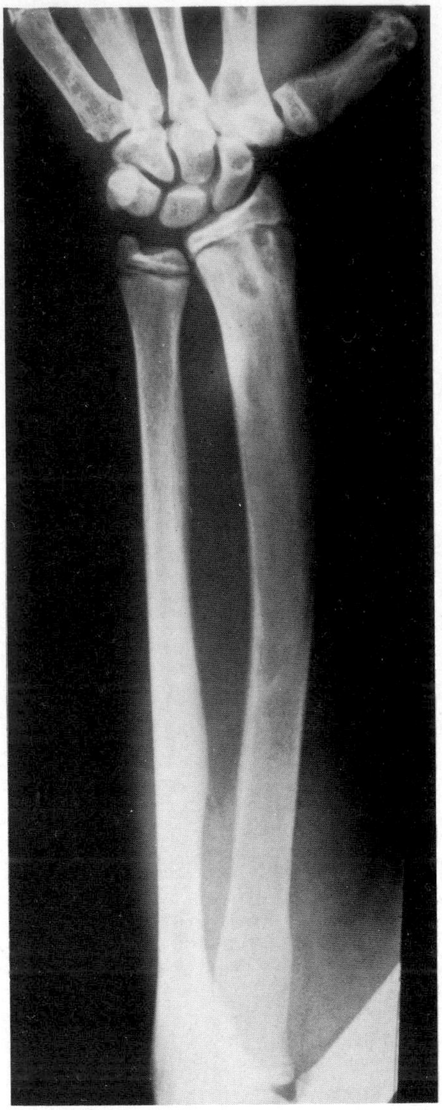   FIG. 3–98 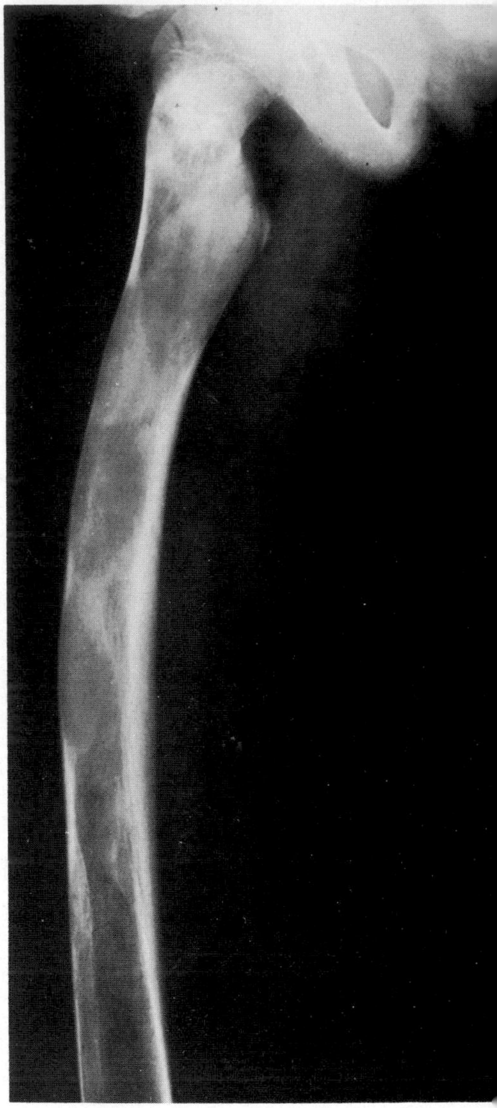   FIG. 3–100

FIG. 3–98. Fibrous dysplasia (humerus). Note the pure radiolucent area with scalloped margins in the shaft of the bone.

FIG. 3–99. Fibrous dysplasia (forearm and wrist). Note several small metaphyseal radiolucencies at the distal radius. There is expansion of the shaft of the radius, with a "ground glass" appearance and cortical thinning, and bowing of the radius. Expansion of the first and fourth metacarpals, with a "ground glass" appearance, cortical thickening of the second metacarpal, and loss of density in the fifth metacarpal, may also be seen.

FIG. 3–100. Fibrous dysplasia (femur)—female, age 12 years, with Albright's syndrome. Note uniform "ground glass" appearance with cortical thinning anteriorly, and cortical thickening posteriorly, in the midshaft. Bowing and slight underconstriction may also be seen.

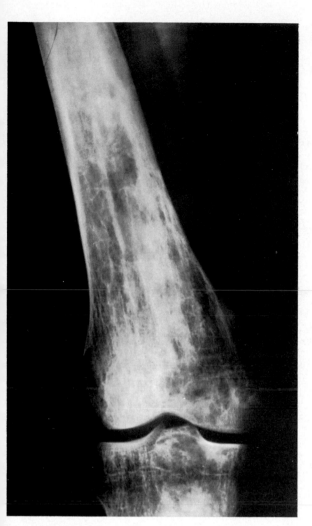

FIG. 3–101. Fibrous dysplasia (distal femur). Note accentuation of the bony trabecular pattern in the distal femur and proximal tibia, a "ground glass" appearance in the femoral shaft, and longitudinal streaks showing increased density in the shaft of the femur.

FIG. 3–102. Fibrous dysplasia (legs)—bilateral involvement—Albright's syndrome. Both tibiae show an undulating margin of the endosteum, with thickening. Scalloping may be noted in the middle of the left shaft, and patches with a "ground glass" appearance are visible in both tibiae and fibulae, with expanded areas in both fibulae.

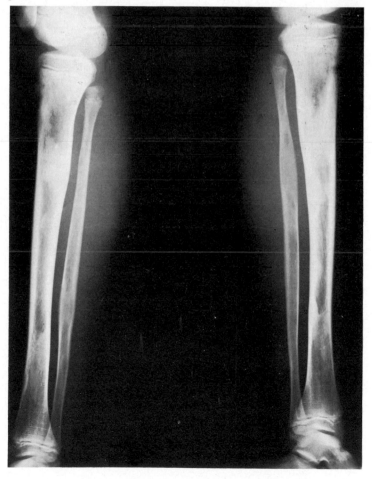

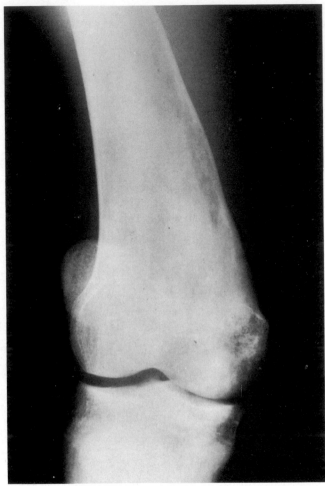

FIG. 3–103. Fibrous dysplasia (distal femur). Note widening of the bone, with an "Erlenmeyer flask" deformity of the distal femur, and increased bone density in the distal femur and proximal tibia.

FIG. 3–104. Fibrous dysplasia (foot). Note marked widening of several metatarsals and phalanges, with a uniformly dense sclerotic appearance. The bones have assumed rectangular and fusiform shapes.

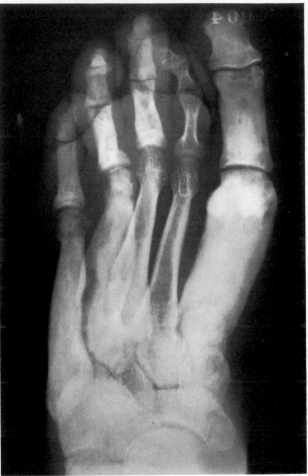

FIG. 3–106. Fibrous dysplasia—Albright's syndrome—pathological fracture of the femoral neck. The proximal femoral shaft is expanded and has a "ground glass" appearance.

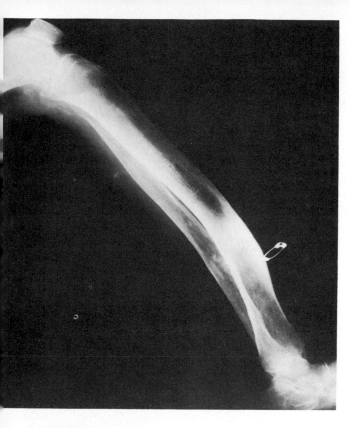

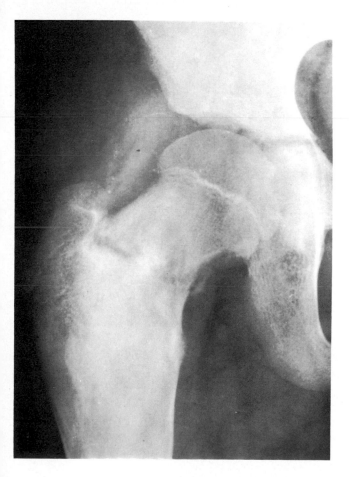

FIG. 3–105. Fibrous dysplasia (tibia). Anterior bowing of the tibia may be noted. Also note widening of the contour of both tibia and fibula, with cortical thinning, loss of bone density, and accentuation of the trabecular pattern.

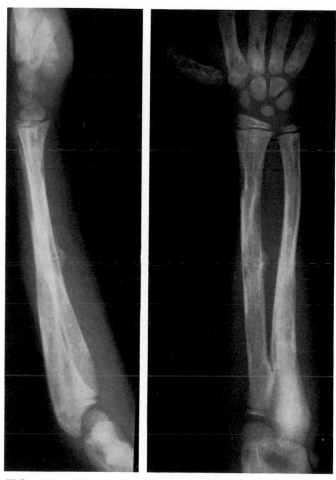

FIG. 3–107. Fibrous dysplasia (left forearm) — male, age 8 years. Characteristic changes of fibrous dysplasia are present, with expansion of bone and "ground glass" appearance. An incomplete fracture with callus formation in the midradial shaft may be seen.

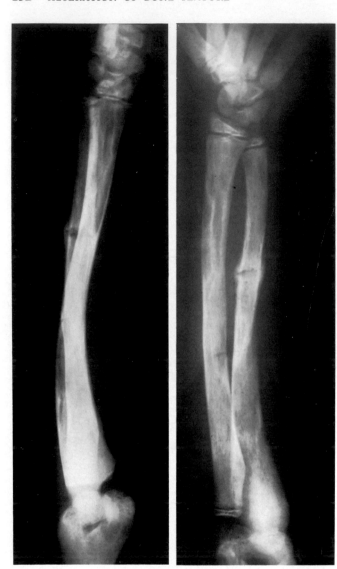

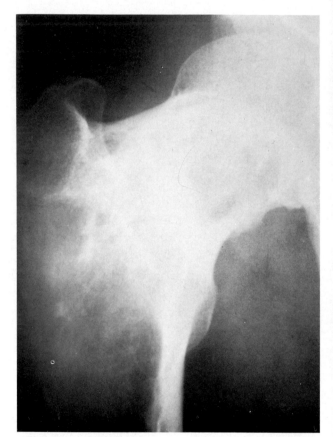

FIG. 3–108. Fibrous dysplasia (left forearm) — male, age 12 years; follow-up on patient in Fig. 3–109, after 4 years. Incomplete fracture of the midradial shaft is still apparent, but there is no callus formation at this site. Another fracture, with callus formation at the distal third shaft of the ulna, can be seen. The changes characteristic of fibrous dysplasia, including bone expansion and the "ground glass" appearance, may also be seen, as on previous film.

FIG. 3–109. Fibrous dysplasia (hip). An incomplete or pseudofracture of the femoral neck within an area of fibrous dysplasia is noted.

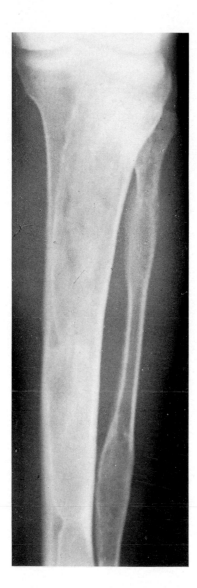

FIG. 3–110. Fibrous dysplasia (leg). An extensive medullary "ground glass" area is seen bounded by a long curvilinear calcific line, reminiscent of a bone infarction.

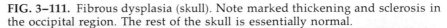

FIG. 3–111. Fibrous dysplasia (skull). Note marked thickening and sclerosis in the occipital region. The rest of the skull is essentially normal.

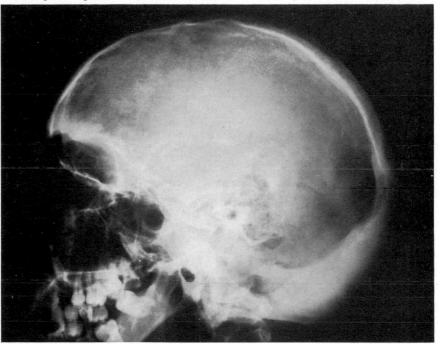

In the skull, a marked sclerotic reaction involving the base and calvarium may be present (Fig. 3–111). Expansion of the outer table may be seen with little involvement of the inner table (Figs. 3–112, 3–113). Multiple, irregular, radiolucent areas in the calvarium may also be present. The sphenoid particularly may be sclerotic and thickened, resulting in displacement of intracerebral vessels. The base of the skull may show similar changes (Fig. 3–114). The paranasal sinuses can be obliterated. Expansion, with a sclerotic or "ground glass" appearance involving the inferior or lateral walls of the antrum, is usually seen. The mandible may be involved with an expansile lesion, sometimes trabeculated, usually in the ramus. Differential diagnosis would include adamantinoma and dentigerous cyst.

Skull changes may be differentiated from those of:

1. Paget's disease (sinuses involved)
2. Meningioma
3. Metastases
4. Thalassemia (ethmoid sinuses not involved)
5. Sickle-cell anemia (sinuses not involved)
6. Other anemias (sinuses not involved)
7. Hyperparathyroidism
8. Acromegaly
9. Leontiasis ossea
10. Localized lesions
11. Cranial hemihypertrophy
12. Craniometaphyseal dysplasia

(Text continues on p. 136)

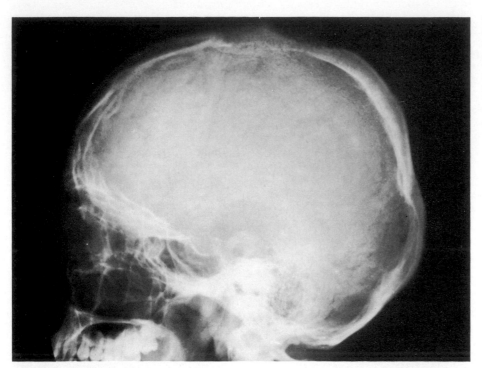

FIG. 3–112. Fibrous dysplasia (skull) — male, age 16 years. There is localized thickening of the parietal bone, with expansion of the outer table and minimal involvement of the inner table. The matrix of this lesion is bony, helping in the differentiation from other processes.

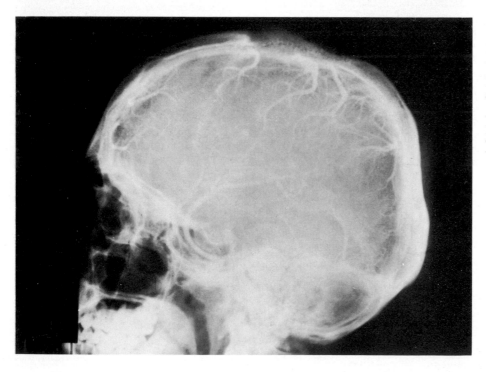

FIG. 3–113. Fibrous dysplasia — arteriogram of skull of patient in Fig. 3–112. There is no new or excess vascularity in the lesional area, and no downward displacement of the dural sinus. This arteriogram demonstrates an avascular area of fibrous dysplasia without an intracranial component. (Courtesy of Dr. Edward Salinas)

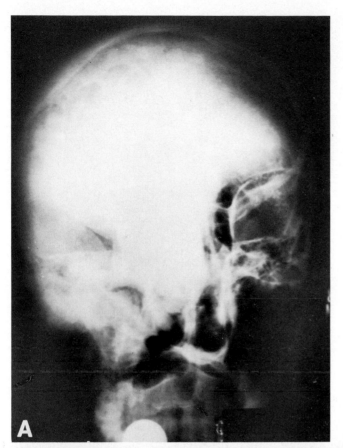

FIG. 3–114. Fibrous dysplasia (skull). **A.** Anteroposterior view shows very extensive bone sclerosis involving the calvarium and the paranasal sinuses on the right as well as the orbits. **B.** Lateral view shows extensive sclerosis involving the frontal sinuses, the calvarium, the sphenoid, and the base of the skull. Basilar invagination is also present.

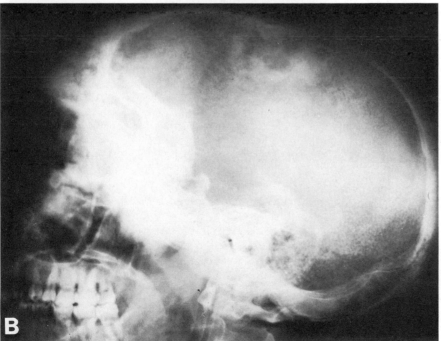

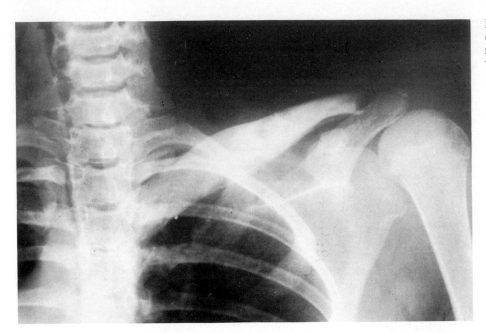

FIG. 3–115. Fibrous dysplasia (clavicle). There is an almost homogeneous sclerosis of the clavicle with fusiform expansion.

It must be kept in mind that sinusitis may supervene and cause changes that may be mistaken for primary involvement. The clavicle may also be involved (Fig. 3–115).

The ribs may show expansile lesions with a "ground glass" or "soap bubble" appearance (Fig. 3–116). The most common cause of an expansile focal rib lesion is fibrous dysplasia. The individual lesions of monostotic and polyostotic fibrous dysplasia tend to differ somewhat.[59] In monostotic disease, the lesions have a well-defined margin which is often sclerotic. The predominant location is the medulla, with the cortex involved as a result of expansion. The lesion is often trabeculated, and bowing is not a prominent feature. Polyostotic disease typically shows fusiform expansion of bone gradually merging with normal areas. A larger segment of bone is usually affected, and gross bending of bone is characteristic as in the "shepherd's crook" deformity of the proximal femora. A "ground glass" appearance is more likely to be found. Pathological fractures are more common.

Malignant degeneration[108] occurs only very rarely in association with fibrous dysplasia. To date, only 16 cases have been reported. The majority were osteosarcoma, with fibrosarcoma, giant-cell tumor, and chondrosarcoma also occurring. Malignant change occurred both in the absence of, and following, radiation therapy.

The lesions tend to stabilize with adulthood. Occasionally, an area may enlarge rapidly after having stabilized. This may represent cystification rather than sarcomatous change.[65]

A newly described entity termed *osteofibrous dysplasia*[27] has been reported by Campanacci. This syndrome chiefly involves the tibia and fibula. The onset is in the first years of life. *Radiologically*, bone enlargement, intracortical osteolytic lesions, thinning or disappearance of the external cortex, sclerosis, and narrowing of the medullary canal may be seen. There may be bowing of bone, pathological fracture, or pseudoarthrosis. Some lesions are reported to heal spontaneously. This condition is claimed to be distinct from fibrous dysplasia.

GAUCHER'S DISEASE

Gaucher's disease[4,49,112] is a hereditary metabolic disturbance characterized by accumulation of cerebrosides (kerasin and phrenosin) in reticuloendothelial cells. The gene is believed to be transmitted as an autosomal recessive. Typical Gaucher's cells are large, 20μ to 80μ in diameter, located in the reticuloendothelial system, and containing cerebrosides. These cells are not found in the peripheral blood without special staining techniques.

The majority of adult cases reported have been in

Jews, although all other ethnic groups can be involved. Both sexes are equally affected.

Clinically, there are two forms of the disease. One-third of patients present with the *acute infantile form,* with predominantly central nervous system and respiratory pathology. Hepatosplenomegaly causes abdominal protrusion. The patient rapidly deteriorates and death usually occurs within a year. Macroscopic bone changes are not found in this form, nor are anemia, purpura, or skin pigmentation. There is a close resemblance to Niemann–Pick disease, but a cherry-red macular spot is not present.

The chronic form has a variable severity and variable age of onset. Cases have been first seen in patients between the ages of 40 to 79 years; however, 50% to 60% of patients have initial symptoms in the first decade of life.

Vague symptoms of weakness and fatigue are present, as well as weight loss. Abdominal discomfort is present. Splenomegaly is almost always present. Hepatomegaly occurs in about 75% of cases. Pulmonary involvement is rare. Anemia and pancytopenia may be present, with hemorrhagic diathesis. There may be a yellow or patchy brown skin pigmentation.

The demonstration of Gaucher's cells in the spleen or sternal marrow establishes the diagnosis. The serum acid phosphatase may be elevated, and the activity of leukocyte and β-glucosidase is greatly decreased.[12] Other laboratory values are usually within normal limits.

Bone symptomatology includes pain and limitation of motion, usually of the hips and knees. Vascular infarction can lead to acute symptoms mimicking osteomyelitis. Pathological fractures occur in 5% to 10% of childhood cases, but rarely in adults. The hips, ribs, and vertebrae are usually involved, and there is prompt callus formation and early union. Very mild or asymptomatic forms of this disease exist.[12]

Radiographically, the most frequent sites of skeletal involvement are the femora, spine, hips, shoulders, tubular bones, and pelvis. The lower extremities are more often involved than the upper. The bone that is the key to the diagnosis of this disease is the femur, with ischemic necrosis of the proximal end, and an "Erlenmeyer flask" deformity at the distal end. The ribs, sternum, scapulae, and mandible may also be involved, as well as any other bone in the body. In multiosseous disease, the skull may be involved.

The basic processes of bone involvement are similar to those of other diseases in which there is proliferation of bone marrow or infiltration of bone marrow with abnormal cells. There may be a loss of bone density, simulating osteoporosis. The spine is often involved. Bone trabeculae are resorbed and the remaining trabeculae stand out in relief to give a picture of an altered or coarsened bony trabecular pattern. Reparative processes may reinforce this picture and lead to bone sclerosis.

Patchy destructive areas may occur in a geographic or "moth-eaten" pattern, giving a picture very similar to that of osteolytic metastases (Fig. 3–117). The margination of these lesions varies. Local-

FIG. 3–116. Fibrous dysplasia (ribs). The ribs show multiple expansile lesions with a "ground glass" appearance.

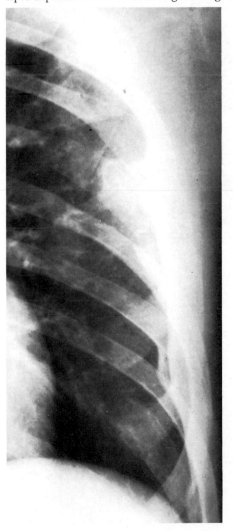

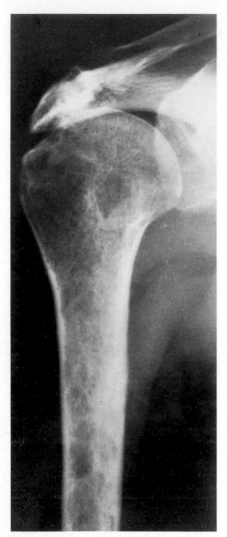

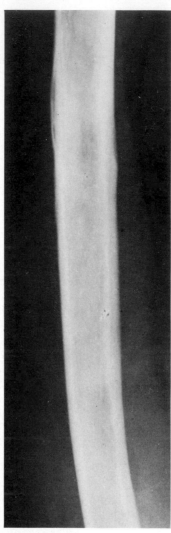

FIG. 3–117. Gaucher's disease (upper humerus)—female, age 77 years. There are patchy destructive osteolytic areas involving the humerus. (From Am J Roentgen 110:800–807, 1970)

FIG. 3–118. Gaucher's disease (femoral shaft). "Splitting" of the cortex into several layers is noted, as well as cortical thickening. (From Am J Roentgen 110: 800–807, 1970)

FIG. 3–117   FIG. 3–118

ized or patchy scleroses may also occur, some of which are due to bone infarction. Ischemic necrosis is one of the most common findings.

The lesions can progress to pathologic fractures, usually in the proximal femora, vertebrae, and ribs. Fractures may occur in areas of normal-appearing bone as well as in altered bone. Ordinarily there are prompt callus formation and early union, although hip fractures may fail to unite. Narrowing of the joint space may occur, although cartilage is not primarily affected. The intervertebral spaces may be narrowed, apparently due to herniation of the nucleus pulposus into a vertebral body.

The cortex is involved in various ways. Destruction of the cortex may be seen, secondary to either infarction or involvement with the primary disease process. Thinning of the cortex is not uncommon. Scalloping of the inner margin of the cortex may also be seen. The cortex may be "split," with an inner layer of new bone formation which does not fuse with the cortex, giving a "bone-within-a-bone" appearance (Fig. 3–118). This finding is also commonly seen in sickle-cell anemia. The cortex may also be thickened (Fig. 3–119).

The periosteum may react with a solid or lacelike type of periosteal new bone formation, particularly in areas of ischemic necrosis, where buttressing is commonly present, owing to subperiosteal hemorrhage or pathologic fracture.

There may be expansion of bone, particularly

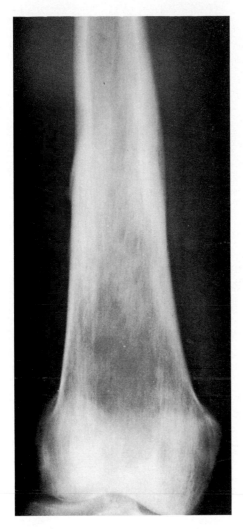

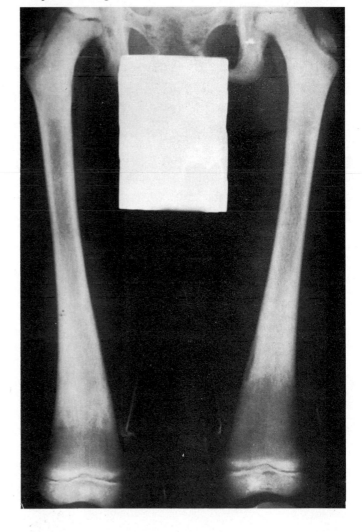

FIG. 3–119. Gaucher's disease (distal femur) — tomogram. Thickening of the cortex can be seen, as well as patchy areas of medullary sclerosis. (From Am J Roentgen 110:800–807, 1970)

FIG. 3–120. Gaucher's disease (femora). Note lack of tubulation of the distal femora, or "Erlenmeyer flask" deformity. Loss of bone density of the distal femora and bone sclerosis at the distal shafts are present. A bony destructive lesion at the distal medial left femoral shaft, its long axis parallel to that of the bone, may also be seen. (Courtesy of Dr. Harvey White, Children's Memorial Hospital, Chicago, IL)

with the characteristic "Erlenmeyer flask" (Fig. 3–120) type of deformity, or expansile trabeculated lesions of the long bones.

The skull is rarely involved, but may show a mottled destruction of the calvarium. Destructive lesions and cystlike areas in the mandible are seen at times. The spine ordinarily shows a generalized loss of bone density. One or more of the vertebrae may collapse, giving a wedgelike or waferlike deformity (Fig. 3–121). Sclerosis of the collapsed vertebra may occur, or the collapsed vertebra may appear osteopenic. In addition, herniation of the nucleus pulposus into a vertebral body may occur, although the appearance of the spine with multiple biconcavities is not seen (Fig. 3–122). Osteosclerotic changes in the spine may also be present. Gibbus formation is rare. Subchondral radiolucent lines may be present, owing to demineralization (Fig. 3–123).

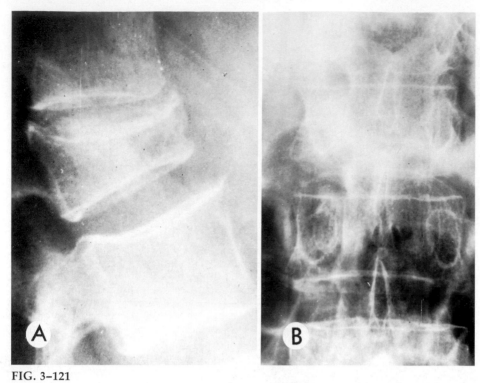

FIG. 3–121

FIG. 3–122

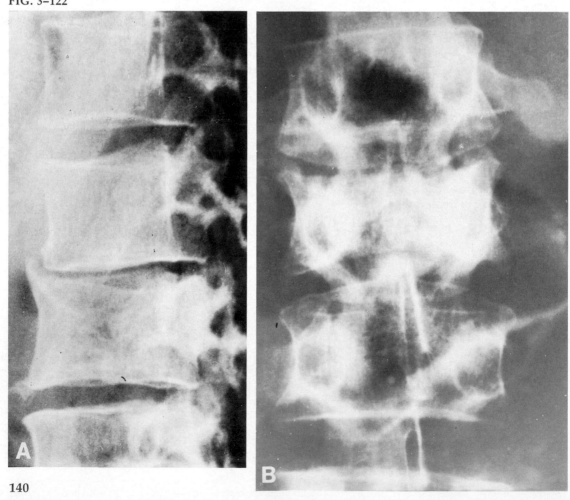

FIG. 3–121. Gaucher's disease (lumbar spine). **A.** Lateral view showing wedgelike collapse of the first lumbar vertebral body. The intervertebral spaces are preserved. **B.** Frontal view showing loss of bone density, which is generalized in the spine. (From Greenfield GB: Bone changes in chronic adult Gaucher's disease. Am J Roentgen 110:800–807, 1970)

FIG. 3–122. Gaucher's disease (lumbar spine). **A.** Lateral view. The intervertebral space between L-1 and L-2 is narrowed, with herniation into the body of L-2. Sclerosis and osteophyte formation are noted. **B.** Frontal view shows sclerosis of the second vertebral body. (From Greenfield GB: Bone changes in chronic adult Gaucher's disease. Am J Roentgen 100:800–807, 1970)

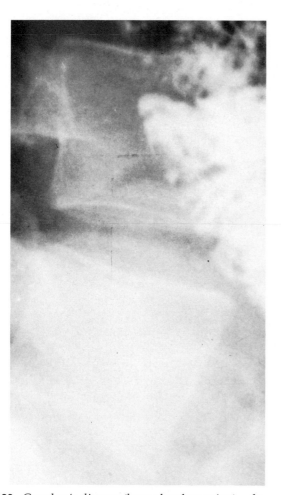

FIG. 3–123. Gaucher's disease (lower lumbar spine)—detail showing loss of bone density with radiolucent lines paralleling the end-plates. (From Greenfield GB: Bone changes in chronic adult Gaucher's disease. Am J Roentgen 110:800–807, 1970)

One area that has not been emphasized in the recent literature is that of the sarcroiliac joints. Marginal sclerosis may be present, and actual obliteration of the sacroiliac joint can be seen (Figs. 3–124, 3–125).

The pelvis may show an alteration of bone texture and also sclerotic changes. The symphysis pubis can also be involved (Fig. 3–126). The most consistent finding in this area is ischemic necrosis of the femoral head (Figs. 3–127, 3–128).

The latter can occur in a wide variety of conditions. The process is basically similar in most etiologies. Initially, there is subchondral sclerosis extending to a large sclerotic area involving the major portion of the femoral head, the so-called "snow-cap" appearance. Structural failure then occurs, initiated by a radiolucent, crescentic subchondral fracture line, at the point of greatest stress. Collapse of the femoral head then follows, with irregularity of contour and patchy sclerotic and radiolucent areas.[4] The cartilage is not primarily involved in Gaucher's disease; however, there can be secondary osteoarthritic changes. Periosteal buttressing along the inferior aspect of the involved site may also be present. Collapse and deformity of subchondral bone in other areas may also occur.

The distal femora show the most characteristic aspects of bone involvement in this disease. There is usually bilateral involvement, although unilateral involvement may occur. The medial border of the distal femur is at first straightened and later assumes a convex contour. Expansion then proceeds to the typical "Erlenmeyer flask" deformity (Fig. 3–129). Expanding lesions may also be seen in the mandible, with a cystlike expansile lesion surrounding the teeth, but not involving the periodontal membrane. The ribs may show expansile lesions, as well as destructive areas with pathologic fractures.

The shoulders also may be involved, with ischemic necrosis of the humeral head similar to femoral head involvement. The phalanges may rarely be involved late in the disease process, with coarsened trabeculation. The spleen is usually enlarged and may be calcified. The liver may be enlarged to a lesser degree. Gallstones have also been reported.

(Text continues on p. 144)

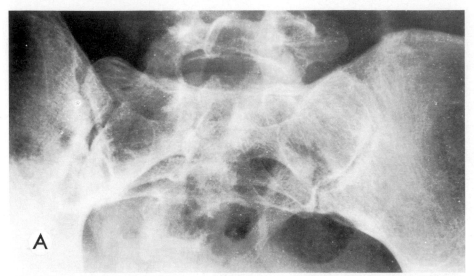

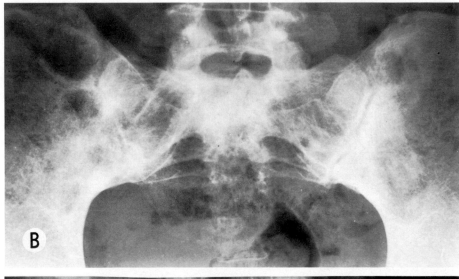

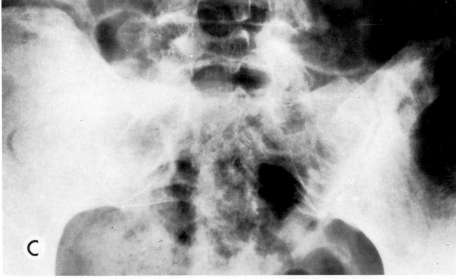

FIG. 3–124. Gaucher's disease (sarcoiliac joints) — female, age 27 years, showing progressive sarcoiliac joint involvement. **A.** Initial roentgenogram taken in 1965, showing both sacroiliac joints to be intact. **B.** Roentgenogram taken in 1967, showing partial obliteration of the right sacroiliac joint, with two distinct areas of sclerosis. The left sacroiliac joint is intact. **C.** Roentgenogram taken in 1970, showing complete obliteration of the right sacroiliac joint. The left sacroiliac joint remains intact. (From Greenfield GB: Bone changes in chronic adult Gaucher's disease. Am J Roentgen 110:800–807, 1970)

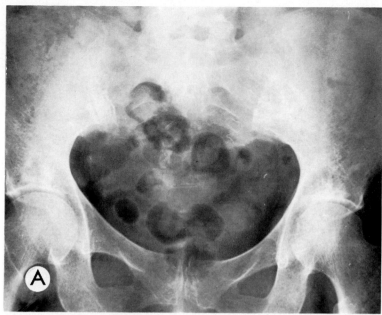

FIG. 3–125. Gaucher's disease (sarcoiliac joint). **A.** Roentgenogram taken in 1961 shows partial obliteration of the left sacroiliac joint with surrounding sclerotic change. The right sacroiliac joint is intact. **B.** Roentgenogram taken in 1966 showing no significant change. Obliteration of the left sacroiliac joint is present, with an intact right sacroiliac joint remaining. (From Greenfield GB: Bone changes in chronic adult Gaucher's disease. Am J Roentgen 110:800–807, 1970)

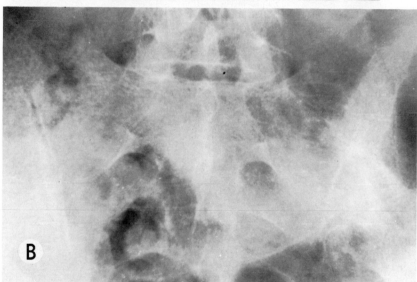

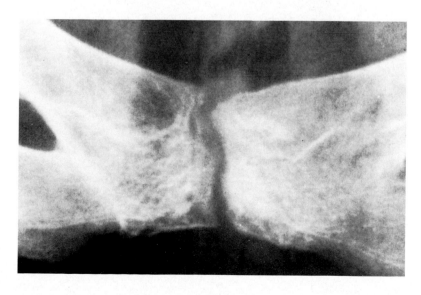

FIG. 3–126. Gaucher's disease (symphysis pubis). There is involvement of the symphysis pubis with sclerosis and destruction; however, the symphysis is not fused.

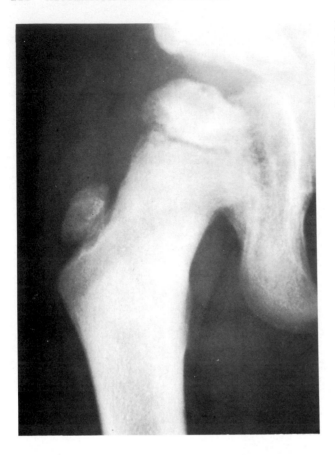

FIG. 3–127. Gaucher's disease (hip). There is ischemic necrosis of the femoral capital epiphysis with collapse, sclerosis, and cyst formation. This picture is indistinguishable from others showing ischemic necrosis of the femoral head from other causes. The joint space is slightly widened. (Courtesy of Dr. Harvey White, Children's Memorial Hospital, Chicago, IL)

FIG. 3–128. Gaucher's disease (hip). There is ischemic necrosis and structural collapse of the femoral head, similar in appearance to ischemic necrosis from other causes. The joint space is preserved. Crumbling of the head and small ill-defined areas of rarefaction in the intertrochanteric region may be seen, as well as thickening or buttressing of the femoral neck at its medial aspect. Mild sclerosis in the ischium is also apparent.

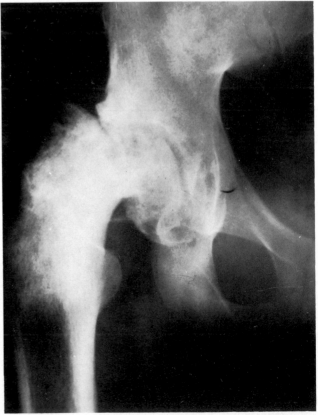

NIEMANN–PICK DISEASE

Niemann–Pick disease is an inherited abnormality of sphingomyelin metabolism in which histiocytes accumulate phospholipids (sphingomyelin and cholesterol). These vacuolated cells are deposited chiefly in the liver, spleen, and lymph nodes. Thirty to 50% of cases reported have been in Jews.

Clinically, the disease has been classified into four groups[50] (Table 3–1).

In Group A, or the "classical" form, the onset of symptoms is usually within the first 6 months of life. Central nervous system and pulmonary involvement, as well as jaundice, are present. The liver and spleen are markedly enlarged. Brown pigmentation of the skin and cutaneous xanthomas are present. In 25% of patients, a cherry-red macular spot is seen, similar to that seen in Tay–Sachs disease. Anemia is present. Vacuoles in the cytoplasm of circulating lymphocytes and monocytes may be seen. The disease is usually rapidly fatal. In other forms, cases have been reported in which death occurred as late as the 19th year. Group B is compatible with long-term survival. Sphingomyelinase de-

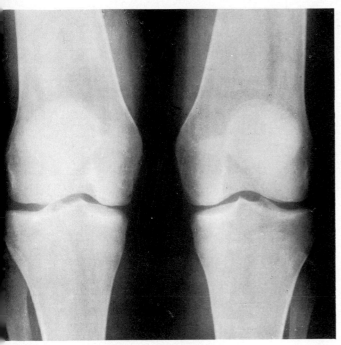

FIG. 3–129. Gaucher's disease (knees). Lack of constriction or modeling of the distal femora and proximal tibiae is noted. This is the so-called "Erlenmeyer flask" deformity.

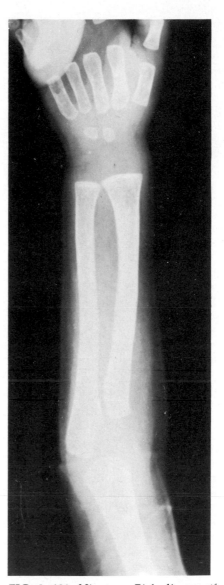

FIG. 3–130. Niemann-Pick disease (forearm and wrist). Widening of the medullary cavity, coarsening of the trabecular pattern, thinning of the cortex, lack of tubulation, particularly of the metacarpals, and loss of bone density may be seen. There is also some nonspecific transverse metaphyseal striping.

TABLE 3–1. Classification of Niemann-Pick Disease*

	Hepatospleno-megaly	Onset of CNS Symptoms	Age at Death (Years)
Group A ("Classical")	Marked	Early infancy	1–2
Group B (Heavy visceral involvement, normal CNS)	Marked	None seen	
Group C (Moderate course)	Moderate	Late infancy	3–7
Group D (Nova Scotian form)	Moderate	Early to middle childhood	12–20

* Modified from Lachman R, Crocker A, Schulman J, Strand R: Radiology 108:659–664, 1973

ficiency in groups A and B has been recently reported.

Radiologically, changes in the bones can be seen in a significant number of cases. The characteristic pattern is widening of the medullary cavity, coarsening of the trabecular pattern, thinning of the cortex, failure of tubulation, and loss of bone density (Figs. 3–130, 3–131, 3–132). Coxa valga is common. Widening of the distal femora and of the metacarpals, with thinning of the cortex, may be seen. In group B patients, progression of marrow cavity expansion has been reported, giving a picture somewhat similar to that of Gaucher's disease. Bone age is usually delayed. Skull changes have not been reported. Bilateral notch defects on the medial aspects of the proximal humeri have been described in a single patient, similar to those seen in Hurler's syndrome. A peculiar phenotype, with symptoms of white hair and diarrhea in infants, has been recorded. Punctate calcific deposits inferior to the sacrum and coccyx, and similar calcifications about the hips and feet, are findings in these patients, along with accentuation of the zones of provisional calcification of the long bones and vertebrae.

The presence of nodular interstitial infiltrations in the lungs in Niemann–Pick disease helps to differentiate it from Gaucher's disease.

GLYCOGEN STORAGE DISEASES

The glycogen storage diseases[99] comprise a group of inborn errors of metabolism as listed in Table 3–2. Either an excess amount of normal glycogen (types I, II, V, VI) or abnormal glycogen (types III, IV) infiltrates organs. Several metabolic changes, particularly hyperuricemia and gout, are associated. The most common type of glycogen storage disease is von Gierke's disease. Types I, III, IV, and VI of glycogen storage disease are associated with skeletal changes. The radiological findings in von Gierke's disease include delayed skeletal maturation, loss of bone density, gout, and miscellaneous bony changes (Fig. 3–133).

Loss of bone density, most probably due to osteoporosis, is universally present. The cortex is thinned and the trabecular pattern is sparse. In addition, widening of the shafts of metatarsals and proximal and middle phalanges may be seen, probably due to marrow hyperplasia. The frequency of the more commonly seen bony abnormalities in this condition has been compiled in a series by Miller *et al*[84] and are summarized in Table 3–3.

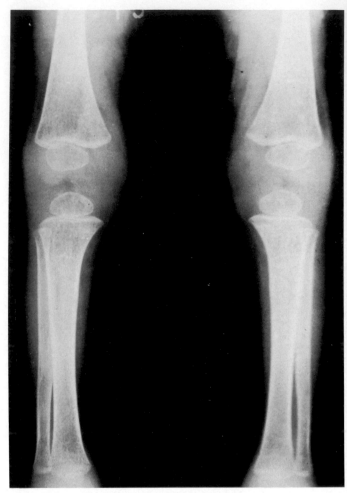

FIG. 3–131. Niemann-Pick disease (lower extremities). Accentuation of the trabecular pattern at the metaphyses and in the epiphyseal ossification centers may be noted bilaterally. There is loss of bone density, cortical thinning, and a slight lack of tubulation, although no marked "Erlenmeyer flask" deformity is present.

FIG. 3–132. Niemann-Pick disease (femora). Loss of bone density, "Erlenmeyer flask" deformities of the distal femora, patchy and sharply marginated radiolucent areas in the distal femora, and a pathological fracture of the proximal right femur are noted.

TABLE 3–2. Glycogen Storage Diseases*

Type	Enzyme Defect	Target Organ	Glycogen Structure	Eponymic Name	Suggested Clinical Name
I	Glucose 6-phosphatase	Liver, kidney, small intestine	Normal	Gierke's disease	Glucose 6-phosphatase deficiency hepato-renal glycogenosis
II	Alpha-1, 4-glucosidase (acid maltase)	Generalized; includes central nervous system, leukocytes, heart	Normal	Pompe's disease	Alpha-1, 4-glucosidase deficiency generalized glycogenosis
III	Amylo-1, 6-glucosidase (debrancher)	Liver, heart, muscle, leukocytes	Abnormal; outer chains missing or very short	Cori's disease	Debrancher deficiency limit dextrinosis
IV	Amylo-1,4–1,6-trans-glucosides (brancher)	Liver, probably other organs	Abnormal; very long inner and outer unbranched chains	Andersen's disease	Brancher deficiency amylopectinosis
V	Muscle glycogen phosphorylase	Skeletal muscle	Normal	McArdle's disease	Myophosphorylase deficiency glycogenosis
VI	Liver glycogen phosphorylase	Liver, leukocytes	Normal	Hers' disease	Hepatophosphorylase deficiency glycogenosis

Bone not affected in types II and V

(Miller JH et al[84]: Am J Roentgen 132:379–387, 1979)

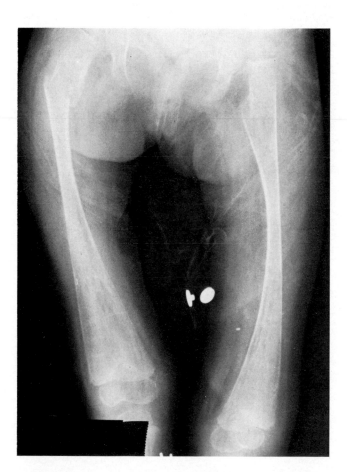

TABLE 3–3. Bone Abnormalities in Glycogen Storage Disease*

Abnormality	Disease Type			
	I	III	IV	VI
Osteopenia	20/30	3/6	0/2	5/5
Retarded maturity	18/29	4/6	1/2	2/5
Multiple growth lines:				
With osteopenia	13/30	0/6	0/2	3/5
Without osteopenia	2/30	0/6	2/2	0/5
Scalloped vertebral bodies	9/30	2/4	1/2	4/5
Multiple fractures	8/30	0/6	0/2	0/5
Prominent nutrient foramina	8/30	1/6	0/2	1/5
Overconstriction of long bones	8/30	0/6	0/2	0/5
Spiculation of the physeal plate	3/30	1/6	1/2	1/5
Subchondral erosions	2/30	0/6	0/2	0/5
Other osseous abnormalities	14/30	0/6	2/2	0/5

Note.—Ratio represents numbers of individuals with positive findings to number of individuals examined. Types II and V do not affect the skeleton.
* (Miller JH et al: Am J Roentgen 132: 379–387, 1979)

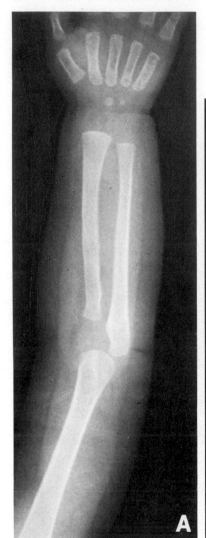

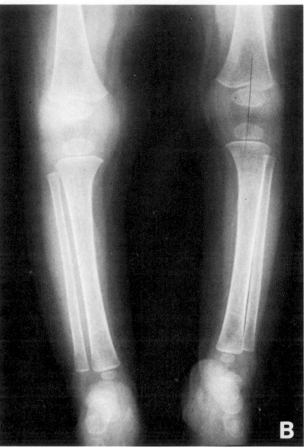

FIG. 3–133. Von Gierke's disease. **A.** Upper extremity. Osteoporosis and lack of modeling are seen. **B.** Lower extremities. Again osteoporosis is seen, with a thin but distinct cortex and lack of modeling and "Erlenmeyer flask" deformities of the distal femora, and lack of constriction of the distal tibiae.

Gout is thought to be due to depression of tubular clearance of uric acid. It has been described in patients as young as 6 years, but is more common in adolescence and early adulthood. The roentgen picture is identical to that of primary gout (Chap. 9).

Miscellaneous changes that have been described include abnormal concavity of the anterior aspects of the vertebral bodies, lumbar kyphosis, delayed union of the vertebral ring epiphyses, Schmorl's nodes, Kirner's deformity, overexpansion of the ribs and sternum, multiple growth centers for metacarpal heads, fibrous cortical defects, radioulnar joint erosions, flaring of lower ribs, multiple growth lines, and a shallow notching of the upper medial humeri, possibly due to abnormal capsule attachments from infiltration by glycogen. A similar change may be seen in Hurler's syndrome.

SARCOIDOSIS

Sarcoidosis is a generalized systemic granulomatous disease of unknown etiology, involving principally the skin, lungs, lymph nodes, and viscera.

Bone involvement occurs in about 10% or more of patients at some time during the course of the disease. A recent worldwide survey of 3676 sarcoidosis patients[94] reported bony lesions in 3%. The bone lesions have a tendency to regress. Blacks are more frequently affected than whites in the United States. Visceral lesions are usually asymptomatic. The diagnosis is usually made when a routine chest radiograph of a young, asymptomatic adult discloses bilateral hilar and right paratracheal lymphadenopathy associated with pulmonary fibrosis. Children are rarely affected.[124] Hypercalcemia,

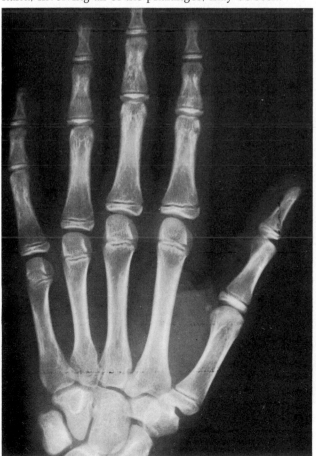

FIG. 3–134. Sarcoidosis (hand). Minimal, diffuse loss of density and accentuation of the trabecular pattern of the hand, involving all of the phalanges, may be seen.

which regresses to normal values following cortisone administration, may be present. The serum alkaline phosphatase levels and the globulin level are frequently elevated. The albumin-globulin ratio may be reversed. The osseous lesions of sarcoidosis are characteristically painless. One patient has been reported as presenting with finger pain. Bone involvement usually occurs in patients with generalized chronic disease and irreversible sarcoidosis in all systems. Bone and chronic skin lesions are often associated.[94]

Radiologically, the bones most often involved are the middle and distal phalanges of the fingers and toes; the metacarpals and metatarsals are involved less frequently. Rarely, a lytic lesion may be seen in the epiphysis of a long bone. A diffuse, coarsened trabecular pattern of long bones or of the scapula may be present less commonly. In the short tubular bones, the disease may take three forms:

1. *The diffuse form.* The contour of the bone is widened with a reticular or honeycomb structure of the spongiosa. There is loss of definition between cortex and medulla. Resorption of the terminal tuft has also been observed in rare cases[51] (Figs. 3–134, 3–135, 3–136, 3–138). Very rarely, resorption of the cortex reminiscent of hyperparathyroidism may be seen (Fig. 3–137).

2. *The circumscribed form.* "Punched-out," cystlike lesions up to 5 mm in diameter with a narrow sclerotic rim may be seen (Figs. 3–139, 3–140, 3–141), as well as small multilocular expanded areas (Fig. 3–142).

3. *The mutilating form.* The "punched-out" areas may coalesce, forming larger areas of destruction. The cortex may be destroyed. No periosteal reaction, new bone formation, or sequestration is present. The three forms may coexist (Fig. 3–143). Areas of sclerosis in the terminal phalanges may also be seen,[80] as well as small nodular densities in the medulla of the phalanges and metacarpals. Destructive changes may also rarely be found in the nasal bones, calvarium, spine, and pelvis.[11] A small number of cases have been reported as involving the spine[22] with only 4 cases to date of sarcoidosis of the cervical spine.[33] One or more vertebra may be involved. The lesions may be destructive, destructive with collapse, destructive with a sclerotic margin, or sclerotic. The bodies with or without the pedicles may be affected. If more than one vertebral body is involved, the lesions may or may not be adjacent. The disk space is usually preserved, although narrowing has been reported.[33] A paraspinal soft-tissue mass may be associated. This picture may mimic tuberculosis.

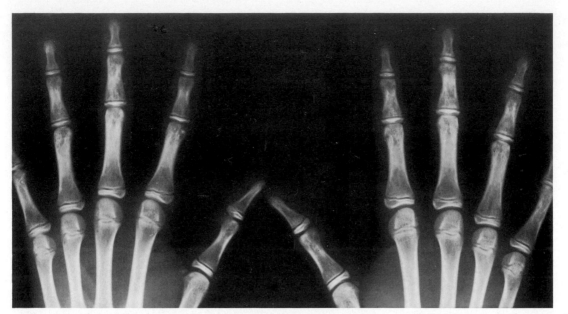

FIG. 3–135. Sarcoidosis (hands)—follow-up on patient in Fig. 3–134 after 7 months. Note progression of diffuse changes of sarcoidosis and definite, multiple, minute areas of radiolucency, with a reticular pattern, particularly in the middle phalanges and the distal aspects of the proximal phalanges.

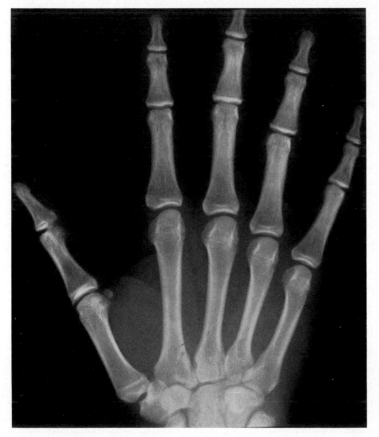

FIG. 3–136. Sarcoidosis (hand)—follow-up on patient in Fig. 3–135 after 2 years. Note complete regression of the bony lesions. The bony structure now appears entirely normal. Normal fusion of ossification centers has occurred.

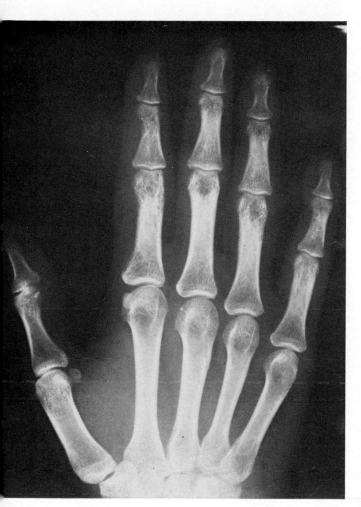

FIG. 3–137. Sarcoidosis (hand). The coarsened trabecular pattern of the digit is noted. In addition, there is loss of the cortex of the radial aspect of the proximal and middle phalanges of the index finger. This is not to be confused with hyperparathyroidism, as the bones are only sporadically involved.

FIG. 3–138. Sarcoidosis (fingers). Subcortical and periarticular cystic dissolutions frequently observed in this disorder. Bone resorption at the terminal tuft of the index finger is also noted, a rare finding. (From Greenfield GB, Escamilla CH, Schorsch HA: The hand as an indicator of generalized disease. Am J Roentgen 99:736–745, 1967)

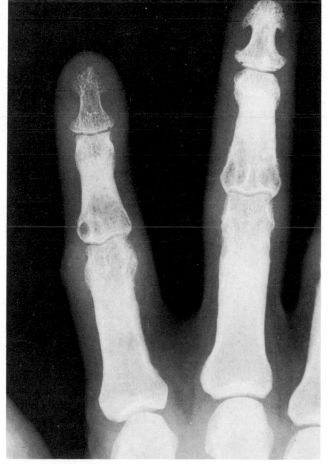

Lesions in the skull[91,125] may occur in association with, or independent of, other bony lesions. The destruction may involve both tables, and may be progressive. The lesions may be single or multiple, are characteristically small in size, and show no sclerotic reaction. Diffuse widening of the cervical spinal cord has been reported.[68] Isolated reports of disseminated osteosclerotic lesions of sarcoidosis in the pelvis, femora, vertebrae, ribs, sphenoid, and a terminal phalanx have been published.[18,75,135] Diffuse osteosclerosis is seen. These changes are rare. Osteosclerosis may be combined with osteolysis. Asymptomatic joint swellings in a child have been reported, as well as joint disease in an adult. Also reported have been patchy disseminated sclerosis-simulating metastases, pathological fracture of the elbow,[130] sarcoid arthritis of the knees with marginal destructive changes, and sarcoid arthritis of the ankle. Involvement of the large joints is very rare.

(Text continued on p. 154)

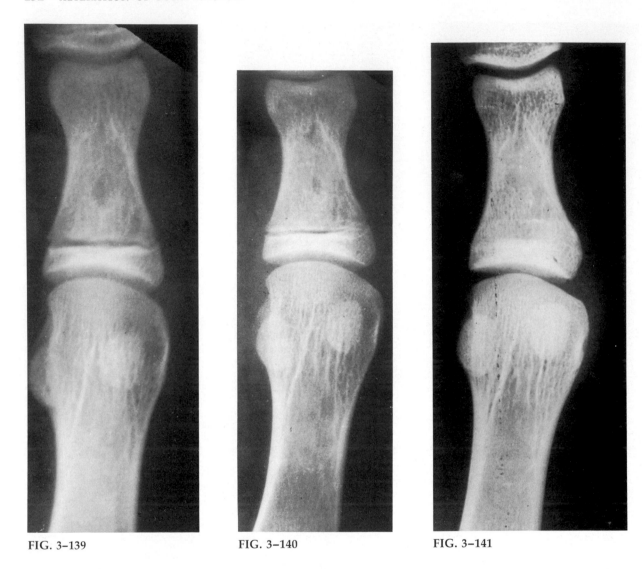

FIG. 3–139   FIG. 3–140   FIG. 3–141

FIG. 3–139. Sarcoidosis (right great toe). A 4 mm cystlike rarefaction in the shaft of the proximal phalanx is present, partially bounded by a faint sclerotic rim. Note a smaller area of radiolucency in the medial metaphyseal region.

FIG. 3–140. Sarcoidosis (right great toe)—follow-up of patient in Fig. 3–130 after 7 months. The radiolucencies have diminished considerably in size.

FIG. 3–141. Sarcoidosis (right great toe)—follow-up on patient in Figs. 3–139 and 3–140 after 2 years. There has been complete healing of the cystlike and radiolucent lesions. The epiphysis has fused normally in the interval.

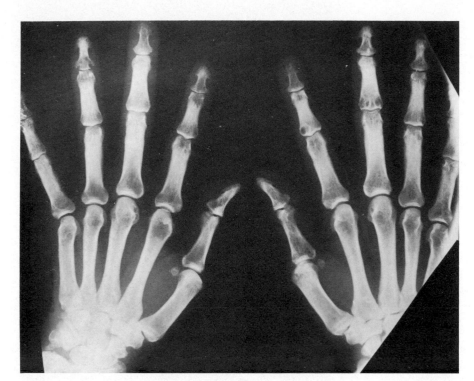

FIG. 3–142. Sarcoidosis (hands)—circumscribed form. Multiple cyst-like, punched-out radiolucencies may be seen in the mid- and distal phalanges, and in several proximal phalanges and several metacarpal heads. Cystlike radiolucencies in the carpal bones are also present. There is an expanded multilocular area at the base of the middle phalanx of the left middle finger.

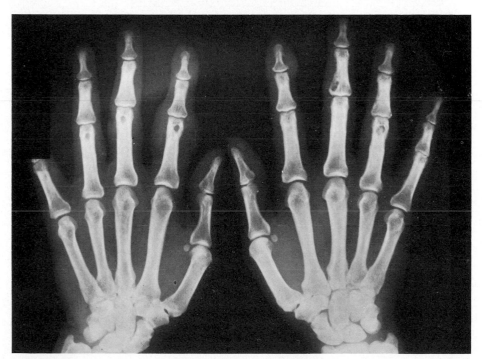

FIG. 3–143. Sarcoidosis (hands). Multiple relatively large, well-demarcated, cystlike radiolucencies at the distal aspects of several phalanges may be seen, some with associated soft-tissue swellings. Note several confluent radiolucencies in the middle phalanx of the left middle finger, causing cortical destruction. The cortex is also partially destroyed at the radial aspect of the middle phalanx of the left ring finger.

PANCREATITIS

Fat necrosis of bone marrow has been reported as occurring in association with acute, relapsing, and chronic calcific pancreatitis, and with traumatic pancreatitis and carcinoma of the head of the pancreas.[18,42,63] The serum or urine amylase levels should be elevated in the acute form.

The radiologically visible bone changes may result from:

1. Calcification and ossification in an area of intramedullary fat necrosis
2. Bone infarction as a result of vascular occlusion caused by fat necrosis

In the acute stage, multiple osteolytic destructive lesions in the long bones and short bones of the hands and feet may be present. There may be endosteal erosion and cortical destruction (Figs. 3–144, 3–145, 3–146, 3–147). Periosteal reaction rarely may be present. In later stages, there are calcified infarcts in the medullary cavity.

The epiphyses may be involved, giving a picture of aseptic necrosis, particularly in the heads of the femur or humerus. Vertebral osteonecrosis leading to collapse of the body, a myelographic defect, and neurological sequella have been reported.[3] Subcutaneous calcifications of soft tissue are also sometimes present.

RADIUM POISONING

Internal deposition of radium salts[6,7,44,78,102] is found chiefly in patients who were former radium watch dial painters prior to 1925, or those who had iatrogenic administration of radium.

The major portion is deposited in the skeletal system. Radium is metabolized in a manner similar to calcium. Long-term alpha radiation exposure causes tissue damage. The principal changes involve the bone and bone marrow. Carcinomas of the paranasal sinuses and mastoids also occur, due to the proximity of the mucosa to bone in these areas. Mandibular changes are more prevalent in patients with mixtures of radium and mesothorium.

Severe effects on the bone marrow include aplastic anemia and leukopenia. Effects on bone and cartilage are usually also present. Bone sarcomas similar to naturally occurring tumors may be induced after many years. The patients frequently present with mandibular complaints. Other "boneseeking" radionuclides, particularly radiostrontium, may induce tumor formation.

154

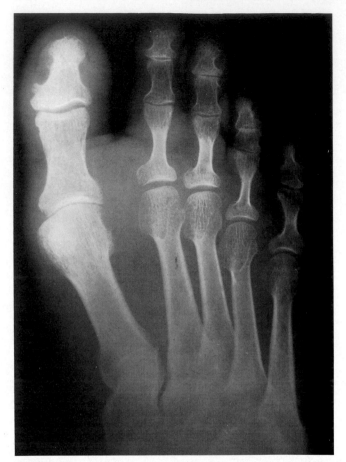

FIG. 3–144

FIG. 3–145

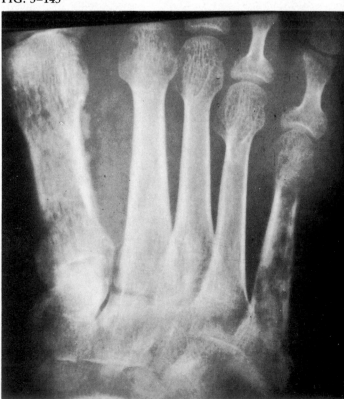

FIG. 3–144. Pancreatitis (right foot)—onset of acute stage. The bony texture and density appear essentially normal.

FIG. 3–145. Pancreatitis (right foot)—follow-up on patient in Fig. 3–144 after 3 weeks. Note extensive bone destruction involving chiefly the first and fifth metatarsals. Multiple radiolucencies, cortical destruction, and periosteal new bone formation may be seen. This area was not tender, and blood cultures were negative. This condition is the result of infarctions.

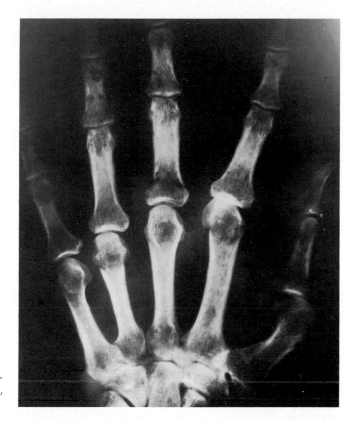

FIG. 3–146. Acute pancreatitis (hand). Note multiple infarctions and areas of radiolucency, cortical destruction, and absence of periosteal reaction.

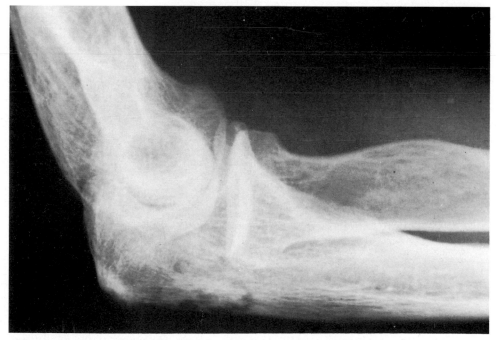

FIG. 3–147. Acute pancreatitis (left proximal ulna). Note small patchy areas of radiolucency, caused by bone infarction.

Radiologically, irregular areas of rarefaction interspersed with areas of sclerosis may be seen. These represent ischemic necrosis and fibrosis. Ischemic necrosis of the femoral and humeral heads may occur. There is involvement of the articular cartilage causing joint space narrowing and secondary osteoarthritic changes, a feature distinguishing radium poisoning from other causes of ischemic necrosis (Fig. 3–148). Pathological fractures, particularly in the vertebra, may occur. Mottled rarefactions in the skull may be seen. Sequestration is common in the mandible, associated with necrosis and infection. Bone that has been included in a radiation treatment field may develop osteoradionecrosis and pathological fractures (Fig. 3–149).

FIBROGENESIS IMPERFECTA OSSIUM[8,46]

Fibrogenesis imperfecta ossium is a rare generalized bone disorder histologically resembling osteomalacia with failure of calcification of matrix. Only 3 living cases and 2 cases from autopsy material have been described. The involved bone contains large amounts of abnormal osteoid tissue, resulting from a defect in collagen formation. Normal mature fibrils do not develop, and the osteoid tissue is not birefringent under polarized light as is normal collagen. The serum calcium and phosphate levels are usually normal, while the serum alkaline phosphatase may be elevated. No associated hematological abnormalities have been reported.

Clinically, the patients are all in late adult life. Both males and females are affected. The patients present with a rapidly progressive course of bone and joint pain, pathological fractures, and disability.

Radiologically, all bones except the skull are diffusely and symmetrically involved, with a general coarsening of the trabecular pattern and increase in bone density. Radiolucent areas may be seen between thick and fuzzy trabeculae.

The cortex is thin or absent, and the bone is not enlarged, in contrast to Paget's disease. Total diffuse involvement or defects in contour or modeling are also not likely to occur. Multiple pathological fractures may be seen, particularly in the spine, ribs, pelvis, and hips.

DIAPHYSEAL AND METAPHYSEAL INFARCTS[24,36]

Infarction of the shaft of a bone is most commonly associated with the following conditions: (1) idiopathic causes, (2) occlusive vascular disease, (3) sickle-cell anemia, (4) caisson disease, (5) infiltrative and collagen diseases, (6) infection.

Infarction is also rarely caused by pancreatitis and has been reported in association with pheochromocytoma.[9] The sites most commonly involved are the distal femur and the proximal tibia. In infants with sickle-cell anemia, dactylitis is most common. A rare case of fibrosarcoma complicating bone infarction in a caisson worker has been reported.[35]

In the initial stages, the roentgenograms show bone rarefaction followed by mottled sclerosis. The cortex may be involved and periosteal reaction may occur. This may be associated with inflammatory signs, particularly in sickle-cell dactylitis. The increased bone density is caused by a combination of the following factors:

1. Crushing of avascular necrotic debris
2. Calcific fat necrosis of marrow
3. Relative increase in density of dead bone owing to osteoporosis of surrounding viable bone
4. Bone apposition caused by revascularization and repair, and
5. Periosteal involucrum formation

Radiologically, a mature infarct appears as a densely calcified area in the medullary cavity, either with serpiginous radiopaque streaks extending from the central region (Fig. 3–150), or sharply limited by a dense sclerotic zone (Figs. 3–151, 3–152, 3–153). This must be differentiated from an enchondroma. The latter shows amorphous, spotty calcifications, is not surrounded by a sclerotic rim, and may expand the bone.

Divers also develop ischemic necrosis of bone in a significant percent,[90] especially if no modern methods of decompression are available. Both medullary bone infarcts and ischemic necrosis of the femoral and humeral heads may be seen.

ALTERATION OF BONE TEXTURE IN THE VERTEBRAL COLUMN

VERTEBRA PLANA

Vertebra plana, or Calvé's disease, is now considered to result from eosinophilic granuloma (Fig. 3–154). Some other causes of vertebral flattening are: (1) Morquio's disease (universal vertebra plana), (2) hyperphosphatasia, (3) Gaucher's disease, (4) metastases, (5) multiple myeloma, and (6) postradiotherapy in childhood.

(Text continues on p. 160)

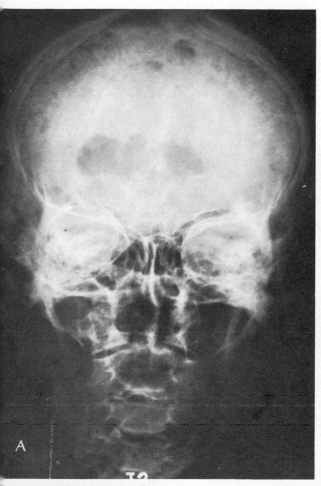

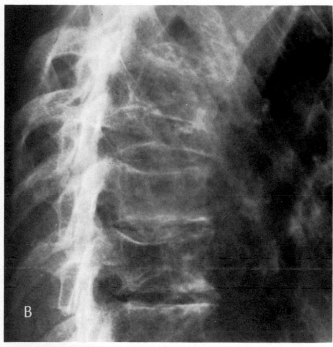

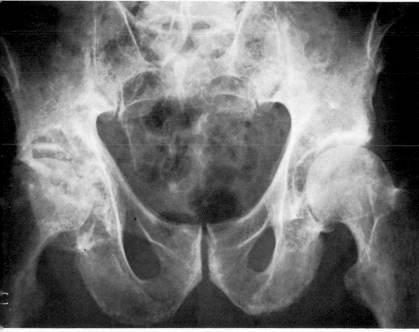

FIG. 3–148. Radium poisoning. A. Skull. Destructive and sclerotic changes of the calvarium can be seen. There has been a hemimandibulectomy for osteoradionecrosis. B. Spine. Collapse of several vertebral bodies can be seen. C. Pelvis. There is a septic necrosis of the right femoral head, with joint space narrowing medially, not at the point of stress. Acetabular cystic dissolutions, cortical thickening and periostitis may also be noted. (Courtesy of Dr. Richard Buenger, Department of Radiology, Presbyterian St. Luke's Hospital, Chicago, IL, Dr. F. Squire, Director)

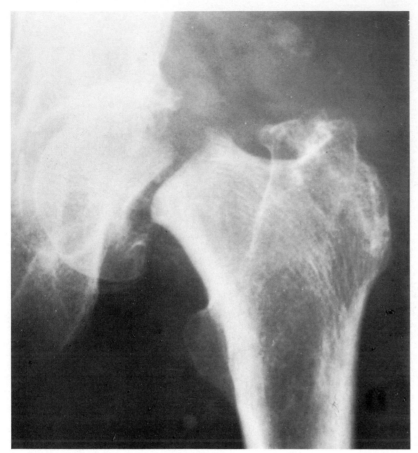

FIG. 3–149. Postradiation changes (hip) — pathological fracture 1 year following radiation therapy for carcinoma of the cervix. Note the smooth transverse fracture of the femoral neck with a well-defined edge.

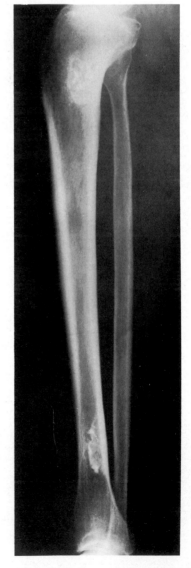

FIG. 3–150. Mature metaphyseal infarcts (tibia). Two infarcts, one at the proximal metaphyses and one near the distal metaphyseal region of the tibia, are present. Note dense area of medullary calcification and serpiginous calcific line, particularly at the distal infarction.

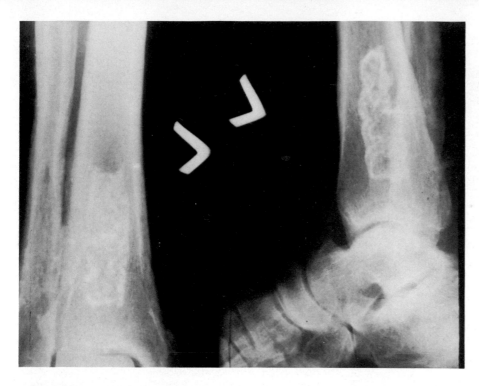

FIG. 3–151. Mature metaphyseal infarct (distal tibia). There is a well-circumscribed, dense area of calcification which is sharply delimited from normal bone. Note serpiginous anterior contour of infarct. Periosteal reaction caused by chronic stasis is incidentally noted.

FIG. 3–152. Medullary bone infarct (proximal femoral shaft). Note the long ovoid area of infarction surrounded by a thin sclerotic margin.

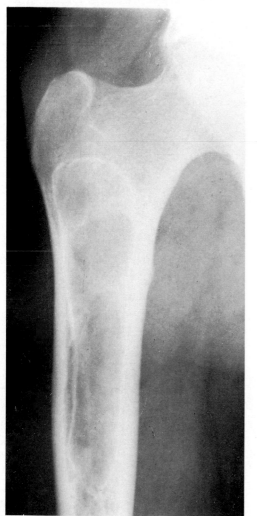

FIG. 3–153. Biopsy-proven bone infarct (distal femur) presenting as a trabeculated radiolucency in the epiphyseal-metaphyseal region.

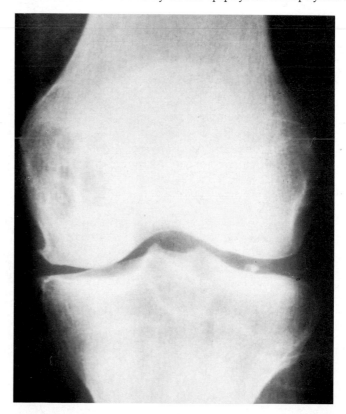

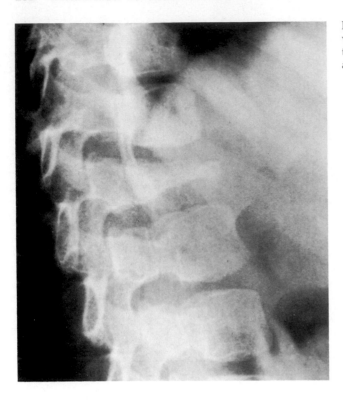

FIG. 3–154. Vertebra plana from eosinophilic granuloma, with flattening of the vertebral body and preservation of the intervertebral spaces. The rest of the vertebral bodies are not involved.

FIG. 3–155. Scheuermann's disease. Note wedging of the vertebral bodies, causing an arcuate kyphosis, and accentuation of the trabecular pattern. The vertebral end-plates are irregular. Multiple Schmorl's nodes and several developing ring epiphyses may also be seen.

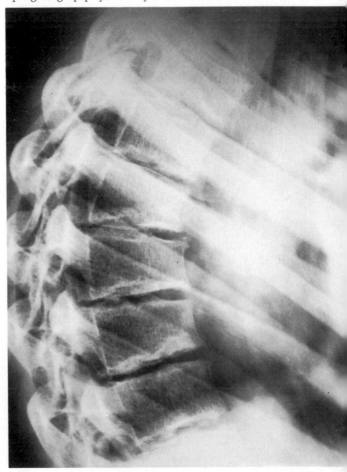

KUEMMELL–VERNEUIL DISEASE

Kuemmell–Verneuil disease[114] is a posttraumatic collapse of one or more vertebral bodies after a variable latent period. The trauma may be minor. The lower dorsal or lumbar spine is usually affected. Initially there is osteoporosis followed by osteosclerosis.

SCHEUERMANN'S DISEASE

Scheuermann's disease refers to osteochondrosis of the secondary ossification centers of the vertebral bodies. It begins at ages 12 to 16 years, is painful, and results in a rounded kyphosis that develops rapidly. The lower dorsal and upper lumbar vertebrae are initially involved, and the process may be limited to several bodies or involve the entire dorsal and lumbar spine (Fig. 3–155). Scoliosis has also been reported. The radiological features consist of wedge-shaped vertebral bodies resulting in an arcuate, rigid kyphosis. There is no gibbus formation. Narrow intervertebral disk spaces with calcifications may be present. Irregularities of the vertebral surfaces are a prominent feature. The vertebral plates are poorly formed and develop multiple herniations of the nucleus pulposus—the Schmorl's nodes. The margins of the vertebral bodies are absent, either from lack of formation, owing to osteochondrosis, or from marginal disk herniations. There is early development of marginal osteophytes. A case of spastic paraplegia secondary to a herniated disk at the apex of the thoracic kyphosis has been reported.[21]

Vertebral epiphysitis is also found in eunuchoidism, ovarian agenesis, and Wilson's disease. The presence of multiple Schmorl's nodes in young people most often indicates Scheuermann's disease, and must be differentiated from osteochondrodystrophy.

HEMANGIOMA OF THE VERTEBRAE[118]

Hemangioma of bone is a primary benign neoplasm. Two histological types have been described, the cavernous and the capillary. The cavernous hemangioma consists of large thin-walled vessels and sinuses lined by a single layer of endothelial cells in intimate relation with the bone trabeculae, causing resorption. Capillary hemangiomas consist of fine capillary hoops that radiate peripherally.

Cavernous hemangiomas are commonly found in the vertebrae. The incidence of hemangiomas of the spine in autopsy material is estimated to be over 10%. The vast majority of these are small, asymptomatic, and cannot be demonstrated on roentgenograms.

Hemangioma of the spine is usually a single lesion, most often involving the lumbar region. Occasionally two or more vertebrae may be involved. The site is usually the body of the vertebra; however, the arch may also be affected.

Clinically, most patients are asymptomatic. There may be ill-defined, intermittent pain. Compression fractures can occur, sometimes complicated by cord compression with resultant neurological symptoms. Blockage of the spinal canal may occasionally occur without a fracture, owing to chronic hemorrhage

FIG. 3–156. Hemangioma of the vertebrae in a paraplegic patient. **A.** Lateral view of the spine showing the typical striated appearance of a vertebral body hemangioma. **B.** Myelogram showing a complete block at the level of the hemangioma. An associated soft-tissue mass in the paraspinal region is also seen. At surgery this patient had meningeal thickening due to repeated small chronic hemorrhages without evidence of a large recent hemorrhage.

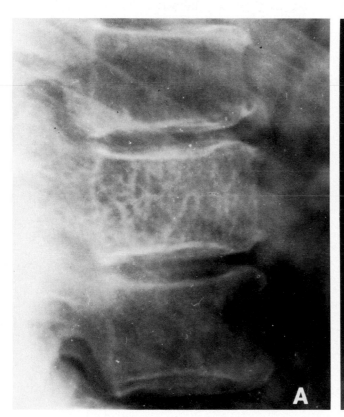

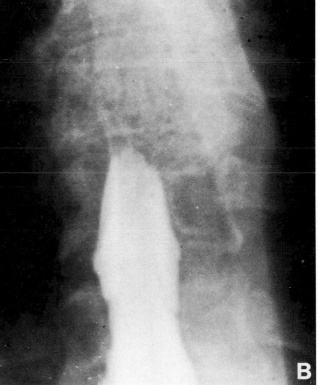

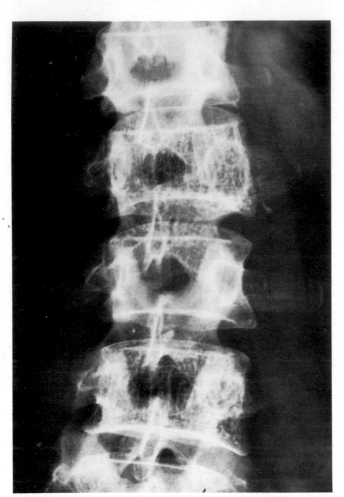

FIG. 3–157. Hemangiomas of the spine involving the second and fourth lumbar vertebrae—anteroposterior view. Note loss of bone density and accentuation of the trabecular pattern, with predominantly vertical stripes. The pedicles are involved and there is expansion of the left transverse process of L-2. The vertebral end-plates are intact.

FIG. 3–158. Hemangiomas of the vertebral bodies—lateral view of spine in Fig. 3–157. Note vertical orientation of accentuated trabeculae in the vertebral bodies, and involvement of the pedicle of L-2. There is decreased bone density of the vertebral bodies, and the anterior vertebral margins are poorly defined.

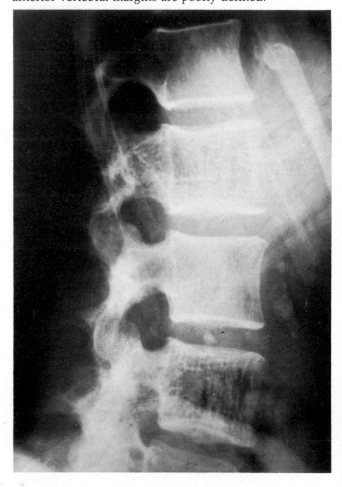

and fibrous reaction. At surgery, only dense fibrosis may be seen (Fig. 3–156).

Radiologically, there is a slight loss of density of the vertebral body. A fine reticulated texture may be seen. The roentgen hallmark is a vertically striped orientation of the bone trabeculae to give a "corduroy cloth" appearance. This is usually best seen on lateral view. The altered texture may extend into the pedicle (Figs. 3–157, 3–158). The cortical margins are usually intact. There may be posterior bulging.

The causes of spinal block associated with a primary bone disorder[89] are summarized as follows:

PRIMARY BONE DISORDERS THAT MAY LEAD TO SPINAL BLOCK[89]

Vertebral hemangioma
Fibrous dysplasia
Paget's disease
Fracture
Osteomyelitis
Chondrosarcoma
Other primary neoplasms
Klippel–Feil syndrome
Achondroplasia
Spinal stenosis

REFERENCES

1. Aegerter E, Kirkpatrick J A Orthopedic diseases, 3d ed. Philadelphia, W B Saunders, 1968

2. Agarwal K N, Dhar, N, Bhardwaj O P: Roentgenolgic changes in iron-deficiency anemia. Am J Roentgen 110:635–637, 1970

3. Allen B L, Jinkins W J: Vertebral osteonecrosis associated with pancreatitis in a child. A case report. J Bone Joint Surg 60 A:985 987, 1978

4. Amstutz H C, Carey E J: Skeletal manifestations and treatment of Gaucher's disease. Review of 20 cases. J Bone Joint Surg 48–A:670–701, 1966

5. Anderson J T, Dehner L P: Osteolytic form of Paget's disease. Differential diagnosis and pathogenesis. J Bone Joint Surg 58–A:994–1000, 1976

6. Ardran G M, Kemp F H: Radium piosoning. Two case reports. Brit J Radiol 31:605–610. 1958

7. Aub J C, Evans R D, Hempelman L H, Martland H S: Late effects of internally deposited radioactive material in man. Medicine 31:221–329, 1952

8. Baker S L, Dent C E, Friedman, M, Watson L: Fibrogenesis imperfecta osseum. J Bone Joint Surg 48–B:804–825, 1966

9. Barton C J, Cockshott W P: Bone changes in hemoglobin SC disease. Am J Roentgen 88:523–532, 1962

10. Becker M H et al: Roentgenographic manifestations of pyruvate kinase deficiency hemolytic anemia. Am J Roentgen 113:491–498, 1971

11. Becker M H, Redisch W, Messina E J: Bone and microcirculatory changes in a child with benign pheochromocytoma. Radiology 88:487–490, 1967

12. Beutler E: Gaucher's disease in an asymptomatic 72-year-old. JAMA 237:2529, 1977

13. Bhate D V et al: Paget's disease and primary hyperparathyroidism. Skel Rad 4:115–118, 1979

14. Bjarnason D F, Forrester D M, Swezey R L: Destructive arthritis of the large joints. A rare manifestation of sarcoidosis. J Bone Joint Surg 55–A:618–622, 1973

15. Bloch S, Movson I J, Seedat Y K: Unusual skeletal manifestations in a case of sarcoidosis. Clin Radiol 19:226–228, 1968

16. Bohrer S P: Acute long bone diaphyseal infarcts in sickle-cell disease. Brit J Radiol 43:685–697, 1970

17. Bohrer S P: Fracture complicating bone infarcts and/or osteomyelitis in sickle-cell disease. Clin Radiol 22:83–88, 1971

18. Bonakdarpour A, Levy W, Aegerter E E: Osteosclerotic changes in sarcoidosis. Am J Roentgen 113:646–649, 1971

19. Boswell S H, Baylin G J: Metastatic fat necrosis and lytic bone lesions in a patient with painless acute pancreatitis. Radiology 106:85–86, 1973

20. Bowerman J W, Altman J, Hughes J L, Zadek R E: Pseudomalignant lesions in Paget's disease of bone. Am J Roentgen 124:57–61, 1975

21. Bradford D S, Garcia A: Neurological complications in Scheuermann's disease. A case report and review of the literature. J Bone Joint Surg 51–A(3):567–572, 1969

22. Brodey P A, Pripstein S, Strange G, Kohout N D: Vertebral sarcoidosis: A case report and review of the literature. Am J Roentgen 126:900–902, 1976

23. Brown H P, LaRocca H, Wickstrom J K: Paget's disease of the atlas and axis. J Bone Joint Surg 53–A:1441–1444, 1971

24. Bullough P G, Kambolis C P, Marcove R C, Jaffe H L: Bone infarctions not associated with caisson disease. J Bone Joint Surg 47–A:477–491, 1965

25. Burgener F A, Perry P E: Pitfalls in the radiographic diagnosis of Paget's disease of the pelvis. Skel Rad 2:231–238, 1978

26. Caffey J, Silverman F N: Pediatric X-ray Diagnosis, 5th ed. Chicago, Year Book Publishers, 1967

27. Campanacci M: Osteofibrous dyaplasia of long bones: A new clinical entity. Ital J Orthop Traumatol 2:221–237, August 1976

28. Cassady J R, Berdon W E, Baker D H: The "typical" spine changes of sickle-cell anemia in a patient with thalassemia major (Cooley's anemia). Radiology 89:1065–1068, 1967

29. Cecil R L, Loeb R F: A Textbook of Medicine, 10th ed. Philadelphia, W B Saunders, 1959

30. Chung S M K, Ralston E L: Necrosis of the femoral head associated with sickle-cell anemia and its genetic variants. J Bone Joint Surg 51–A:33–58, 1969

31. Cockshott P W: Dactylitis and growth disorders. Brit J Radiol 3619–26, 1963

32. Cornelius E A, McClendon J L: Cherubism—hereditary fibrous dysplasia of the jaws. Roentgenographic features. Am J Roentgen 106:136–143, 1969

33. Cutler S S, Sankaran G: Vertebral sarcoidosis. JAMA 240:557–558, 1978

34. Dines D M, Canale V L, Arnold W D: Fractures in thalassemia. J Bone Joint Surg 58–A 662–670, 1976

35. Dorfman H D, Norman A, Wolff H: Fibrosarcoma complicating bone infarction in a caisson worker. A case report. J Bone Joint Surg 48–A:528–532, 1966

36. Edeiken J, Hodes P J, Libshitz H I, Weller M H: Bone ischemia. Radiol Clin N Amer 5:515–529, 1967

37. Engh C A, Hughes J L, Abrams R C, Bowerman J W: Osteomyelitis in the patient with sickle-cell disease. Diagnosis and management. J Bone Joint Surg 53–A:1–15, 1971

38. Feldman F, Seaman W B: The neurologic complications of Paget's disease in the cervical spine. Am J Roentgen 105:375–382, 1969

39. Fellows K E, Rosenthal A: Extracardiac roentgenographic abnormalities in cyanotic congenital heart disease. Am J Roentgen 114:371–379, 1972

40. Friedrich M, Gerstenberg E, Cochanek M, Rost A: An analysis of the radiological appearance of osteoblastic metastases and osteitis deformans (Paget's disease). Fortschr Roentgenstr 125:404–413 1976

41. Gelpi A P, Perrine R P: Sickle-cell disease and trait in white populations. JAMA 224:605–608, 1973

42. Gerle R D, Walker L A, Arnold J L, Weens H S: Osseous changes in chronic pancreatitis. Radiology 85:330–337, 1965

43. Gibson M J, Middlemiss J H: Fibrous dysplasia of bone. Brit J Radiol 44(517):1–13, 1971

44. Glasser O, Quimby, E H, Taylor L S, Weatherwax J L: Physical Foundations of Radiology, 2nd ed. New York, Paul B Hoeber, 1952

45. Godine E, Capesius P, Kemp F: Acroosteosclerosis in the course of sarcoidosis. J Radiol Electrol 58:115–118, 1977

46. Golde D, Greipp P, Sanzenbacher L, Gralnick H R: Hematological abnormalities in fibrogenesis imperfecta ossium. J Bone Joint Surg 53–A:365–370, 1971

47. Goldman A B, Bullough P, Kammerman S, Ambos M: Osteitis deformans of the hip joint. Am J Roentgen 128:601–606, 1977

48. Graham J, Harris W H: Paget's disease involving the hip joint. J Bone Joint Surg 53–B:650–659, 1971

49. Greenfield G B: Bone changes in chronic adult Gaucher's disease. Am J Roentgen 110:800–807, 1970

50. Greenfield G B Miscellaneous diseases related to the hematologic system. Seminars in Roent 9:241–249, 1974

51. Greenfield G B, Escamilla C H, Schorsch H A: The hand as an indicator of generalized disease. Am J Roentgen 99:736–745, 1967

52. Greenspan A, Norman A, Sterling A P: Precocious onset of Paget's disease: A report of 3 cases and review of the literature. J Canad Assn of Rad 28:69–72, 1977

53. Grundy M: Fractures of the femur in Paget's disease of bone. J Bone Joint Surg 52–B:252–263, 1970

54. Grundy M, Patton J T: Hand in Paget's disease. Brit J Radiol 42:748–752, 1969

55. Grunebaum M: The roentgenographic findings in the acute neuronopathic form of Niemann–Pick disease. Brit J Roent 49:1018–1022, 1976

56. Guyer P B, Debury K C: The hip joint in Paget's disease (Paget's coxopathy). Brit J Radiol 51:574–578, 1978

57. Harper H A: Review of Physiological Chemistry, 11th ed. Los Altos, C A, Lange Medical Publications, 1967

58. Hasterlik R J, Miller C E, Finkel A J: Radiographic development of skeletal lesions in man many years after acquisition of radium burden. Radiology 93:599–604, 1969

59. Henry A: Monostotic fibrous dysplasia. J Bone Joint Surg 51–B:300–306, 1969

60. Hill M C, Oh K, Bowerman J W, Siegelman S S, James A E: Abnormal epiphyses in the sickling disorders. Am J Roentgen 124:34–43, 1975

61. Hsia Y D: Inborn Errors of Metabolism. Part I: Clinical Aspects, 2nd ed. Chicago, Year Book Publishers, 1966

62. Hutter R V P, Foote F W, Frazell E. L, Francis, K C: Giant-cell tumors complicating Paget's disease of bone. Cancer 16:1044–1056, 1963

63. Immelman E J, Bank S, Krige H, Marks I N: Roentgenological and clinical features of intramedullary fat necrosis in bones in acute and chronic pancreatitis. Am J Med 36:96–105, January 1964

64. Jacobs P: Osteolytic Paget's disease. Clin Rad 25:137–144, 1974

65. Jaffe H L: Tumors and Tumorous Conditions of the Bones and Joints. Philadelphia, Lea & Febiger, 1958

66. Kadir S, Kalisher L Schiller A L: Extramedullary hematopoiesis in Paget's disease of bone. Am J Roentgen 129:493–495, 1977

67. Karpathios R et al: The hand-foot syndrome in sickle-cell β-thalassemia disease. JAMA 238:1540–1541, 1977

68. Kirks D R, Newton T H: Sarcoidosis: A rare cause of spinal cord widening. Radiology 102:643, 1972

69. Korsten J, Grossman H, Winchester P H, Canale V C: Extramedullary hematopoiesis in patients with thalassemia anemia. Radiology 95:257–264, 1970

70. Kulowski J: Gaucher's disease in bone. Am J Roentgen 63:840–850, 1950

71. Lachman R, Crocker A, Schulman J, Strand R: Radiological findings in Neimann–Pick disease. Radiology 108:659–664, 1973

72. Leichtman D A, Bigongiari L R, Wicks J D: The incidence and significance of tibiotalar slant in sickle-cell anemia. Skel Rad 3:99–101, 1978

73. Levin B: Gaucher's disease: Clinical and roentgenologic manifestations. Am J Roentgen 85:685–696, 1961

74. Lin J P, Goodkin R, Chase N E, Kricheff II: The angiographic features of fibrous dysplasia of the skull. Radiology 92:1275–1280, 1969

75. Lin S R et al: Unusual osteosclerotic changes in sarcoidosis simulating osteoblastic metastases. Radiology 106:311–312, 1973

76. Littman M S, Kirsh I, Keane A T: Radium-induced malignant tumors of the mastoid and paranasal sinuses. Am J Roentgen 131:773–785, 1978

77. Looney W B: Late effects (25 to 40 years) of the early medical and industrial use of radioactive materials. Their relation to the more accurate establishment of maximum permissible amounts of radioactive elements in the body. J Bone Joint Surg 37–A:1169–1187, 1955; 38–A:175–218, 1956; 38–A:392–406, 1956

78. Looney W B, Hasterlik R J, Brues A M, Skirmont E: Clinical investigation of chronic effects of radium salts administered therapeutically (1915–1931). Am J Roentgen 73:1006–1037, 1955

79. Mandell G, Kricun M E: Exaggerated anterior vertebral notching. Radiology 131:367–369, 1979

80. McBrine G S, Fisher M S: Acrosclerosis in sarcoidosis. Radiology 115:279–281, 1975

81. Meschan I, Farrer-Meschan R M F: Roentgen Signs in Clinical Practice, Vol 1. Philadelphia, W B Saunders, 1966

82. Meyers P H, Roy M, Nice C M: Differential Diagnosis of Cardiovascular Disease by X-ray. New York, Hoeber Medical Division (Harper & Row), 1966

83. Middlemiss J H, Raper A B: Skeletal changes in the hemoglobinopathies. J Bone Joint Surg 48–B:693–702, 1966

84. Miller J H, Stanley P, Gates G F: Radiography of glycogen storage diseases. Am J Roentgen 132:379–387, 1979

85. Moseley J E: Bone Changes in Hematologic Disorders (Roentgen Aspects). New York, Grune & Stratton, 1963

86. Moseley J E: The paleopathologic riddle of "symmetrical osteoporosis." Am J Roentgen 95:135–142, 1965

87. Myers H S, Cremin B J, Beighton P, Sacks S: Chronic Gaucher's disease: Radiological findings in 17 South African cases. Brit J Radiol 48:465–469, 1975

88. Nixon G W, Condon V R: Epiphyseal involvement in polyostotic fibrous dysplasia. A report of 2 cases. Radiology 106:167–170, 1973

89. O'Carroll M P, Witcombe J B: Primary disorders of bone with "spinal block." Clin Rad 30:299–306, 1979

90. Ohta Y, Matsunaga H: Bone lesions in divers. J Bone Joint Surg 56–B:3–16, 1974

91. Olsen T G: Sarcoidosis of the skull. Radiology 80:232–234, 1963

92. Pavlica P et al: Osteosclerosis in the phalanges in sarcoidosis. J Radiol Electrol 58:603–604, 1977

93. Petasnick J P: Tomography of the temporal bone in Paget's disease. Am J Roentgen 105:838–843, 1969

94. Pierson D J, Willett S: Sarcoidosis presenting with finger pain. JAMA 239:2023–2024, 1978

95. Porat S, Brezis M, Kopolovic J: *Salmonella typhi* osteomyelitis long after a fracture. J Bone Joint Surg 59–A:687–689, 1977

96. Poser V H, Gabriel–Jurgens P: Bone and joint changes due to compressed air in divers and caisson workers. Fortschr Roentgenstr 126:156–160, 1970

97. Powell J W, Weens H S, Wenger N K: The skull roentgenogram in iron-deficiency anemia and in secondary polycythemia. Am J Roentgen 95:143–147, 1965

98. Pratt A D, Felson B, Wiot J F, Paige M: Sequestrum formation in fibrous dysplasia. Am J Roentgen 106:162–165, 1969

99. Preger L et al: Roentgenographc skeletal changes in the glycogen storage diseases. Am J Roentgen 107:840–847, 1969

100. Price C H G: Myeloma occurring with Paget's disease of bone. Skel Rad 1:15–20, 1976

101. Price C H G, Goldie W: Paget's sarcoma of bone. J Bone Joint Surg, 51–B:205–224, 1969

102. Public Health Service: Radiological Health Handbook, rev ed. U.S. Department of Health, Education, and Welfare, September 1960

103. Ratcliff R G, Wolf M D: Avascular necrosis of the femoral head associated with sickle-cell trait (AS hemoglobin). Ann Intern Med 57:299–304, 1962

104. Reimann F et al: Behaviour of the sella turcica in juveniles with severe iron deficiency. Fortschr Roentgenstr 129:598–604, 1978

105. Reynolds J: A reevaluation of the "fish-vertebra" sign in sickle-cell hemoglobinopathy. Am J Roentgen 97:693–707, 1966

106. Reynolds J: Radiologic manifestations of sickle-cell hemoglobinopathy. JAMA 238:247–250, 1977

107. Reynolds J, Pritchard J A, Ludders D, Mason R A: Roentgenographic and clinical appraisal of sickle-cell β-thalassemia disease. Am J Roentgen 118:378–400, 1973

108. Riddell D M: Malignant change in fibrous dysplasia. J Bone Joint Surg 46–B:251–255, 1964

109. Rohlfing B M: Vertebral end-plate depression. Report of 2 patients without hemoglobinopathy. Am J Roentgen 128:599–600, 1977

110. Rosenbaum H D, Hanson D J: Geographic variation in the prevalence of Paget's disease of bone. Radiology 92:959–963, 1969

111. Ross P, Logan W: Roentgen findings in extramedullary hematopoiesis. Am J Roentgen 106:604–613, 1969

112. Rourke J A, Heslin D J: Gaucher's disease. Roentgenologic bone changes over 20–year interval. Am J Roentgen 94:621–630, 1965

113. Schajowicz F, Slullite I: Giant-cell tumor associated with Paget's disease of bone. J Bone Joint Surg 48–A:1340–1349, 1966

114. Schinz H R, Baensch W E, Fridl E, Uehlinger E: Roentgen Diagnostics. New York, Grune & Stratton, 1952

115. Seaman W B: The roentgen appearance of early Paget's disease. Am J Roentgen 66:587–594, 1951

116. Sebes J I, Diggs L W: Radiographic changes of the skull in sickle-cell anemia. Am J Roentgen 132:373–377, 1979

117. Shaub M S, Rosen R, Boswell W, Gordonson J: Tibiotalar slant: A new observation in sickle-cell anemia. Radiology 117:551–552, 1975

118. Sherman R S, Wilner D: Roentgen diagnosis of hemangioma of bone. Am J Roentgen 66:587–594, 1951

119. Silverstein M N, Kelly P J: Osteoarticular manifestations of Gaucher's disease. Am J Med Sci 253:569–577, 1967

120. Steinberg M H, Dreiling B J, Morrison R S, Necheles T F: Mild sickle-cell disease. Clinical and laboratory studies. JAMA 224:317–321, 1973

121. Stump M S, Spock A, Grossman H: Vertebral sarcoidosis in adolescents. Radiology 121:153–155, 1976

122. Tchang S, Tyrrell M J, Bharadwai B: Skeletal change in cyanotic heart disease simulating Cooley's anemia: Report of a case with regression of bony changes following palliative cardiac surgery. J Canad Assn Rad 24:275–280, 1973

123. Teplick G J, Haskin M E, Schimert A P: Roentgenologic Diagnosis: A Complement in Radiology to the Beeson and McDermott Textbook of Medicine. Philadelphia, W B Saunders, 1967

124. Toomey F, Bautista A: Rare manifestations of sarcoidosis in children. Radiology 94:569–574, 1970

125. Turner O A, Weiss S R: Sarcoidosis of the skull: Report of a case. Am J Roentgen 105:322–325, 1969

126. Uehlinger E, Wurm K: Sarcoidosis of the skeleton. Review of the literature and case report. Fortschr Roentgenstr 125:111–122, 1976

127. Valderma J A F, Mathews J M: The hemophilic pseudotumour or hemophilic subperiosteal hematoma. J Bone Joint Surg 47–B:256–265, 1965

128. Vogelsang H, Stöppler L, Thiede G: Fibröse Dysplasie des Schädels. Fortschr Roentgenstr 128:253–257, 1978

129. Warrick C K: Some aspects of polyostotic fibrous dysplasia. Possible hypothesis to account for the associated endocrinological changes. Clin Radiol 24:125–138, 1973

130. Watson R C, Cahen I: Pathological fracture in long bone sarcoidosis. Report of a case. J Bone Joint Surg 55–A:613–617, 1973

131. Westerman M P, Greenfield G B, Wong, P W K: "Fish vertebrae," homocystinurea, and sickle-cell anemia. JAMA 230:261–262, 1974

132. Williams W J, Beutler E, Ersley A J, Rundles R W: Hematology, 2nd ed. New York, McGraw–Hill, 1977

133. Winchester P H, Cerwin R, Dische R, Canale V: Hemosiderin-laden lymph nodes: An unusual roentgenographic manifestation of homozygous thalassemia. Am J Roentgen 118:222–226, 1973

134. Worral V T, Butera V: Sickle-cell dactylitis. J Bone Joint Surg 58–A:1161–1163, 1976

135. Young D A, Laman M L: Radiodense skeletal lesions in Boeck's sarcoid. Am J Roentgen 114:553–558, 1972

136. Zadek R E, Milgram J W: Progression of Paget's disease in the tibia. J Bone Joint Surg 58–A:876–878, 1977

137. Ziter F M H: Central vertebral end-plate depression in chronic renal disease. Report of 2 cases. Am J Roentgen 132:809–811, 1979

The end of a tubular bone is composed of a complex of component parts, definitions of which have been adapted from Rubin* as follows:

1. The epiphysis is a cap of bone that is covered by articular cartilage and serves to protect the growth plate from the stress of joint action. It contributes little to the growth in length of a long bone. The epiphysis grows in two directions, forming the scaffold for the bony epiphysis and replenishing the articular cartilage. Its growth is largely hemispheric. Failure of normal epiphyseal growth leads to failure of development of the ossification center, as well as of articular cartilage.

2. The growth plate or physis is the area in which both horizontal and vertical growth occurs. Cartilaginous growth is the major factor of growth in tubular bones. Bone growth is a substitution phenomenon after cartilage growth. The transverse diameter is increased by appositional growth, and the vertical dimension by interstitial growth.

3. The metaphysis is the zone of transformation of cartilage into bone. It is the area between the growth plate and the diaphysis in which active bone absorption occurs. The normal tendency is toward a progressive reduction in shaft caliber. The metaphysis is shaped like a funnel. The primary and secondary spongiosa are absorbed due to osteoclasis and vascular mesenchyme. This serves to reduce the transverse diameter of the shaft.

HISTOLOGY OF THE EPIPHYSEAL CARTILAGE PLATE

The basic process of enchondral bone formation is proliferation and degeneration of hyaline cartilage, which is eroded by capillaries and osteocytes and replaced by bone (Fig. 4–1). There are zones of resting cartilage, proliferating cartilage, degenerating cartilage, and provisional calcification. The proliferating chondrocytes line up in columns perpendicular to the growth plate, as opposed to the irregular distribution found in the resting zone. Proceeding toward the metaphysis, the cells become vacuolated and hypertrophic, and degenerate. The regional matrix becomes calcified. In the presence of sufficient serum concentrations of calcium and phosphorus, the cartilage bands between the columns of cells become calcified. This is the zone of provisional calcification, situated between hyaline cartilage and the primary spongiosa. Ordinarily, this is only several cartilage cells thick.

Blood vessels and connective tissue invade the cartilage, destroy the vacuolated cells, form communicative canals, and lyse the septa. Those connective tissue cells that touch the cartilage matrix turn into osteoblasts. A new tissue (osteoid) that can be calcified is laid down. Under physiological conditions, calcification of osteoid may lag, owing to a local shortage of mineral. Upon calcification, this tissue becomes the zone of primary spongiosa.

HISTOLOGY OF THE METAPHYSIS

Two zones are present in the metaphysis—the primary and the secondary spongiosa. The primary spongiosa grows by osteoblastic activity, extending into the zone of provisional calcification. This is the mechanism of lengthening of bone. Bone resorption by osteoclasts takes place at the free trabecular ends, giving a relatively constant thickness to the spongiosa. In addition, osteoclasts are present about the periphery of the metaphysis in the "ossification groove," causing a reduction of the transverse diameter of the bone. This concept has been challenged by Whalen et al with the claim that osteocytic osteolysis is the major mechanism of shaft diameter reduction.[120]

The secondary spongiosa is a layer of remodeled trabeculae blending with the cancellous bone of the marrow cavity. Remodeling takes place by a complex process. At the periphery the cancellous bone forms compacta through the lack of resorption at the free ends. The transverse diameter is further reduced in this zone so that the metaphysis blends with the diaphysis.

* From Rubin P: Dynamic Classification of Bone Dysplasias. Chicago, Year Book Publishers, 1964

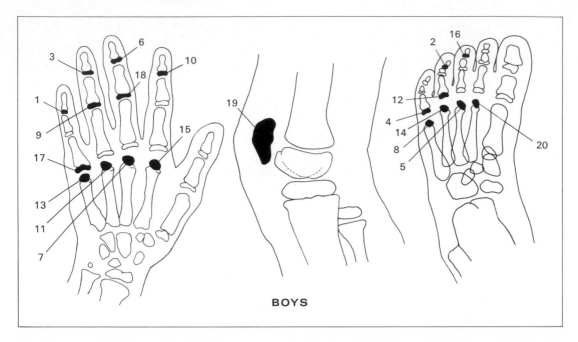

BOYS

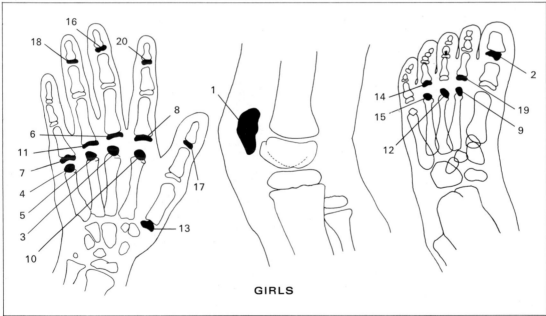

GIRLS

DIAGRAM 4–1. The 20 centers of maximum predictive value in boys and in girls. The postnatal ossification centers that have the highest statistical "communality" and hence the greatest predictive value in skeletal assessment are located in the hand, the foot, and the knee. Thus, three radiographs can actually provide more diagnostically useful information than the larger number often made. (From Garn SM, Rohmann CG, Silverman FN: Radiographic standards for postnatal ossification and tooth calcification. Medical Radiography and Photography 43(2):45–66, 1967. Published by Radiography Markets Division, Eastman Kodak Company)

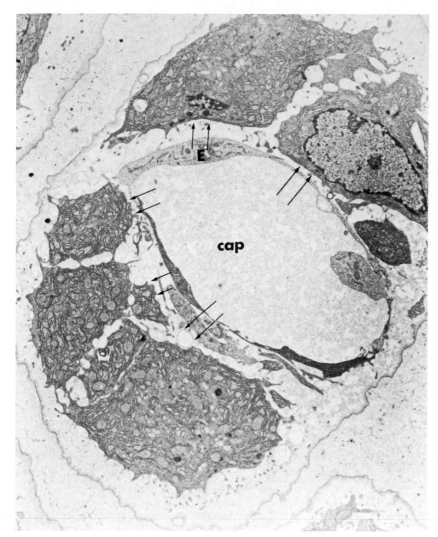

FIG. 4–1. Epiphyseal capillary loop of normal rat (electron micrograph, × 5000)—decalcified section; cross section through an epiphyseal capillary in the zone of vascular resorption. The zone of provisional calcification surrounds the osteoblasts, which are beginning to lay down collagen to form true bone. The darker intracellular membranes filling most of the osteoblasts are rough-surfaced endoplasmic reticulum. Their prominence indicates that these cells are very active in protein (collagen) synthesis. E, endothelial cells; cap, capillary lumen; arrows point to osteoblasts (the large cells). (Courtesy of Dr. Reuben Eisenstein, Associate Attending Pathologist, Presbyterian St. Luke's Hospital, Chicago, IL)

At the end of the period of growth, proliferation of cartilage cells terminates. Bone replaces the epiphyseal plate and the epiphyseal ossification center fuses with the shaft. Longitudinal growth is no longer possible at this site.

The disturbance of any of the above mechanisms by a specific factor results in a specific clinical-pathological entity. Rubin defines three types of disturbances of bone form or modeling as follows:*

1. Dysplasia—a disturbance in growth, intrinsic to bone
2. Dystrophy—a disturbance in nutrition or metabolism, extrinsic to bone
3. Dysostosis—a disturbance or defect in developmental ectodermal or mesenchymal tissues

* From Rubin P: Dynamic Classification of Bone Dysplasias. Chicago, Year Book Publishers, 1964

These conditions can affect the epiphysis, physis, metaphysis, or diaphysis. A classification of bone dysplasias based on growth mechanisms has been proposed by Rubin,[102] which is still useful and is presented below.

DYNAMIC CLASSIFICATION OF BONE DYSPLASIAS

 I. Epiphyseal Dysplasias
    A. Epiphyseal hypoplasias
       1. Failure of articular cartilage: spondyloepiphyseal dysplasia, congenita and tarda
       2. Failure of ossification of center: multiple epiphyseal dysplasia, congenita and tarda
    B. Epiphyseal hyperplasia
       1. Excess of articular cartilage: dysplasia epiphysialis hemimelica

(Text continued on p. 172)

II. Physeal Dysplasias
 A. Cartilage hypoplasias
  1. Failure of proliferating cartilage: achondroplasia, congenita and tarda
  2. Failure of hypertrophic cartilage: metaphyseal dyostosis, congenita and tarda
 B. Cartilage hyperplasias
  1. Excess of proliferating cartilage: hyperchondroplasia
  2. Excess of hypertrophic cartilage: enchondromatosis
III. Metaphyseal Dysplasias
 A. Metaphyseal hypoplasias
  1. Failure to form primary spongiosa: hypophosphatasia, congenita and tarda
  2. Failure to absorb primary spongiosa: osteopetrosis, congenita and tarda
  3. Failure to absorb secondary spongiosa: craniometaphyseal dysplasia, congenita and tarda
 B. Metaphyseal hyperplasias
  1. Excessive spongiosa: multiple exostoses
IV. Diaphyseal Dysplasias
 A. Diaphyseal hypoplasias
  1. Failure of periosteal bone formation: osteogenesis imperfecta, congenita and tarda
  2. Failure of endosteal bone formation: idiopathic osteoporosis, congenita and tarda
 B. Diaphyseal hyperplasias
  1. Excessive periosteal bone formation: progressive diaphyseal dysplasia
  2. Excessive endosteal bone formation: hyperphosphatasemia

MATURATION OF BONE

Somatic maturation is represented by the developmental increments that appear along the pathway to adult status. An objective indicator of this progress is the development of the skeletal system.[36,42,44] Growth and maturation are separate phenomena. It is skeletal maturation, not growth, that correlates with physical and sexual maturity. Skeletal maturation, however, does not correlate with mental development.

Maturation of bone refers only to the times and the sequence of the appearance and fusion of the various ossification centers. Normal development is under the control of endocrine stimuli—pituitary, thyroid, adrenal cortical, and gonadal hormones chiefly instigate epiphyseal closure. Failure or delay in the appearance of the ossification centers occurs also in abnormalities that involve protein metabolism, deranged mineral metabolism, and intrinsic bone disease. Excessive hormonal stimulation is responsible for generalized, accelerated bone maturation. Localized disturbances, in particular hyperemia, produce accelerated maturation in the affected area. Cooley's anemia (thalassemia) causes a paradoxical situation in which the appearance of the epiphyseal ossification centers is delayed but their fusion is premature.[20]

"Skeletal imbalance" means derangement of the normal sequence of ossification. An ossification center may fail to appear at the proper time if an individual is suffering from severe, generalized illness. Upon recovery, subsequent centers appear on schedule, before the interrupted center makes its delayed appearance. The sequence of skeletal ossification thus provides a record of the time and severity of previous illnesses.

There is a large, normal, individual, genotypic variation in the maturation process. Centers appear and fuse earlier in females than in males. The norms vary according to race, environment, and family. Standards compiled from data on previous generations are not currently valid. In contrast to bone development, dental development is not significantly affected by hormonal or nutritional influences.

The age-at-appearance percentiles for major ossification centers tabulated from current standards[36] are presented in Table 4–1. The ossification centers of greatest predictive value[36] are presented in Table 4–2. Causes of altered skeletal maturation are presented below.

CAUSES OF ALTERED BONE MATURATION

A. Generalized Accelerated Maturation
 1. Maternal hyperthyroidism
 2. Hypergonadism
 3. Adrenocortical tumors or hyperplasia
 4. McCune-Albright syndrome
 5. Pinealoma
 6. Intracranial masses
 7. Hepatoma
 8. Obesity
 9. Ellis-van Creveld syndrome
 10. Precocious sexual development
 11. Hyperthyroidism (rare in children)
 12. Intrinsic bone disease
 13. Ovarian neoplasm

14. Hormonogenic teratomas[45]
B. Localized Accelerated Maturation
    1. Rheumatoid arthritis
    2. Hemophilia
    3. Hyperemia
    4. Chronic infections
    5. Healing fractures
    6. Arteriovenous fistula
C. Generalized Retarded Maturation
    1. Hypothyroidism
    2. Diabetes mellitus
    3. Severe constitutional diseases
    4. Anemia
    5. Congenital heart disease
    6. Chronic malnutrition
    7. Nephrosis
    8. Cerebral hypoplasia
    9. Craniopharyngioma
    10. Rachitic states
    11. Hypogonadism
    12. Addison's disease
    13. Cushing's syndrome
    14. Celiac disease
    15. Congenital syndromes of dwarfism or mental retardation
    16. Nonspecific retardation
D. Localized Retarded Maturation
    1. Infections, including tuberculosis
    2. Infarcts
    3. Trauma
    4. Radiation
    5. Neoplasms

The determination of gestational age in the neonate[62,68,69,100,101] shows better correlation with mandibular tooth age than with knee ossification, when a history of intrauterine disorders is present. Second deciduous molar teeth do not appear radiographically before 36 to 37 fetal weeks, and first deciduous molars do not appear before 33 to 34 weeks of gestation. Retarded epiphyseal ossification, as compared with tooth development in the newborn, suggests an abnormality in intrauterine development.

The humeral head epiphyses provide a more accessible indication of gestational age, being readily visible on a routine chest film. If the humeral head is not seen, no conclusions about maturity can be drawn. The coracoid epiphysis is more variable than the humeral head in its ossification.

The humeral head is almost never ossified before 38 weeks of gestational age. It is visible in 15% of newborns at 38 to 39 weeks, in 40% at 40 to 41 weeks, and in 82% at 42 weeks or more of gestational age.

The newborn with dyspnea whose chest radiograph demonstrates ossified humeral heads has less than a 1% chance of being involved with the respiratory distress syndrome of prematurity. Meconium aspiration should then be suspected. Neonates with cyanotic congenital heart disease, particularly with uncorrected transportation of the great vessels, have a high correlation with ossified epiphyses of the humeral heads at birth. If the humeral heads are radiographically visible, prematurity is virtually excluded.

DISEASES MANIFESTED BY ROENTGEN CHANGES OF THE EPIPHYSIS

ENDOCRINE DISEASES ALTERING SKELETAL MATURATION

The principal endocrine glands exerting effects on developing bone are the pituitary, thyroid, adrenal, and gonads. *Deficiency of pituitary hormone* in preadolescents leads to the Lorraine–Levi type of proportional dwarfism, in which epiphyseal closure may not occur until the fifth decade. An enlarged sella turcica may be seen if a pituitary tumor is involved (Figs. 4–2, 4–3). *Excess growth hormone* is caused by an eosinophilic adenoma or hyperplasia of the anterior lobe of the pituitary gland. Prepubertal hyperpituitarism results in giantism, with a great increase in length and caliber of the long bones. Bone maturation may be normal or delayed. Hyperpituitarism taking place after closure of the epiphyses results in acromegaly (see Chap. 5).

HYPOTHYROIDISM

Hypothyroidism[122] in childhood may be congenital (cretinism) or acquired (juvenile myxedema). *Cretinism* usually results in more severe symptomatology, but similar effects are present in the acquired form. There is delayed appearance and fusion of all epiphyses (Fig. 4–4). The epiphyseal ossification centers may also be deformed in the following ways:

1. Slight granular lack of homogeneity (Fig. 4–5)
2. Fine stippling (Fig. 4–6)
3. Coarse stippling
4. Fragmentation with or without coherence (Fig. 4–7)

(*Text continued on p. 179*)

TABLE 4–1. Age-at-Appearance Percentiles for Major Postnatal Ossification Centers (in Years)*

	Percentiles					
	Boys			Girls		
Ossification Center	5th	50th	95th	5th	50th	95th
1. Head of humerus	—	.03	.32	—	.03	.30
2. Proximal epiphysis of tibia	—	.04	.10	—	.01	.04
3. Coracoid process of scapula	—	.04	.36	—	.03	.42
4. Cuboid of tarsus	—	.07	.30	—	.05	.16
5. Capitate of carpus	—	.25	.60	—	.15	.56
6. Hamate of carpus	.03	.31	.82	—	.18	.59
7. Capitulum of humerus	.06	.33	1.07	.05	.26	.77
8. Head of femur	.06	.35	.64	.04	.33	.62
9. Third cuneiform of tarsus	.05	.46	1.58	—	.23	1.23
10. Greater tubercle of humerus	.25	.83	2.33	.20	.51	1.14
11. Primary center, middle segment of 5th toe	—	1.04	3.81	—	.74	2.08
12. Distal epiphysis of radius	.53	1.10	2.30	.38	.82	1.70
13. Epiphysis, distal segment of 1st toe	.71	1.21	2.10	.39	.78	1.68
14. Epiphysis, middle segment of 4th toe	.40	1.21	2.88	.40	.92	3.00
15. Epiphysis, proximal segment of 3rd finger	.77	1.37	2.15	.41	.85	1.61
16. Epiphysis, middle segment of 3rd toe	.41	1.40	4.27	.21	1.02	2.47
17. Epiphysis, proximal segment of 2nd finger	.78	1.41	2.17	.40	.87	1.64
18. Epiphysis, proximal segment of 4th finger	.80	1.49	2.40	.41	.90	1.66
19. Epiphysis, distal segment of 1st finger	.75	1.51	2.70	.42	.99	1.73
20. Epiphysis, proximal segment of 3rd toe	.90	1.58	2.52	.51	1.05	1.88
21. Epiphysis of 2nd metacarpal	.93	1.61	2.82	.64	1.09	1.69
22. Epiphysis, proximal segment of 4th toe	.95	1.64	2.65	.61	1.24	2.06
23. Epiphysis, proximal segment of 2nd toe	.97	1.74	2.65	.63	1.19	2.05
24. Epiphysis of 3rd metacarpal	.95	1.79	3.01	.65	1.13	1.94
25. Epiphysis, proximal segment of 5th finger	1.00	1.85	2.82	.65	1.19	2.07
26. Epiphysis, middle segment of 3rd finger	1.01	1.97	3.31	.63	1.28	2.36
27. Epiphysis of 4th metacarpal	1.09	2.03	3.60	.75	1.29	2.17
28. Epiphysis, middle segment of 2nd toe	.89	2.04	4.05	.49	1.18	2.24
29. Epiphysis, middle segment of 4th finger	1.00	2.05	3.24	.63	1.24	2.43
30. Epiphysis of 5th metacarpal	1.27	2.17	3.82	.86	1.37	2.35
31. First cuneiform of tarsus	.89	2.17	3.77	.50	1.43	2.82
32. Epiphysis of 1st metatarsal	1.39	2.18	3.12	.96	1.58	2.23
33. Epiphysis, middle segment of 2nd finger	1.30	2.19	3.31	.67	1.36	2.54
34. Epiphysis, proximal segment of 1st toe	1.45	2.35	3.31	.89	1.55	2.47
35. Epiphysis, distal segment of 3rd finger	1.31	2.41	3.72	.72	1.46	2.69
36. Triquetral of carpus	.49	2.43	5.47	.29	1.70	3.73
37. Epiphysis, distal segment of 4th finger	1.37	2.44	3.73	.73	1.52	2.82
38. Epiphysis, proximal segment of 5th toe	1.53	2.45	3.65	.97	1.73	2.67
39. Epiphysis of 1st metacarpal	1.45	2.59	4.32	.92	1.60	2.67
40. Second cuneiform of tarsus	1.19	2.65	4.21	.81	1.80	3.00
41. Epiphysis of 2nd metatarsal	1.93	2.86	4.33	1.22	2.14	3.43
42. Greater trochanter of femur	1.92	2.96	4.35	.96	1.85	3.03
43. Epiphysis, proximal segment of 1st finger	1.84	3.00	4.57	.93	1.71	2.84
44. Navicular of tarsus	1.12	3.02	5.40	.77	1.94	3.58
45. Epiphysis, distal segment of 2nd finger	1.80	3.17	4.97	1.06	2.50	3.29
46. Epiphysis, distal segment of 5th finger	2.06	3.29	4.98	1.01	1.96	3.45
47. Epiphysis, middle segment of 5th finger	1.94	3.40	5.84	.88	1.97	3.54
48. Proximal epiphysis of fibula	1.86	3.47	5.24	1.33	2.61	3.92
49. Epiphysis of 3rd metatarsal	2.33	3.48	5.00	1.42	2.48	3.68
50. Epiphysis, distal segment of 5th toe	2.34	3.94	6.30	1.17	2.31	4.07
51. Patella of knee	2.55	4.00	5.96	1.47	2.48	4.01
52. Epiphysis of 4th metatarsal	2.92	4.02	5.74	1.77	2.84	4.05
53. Lunate of carpus	1.53	4.07	6.77	1.08	2.62	5.65
54. Epiphysis, distal segment of 3rd toe	2.99	4.36	6.19	1.37	2.73	4.11
55. Epiphysis of 5th metatarsal	3.12	4.37	6.34	2.08	3.24	4.93
56. Epiphysis, distal segment of 4th toe	2.95	4.38	6.40	1.36	2.58	4.09
57. Epiphysis, distal segment of 2nd toe	3.25	4.64	6.75	1.50	2.93	4.50

| Ossification Center | Percentiles | | | | | |
| | Boys | | | Girls | | |
	5th	50th	95th	5th	50th	95th
58. Capitulum of radius	3.00	5.21	7.97	2.26	3.87	6.28
59. Navicular of carpus	3.59	5.63	7.81	2.35	4.12	5.99
60. Greater multangular of carpus	3.53	5.87	8.97	1.94	4.08	6.36
61. Lesser multangular of carpus	3.12	6.22	8.50	2.38	4.17	6.01
62. Medial epicondyle of humerus	4.27	6.25	8.41	2.05	3.40	5.07
63. Distal epiphysis of ulna	5.25	7.10	9.07	3.29	5.37	7.63
64. Epiphysis of calcaneus	5.17	7.59	9.55	3.54	5.37	7.30
65. Olecranon of ulna	7.78	9.67	11.90	5.62	8.01	9.93
66. Lateral epicondyle of humerus	9.23	11.24	13.70	7.14	9.24	11.28
67. Tubercle of tibia	9.92	11.81	13.38	7.89	10.25	11.82
68. Adductor sesamoid of 1st finger	11.03	12.76	14.62	8.67	10.72	12.68
69. Os acetabulum of hip	11.90	13.54	15.32	9.60	11.47	13.39
70. Acromion of clavicle	12.15	13.74	15.48	10.32	11.92	13.79
71. Epiphysis, iliac crest of hip	12.03	14.03	15.91	10.81	12.79	15.31
72. Accessory epiphysis, coracoid process of scapula	12.74	14.35	16.31	10.37	12.21	14.37
73. Ischial tuberosity of hip	13.57	15.26	17.08	11.71	13.89	16.00

* Garn S M, Rohmann C G, Silverman F N: Radiographic standards for postnatal ossification and tooth calcification. Medical Radiography and Photography 43(2):45–66, 1967. (Published by Radiography Markets Division, Eastman Kodak Company.)

TABLE 4–2 The 20 Ossification Centers of Greatest Predictive Value and Their Communalities*

| Boys | | Girls | |
Ossification Center	Internal Communality† (intra se)	Ossification Center	Internal Communality† (intra se)
Distal V, hand	0.637	Patella knee	0.625
Distal IV, foot	0.650	Distal I, foot	0.663
Distal IV, hand	0.660	Metacarpal III, hand	0.696
Proximal V, foot	0.586	Metacarpal V, hand	0.652
Metatarsal III, foot	0.623	Metacarpal IV, hand	0.653
Distal III, hand	0.650	Proximal III, hand	0.685
Metacarpal III, hand	0.621	Proximal V, hand	0.668
Metatarsal V, foot	0.589	Proximal II, hand	0.689
Middle IV, hand	0.607	Metatarsal II, foot	0.636
Distal II, hand	0.602	Metacarpal II, hand	0.641
Metacarpal IV, hand	0.598	Proximal IV, hand	0.696
Proximal IV, foot	0.550	Metatarsal III, foot	0.616
Metacarpal V, hand	0.601	Metacarpal I, hand	0.596
Metatarsal IV, foot	0.592	Proximal IV, foot	0.623
Metacarpal II, hand	0.570	Metatarsal IV, foot	0.615
Distal III, foot	0.587	Distal III, hand	0.659
Proximal V, hand	0.551	Distal I, hand	0.619
Middle III, hand	0.583	Distal IV, hand	0.636
Patella, knee	0.477	Proximal II, foot	0.589
Metatarsal II, foot	0.542	Distal II, hand	0.620
Mean internal communality	0.595	Mean internal communality	0.645

* Garn SM, Rohmann CG, Silverman FN: Radiographic standards for postnatal ossification and tooth calcification. Medical Radiography and Photography 43(2):45–66, 1967.

† The term "internal communality" is defined as the mean of correlations involving a given center, or group of centers, with the other centers in a given group.

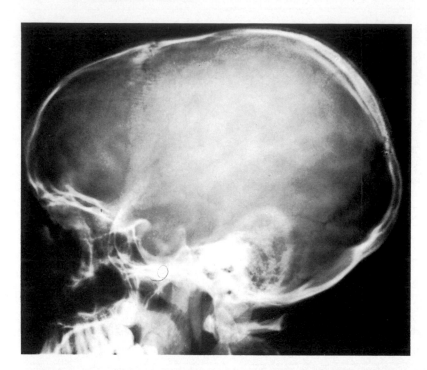

FIG. 4–2. Pituitary dwarfism due to chromophobe adenoma (skull)—female, age 16 years—lateral view. There is marked enlargement of the sella turcica. The skull shows no other significant abnormalities.

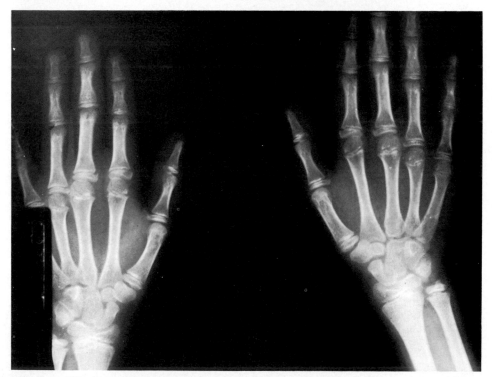

FIG. 4–3. Pituitary dwarfism due to chromophobe adenoma (hands)—same patient as in Fig 4–2. The hands are of small size but the bone structure is otherwise normal. The patient is proportionally small in stature.

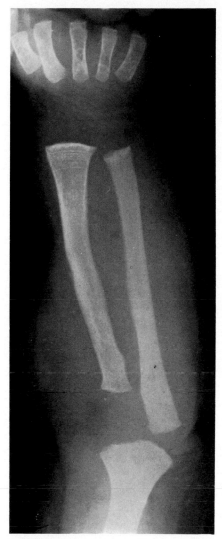

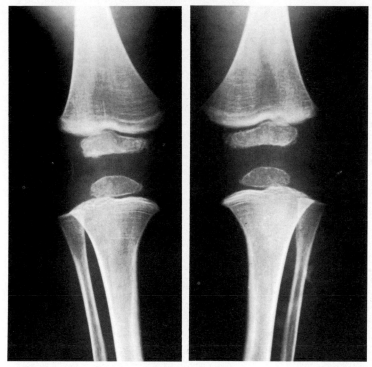

FIG. 4–5. Cretinism (knees). There is a lack of homogeneity of the epiphyseal ossification centers, with granularity and marginal irregularities. Nonspecific metaphyseal transverse striping may also be noted.

FIG. 4–6. Cretinism (hands). Note stippling of the secondary epiphyseal ossification centers, with a fine stippled pattern.

FIG. 4–4. Cretinism (forearm and wrist)—female, age 3½ years. Note complete absence of all secondary ossification centers and carpal centers.

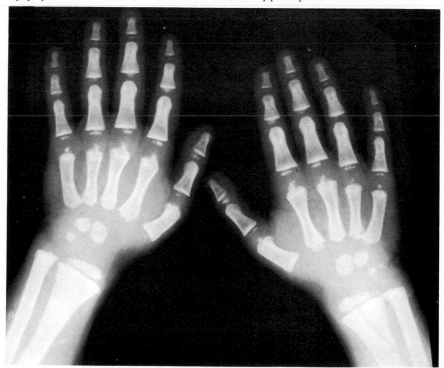

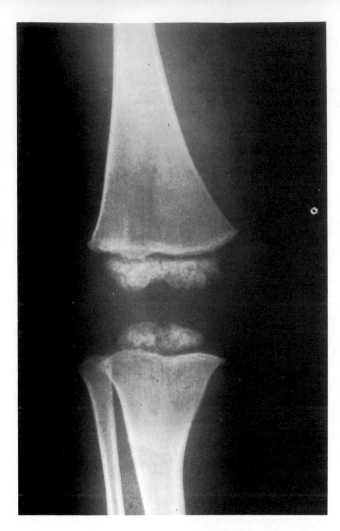

FIG. 4–7. Cretinism (knee). Note fragmentation of the epiphyseal ossification centers with coherence of fragments.

FIG. 4–8. Cretinism (pelvis and hips)—age 3½ years. Neither the femoral capital epiphyses nor the ossification centers of the greater trochanter have appeared as yet. A decreased angle between the neck and the shaft may be seen, indicating coxa vara.

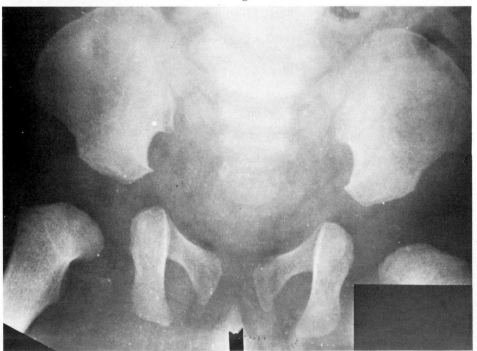

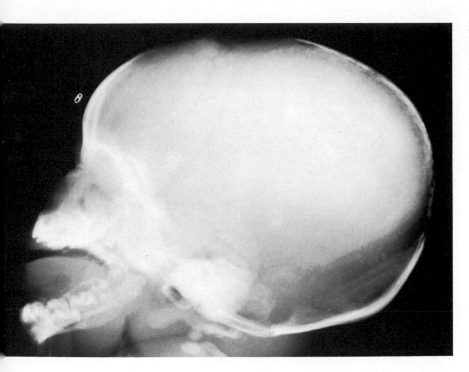

FIG. 4–9. Cretinism (skull). Multiple wormian bones and widening of the lambdoid suture may be seen. Also note increased density of the frontal and occipital bones. This patient had aplasia of the thyroid gland.

These changes must be differentiated from those of multiple epiphyseal dysplasia and chondrodystrophia calcificans congenita. The effects of cretinism are not present at birth because of the presence of maternal thyroid hormone.

The hips show characteristic deformities. Delayed and spotty ossification of the femoral capital epiphysis is common, leading to fragmentation that divides the center into outer and inner halves. Secondary changes in the acetabulum follow. The femoral neck is shortened and coxa vara with elevated position of the trochanter results (Fig. 4–8).

The skull is usually brachycephalic with a short base. Hypertelorism, small facial bones, and prognathism are common. There is decreased pneumatization of the paranasal sinuses and the mastoids. Dentition is delayed and dental caries are present. The calvarium shows wormian bones and may be increased in density (Fig. 4–9). The internal and external tables are poorly differentiated. Closure of the sutures and fontanelles is delayed. The sella turcica is often enlarged, having a round, sharply marginated appearance (Fig. 4–10). There may be thickening of the greater wings of the sphenoid.

The vertebral column shows kyphosis and flattening of the bodies with an increase in the width of the intervertebral spaces (Fig. 4–11). There may be a "sail" upper lumbar vertebra with a wedge or hook configuration, which is also common in Hurler's syndrome, achondroplasia, and Morquio's syndrome. This configuration is thought to result from stress rather than from a specific genetic abnormality.

The long bones show shortening, slender shafts with endosteal thickening, dense transverse bands at the metaphyseal ends (Fig. 4–12), and thick, irregular epiphyses. Humerus varus may be present. The hands present as one of three types: (1) normal, (2) short and stubby (Fig. 4–13), and (3) long and slender (Fig. 4–14). Short, thick metacarpals and hypoplastic middle and terminal phalanges of the fifth finger are present in the short and stubby type. The distal phalanges may show a central dense area in the epiphyseal cartilage plate.[54]

The bone changes may have completely regressed in adult cretins.

HYPERTHYROIDISM

Hyperthyroidism in the chronic form in children accelerates the appearance and growth of the secondary ossification centers. Osteoporosis is commonly present. Cases of neonatal hyperthyroidism have been reported, with markedly advanced bone age at birth, and development of craniosynostosis and brachydactyly.[8,99] Cone-shaped epiphyses were sometimes present, and asymmetrical shortening of metacarpals and phalanges was seen.

(Text continued on p. 182)

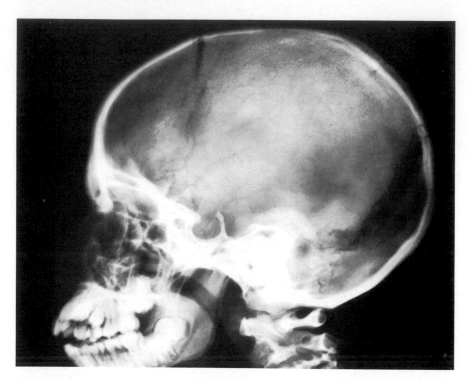

FIG. 4–10. Cretinism (skull)—female, age 18 years. There is enlargement of the sella turcica, with a rounded, sharply marginated appearance. A positive "double floor" sign is present. Note that the inner and outer tables and diploë of the calvarium in the frontal region appear undifferentiated; normal differentiation may be seen in the posterior parietal and occipital regions.

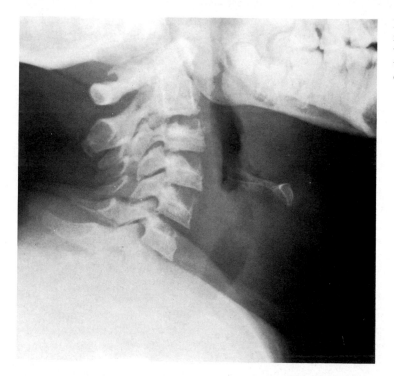

FIG. 4–11. Hypothyroidism (cervical spine)—female, age 19 years. Lack of height of the cervical vertebral bodies is present, with wide intervertebral spaces. Note large goiter. Periapical abscess of the second molar is noted in the mandible.

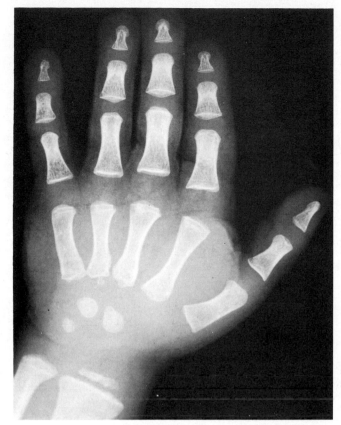

FIG. 4–13. Cretinism (hand)—short, stubby type.

FIG. 4–14. Cretinism (hands)—long, slender type.

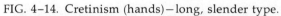

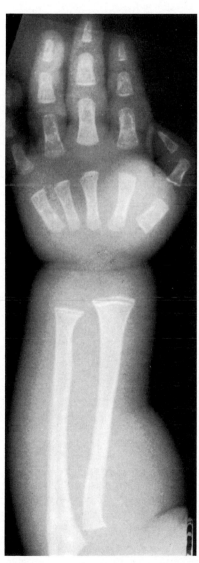

FIG. 4–12. Cretinism (forearm and hand)—aplasia of the thyroid; same patient as in Fig. 4–9. Nonspecific, dense horizontal metaphyseal striping may be noted.

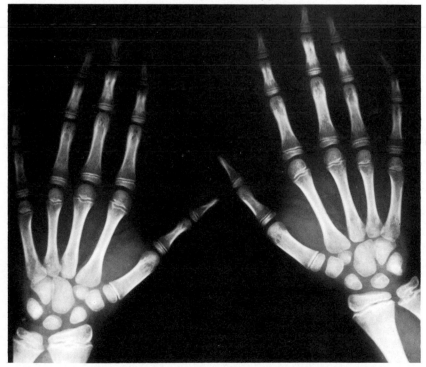

HYPOGONADISM

Hypogonadism may be caused by a deficiency of pituitary gonadotropins with a lack of LH and FSH, or by a primary gonadal deficiency accompanied by normal or increased levels of urinary gonadotropin. Skeletal maturation is delayed with respect to the fusion of centers.

EUNUCHOIDISM

Eunuchoidism is a primary gonadal deficiency. Fusion of the epiphyses is delayed, resulting in a long slender bone. Osteoporosis may also be present. The typical proportions are abnormally long limbs with a relatively short trunk.

OVARIAN AGENESIS AND KLINEFELTER'S SYNDROME

Ovarian agenesis and Klinefelter's syndrome are inherited sex-linked disorders involving the gonads. In Turner's syndrome, characteristic bone changes other than maturation effects are present (see Chap. 5).

CUSHING'S SYNDROME

Cushing's syndrome is caused by overproduction of steroid hormones by the adrenal cortex or by iatrogenic administration of exogenous steroids. In adults, adrenal hyperplasia causes approximately 75% of endogenous disease. In children, carcinoma of the adrenal cortex accounts for approximately two-thirds of the cases.

Delayed skeletal maturation occurs. Osteoporosis with resultant pathological fractures, particularly in the spine, is present. The vertebral bodies may show wedging or biconcavity. Horizontal sclerotic bands adjacent to the vertebral end-plates are evident, due to excessive callus formation at infraction sites. The anterior ribs and pubic and ischial rami are common sites of fracture. Abundant callus may be present at all fracture sites. Features that are not usually found in osteoporosis, such as partial absence of the lamina dura[86] and bending of bones, have been reported. Ischemic necrosis, particularly of the femoral and humeral heads, and septic arthritis are common. Premature vascular calcification also may occur. Very rarely, in a case of pituitary basophilic adenoma, the sella turcica is enlarged. Laboratory diagnosis is established on the basis of steroid analysis. A differentiation between hyperplasia, adenoma, and carcinoma can often be made.

ADRENOGENITAL SYNDROME

The *adrenogenital syndrome*[45] may be congenital or acquired. The congenital form is due to adrenal cortical hyperplasia, a result of faulty cortisol production that does not suppress the release of corticotropin by the pituitary. The acquired form is usually due to adrenal adenoma or carcinoma. In the congenital form, virilization of the female may be present at birth or may develop at a later age. In the male, precocious sexual and somatic development is usually noted between the ages of 2 and 4 years.

Osseous changes that are radiologically detectable include accelerated skeletal maturation, usually evident in the second half of the first year of life. Premature fusion of epiphyseal centers follows, resulting in dwarfism. Dentition is accelerated. Prominent muscular development is present, associated with osseous prominences. Accelerated development of the paranasal sinuses and mastoids, as well as thickening of the calvarium, may be seen in the skull. Premature calcification of rib and laryngeal cartilages may also occur.

ADDISON'S DISEASE

Addison's disease[77] or primary adrenocortical insufficiency of the chronic type, may reflect changes in the osseous system radiologically. This is uncommon in infants and young children. Approximately 90% of the adrenal cortex must be destroyed in order to produce symptoms. The various etiologies of Addison's disease are:

1. Idiopathic
2. Tumors or leukemia
3. Tuberculosis or other granulomas
4. Thrombosis or hemorrhage
5. Hemochromatosis
6. Amyloidosis
7. Postsurgical

Approximately 25% of all patients have unilateral or bilateral adrenal calcifications.

Skeletal maturation and growth are delayed. Calcifications of the pinnae of the ear and the rib cartilage are present. Bone tuberculosis may occasionally be a complicating condition.

EPIPHYSEAL ISCHEMIC NECROSES

Many localized areas of ischemic necrosis have been described. This condition is now considered to be caused by local loss of blood supply,[25] which can result from thrombosis, disease of the arterial

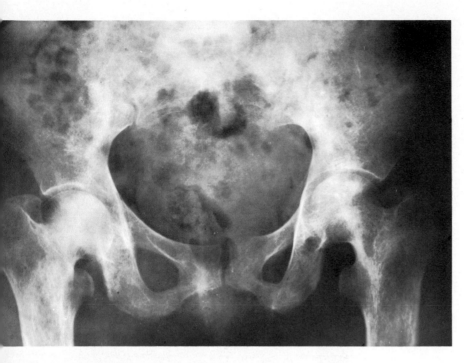

FIG. 4–15. Ischemic necrosis (hips) due to sickle-cell anemia — epiphyseal infarctions. Note dense areas of both femoral heads and necks, more marked on the right. This is the initial stage of ischemic necrosis; structural collapse has not occurred as yet. The contours of the femoral heads are normal.

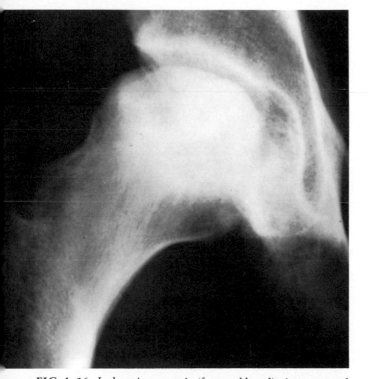

FIG. 4–16. Ischemic necrosis (femoral head). A segmental spherical radiopacity involving the major portion of the head may be noted, with beginning cyst formation. The contour of the femoral head is essentially intact.

wall, disease of surrounding bone, inadequate blood supply, or trauma causing disruption of the blood supply. The cortex of a bone is unyielding, and any infiltrative or purulent process increasing the pressure within the medullary cavity effectively diminishes the regional blood supply. In general, the affected part shows a change in density, loss of contour, and fragmentation.

A tabulation of idiopathic ischemic necroses[15] is presented below.

IDIOPATHIC ISCHEMIC NECROSES*

1. Head of humerus	Hass 1921
2. Capitulum of humerus	Panner 1927
3. Lower ulna	Burns 1921
4. Carpal navicular	Preiser 1911
5. Carpal semilunar	Kienböck 1910
6. Entire carpus bilateral	Caffey 1945
7. Heads of metacarpals	Mauclaire 1927
8. Basal phalanges	Thiemann 1909[18]
9. Vertebral epiphyses	Scheuermann 1921
10. Vertebral body	Calvé 1925
	Kümmel–Verneuil
	disease (posttraumatic)

11. Iliac crest	Buchman 1927
12. Symphysis pubis	Pierson 1929
13. Ischial apophysis	Milch 1953
14. Ischiopubic synchondrosis	Van Neck 1924
15. Femoral epiphysis	Legg–Calvé–Perthes 1910
16. Greater trochanter	Mandl 1922
17. Primary patellar center	Köhler 1908
18. Secondary patellar center	Sinding–Larsen 1921
19. Intercondyloid spines	Caffey 1956
20. Medial tibial condyle	Blount 1937
21. Tibial tubercle	Osgood–Schlatter 1903
22. Distal tibial center	Liffert and Arkin 1950
23. Epiphysis of calcaneus	Sever 1912[50]
24. Astragalus	Diaz 1928
25. Os tibiale externum	Haglund 1908
26. Tarsal navicular	Köhler 1908
27. Fifth metatarsal base	Iselin 1912
28. Second metatarsal head	Freiberg 1914
29. Osteochondritis dissecans	Koenig 1887

A traumatic ischemic necrosis of the talus in adults, associated with alcoholism and cortisone therapy, has been described.

IMPORTANT SITES AND CONDITIONS OF ISCHEMIC NECROSES[74]

Ischemic necrosis of the *femoral capital epiphysis* is associated with a vast variety of diseases. The sequence of roentgen changes in various diseases and at other sites is largely similar. Changes in the femoral head demonstrate the general process to good advantage.

The lesions are juxta-articular. There is no initial involvement of the joint cartilage, thus distinguishing this process from subchondral sclerosis caused by arthritis or radium poisoning.

Initially, dense areas in the femoral head appear (Fig. 4–15). These areas may take the form of a bandlike linear opacity along the articular surface (up to two-thirds of the joint), or may follow the epiphyseal line. Widening of the epiphyseal cartilage plate may then occur. Spherical segmental opacities then appear, giving the so-called "snow-cap" appearance (Fig. 4–16).

Structural failure occurs next, the first sign of which is a radiolucent subcortical band that repre-

sents a fracture line[88](Figs. 4–17, 4–18). The subcortical fracture line may precede the sclerosis. Then, the articular cortex in the weight-bearing area—the superior lateral aspect of the femoral head—collapses. "Step-formation" occurs at the junction with normal cortex. There is sequestration of this portion of the cortex (Fig. 4–19). A fibrosis band surrounds the lesion. Mottled cystic areas are present. A zone of sclerosis surrounds the entire process, giving a geographical appearance (Fig. 4–20). Advance destructive and resorptive changes follow (Fig. 4–21). Periosteal bone apposition along the femoral neck is a prominent feature.

The *radiologic* manifestations of ischemic epiphyseal necrosis are a consequence of fragmentation, compression, and resorption of dead bone, along with proliferation of granulation tissue, revascularization, and production of new bone.

The subchondral radiolucent fracture line, or "rim sign," may be shown more readily if traction

(Text continued on p. 187)

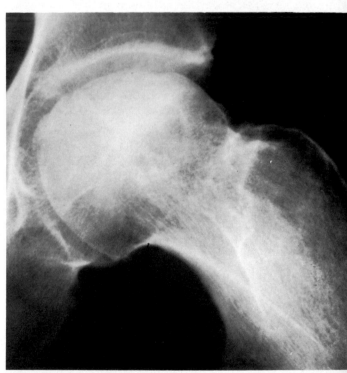

FIG. 4–17. Idiopathic ischemic necrosis (femoral head). Note radiolucent subcortical band involving the major portion of the femoral head; this is the first roentgen sign of structural failure. A "snow-cap" appearance is also present.

* From Caffey J, Silverman FN: Pediatric X-ray Diagnosis, 5th ed. Chicago, Year Book Publishers, 1967

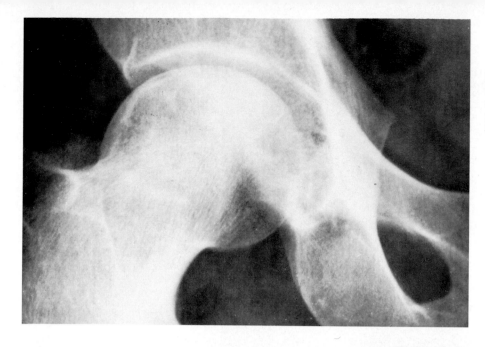

FIG. 4–18. Ischemic necrosis (hip). Appearance of radiolucent subcortical line or "crescent sign" prior to appearance of significant amount of sclerosis is noted.

FIG. 4–19. Ischemic necrosis (femoral head) showing collapse of the articular surface in the weight-bearing area at the superior portion of the femoral head. Note sharp demarcation or "step" formed with the normal cortex. A surrounding radiolucent zone sequesters the involved area.

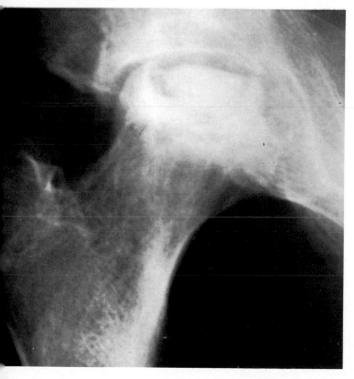

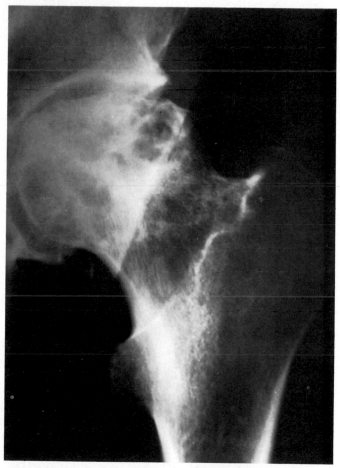

FIG. 4–20. Ischemic necrosis (femoral head). Note flattening of the contour of the head, and many mottled cystlike areas. A sclerotic zone surrounds the involved area.

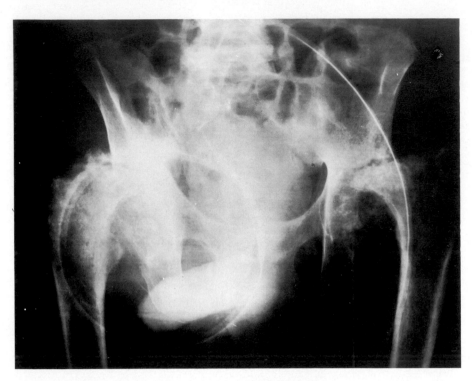

FIG. 4–21. Ischemic necrosis (pelvis and hip joints) due to systemic lupus erythematosus. Note advanced ischemic necrosis of both hips and marked destructive and resorptive changes of both femoral heads. In spite of advanced destruction, the joint space is preserved.

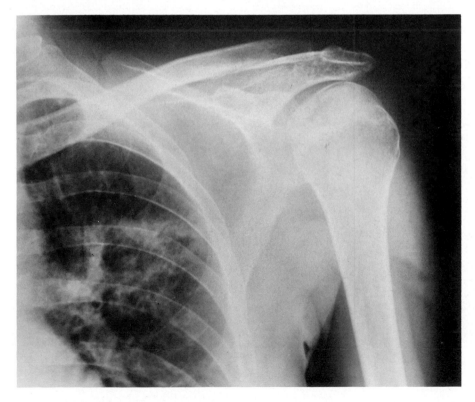

FIG. 4–22. Systemic lupus erythematosus (shoulder). Note the ischemic necrosis of the humeral head. A tuberculous infiltration in the left lung is also seen. This patient was on steroids which reactivated pulmonary tuberculosis.

is applied to the hip during radiography.[73] Gas collects in the subchondral area due to a vacuum phenomenon. Thirty to 40 pounds of manual traction are applied in an adult. Subluxation may also result, permitted by joint effusion.

A fragmented appearance of the femoral head has been associated with the diseases listed below. The humeral head is not uncommonly involved, (Fig. 4–22).

CONDITIONS ASSOCIATED WITH A FRAGMENTED FEMORAL HEAD

1. Fairbank's disease
2. Trevor's disease
3. Cretinism
4. Legg–Calvé–Perthes' disease[13]
5. Congenital dislocation of the hip
6. Traumatic dislocation
7. Postslipped capital femoral epiphysis
8. Rickets
9. Gaucher's disease
10. Hemophilia
11. Christmas disease
12. Sickle-cell anemia
13. Sickle-cell hemoglobin C disease
14. Sickle-cell thalassemia
15. Sickle-cell trait
16. Achondroplasia
17. Hurler's syndrome
18. Morquio's syndrome
19. Adrenogenital syndrome
20. Cushing's syndrome[86]
21. Excess steroid therapy[30]
22. Lupus erythematosus
23. Rheumatoid arthritis
24. Diabetes mellitus
25. Celiac disease
26. Carcinoma of the thyroid
27. Aregenerative anemia
28. Familial fibrosis of jaws
29. Chondrodystrophia calcificans congenita
30. Ollier's disease
31. Osteochondrosis dissecans
32. Pancreatitis, acute[58]
33. Pancreatitis, chronic calcific
34. Traumatic pancreatitis
35. Carcinoma of the head of the pancreas
36. Thromboemobolic disease
37. Caisson disease[78, 87]
38. Radium poisoning

(Text continued on p. 190)

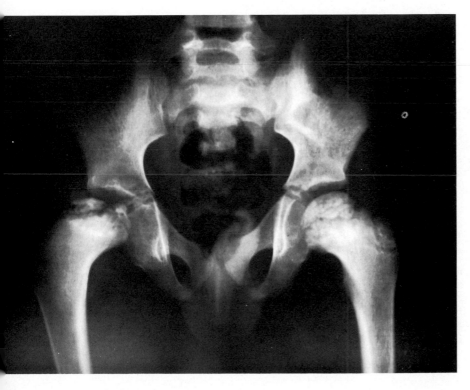

FIG. 4–23. Legg-Perthes' disease (initial picture, 1961) in male, age 8 years. There is structural collapse and fragmentation of the head of the right femur, with cyst formation. Widening of the right femoral neck may also be seen. The contour of the left femoral head is maintained. Note textural irregularities about the femoral capital epiphyseal plate and the epiphysis of the greater trochanter. The joint spaces are widened.

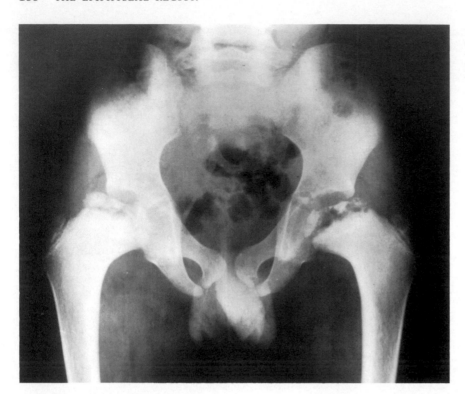

FIG. 4–24. Legg-Perthes' disease—
same patient as in Fig. 4–23 (picture
taken in 1962). The left femoral head
has collapsed. Note fragmentation of
both femoral heads, with multiple
cystic radiolucencies and widening
of both femoral necks.

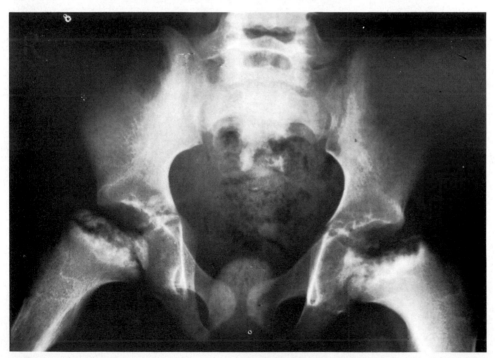

FIG. 4–25. Legg-Perthes' disease—same patient as in Figs. 4–23 and 4–24. Note progression of fragmentation of the femoral capital epiphyses, particularly on the left; here a
steplike formation involving the major portion of the femoral head is visible, with loss of
bone substance. The necrotic area is surrounded by a zone of sclerosis.

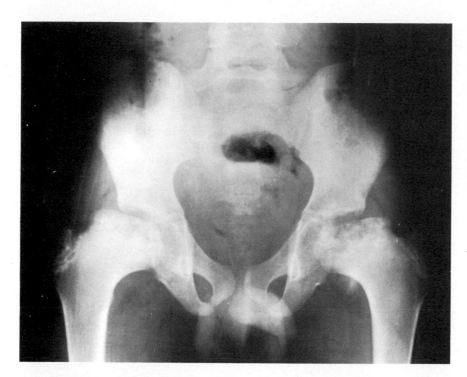

FIG. 4–26. Legg-Perthes' disease — same patient as in previous three figures (picture taken in 1964). Reconstruction of the texture of the right femoral capital epiphysis may be noted, with residual "mushroom" deformity and wide femoral neck. Sclerotic changes at the metaphyses are also apparent. Partial reconstruction of the left femoral head may be seen, with areas of radiolucency bounded by sclerotic margins.

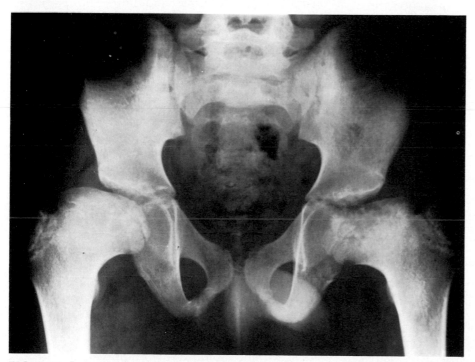

FIG. 4–27. Legg-Perthes' disease — same patient as in previous four figures (picture taken in 1966). Note reconstruction of the bone texture — now almost normal — in the right femoral head, with flattening of the head and widening of the neck to give a mushroomlike deformity. The epiphyseal plate is still intact. Partial reconstruction with diminution of the radiolucent and sclerotic areas has occurred in the left femoral head since last picture was taken. The joint spaces are preserved.

39. Postfracture of the femoral neck
40. Surgical trauma
41. Manipulative trauma
42. Poikiloderma congenitale[24]
43. Idiopathic ischemic necrosis[94]
44. Wilson's disease
45. Alcholism
46. Arteriosclerotic infarcts
47. Histiocytosis
48. Sarcoidosis
49. Infections
50. Gout
51. Leukemia
52. Following renal transplantation[49]
53. Fabry's disease
54. Hyperlipidemia

Legg–Perthes' Disease

Legg–Perthes' disease[13] (osteochondrosis of the femoral head, coxa plana) is a condition of necrosis of the femoral capital epiphyseal ossification center. It occurs at a peak age of 4 to 8 years, involves males in a ratio of 4 to 1, and is virtually absent in blacks. It occurs earlier in females. Most male patients have a bone age more than 2 standard deviations below the mean. The etiology is not determined; concepts proposed include ischemic necrosis, direct compression injury, synovitis, or a generalized constitutional disorder. Symptoms include groin pain, spasm, limp, atrophy of the thigh and buttock, and decreased internal rotation.

*Radiologically,*the earliest changes include slight lateral displacement of the femur and widening of the joint space. In many cases the involved epiphyseal ossification center is smaller than on the normal side. The next stage is a subchondral fracture prior to flattening of the femoral head contour. This is manifested by a subcortical radiolucent crescent in the anterolateral superior segment, and can often be visualized only in the frog-leg position. Flattening of the head follows fracture in the same segment in the vast majority of cases, or the two may develop simultaneously. Sclerosis of the epiphysis subsequently occurs, or it may precede the fracture. Radiolucent metaphyseal defects appear later. The entire center or a portion, usually the anterolateral superior quadrant, may be involved, with an irregular dense sclerosis which proceeds to fragmentation. In Legg–Perthes' disease reossification always occurs with reconstruction and remodeling to either a spherically shaped head, or a "mushroom shape" with flattening of the head and a broad neck. A widened joint space consistently persists in late stages of the disease. Premature fusion of the ossification center may occur as well as "trochanteric overgrowth" which refers to a disproportionately larger greater trochanter owing to shortening of the femoral neck.[91] Osteochondrosis dissecans of the femoral head may be seen with separation of an osteochondral fragment. Recurrence of infarction is said to be uncommon. Significant residual disability on long-term follow-up after treatment is said to be rare. Legg–Perthes' disease follows a different course from ischemic necrosis in later life, with respect to reconstruction. Ten to 15% of patients show bilateral involvement, with a relatively high proportion of female patients, and a younger age group (Figs. 4–23, 4–24, 4–25, 4–26, 4–27).

Slipped Capital Femoral Epiphysis

"Slipping," or a Salter–Harris type 1 fracture through the proximal epiphyseal cartilage plate of the femur, is a distinct clinical entity. The age range is between 9 and 17 years, with a peak of 13 years in males and 12 years in females. A history of a definitive traumatic episode is seldom found. This condition, slightly more frequent in males, is usually unilateral. In 20% to 30% of patients it is bilateral. The symptoms consist of pain and limp. The conditions which may predispose to slippage are:

Trauma
Obesity
Nutrition
Radiation therapy[126]
Hypothyroidism[85]
Mechanical stress
Rapid growth spurt[29]
Renal osteodystrophy[40]

Radiologically, the epiphyseal cartilage plate is widened, with irregularity and rarefaction of the metaphysis. The epiphyseal ossification center is usually displaced medially and dorsally, but only one or the other displacement may occur. The displacement may show slow progression. A frog-leg view should be obtained.

A rare but severe sequel to slipped capital femoral epiphysis is *acute chondrolysis*. This occurs after treatment but may rarely occur spontaneously. The black population has a much higher incidence.

The *clinical* manifestations are severe pain and limitation of motion in the involved joint. *Radiologically*, rapid narrowing of the joint space is seen associated with osteoporosis and subchondral erosions. The etiology is unknown. A pannuslike granulation tissue is found at surgery, which erodes articular cartilage. The joint space may reconstitute, but a full range of motion may never return (Fig. 4–28).

Osgood–Schlatter's Disease

Osgood–Schlatter's disease, or osteochondrosis of the tibial tuberosity, is best diagnosed clinically rather than radiologically. It is found most frequently in boys between 10 and 15 years of age. It is considered to result chiefly from trauma to the tibial tuberosity. Pain and soft-tissue swelling are requisites for this diagnosis. These findings may be present without initial fragmentation of the ossification centers of the tibial tuberosity; fragmentation may develop up to several years later (Fig. 4–29). Because the normal appearance of the developing tibial tuberosity may vary widely, this disease cannot be diagnosed from an irregular epiphyseal appearance alone.

Osteochondrosis Dissecans

Osteochondrosis dissecans, or segmental ischemic necrosis, most commonly occurs in males, in the knee on the lateral aspect of the medial femoral condyle (Figs. 4–30, 4–31). The lateral condyle may rarely be involved (Fig. 4–32). Other areas that may be involved are the femoral head, elbow, shoulder, patella,[92] and ankle (Fig. 4–33). A small necrotic segment of bone with its articular cartilage detaches and lies in a depression in the joint surface. It may be denser than surrounding bone. It is demarcated by a crescentic radiolucent zone, and may separate from the surface to form a loose osteocartilaginous body in the joint space. A residual pit in the articular surface remains. The loose body may subsequently become resorbed. The regional articular surface may become sclerotic. The specimens may contain only articular cartilage and no subchondral bone. This suggests a traumatic etiology. Many islands of calcification within the articular cartilage may sometimes be seen. Adolescents are chiefly affected. A distinct clinical entity, termed *spontaneous osteonecrosis of the knee,*[124] has been described as occurring in patients over 50 years of age. The weight-bearing portion of the medial femoral condyle

(Text continued on p. 194)

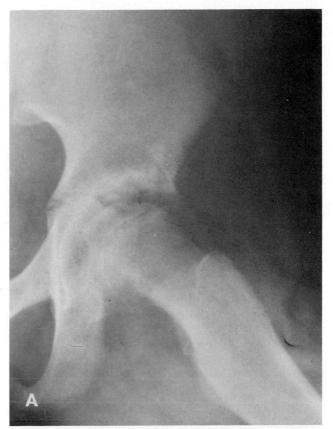

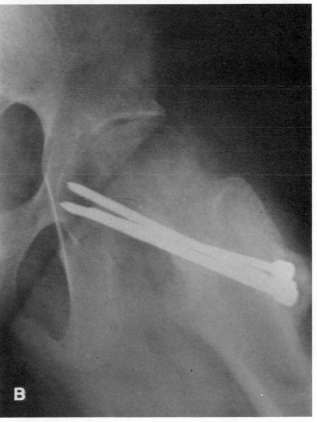

FIG. 4–28. Slipped capital femoral epiphysis. There is rotation of the femoral epiphyseal ossification center posteriorly and medially. **A.** Widening of the epiphyseal cartilage plate is seen secondary to the fracture. The joint space appears normal. **B.** Same patient after fixation of the femoral epiphyseal ossification center with three metallic screws. There is marked narrowing of the hip joint space.

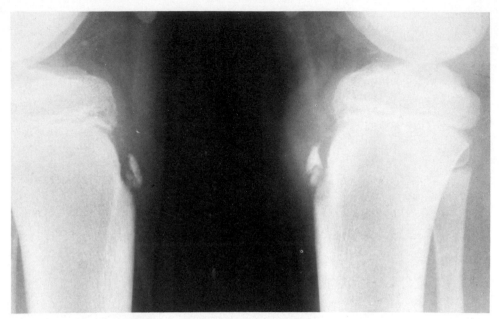

FIG. 4–29. Osgood-Schlatter's disease. Pain, tenderness, and swelling over the left tibial tuberosity were present. Note fragmentation of the left tibial tuberosity. The normal right tibial tuberosity is shown for comparison.

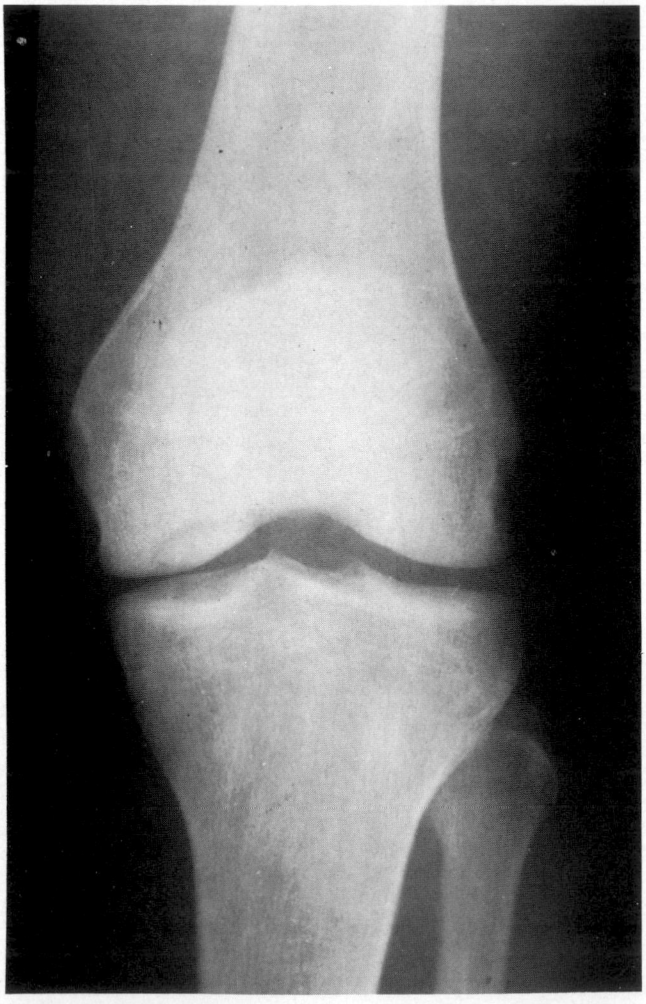

FIG. 4–30. Osteochondrosis dissecans (knee). An ovoid segment of bone surrounded by radiolucent zone may be seen at the lateral aspect of the medial femoral condylar articulating surface. The knee appears otherwise normal.

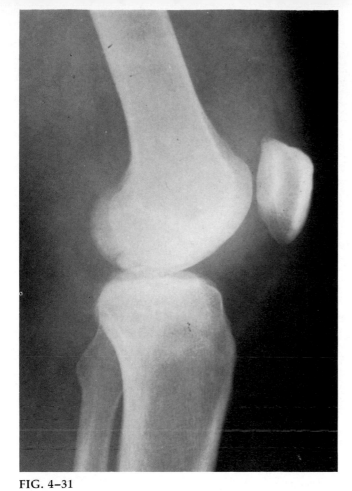

FIG. 4–31

FIG. 4–31. Osteochondrosis dissecans—lateral view of knee in Fig. 4–30. Note radiolucent zone surrounding bony segment at medial femoral condyle in the posterior aspect.

FIG. 4–32. Osteochondrosis dissecans (knee). A radiolucent area with a central bony density is noted involving the lateral condyle of the knee.

FIG. 4–33. Osteochondrosis dissecans (ankle). A small, dissected segment of bone surrounded by a radiolucent area may be seen at the articular surface of the talus.

FIG. 4–32

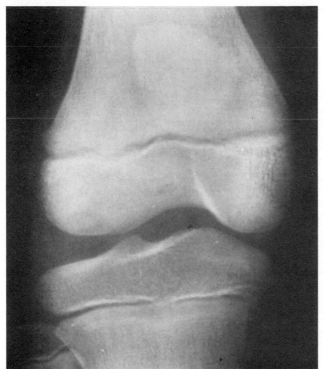

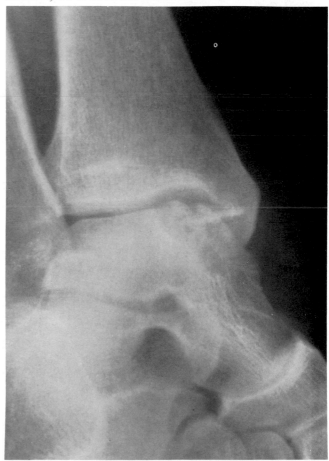

shows changes similar to those of conventional osteochondrosis dissecans. The onset occurs at a much older age. Many patients received steroids either parenterally or by intra-articular injection. Medial meniscal tears are very common in this group. It is postulated that medial meniscal tears in older patients may lead to osteonecrosis.[89]

Koehler's Disease

Koehler's disease refers to ischemic necrosis of the tarsal navicular. Males are most commonly affected, with peak incidence at 5 to 6 years of age. Pain and swelling are often present. The lesion progresses from an irregularity (Fig. 4–34) to fragmentation, compression with increased density, and a disklike shape (Fig. 4–35). The joint spaces are preserved. Recovery occurs and the bone may assume a normal appearance. This is a rare condition. Ischemic necrosis of other small bones generally follows the same pattern (Fig. 4–36).

Kienböck's Disease

Kienböck's disease refers to ischemic necrosis of the carpal lunate. A traumatic etiology has been postulated but not proven. The patient complains of localized pain and tenderness. Radiographs early in the disease may show no findings. The lunate then shows increased density outstanding as compared to the disuse osteoporosis of the surrounding carpus. Irregular radiolucencies develop and the lunate becomes fragmented and compressed (Fig. 4–37). A relationship is claimed between the relative lengths of the radius and ulna and the incidence of Kienböck's disease.[37] If the ulna is shorter than the radius (negative ulnar variance), then there may be pressure on the lunate from the medial corner of the radius, predisposing it to necrosis.

Blount's Disease

Blount's disease[70] refers to osteochondrosis of the medial tibial metaphysis, which may develop during infancy or childhood. The infantile type is usually bilateral, but the childhood type is usually unilateral. Metaphyseal irregularlity is evident in the radiograph, with enlargement and a beaklike projection pointed medially and distally (Fig. 4–38). The medial aspect of the epiphysis may also be deformed (Fig. 4–39). This is associated with bowing. Caffey believes that the Blount lesion is a sequel to bowing rather than a forerunner or cause.

Sever's Disease

Sever's disease or ischemic necrosis of the secondary calcaneal ossification center, may not truly exist as a distinct entity. The normal ossification center varies widely in appearance and coherence. The secondary center normally has a greater density than the body of the calcaneus. In the event of interference with the normal weight-bearing of a limb, this normal increased density is not present[107] (Fig. 4–40).

CHONDRODYSTROPHIA CALCIFICANS CONGENITA

Chrondrodystrophia calcificans congenita[9,75] (stippled epiphysis) is a rare epiphyseal dysplasia characterized by multiple discrete punctate areas of calcification in the epiphyses. The most commonly involved sites are the hips, knees, shoulders, and wrists; other areas are less commonly affected. The involved bone may be shortened or the process may regress and leave no deformity. The diagnosis is usually made during the first year of life. Associated abnormalities that have been reported are flexion deformities, clubfoot, congenital dislocation of the hips, monomelic shortening, saddle nose, microcephaly, oxycephaly, dwarfism, mental deficiency, cleft palate, cardiac defects, cataracts, poor resistance to infections, calcification of the synovial tissues, hemivertebrae, cutaneous thickenings, and tracheal ring calcifications. The disease has been classified into two types: (1) the lethal rhizomelic type, and (2) the mild Conradi–Hünermann type (Spranger *et al*). The rhizomelic type includes gross shortening of bone.

Anatomically, there is an extreme vascularity of the epiphyseal cartilage with mottled mucous degeneration and fragmentation. These fragments become foci for calcareous deposits. An elevated serum alkaline phosphatase has been noted in some cases. Other biochemical studies are normal.

Radiologically, this condition is characterized by fine calcific punctate stippling of the involved epiphyses prior to the normal time of appearance of epiphyseal ossification centers (Fig. 4–41). The densities may disappear by the age of 3 years or coalesce to form a normal ossification center (Fig. 4–42). Stippled calcifications of the laryngeal cartilages may also be noted. Usually there is no shortening of the tubular bones, although asymmetrical shortening may occur, not to be confused with achondroplasia which shows irregular calcifications. Accelerated maturation occurs. The flat bones

(Text continued on p. 198)

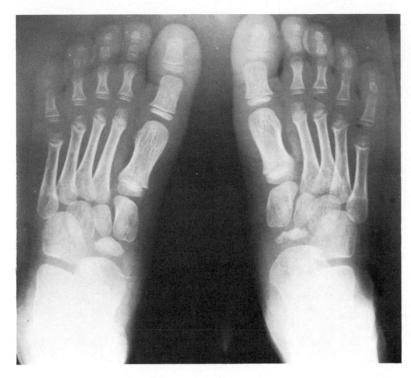

FIG. 4–34. Koehler's disease (feet). Note irregularity and slight increase in density of the left tarsal navicular, with slight flattening.

FIG. 4–36. Freiberg's disease (third metatarsal). Note flattening of the third metatarsal head.

FIG. 4–35. Koehler's disease (feet). Note fragmentation and marked flattening of the left tarsal navicular, with increase in density.

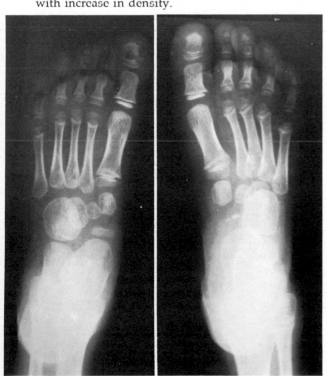

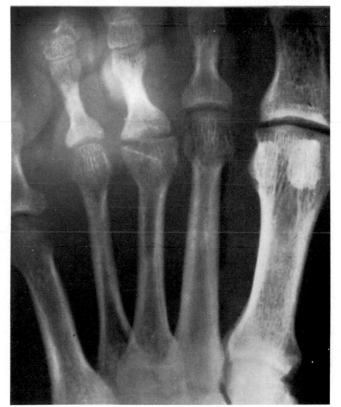

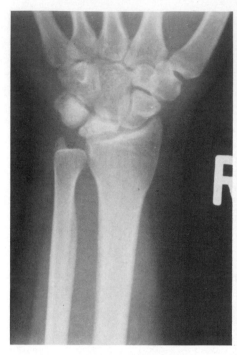
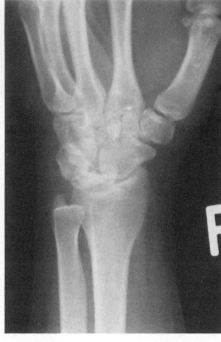

FIG. 4–37. Kienböck's disease. Ischemic necrosis of the lunate is noted, as well as relative shortening of the ulna, or negative ulnar variance.

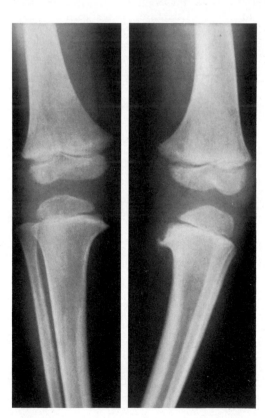

FIG. 4–38. Blount's disease (knees)—unilateral. Irregularity of the medial metaphysis of the left tibia is shown. A small beaklike projection may be seen pointing medially and distally.

FIG. 4–39. Blount's disease (knee)—anteroposterior and lateral view—reconstructed stage. Note residual beaking of the medial tibial metaphyses, and deformity of the medial aspect of the tibial epiphyses. Genu varum is present.

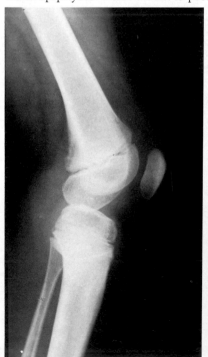
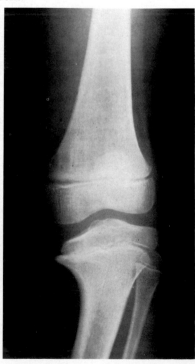

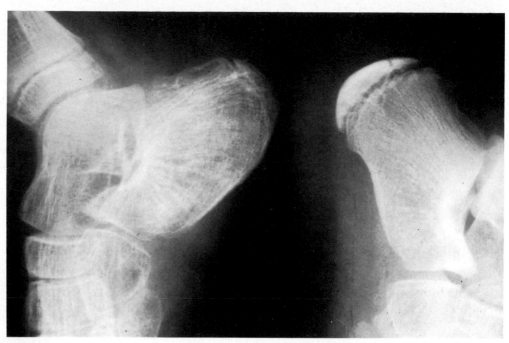

FIG. 4–40. Normal increased density of the secondary calcaneal ossification center on the left. Function in the right leg is impaired due to paralytic poliomyelitis. Note lack of density of the epiphysis, and osteoporosis.

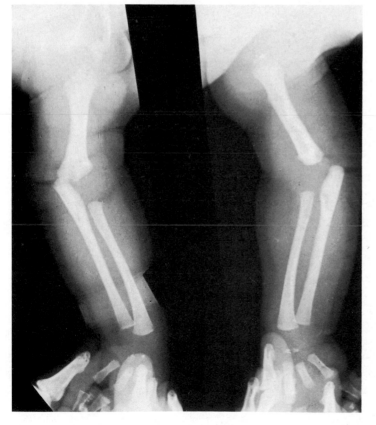

FIG. 4–41. Chondrodystrophia calcificans congenita (arms)—infant, 5 days of age. Note stippled calcification of the proximal humeral epiphyseal ossification center, a small stippled calcification in the capitulum, and stippled carpal ossification centers. This represents precocious appearance as well as stippling.

and vertebrae may be involved; the mandible and clavicle are not. Wormian bones may also be seen (Fig. 4–43). Universal coronal cleft vertebrae as well as hemivertebrae, butterfly vertebrae, and scoliosis have been reported in association with this condition. Stippling of the vertebral body may also be seen at birth (Fig. 4–44). Atlantoaxial dislocation has been reported, with death occurring due to cord compression.[2] Bilateral femoral artery calcification has also been observed.

The punctate stippling is finer than the fragmented epiphyses seen in cretinism or mutiple epiphyseal dysplasia.

CEREBROHEPATORENAL SYNDROME OF ZELLWEGER

The cerebrohepatorenal syndrome of Zellweger[95, 100] consists of flaccidity, abnormal facies, cataracts, flexion contractures, small cortical renal cysts, and liver fibrosis. Bone changes are said to be pathognomonic, consisting of a stippled acetabular "Y" cartilage and a stippled scimitar-shaped calcification of the inferior margin of the patella. Calcifications of the hyoid bone and thyroid cartilages may also be present. Dolichocephaly and wormian bones are also seen, as well as deformities of the hands and feet. Bone maturation is retarded. Seizures occur, and the patients generally die in infancy. The pattern of stippling is similar to that seen in chondrodystrophia calcificans congenita; however, the epiphyses are not affected. The term *Conradi's disease* has been proposed to designate a spectrum of epiphyseal stippling with or without other organic defects. This condition may possibly lie in that spectrum.

MULTIPLE EPIPHYSEAL DYPLASIA

Multiple epiphyseal dysplasia[28,35,57] (Fairbank's disease) is considered by Rubin[102] to be the tarda form of chondrodystrophia calcificans congenita. Fairbank considers it to be a distinct entity. The roentgen characteristic is an irregular, mottled ossification of the epiphyses. Maturition is delayed. The findings are bilateral and symmetrical.

Clinically, the disease has not been seen either in neonates or in infants. The earliest onset is 3 years of age and most cases are in the 5- to 14-year age groups. Some of the reported cases have a familial tendency. There may be mild dwarfism of the short-limb type. Chief complaints are pain and stiffness of the hips and knees. Flexion deformities and coxa

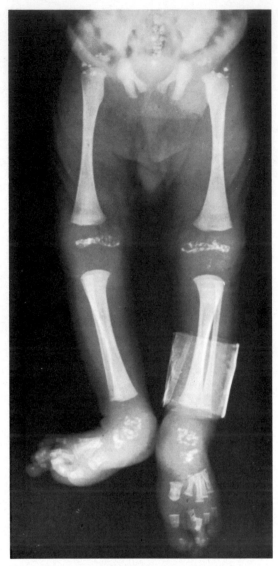

FIG. 4–42. Chondrodystrophia calcificans congenita (lower extremities)—infant. Note stippled calcific ossification centers of the sacrum, femoral heads, greater trochanters, distal femora, and tarsus. The distal femoral ossification centers have a tendency to coalesce.

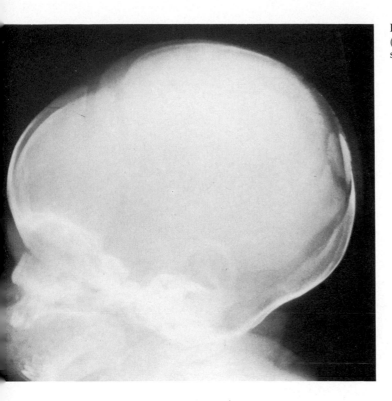

FIG. 4–43. Chondrodystrophia calcificans congenita (skull)—female, age 5 days. Wormian bones may be seen.

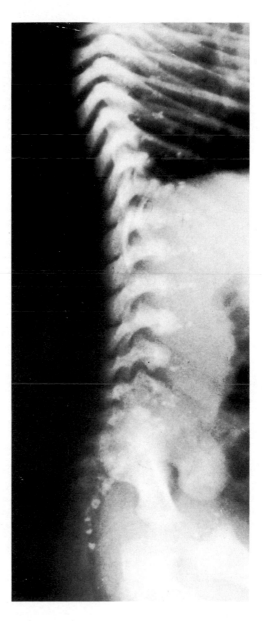

vara may be present. Early and severe degenerative arthritis occurs, owing to epiphyseal deformities. The laboratory values are usually within normal limits.

Radiologically, there is bilateral symmetrical irregularity and mottling of the epiphyseal ossification centers without sclerosis. The appearance and growth of the center are delayed, but the time of fusion is usually normal. Associated metaphyseal irregularity may occasionally occur. Involvement of the primary ossification centers of the carpals and tarsals is common.

The sites most frequently involved are the hips (Fig. 4–45), knees (Fig. 4–46), and ankles; the shoulders, wrists, and elbows show the least involvement. A deficiency of the lateral aspect of the distal tibial epiphysis, producing a tibiotalar slant, is a common deformity in this disease (Fig. 4–47). This

FIG. 4–44. Chondrodystrophia calcificans congenita (spine)—female, age 5 days. Note stippled calcifications of the vertebral bodies (particularly at the anterior aspects), and stippled calcifications of the femoral capital epiphyses.

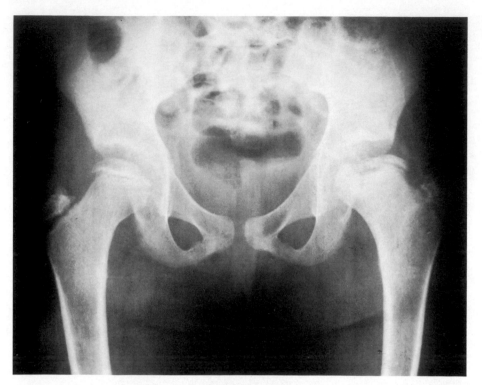

FIG. 4–45. Multiple epiphyseal dysplasia or Fairbank's disease (pelvis and hips). Note irregularity of the epiphyseal ossification centers of the femoral heads and of the greater trochanters. Flattening of the left femoral capital epiphysis is also present. The changes are somewhat similar to those occurring in Legg-Perthes' disease. Involvement of other ossification centers and age of onset establishes the diagnosis.

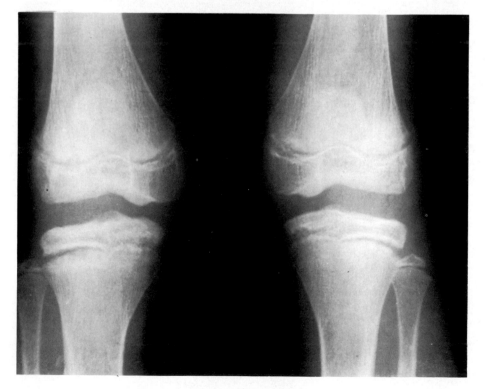

FIG. 4–46. Multiple epiphyseal dysplasia or Fairbank's disease (knees)—same patient as in Fig. 4–45. Irregularities of the epiphyses with slight associated metaphyseal irregularities are noted.

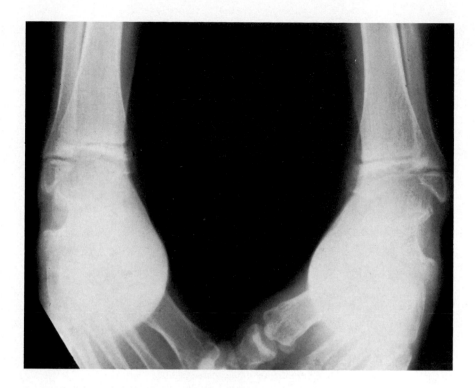

FIG. 4–47. Multiple epiphyseal dysplasia or Fairbank's disease (ankles). Note irregularity of the distal tibial epiphyses, bilaterally and symmetrically, with deficiency of the ossification center at the lateral aspects. This results in a tibio-talar slant.

is also seen in hemophilia and juvenile rheumatoid arthritis. The skull, mandible, clavicles, ribs, scapula, and sternum are not involved. Short stubby digits and metacarpals are also sometimes present, but the feet are less frequently involved. The vertebrae are usually normal; however, the following changes have been reported:

1. Hemivertebra
2. Osteochondrosis
3. Platyspondyly
4. Irregular surfaces with Schmorl's nodes
5. Anterior wedging
6. Anterior rounding of edges
7. Narrowing of intervertebral disk spaces
8. Osteoarthrosis of the spine

In the adult, residual epiphyseal irregularities and degenerative joint changes are most commonly seen, and less frequently, bone shortening. The conditions associated with irregular epiphyses are summarized below.

CONDITIONS ASSOCIATED WITH IRREGULARITIES OR STIPPLING OF THE EPIPHYSEAL OSSIFICATION CENTERS

1. Cretinism
2. Osteochondroses or ischemic necroses
3. Pituitary giantism

4. Chondrodystrophia calcificans congenita
5. Multiple epiphyseal dysplasia
6. Osteopoikilosis ⎫
7. Osteopetrosis ⎭ with sclerosis

A classification of multiple epiphyseal dysplasias[4] follows.

CLASSIFICATION OF THE MULTIPLE EPIPHYSEAL DYSPLASIAS (MED)*

Multiple epiphyseal dysplasia congenita (MEDC)
1. MEDC I (short wrist)
2. MEDC II (stunted growth and mild skeletal changes)
3. MEDC III (stunted growth, rhizomelia, "saddle nose")
4. MEDC IV (ectodermal dysplasia, scoliosis, short legs)
5. MEDC V (mental retardation, cataracts, early death)

Multiple epiphyseal dysplasia tarda (MEDT)
1. Type I (lower limb, spine, and upper limb involvement)
   A. Fairbanks MEDT

*Modified from Bailey JA: Disproportionate Short Stature. Diagnosis and Management. Philadelphia, WB Saunders, 1973.

    B. Pseudoachondroplastic form of MEDT
    C. Ribbing's MEDT (particularly in greater trochanter)
    D. Maroteaux's MEDT
    E. Juberg's MEDT
2. Type II (lower limb and spine involvement)
    A. Weinberg's MEDT
3. Type III (lower limb and upper limb involvement)
    A. Thiemann's diease
    B. Dietrich's disease
    C. Elbow-knee MEDT
    D. Elsbach's dysplasia
4. Type IV (lower limb involvement)
    A. Orkel's MEDT

DYSPLASIA EPIPHYSEALIS HEMIMELICA

Dysplasia epiphysealis hemimelica[65] (Trevor's disease) is a rare unilateral asymmetrical hyperplasia of the epiphyses leading to swelling, deformities, and functional impairment of the involved joints. The knees and ankles are most commonly involved, limitation of motion, knock-knee, bowed legs, and flat feet. The patient may complain of pain and "locking" of the knee. Regional muscular atrophy has been reported.

    Radiologically, the lesion is limited to one-half of the epiphysis. There may be irregular cartilage overgrowth or an epiphyseal osteocartilaginous exostosis (Fig. 4–48). Rarely, the affected limb may be longer or shorter than normal with varus or valgus deformity. The most frequent sites of involvement are the talus, the distal femur, and the distal tibia. This condition may very rarely be associated with a variety of cartilaginous tumors, including intracapsular chondroma, extraskeletal osteochondroma, and typical osteochondroma.[52]

EPIPHYSEAL DYSOSTOSIS

Epiphyseal dysostosis[98,113] without dwarfism is a rare hereditary syndrome with peripheral changes somewhat similar to those of diastrophic dwarfism (see Chap. 5), but without shortening of stature, scoliosis, or dislocations. This disorder is characterized by multiple deformities of the hands and feet. Brachydactyly with asymmetrical short phalanges and metacarpals, accessory ossification centers, and deformities may be seen. The spine may show fusions of vertebral bodies and arches, irregularities of end-plates, and narrowing of the lumbar interpedicular distances. Shallow acetabula and bulbous femoral heads may also be present.

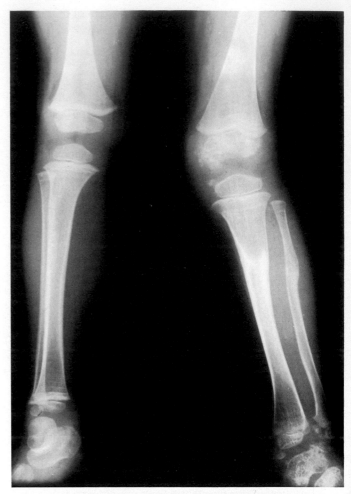

FIG. 4–48. Dysplasia epiphysealis hemimelica or Trevor's disease (lower extremities)—unilateral involvement. Osteotomy has been performed on the involved side. There is hyperplasia of the medial distal femoral ossification center, the medial distal fibular ossification center, and the ossification center of the talus. A small area of calcification medial to the proximal tibial ossification center may also be seen.

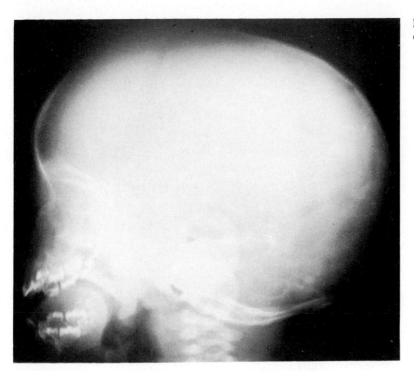

FIG. 4–49. Rickets (skull). Marked thinning of the calvarium is noted.

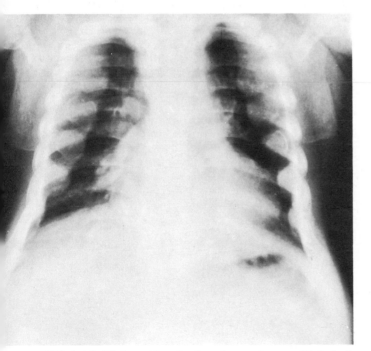

FIG. 4–50. Rickets (chest) — female, age 2 years. Note bulbous widening of the distal ends of the ribs to form the "rachitic rosary." Periosteal elevation and new bone formation of the shafts of the ribs may also be seen.

DISEASES MANIFESTED BY ROENTGEN CHANGES AT THE METAPHYSIS

RICKETS

Rickets[15,93,114] is a systemic disease of infancy and childhood in which the calcification of growing skeletal elements is deficient. It is the equivalent of osteomalacia (see Chap. 2) in the mature skeleton. Prematurity is a predisposing factor.

Clinically, infantile vitamin D-deficient rickets usually develops between 6 months and 1 year of age. It may rarely be seen at birth in children of osteomalacic mothers. Softening of the skull bones, or craniotabes, may be present initially (Fig. 4–49), followed by frontal and parietal bossing in later stages of the disease. Premature fusion of cranial sutures may occur. The ribs show enlargement of the costochondral junctions — the "rachitic rosary" (Fig. 4–50). Epiphyseal swellings and limb deformities are present. Increased irritability and sweating also occur.

The serum calcium level ranges from normal to slightly lowered and the serum phosphorus concentration is slightly lowered. The serum alkaline phosphatase level is elevated.

Radiologically, the characteristic changes occur in the ends of the long bones; these changes are similar for rickets of all etiologies. Normal calcification of cartilage matrix is lacking in the zone of provisional calcification of the epiphyseal cartilage plate. Cartilage cells continue to proliferate in an irregular manner. This may be seen as widening of the epiphyseal plate and irregularity of the provisional zone of calcification (Fig. 4–51). Uncalcified osteoid is also present, causing softening of the bone. Metaphyseal cupping and widening then follows, due to the pull of muscular and ligamentous attachments (Fig. 4–52). Cupping is not pathognomonic of rickets; it may occur in other diseases and as a normal variant in early life. The changes are most marked in the sternal ends of the ribs, the proximal tibia and humerus, and the distal radius and ulna. Changes in the ulna often develop before changes in the radius.

In the shafts of long bones, uncalcified subperiosteal osteoid is present, causing the loss of the sharp cortical outline (Fig. 4–53), and allowing the development of bowing deformities, particularly in the tibia. Bone texture is also coarsened. Greenstick fractures are common (Fig. 4–54). Pseudofractures are rarely present (Fig. 4–55). The appearance of ossification centers in the epiphyses and small bones is delayed because of the lack of calcification. The ossification centers may regress during the active stage of rickets. They are poorly marginated. The iliac crests may show irregular mineralization. Concavity of the inferior border of the scapula, rather than its normal convex contour, may also be seen.[119]

Healing changes begin with mineralization of the zone of provisional calcification (Fig. 4–56), which widens. It appears as a dense line in the epiphyseal cartilage separated from the metaphysis. The cupping increases. Remineralization of subperiosteal osteoid appears as periosteal new bone formation, which may be solid or laminated (Fig. 4–57). The ribs may also show this finding. Calcification of ossification centers occurs with a marginal ring shadow that eventually fuses with the center.

Although complete healing usually occurs, residual deformities may persist (Fig. 4–58). Severe residual pelvic deformities may cause dystocia in the female. Metaphyseal zones of increased density and undertubulation sometimes persist as residual changes.

Juvenile rickets presents with changes basically similar to those of infantile rickets, showing metaphyseal irregularities and widening of the physis (Fig. 4–59). The various etiologies of rickets cannot be differentiated by the roentgen pattern (Figs. 4–60, 4–61), except in the glomerular type of renal rickets, in which changes of secondary hyper-

(Text continued on p. 210)

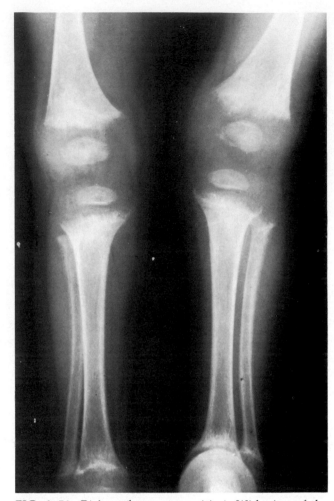

FIG. 4–51. Rickets (lower extremities). Widening of the epiphyseal cartilage plate and irregular mineralization of the zone of provisional calcification, causing "fraying," are prominent. Note bowing deformities caused by softening of the bone and loss of sharp outline of the proximal fibular cortices. Metaphyseal cupping at the distal ends is also visible.

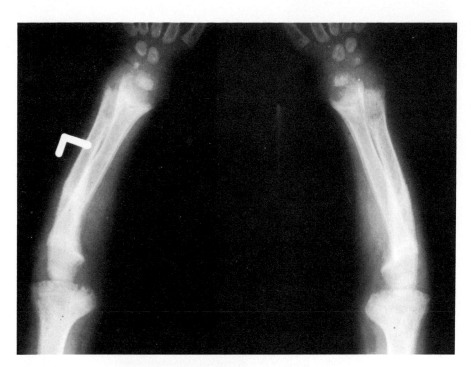

FIG. 4–52. Rickets (forearms and wrists). Note marked metaphyseal cupping of both distal radius and ulna, and loss of definition of the distal radial epiphyseal ossification center. Pseudofractures of the midshafts of both ulnae are present, and there is a solid type of periosteal reaction.

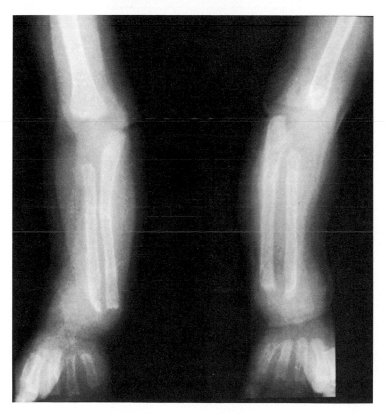

FIG. 4–53. Biliary rickets (upper extremities). There is loss of sharp cortical outline and marked deossification of bone due to both osteomalacic and osteoporotic processes. No secondary ossification centers are visible. Note apparent radial carpal subluxations and greenstick fracture of the midshaft of the right ulna.

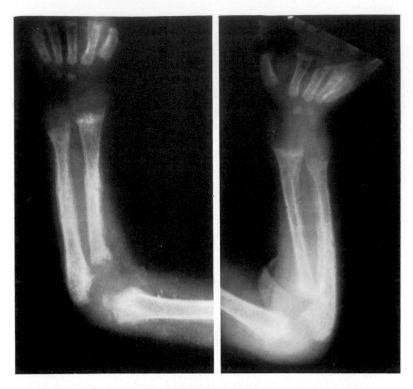

FIG. 4-54. Rickets (forearms and wrists). Note greenstick fracture of the distal left radius, and pseudofractures in both ulnae and in the right midradial shaft. Loss of bone density, metaphyseal cupping and fraying, and periosteal reaction may also be seen.

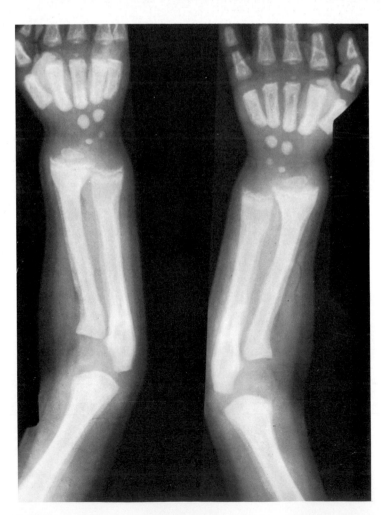

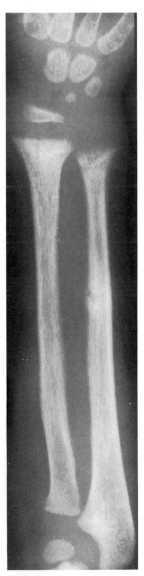

FIG. 4-55

FIG. 4-56

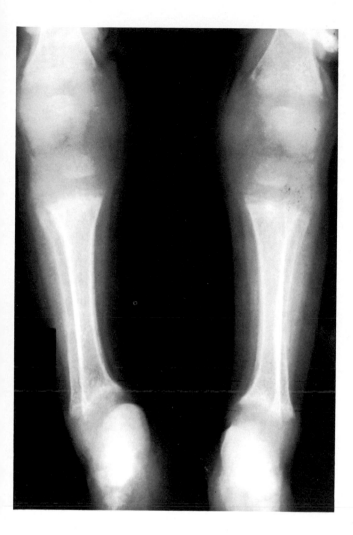

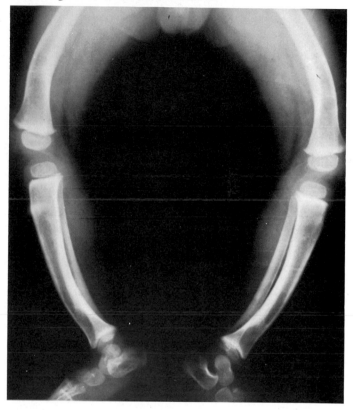

FIG. 4–57. Rickets (legs)—active stage. A laminated or "onionskin" type of periosteal new bone formation at the medial aspects of both tibiae may be seen. Note the characteristic signs of rickets, including metaphyseal fraying, widening of the epiphyseal cartilage plate, cupping, and bowing of the distal tibiae.

FIG. 4–58. Rickets (lower extremities). Note residual deformity, marked bowing of legs, and zones of increased density at the metaphyses. Cortical thickening along the sides of greatest stress is also visible.

FIG. 4–55. Rickets (forearm and wrist)—female, age 5 years. A pseudofracture at the distal third of the shaft of the ulna may be seen. There is marked widening of the epiphyseal cartilage plate at the distal radius.

FIG. 4–56. Rickets (upper extremities)—healing stage. There is mineralization of the zone of provisional calcification in the distal radii and ulnae, which is separated from the metaphyses by a radiolucent area. Widening and cupping of the metaphyses are also visible, and periosteal new bone formation is present in the long bones and metacarpals. A marginal condensation of density about the secondary ossification centers of the distal radii may be seen.

207

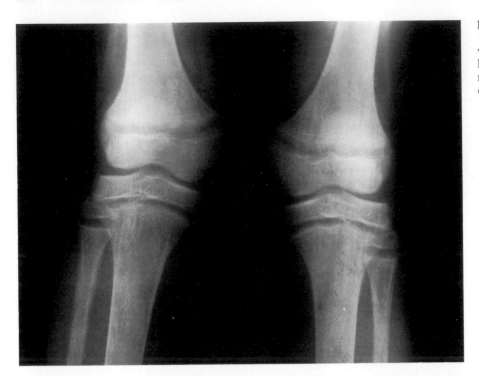

FIG. 4–59. Vitamin D deficiency —juvenile rickets (knees). Note widening of the epiphyseal cartilage plate, lack of definition of the metaphyses, and loss of bone density.

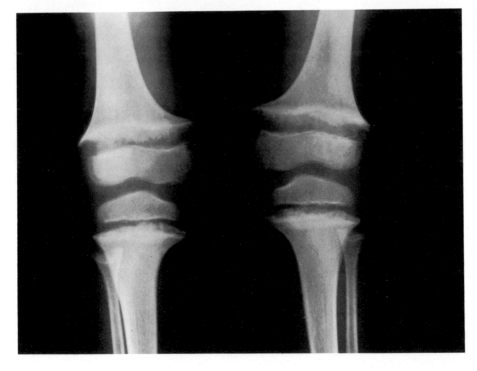

FIG. 4–60. Vitamin D-resistant rickets (knees). There are widening of the epiphyseal cartilage plate and metaphyseal irregularity.

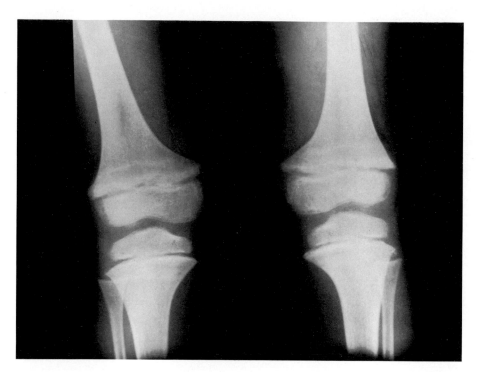

FIG. 4–61. Vitamin D-resistant rickets (knees) — same patient as in Fig. 4–60, 3 months later, after intensive treatment with high dosage of vitamin D. There has been remineralization of the epiphyseal cartilage plate, with mild residual metaphyseal irregularities. The bone density appears normal.

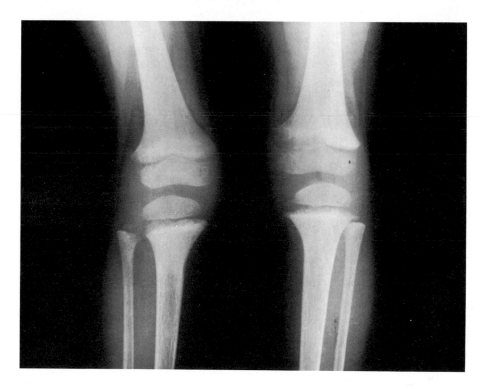

FIG. 4–62. Renal glomerular rickets (knees). Note widening of the epiphyseal cartilage plate, with metaphyseal irregularity. In addition, there is loss of cortex of the upper medial aspects of both tibiae due to subperiosteal resorption from secondary hyperparathyroidism. Loss of bone density and slight accentuation of the trabecular pattern may also be seen.

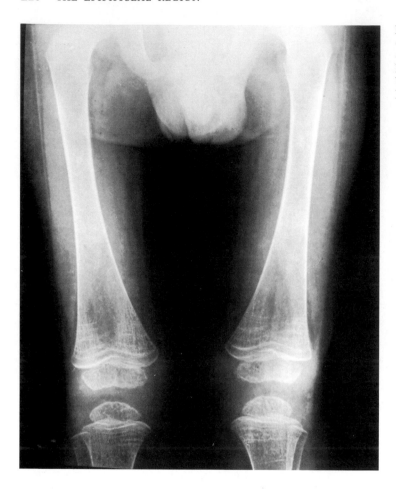

FIG. 4–63. Celiac disease (lower extremities). The cortex is thinned and there is marked loss of bone density. The metaphyses are relatively dense. Nonspecific multiple transverse metaphyseal bands are visible. Note sparsity of bone trabeculae.

parathyroidism are superimposed (Fig. 4–62). In biliary disease or celiac disease (Fig. 4–63), osteoporosis may be concurrent.

BILIARY ATRESIA

Biliary atresia is a congenital malformation of the bile ducts. It occurs in two forms, extrahepatic and the much less common intrahepatic form.

EXTRAHEPATIC BILIARY ATRESIA

Patients with *extrahepatic biliary atresia*, or congenital absence of the biliary system, have clinical features of progressive obstructive jaundice, hepatosplenomegaly, gastrointestinal bleeding, and cachexia. Rickets is frequently seen during the period of rapid growth, commonly in the second half of the first year. Marked osteoporosis, thin cortices with prominent bone trabeculae, and multiple fractures may also be seen. Spiculated periosteal

new bone formation has been reported.[64] Undertubulation with a widened medullary cavity and square-shaped femoral necks also occur. The condition usually terminates fatally within 1 or 2 years, unless it is corrected surgically.

INTRAHEPATIC BILIARY ATRESIA

Intrahepatic biliary atresia,[5] or congenital absence of the intrahepatic bile ducts, is a rare anomaly. The defect may be caused by a progressive loss of intrahepatic bile ducts owing to preductal bile stasis. *Clinically,* early obstructive jaundice is present, with elevation of the serum lipids, cutaneous xanthoma, pruritis, and later hypersplenism and portal hypertension. These patients live longer than patients with extrahepatic biliary atresia.

A specific roentgen picture is claimed for this condition.[5] The skeleton is normal at birth, and shows progressive loss of density. Lack of normal modeling results in "Erlenmeyer flask" deformities

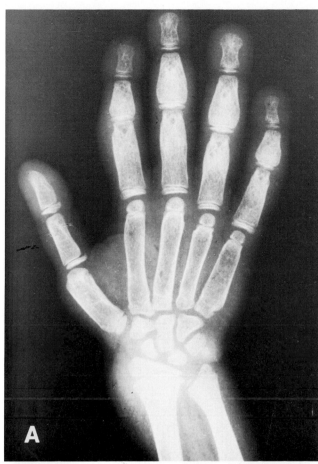

A

and widening of the shafts of long and short bones. Marked swellings about joints, particularly the knees, is seen, resulting from hemarthrosis. Periosteal new bone formation may also be present owing to subperiosteal hemorrhage. Growth and maturation are retarded. Rickets is not a prominent feature of this disorder, possibly because the patients do not show periods of rapid growth. Esophageal varices occur in about one-half of patients. The skull remains normal. Pathological fractures may occur.

Although these features are claimed to be specific, we have observed an identical clinical and radiological picture in a patient who had proven extrahepatic biliary atresia and survived to the age of 12 years (Fig. 4–64). This case suggests that the ensuing picture depends upon the length of survival rather than the specific site of obstruction of the biliary tree.

TYROSINOSIS

Tyrosinosis, an inborn error of tyrosine metabolism, results from the absence of the enzyme p-hydroxyphenylpyruvic oxidase. P-hydroxyphenylpyruvic

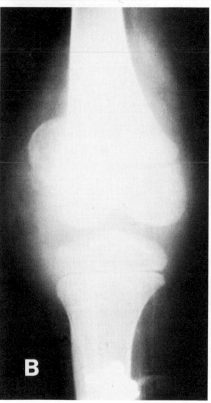

B

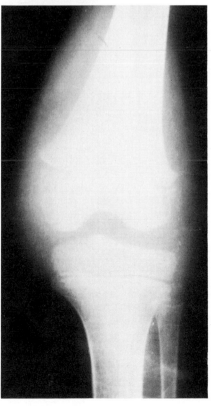

FIG. 4–64. Biliary atresia. A. Hand. Autopsy-proven extrahepatic biliary atresia with findings usually attributed to intrahepatic biliary atresia; bulbous widening of the phalanges is seen, with loss of density and accentuation of the trabecular pattern. Soft-tissue swelling, particularly about the wrist joint, is noted. The epiphyseal cartilage plates are not markedly widened. B. Knees. There is marked swelling of the soft tissues about the knee joint due to hemarthrosis. Only minimal widening of the epiphyseal cartilage plates is present.

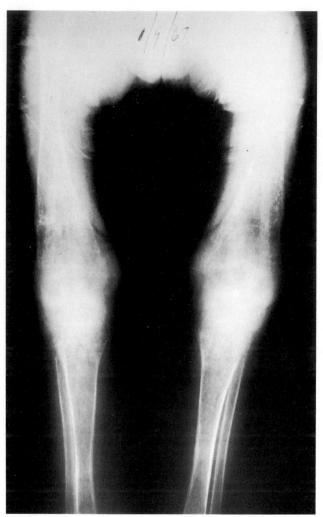

FIG. 4–65. Tyrosinosis (lower extremities). A severe rachitic picture is apparent, with marked loss of bone density about the knees, widening of the epiphyseal cartilage plate, and loss of bone definition. Underconstriction in the distal femora may also be noted.

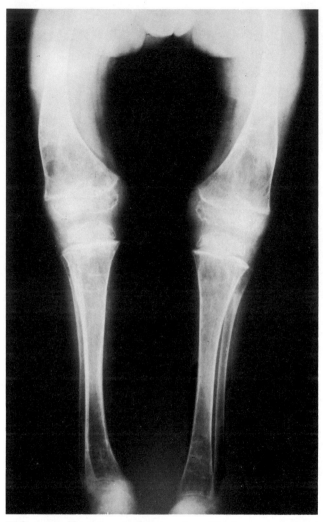

FIG. 4–66. Tyrosinosis (lower extremities)—same patient as in Fig. 4–65, 13 months later, after treatment. Note restoration of definition of bone and return of epiphyseal cartilage plate to normal width. There are residual loss of bone density, residual bowing of the distal femora, and residual underconstriction at this site.

FIG. 4–67. Scurvy (wrist), early changes. There is loss of bone density, with "ground glass" appearance of the distal radius and ulna. Minimal spurring at the margins of the ulnar metaphysis (Pelken's sign) may be noted. Also note increased density at the metaphyses, indicating slight widening of the zone of provisional calcification. There is faint ring formation (Wimberger's sign) at the periphery of secondary ossification centers.

acid is present in the urine. *Clinically*, hepatosplenomegaly is present in early infancy. A Fanconi syndrome with phosphaturia and aminoaciduria is present. The disease is familial and is treated with a diet free of phenylalanine and tyrosine. *Radiologically*, a severe rachitic picture is present (Fig. 4–65, 4–66).

CYSTINOSIS

Cystinosis is a metabolic disease characterized by the abnormal accumulation of cystine in tissues and organs. This is a disease of children. Usually the patients die of renal failure in the first or second decade of life, owing to the deposition of cystine in the kidney. Early in the disease the principal bone changes are those of rickets. The thyroid gland also is a target organ for cystine crystal deposition. This leads to hypothyroidism with resultant retardation of skeletal growth and maturation.[46] If the patient is treated with thyroid hormone, the rickets previously controlled by vitamin D therapy may exacerbate because of the new growth spurt.

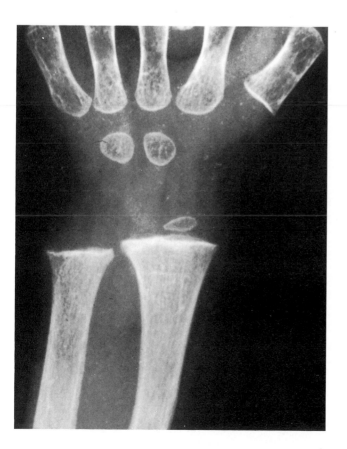

SCURVY

Scurvy[10,79,108] is the result of vitamin C deficiency. Infantile scurvy (Barlow's disease) is found in infants fed on pasteurized or boiled milk formulas, since the pasteurization and boiling processes destroy the vitamin C content. Scurvy is not seen under 3 months of age, and usually occurs in the 6-month to 2-year age group. It is much less frequently seen than rickets.

Clinically, there is progressive irritability. The legs are very tender and edematous and are held in the "frog position." Pseudoparalysis may be present. Subcutaneous and mucous membrane hemorrhages occur. Bulges at the costochondral junctions (rosary) and sternal depression are also present. A secondary anemia develops. Clinical improvement may begin 48 hours after initation of treatment.

Pathophysiologically, the basic defect is the inability of the supporting tissues to produce and maintain intercellular substances. This includes bone, cartilage, and vascular endothelium. Although bone formation ceases, absorption proceeds, resulting in osteoporosis. Osteoblasts assume the appearance of fibroblasts and proliferate subperiosteally forming a thick cellular layer in which hemorrhages occur.

Cartilage cells in the epiphyseal plate stop proliferating. Vascular invasion of the zone of provisional calcification is arrested. Cartilage mineralization is not arrested and, as a result, there is marked widening and density of the zone of provisional calcification. The margins of this zone project outward beyond the limits of bone to form spurs. Spurs are also formed by ossification at periosteal attachments owing to lifting of the periosteum by hemorrhages. The primary spongiosa of the metaphysis is sparse and is seen as a radiolucent stripe called the "scurvy line" or the Truemmerfeld zone (zone of debris). Fracture may occur at this site.

Radiologically, generalized osteoporosis and a "ground glass" appearance with cortical thinning are seen (Fig. 4–67). The earliest metaphyseal changes may be seen at the knees, followed shortly thereafter by changes at the ends of other long bones. There is widening and increased density of the zone of provisional calcification. Increased brittleness of this zone may result in infractions, giving the appearance of metaphyseal cupping, or longitudinal fractures. Marginal spur formation (Pelken's sign) occurs. A zone of radiolucency (Truemmerfeld zone) forms, giving the appearance of a double epiphysis. Separation at this zone occurs, resulting in displacement of an intact epiphysis and plate (Fig. 4–68). Healing occurs with little

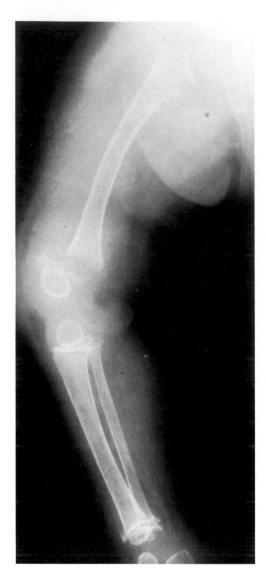

FIG. 4–68. Scurvy (lower extremity). Note submetaphyseal zones of radiolucency at the proximal femur and distal tibia, the so-called Truemmerfeld zone. There has been separation, with anterior displacement at the Truemmerfeld zone at the distal femoral metaphysis. Loss of bone density, "ground glass" appearance, Winberger's sign—or rings about the epiphyseal ossification centers—and Pelken's sign at the distal tibial metaphyses are well demonstrated.

FIG. 4–69. Scurvy (lower extremity)—healing changes with calcification of subperiosteal hemorrhages. Note cupping at the distal tibia and fibula, and Wimberger's sign.

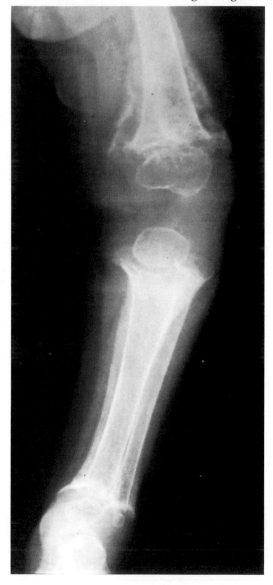

deformity after treatment. Initially, the Truemmerfeld zone may be present only at the margins (Corner sign). The epiphyseal ossification centers and the ossification centers of small bones show a dense marginal ring of calcification that is sharply demarcated (Wimberger's sign of scurvy). Large subperiosteal hemorrhages resulting in soft-tissue edema occur in later stages of the disease.

Upon healing, the subperiosteal hemorrhages clacify, beginning with a shell of subperiosteal bone (Figs. 4–69, 4–70, 4–71). When resorption of the hematoma occurs, this layer of bone thickens, blends with the cortex, and can persist as residual cortical thickening for many years. The metaphyseal fractures heal spontaneously. The zone of provisional calcification resumes normal width, and the bone resumes normal density. Premature fusion of the central portion of the epiphysis may result as a sequel to fracture with the appearance of a "ball-and-socket" formation that may later heal with minimal tenting of the intercondylar notch.

HYPOPHOSPHATASIA

Hypophosphatasia[21,34,102] is a metaphyseal dysplasia in which primary spongiosa fails to form. It is a genetically determined error of metabolism. Alkaline phosphatase activity is decreased, associated with a disturbance of normal bone formation. The defect has been localized to proliferating osteoblasts and hypertrophic chondrocytes.

Laboratory values are characterized by a low serum alkaline phosphate that can be about 25% of the normal low value. Hypercalcemia is present in severe cases in infants. The level of serum calcium may reach 14 mg%. Phosphorylethanolamine is constantly excreted in the urine, although this may be found also in patients with celiac disease and in some normal adults. Serum phosphorus levels are normal.

The pathological features are similar to those of rickets. There is an identical disturbance of enchondral bone formation in the epiphyseal cartilage plate. There is an excess of osteoid tissue, particularly subperiosteally. A deficiency of osteoblasts, which is believed to be a secondary phenomenon, is found.

Clinical features have been categorized into four age groups, with the most severe symptoms occurring in earlier life. Radiological appearance correlates with the four clinical groups.

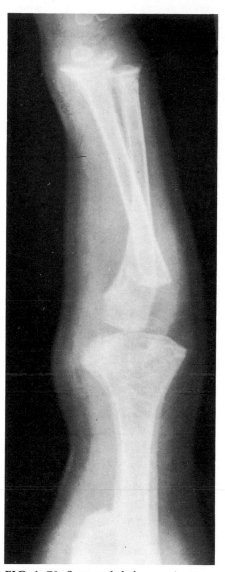

FIG. 4–70. Scurvy (left forearm)—same patient as in Fig. 4–69. Note Truemmerfeld zones at the distal radius and ulna, and increased density of the zone of provisional calcification. Calcification of subperiosteal hemorrhage, seen as lines of periosteal new bone formation, may also be noted. A large calcified hematoma at the midshaft of the humerus is present.

CONGENITAL NEONATAL HYPOPHOSPHATASIA

Stillbirth is common in this condition. Respiratory distress and cyanosis frequently occur. The skeleton is soft and severe deformities may be seen. Fever, convulsions, anorexia, vomiting, and constipation occasionally are present. Death may rapidly ensue. *Radiologically*, there may be extreme deficiency of bone mineralization, with only a minimal amount of calcification visible in the entire skeleton (Fig. 4–72). Long bones show cupping of the metaphyses and metaphyseal irregularities similar to those of rickets. The skull demonstrates a lack of ossification similar to that seen in osteogenesis imperfecta. A rachitic rosary, as well as fracture of the shafts of bone with abundant callus formation may be present.

INFANTILE HYPOPHOSPHATASIA

The infant with this condition not only fails to thrive, but also shows an actual loss of height and weight. Fever, irritability, cyanosis, and gastrointestinal symptoms occur. The sutures separate and the fontanelles bulge. Many patients may die, but if the infant survives, the clinical picture gradually improves. *Radiologically*, the changes are less severe than, but similar to, those of the neonatal form. Soft-tissue calcification due to hypercalcemia may also occur.

CHILDHOOD HYPOPHOSPHATASIA

These patients present with defective gait, short stature, and painful extremities. Rachitic rosary, enlarged bone ends, and defective dentition are also present, with early loss of deciduous teeth. Rarely, craniostenosis is seen. *Radiologically*, poorly calcified metaphyses (Fig. 4–73) with occasional large "punched-out" central defects of uncalcified osteoid are the features most diagnostic of this condition (Fig. 4–74). Bowing deformities and genu valgum are commonly observed. The skull may show changes of craniostenosis and increased intracranial pressure (Fig. 4–75), which can be associated with mental retardation.

ADULT HYPOPHOSPHATASIA[61]

The mildest changes are found in this group. Increased bone fragility, decreased stature, and bone deformities are seen. An "Erlenmeyer flask" deformity may also be present. Pseudofractures and bowing of the femora are present, as well as cortical thickening and multiple fractures at various sites.

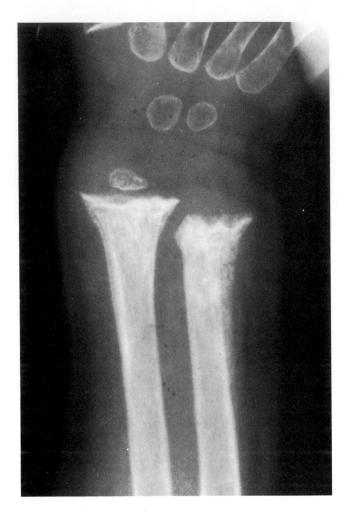

The spine shows calcification of the spinal ligaments, and Schmorl's nodes. Scoliosis and posterior scalloping of the vertebral bodies have been reported, as well as narrowing of the intervertebral spaces. The biochemical findings of low serum alkaline phosphatase and phosphorylethanolamine in the urine establish the diagnosis. A previous rachitic history may be elicited. Early tooth loss may occur.

METAPHYSEAL DYSOSTOSIS (METAPHYSEAL CHONDRODYSPLASIA)

Metaphyseal dysostosis[22,38,60,84] is a rare cartilage dysplasia characterized by cupping, spreading, and defective irregular mineralization of the metaphyses of the tubular bones. The term describes several different and probably unrelated conditions

FIG. 4–71. Scurvy (forearm and wrist) —healing stage. Note spurring, or Pelken's sign, at the distal radius and ulna, increased metaphyseal density, and calcification of subperiosteal hemorrhage, particularly at the distal ulna.

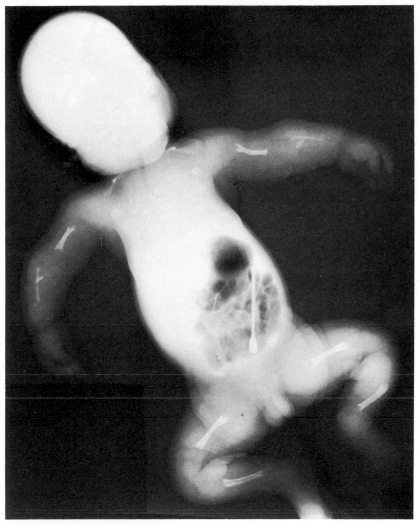

FIG. 4–72. Congenital neonatal hypophosphatasia. There is extreme lack of mineralization of the entire skeleton.

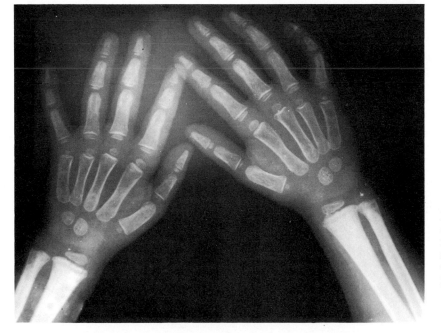

FIG. 4–73. Childhood hypophosphatasia (wrists). Note bilateral radiolucent submetaphyseal bands, and radiolucent defects in the metaphyses of the distal ulnae. Loss of density of the bones of the hand is apparent.

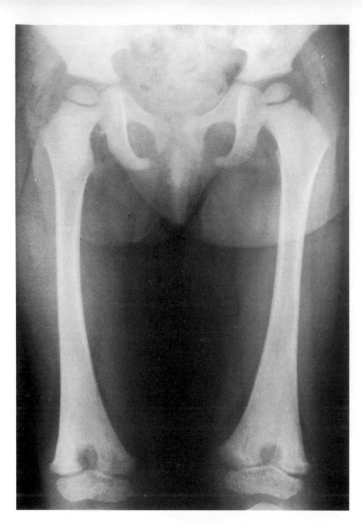

FIG. 4–74. Hypophosphatasia (femora) — same patient as in Fig. 4–13. Note large central, lytic, metaphyseal, "punched-out" defects in the distal femora, bilaterally and symmetrically; this is the most pathognomonic feature of hypophosphatasia. Minimal submetaphyseal radiolucent bands in the proximal femoral metaphyses may also be noted. Bone density of the pelvis and femora appears normal.

FIG. 4–75. Hypophosphatasia (skull). Premature fusion of the cranial sutures with resultant increased intracranial pressure, as evidenced by the "beaten copper" effect, is noted. (Courtesy of Dr. Harvey White, Children's Memorial Hospital, Chicago, IL)

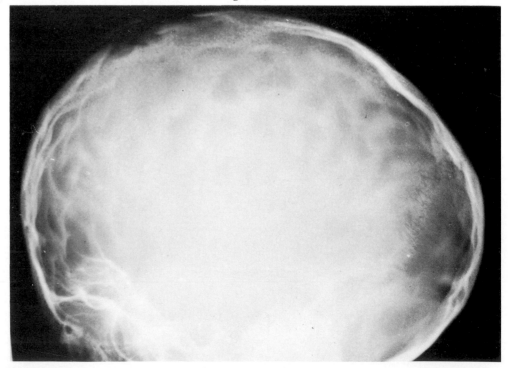

TABLE 4–3. Classification of Metaphyseal Dysostoses (Chondrodysplasia)*

Types of Metaphyseal Chondrodysplasia

Name of 1st Describing Author	Incidence	Heredity	Growth Retardation	Bony Changes			
				Distribution	Severity	Coxa Vara	Vertebrae
Jansen, 1934	Extremely rare	?	++	Generalized	+++	+	+
Schmid, 1949	Relatively frequent	Autosomal dominant	+ +	Generalized (extremities)	+–++	+ (Typical)	–
Spahr, 1961	?	Autosomal recessive ?	+	Generalized (extremities)	+–++	+	–
Maroteaux, 1963 (Partial form)	Relatively frequent ?	Autosomal recessive	++	Mainly knee	(+)–+	–	–
McKusick, 1964 (Cartilage-hair hypoplasia [CHH])	"Amish" 0.1–0.2% (gastrointestinal symptoms)	Autosomal recessive	++	Mainly knee	+	–	–
Burke et al, 1967 (Pancreatic insufficiency, chronic neutropenia and dysostosis)	?	?	+	Mainly knees and ribs	+	–	–
Kozlowski, 1962 ("Intermediate type")	Rare	?	+	Generalized epimetaphyseal mixed form	++	–	–
Sutcliffe (Case 3, 1965) (Spondylometaphyseal dysostosis)	Rare	?	?	Generalized epimetaphyseal	++	+	+
Schmidt, 1963 (Spondylometaphyseal dysostosis)	Rare	?	+	Variable	+–++	+	++
Kozlowski et al, 1966 (Spondylometaphyseal dysostosis)	Rare	?	+	Generalized	++	+	+

(Also described by Rimoin, Davis, Schwachman, Pena, Murdock)

* Modified from Giedion A et al: Fortschr Roentgenstr 108:51–57, 1968

having only some radiological features in common. Radiographic similarities to rickets or achondroplasia are typical. There are several forms; the severe form (Jansen type)[90] is extremely rare. It can lead to rhizomelic dwarfism, severe deformity and disability, and early death. The milder form (Schmid type)[105] is more common. Only the metaphyses of the major long bones show involvement. Reduced stature may result. A partial form (Maroteaux type) has also been reported, which is identical to cartilage-hair hypoplasia (McKusick type). Metaphyseal dysostosis may be associated with the syndrome of exocrine pancreatic insufficiency and chronic neutropenia. The Spahr form is recessive, with features similar to those of the Schmid (dominant) type. A classification of metaphyseal dysostoses[38] is presented in Table 4–3.

Pathologically, the metaphysis is composed of irregular masses of cartilage without column formation. Hypertrophied cartilage cells are found in peripheral clusters. No excess osteoid is present.

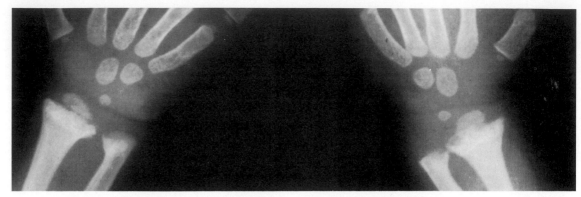

FIG. 4–76. Metaphyseal dysostosis (wrists)—Schmid type. Irregularity in outline and calcification of the distal radial and ulnar metaphyses may be seen. The epiphyseal ossification centers and carpal ossification centers appear normal. Bone density of the shafts of the distal radius and ulna is maintained. There is no evidence of periosteal new bone formation.

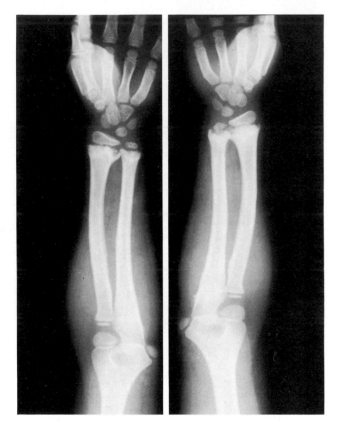

FIG. 4–77. Metaphyseal dysostosis (wrists)—same patient as in Fig. 4–76, 3½ years later. The secondary and carpal ossification centers appear normal. Cupping of the distal metaphyses of the radius and ulna may be noted. The metaphyses of the short tubular bones, and those about the elbow, appear normal. Irregular mineralization of the involved metaphyses is present. The irregularity of mineralization and cupping are more pronounced than in earlier pictures.

Radiologically, the tubular bones show metaphyseal cupping, radiolucent streaking, and sometimes stippled calcification (Figs. 4–76, 4–77, 4–78, 4–79). This epiphysis appears normal but its ossification may be delayed. The diaphysis has a normal texture and caliber, but is shortened. The pelvis

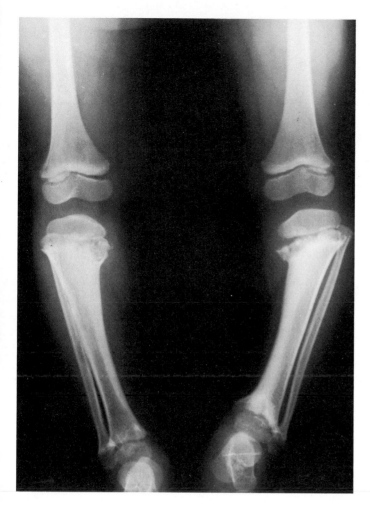

FIG. 4–78. Metaphyseal dysostosis (lower extremities). There is minimal involvement of the distal femoral metaphyses. There is marked irregularity of contour and mineralization of the proximal tibial metaphyses, with bilateral genu vara. The medial aspects of the tibial metaphyses appear more involved. There are metaphyseal irregularity and cupping of the distal tibial metaphyses. The cupping is more marked on the left.

FIG. 4–79. Metaphyseal dysostosis (lower extremities)—same patient as in Fig. 4–78, 5 years later, following bilateral osteotomies. There has been marked improvement in the appearance of the tibial metaphyses. The alignment of the legs has been corrected. Metaphyseal irregularities are greatest at the distal tibial and fibular metaphyses.

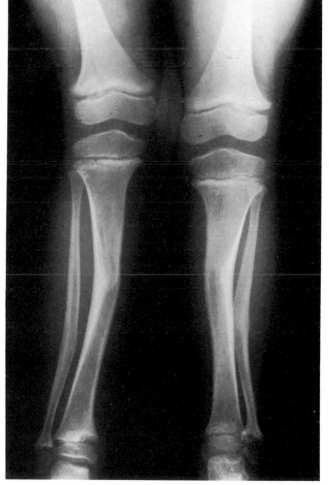

may be hypoplastic with cystic changes. Coxa vara with resorption of the femoral necks is sometimes present (Fig. 4–80). The rib ends show changes similar to those of the long bones (Fig. 4–81), and the shafts may be deformed. The cuboid bones and spine are usually normal. In the skull, the calvarium is normal but the base is underdeveloped. The joints show flexion deformities, particularly in the hips, knees, and ankles.

The mild forms may show only metaphyseal cupping and irregularities similar to those of rickets and hypophosphatasia. The epiphyseal ossification centers are normal and sharply outlined. This factor serves as a differential point from rickets.

The patient originally described by Jansen at the age of 10½ years was reexamined at the age of 44 years. The bones had developed to normal texture, but there was marked deformity and dwarfing. Joint surfaces remained intact.[22]

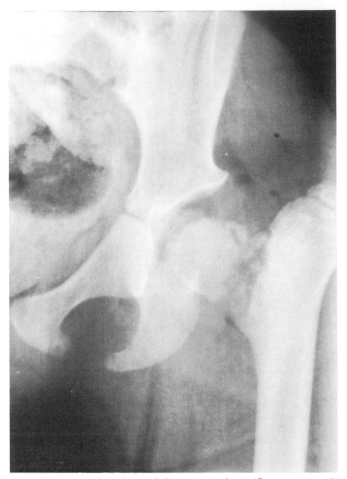

FIG. 4–80. Metaphyseal dysostosis (hip). Coxa vara with resorption of the femoral neck is noted.

PHENYLKETONURIA

Phenylketonuria[27] is a genetically determined error of metabolism in which a deficiency of the enzyme phenylalanine hydroxylase in the liver prevents the conversion of phenylalanine to tyrosine. Phenylalanine accumulates in the blood and, together with its metabolites, is excreted in the urine. Deamination produces the keto acid phenylpyruvic acid that, when conjugated with glutamine,[48] is prominent in the urine. A defect in tryptophan metabolism may also be involved. Tyrosine metabolism is reduced, leading to underproduction of melanin, which accounts for the light complexions of these patients.

Clinically, the incidence is about 1 in 50,000 births. About 1% of mental defectives in state institutions are affected with phenylketonuria. The majority of patients are light-complexioned, blond-haired and blue-eyed, and were normal at birth.

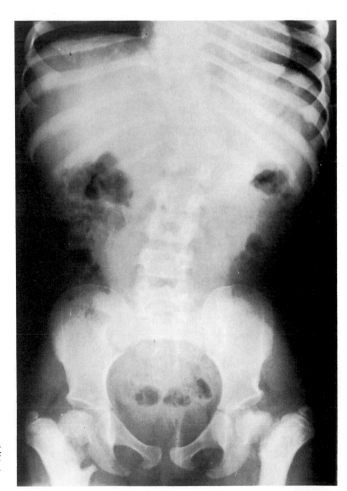

FIG. 4–81. Metaphyseal dysostosis. The ends of the ribs show widening and fraying. Note congenital scoliosis with hemivertebrae, and bilateral coxa vara with resorption of the femoral necks. The iliac wings do not show normal flaring.

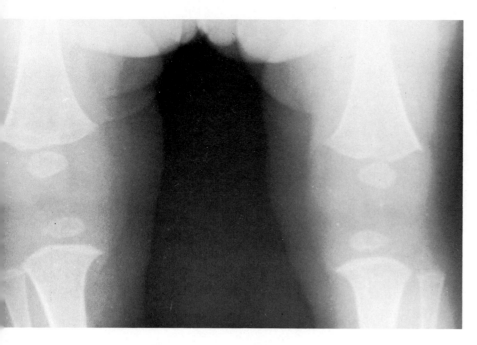

Profound mental retardation is the rule, although 1% of patients are mentally normal. Eczema and convulsions occur, decreasing with age. Biochemical changes can be detected at 3 to 6 days of age.

Radiologically, cupping and beaking of the distal metaphyses of the radius and ulna are present (Fig. 4–82). Fine opaque spicules project from the metaphysis into epiphyseal cartilage (Fig. 4–83). With growth, spicules continue to form and the original portions are incorporated into the osseous metaphysis. Remnants of these may be found in the metaphysis as striations. The zone of provisional calcification is not demineralized, thus differentiating this process from rickets.

There is no evidence to show that the changes seen radiographically are caused by the therapeutic diet rather than the disease process.

BATTERED CHILD SYNDROME[55,109]

Traumatic metaphyseal fragmentation and cortical thickening without fractures or dislocations should be considered in the differential diagnosis of metaphyseal lesions, even in the absence of a history of trauma. These are common findings and they do not represent deliberate trauma to the infant in all instances. Some cases may be due to birth injury.

In infants, the periosteum and perichondrium are tightly attached at the terminal end of the metaphysis, and loosely attached to the shaft. This arrangement permits large and frequent subperiosteal

FIG. 4–83. Phenylketonuria (wrist). Cupping with several small, ill-defined bony projections into the epiphyseal cartilage plate may be seen. (Courtesy of Dr. Harvey White, Children's Memorial Hospital, Chicago, IL)

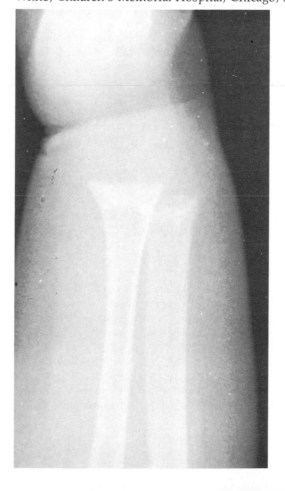

hemorrhages in this age group. Metaphyseal fragmentation can be seen immediately following trauma.

Roentgen findings consist of metaphyseal fragmentation at the periphery of the cartilage-shaft junctions (Figs. 4–84, 4–85). A large single fragment may be avulsed, giving a "bucket handle" appearance. Fragments may migrate into the soft tissues. The corners of the shaft may become initially involved. The healing process then exaggerates the abnormalities. Epiphyseal separations also occur. These changes are present immediately after injury. A shell of periosteal new bone formation surrounding a subperiosteal hematoma may be seen 10 to 20 days following trauma (Fig. 4–86). This shell gradually merges with the cortex and persists as an area of cortical thickening (Fig. 4–87). Fractures may be present, characterized by their variability in both location and age. The classic metaphyseal fractures may not be present in a large percentage of patients.[67] Spiral and transverse fractures of the long bones are reported to be more common, with multiple fractures less common than previously supposed. Skull fractures and spread of the cranial sutures are frequent injuries. Fracture sites that raise a suspicion of child abuse are the lateral end of the clavicle, the ribs, the scapula, the sternum, and the spine.[67] Metaphyseal cupping with shortening of the shaft and a "ball-and-socket" configuration may develop as a late sequel. Isolated bony sclerosis has been described.[23] The child may develop traumatic pancreatitis with resultant medullary necrosis and periosteal new bone formation.[111] There may be associated subdural hematoma or visceral injury, as well as spinal injury. Metaphyseal fractures may also be seen in osteogenesis imperfecta and should not be confused with this condition.[3]

PRIMARY HYPEROXALURIA (OXALOSIS)

Primary hyperoxaluria[118] is a rare inherited error of metabolism due to lack of the enzyme glutamic glyoxylic transaminase, which converts glyoxylate to glycine. The excess glyoxylate is oxidized to oxalate, which is found continuously in the urine. This causes calcium oxalate nephrolithiasis and nephrocalcinosis, leading to recurrent urinary tract infections, hypertension, renal failure, and early death. Oxalate deposits are found in other organs of the body in addition to the kidneys, including the bones. Irregular radiolucent metaphyseal defects in the long bones have been described radiologically. Caffey's case[15] was a 10-year-old girl with cystic rarefaction of the tubular bones situated near the met-

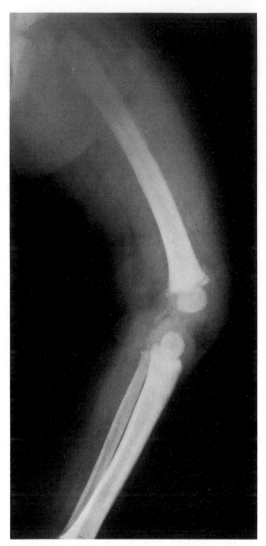

FIG. 4–84. Battered child syndrome (lower extremity). Metaphyseal fragmentation at the distal femur may be noted. There is periosteal elevation along the femoral shaft and a fracture at the femoral capital epiphysis. Bone density and ossification centers appear normal.

FIG. 4–85. Battered child syndrome (knee). Metaphyseal fragmentation is noted, as well as periosteal reaction at the distal femur.

aphyseal ends. The epiphyseal ossification centers appeared relatively sclerotic. There was generalized coarse rarefaction of the shafts, subperiosteal resorption, and symmetrical Milkman's clefts. Some of these changes may have been due to renal osteodystrophy.

More commonly, oxalosis is secondary to another condition. The possible mechanisms are excessive oxalate intake, deficiency of a cofactor involved in oxalate metabolism, or chronic renal failure. Decreased excretion of oxalate is cited as the cause in chronic renal failure, and bone involvement is very rare.[83]

The sites of oxalate crystal deposition are the hypertrophic zone of the epiphyseal plates, the bone marrow in the metaphyses, and areas around disc degeneration. *Radiological findings* include metaphyseal radiolucent bands with focal zones of radiodensity, as well as changes of rickets and renal osteodystrophy.[83]

ACHONDROPLASIA

Achondroplasia (see Chap. 5) is a defect in enchondral bone formation. Metaphyseal changes similar to those seen in rickets associated with bone shortening take place.

ENCHONDROMATOSIS

According to Rubin,[102] *enchondromatosis* is an osseous dysplasia characterized by an excess of hy-

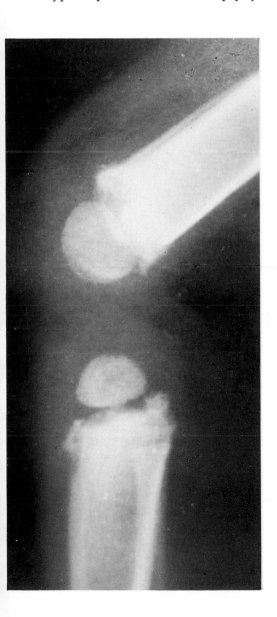

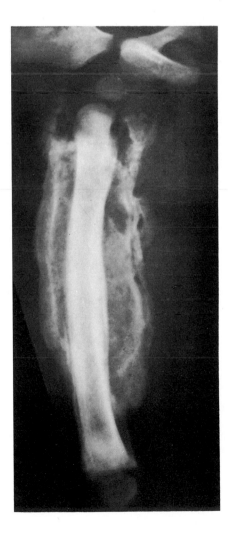

FIG. 4–86. Battered child syndrome (femur). A large calcified shell of new bone formation in a subperiosteal hematoma may be seen. Also note fragmented distal femoral metaphysis.

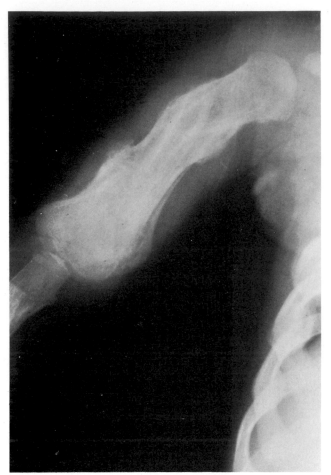

FIG. 4–87. Battered child syndrome (humerus) showing healed fracture of the shaft with callus formation and calcified subperiosteal hematoma persisting as marked cortical thickening. Healing fractures of the ribs may also be noted.

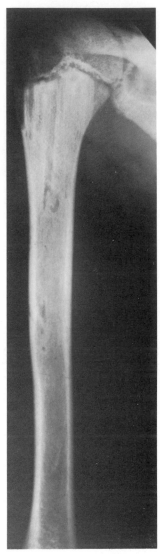

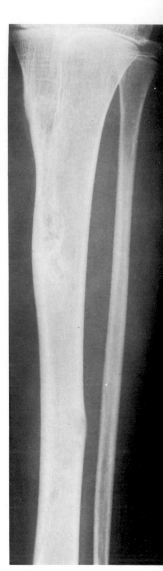

FIG. 4–88   **FIG. 4–89**

pertrophic cartilage that has not been resorbed and ossified in normal fashion at the growing ends of bones. Aegerter considers this condition a hamartomatous proliferation of cartilage cells within the metaphysis.[1] This condition is probably not hereditary, familial, or congenital.

Clinically, the disease is usually discovered between the second and tenth years, although it has been seen as early as 6 months of age. There may be marked shortening of an extremity or severe deformity. Deforming masses may be present. Facial asymmetry has been reported. The disease may be associated with multiple hemangiomas, in which case it is called Maffucci's syndrome. Laboratory values are within normal limits.

Radiologically, rounded or columnar radiolucencies in the metaphyses and shafts of the tubular bones are characteristic (Figs. 4–88, 4–89). The lesions may be expansile or show stippled central calcification (Figs. 4–90, 4–91). Shortening of the bone and deformities due to eccentric growth and undertubulation are commonly seen (Fig. 4–92). Linear radiolucencies extending from the metaphyses to the shaft, interspersed with normal bone, result from failure of enchondral bone formation. Rarely, the flat bones are involved (Fig. 4–93). The iliac crest may have a scalloped appearance and bands of cartilage may radiate to the crest.

The disease has been classified into five types to show its distribution:

FIG. 4–88. Enchondromatosis (humerus). Linear radiolucencies at the proximal humeral metaphysis are present; the epiphysis is spared. Note radiolucencies at the midshaft of the humerus, and a rounded radiolucency with a well-defined margin in the scapula.

FIG. 4–89. Enchondromatosis (tibia). Note rounded radiolucencies in the shaft—some expansile and some containing calcifications.

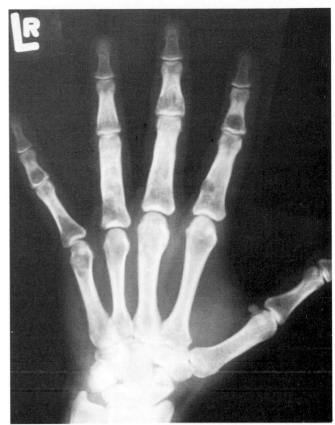

FIG. 4–91. Enchondromatosis (hand). Several well-circumscribed radiolucent lesions, some of them expansile, are noted in the phalanges and metacarpals.

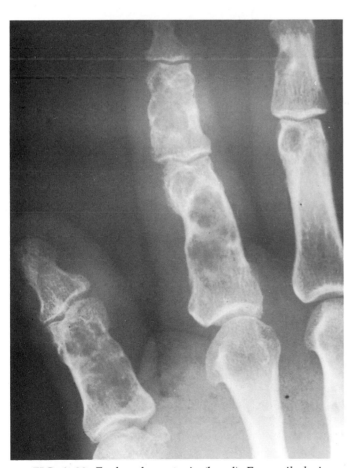

FIG. 4–90. Enchondromatosis (hand). Expansile lesions, several containing amorphous calcifications, may be seen.

1. Acroform (involving hands and feet)
2. Ray form
3. Unilateral form (Ollier's disease)
4. Oligotopic (few chondromas, near a joint)
5. Generalized form

Malignant degeneration occurs, but precise statistics on this condition are lacking.

OSSEOUS CHANGES IN RUBELLA EMBRYOPATHY

Maternal rubella infection during the first trimester of pregnancy may result in such defects as neonatal dwarfism, thrombocytopenic purpura, congenital heart disease, cataracts, chorioretinitis, deafness, hepatosplenomegaly, and unique osseous roentgen changes.[96,110,123]

All long bones may be involved; however, there is a predilection for the distal femoral and the proximal tibial metaphyses. The zones of provisional calcification are absent. The metaphyseal ends are irregular but not cupped (Fig. 4–94). The architecture of the metaphysis and adjacent diaphysis is disorganized with longitudinal or ovoid radiolucencies and sclerosis alternating with coarse bony trabeculae, giving a "celery stick" appearance. Similar changes have been described in *cytomegalic inclusion disease*.

The entire metaphyseal region may occasionally show loss of density. Metaphyseal bands of radiolucency parallel to the growth plate may develop after the neonatal period, as well as small beaklike projections, most pronounced at the medial aspect of the distal femoral metaphysis (Fig. 4–95).

The epiphyseal ossification centers may be irregular, with frayed margins. The sternal ossification centers may be absent. No periosteal reaction is present, an important differential point from congenital lues. The shaft may show failure of modeling. The anterior ends of the ribs may be similarly involved. The osseous changes regress in those infants who grow normally, but persist in those who fail to thrive. Normal diaphyseal modeling is achieved within 2 months, coincident with correction of the metaphyseal changes.[121]

Similar changes have been reported in 2 cases of cytomegalic inclusion disease, along with cerebral periventricular calcifications, osteosclerosis, and metaphyseal bands.[43,80]

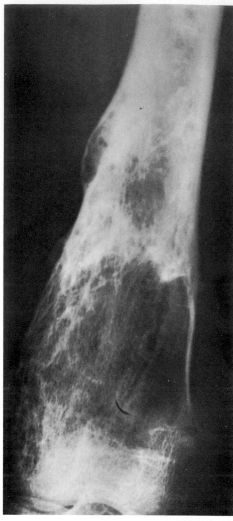

FIG. 4–92

FIG. 4–93

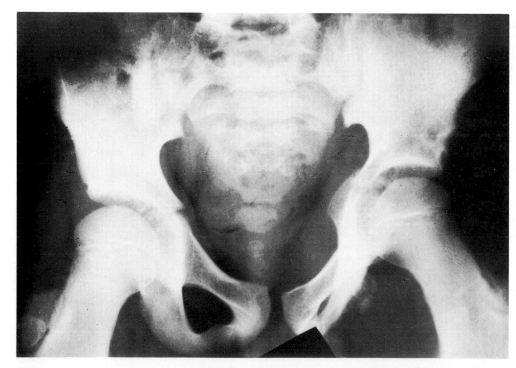

◀ **FIG. 4–92.** Enchondromatosis (distal femur). Radiolucency of the distal femoral shaft may be seen with lack of tubulation, giving an "Erlenmeyer flask" configuration. Note small expansile lesion in the shaft, and calcific medullary stippling.

◀ **FIG. 4–93.** Ollier's disease (pelvis). Hypoplasia of the right side of the pelvis is seen with enchondromas in the supra-acetabular area and the ischium.

FIG. 4–94. Rubella (leg). Note irregularity of the metaphyses, most pronounced at the distal femur. No cupping is evident. There is loss of outline of the zone of provisional calcification. Radiolucent streaks in the distal femur and distal tibia may be seen. No periosteal new bone formation is present.

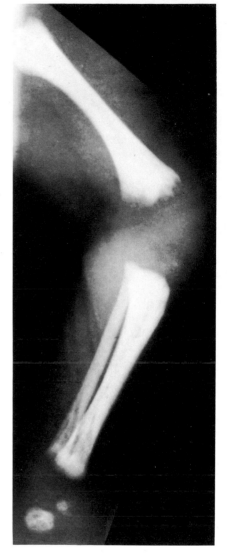

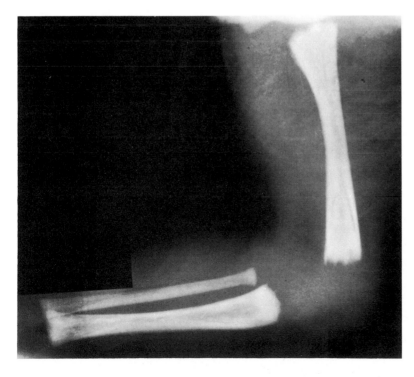

FIG. 4–95. Rubella (leg). Note metaphyseal irregularity of the distal femur with a beaked projection. No periosteal reaction is visible.

INFANTILE SYPHILIS OF BONE

Syphilis of the bone[12,32,72] occurs in the infant or adolescent age groups if congenital, or in adults if acquired. The child may be stillborn with well-marked evidence of lues, may be born alive with luetic changes, or may appear healthy with the lesions developing subsequently.

Neonatal or infantile syphilis may manifest osseous changes caused not only be luetic metaphyseal and diaphyseal osteomyelitis, but also by nonspecific trophic disturbances in enchondral bone formation. The disease is characterized by symmetrical involvement of multiple bones. The extent can vary from minimal to almost total involvement of the bones.

Pathophysiologically, spirochetes in the metaphyses and diaphyses produce destructive and productive changes, with the formation of granulation tissue replacing bone and marrow. A broad irregular yellow epiphyseal plate is characteristic on gross inspection.

Radiologically, the metaphyses and the disphyses show changes, but the epiphyseal ossification centers are not involved even when the most severe disease involves the adjacent bone.

In the metaphysis, transverse striping due to trophic changes may be the earliest finding (Fig. 4–96). There is widening of the zone of provisional calcification, widening of the epiphyseal cartilage plate, and cupping (Fig. 4–97).

Destructive lesions occur in moderately severe cases. They initially involve the corners of the metaphysis adjacent to the cartilage plate, partially sparing the widened zone of provisional calcification. Distribution is remarkably symmetrical. The most characteristic location is at the proximal medial tibial metaphysis, which is known as Wimberger's sign of syphilis (Fig. 4–98). The destructive area may extend across the width of the shaft, leading to pathological fractures with epiphyseal displacement or impaction (Figs. 4–99, 4–100). Another characteristic location is the sigmoid (semilunar) notch of the proximal ulna, with gross erosion of the articular surface. Calcifications may extend from the metaphyseal margin into the epiphyseal cartilage plate, causing a frayed appearance similar to that of rickets.

In the diaphysis, focal areas of patchy rarefaction of the spongiosa and cortex occur. There may be expansion, particularly fusiform expansion of the short tubular bones that gives the "spina ventosa luetica." Periosteal elevation, either solid or lamellated, may occur with or without destructive bony

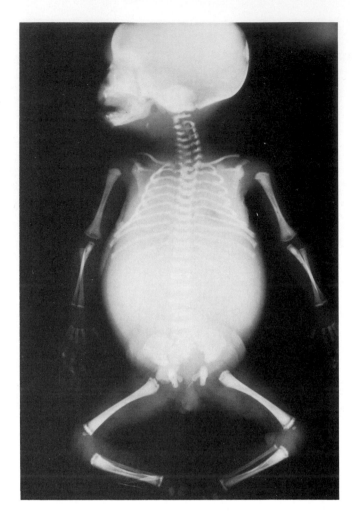

lesions. Destructive areas in the calvarium may also be present.

After initiation of therapy, the changes completely regress with only a minimum of residual cortical thickening. Residual thickening of the anterior tibial cortex to produce the "sabre shin" appearance is common. This finding can be present in both congenital and acquired syphilis (Fig. 4–101).

ERYTHROBLASTOSIS FETALIS

Erythroblastosis fetalis is a congenital hemolytic anemia that results from Rh factor incompatibility. Hydrops fetalis is the most severe form. Bone changes that consist of transverse metaphyseal bands of increased and decreased densities may be present. Diffuse sclerosis of the diaphysis has also been reported. The normal spinal curvature is obliterated by hepatosplenomegaly and ascites.

◀ **FIG. 4–96.** Congenital lues (stillborn infant)— air in the heart and vascular system. Transverse metaphyseal striping is generally noted. Note metapyseal irregularities with small spicules of bone extending into the epiphyseal cartilage plate (fraying), more pronounced in the lower extremities.

FIG. 4–97. Congenital lues (lower extremities). Note marked metaphyseal cupping and generalized periosteal elevated new bone formation. Small calcific densities separated from the metaphyses by a radiolucent line, best seen in the proximal femora, represent widening of the zone of provisional calcification.

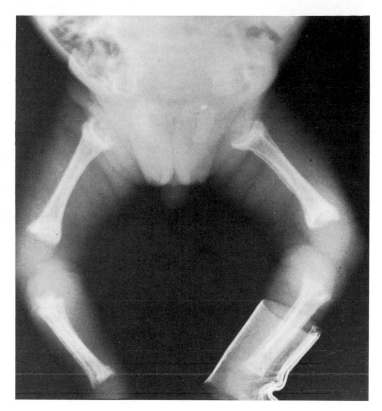

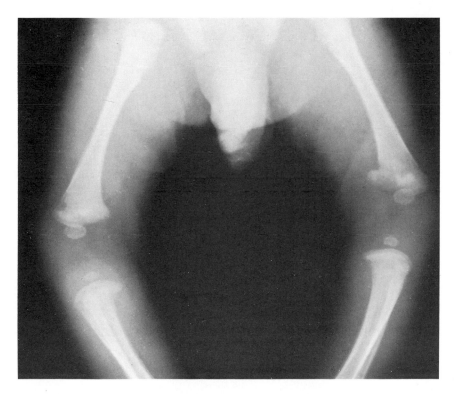

FIG. 4–98. Congenital lues (lower extremities). Destructive metaphyseal changes may be seen, involving the distal femoral medial metaphyses and the medial aspects of the proximal tibial metaphyses. The latter findings are known as Wimberger's sign of syphilis. Mild periosteal new bone formation is also present.

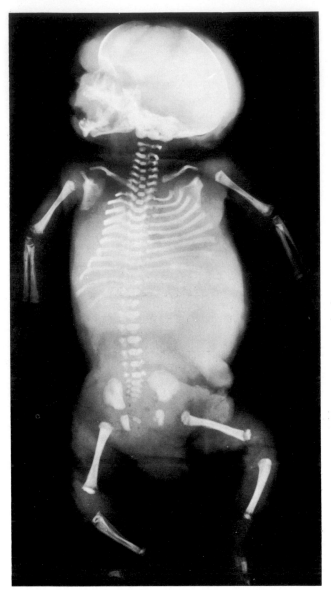

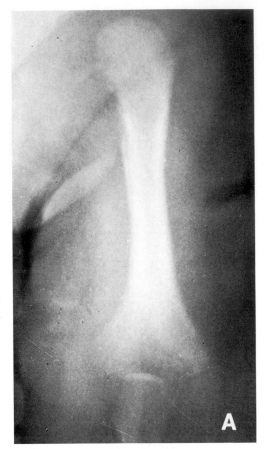

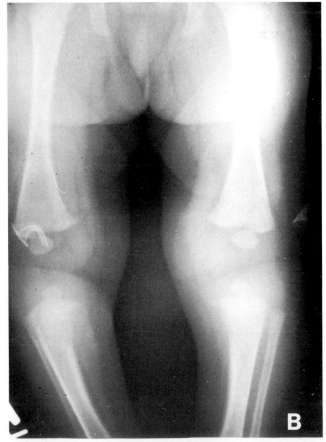

FIG. 4–99. Congenital lues (stillborn infant). Note calcifications of the kidneys. Transverse metaphyseal bands that have proceeded to areas of destruction are generally seen. Pathological fractures have occurred across the metaphyseal bands, particularly at the left femur.

◀ FIG. 4–100. Congenital lues. **A.** Humerus. Periosteal new bone formation along the diaphysis is seen without destructive changes. **B.** Lower extremities. Periosteal new bone formation along the femoral shaft is seen bilaterally. Periosteal new bone formation is also seen along the medial aspect of both tibiae. Destructive lesions at the medial tibial metaphysis, the so-called Wimberger's sign of syphilis, are present.

LEUKEMIA

Leukemia frequently produces bone changes in children. Rarely, congenital leukemia occurs. In early stages of the disease, leukemic cells infiltrate the bone marrow causing pain without producing radiographically discernible changes. The earliest changes take place in the metaphyses. There is a transverse band of radiolucency formed, caused by proliferation of leukemic cells and followed by destruction and periostitis (see Chaps. 3 and 6).

LEAD INTOXICATION

Lead intoxication[71] in infants and children is still commonly seen. Cerebral edema and its effects are encountered in acute lead intoxication. Radiographic aid in diagnosis is limited to demonstrating lead particles in the gastrointestinal tract and separation of the cranial sutures. Chronic lead poisoning of about one month's duration may be expected to show radiographic changes in growing bones. The characteristic finding is the lead line, a dense metaphyseal band resulting from the deposition of lead, which interferes with the normal resorption of the primary spongiosa (Figs. 4–102, 4–103, 4–104). The margins of flat bones may also show an increase in density, and concentric bands paralleling the iliac crests can be seen. The **density** of the bands depends on the concentration of lead ingested, the **width,** on the duration of intoxication, and the **number,** on the number of episodes of lead ingestion. The bands interfere with normal modeling, and an "Erlenmeyer flask" deformity can result (Fig. 4–105). Periosteal reaction is not present in this condition.

Laboratory diagnosis is usually possible before lead lines are seen. Anemia, basophilic stippling of erythrocytes, and increased excretion of coproporphyrins and lead in the urine are present. The blood lead level is elevated (normal is less than 3 μg%).

This is a grave condition in which the mortality rate can reach 25% in children under 2 years of age.

Dense metaphyseal bands are not pathognomonic of lead poisoning. Normally, the metaphysis is dense in children under 4 years of age, and may be markedly conspicuous in an unusual case. Bismuth, mercury, and phosphorus ingestion or injection can cause densities indistinguishable from lead lines on the radiograph. Healed rickets may show zones of increased density, as can osteopetrosis. Vitamin D intoxication may show a series of metaphyseal radiopaque and radiolucent transverse bands. Dense bands are also seen in cretinism.

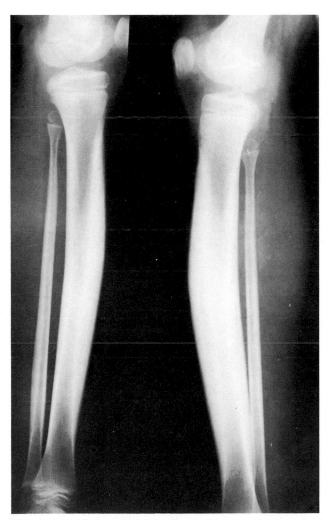

FIG. 4–101. Congenital lues (legs). Note marked cortical thickening, particularly of the left anterior tibial cortex, giving a "sabre shin" appearance.

PHOSPHORUS INTOXICATION

In the past years, children with tuberculosis and rickets were treated with phosphorized cod liver oil. This treatment left a residue of deep stratified transverse metaphyseal bands of increased density in the long bones and curvilinear bands of increased density in the flat bones, which parallel the iliac crest in the pelvis. Similar changes can be seen after ingestion of yellow phosphorus. This condition is now rare. The bands of increased density gradually fade out after ingestion of phosphorus has ceased. In severe cases of yellow phosphorus poisoning the mandible may be involved. The process begins as gingivitis and periostitis and progresses to osteomyelitis, sequestration, and occasionally destruction of the entire mandible.

The dense bands of phosphorus intoxication are radiologically indistinguishable from those of lead and bismuth poisoning (Fig. 4–106).

TRANSVERSE LINES AND ZONES

Fine symmetrical opaque transverse lines or dense zones (complete or incomplete) across the ends of growing long bones, and marginal lines in the flat bones and cuboid bones, may be seen in the normal

FIG. 4–102

FIG. 4–103

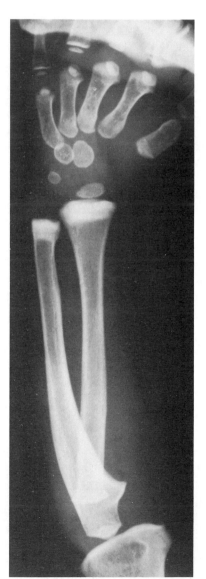

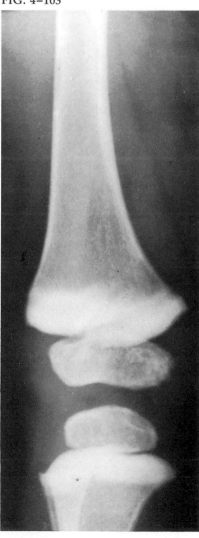

FIG. 4–102. Chronic lead poisoning. Note wide, dense metaphyseal bands at the distal radius and ulna, a narrower band of increased density at the distal humerus, and still narrower bands of increased density at the metaphyses of the phalanges.

FIG. 4–103. Lead intoxication (knee). Dense metaphyseal bands of increased density may be seen at the distal femur, proximal tibia, and proximal fibula. The epiphyseal ossification centers appear normal.

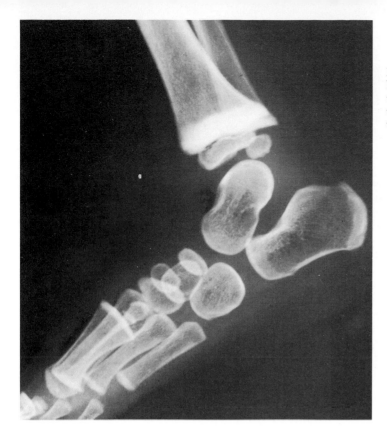

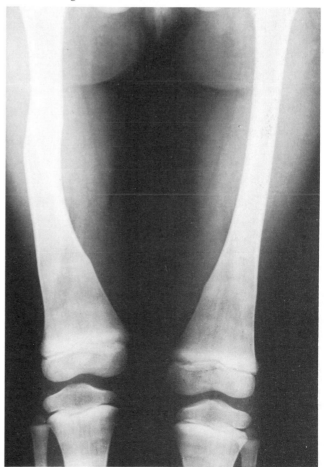

FIG. 4–104. Chronic lead intoxication (ankle). Dense metaphyseal bands may be noted at the distal tibia and fibula. Also note dense margins of the tarsal bones and increased metaphyseal densities in the short tubular bones.

FIG. 4–105. Chronic lead poisoning—recovery phase. Slight residual metaphyseal increase in density may be noted. There is underconstriction of the shaft of bone, causing an "Erlenmeyer flask" deformity. Healed fracture of the right femoral shaft is visible.

skeleton. They may be single or multiple and vary in thickness and number. They parallel the contour of the provisional zone of calcification. The formation of these lines is related to stresses such as malnutrition or disease. Follis and Park[33] state that dense zones result from overproduction of, and failure to destroy, calcified cartilage matrix. Dense lines are formed by bone formation in a horizontal plane along the undersurface of cartilage (Figs. 4–107, 4–108). Transverse radiolucent metaphyseal bands indicate a nonspecific insult to the system. In newborn infants, they may also be associated with fetal meconium peritonitis.

DIFFERENTIAL DIAGNOSIS OF METAPHYSEAL CHANGES

TIME OF APPEARANCE OF DISEASE

Certain trophic disturbances are not present in the neonate—notably rickets and scurvy. A rachitiform picture in the newborn may represent hypophosphatasia or metaphyseal dysostosis. Alkaline phosphatase determination, low in the former condition and normal in the latter, will establish the diagnosis. A radiolucent metaphyseal band in the new-

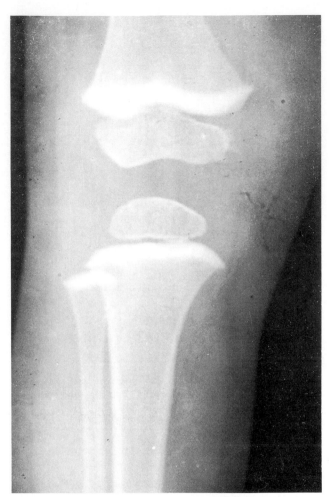

FIG. 4–106. Phosphorus intoxication (knee). Note dense metaphyseal bands, indistinguishable radiologically from heavy metal intoxication. (Courtesy of Dr. Harvey White, Children's Memorial Hospital, Chicago, IL)

born could not represent scurvy; however, congenital lues, rubella syndrome, congenital leukemia, or erythroblastosis fetalis are possibilities. Serological and blood studies would indicate the correct diagnosis.

OBSERVATION OF SPECIFIC STRUCTURAL COMPONENTS

The epiphysis, the epiphyseal cartilage plate, the zone of provisional calcification, and the primary and secondary spongiosa react differently to the various disease processes. Epiphyseal changes are indicators of maturation disturbances. Physeal disturbances lead to growth changes.

The epiphysis is well marginated and sharply defined in metaphyseal dysostosis and congenital lues, but has a dense ringlike margin in scurvy. The epiphysis is poorly and fuzzily marginated in rubella and the rachitiform diseases; this finding may also be present in leukemia.

Destructive metaphyseal changes caused by rubella syndrome could be confused with those of congenital lues; however, lack of periosteal reaction and a negative serology would indicate rubella. The inborn errors of metabolism are best diagnosed by demonstration of their specific metabolite in the urine. The principal changes are summarized in Table 4–4.

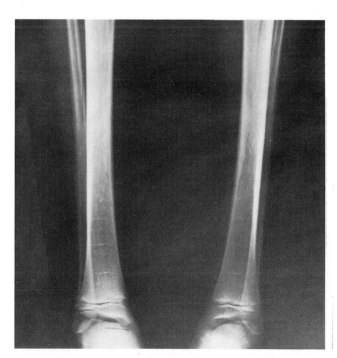

FIG. 4–107. Growth lines (tibia). Horizontal lines run parallel to the metaphysis at the distal tibia. This is a normal finding.

TABLE 4-4. Differential Diagnosis of Metaphyseal Disturbances

Disturbance	Epiphysis	Physis	Zone of Provisional Calcification	Fraying	Cupping	Radiolucent Metaphyseal Band	Metaphyseal Fracture	Periosteal Reaction	Age of Onset (May be Present)
Rickets	Ill-defined	Widened	Early stage—Ill-defined Healing stage—Widened	+	+	−	−	+	6 months—rarely at birth (Osteomalacic mothers)
Scurvy	Ringed	Narrow, normal	Widened	−	From infraction	+	+	+	3 months
Hypo-phosphatasia	Ill-defined	Widened	Ill-defined	+	+	−	−	+	Birth
Metaphyseal dysostosis	Normal	Widened	Ill-defined	+	+	−	−	−	Birth
Phenylketonuria	May be retarded	Spicules of calcium protrude	Normal	−	+	−	−	−	1 month
Infantile trauma	Normal	Normal	Normal	−	−	−	+	+	Birth injury
Rubella	Ill-defined	Normal	Absent	+	−	+	−	−	Birth
Lues	Normal	Widened	Widened	+	+	+	+	+	Birth
Leukemia	Ill-defined, destructive foci	Normal	Normal	−	−	+	−	+	Birth

[237]

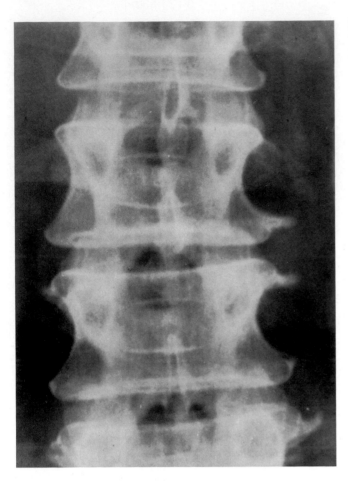

FIG. 4–108. Growth lines (spine). Note fine dense lines within the lumbar vertebral bodies parallel to the endplates. This is a normal variant.

REFERENCES

1. Aegerter E, Kirkpatrick J A: Orthopedic Diseases, 3rd ed. Philadelphia, W B Saunders, 1968

2. Afshani E, Girdany B R: Atlanto-axial dislocation in chondrodysplasia punctata. Report of findings in 2 brothers. Radiology 102:399–401, 1072

3. Astley R: Metaphyseal fractures in osteogenesis imperfecta. Brit J Radiol 52:441–443, 1979

4. Bailey J A: Disproportionate Short Stature. Diagnosis and Management. Philadelphia, W B Saunders, 1973

5. Baker D H, Harris R C: Congenital absence of the intrahepatic bile ducts. Am J Roentgen 91:875–884, 1964

6. Bartoletti S, Armfield S L, Ledesma–Medina J: The cerebrohepatorenal (Zellweger's) syndrome. Radiology 127:741–745, 1978

7. Boettscher W G, Bonfiglio M, Hamilton H H, Sheets R F, Smith K: Nontraumatic necrosis of the femoral head. Part I: Relation of altered hemostasis to etiology. J Bone Joint Surg 52-A:312–321, 1970

8. Bonakdarpour A, Kirkpatrick J A, Renze A, Kendall N: Skeletal changes in neonatal thyrotoxicosis. Radiology 102:149–150, 1972

9. Brogdon B G, Grow N E: Chondrodystrophia calcifications congenita. Am J Roentgen 80:443–448, 1958

10. Bromer R S: A critical analysis of the roentgen signs of infantile scurvy. Am J Roentgen 49:575–579, 1943

11. Buchignani J S, Cook A J, Anderson L G: Roentgenographic findings in familial osteodysplasia. Am J Roentgen 116:602–608, 1972

12. Caffey J: Syphilis of the skeleton in early infancy: The nonspecificity of many of the roentgenographic changes. Am J Roentgen 42:637–655, 1939

13. Caffey J: The early roentgenographic changes in essential coxa plana—their significance in pathogenesis. Am J Roentgen 103:620–634, 1968

14. Caffey J: Traumatic cupping of the metaphysis of growing bones. Am J Roentgen 108:451–460, 1970

15. Caffey J, Silverman F N: Pediatric X-ray Diagnosis, 5th ed. Chicago, Year Book Publishers, 1967

16. Carsen G M, Radkowski M D: Calcium oxalosis. A case report. Radiology 113:165–166, 1974

17. Cooper R R, Ponseti I V, Maynard J A: Pseudoachondro-

plastic dwarfism. A rough-surfaced endoplasmic reticulum storage disorder. J Bone Joint Surg 55–A:475–484, 1973

18. Cullen J C: Thiemann's disease. J Bone Joint Surg 52–B:532–534, 1970

19. Cullen J C: Spinal lesions in battered babies. J Bone Joint Surg 57–B:364–366, 1975

20. Currarino G, Erlandson M E: Premature fusion of the epiphyses in Cooley's anemia. Radiology 83:656–664, 1964

21. Currarino G, Neuhauser E B D, Reyersbach G C, Soble E H: Hypophosphatasia. Am J Roentgen 78:392–419, 1957

22. De Haas W H D, De Boer W, Griffoen F: Metaphyseal dysostosis. A late follow-up of the first reported case. J Bone Joint Surg 51–B:290–299, 1969

23. DeSmet A A, Kuhns L R, Kaufman R A, Holt J F: Bony sclerosis and the battered child. Skel Rad 2:39–41, 1977

24. Dunn A: Avascular necrosis of capital femoral epiphysis and poikiloderma congenitale. JAMA 193:852–853, 1965

25. Edeiken J, Hodes P J, Libshitz H I, Weller M H: Bone ischemia. Radiol Clin N Amer 5:515–529, 1967

26. Fairbank H A T: Dysplasia epiphysealis punctata. J Bone Joint Surg 31–B:114–117, 1949

27. Feinberg S B, Fisch R O: Roentgen findings in growing long bones in phenylketonuria. Radiology 78:394–398, 1962

28. Felman A H: Multiple epiphyseal dysplasia: Three cases with unusual vertebral anomalies. Radiology 93:119–125, 1969

29. Fidler M W, Brook C G D: Slipped upper femoral epiphysis following treatment with human growth hormone. J Bone Joint Surg 56–A:1719–1722, 1974

30. Fisher D E, Bickel W H: Corticosteroid-induced avascular necrosis. A clinical study of 77 patients. J Bone Joint Surg 53–A:859–873, 1971

31. Fisher R L: An epidemiological study of Legg–Perthes' disease. J Bone Joint Surg 54–A:769–778, 1972

32. Fleming T C, Bardenstein M B: Brief note. Congenital syphilis. J Bone Joint Surg 53–A:1648–1651, 1971

33. Follis R H, Park E A: Some observations on bone growth with particular respect to zones and transverse lines of increased density in the metaphysis. Am J Roentgen 68:709–724, 1952

34. Fraser D: Hypophosphatasia. Am J Med 22:730–746, 1957

35. Freiberger R H: Multiple epiphyseal dysplasia: A report of 3 cases. Radiology 70:379–385, 1958

36. Garn S M, Rohmann C G, Silverman F N: Radiographic standards for postnatal ossification and tooth calcification. Med Radiog Photog 43(2):66, 1967

37. Gelberman R H, Salomon P B, Jurist J M, Pusch J L: Ulnar variance in Kienbock's disease. J Bone Joint Surg 57–A:674–676, 1975

38. Giedion A et al: Metaphyseal dysostosis and congenital pancreatic insufficiency. Fortschr Roentgenstr 108:51–57, 1968

39. Goldman A B, Hallel T, Salvati E M, Freiberger R H: Osteochondritis dissecans complicating Legg–Perthes' disease. A report of 4 cases. Radiology 121:561–566, 1976

40. Goldman A B, Lane J M, Salvati E: Slipped capital femoral epiphyses complicating renal osteodystrophy. Radiology 126:333–339, 1978

41. Gower W E, Johnston R C: Legg–Perthes' disease. Long-term follow-up of 36 patients. J Bone Joint Surg 53–A:759–768, 1971

42. Graham C B: Assessment of bone maturation—methods and pitfalls. Radiol Clin N Amer 10:185–202, 1972

43. Graham C B, Thal A, Wassum C S: Rubella-like bone changes in congenital cytomegalic inclusion disease. Radiology 94:39–43, 1970

44. Greulich W W, Pyle S I: Radiographic Atlas of Skeletal Development of Hand and Wrist, 2nd ed. Stanford, CA, Stanford University Press; London, Oxford University Press, 1959

45. Grossman H, New M: Precocious sexual development—roentgenographic aspects. Am J Roentgen 100:48–62, 1967

46. Grunebaum M, Lebowitz R L: Hypothyroidism in cystinosis. Am J Roentgen 129:629–630, 1977

47. Hallel T, Salvati E A: Osteochondritis dissecans following Legg–Calve–Perthes' disease. J Bone Joint Surg 58–B:37–40, 1976

48. Harper H A: Review of Physiological Chemistry, 14th ed. Los Altos, CA, Lange Medical Publications, 1973

49. Harrington K D, Murray W R, Kountz S L, Belzer F D: Avascular necrosis of bone after renal transplantation. J Bone Joint Surg 53–A:203–215, 1971

50. Harris R D, Silver R A: Atraumatic aseptic necrosis of the talus. Radiology 106:81–83, 1973

51. Harrison M H M, Turner M H, Jacobs P: Skeletal immaturity in Perthes' disease. J Bone Joint Surg 58–B:37–40, 1976

52. Hensinger R N, Cowell H R, Ramsey P L, Leopold R G: Familial dysplasia epiphysealis hemimelica, associated with chondromas and osteochondromas. Report of a kindred with variable presentations. J Bone Joint Surg 56–A:1513–1516, 1974

53. Hermon R: Two cases of osteochondral hypothyroidism. Brit J Radiol 16:208–211, 1943

54. Hernandez R J, Poznanski A K: Distinctive appearance of the distal phalanges in children with primary hypothyroidism. Radiology 132:83–84, 1979

55. Hiller H G: Battered or not—a reappraisal of metaphyseal fragility. Am J Roentgen 114:241–246, 1972

56. Hug I, Mihatsch J M: Primary oxalosis. Report of a case with radiologic-pathological-anatomical correlation, and review of the literature. Fortschr Roentgenstr 123:154–162, 1975

57. Hulvey J T, Keats T: Multiple epiphyseal dysplasia: A contribution to the problem of spinal involvement. Am J Roentgen 106:170–177, 1969

58. Immelman E J, Bank S, Krige H, Marks I N: Roentgenological and clinical features of intramedullary fat necrosis in bones in acute and chronic pancreatitis. Am J Med 36:96–105, 1964

59. Inove A, Freeman M A R, Vernon-Roberts B, Mizuno S: The pathogenesis of Perthes' disease. J Bone Joint Surg 58–B:453–461, 1976

60. Jansen M: Über atypische Chondrodystrophie (Achondroplasie) und über eine noch nicht beschriebene angeborene Wachstumsstörung des Knochensystems: Metaphysäre Dysostosis. Z Orthop Chir 61:255, 1934

61. Jardon O M, Burney D W, Fink R L: Hypophosphatasia in the adult. J Bone Joint Surg 52–A:1477–1484, 1970

62. Johnson G F et al: Reliability of skeletal age assessments. Am J Roentgen 118:320–327, 1973

63. Kahmi E, MacEwen G D: Osteochondritis dissecans in Legg–Calve–Perthes' disease. J Bone Joint Surg 57–A:506–509, 1975

64. Katayama H, Suruga K, Kurashige T, Kimoto T: Bone changes in congenital biliary atresia: Radiological observation of 8 cases. Am J Roentgen 124:107–112, 1975

65. Kellekamp D B, Campbell C J, Bonfiglio M: Dysplasia epiphysealis hemimelica. A report of 15 cases and a review of the literature. J Bone Joint Surg 48–A:746–766, 1966

66. Koehler A, Zimmer E A: Borderlands of the Normal and Early Pathologic in Skeletal Roentgenology, 10th ed. New York, Grune & Stratton, 1961

67. Kogutt M S, Swischuk L E, Fagan C J: Patterns of injury and significance of uncommon fractures in the battered child syndrome. Am J Roentgen 121:143–149, 1974

68. Kuhns L R, Sherman M P, Poznanski A K: Determination of neonatal maturation on the chest radiograph. Radiology 102:597–604, 1972

69. Kuhns L R, Sherman M P, Poznanski A K, Holt J F: Humeral head and coracoid ossification in the newborn. Radiology 107:145–150, 1973

70. Langenskiold A, Riska E B: Tibia vara (osteochondrosis deformans tibiae). A survey of 71 cases. J Bone Joint Surg 46–A:1405–1420, 1964

71. Leone A J: On lead lines. Am J Roentgen 103:165–167, 1968

72. Levin E J: Healing in congenital osseous syphilis. Am J Roentgen 110:591–597, 1970

73. Martel W, Poznanski A K: The effect of traction on the hip in osteonecrosis: A comment on the "radiolucent crescent line." Radiology 94:505–508, 1970

74. Martel W, Sitterley B H: Roentgenologic manifestations of osteonecrosis. Am J Roentgen 106:509–522, 1969

75. Mason R C, Kozlowski K: Chondrodysplasia punctata. Radiology 109:145–150, 1973

76. Maximow A A, Bloom W: A Textbook of Histology, 6th ed. Philadelphia, W B Saunders, 1952

77. McAlister W H, Koehler P R: Diseases of the adrenal. Radiol Clin N Amer 5:205–220, 1967

78. McCallum R I et al: Bone lesions in compressed air workers, with special reference to men who worked on the Clyde Tunnels, 1958–1963. Report of decompression sickness panel. Medical Research Council. J Bone Joint Surg 48–B:207–235, 1966

79. McCann F: The incidence and value of radiological signs of scurvy. Brit J Radiol 35:683–686, 1962

80. Merten D F, Gooding C A: Skeletal manifestations of congenital cytomegalic inclusion disease. Radiology 95:333–334, 1970

81. Meschan I, Farrer–Meschan R M F: Roentgen Signs in Clinical Practice, Vol 1. Philadelphia, W B Saunders, 1966

82. Milgram J W: Radiological and pathological manifestations of osteochondritis dissecans of the distal femur. Radiology 126:305–311, 1978

83. Milgram J W, Salyer W R: Secondary oxalosis of bone in chronic renal failure. A histopathological study of 3 cases. J Bone Joint Surg 56–A:387–395, 1974

84. Miller S M, Paul L W: Roentgen observations in familial metaphyseal dysostosis. Radiology 83:665–673, 1964

85. Moorefield W B et al: Acquired hypothyroidism and slipped capital femoral epiphysis. Report of 3 cases. J Bone Joint Surg 58–A:705–708, 1976

86. Murray R O: Radiological bone changes in Cushing's syndrome and steroid therapy. Brit J Radiol 33:1–19, 1960

87. Nellen J R, Kindwall E P: Aseptic necrosis of bone secondary to occupational exposure to compressed air: Roentgenologic findings in 59 cases. Am J Roentgen 115:512–524, 1972

88. Norman A: Radiolucent crescent line: Early diagnostic sign of avascular necrosis of femoral head. Bull Hosp Joint Dis 24:99–104, 1963

89. Norman A, Baker N D: Spontaneous osteonecrosis of the knee and medial meniscal tears. Radiology 129:653–656, 1978

90. Ozonoff M B: Metaphyseal dysostosis of Jansen. Radiology 93:99–104, 1969

91. Ozonoff M B: Pediatric Orthopedic Radiology. Philadelphia, W B Saunders, 1979

92. Pantazoupolos T, Exarchou E: Osteochondritis dissecans of the patella. Report of 4 cases. J Bone Joint Surg 53–A:1205–1207, 1971

93. Park E A: Observations on the pathology of rickets with particular reference to the changes at the cartilage-shaft junctions of growing bones. Harvey Lect 34:157, 1938–1939

94. Patterson R J, Bickel W H, Dahlin D C: Idiopathic avascular necrosis of the head of the femur: A study of 52 cases. J Bone Joint Surg 46–A:267–282, 1964

95. Poznanski A K, Nosanchuk J S, Baublis, J, Holt J F: The cerebrohepatorenal syndrome (CHRS) (Zellweger's syndrome). Am J Roentgen 109:313–322, 1970

96. Rabinowitz J G, Wolf B S, Greenberg E I, Rausen A R: Osseous changes in rubella embryopathy. Radiology 85:494–499, 1965

97. Raghavendra B N, Genieser N B: Bone changes in intrahepatic biliary atresia. Brit J Radiol 49:181–183, 1976

98. Rennel C, Steinbach H L: Epiphyseal dysostosis without dwarfism. Am J Roentgen 108:481–487, 1970

99. Riggs W, Wilroy R S, Etteldorf J N: Neonatal hyperthyroidism with accelerated skeletal maturation, craniosynostosis, and brachydactyly. Radiology 105:621–625, 1972

100. Roche A F, Davila G H, Pasternak B A, Walton M J: Some factors influencing the replicability of assessments of skeletal maturity (Greulich–Pyle). Am J Roentgen 109:299–306, 1970

101. Roche A F, French N Y: Differences in skeletal maturity

levels between the knee and hand. Am J Roentgen 109:307–312, 1970

102. Rubin P: Dynamic Classification of Bone Dysplasias. Chicago, Year Book Publishers, 1964

103. Russell J G B, Hill L F: True fetal rickets. Brit J Radiol 47:732–734, 1974

104. Schintz H R, Baensch W E, Fridl E, Uehlinger E: Roentgen Diagnostics. New York, Grune & Stratton, 1952

105. Schmid F: Beitrag zur Dysostosis Enchondralis Metaphysaria. Mschr Kinderheilk 97:393–397, 1949

106. Shea D, Mankin H J: Slipped capital femoral epiphysis in renal rickets. Report on 3 cases. J Bone Joint Surg 48–A:349–355, 1966

107. Shopfner C E, Coin C G: Effect of weight bearing on appearance and development of the secondary calcaneal epiphysis. Radiology 86:201–206, 1966

108. Silverman F N: Recovery from epiphyseal invagination: Sequel to an unusual complication of scurvy. J Bone Joint Surg 52–A:384–390, 1970

109. Silverman F N: Unrecognized trauma in infants, the battered child syndrome, and the syndrome of Ambroise Tardieu. Rigler lecture. Radiology 104:337–356, 1972

110. Singleton E B, Rudolph A J, Rosenberg H S, Singer D B: The roentgenographic manifestations of the rubella syndrome in newborn infants. Am J Roentgen 97:82–91, 1966

111. Slovis T L, Berdon W E, Haller J D, Baker D H, Rosen L: Pancreatitis and the battered child syndrome. Am J Roentgen 125:456–461, 1975

112. Somerville E W: Perthes' disease of the hip. J Bone Joint Surg 53–B:639–649, 1971

113. Steinbach H L, Brown R A: Epiphyseal dysostosis. Am J Roentgen 105:860–869, 1969

114. Tapia J, Stearns G, Ponseti I V: Vitamin D-resistant rickets: A long-term clinical study of 11 patients. J Bone Joint Surg 46–A:935–958, 1964

115. Taybi H, Mitchell A D, Friedman G D: Metaphyseal dysostosis and the associated syndrome of pancreatic insufficiency and blood disorders. Radiology 93:563–571, 1969

116. Theander G, Pettersson H: Calcification in chondrodysplasia punctata. Relation to ossification and skeletal growth. ACTA Rad Diag 19:205–222, 1978

117. Thomas P S, Glasgow J F T: The "mandibular mantle"—a sign of rickets in very low birth rate infants. Brit J Radiol 51:93–98, 1978

118. Weber A L: Primary hyperoxaluria. Roentgenographic clinical, and pathological findings. Am J Roentgen 100:155–161, 1967

119. Weiss A: The scapular sign in rickets. Radiology 98:633–636, 1971

120. Whalen J P, Winchester P, Krook L, Dische R, Nunez E: Mechanisms of bone resorption in human metaphyseal remodeling. Am J Roentgen 112:526–531, 1971

121. Whalen J P, Winchester P, Krook L, O'Donohue N, Dische R, Nunez E: Neonatal transplacental rubella syndrome: Its effect on normal maturation of the diaphysis. Am J Roentgen 121:166–172, 1974

122. Wietersen F K, Balow R M: The radiological aspects of thyroid disease. Radiol Clin N Amer 5:255–266, 1967

123. Williams H J, Carey L S: Rubella embryopathy. Roentgenologic features. Am J Roentgen 97:92–99, 1966

124. Williams J L, Cliff A M, Bonakdarpour A: Spontaneous osteonecrosis of the knee. Radiology 107:15–19, 1973

125. Williams J P, Secrist L, Fowler G W, Gwinn J L, Dumars K C: Roentgenographic features of the cerebrohepatorenal syndrome of Zellweger. Am J Roentgen 115:607–610, 1972

126. Wolf E L: Slipped femoral capital epiphysis as a sequela to childhood irradiation for malignant tumors. Radiology 125:781–784, 1977

127. Wolfson J J, Engel R R: Anticipating meconium peritonitis from metaphyseal bands. Radiology 92:1055–1060, 1969

A bone can exhibit excessive or diminished growth or tubulation, or a characteristic deformity. These features form the basis of a radiological classification that is correlated with a specific clinicopathological entity. Generalized undergrowth with or without deformity constitutes dwarfism.

The classification of dwarfism[53,68,89] is still in a state of flux. Historically, the two basic types are proportionate and disproportionate short stature.[13] The disproportionate type is basically divided into short-trunk dwarfism and short-limb dwarfism. Transitional forms, with features common to both, also exist. New syndromes are constantly being discovered. New biochemical knowledge of known syndromes allows reclassification of some. Terms which were general in the older literature (e.g., Morquio's syndrome) have evolved to denote rigidly specific conditions.

The latest generally accepted classification of dwarfism was established by the European Society for Pediatric Radiology and the National Foundation–March of Dimes. They set forth the "International Nomenclature of Constitutional Diseases of Bone," revised in 1977. The term "dwarfism" has been eliminated from the nomenclature because it seemed offensive. It is now replaced by other terms, such as dysplasia. (See Table 5–5 pp 348–357).

The seemingly never-ending reclassification and subclassification of dwarfism does serve a purpose other than sheer mental exercise in the description of incurable conditions. It is of prime fundamental importance to be able to predict for the parent of a child with this affliction the probability for the occurrence of a similar defect in subsequent children. They must know whether the affected child will be mentally retarded or normal, what physical deformities he will have, and how long he is expected to live. Also, the treatment must be planned.

A radiological classification of dwarfism can be only partially complete. A vast spectrum of intermediate and mild forms exist, some of which are not as yet well enough defined. One disease may show radiological similarities to another, and share many specific features. Each disease may vary greatly in its roentgen manifestations. In addition, phenocopies (nongenetic simulation of genetic diseases) may occur. Because of this, only the major types of dwarfism and those types that have received attention in the radiological literature are included in this chapter. Some of the minor syndromes are summarized in Table 5–5.

The radiological classification of short-limb dwarfism based on the segment of bone that shows the greatest shortening is currently widely accepted. Rhizomelic dwarfism is predominantly shortening of the proximal segment (of the humerus and femur); mesomelic dwarfism, shortening of the middle segment (of the forearm and leg); and acromelic dwarfism, shortening of the distal segment (of the hands and feet). Other forms include a deformed type of dwarfism, a proportional shortening, and a large group of syndromes composed of bone shortening and deformity combined with other specific features that can best be classified as miscellaneous. Moreover, many disturbances in the epiphyseal region also cause shortening of bone. This classification is summarized below.

CLASSIFICATION OF CONDITIONS AFFECTING SIZE AND SHAPE OF BONE

I. Generalized Undergrowth of Bone (Dwarfism) —Major Syndromes of Short-Limb Dwarfism
   1. Rhizomelic Dwarfism
     A. Achondroplasia
     B. Thanatophoric dwarfism (dysplasia)
     C. Achondrogenesis
     D. Pseudoachondroplastic dysplasia
     E. Metatropic dwarfism (dysplasia)
   2. Mesomelic Dwarfism
     A. Chondroectodermal dysplasia
     B. Dyschondrosteosis
   3. Acromelic Dwarfism
     A. Peripheral dysostosis
     B. Asphyxiating thoracic dysplasia
   4. Deformed Type of Dwarfism
     A. Diastrophic dwarfism (dysplasia)
II. Minor Dwarfism syndromes (see Table 5–5)

III. The Genetic Mucopolysaccharidoses
1. Hurler's syndrome
2. Hunter's syndrome
3. Sanfilippo's syndrome
4. Morquio's syndrome
5. Scheie's syndrome
6. Maroteaux–Lamy syndrome
7. Other mucopolysaccharidoses
IV. Mucolipidoses
1. GM$_1$ gangliosidosis
2. Mannosidosis
3. Type I mucolipidosis (Spranger and Wiedmann)
4. Type II mucolipidosis (I-cell disease of Leroy)
5. Type III mucolipidosis (Pseudo-Hurler polydystrophy)
V. Miscellaneous Syndromes of Growth Disturbance or Deformity of Bone
1. Progeria
2. Cornelia de Lange syndrome
3. Craniostenosis-syndactylism syndromes
a. Apert's syndrome
b. Seathre–Chotzen syndrome
c. Carpenter's syndrome
d. Pfeiffer's syndrome
4. Cleidocranial dysostosis
5. Hereditary onychoosteodysplasia
6. Pseudohypoparathyroidism and pseudo-pseudohypoparathyroidism
7. Chromosomal abnormalities
A. Autosomal syndromes
1) Mongoloidism
2) Trisomy 17–syndrome
3) Trisomy 13–15 syndrome
4) Cri-du-chat syndrome
5) Wolf syndrome
6) Trisomy 9$_p$
7) Basal-cell nevus syndrome
B. Sex-linked syndromes (Gonadal dysgenesis)
1) Turner's Syndrome
2) Pseudo-Turner's syndrome
3) Klinefelter's syndrome and Klinefelter variants
4) Polysyndromes
8. Fanconi's anemia
9. Erythrogenesis imperfecta
10. Congenital hypoplastic thrombocytopenia
11. Holt–Oram syndrome
12. Myositis ossificans progressiva
13. Effect of radiation on growing bone
14. Acromegaly and giantism
15. Homocystinuria
16. Marfan's syndrome
17. Macrodactyly
18. Idiopathic hemihypertrophy
19. Neurofibromatosis
20. Osteogenesis imperfecta
21. Pyle's disease
22. Craniometaphyseal dysplasia
23. Weismann–Netter syndrome
24. Aplasia, hypoplasia, and malsegmentation

GENERALIZED UNDERGROWTH OF BONE (DWARFISM)

RHIZOMELIC DWARFISM

ACHONDROPLASIA (CHONDRODYSPLASIA FETALIS, CHONDRODYSTROPHIA FETALIS, CHONDRODYSTROPHIC DWARFISM, MICROMELIA)

Achondroplasia[182] is a bone dysplasia in which the primary defect is enchondral bone formation. It is transmitted as a mendelian dominant. Ninety percent of cases are sporadic, although familial histories have been reported, indicating that the majority are caused by mutations. There is a generalized shortening of bone of the rhizomelic type.

Clinically, this is the most common form of dwarfism. Bone deformities are present at birth. The majority of stillbirths are due to hydrocephalus. A large percentage of achondroplasts die within the first year. Neurological complications and paraplegias may ensue. If the infant survives the first year, life expectancy is good, unlike in most other forms of dwarfism. Mental and sexual development are not retarded.

Although clinical diagnosis in the newborn may be difficult, the older child and the adult achondroplast show characteristic features. The extremities are shortened. There is a lordotic spine with a protuberant abdomen. The thorax is shallow. The head is enlarged by nonprogressive hydrocephalus.

The forehead is prominent and the bridge of the nose is recessed, through brachycephaly. The mandible is prominent and the lips and tongue are enlarged.

The major *pathological* change is a failure of normal cartilage growth in the physis. Only a thin zone of chondrocytes is present, without normal column formation or vacuolization. There is interference with the formation of the zone of provisional calcification and the primary spongiosa of the metaphysis. Periosteal strips of fibrous tissue may seal the epiphyseal line, thus preventing further growth in length. Articular cartilage formation and periosteal ossification are normal.

No abnormal biochemical values have been found. No causal endocrine disorders have been discovered.

Radiologically, three types of achondroplasia have been recognized. The *hypoplastic* type is the most common and represents true achondroplasia. The *hyperplastic* type shows irregular epiphyses and broad terminal bony segments. This appearance is most consistent with pseudoachondroplasia or metatropic dwarfism. The *malacic* type most probably represents superimposed rickets.

There is symmetrical shortening of all tubular bones with a proportional rhizomelic predominance. Periosteal growth proceeds normally, resulting in relative thickening of bone. The bone ends are splayed, with metaphyseal cupping and loss of the provisional zone of calcification (Figs. 5–1, 5–2). The bones tend to be rectangular in shape, with normal thickness of the cortex and medulla.

Shortening of digits leads to an appearance of thick bones in the hands and feet. The fingers are all of the same length. Separation of the ring and middle fingers results in a trident hand.

Disproportionate shortening of the long bones results in the ulna being shorter than the radius, and the tibia shorter than the fibula (Fig. 5–3).

At birth, the spine shows flattened vertebral bodies and an increase in the height of the intervertebral spaces. Residual changes usually persist in later life. The spinal canal is narrowed in both dimensions. The interpediculate distances progressively narrow without the normal lumbar bulge. Angular kyphosis with a hypoplastic upper lumbar vertebra is sometimes seen (Fig. 5–4). There may be partial beaking of the lumbar vertebral bodies and scalloping of their posterior margins. The foramen magnum is small and flat.

The skull is enlarged, usually because of communicating hydrocephalus. Brachycephaly is present. The frontal bones are prominent. The ribs are markedly shortened and do not extend normally around the chest. The mandible and clavicles are only minimally affected. The scapula appears flattened at its inferior aspect. The pelvis is smaller than normal with shortening of the ilia and narrowing of the sacrum. This results in the reduction of the greater sciatic notch to a small slit, low sacroiliac articulations, squaring of the iliac wings, and flattening of the acetabular angles. Excessive cartilage at the Y-articulations of the acetabula is also present (Figs. 5–5, 5–6). The tarsal bones, the carpal bones, and the joints are normal or minimally involved.

Mild forms,[200] called *chondrohypoplasia* (Ravenna) and *hypochondroplasia*[83] (Leri and Linossier) have been reported. Chondrodystrophia calcificans congenita gives an appearance suggesting asymmetrical or unilateral achondroplastic changes. *Cartilage-hair hypoplasia* (McKusick *et al*[150]) is a variant form described in the Amish.

(Text continued on p. 250)

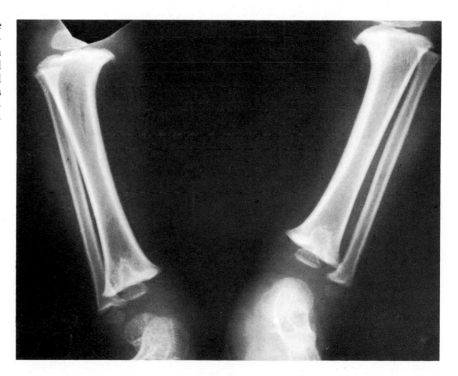

FIG. 5–1. Achondroplasia (legs). The distal tibial metaphyses show a central defect, which is the transition from a cupping form to a V-shaped metaphysis. All bones are shorter and relatively thicker, and the fibula is longer than the tibia. There is irregularity at the proximal tibial metaphysis, with central beaking.

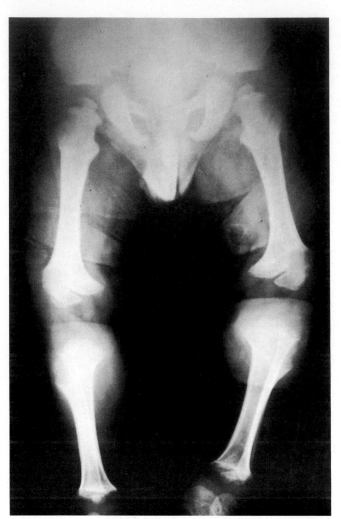

FIG. 5–2. Achondroplasia (lower extremities). Note shortening of all bones, with greater proportional shortening of the femora, or rhizomelic predominance. Irregularities and splaying of the metaphyses may be noted, with a tendency of the distal femoral metaphysis to become V-shaped, and of the distal tibial metaphysis to become cup-shaped. Also note lateral position of the distal femoral ossification centers, a characteristic finding.

FIG. 5–3. Achondroplasia (lower extremities). The bones are all shortened. The tibiae are shorter than the fibulae. There is a hyperplastic type of configuration of the distal femoral metaphyses. Splaying and cupping of the tibial and fibular metaphyses are present.

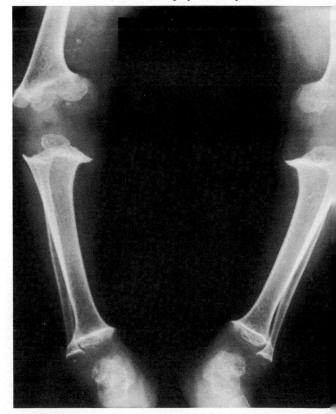

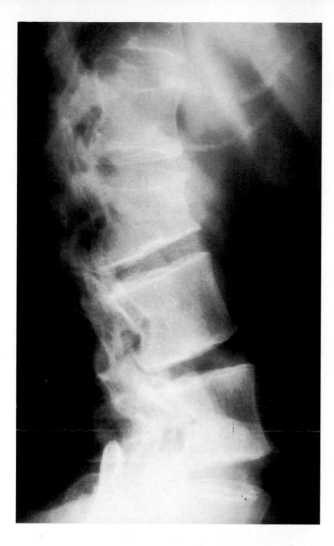

FIG. 5–4. Achondroplasia (lumbar spine)—female, age 38 years. Note hypoplastic first lumbar vertebra with wedging. There is also a decrease in the anteroposterior dimension of the vertebral bodies, and scalloping of their posterior margins.

FIG. 5–5. Achondroplasia (pelvis)—male, age 7 years. There is narrowing of the sacrosciatic notches to give the pelvic opening a "champagne glass" appearance. Note large amount of residual cartilage at the ilioischiac junctions, and wide separation at the ischiopubic synchondrosis. The presence of ossification centers in the femoral capital epiphyses, and the narrow sacrosciatic notches, help differentiate this picture from one of Morquio's syndrome.

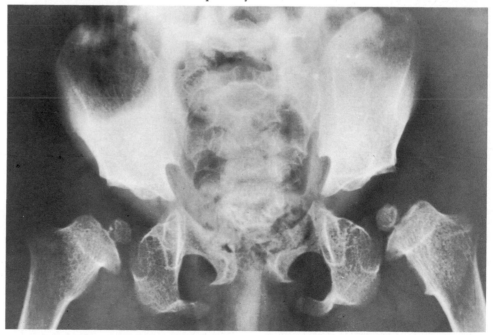

THANATOPHORIC DWARFISM

Thanatophoric dwarfism (thanatophoric dysplasia)[39,109,130,145] is a short-limb dwarf condition resulting either in stillbirth or death in the neonatal period.

Clinically, marked short-limb dwarfism is obvious at birth. The condition has been demonstrated radiographically *in utero.* Hydramnios is common. The trunk is essentially of normal length. The head is relatively large. The abdomen is distended. The microextremities are held in an extended position. The thorax is small in its anteroposterior diameter. If the child is born alive, respiratory distress is a constant feature and the most common cause of death. The forehead is prominent, the eyes may bulge, and the bridge of the nose is depressed. Hypotonia and absence of primitive reflexes occur. The longest reported survivor died at the age of 25 days. The mode of inheritance is unknown.

Radiologically, the entire skeleton is involved. There is a striking discrepancy between the short extremities and the relatively longer trunk. The calvarium may be well mineralized with large fontanelles, frontal bossing, and depressed nasal bridge. The size of the calvarium is large in comparison to the facial bones. The base of the skull may be short, and the foramen magnum narrow.

A frequently associated finding is the presence of a "cloverleaf" skull deformity (Kleeblattschädel).[248] This refers to a grotesque trilobed deformity of the skull owing to fusion of the coronal and lambdoid sutures, downward depression of the middle cranial fossa, and defects in the frontal, temporal, and occipital squamosa. Calvarial bulging at the frontal squamosa, and laterad at the temporal squamosa produce a trilobed deformity in the frontal projection (Fig. 5–7). The long bones of the extremities are very short, with a rhizomelic distribution. They are relatively broad, with flaring of the metaphyses, and possibly cupping. Marked curvature may be present, with a configuration likened to a "telephone receiver," which is said to be characteristic, particularly in the lower extremities. An exostosis-like projection of the inner proximal margin of the bowed femur is characteristic (Fig. 5–8).

The small bones are short and broad, with particular shortening of the first metacarpals, first meta-

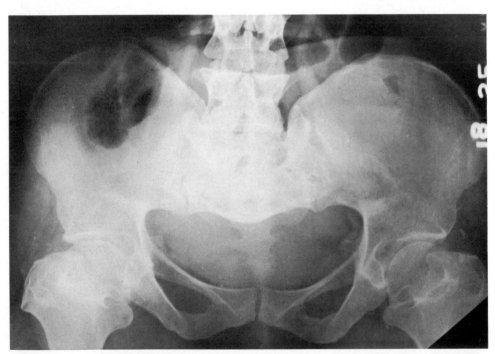

FIG. 5–6. Achondroplasia (pelvis)—small pelvis with a kidney-shaped pelvic inlet. There is narrowing of the sacrum. The interpediculate distances of the lower lumbar vertebrae are also visibly narrowed.

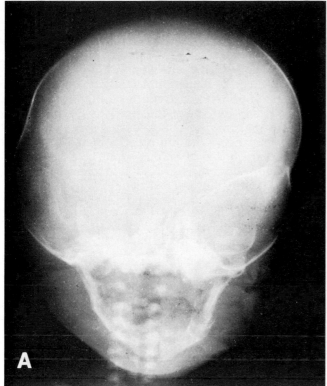

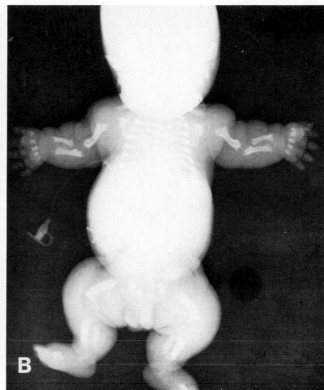

FIG. 5–7. Thanatophoric dwarfism with "cloverleaf" skull. **A.** Skull, frontal view. A defect in the frontal squamosa with soft-tissue bulging and lateral bulging of the temporal squamosa produces a trilobed deformity. **B.** Trunk and extremities. Shortening of the long bones in rhizomelic proportion with cupping and flaring of the metaphyses is present, as well as curvature, particularly of the humeri and femora. An exostosis-like projection at the inner proximal margin of the femora is noted bilaterally. The metacarpals and phalanges are short and broad and all of the same length. The middle phalanges are triangular-shaped. The spine shows flattening of the vertebral bodies with an "H" or "U" configuration. There is widening of the intervertebral spaces. The normal widening of the interpediculate distances is not present. The iliac bones are short with horizontal inferior margins and a narrow sacrosciatic notch. The pubis and ischium are present. The ribs are shortened with a horizontal pitch.

tarsals, and proximal phalanges of the hands. The middle phalanges may be triangular-shaped.

The spine shows a characteristic flattening of the vertebral bodies in their midportions, resulting in an inverted "U" or an "H" configuration when superimposed over well-mineralized posterior elements. This is associated with marked increase in height of the intervertebral disk space. The interpediculate distances are narrowed, usually narrowest at the L–3 or L–4 level.

The iliac bones are short in their vertical diameter, with horizontal inferior margins. The sacrosciatic notch is narrow. The pubis and ischium are short and thick, but present. The pelvis is short and broad overall.

The thorax is narrow due to short ribs that do not extend around the anterior chest wall, and have a horizontal pitch. The rib ends are flared and may be cupped. The scapulae are small. The clavicles appear normal. Subcutaneous fat is increased.

The condition that thanatophoric dwarfism most closely resembles is homozygous achondroplasia. A history of both parents being achondroplastic would establish the diagnosis.

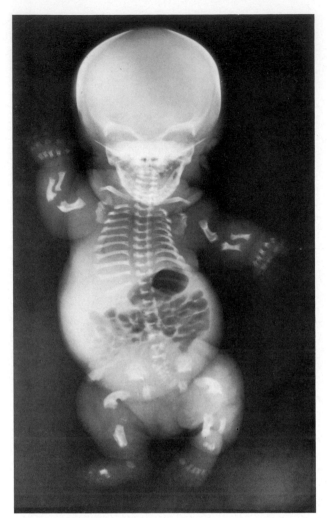

FIG. 5-8. Thanatophoric dwarfism—newborn infant. Note enlargement of the calvarium due to hydrocephalus. There is shortening of the ribs, which do not extend around the anterior thorax. The pelvis shows iliac underdevelopment, narrow sacrosciatic angles, and flat acetabular roofs. The spine shows flattening of all of the vertebral bodies and wide intervertebral spaces. There is diminution of the interpediculate distances, particularly in the lumbar region. The bones show shortening, curved deformities, and relative thickening. Irregularity and cupping of the metaphyses may be seen. The metacarpals tend to be of uniform length, as do the other short tubular bones.

ACHONDROGENESIS

Achondrogenesis[204] is a short-limb dwarf condition, classified into 2 types: a lethal type (type 1 or Parenti–Fraccaro), and a nonlethal type. The lethal type is incompatible with life. The clinical features overlap those of thanatophoric dwarfism, with extreme shortening of extremities and a usually enlarged head size. The overall body length is shorter than in thanatophoric dwarfism. There is a short chest, short neck, and rotund abdomen. The condition is transmitted as an autosomal recessive.

Radiologically, the disease is characterized by severe micromelia and extreme delay in ossification. The tubular bones are shortened with a rhizomelic distribution. The humeri and femora are short and wide but not bowed, a differential point from thanatophoric dwarfism. Short, sharp periosteal spicules of bone project from the ends of the femur, producing a faint "hairbrush" pattern.

The bones of the arms and the legs are also shortened, with irregular, poorly outlined, and cupped metaphyseal margins. Slight bowing of these bones is possible. The short tubular bones are shorter and wider than normal. The most striking radiologic feature is failure of ossification. This does not occur in thanatophoric dwarfism, and should be differentiated also from hypophosphatasia. The cervical and lumbar spine may not ossify, nor may the sacrum, ischia, pubis, calcaneus, and talus. The intervertebral disk spaces show a moderate increase in height. The interpediculate distances are normal (Fig. 5–9).

The shape of the ilia is distinctive, with diminished height, flat acetabular roofs, and poorly outlined lateral margins. The medial margins form a single large arc.

The skull may be normal, or enlarged with a normal base. The facial bones are disproportionately small.

The ribs are short with a horizontal pitch, and show flaring and irregularity at the anterior margins. Sternal ossification centers are absent. The scapulae are small and irregular, while the clavicles appear normal. The soft tissues are prominent.

There are many syndromes of neonatal dwarfism that are not compatible with life, and some that in their severe forms are not compatible with life. These are presented below.

NEONATAL DEATH DWARFISM[118]

Thanatophoric dwarfism
Chondrodysplasia punctata
Osteogenesis imperfecta congenita

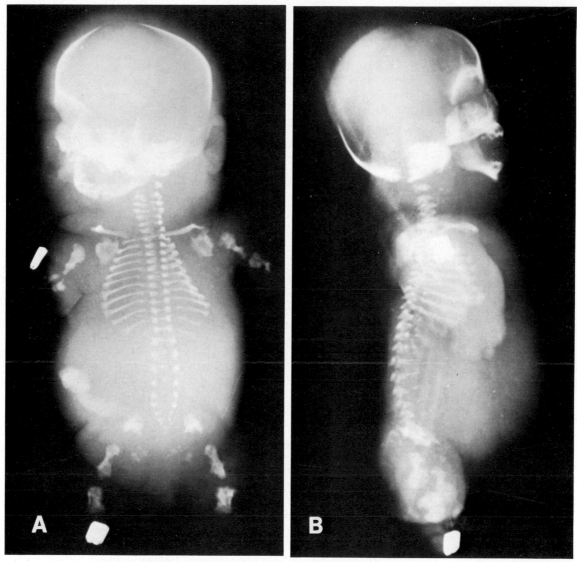

FIG. 5–9. Achondrogenesis. **A.** Anteroposterior view. There is shortening of both trunk and extremities, with extreme shortening of the tubular bones and irregular ossification. Metaphyseal widening giving a knobby appearance is present, but no bowing is seen. The ends of the bones, particularly the tibiae, have a radiating appearance. The ribs are shortened, and there is extreme narrowing of the vertebral bodies and widening of the intervertebral spaces. Normal widening of the interpediculate distances in the cervical and lumbar region is present. There is lack of ossification, most marked in the pelvis, with only rudimentary ossification of the ischia and pubes and minimal ossification of the ilia and sacrum. Ossification defects in the calvarium are also seen. The medial margins of the ilia form a single large arc. Prominence of the soft tissues is present. **B.** Lateral view shows extremely narrow vertebral bodies and wide intervertebral spaces, markedly shortened extremities, and ossification defects. The soft tissues are markedly prominent.

Asphyxiating thoracic dystrophy
Diastrophic dwarfism
Achondrogenesis lethal type
Hypophosphotasia — lethal form
Achondroplasia — homozygous
Unclassified lethal bone dysplasias

PSEUDOACHONDROPLASTIC DYSPLASIA (SPONDYLOEPIPHYSEAL DYSPLASIA, PSEUDOACHONDROPLASTIC TYPE, PSEUDOACHONDROPLASIA)

Pseudoachondroplastic dysplasia[69,144] is a rare short-limb bone dysplasia comprising dwarfism and rhizomelic shortening. It is transmitted as a mendelian dominant. A tarda form exists that is recessive. It is largely similar to achondroplasia except that:

1. It is not present at birth. Dwarfism usually becomes evident after the end of the second year. A late form with onset in the second decade has been reported.
2. The skull is not involved. The characteristic facial features of achondroplasia are lacking (Fig. 5–10).
3. The epiphyseal and metaphyseal portions of tubular bones show the changes that are ascribed to the hyperplastic type of achondropla-

sia. There are flaring, gross irregularities, fragmentation, and widening of the bone ends (Figs. 5–11, 5–12, 5–13). The hands and feet are short and stubby.

4. The spine shows changes similar to those of Morquio's disease. There are platyspondyly, hypoplasia of an upper lumbar vertebra, and anterior central tonguing of the vertebral bodies. Scoliosis may be present. The interpediculate distances are normal (Fig. 5–14). Posterior arch defects are common.
5. Initially, the pelvis is normal. There is no narrowing of the sacrosciatic notch. Marked irregularity of the acetabulum and femoral capital epiphysis develops. Hip dislocation, destruction of the hip joint, acetabular protrusion, and coxa vara may follow.
6. The ribs may be normal.

Electron microscopic studies indicate a specific ultrastructural defect of storage in the rough-surfaced endoplasmic reticulum of inclusions and whorls with alternate electron-dense and electron-lucent layers. The investigators suggest that the material may be abnormal protein — perhaps lipoprotein or glycoprotein. They theorize that a marked alteration in metabolism produces soft cartilage that deforms markedly under stress, and explain the

(Text continued on p. 257)

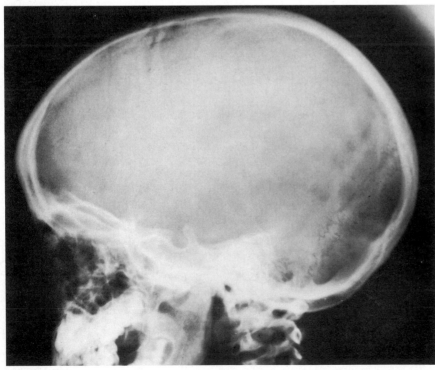

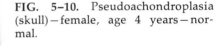

FIG. 5–10. Pseudoachondroplasia (skull) — female, age 4 years — normal.

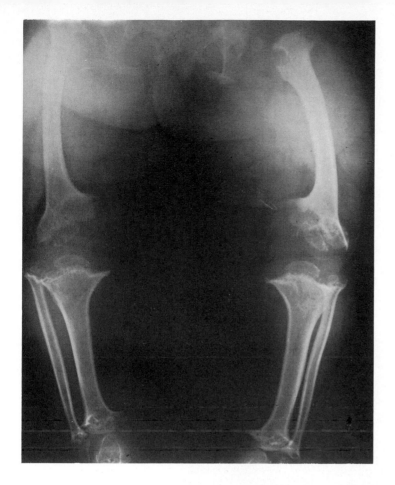

FIG. 5–11. Pseudoachondroplasia (lower extremities)—same patient as in Fig. 5–10, at age 6 years. Note shortening of all bones, fragmentation and irregularity of the metaphyses, and splaying of the ends. Small medially placed ossification centers at the femoral heads, and marked irregularity with slanting and deformity at the distal femoral metaphyses, may also be seen.

FIG. 5–12. Pseudoachondroplasia (lower extremities)—same patient as in Figs. 5–10 and 5–11, 4 years later. The appearance of the legs suggests the hyperplastic form of achondroplasia. There has been smoothening of the distal tibial and fibular epiphyses, with overgrowth at the malleoli. Residual irregularity at the proximal tibial metaphyses is present, and the previously seen splaying has now assumed a hyperplastic form. Shortening and relative thickening of the bones are prominent; the metatarsals, however, show thinning of the shafts and deformity.

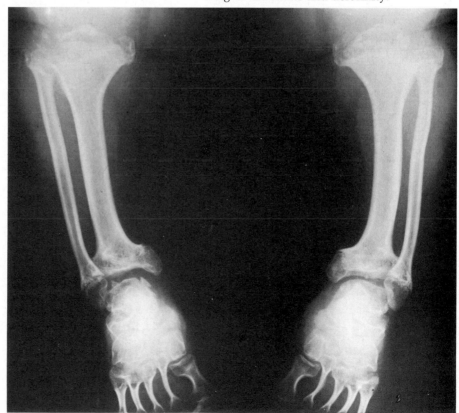

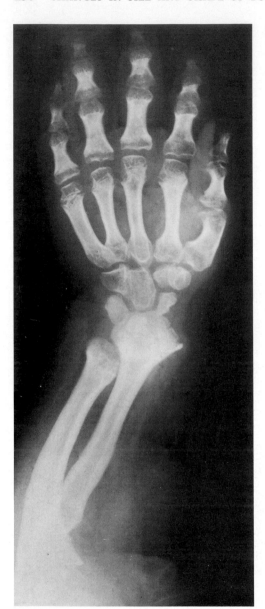

FIG. 5–13. Pseudoachondroplasia (left forearm)—same patient as in Figs. 5–10 to 5–12 at age 10 years. Note rectangular shape of bones with considerable shortening of radius and ulna. Prominence of distal radius and ulna is seen, with metaphyseal irregularity, indicative of pseudoachondroplasia.

FIG. 5–14. Pseudoachondroplasia (dorsolumbar spine)—same patient as in Figs. 5–10 to 5–13 at age 5 years. Platyspondylia with a central peg most marked in the lumbar spine, but also extending into the dorsal spine, can be seen.

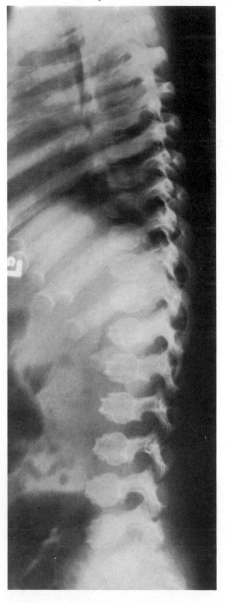

skeletal lesions as deformations which result when normal forces are applied to the soft epiphyseal cartilage. Normal ossification seems to prevail at sites protected from excessive stress such as the base of the skull, the face, and the sacrum. The skeletal abnormalities progress throughout childhood but improve with skeletal maturity. The disease has been classified into types I through IV, depending on severity and mode of genetic transmission.

METATROPIC DWARFISM

Metatropic dwarfism (metatropic dysplasia)[131] is a short-limb dwarfism with rhizomelic distribution and progressive kyphoscoliosis. At birth no clinical abnormalities may be recognized, or changes of achondroplasia may be suggested, with relatively short limbs, joint enlargement, and a relatively long trunk. The condition transforms itself, in time, to the opposite proportions with a short trunk and relatively long extremities, resembling Morquio's syndrome. It is transmitted as an autosomal recessive. No urinary mucopolysaccharides or corneal opacities have been reported.

Radiologically, in early life, the long tubular bones are shortened and thickened with a "dumbbell" shape owing to hyperplastic metaphyses, best seen at the lesser femoral trochanters. Platyspondyly and a "sail" vertebra may be present. The skull is generally normal. The hands are short and stubby. The ribs are short. The pelvis shows squared ilia, flattened acetabular roofs, and small sacroiliac notches, similar to those seen in achondroplasia. There is frequently a tail-like appendage at the cephalic end of the gluteal cleft, produced by a linear fold of skin extending over the coccyx. Ossification is delayed.

Kyphoscoliosis, which may be present at birth, progresses markedly, as does platyspondyly. The vertebral bodies are flattened, and in the lumbar area show posterior ossification defects and concavity. The interpediculate distances are usually normal. The base of the skull remains normal.

As the disease progresses, the extremities grow longer than would be expected in achondroplasia, and the proportions between the limbs and trunk reverse themselves (Fig. 5–15).

MESOMELIC DWARFISM

CHONDROECTODERMAL DYSPLASIA
(ELLIS–VAN CREVELD SYNDROME)

Chondroectodermal dysplasia[61] is a dysostosis caused by a defect in development of ectodermal and mesenchymal tissues. This leads to mesomelic dwarf-

ism associated with polydactyly, defects in hair, teeth and nails, and congenital heart disease, most commonly septal defects.

Clinically, the disease is manifest at birth. There is a narrow thorax and dwarfism, with the greatest shortening distal to the knees and elbows. The hands are short and stubby, with polydactyly or syndactyly; dentition is delayed and defective; and the scalp shows hypotrichosis. The nails are small, deformed, or absent. No constant biochemical abnormalities have been found. A high incidence in Amish populations of Pennsylvania and Ohio have been reported. The transmission is autosomal recessive.

Radiologically, there is shortening of the long bones, principally of the radius, ulna (Fig. 5–16), tibia, and fibula. Radioulnar dislocation is frequently present at the proximal end. The humerus and femur are of relatively normal length, although bowing and shortening may be present. According to Caffey,[38] the most characteristic findings in this disease are hypoplasia and medial position of the proximal tibial ossification center. There is ridging of the proximal shaft, and the lateral aspect of the ossification center does not develop (Fig. 5–17). A small exostosis may also be present. There is massive fusion of the carpal bones. Syndactyly and polydactyly are usually present (Fig. 5–18), associated with shortening of the digits, most pronounced in the distal and midphalanges. Maturation is accelerated. The ribs are shortened (Fig. 5–19). The pelvis is inconstantly involved, but may be underdeveloped in the supra-acetabular region. (Fig. 5–20). The skull and spine are normal. The joints are affected by dysplastic changes in the articular cartilage and bone deformities.

DYSCHONDROSTEOSIS

Dyschondrosteosis[119,125] is a rare congenital mesomelic dwarfism characterized by Madelung's deformity of the forearms and wrists, short forearms, and short lower legs. The disease is transmitted as an autosomal dominant with female preponderance.

Clinically, short stature, bowing of the radius, wrist drop, and limitation of movement at the wrist are noted. Intelligence is normal. No abnormal biochemical or endocrine values have been found.

Radiologically, Madelung's deformity is the hallmark of this disease. The process usually begins in adolescence with premature fusion of the medial aspect of the distal radial epiphysis, resulting in asymmetrical growth. The distal radial epiphysis assumes a triangular configuration prior to com-

(Text continued on p. 261)

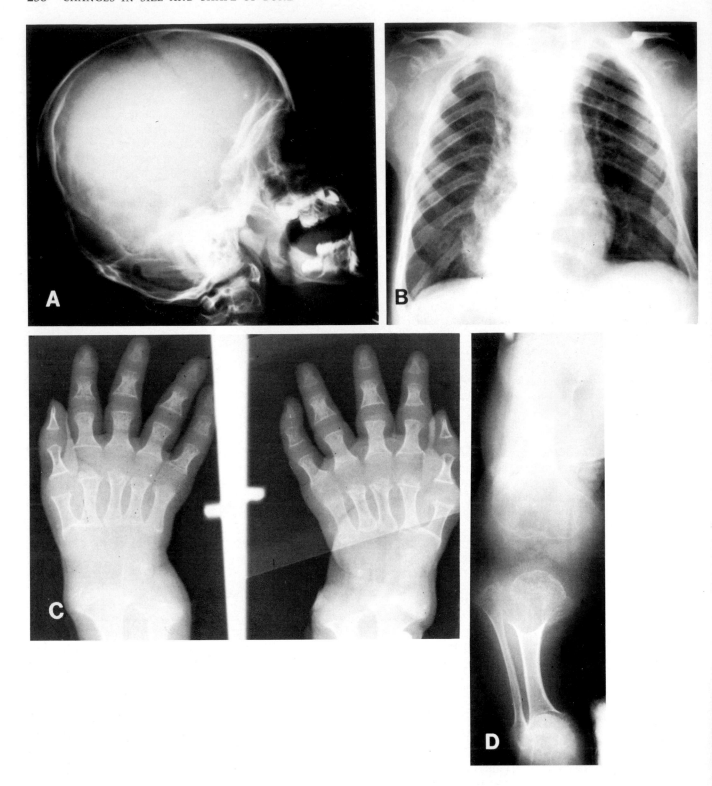

FIG. 5–15. Metatropic dwarfism—late kyphoscoliotic period. **A.** Skull. Brachycephaly with a shortened base and vertical clivus is noted. Hypoplasia of the odontoid process with atlantoaxial subluxation is also seen. **B.** Chest. Dorsal scoliosis, short and square scapulae, high clavicles, and bulbous ends of ribs are seen. **C.** Hands. Shortened metacarpals and phalanges with widened and cupped metaphyses are seen, as well as widening of the distal radius and ulna. **D.** Lower extremity. Shortening of the femur and tibia, and to a lesser extent the fibula, is noted. The metaphyses are broad and misshapen. The proximal femur is characteristically shaped like a battle-axe (halberd). (Courtesy of Dr. Harold Rosenbaum, Lexington, KY)

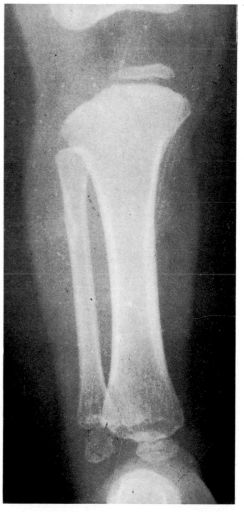

FIG. 5–17. Chondroectodermal dysplasia (leg). Note shortening of both tibia and fibula. The epiphyseal ossification center of the proximal tibia is hypoplastic and medially situated. There is a deficiency of the ossification center at the lateral aspect, and the metaphyseal line slopes laterally and distally. (Courtesy of Dr. Harvey White, Children's Memorial Hospital, Chicago, IL)

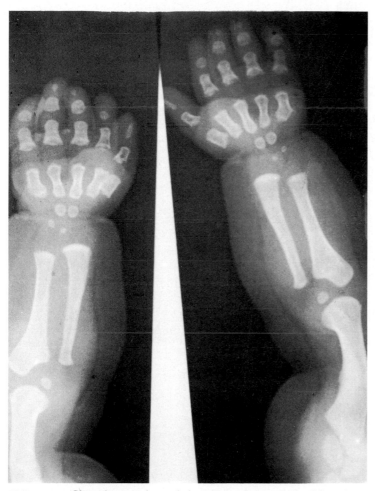

FIG. 5–16. Chondroectodermal dysplasia (forearms and hands). There is a mesomelic type of dwarfism, with shortening of the radius and ulna. Shortening of the small bones of the hand and of the humerus is also present. (Courtesy of Dr. Harvey White, Children's Memorial Hospital, Chicago, IL)

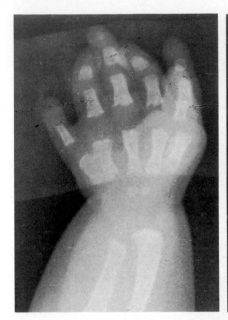

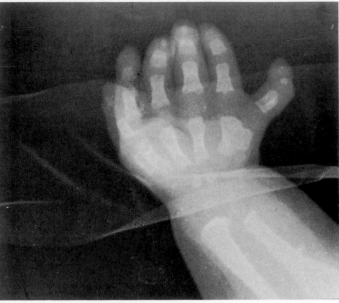

FIG. 5–18. Chondroectodermal dysplasia (hands). There is polydactylia with six digits bilaterally. Fusion of the fifth metacarpal with the supernumerary metacarpal bilaterally, and shortening of the tubular bones may also be noted. (Courtesy of Dr. Harvey White, Children's Memorial Hospital, Chicago, IL)

FIG. 5–19. Chondroectodermal dysplasia (ribs). Note shortening of all the ribs. (Courtesy of Dr. Harvey White, Children's Memorial Hospital, Chicago, IL)

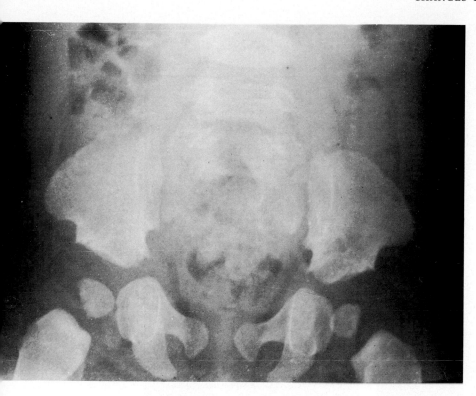

FIG. 5–20. Chondroectodermal dysplasia (pelvis). Enlargement of the acetabula bilaterally, a low sacral articulation, and hypoplasia of the ilia may be seen. (Courtesy of Dr. Harvey White, Children's Memorial Hospital, Chicago, IL)

plete fusion. The radius becomes bowed and decreased in length. A localized area of radiolucency at the ulnar aspect of the radial metaphysis may be present. A small exostosis may also be seen in this region. There is ulnar and volar angulation of the distal radial articular surface. The distal ulna is subluxed dorsally, with deformity of the ulnar head. The ulnar length may be decreased (Fig. 5–21). Partial dislocation of the elbow may also be present. The carpal bones become wedged between the deformed radius and ulna, and assume a triangular configuration with the lunate at the apex.

Additional findings are shortening and curvature of the tibia, and shortening of the fibula. The tibial metaphysis may be deformed, with valgus deformity of the knee, flattening of the medial epiphysis, and exostosis formation medially, reminiscent of Turner's syndrome.

The skull and axial skeleton are characteristically normal.

Madelung's deformity was first described in 1878, prior to dyschondrosteosis. Not all patients with Madelung's deformity have short stature, and the deformity may be unilateral.[67]

ACROMELIC DWARFISM

PERIPHERAL DYSOSTOSIS

Peripheral dysostosis[164,219] is a rare defect in enchondral bone formation limited to the hands and feet, leading to acromelic dwarfism.

Radiologically, there is shortening of the metacarpals, metatarsals, and phalanges. The epiphyses are cone-shaped or triangular-shaped, and extend into the central portions of the metaphyses (Fig. 5–22). Rarely the ossification centers may be sclerotic or ill-defined. The changes are most severe in the proximal phalangeal row. Accessory epiphyseal ossification centers may be present at the distal ends of the proximal phalanges and the proximal ends of the second and fifth metacarpals. A "ball-and-socket" configuration may also be present. The short tubular bones are short and broad. Several entities show these findings (also see pp 344–348), including: acrodysostosis, Brailsford's peripheral dysostosis, Ellis–van Creveld syndrome, Steinbach's epiphyseal dysostosis, trichorhinophalangeal syndrome, and pycnodysostosis.

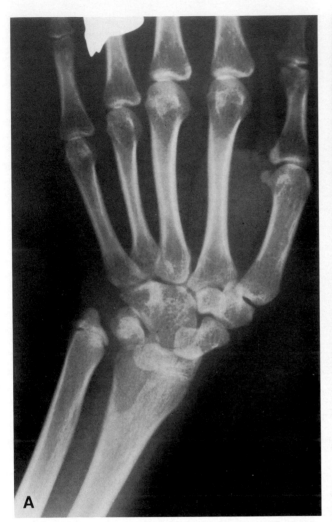 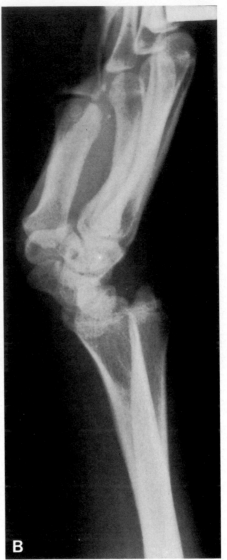

FIG. 5–21. Madelung's deformity, which may be seen in dyschondrosteosis. **A.** There is an increase in the interosseous space between the radius and the ulna, with a central obliquity giving a ''V''shape to the radiocarpal articulation. **B.** Lateral view of wrist. There is anterior curvature of the radius and posterior curvature of the distal ulna.

ASPHYXIATING THORACIC DYSPLASIA

Asphyxiating thoracic dysplasia (Jeune syndrome [99,115,180] or familial asphyxiating thoracic dystrophy) is a disturbance of formation of the ribs and distal phalanges. The patients die at an early age from pulmonary infections. There is no thoracic mobility during respiration.

Milder forms may occur, with longer survival. Progressive renal disease is reported if the patient survives infancy. The disease is transmitted as an autosomal recessive.

Radiologically, there is hypoplasia of the distal phalanges, similar to that in Ellis–van Creveld syndrome, causing an acromelic dwarfism. The thoracic cage is too small, with the ribs ending at the midaxillary line with bulbous expansion. The clavicles are horizontal and highly situated. There is flaring of the iliac bone, with irregular acetabular roofs and prominent spurs, and hypertrophy of the glenoid fossa. Jeune syndrome differs chiefly from Ellis–van Creveld syndrome by the absence of tibial plateau changes and the absence of carpal fusion (Fig. 5–23).

DEFORMED TYPE OF DWARFISM

DIASTROPHIC DWARFISM

Diastrophic dwarfism (diastrophic dysplasia)[6,122,124,333] is a congenital, autosomal recessive, skeletal abnormality which is present at birth. The principal changes are short-limb dwarfism combined with clubfoot and scoliosis, giving a deformed or twisted appearance. This is caused by a neuromesodermal defect. Restricted joint motion and dislocations — particularly of the hips — are common. There is a thickened earlobe and reduced auditory canal. Cleft palate may also be present. The clubfoot deformities are said to resist correction. No abnormal laboratory values have been found. Mentation is normal. The sex incidence is equal.

Radiologically, the long bones are shortened, usu-ally most pronouncedly in the forearms. Bowing may be present. The appearance of the epiphyses is delayed. The bone ends are enlarged. The femoral heads may be larger than the acetabula. The metaphyses are wide and flared, and occasional cystic changes may be present. Cupping may occur. Talipes equinovarus is present (Fig. 5–24). The hands show uneven brachydactyly, deformities, and abducted thumbs, the so-called "hitchhiker" thumb (Fig. 5–25). The first metacarpal may have a triangular shape. The skull is normal and no hydrocephalus is present. There may be hypertelorism and protruding upper teeth. The vertebral column shows scoliosis and lumbar lordosis with posterior tilt of the sacrum. Kyphosis may also be present. The interpediculate distances have been reported as narrowed. The vertebral bodies are normal (Figs. 5–26, 5–27). Subluxations in the cervical spine may be present. The pelvis, scapula, and ribs are essentially normal, except for secondary changes.

(Text continued on p. 266)

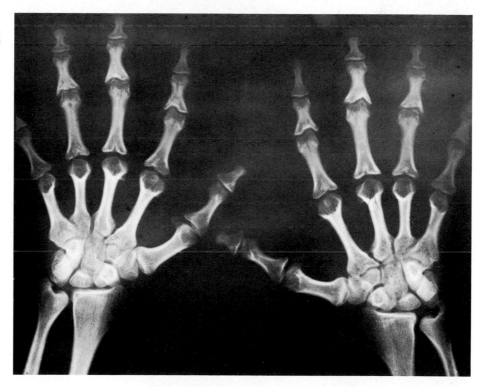

FIG. 5–22. Peripheral dysostosis (hands). Note shortening of all the short tubular bones of the hands, with the typical cup-shaped metaphyses.

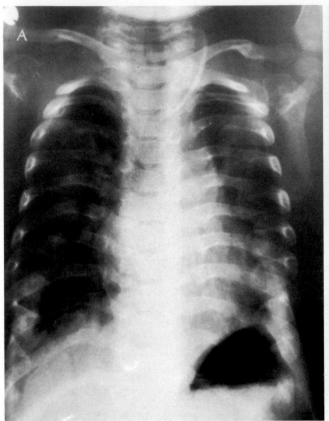

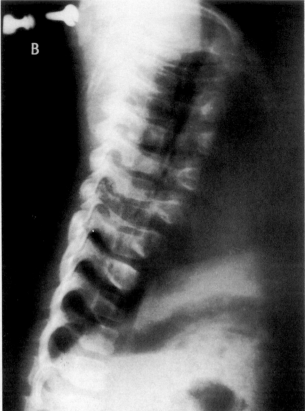

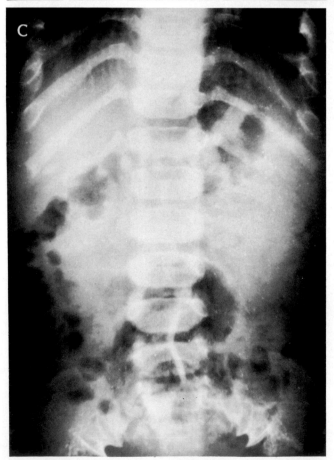

FIG. 5–23. Familial asphyxiating thoracic dystrophy —male, age 13 months, who died of respiratory causes. **A,B.** The ribs are short, do not extend around the chest, and have a horizontal pitch. The spine is normal. **C.** The ilia are flared and the acetabular roofs are flattened. (Obliquity has also been reported.) A "hooklike" configuration at the greater sciatic notch is present.

The hands and feet in this case are normal. Polydactyly has been reported in infants, as well as cone-shaped epiphyses and early fusion of epiphyses of the hands and feet. Early ossification of the femoral capital epiphyses may be present. (Courtesy of Dr. Antonio Pizarro, Mount Sinai Hospital, Chicago, IL) Data from: Langer LO: Thoracic pelvic-phalangeal dystrophy. Radiology 91:447–456, 1968)

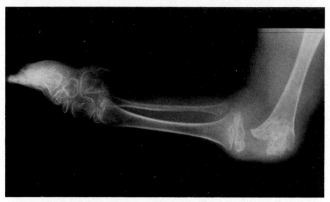

FIG. 5–24. Diastrophic dwarfism (leg and foot). Note shortening of the bones with flaring of the epiphysis and a cup-shaped distal femoral metaphysis, and equinus deformity of the foot. (From Amuso SJ: Diastrophic dwarfism. J Bone Joint Surg 50-A:113–122, 1968)

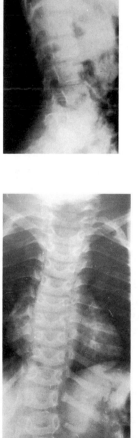

FIG. 5–26. Diastrophic dwarfism (spine, lateral view). The vertebral bodies and the intervertebral spaces are normal. (From Amuso SJ: Diastrophic dwarfism. J Bone Joint Surg 50-A:113–122, 1968)

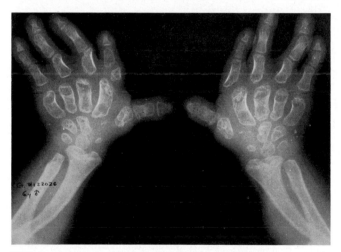

FIG. 5–25. Diastrophic dwarfism (hands). The metacarpals and phalanges are short, thick, and irregularly ossified. The deformed carpal bones have sharp, dense borders. The first metacarpal is particularly short and is oval or triangular in shape. The position of the thumbs is characteristically abducted. (From Amuso SJ: Diastrophic dwarfism. J Bone Joint Surg 50-A:113–122, 1968)

FIG. 5–27. Diastrophic dwarfism (dorsolumbar spine). Thoracic scoliosis is present. The interpediculate spaces of the lumbar spine are normal or only slightly narrower. (From Amuso SJ: Diastrophic dwarfism. J Bone Joint Surg 50-A:113–122, 1968)

THE GENETIC MUCOPOLYSACCHARIDOSES[77,80,162]

Mucopolysaccharides are widely distributed tissue structural components. The mucopolysaccharide molecule consists of a protein core from which polysaccharide side chains arise. These side chains are composed of repeating disaccharide units, each consisting of a uronic acid and a sulfated hexoxamine residue. The differences between the various types are determined by different constituents in their disaccharide units. The various mucopolysaccharides have been summarized by Groover et al[77] and are presented below.

NOMENCLATURE OF MUCOPOLYSACCHARIDES*

Old Term	New Term
Acid mucopolysaccharide	Glycosaminoglycuronoglycan
Chondroitin sulfate A	Chondroitin 4-sulfate
Chondroitin sulfate C	Chondroitin 6-sulfate
Chondroitin sulfate B	Dermatan sulfate
Heparatin sulfate	Heparan sulfate
Keratosulfate	Keratan sulfate

Mucopolysaccharides are normally excreted in the urine in amounts less than 15 mg per 24 hours. In the genetic mucopolysaccharidoses, patients often excrete more than 100 mg per 24 hours. Each disease is characterized by a predominant urinary mucopolysaccharide, with some others present as well, and also partly degraded forms.

The basic defect in these diseases is impairment of the breakdown of the side chains due to specific enzyme defects. Electron microscopy has shown that the intracellular accumulations are within lysosomes that are packed with particles of only partly degraded mucopolysaccharide. Intracellular accumulation of gangliosides also occurs in some of these disorders. The diseases have been classified on the basis of clinical features and the predominantly excreted acid mucopolysaccharide,[150] and are presented in Table 5–1.

The mucopolysaccharidoses (except Morquio's syndrome) and the mucolipidoses all show a somewhat similar roentgen appearance and cannot be differentiated on roentgen examination alone.

* From Groover RV, Burke EC, Berdon WE: Seminars Hemat 9:371–402, 1972

HURLER'S SYNDROME[28,88] (GARGOYLISM, DYSOSTOSIS MULTIPLEX, LIPOCHONDRODYSTROPHY, HURLER–PFAUNDLER SYNDROME)

The patients with this disease excrete heparan sulfate and dermatan sulfate in the urine.

The disease is not seen at birth, and usually becomes evident at the end of the first year of life. In rare cases bone changes may be seen as early as 2 months of age. It is transmitted as an autosomal recessive.

Clinical features include dwarfism, infantilism, mental retardation, coarse facial features, large bulging head, flat bridge of the nose, flared nostrils, large tongue and lips, hypertelorism, corneal opacities, deformed teeth, hepatosplenomegaly, short neck, kyphosis with dorsolumbar gibbus, and limited extension of joints. Respiratory infections and cardiac failure commonly occur, usually causing death within the first decade.

Histologically, a cell distended with cytoplasmic polysaccharide deposition, called a "clear cell" or "gargoyle cell," is present in the lesions. Heavy granulations in the protoplasm of polymorphonuclear leukocytes and lymphocytes have been found in many cases.

Radiologically, there is a marked degree of variation in the involvement of the extremities. The long bones usually show thickening and sclerosis; however, an osteoporotic type of variation may be present. The upper extremities are usually more affected than the lower, and either end of a bone may show involvement. The principal change is thickening of the shafts of bone, tapering toward the ends. The diaphysis may have an irregular, wavy contour. The cortex may be thickened or thinned. There is an angulated obliquity of the growth plates. The radius and ulna may be tipped toward each other (Figs. 5–28, 5–29). Dorsal angulation of the proximal humeral segment may also be present, causing limited motion in the shoulder. Coxa valga is common. The proximal femora are usually constricted and narrowed in caliber. Genu valgum is constantly present (Fig. 5–30). The hands are trident and show coarse trabeculation. The most characteristic change in the hands is proximal tapering of the metacarpals (Fig. 5–31). The metacarpals and phalanges do not have a normal diaphyseal constriction.

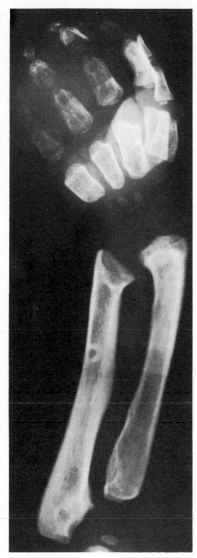

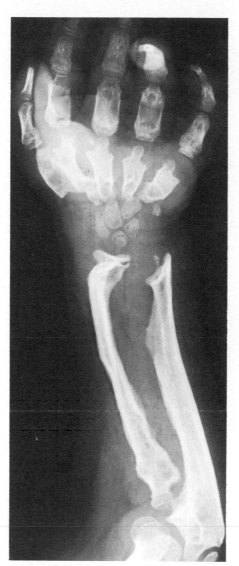

FIG. 5–28. Hurler's syndrome (forearm, wrist, and hand). Note thickening of the shafts of the long and short bones, with tapering at the ends. The inner aspects of the radius and ulna show an irregular wavy contour. The metaphyses are obliquely slanted, the distal radial and ulnar metaphyses tilting toward each other.

FIG. 5–29. Hurler's syndrome (forearm and hand). There is an irregular wavy contour of the diaphyses of both radius and ulna, with tapering of the distal ulna and shortening and proximal tapering of the metacarpals. Note the notchlike configuration of the distal metacarpals and a "cut corner" appearance of several proximal phalanges. (Courtesy of Dr. Harvey White, Children's Memorial Hospital, Chicago IL)

FIG. 5–28   FIG. 5–29

TABLE 5–1. Classification of the Genetic Mucopolysaccharidoses

McKusick's	Name Other Names	Genetics*	Predominant Mucopolysaccharide in Urine
Type I	Hurler	AR	Heparan sulfate Dermatan sulfate
Type II	Hunter	XR	Heparan sulfate Dermatan sulfate
Type III	Sanfilippo: polydystrophic oligophrenia	AR	Heparan sulfate
Type IV	Morquio Morquio–Brailsford	AR	Keratan sulfate
Type V	Scheie	AR	Heparan sulfate
Type VI	Maroteaux–Lamy: polydystrophic dwarfism	AR	Dermatan sulfate
Others:			

* AR, autosomal recessive; XR, X-linked recessive.

The skull is larger than normal, usually dolichocephalic (Fig. 5–32) because of premature fusion of the sagittal suture, although acrocephaly, oxycephaly, brachycephaly, and hydrocephalus have been reported. Prominence of the frontal bones is common. A "J-shaped" sella turcica is characteristic (*i.e.,* a shallow elongated sella with a long anterior recess extending under the anterior clinoid processes) (Fig. 5–33). There is a broad mandible, poorly developed dentition, and widely separated teeth. The mandibular condyle shows flattening or concavity of the articular surface. The ribs are typically widened at the shafts, causing a decrease in the intercostal space. There is a spatulalike narrow origin and a "bullet nose" appearance of the termination, resulting in "canoe paddle" ribs (Fig. 5–34). The pelvis shows variable involvement, with flaring of the iliac wings and tapering or constriction of the ilia near the acetabulum (Fig. 5–35). There may be shallow acetabula, or acetabular protrusion. The clavicle may show resorption, sclerosis, and tapering.

The spine shows distinctive changes. Oval centra with an anterior inferior beak are present (Fig. 5–36). A hypoplastic ("sail") vertebra in the upper lumbar region is present, with an inferior beak, causing sharp angular kyphosis (Fig. 5–37). Deep

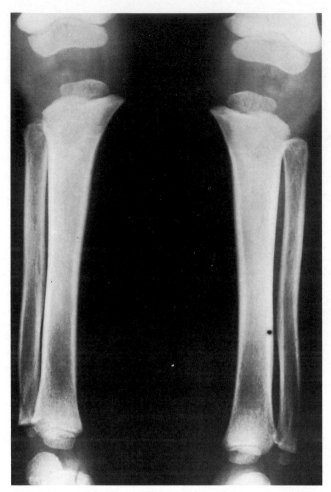

FIG. 5–30. Hurler's syndrome (knees and legs). Note underconstriction of the shafts of both tibiae and fibulae. The distal femoral metaphyses and growth plates tilt medially, associated with a marked lateral tilt of the proximal tibial epiphyseal plates, resulting in a genu valgum.

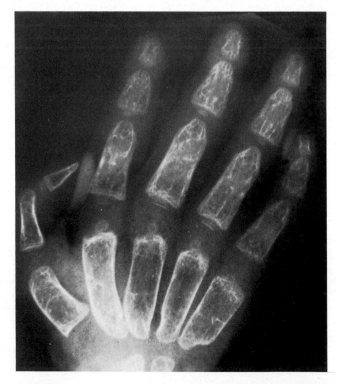

FIG. 5–31. Hurler's syndrome (hand). There is severe osteoporosis with cortical thinning. The characteristic proximal tapering of the metacarpals is prominent.

FIG. 5–32. Hurler's syndrome (skull). Note dolichocephaly and "J-shaped" sella turcica with a shallow configuration and a very long anterior recess.

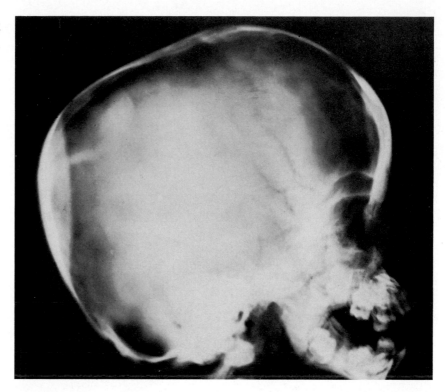

FIG. 5–33. Hurler's syndrome (skull)—enlargement of the skull due to hydrocephalus. Note burr holes posteriorly and residual contrast material. A "J-shaped" sella turcica is well demonstrated, with an anterior recess extending under the anterior clinoid processes.

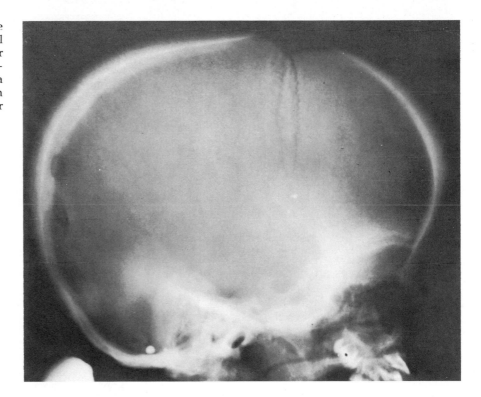

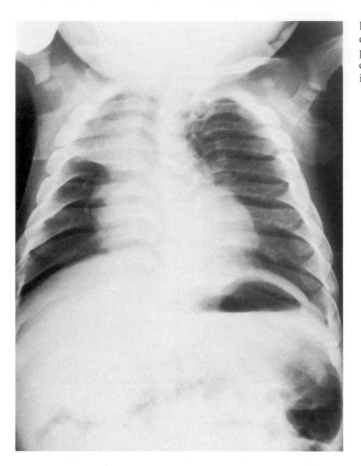

FIG. 5–34. Hurler's syndrome (chest). There is widening of the middle and distal aspects of the ribs, with a narrow proximal segment, giving the so-called "canoe paddle" rib configuration. A right upper lobe atelectasis may be noted incidentally.

FIG. 5–35. Hurler's syndrome (pelvis and upper femora). Note flaring of the iliac wings with tapering of the distal ilia, and the characteristic bilateral constriction superior to the acetabula. There is widening of the sacroiliac joints bilaterally. Both acetabula are shallow. Bilateral coxa valga and constrictions of the proximal femora are present.

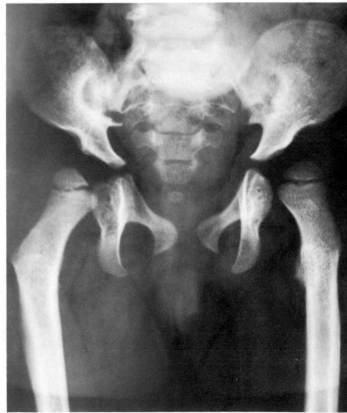

indentations, or scalloping of the lateral aspects of the sacral vertebrae, are sometimes seen. There may be hypoplasia and demineralization of the pedicles with widening of the interpediculate spaces and posterior scalloping of the vertebral bodies, giving a false impression of an intraspinal mass (Fig. 5–38).

Differentiation from Morquio's syndrome can best be determined in the spine. Ovoid bodies with inferior beaking can be easily distinguished from the typical universal vertebra plana with central beaking of Morquio's syndrome. In addition, acetabular irregularities are more pronounced in Morquio's syndrome.

Patients showing the features of Hurler's syndrome but without mucopolysacchariduria have been reported.[226]

HUNTER'S SYNDROME

Hunter's syndrome is similar clinically and radiologically to Hurler's syndrome, but has a slower rate

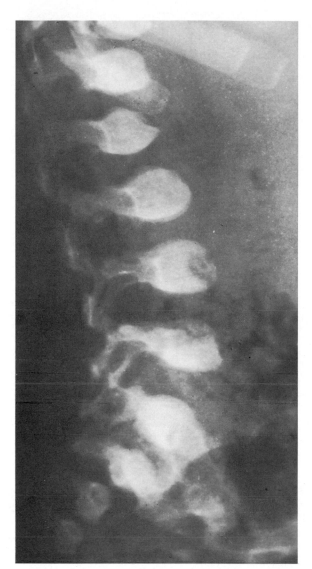

FIG. 5–36. Hurler's syndrome (lumbar spine). Note oval centra with inferior beaking. There is hypoplasia of the second lumbar vertebra with an inferior beak, the so-called "sail" vertebra. Hypoplasia of an upper lumbar vertebra is not limited to this condition. (See Table 5–8 for differential diagnoses.) Posterior scalloping of the lumbar vertebral bodies is also visible with an apparent increase in the depth of the spinal canal.

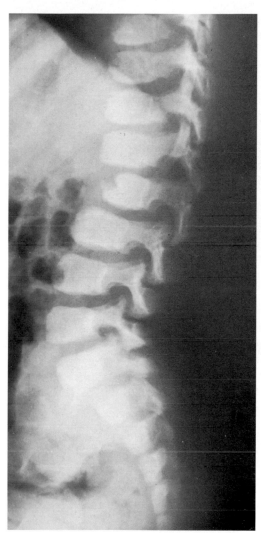

FIG. 5–37. Hurler's syndrome (spine). Note hypoplastic second lumbar vertebral body or "sail" vertebra, with sharp inferior beak.

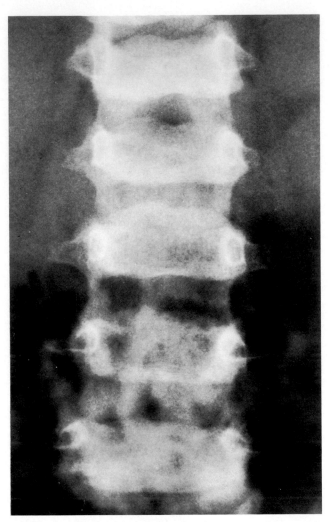

FIG. 5–38. Hurler's syndrome (lumbar spine). Note widening of the interpediculate spaces, giving the false impression of an intraspinal mass.

of progression. The disease is usually detected between the ages of 2 and 6 years. Mental retardation occurs. Corneal clouding is absent. It is transmitted as an X-linked recessive. Death usually occurs in the second or third decade. All reported cases are in males[13] (Figs. 5–39, 5–40, 5–41).

SANFILIPPO'S SYNDROME

Patients with this syndrome show signs of mental retardation toward the end of the second year of life. There is progressive coarsening of facial features and hypertrichosis. Dwarfism does not occur and skeletal abnormalities are minimal. Significant heart disease is rare. Progressive spastic quadriparesis occurs, resulting in death usually in the first or second decade (Fig. 5–42).

SCHEIE'S SYNDROME

The manifestations of *Scheie's syndrome* are variable. Corneal clouding usually occurs at about 6 years of age, but the age of occurrence may range from infancy to adolescence. Mentation is not usually impaired. Mild visceral and skeletal abnormalities are seen. Aortic regurgitation may occur. The patients reported have survived to adulthood.[13]

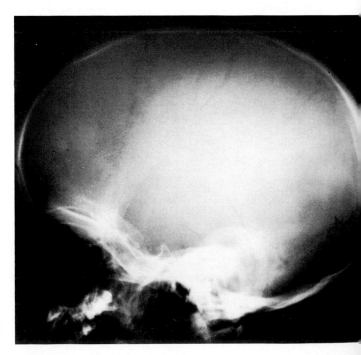

FIG. 5–39. Hunter's syndrome (skull). Enlargement of the skull and a "J-shaped" sella turcica are noted.

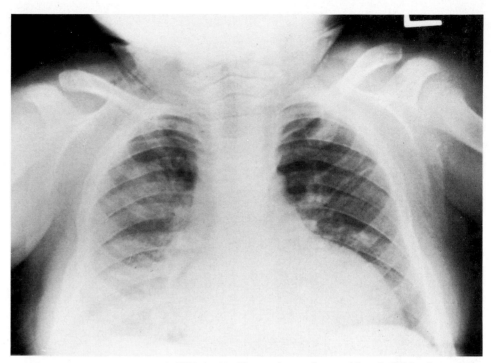

FIG. 5–40. Hunter's syndrome (chest). Widening of the ribs with a narrow margin giving a "canoe paddle" appearance is noted.

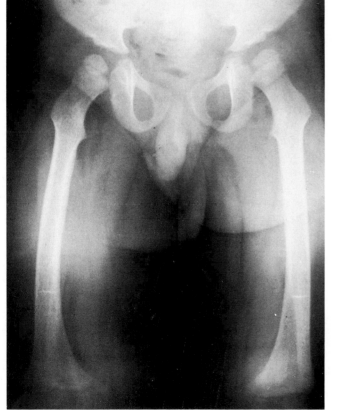

FIG. 5–41. Hunter's syndrome (pelvis and femora). There is flaring of the ilia with constriction and a notch superior to the acetabula. The acetabula are shallow. Bilateral coxa valga is present as well as osteoporosis of the femora and lack of constriction. Nonspecific transverse growth lines in the distal femora are also seen.

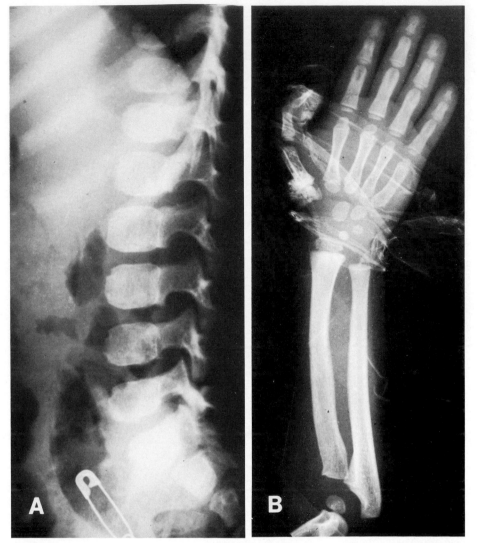

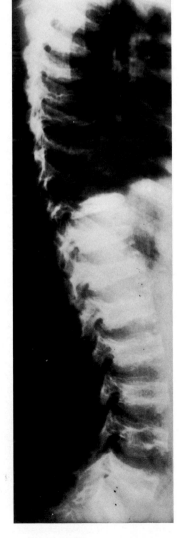

FIG. 5–42. Sanfilippo's syndrome. **A.** Lumbar spine. Oval vertebral bodies with beaking, some of which are inferior and some of which are central, are noted. **B.** Forearm, wrist, and hand. Loss of bone density with slight coarsening of the trabecular pattern is present. There is no evidence of proximal tapering.

FIG. 5–43. Morquio's syndrome (spine)—universal vertebra plana. Central beaking of the fourth and fifth lumbar vertebral bodies may be noted, in contrast to the inferior beaking seen in Hurler's syndrome.

MAROTEAUX–LAMY SYNDROME

Patients with this syndrome develop skeletal dysplasia between the ages of 2 and 5 years. Corneal clouding develops early. The intellect is normal. Progressive bony changes similar to those of Hurler's syndrome ensue, leading to dwarfism and flexion contractures of joints. Macrocrania and hydrocephalus may occur. Hepatomegaly and cardiac lesions are frequent, as is hearing loss. The patients reported have survived to early adulthood.[13]

OTHER MUCOPOLYSACCHARIDOSES

Winchester et al[245] have described a condition with a roentgen appearance simulating that of rheumatoid arthritis. Horton and Schimke have described a condition with progressive joint contractures.[245] A concept of focal mucopolysaccharidosis has been proposed for several syndromes. Genetic compound syndromes, such as Hurler–Scheie, have also been reported.

MORQUIO'S SYNDROME
(MORQUIO–BRAILSFORD DISEASE)[128,211]

Morquio's syndrome now has rigid diagnostic criteria, and is restricted to those patients having mucopolysacchariduria. Mucopolysaccharide excretion may decrease with age. Clinical manifestations are generally first seen during the second year of life, with slowing of linear growth and progressive skeletal deformity. Corneal opacities are present. Hepatomegaly, cardiac lesions, and deafness may occur.

The body proportions are the opposite of those seen in achondroplasia, with a short trunk and extremities of relatively normal length. The head is relatively large, but it has a normal shape, and the facies are normal. There is usually no mental retardation. There are dorsolumbar kyphosis and multiple deformities of the extremities, with flexion deformities of both knees and hips resulting in a semicrouching stance, knock knees, swelling at the knees and elbows, and flat feet. A short deep thorax with a pigeon breast deformity is present. Weakness of the arms and legs is associated with a clumsy gait. Death may occur in the first or second decade, although some patients survive longer. Many patients have dysplasia of the odontoid process with resultant atlantoaxial instability. These patients are at risk of acute traumatic quadriparesis, chronic myelopathy, and sudden death by respiratory arrest. The external proportions described above must be present in order to diagnose this condition, regardless of the roentgen appearance.

Radiologically, the most important changes are seen in the spine, and consist of universal vertebra plana which is the principal cause of loss of stature (Fig. 5–43). There may be a hypoplastic dens, which gives rise to neurological symptoms (Fig. 5–44). A hypoplastic upper lumbar vertebra may also be present. The vertebral bodies show a central anterior beak in contrast to the inferior anterior beak seen in Hurler's disease. The intervertebral spaces initially are widened, and later become narrowed. There is shortening of the neck, dorsal rotary scoliosis, and dorsolumbar kyphosis. Wide interpediculate spaces may also be seen (Fig. 5–45).

In the long bones, according to Caffey,[38] the most diagnostic finding is defective and irregular ossification of the femoral capital epiphyses with flattening. The femoral neck is short and thick, and there may be varus or valgus deformity (Fig. 5–46).

There is delay in appearance of the epiphyseal ossification centers and carpal and tarsal bones, as well as irregularity and multiple centers. The appearance of the long bones is very variable. Some cases resemble achondroplasia, and others resemble rickets with metaphyseal flaring (Fig. 5–47). The length and caliber of the diaphysis varies.

The hands show brachydactyly, and the metacarpal ends may have an irregular conical appearance. An accentuated trabecular pattern is sometimes present (Fig. 5–48).

The skull and facial bones are normal. The ribs may be thickened or thinned, and are often associated with a barrel chest. The mandible, clavicle, and teeth are normal. The pelvis shows rounding of the iliac crests and tapering of the distal ilia. The acetabulum is deep, enlarged, and has an irregular contour. The sacrum is small and may articulate low on the ilia (Fig. 5–49), with a narrow ovoid pelvic inlet and a wide pubic synchrondrosis.

There is marked degeneration involving all of the articular surfaces. The wrists and ankles develop irregularities and angulations. Hyperlaxity of joints is present, progressing to limitation of motion.

Morquio's syndrome should be differentiated from:

1. Spondyloepiphyseal dysplasia congenita
2. Spondyloepiphyseal dysplasia tarda
3. Metatropic dwarfism (see p. 256)
4. Parastremmatic dwarfism (see Table 5–5, p. 354)
5. Kniest's dwarfism (see Table 5–5, p. 355)
6. Diastrophic dwarfism (see p. 263)

(Text continued on p. 279)

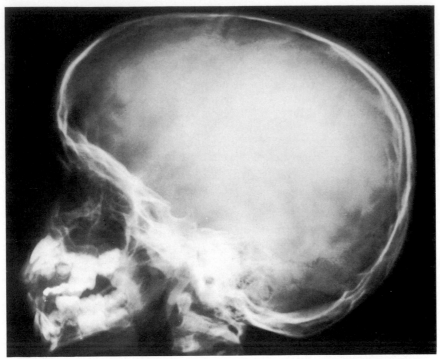

FIG. 5–44. Morquio's syndrome (skull and upper cervical spine). There is hypoplasia of the odontoid process of C-2, which does not articulate with the atlas. The skull appears normal.

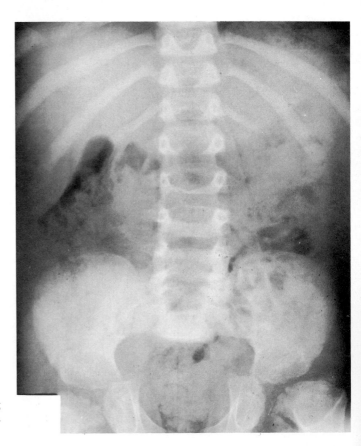

FIG. 5–45. Morquio's syndrome (lumbar spine). Widening of the lumbar interpediculate spaces, similar to that seen in Hurler's syndrome, is noted.

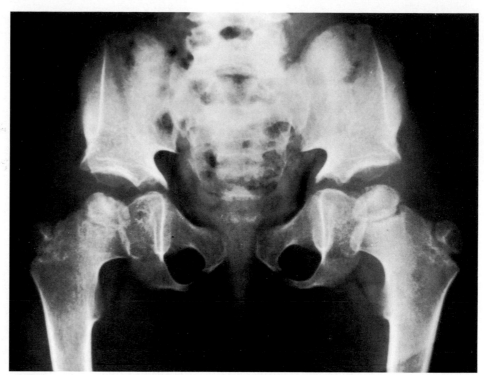

FIG. 5–46. Morquio's syndrome (pelvis and upper femora). Note irregularity and flattening of the femoral capital epiphyses, and irregularity of the ossification centers of the greater trochanter. Shortening and thickening of both femoral necks may be seen, and there is enlargement of the acetabula.

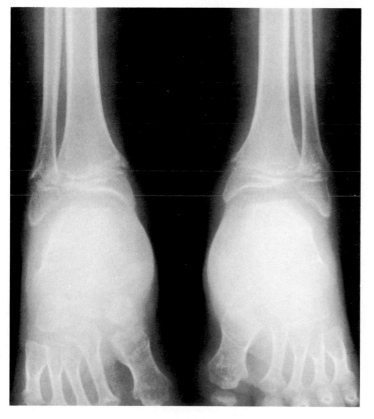

FIG. 5–47. Morquio's syndrome (ankles). Note metaphyseal irregularity. The contour and density of the distal tibial and fibular shafts appear normal.

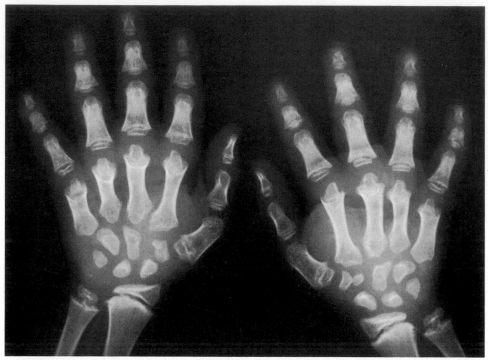

FIG. 5–48. Morquio's syndrome (hands). Note brachydactyly and irregular conical appearance of the distal metacarpals bilaterally. Metaphyseal cupping and metaphyseal irregularities of the distal radii and ulnae may also be seen. Slight accentuation of the trabecular pattern of the phalanges is apparent.

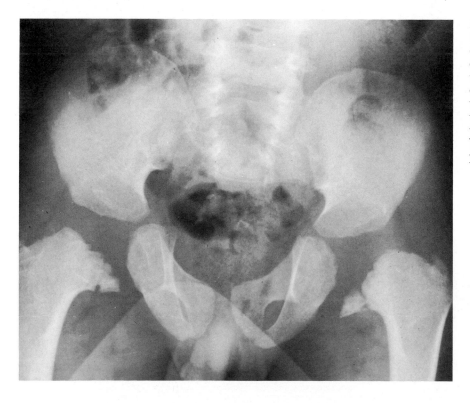

FIG. 5–49. Morquio's syndrome (pelvis). There is marked widening of the acetabula with irregularity of contour. The sacrum is set low on the ilia. Note defective ossification of the femoral capital epiphyses, with metaphyseal irregularity and thick femoral necks, and some thickening of the femoral shafts. Widening of the lumbar interpediculate spaces is present.

TABLE 5–2. The Mucolipidoses*

Disease	Enzyme Deficiency	Mucopolysacchariduria
GM$_1$ gangliosidosis I	β-Galactosidases A, B, and C	No
GM$_1$ gangliosidosis II	β-Galactosidases B and C	No
Fucosidosis	α-Fucosidase	No
Mannosidosis	α-Mannosidase	No
Sulfatide lipidosis with mucopolysaccharidosis (Austin)	Arylsulfatases A, B, and C	Yes
Mucolipidosis I (lipomucopolysaccharidosis—Spranger and Wiedemann)	?	No
Mucolipidosis II (I-cell disease of Leroy)	?	No
Mucolipidosis III (pseudopolydystrophy)[12, 154]	?	No

* Modified from Groover RV, Burke EC, Gordon H, Berdon WE: Seminars Hemat 9:371–402, 1972

Spondyloepiphyseal dysplasia congenita[224] is a heritable bone dysplasia with probable autosomal dominant transmission. It is manifest at birth, with short stature and retarded ossification of the vertebral bodies, pelvis, and extremities. In later life flattening and dysplasia of the vertebral bodies, hypoplasia of the odontoid process, pelvic dysplasia with a low square ilium and a horizontal deep acetabulum, underossified femoral head and neck with varus deformity, shortening of the long bones with rhizomelic distribution, and epiphyseal and metaphyseal dysplasia are seen. The hands and feet are relatively normal. Myopia and retinal detachment are common. Dorsal kyphosis is constant, and scoliosis may develop.

This condition may be differentiated from Morquio's syndrome by absence of corneal clouding and mucopolysacchariduria, and by manifestations present at birth. Radiological differences in the pelvis are significant. Morquio's syndrome, unlike this condition, shows severe changes in the hands and feet.

Spondyloepiphyseal dysplasia tarda is a short-trunk type of dwarfism transmitted as an X-linked recessive. Only males are affected, and the condition is rarely discovered before the tenth year. Platyspondyly and a hump-shaped mound on the superior and inferior surfaces of the lumbar vertebral bodies may be seen. A deep narrow pelvic configuration has been described, with later development of osteoarthritic changes in the hips.

THE MUCOLIPIDOSES

The mucolipidoses are a group of disorders in which excess materials are stored in lysosomes. The materials may be acid mucopolysaccharides, glycolipids, or sphingolipids. Mucopolysacchariduria does not occur in most of these conditions. A classification has been suggested by Groover *et al*[77] and is presented in Table 5–2.

Clinically and radiologically, the mucolipidoses resemble the mucopolysaccharidoses, with a wide spectrum of severity in the various forms.

GM$_1$ gangliosidosis is characterized by the accumulation of 10 times the normal amount of GM$_1$ ganglioside (monosialoganglioside) in the brain. There is a deficiency of the enzyme B-galactosidase, required for the normal catalysis of ganglioside (GM) and mucopolysaccharide. Visceral histiocytosis is present and contains a mucopolysaccharide that is structurally similar to keratin sulfate. The quantity of mucopolysaccharides in the urine is usually normal. The patients show psychomotor retardation, hepatosplenomegaly, and many of the clinical and radiological features of Hurler's syndrome. The characteristic upper lumbar kyphosis and beaking is present due to an abnormal growth process.[193]

Mannosidosis[223] is a lysosomal storage disorder owing to a defect in the enzyme α-D-mannosidase. This results in intracellular accumulation and excessive urinary excretion of mannose-containing oligosaccharides.

Clinically, the disease manifests itself between 1 and 3 years of age. Slow psychomotor development, impaired speech, coarse facial features, hepatosplenomegaly, hearing loss, cataracts, and umbilical or inguinal hernias are the principal findings.

Radiologically, the picture is of a moderate dysostosis multiplex pattern, with thickened calvaria, ovoid, flat, or beaked deformity of the vertebral bodies, and expansion of the short tubular bones.

No canoe-paddle ribs are noted. The long bones are normal.

Type I Mucolipidosis (Spranger and Wiedemann) is characterized by excess accumulation of mucopolysaccharides and glycolipids. No excess mucopolysacchariduria is present. The patients show mild mental retardation, neurological deterioration, hypotonia, and cherry-red macular spots. The clinical features resemble those of Hurler's syndrome. The disease is transmitted as an autosomal recessive. Radiologic changes are similar to those of the Sanfilippo syndrome.

Type II Mucolipidosis (I-Cell Disease of Leroy)[174, 232] resembles Hurler's syndrome clinically, except that these patients excrete a normal amount of urinary acid mucopolysaccharides. Fibroblasts grown from skin biopsies contain a large number of dark inclusions in the cytoplasm, hence the term *inclusion* or *I-cell disease.*

These inclusions have unusual staining properties. Clinical findings include congenital dislocation of the hips, mental retardation, dwarfism, limited joint mobility, possible hepatosplenomegaly, and tightness of the skin. The mode of transmission is probably autosomal recessive. The condition is apparent within the first 6 months of life. No corneal clouding is present. The radiological features are similar to those found in Hurler's sydrome.

Three cases of I-cell disease in neonates with unusual features have been reported.[174] These included subperiosteal bone resorption, periosteal new bone formation, and metaphyseal irregularities. Premature synostosis of the cranial sutures also occurred. At 10 months of age, the features become similar to those of dysostosis multiplex.

Type III Mucolipidosis (Pseudo-Hurler Polydystrophy)[12] may be the most common type. Clinical features of Hurler's syndrome are present, but with a slower evolution, stiff joints, and no excess mucopolysacchariduria. The disease first becomes apparent at the age of about 18 months, with joint contractures. Dwarfism ensues, as well as corneal clouding. Mental retardation often occurs, as well as aortic regurgitation and hepatosplenomegaly. Skin fibroblasts exhibit metachromasia and an increased uronic acid content. The disease is inherited as an autosomal recessive.

Radiological changes are very variable. They include mandibular prognathism, absence of the dens, short and wide clavicles, short and plump tubular bones with cystic defects in their distal ends, clawhands with nonunion of the radial sty-

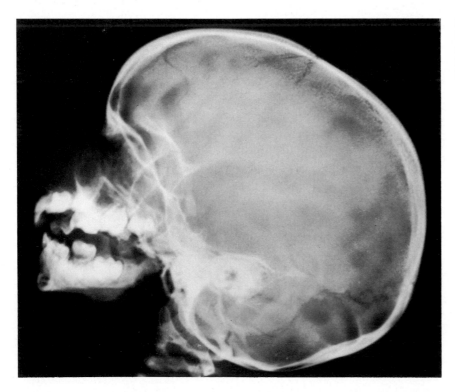

FIG. 5–50. Progeria (skull). The fontanelles are closed. The maxilla and mandibles are small, with overcrowding of teeth. Wormian bones in the lambdoid suture may be noted.

loid, canoe-paddle ribs, and disappearance of the lamina dura of the tooth sockets. The skull shows premature fusion of the sutures in some patients. Shortening of the metacarpals and phalanges is uniformly present. An important point of differentiation from Hurler's syndrome is preservation of some degree of diaphyseal constriction in the metacarpals.

MISCELLANEOUS SYNDROMES OF GROWTH DISTURBANCE OR DEFORMITY OF BONE

PROGERIA (HUTCHINSON–GILFORD SYNDROME)

Progeria[143, 213] is a rare disease of unknown etiology, characterized by dwarfism, premature aging, and early death, which in all reported cases has occurred under the age of 27 years.

The child is normal at birth and until the end of the first year of life, when a failure of normal weight

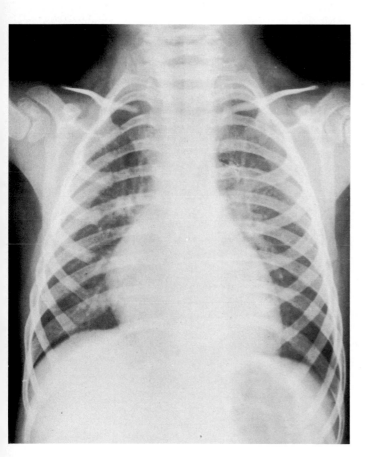

gain and development is noted. There is rapid aging. A facial configuration with beaked nose, receded chin and baldness is typical. Sclerodermalike changes of the skin, prominent veins, and brown pigmented areas are present, as well as severe arteriosclerosis. Intelligence is not affected. Bone maturation is normal.

Radiologically, the calvarium is thin, with either open or closed fontanelles and wormian bone formation (Fig. 5–50). The facial bones and mandible are disproportionately small. The sella turcica may be enlarged. The chest is narrow. The clavicles are small in caliber, rarefy, resorb, and may disappear completely (Fig. 5–51). The vertebral bodies retain their infantile central notching (Fig. 5–52). Bilateral coxa valga is constantly present. The long bones are overconstricted. The knees are prominent (Fig. 5–53). The elbow shows a characteristic deformity, with enlargement of the capitulum and head of the radius (Fig. 5–54). The hands show resorption of the terminal tufts, with a pointed end (Fig. 5–55). There may be arthritic changes of the distal interphalangeal joints. Generalized osteoporosis is present, as well as lack of subcutaneous fat.

Progressive resorption of the clavicles and ribs leading to their complete disappearance has been reported, as well as constriction of the proximal humeral shafts resulting in pathological fractures.[169]

CORNELIA DE LANGE SYNDROME (TYPUS DEGENERATIVUS AMSTELODAMENSIS)

The Cornelia de Lange syndrome[132] is composed of dwarfism and severe mental retardation, associated with a characteristic facies and skeletal abnormalities. It is estimated to occur once in every 10,000 births, and is probably transmitted as an autosomal recessive. The majority of patients have normal karyotypes. No consistent biochemical abnormalities have been found.

The typical facies shows a low hairline and strikingly heavy eyebrows that are confluent medially. The upper lip is thin with an upward curve, giving a grim masklike appearance.

There is marked dwarfism and retarded maturation. Severe mental retardation is present, with I.Q.'s in the 30 to 50 range. Symmetrical deformities

FIG. 5–51. Progeria (chest). The chest is narrow. Resorption of the distal ends of the clavicles and sclerosis of the clavicles are visible.

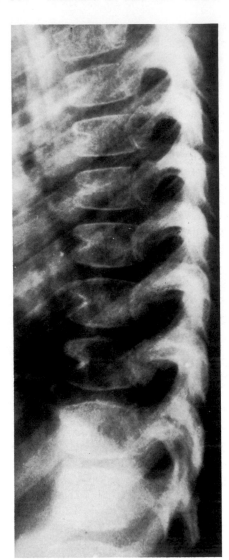

FIG. 5–52. Progeria (dorsolumbar spine). Note central notching of the vertebral bodies—the infantile configuration.

FIG. 5–53. Progeria (lower extremity)—marked coxa valga deformity. Note overconstriction of the shafts, prominence of the knees, and osteoporosis, particularly about the knee joints. Marked soft-tissue atrophy is also apparent.

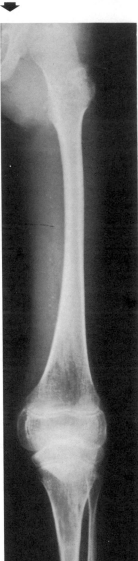

FIG. 5–54. Progeria (elbow). Note enlargement of the lateral humeral ossification center or capitulum, and of the head of the radius. This is a characteristic deformity.

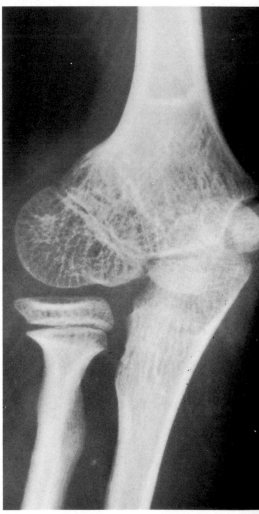

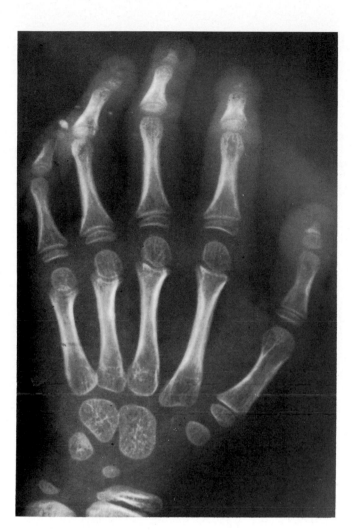

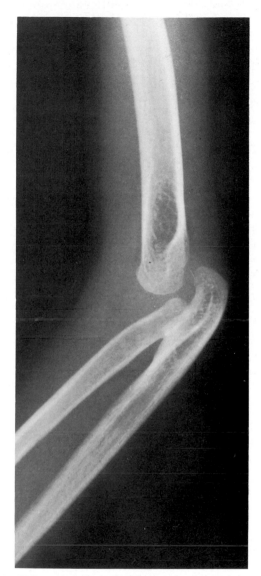

FIG. 5–56. Cornelia de Lange syndrome (elbow). There is subluxation of the radial head. (Courtesy of Dr. Harvey White, Children's Memorial Hospital, Chicago, IL)

of the extremities are constantly present, as is generalized hirsutism. Several cases have revealed a history of maternal exposure to drugs or radiation during gestation.

Radiologically, the skull is microcephalic, but no other consistent changes are seen. The vertebral column is normal. The sternum is short and the ribs have a horizontal pitch. The pelvis shows low acetabular angles during the first year of life, after which it appears normal. Hip dislocations have been reported, but are not a constant finding.

The most pronounced roentgen changes appear in the upper extremities, at times symmetrically distributed. The elbows and the hands are characteristically involved. There may be hypoplasia and tapering of the proximal radius or dorsal subluxation of the radial head (Fig. 5–56). The hands show hypoplasia of the first metacarpal, and clinodactyly or incurving of the little finger due to hypoplasia of the middle phalanx (Fig. 5–57). The above triad is said to be characteristic. Marked retardation of bone maturation is present. Segmentation anomalies may also occur (Fig. 5–58). A unilateral supracondylar spur, as well as a spur at the inferior anterior surface of the midline of the mandible in infants, may be seen.[49]

CRANIOSTENOSIS–SYNDACTYLISM SYNDROMES[172]

The classification of these conditions is complex owing to a great number of variables in the appearance of the face and hands. McKusick subdivided them into five groups:[151]

Type I   Apert
Type II Apert–Crouzon or Vogt, similar to Apert but changes in the face having more the appearance of Crouzon disease.
Type III Saethre–Chotzen
Type IV Waardenburg, with asymmetry, bifid digits, and absence of the first metatarsals
Type V   Pfeiffer

Cephelometric analysis according to the method of Bjork[63] is said to be of value in differentiating these and other syndromes. Many points are differentiated on radiographs of the skull, such as the sella, nasion, gonion, basion, anterior nasal spine, and so forth. Angular and linear measurements are made and compared to standards. The site of skeletal malformations can be objectively localized.

APERT'S SYNDROME (ACROCEPHALOSYNDACTYLY)

Apert's syndrome is a congenital autosomal dominant hereditary condition in which there is scaphocephaly and syndactylism of the hands and feet. Synostoses in the cervical spine are also present. The bone fusions may be progressive.[210] There is a characteristic appearance of a vertically elongated head, wide face, and parallel planes of the face and back of the skull, high forehead, widely spaced bulging eyes, and short nose. Deformities of the shoulders and elbows may also be present. Most patients are mentally retarded.

Radiologically, changes are seen in the skull, hands, feet, and cervical spine. The skull shows premature closure of the sutures with resultant

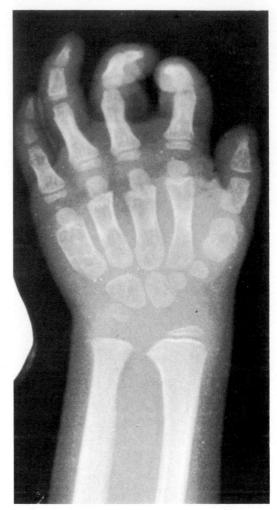

FIG. 5–57. Cornelia de Lange syndrome (hand). There is hypoplasia of the first and third metacarpals, with widening of the first and fifth metacarpals. Clinodactyly of the fifth finger with slanting of the middle phalanx is also present. (Courtesy of Dr. Harvey White, Children's Memorial Hospital, Chicago, IL)

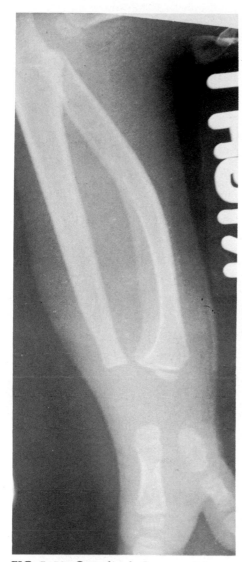

FIG. 5–58. Cornelia de Lange syndrome —same patient as in Figs. 5–56 and 5–57. Segmentation anomaly of right hand, with development of only two radials, is noted. (Courtesy of Dr. Harvey White, Children's Memorial Hospital, Chicago, IL)

FIG. 5–59. Apert's syndrome. Premature closure of the sutures with brachycephaly, and hypoplasia of the maxilla, may be seen.

deformities, convolutional atrophy, and hypoplasia of the maxilla (Figs. 5–59, 5–60). The hands and feet show fusion of digits, metacarpals and metatarsals, carpals and tarsals, and marked deformities in shape of the various involved bones. The digits may be fused proximally or distally. There may be failure of tubulation, and pseudoarthrosis formation (Fig. 5–61). Calcaneocuboid fusions and metatarsal-tarsal fusions occur (Figs. 5–62, 5–63). These changes are similar to those caused by burns (Fig. 5–64). Fusions of the bodies and spinous processes in the cervical spine have also been reported.

SAETHRE–CHOTZEN SYNDROME

Saethre–Chotzen syndrome[63] is characterized by acrocephalosyndactyly with mild or absent osseous changes. The thumbs appear normal. There may only be cutaneous syndactyly.[183] The skull changes consist chiefly of malformations in the cranial base. The sella turcica is positioned abnormally low and the posterior cranial base is short and vertically oriented. This may be due to premature and asymmetric closure of the sphenoido-occipital synchon-

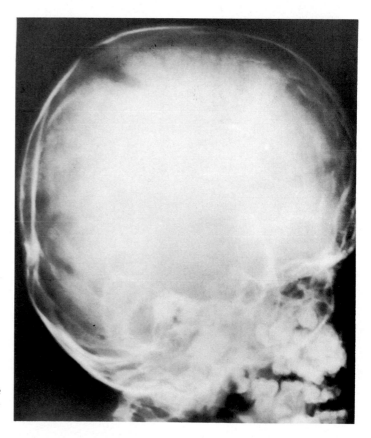

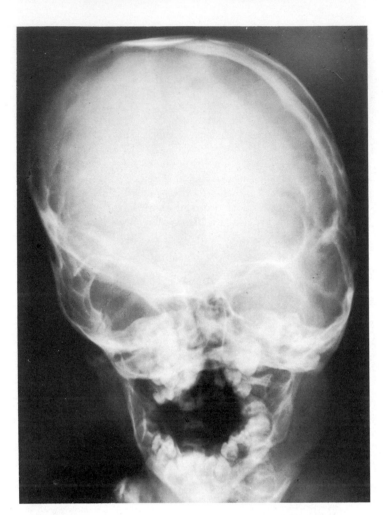

FIG. 5–60. Apert's syndrome (skull). Note marked deformity resulting from premature fusion of sutures, and maxillary hypoplasia.

FIG. 5–61. Apert's syndrome. **A.** Skull. Brachycephaly is present. **B.** Hand. Soft-tissue and bony syndactylism are seen.

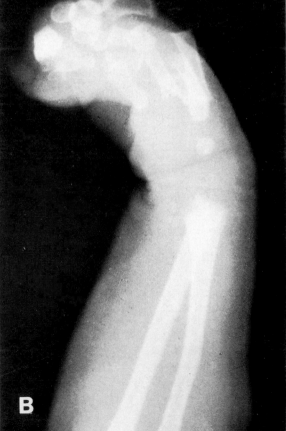

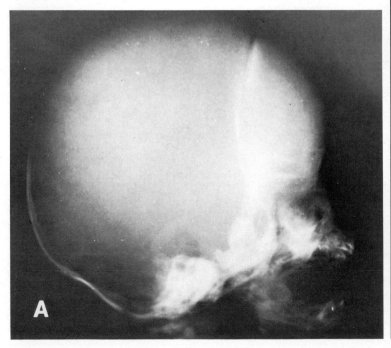

A

B

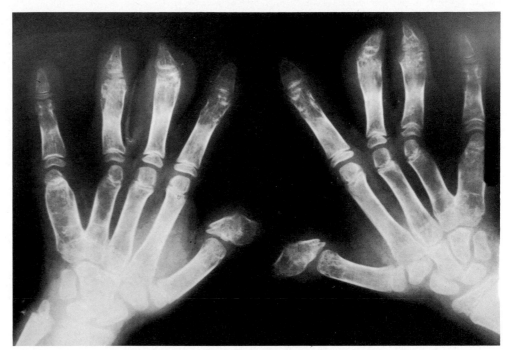

FIG. 5–62. Apert's syndrome (hands). Note fusions of all the proximal interphalangeal joints, and at the bases of the fourth and fifth metacarpals bilaterally. Tapering of the distal phalanges and widening of the shafts of the middle phalanges and fifth metacarpals may also be noted. There is fusion of the capitate and hamate on the right. Osteoporosis at the distal aspects of the phalanges is present.

FIG. 5–63. Apert's syndrome (feet). Note marked deformity, particularly of the great toes, with fusions and pseudarthroses between the first and second metatarsals. Resorption of the terminal tufts of the distal phalanges and fusions of the interphalangeal joints may be seen. Triangular deformities of the phalanges of the great toes are also visible.

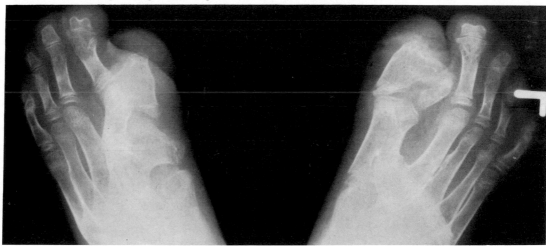

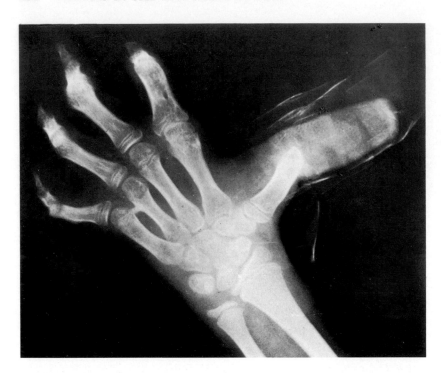

FIG. 5–64. Burns (hand). Changes reminiscent of Apert's syndrome are noted. There is syndactyly with bony bridging between the fourth and fifth metacarpals. Soft-tissue syndactyly is seen at the middle and ring fingers, at their bases. Loss of density and deformity of the bones are present. However, there is loss of phalanges of the thumb and index finger.

drosis. The mandibular plane angle is steep with a short mandibular ramus. Growth retardation occurs. The frontal and mastoid sinuses are absent or reduced in size.

CARPENTER'S SYNDROME (ACROCEPHALOPOLYSYNDACTYLY)

Carpenter's syndrome is a rare condition characterized by craniosynostosis, polydactyly, syndactyly, variable short stature, and obesity. Clinical features include a peculiar facies with skull asymmetry, hypogenitalism, short broad thumbs, clinodactyly, and mental retardation. Congenital heart disease and diabetes mellitus may be associated with this syndrome. The transmission is autosomal recessive; autosomal dominant transmission of these features is referred to as *Noack's syndrome.*

Radiologically, the skull changes are not as severe as in Apert's syndrome. Trigonocephaly and dolichocephaly may be present. Polydactyly is present, usually involving the thumbs and great toes (Fig. 5–65). Exostoses at these sites may also be seen. Only soft-tissue syndactyly occurs in this syndrome. Shortening of the middle phalanges is common, with clinodactyly. The changes in the hands and feet are also not as severe as may be seen in Apert's syndrome, and there are no interdigital osseous fusions.

PFEIFFER'S SYNDROME (FAMILIAL ACROCEPHALOSYNDACTYLY)

Pfeiffer's syndrome[205] is an autosomal dominant familial variety of acrocephalosyndactyly, caused by a gene distinct from that which causes Apert's syndrome. Acrocephaly is present, along with broad thumbs and great toes, and mild soft-tissue syndactyly. Intelligence is normal.

Radiologically, the skull shows changes similar to those seen in Apert's syndrome. Other findings include a flat nasal bridge, hypertelorism, varus deformities of the great toes, brachymesophalangia, trapezoidal shape of the proximal phalanx of the thumb, and a deformed wide first metatarsal. There may be congenital fusions in the cervical and lumbar spine, coxa valga, and widening of the symphysis pubis. Coalition of the tarsal bones may also occur, as well as hypoplasia of the elbow and shoulder joints, fusion of the interphalangeal joints of the thumbs, and selective shortening of the middle phalanges of the index and little fingers.

The chief radiological point of differentiation from Apert's syndrome is the lack of interdigital osseous fusions in Pfeiffer's syndrome.

FIG. 5–65. Carpenter's syndrome. Polydactyly of the great toes, as well as multiple deformities of the phalanges and metatarsals, are seen.

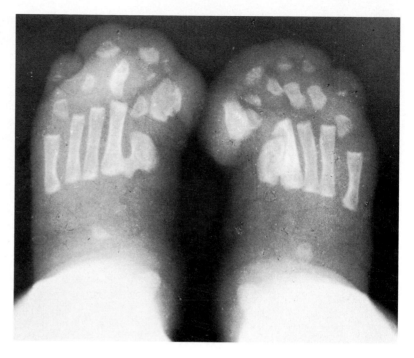

CLEIDOCRANIAL DYSOSTOSIS

Cleidocranial dysostosis[98,105] is a congenital hereditary dysostosis caused by a germ plasm defect. There is faulty intramembranous bone formation, involving principally the calvarium and the clavicle. Multiple associated abnormalities of enchondral bone formation may also be present.

Clinically, the patient has a large head, disproportionately small facial bones, narrow chest, and sagging shoulders. Dwarfism has been reported. Defective or delayed dentition is often seen. There is no mental retardation. Mild hydrocephalus may rarely be present. Hearing loss has been reported.[82] Laboratory values are normal.

Radiologically, the three most constant findings are in the skull, clavicles, and pelvis.

The principal change in the skull is defective ossification of the calvarium, with wide sutures and wormian bone formation (Figs. 5–66, 5–67). The metopic suture may remain open. Localized thickening in the supraorbital regions, temporal squama, and the occipital bone may produce eminences. The base of the skull may be flattened. There may be marked brachycephaly. The foramen magnum is large and often deformed. Underdevelopment of the maxilla and facial bones with deficiency of the zygoma and the lacrimal and nasal bones occurs. Hypoplasia of the paranasal sinuses and a high cleft palate are sometimes seen. A prominent mandible is present, with delayed or defective dentition. Keats has reported a case in which the base of the skull was flattened and the foramen magnum deformed.[105]

The clavicle is formed from three separate ossification centers: the sternal, the middle, and the distal. One or more segments in any combination may be absent in this condition. In 10% of cases, the clavicles are completely lacking (Figs. 5–68, 5–69). The medial third may show flaring. The medial fragment is larger when two separate fragments are present. Pseudarthrosis may occur. A cone-shaped thorax is usually seen. The ribs are normal.

The pelvis is invariably involved and most frequently shows separation of the pubic symphysis (Fig. 5–70). There is also defective ossification of the ischia, pubis, and hypoplasia of the iliac wings. Also seen is widening of the sacroiliac joints giving a "see-through" appearance, poorly formed sacrum and coccyx, and deformity of the pelvic inlet. The hips show a distinctive lateral notching of the proximal femoral ossification center. Widening of the femoral neck may also occur.

The long bones occasionally show changes. There may be hypoplasia or, rarely, absence of the radius. Coxa vara is often present. Also, the femoral necks may be deformed or absent. Undertubulation of the tibia, fibula, and radius has been reported, with increased obliquity of the distal radial articulating surface.

(Text continued on p. 293)

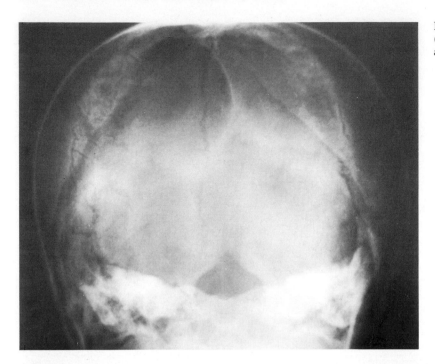

FIG. 5–66. Cleidocranial dysostosis (skull). Marked wormian bone formation about the lambdoid suture is noted.

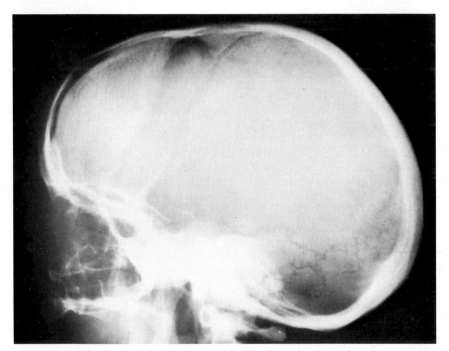

FIG. 5–67. Cleidocranial dysostosis (skull)—lateral view; female, age 23 years. The patient is edentulous. Wormian bone formation along the lambdoid suture is present. Hypoplasia of the frontal sinus is seen. There is no brachycephaly.

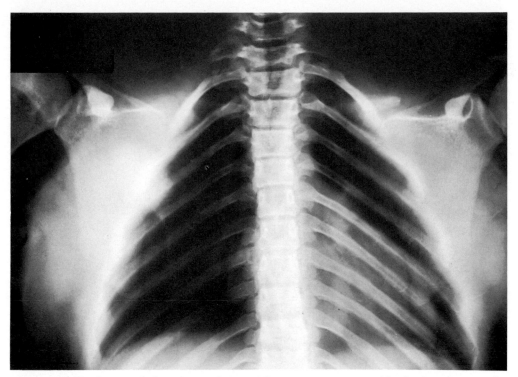

FIG. 5–68. Cleidocranial dysostosis (thorax). The major portions of both clavicles are absent; only rudimentary sternal portions remain.

FIG. 5–69. Cleidocranial dysostosis (shoulder). Only rudimentary proximal and midportions of the clavicle are present. Lack of fusion of the cervical and upper dorsal spinous processes is also noted.

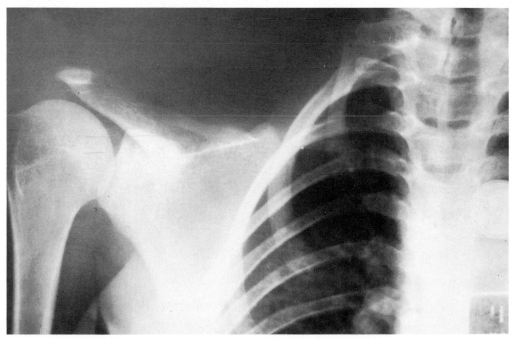

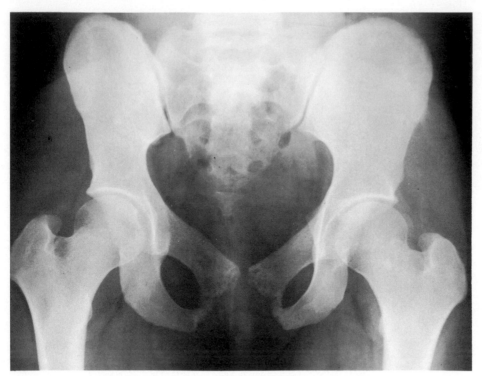

FIG. 5–70. Cleidocranial dysostosis (pelvis). Widening of the symphysis pubis with defective ossification is seen. Note triangular deformity of the pelvic inlet and an ununited spinous process of the first sacral segment.

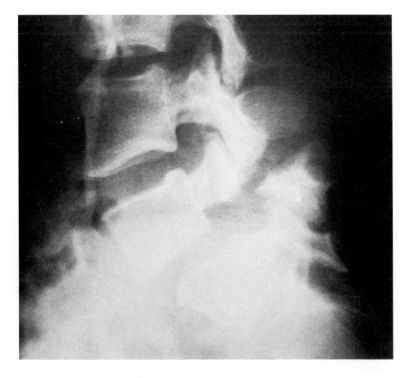

FIG. 5–71. Cleidocranial dysostosis (lumbosacral spine). Wide defect in the pars interarticularis of L-5 is noted.

The hands show multiple accessory ossification centers of the metacarpals and phalanges. The second metacarpal can be excessive in length. Transverse clefts in the distal phalanges may also be present. The terminal tufts may show excessive pointing.

The spine, if involved, shows defective fusion of multiple neural arches (Fig. 5–71). Kyphosis, lordosis, or scoliosis may be present. Defective ossification of the vertebral bodies and a "bone-within-a-bone" appearance has also been reported. Posterior wedging of the thoracic vertebrae, as well as hemivertebrae may be seen. Right clavicular selectivity has been reported.[98]

HEREDITARY ONYCHO-OSTEODYSPLASIA (H.O.O.D. SYNDROME)

Hereditary onycho-osteodysplasia[40,52,55,191] is an autosomal dominant disorder involving ectodermal and mesodermal elements. It is transmitted autosomally on the same chromosome as ABO blood groups. The chromosome count and karyotype are normal. The principal anatomic sites involved are the nails, pelvis, knees, and elbows. Associated anomalies that have been reported are renal dysplasia and proteinuria, abnormal pigmentation of the iris, Plummer–Vinson syndrome, foot deformities, and congenital contraction of the little finger. The severity of involvement at each site may vary. The fingernails and toenails show hypoplasia, dyspla-sia, or complete absence. The thumbs and index fingers are not severely affected. Hypoplasia of the skin folds of the interphalangeal joints is also a common occurrence.

Radiologically, iliac horns are seen. These may be observed in some infants during the first 2 months of life, permitting early diagnosis. They represent osteocartilaginous exostoses, bilateral and symmetrical, extending posteriorly from the iliac wings (Fig. 5–72). They may also occur as an isolated finding *(Fong's disease)*. A unilateral iliac horn has also been reported, without associated abnormalities. Flaring of the iliac crests also occurs.

The patella may show lateral subluxation (Fig. 5–73), hypoplasia, or aplasia. The lateral femoral condyles are small and flattened, while the medial condyle is enlarged. Sloping of the medial tibial plateau may also be seen. The radial head is usually hypoplastic, leading to increase in the radial carrying angle. Posterior dislocation or subluxation of the radial head is frequently seen. Hyperplasia of the medial condyle of the humerus, as well as other bones, has been reported (Fig. 5–74). The soft tissues show flexion contractures of various joints, web formation about the elbows and axillae, and muscular hypoplasias. Contractures of the interphalangeal joints may also be seen.

Nephropathy[59] is a frequent accompanying condition. Proteinuria may be detected in infancy, and renal impairment in adulthood. One case has been reported of renal osteodystrophy with rachitic changes in an 11-year-old boy with this condition.

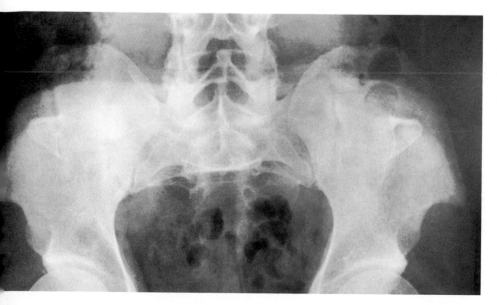

FIG. 5–72. Hereditary onycho-osteodysplasia (pelvis). Note iliac horns bilaterally, and deformity of the iliac crest with a breaking contour pointed inferiorly. (Courtesy of Dr. Miguel Garces, Chicago, IL)

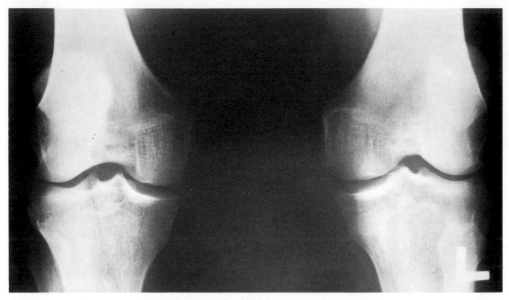

FIG. 5–73. Hereditary onycho-osteodysplasia (knees)—same patient as in previous figure. Note lateral subluxations of both patellae.

FIG. 5–74. Hereditary onycho-osteodysplasia (elbow)—same patient as in previous two figures. There is posterior luxation of the radial head.

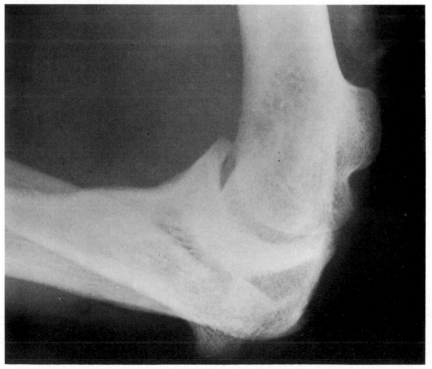

PSEUDOHYPOPARATHYROIDISM (PH) AND PSEUDOPSEUDOHYPOPARATHYROIDISM (PPH)

Pseudohypoparathyroidism (PH)[190,227,228] is a congenital syndrome consisting of dwarfism and brachydactyly, biochemical disturbances, and soft-tissue calcification. The patients appear short and obese with round facies, and they may have corneal and lens opacities. They are mentally retarded. Because the renal tubules cannot respond to parathyroid hormone, there is a low serum calcium level and a high serum phosphorus level. The failure of response to parathormone resides in the renal cortical tubular tissue where the hormone fails to activate adenyl cyclase, resulting in defective renal excretion of cyclic 3′,5′-adenosine monophosphate (AMP) or second messenger.[75] Cyclic AMP has been found to influence a number of metabolic processes, including the induction of secretion or activation of intracellular enzymes, and release of other hormones. This mechanism may account for the various changes that are present in PH. The parathyroid glands may hypertrophy, and in some cases osseous changes of hyperparathyroidism may be seen in the roentgenogram, a condition to which the term *pseudohypohyperparathyroidism* has been applied. *Pseudopseudohypoparathyroidism* (PPH) is an incomplete genetic manifestation of PH in which the blood chemistries are normal and eye calcifications are lacking. The physical appearance and bony roentgen features may be identical to those of PH. Both conditions affect twice as many females as males.

Radiologically, calcification of the basal ganglia and other parts of the brain may be seen (Fig. 5–75). This finding is also present in idiopathic hypoparathyroidism, and develops in late childhood or early adult life. It is independent of other soft-tissue calcification. Thickening of the calvarium and abnormal dentition also occur.

The hands show the most commonly known feature of this condition: a disproportionate shortening of metacarpals and phalanges, sometimes but not always symmetrical (Fig. 5–76). Brachydactyly can be seen in many other diseases and is not pathognomonic of this condition (see pp 344–348). Analysis of metacarpal profile patterns in PHP and PPHP show changes that are almost identical.[190] Brachydactyly E is indistinguishable radiologically from the above syndromes. The changes in Turner syndrome are less severe. *Acrodysostosis*, a condition of marked shortening of the bones of the hands and feet with mental retardation and nasal dysplasia, shows a somewhat similar pattern to the above. The fourth and fifth metacarpals are shortened in over 90% of cases. Shortening of the distal first

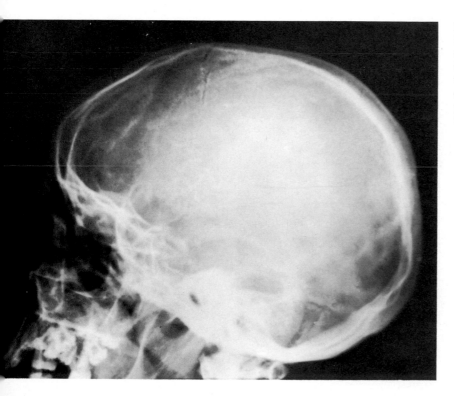

FIG. 5–75. Pseudohypoparathyroidism (skull)—female, age 23 years, complaining of convulsions of 10 years' duration. Physically, the patient was short and thick-set, with an unusually round facies. Her serum calcium level was 6.0 mg% and the serum phosphorus was 8.8 mg%. Note calcifications in the basal ganglia.

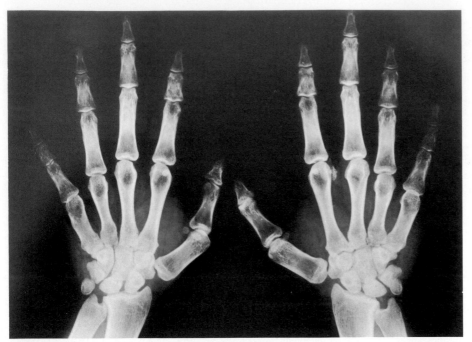

FIG. 5–76. Pseudohypoparathyroidism (hands). Same patient as in previous figure. Note brachydactyly involving the distal phalanges of the thumbs, the distal phalanges of the index fingers, the middle phalanges of the index fingers, and, to a slight degree, both the fourth and fifth metacarpals.

FIG. 5–77. Pseudohypoparathyroidism (lower extremities)—same patient as in previous two figures. Soft-tissue calcifications and ossification in the thighs, most marked in the medial aspect of the right thigh, may be seen.

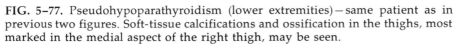

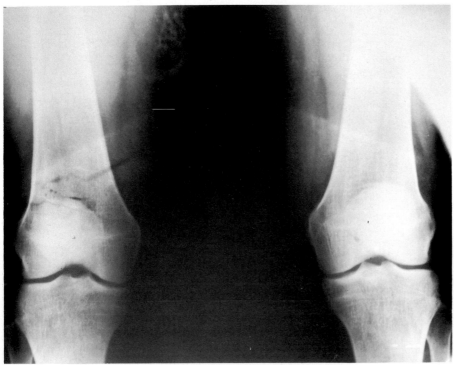

phalanx is common. The feet show similar changes. There is uniform shortening of bones in patients with short stature. Maturation is accelerated. Single or multiple exostoses may be seen, not in the metaphyseal region as in osteochondromas, but at the diaphysis. Some or possibly all of these lesions begin as soft-tissue ossifications and fuse with the shaft. Bowing of the long bones has also been reported. The hips may show coxa valga or coxa vara. Defective metaphyseal ossification with a rachitiform appearance and slipped femoral capital epiphyses may be associated with coxa vara. Osteoporosis, or more rarely osteosclerosis, may be seen. Secondary hyperparathyroidism with subperiosteal bony resorption is present in 10% of cases of PH, but not in PPH.

Soft-tissue ossification and calcification are present in both PH and PPH in a high percentage of cases, and may be present at birth. These are distributed in subcutaneous tissues (Fig. 5–77), periarticular areas, ligaments, tendons, and fascial planes. These formations are not related to altered blood chemistry.

CHROMOSOMAL ABNORMALITIES[18,46,57,220]

The fundamental unit of inheritance is the gene, composed of desoxyribonucleic acid. About 50,000 structural genes have been postulated for humans. Progress has been made on a gene map of the human chromosomes, which now shows assignment of at least one structural gene locus to all 22 autosomes as well as the X and Y chromosomes.[152] For example, the ABO blood group is in chromosome 9. The precise locus for hemophilia A on the X chromosome is known. Genes are located on chromosomes at specific locations. Human somatic cells normally have 23 pairs of chromosomes: 22 autosomes and one pair of chromosomes that determine genetic sex.[237] The sex chromosomes are homologous in the female (XX), but not in the male (XY).

Darkly staining chromatin material (Barr body) is present in female cells but not in male cells. This material originates from the second X chromosome. Thus the female genotype is chromatin-positive and the male genotype is chromatin-negative. The presence, in abnormal states, of one X chromosome will cause a chromatin-negative genotype while two X chromosomes will result in a chromatin-positive genotype. Three X chromosomes will form two chromatin bodies in a single cell.

Chromosomal studies are performed by incubating white blood cells in a culture medium. The Denver system of karyotype analysis is used. The chromosomes are photographed, paired, and numbered in groups according to their length and location of the centromere. The groups are 1–3, 4–5, 6–12, 13–15, 16–18, 19–20, 21–22, and sex chromosomes.

The chromosomes contain only the genetic information of their genes, and are the physical containers for these genes. Genetic defects and chromosomal abnormalities are usually not directly related, because many chromosomal abnormalities lead to infertility. Genetic diseases are manifested at the molecular level and are not microscopically demonstrable. Genetic disposition to chromosomal abnormalities in humans, however, may occur, and account for familial tendencies in this direction.

Chromosomal defects appear as abnormalities in the number or configuration of chromosomes. In the reduction division of gamete cells (meiosis), the normal diploid number of chromosomes (46) is reduced to 23 (haploid) in the sperm cell or ovum. The process of splitting a chromosome pair is called disjunction. If one pair does not split (nondisjunction), then a germ cell is formed with either 22 or 24 chromosomes. If fertilization occurs in this case, the individual will have either 45 chromosomes (monosomy of one pair) or 47 chromosomes (trisomy of one pair). This may involve the sex chromosomes or the other 22 pairs (autosomes). Loss or gain of a sex chromosome is compatible with life, and leads to a specific syndrome. Autosomal monosomy is usually fatal, as is autosomal trisomy of the larger chromosomes. Trisomy of the smaller groups is compatible with life and occurs with specific features.

Other mechanisms of chromosomal abnormality are: translocation, resulting from the fracture of two chromatids and the reunion of fragments with the wrong chromosomes; mosaicism, or an individual composed of different genotypic tissues, such as XX/XO; deletion (loss) of genetic material; isochromosomes, or transverse instead of longitudinal division of a centromere; inversion of fragments; and ring chromosomes. Newer chromosomal banding techniques permit better definition of aberrations.

The etiology of chromosomal defects is thought to be related to advanced maternal age (but not paternal age), chronic disease, radiation, genetic influences, or mutagenic viruses. Acquired chromosomal abnormalities in chronic myeloid leukemia have been demonstrated.

The principal autosomal syndromes now recognized are:

1. Trisomy G 21–22 (mongoloidism; 47 chromosomes)

2. Trisomy E 17–18 (47 chromosomes)
3. Trisomy F 13–15 (47 chromosomes)
4. Cri-du-chat syndrome (deletion of a short arm of a 4–5 chromosome).
5. Wolf syndrome (B 4/G22 Translocation)
6. Trisomy 9$_p$

Mongoloidism may also be caused by translocation or mosaicism.

The principle sex chromosome disorders are:

1. Turner's syndrome XO (chromatin-negative; female)
2. Klinefelter's syndrome XXY (chromatin-positive; male)

Other sex chromosome disorders of lesser frequency are:

1. Superfemale XXX (no specific radiological findings)
2. Klinefelter variants XXXY, XXXXY, XXYY (radioulnar synostosis and delayed bony maturation are the only consistent radiological findings).

Combinations, or polysyndromes, also exist.

AUTOSOMAL SYNDROMES

Mongoloidism (Down's Syndrome)[97]

Mongoloidism is the clinical manifestation of a trisomy at the G 21–22 group, due to nondisjunction, mosaicism, or, in rare cases, to translocation. A bimodal maternal age peak at 27 and 40 years has been reported. It is the most common of the autosomal syndromes, occurring once in every 600 births. The condition is clinically recognizable at birth by eyes that slant upward, a small brachycephalic head, a small nose with flat bridge, and a protruding tongue. The hands are broad, with incurving of the fifth finger. Mental retardation is constantly present. The earlobes are small or absent and there is a high arched palate. Brushfield spots (circle of silver-gray spots near the periphery of the iris) are seen in young infants. There are characteristic dermatoglyphic findings.[18]

Congenital heart disease is common. Mongoloids have a higher incidence of leukemia than the normal population. Hypothyroidism may coexist. Hyperuricemia has also been reported.[104]

Radiologically, the most characteristic findings are in the pelvis,[160] which shows flaring of the iliac wings, flattening of the roofs of the acetabula, and ischial tapering. The iliac index (half the sum of both iliac and acetabular angles) is reduced; this index is valid only during the first year of life (Figs. 5–78, 5–79). The mean normal value in the newborn is 81° with a range of 65° to 97°. The mean value in mongoloids is 62° with a range of 49° to 87°.

In the hands, hypoplasia of the middle phalanx of the fifth finger with clinodactyly is seen. This is not specific and may be seen in other conditions (see pp 344–348). The abnormal phalanx is shortened, disproportionately wide, and frequently wedge-shaped. This is in contrast to the shape of a hypoplastic phalanx that may be seen as a variation in normal individuals, particularly of Asiatic ethnology, where a concave defect in the base of the shaft without clinodactyly has been reported.[76] Accessory epiphyses at the first and second metacarpals may also be present, again a nonpathognomonic finding. Bone maturation is accelerated. There may be hypoplasia of the fingers, toes, and mandible.

The skull may show brachycephaly and microcephaly, with thinning of the calvarium and loss of the diploic space. Delayed closure of sutures is common. A high arched palate is present, resulting from maxillary hypoplasia. A short, hard palate in the newborn, with a length of 26 mm or less, is reported to be characteristic.[11] Pneumatization of paranasal sinuses and mastoids is retarded. There is undergrowth at the spheno-occipital synchondrosis, leading to shortening of the base of the skull. The sphenoid is rotated upward and backward in relation to the clivus.

The cribriform plate is highly placed. Hypoplasia of the nasal bones is a constant finding (Fig. 5–80). There is persistence of the metopic suture (Fig. 5–81).

Dentition is defective, with teeth that are small and deformed, or absent. Only 11 pairs of ribs are present in some patients, but this is not a specific finding.

Dislocations of the atlas have been reported as occurring in a significant percentage of mongoloids, caused by a congenital anomaly of the transverse portion of the cruciate ligament.[146,215,236] Congenital heart disease, usually atrioventricular commune, and duodenal atresia are commonly associated anomalies.

Trisomy 17–18 Syndrome (E₁ Group Trisomy)

Trisomy E 17–18 syndrome[95,161,240] is a specific clinical manifestation of trisomy—probably of the 18 group—caused by nondisjunction, with a definite pattern of developmental disturbances that is more constant than that of the other two recognized trisomies.

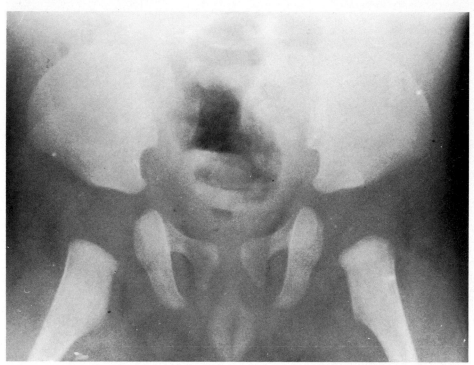

FIG. 5–78. Mongoloidism (pelvis). There is flaring of the iliac wings, flattening of the acetabular roofs, and tapering of the ischia. (Courtesy of Dr. Harvey White, Children's Memorial Hospital, Chicago, IL)

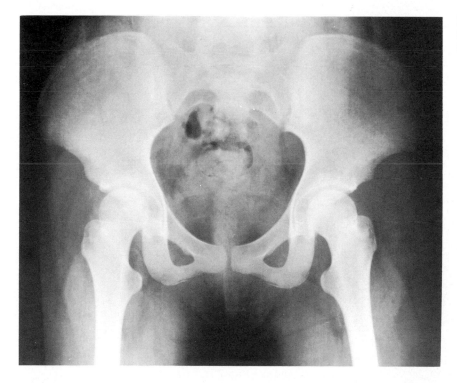

FIG. 5–79. Mongoloidism (pelvis)— female, age 15 years. There is wide flaring of the iliac wings.

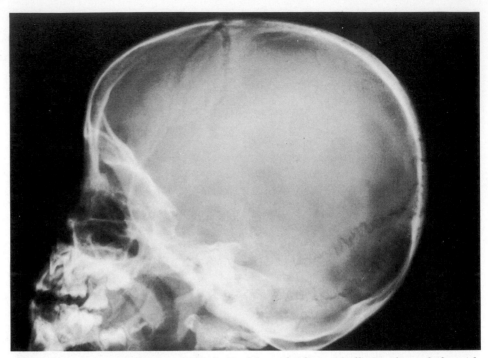

FIG. 5–80. Mongoloidism (skull). Brachycephaly with shortening of the base of the skull, and thinning of the calvarium in the frontal region, with partial loss of the diploic space, may be noted. A high sloping contour of the lesser wing of the sphenoid is visible. The nasal bones are hypoplastic.

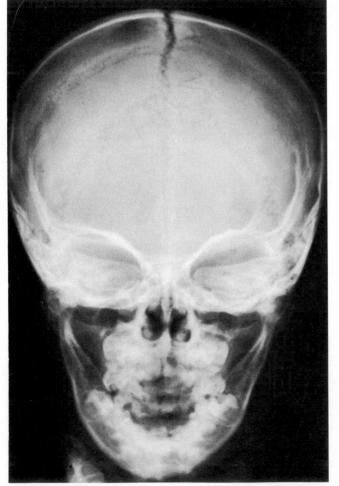

FIG. 5–81. Mongoloidism (skull) — frontal view; same patient as in Fig. 5–80. Wormian bones may be seen. There is lack of development of the frontal sinuses and a persistent metopic suture.

The patients are mentally retarded. The longest reported duration of life has been 16 months. Clinically, there are low-set, misshapen ears, receding chin, a small triangular mouth, prominent occiput, short sternum, flexion deformity of fingers with the index finger over the third finger, "rocker-bottom" feet, "hammer" great toe, cardiac malformations (chiefly interventricular septal defect and patent ductus arteriosus), and renal and skeletal anomalies. A mean maternal age of 34.8 years in reported cases has been calculated by Moseley. The infants are small at birth and fail to thrive and mature.

Radiologically, the fingers are held in flexion with the index finger overlapping the third finger. Ulnar deviation of the third, fourth, and fifth fingers results in a gap between the index and middle fingers. The first metacarpal is hypoplastic. The feet show a "rocker-bottom" or equinovarus deformity. The phalangeal ossification centers may be absent. The great toe is dorsiflexed and shortened. Triangular, hypoplastic distal phalanges may be seen. Soft-tissue syndactyly may be present. Three cases have been reported with absent radius and rudimentary humerus (Fig. 5–82).

The mandible is constantly hypoplastic, as is the maxilla. There is elongation of the posterior fossa and of the sella turcica (Fig. 5–83). The sternum is short and the ribs are thin and deformed in the presence of a full chest and enlarged cardiac silhouette with prominent pulmonary vascularity (Fig. 5–84). Eventration of the diaphragm and hypoplasia of the medial clavicles have been reported. The pelvis is small and has an antimongoloid configuration with increased slope of the acetabulum, dislocated hips, and thin ilia (Figs. 5–85, 5–86). A case of mosaic trisomy 18 with 14 thoracic complete segments and coronal cleft vertebrae has been reported.[198]

Trisomy 13–15 Syndrome (D₁ Group Trisomy, Patou Syndrome)[96]

Trisomy D 13–15 is less distinctive radiologically than trisomy 17–28. There are many features that are common to both. This condition is also caused by nondisjunction during meiosis, and is more frequent in advanced maternal age.

Clinically, microphthalmos, colobomas, mental retardation, seizures, and deafness are present. Abnormal calcification of the skull has been cited. Arhinencephaly and hypoplasia of the frontal lobes may be seen. A cleft lip and palate are present. The fingernails are narrow and hyperconvex. Polydactyly and capillary hemangiomas may be present.

(*Text continued on p. 304*)

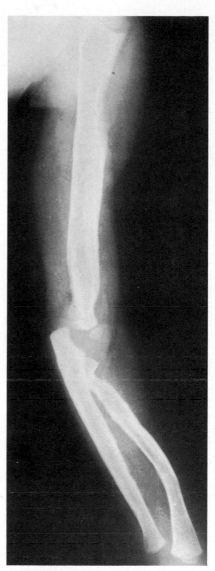

FIG. 5–82. Trisomy 17–18 syndrome (upper extremity). There is hyperplasia and curvature of the radius, with deformity at the radial neck. Note "scooped out" depression at the lateral aspect of the proximal humerus and underconstriction of the humeral shaft, with an abrupt ridge formation at the distal aspect. (Courtesy of Dr. Miguel Garces, Chicago, IL)

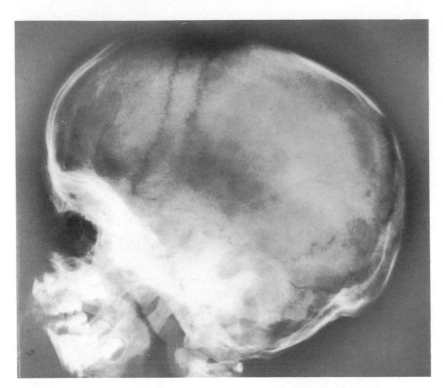

FIG. 5–83. Trisomy 17–18 syndrome (skull). Note marked hypoplasia of the mandible. There is sloping of the base of the skull and enlargement of the posterior cranial fossa. The sella turcica is elongated. A wide anterior fontanelle is also apparent. (Courtesy of Dr. Miguel Garces, Chicago, IL)

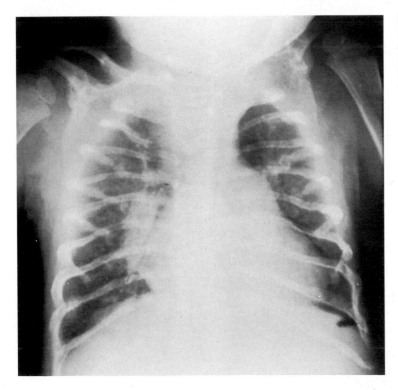

FIG. 5–84. Trisomy 17–18 (chest)—same patient as in Fig. 5–83. Thinning and deformities of the ribs and clavicles may be seen. The heart is enlarged and there is an increase in pulmonary vascularity. (Courtesy of Dr. Miguel Garces, Chicago, IL)

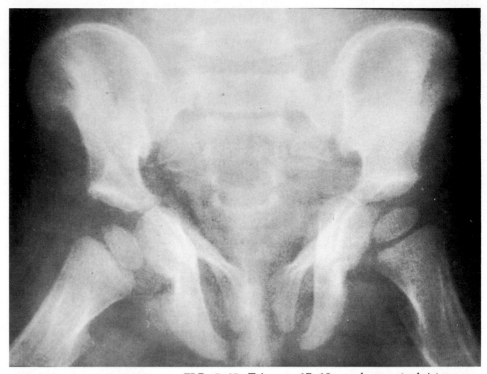

FIG. 5–85. Trisomy 17–18 syndrome (pelvis)—same patient as in Figs. 5–83 and 5–84. The pelvis is small, and the ilia have a peculiar, constricted contour. Increased sloping and widening of both acetabulae may be noted.

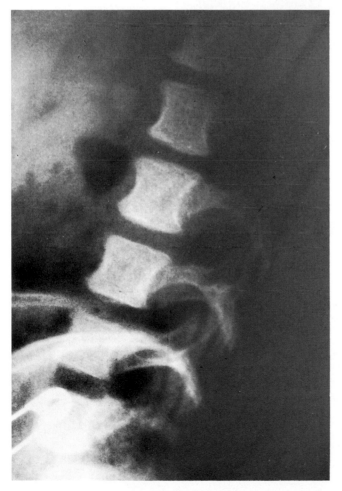

FIG. 5–86. Trisomy 17–18 syndrome (lumbar spine)—lateral view; same patient as in Fig. 5–82. There is increased height of the vertebral bodies, with posterior scalloping. (Courtesy of Dr. Miguel Garces, Chicago, IL)

There is failure to thrive. Females are more frequently seen to be affected than males, owing to early death in the individual with an XY constitution.

Radiologically, the skull shows sloping of the forehead, small orbits with hypertelorism, poor ossification, and widened sutures. The mandible is hypoplastic, in common with trisomy 17–18. Interpediculate distances in the cervical spine are increased. Polydactyly, syndactyly, and prominent calcaneii may be seen in the extremities. "Ribbonlike" ribs may also be seen. An antimongoloid configuration of the pelvis has not been described in this condition. Congenital cardiac malformations are present. Renal anomalies, intestinal malrotation, horseshoe kidney, and umbilical hernia are also said to occur. Only 11 pairs of ribs may be present (Fig. 5–87).

Cri-du-Chat Syndrome (Cat-Cry Syndrome)

Cri-du-chat syndrome[94, 148] is characterized by the catlike wail of the infant. The condition is caused by deletion of a short arm of a B 5-group chromosome, and it occurs more frequently in advanced maternal age. There are deformity of the larynx, mental retardation, "moonlike" facies, and failure to thrive.

Radiologically, microcephaly and hypertelorism are seen combined with microretrognathia. The pelvis is said to show an increase of the iliac angles. There is no congenital heart disease.

Wolf Syndrome (deletion 4$_p$-Syndrome)[54]

Wolf Syndrome results from the translocation of a G22 chromosome onto a B4 chromosome. Approximately two-thirds of the short arm of the B4 chromosome is lost, causing the deletion 4$_p$-syndrome.

Some features are in common with the cri-du-chat syndrome, including retarded growth and development, microcephaly, and hypertelorism. The kitten cry of cri-du-chat is not usually heard in this syndrome.

Radiological findings include polydactyly, cervical ribs, and fusion defects of the elbows, ribs, and spine. Hip dislocation may also be seen.

Trisomy 9$_p$ Syndrome

Trisomy 9$_p$[209] is a syndrome due to trisomy of the short arm of chromosome 9. About 100 cases have been reported, and the pattern of radiographic findings appears to be unique.

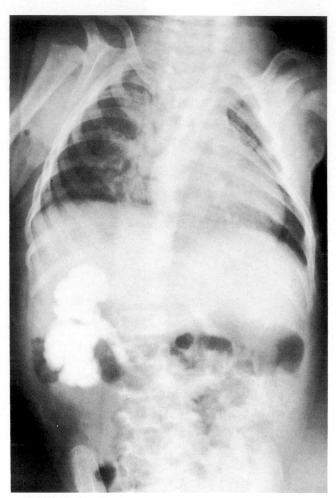

FIG. 5–87. Trisomy 13–15, or Patou syndrome (ribs)—hypoplasia of the left fourth rib. Only eleven pairs of ribs are present, and the eleventh ribs are hypoplastic. There is marked hydronephrosis on the right, with the possibility of a retrocaval ureter. (Courtesy of Dr. Antonio Pizarro, Mount Sinai Hospital, Chicago, IL)

Clinical features include growth and mental retardation, hypertelorism with antimongoloid features, large nose, cup-shaped ears, and kyphoscoliosis. This is not to be confused with trisomy of the entire chromosome 9, which has only short survival.

Radiologically, the hands, feet, and pelvis are chiefly involved. Delayed maturation is present. pseudoepiphyses, clinodactyly, transverse notches of the phalanges, and shortening of the phalanges of the thumb and little finger are seen. The pelvis shows delayed ossification of the pubic bones and ischiopubic synchondroses, broad ischeal tuberosities, wide pubic symphysis, hip dislocations, narrow iliac wings, and anomalies of the sacrum and lumbar spine.

Basal-Cell Nevus Syndrome (Gorlin's Syndrome)

Basal-cell nevus syndrome[137] consists of a combination of multiple basal-cell epitheliomas (there may be up to 1,000), mandibular cysts, brachydactyly, bifid rids, scoliosis, extensive calcification of the falx cerebri, and multiple calcified mesenteric cysts. Cytogenetic abnormalities have been found in several patients that consisted of deletions in the F 19–20 group and marker chromosomes in the same group. (A marker chromosome has an unusually long pair of secondary constrictions in one of its pairs of arms, giving a satellited appearance.)

SEX-LINKED SYNDROMES (GONADAL DYSGENESIS)

Gonadal dysgenesis[108] indicates a group of syndromes featuring gonadal abnormalities or aplasia. Included in this group are Turner's syndrome, Klinefelter's syndrome, and myotonia dystrophica. Patients with Turner's or Klinefelter's syndrome have sex-chromosome abnormalities. Three clinical types of gonadal dysgeneses have been described in females:

1. Isolated gonadal dysgenesis with normal stature and without anomalies
2. Gonadal dysgenesis with short stature and without anomalies
3. Gonadal dysgenesis with short stature and with somatic anomalies (Turner's syndrome)

Turner's Syndrome

Turner's syndrome[14, 192] results from nondisjunction of the sex chromosomes, causing monosomy of the X chromosome in the zygote, or XO. There is a male chromatin-negative pattern and a female phenotype. A total of 45 chromosomes is present. Mosaicism or partial deletion of an X chromosome may also result in ovarian agenesis.

Turner's original triad of signs comprised infantilism, congenital webbed neck, and cubitus valgus. Other clinical features include short stature, primary amenorrhea, absence of secondary sexual characteristics, infantile internal female genitalia, shield chest, coarctation of the aorta (in less than 10% of patients), hypertension, and skeletal changes, most often short metacarpals. The infantile

form may exhibit lymphedema of the hands and feet, congenital webbed neck or loose skin folds of the neck, and broad-spaced nipples (Bonnevie–Ullrich syndrome).

Mental retardation is rare.

Hypertelorism and eighth nerve deafness may be present. There may be multiple pigmented nevi and a tendency to keloid formation. The facies is usually normal. The ovaries are represented by white streaks in the broad ligaments. Partial agenesis of the ovaries may occur rarely.

The majority of patients with Turner's syndrome have no roentgen abnormalities.

Radiological findings consist of osteoporosis and delay of fusion of epiphyseal ossification centers, particularly the epiphyses of the iliac crests (Fig. 5–88). Skeletal maturation is normal up to the age of about 15 years.

The most characteristic findings are in the hands,[117] wrists, and knees. It must be emphasized that these signs occur in a minority of patients. "Drumstick" distal phalanges as well as overconstriction of the proximal and midphalanges are present in about one-third of patients. The heads of the third and fourth metacarpals may be flattened. Shortening of some phalanges and thickening of the soft tissues of the fingers may also be seen. The hands show undergrowth of the fourth and fifth metacarpals (Fig. 5–89). A metacarpal sign has been devised in which a line drawn tangential to the heads of the fourth and fifth metacarpals passes through the head of the third metacarpal if the sign is positive, instead of distal to it, if proportions are normal. Normally, the total length of the distal and proximal phalanges equals the length of the metacarpal, best seen in the fourth ray. If the metacarpal is shortened, the combined phalangeal length exceeds the metacarpal length by 3 or more mm, and this disproportion is referred to as phalangeal preponderance. Shortening of the metacarpals can be seen in many other conditions (see pp 344–348, Brachydactyly). More detailed methods for metacarpophalangeal evaluation have evolved (p. 345). Sloping of the radial surface with a decrease of the carpal angle may also be seen in this condition (Fig. 5–90). Cubitus valgus is often present but is more apparent clinically than radiologically.

The knees show depression of the medial tibial plateau, the most common skeletal sign in this disorder, sometimes associated with medial tibial exostosis formation (Fig. 5–91). Overgrowth of the medial femoral condyle also occurs.

Baker[14] stresses that other findings such as spina bifida occulta, pes planus, and vertebral apophy-

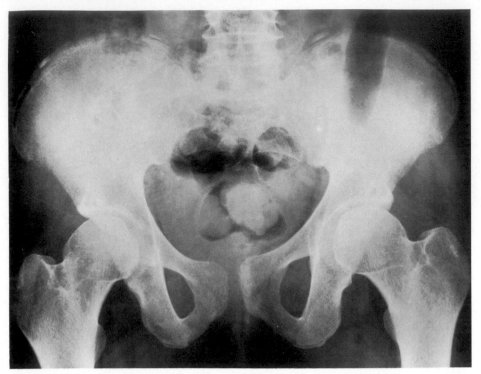

FIG. 5–88. Turner's syndrome (pelvis)—female, age 44 years, who is short in stature and has never menstruated. The secondary ossification centers of the iliac crests and the ischial apophyses have not fused.

FIG. 5–89. Turner's syndrome (hands)—same patient as in Fig. 5–88. Note shortening of the right fourth metacarpal and first metacarpal. Osteoporosis is also apparent.

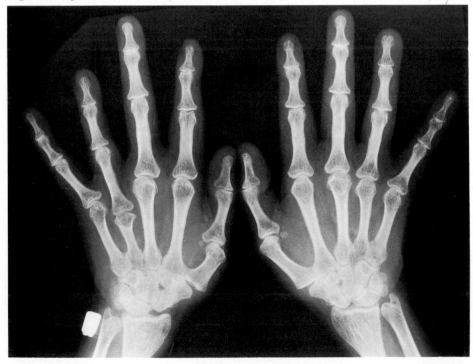

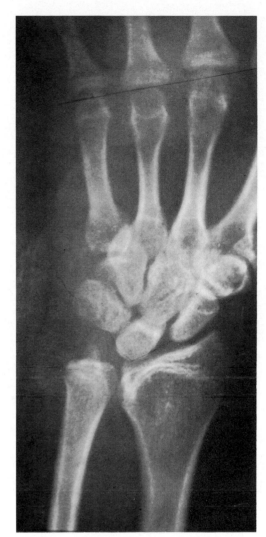

FIG. 5–90. Turner's syndrome (wrist). Sloping of the radial surface, with a decrease in the carpal angle, is present. There is also a positive metacarpal sign.

sitis do not occur in these patients in any greater proportion than in the normal population. Malrotated and horseshoe kidneys, vesicoureteral reflux, and ureteropelvic obstruction have been found.

Less common roentgen findings include hypoplasia of the first cervical vertebra, maldevelopment of the odontoid process, hypoplasia of the outer clavicles, notched and narrow ribs, an android pelvic inlet, small sella turcica, basilar impression, and hypertelorism.

The most characteristic laboratory value is elevation of the urinary gonadotropins in the adult female.

Pseudo-Turner's Syndrome (Noonan's Syndrome)[94]

Pseudo-Turner's syndrome[14] can occur in both males and females and has been reported as "Turner's phenotype in the male." Chromosomal studies and chromatin smears in these patients are normal. Mental retardation is common. There is a characteristic facies with prominent brow, hypertelorism,

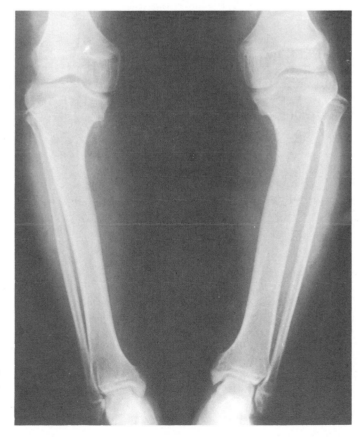

FIG. 5–91. Turner's syndrome (knees). Bilateral genu varum may be noted, with depressions of the medial tibial plateaus and overgrowth of the medial tibial condyles. Exostosis formation at the medial tibial metaphyses and at the proximal fibulae is also visible.

antimongoloid slant, depressed bridge of the nose and low-set abnormal ears. Short stature and webbed neck contribute to the resemblance to Turner's syndrome. Cardiac malformations are present, most commonly atrial septal defect or pulmonic stenosis, as opposed to coarctation of the aorta most commonly seen in Turner's syndrome. Neither the skeletal signs of short metacarpals or large medial tibial condyles, nor the renal anomalies of malrotated or horseshoe kidney, are found in this condition. Pectus cavus or pectus carinatum may occur with equal frequency. Osteoporosis and retardation of bone age may be seen. The skull may show steep inclination of the anterior fossa and hypoplasia of the mandible.

Turner–Mongolism Polysyndrome

Turner–Mongolism polysyndrome[239] (Villaverde syndrome) is, as the name implies, a rare combination of Turner and mongoloidism. This may not be coincidence, but may be a result of a common pathogenesis. Usually the karyotype is mosaic XO/G+. The clinical features include retarded growth, shield chest, short neck with folds, low hairline, oblique eyes with epicanthal folds, squat nose, high or cleft palate, short hands and feet, cubitus valgus, and mental retardation.

Other combinations that may be seen are *Klinefelter–Mongoloidism*, and *Mixed Gonadal Dysgenesis*. The latter may have ambiguous gonads.[247]

Klinefelter's Syndrome

Klinefelter's syndrome[167] is believed to be the most frequent of all chromosomal disorders. It is due to nondisjunction of sex chromosomes and has an XXY genotype (47 chromosomes). The double X leads to a chromatin-positive (female) pattern in a male phenotype. Chromosomal variants with additional sex chromosomes have been reported. Radioulnar synostosis has been described in these variants (Fig. 5–92). The principal pathological lesion is fibrosis of the seminiferous tubules. The features were summarized in the original article in 1942 as "Syndrome Characterized by Gynecomastia, Aspermatogenesis without A–Leydigism and Increased Excretion of Follicle-Stimulating Hormone." Infertility is present. "False" or chromatin-negative Klinefelter's syndrome, probably on the basis of hypogonadism, also occurs.

Clinically, the patients have small testes, a eunuchoid habitus, and gynecomastia. There is an increase in urinary gonadotropin excretion after puberty.

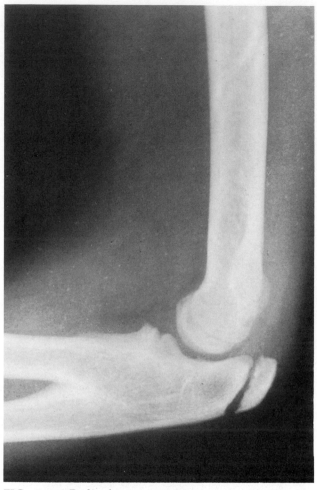

FIG. 5–92. Radioulnar synostosis, as may be seen in Klinefelter variants (elbow).

FIG. 5–93. Hypoplasia of the thumb and first metacarpal, as seen in Fanconi's anemia, myositis ossificans progressiva, and other conditions (see pp. 344–348).

Radiologically, a positive metacarpal sign, brachymesophalangia with clinodactyly of the little finger, or a small bridged sella turcica may be present, although rarely. No specific roentgen signs have been described. Bone density and maturation are normal. Findings that have been described in a small minority of patients include flattening of the ulnar styloid process, accessory epiphysis of the second metacarpal, rib anomalies (minor), and retarded bone age.

FANCONI'S ANEMIA

Fanconi's anemia[101, 157] represents a rare triad of signs of severe aplastic anemia and pancytopenia, skin pigmentation, and multiple congenital anomalies. It is transmitted as an autosomal recessive. The congenital anomalies are present at birth, thus preceding the blood dyscrasia that often manifests itself near the end of the first decade of life and rarely

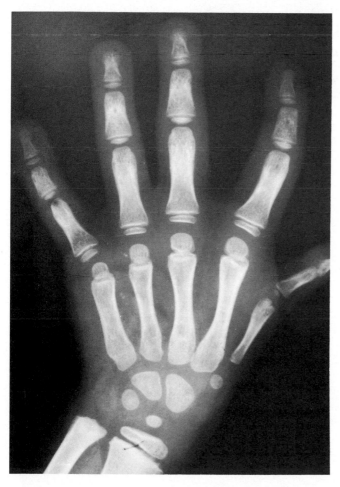

at the beginning of the third. The median age of onset is 7 years. Men are more often affected than women.

Clinically, symptoms of anemia are present, and there is increased bleeding tendency and increased susceptibility to infection. The erythrocytes are macrocytic and hyperchromic. Varying degrees of leukopenia and thrombocytopenia are present. Brown pigmentation of the skin frequently occurs from melanin deposition. The congenital anomalies that occur most frequently are skeletal anomalies, retarded growth, hypogonadism, renal anomalies (most often aplasia, ectopia, and horseshoe kidney), strabismus, and deafness. The disease is slowly progressive, with a fatal outcome usually within 5 years after onset.

Radiologically, the skeletal deformities are diagnostic indicators. Mild to moderate growth retardation and microcephaly are seen. Bone maturation is retarded. Osteoporosis is occasionally present.

The most characteristic features are hypoplasia or aplasia of the radius, the greater multangular and navicular bones, the first metacarpal, and the phalanges of the thumb (Fig. 5–93). The involvement may range from minor shortening of the bone to complete absence. Radial deviation of the hands often is present. Hypoplasia of the middle phalanges of the little finger may also occur, leading to clinodactyly. Dislocation of the radial head has also been reported. Triphalangeal thumbs may also be seen (Fig. 5–94). Hypoplasia of the thumb is not pathognomonic of this condition and also occurs in several other diseases (see pp 344–348).

ERYTHROGENESIS IMPERFECTA (CONGENITAL HYPOPLASTIC ANEMIA, PURE RED-CELL ANEMIA, CONGENITAL AREGENERATIVE ANEMIA)

Erythrogenesis imperfecta[157] is a congenital normocytic, normochromic anemia. The erythrocytes are involved selectively and there is no leukopenia, thrombocytopenia, or jaundice. The onset is in infancy, with slow progression and periods of remission. A disturbance of tryptophan metabolism has been reported, with identification of anthranilic acid in the urine.

One-third of the patients affected show at least one congenital anomaly. The most common are retarded growth, mental retardation, congenital heart disease, skeletal anomalies, and renal anomalies.

There may be hypoplasia of the middle phalanx of the little finger with clinodactyly. An extra phalanx of one thumb and a supernumerary thumb

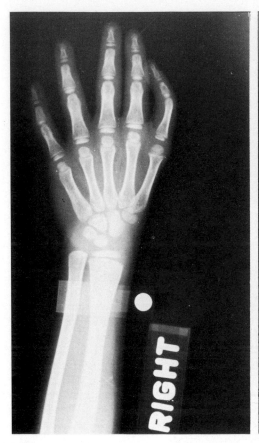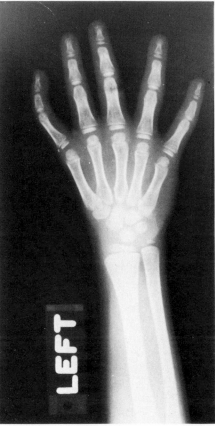

FIG. 5–94. Fanconi's anemia (hands and wrists). Triphalangeal thumbs, as well as bilateral absence of the scaphoid, and loss of bone density are noted.

have also been reported. Skeletal anomalies in this disease are less frequent and less marked than in Fanconi's anemia.

CONGENITAL HYPOPLASTIC THROMBOCYTOPENIA

Congenital hypoplastic thrombocytopenia[116] is a rare condition of isolated deficiency of megakaryocytes in an otherwise normal bone marrow. The outcome is usually fatal, and the disease is associated with other congenital defects. The most constant anomaly is bilateral absence of the radii (Fig. 5–95). Other findings may include cleft palate, micrognathia, mental retardation, congenital heart disease, and renal malformations. One case report of association with maternal rubella has been documented. Bilateral absence of the radii may also occur, in association with *congenital leukemia.*

HOLT–ORAM SYNDROME (UPPER LIMB–CARDIOVASCULAR SYNDROME)

Holt–Oram syndrome[136, 185] consists of a rare combination of upper extremity skeletal anomalies with congenital heart disease, most often atrial septal defect. The disease is transmitted as an autosomal dominant.

Radiologically, the findings may range from hypoplasia of the thumbs (Fig. 5–96) to phocomelia of the upper extremities. The most distinctive finding is the presence of extra carpal bones, the residual of a primitive central carpal row. An os centrale, isolated or partly fused to the scaphoid, may be seen (Fig. 5–97). There may be an elongated slender first metacarpal situated more distally than normal with radial deviation of the proximal phalanx of the thumb. The phalanges of the thumb may be hypoplastic with clinodactyly, or supernumerary phalanges of the thumb may be present. A short middle phalanx of the little finger with clinodactyly is often present. Shoulder and clavicular abnormalities, as well as a prominent medial epicondyle of the elbow with posterior projection, are frequent. Other anomalies include: dislocation of the greater multangular; carpal fusion; hypoplasia of the ulna, humerus, scapula, and clavicles; and abnormalities of the sternum. Coracoclavicular articulations and upwardly rotated scapulae may also be seen. There is no retardation of bone age, no microcephaly, nor shortness of stature.

MYOSITIS OSSIFICANS PROGRESSIVA

Myositis ossificans progressiva[64] is a syndrome caused by a mesodermal disorder, is which inflammatory foci occur in fascia, tendons, and ligaments, followed by ossification. Also present are congenital anomalies of the hands and feet. The bone anomalies, which chiefly involve the thumbs and great toes, are present at birth and precede the soft-tissue changes.

The etiology is unknown and there is no known effective treatment. There is an inexorable slowly progressive course of ossification leading to complete disability. The tongue, heart, larynx, diaphragm, and sphincters are not involved. Muscle phosphatase activity is greatly increased, but other laboratory values are not significantly altered.

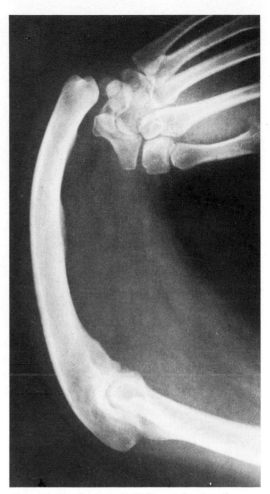

FIG. 5–95. Congenital hypoplastic thrombocytopenia (forearm). Absence of the radius and curvature of the ulna are noted. This finding was present bilaterally.

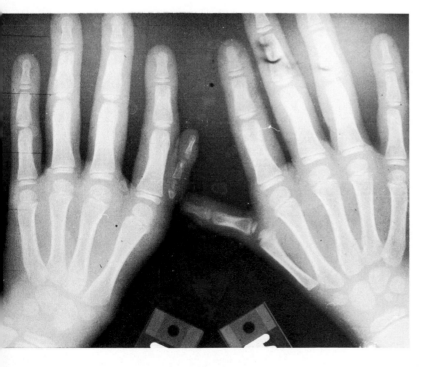

FIG. 5–96. Holt-Oram syndrome (hands). Hypoplasia of both thumbs and absence of the first left metacarpal are noted.

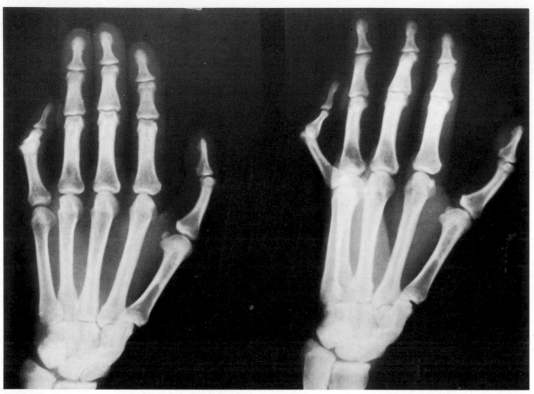

FIG. 5–97. Holt-Oram syndrome (hand and wrist). There is fusion of the lunate to the trapezium with partial fusion of the scaphoid and the trapezoid. Camptodactyly of the little finger is also present. This patient had both atrial septal defect and ventricular septal defect.

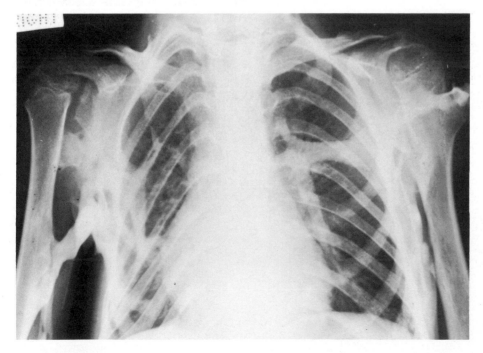

FIG. 5–98. Myositis ossificans progressiva (chest). Extensive new bone formation in the soft tissues with severe limitation of arm motion is present. Note exostosis at the left proximal humerus, due to blending of the ossific foci with the cortex of the bone. (Courtesy of Dr. Harvey White, Children's Memorial Hospital, Chicago, IL)

FIG. 5–99. Myositis ossificans progressiva (knees). Note exostosis-like projections at the distal femora and proximal tibia medially, caused by blending of ossific soft-tissue foci with the bone cortex. (Courtesy of Dr. Harvey White, Children's Memorial Hospital, Chicago, IL)

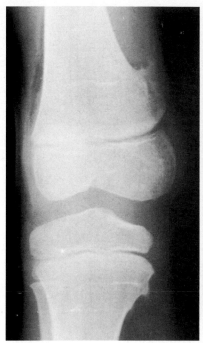
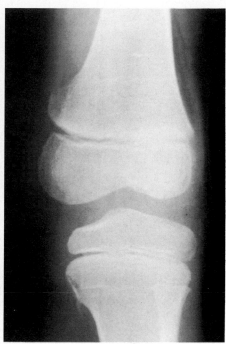

The soft-tissue changes begin as localized areas of edema that are tender and warm. These may be present in the first month of life and usually involve the neck and back initially. The inflammatory reaction subsides and ossification commences. The muscles are involved secondarily to the fibrous tissue. New areas continue to show the same cycle of inflammation and ossification. Initially a cloudlike calcific density may be seen radiographically, which becomes organized into cortex and trabeculae, the recognizable structure of bone (Fig. 5–98). Exostosis-like projections may be seen, because of blending of ossified foci with the cortex (Fig. 5–99).

The skeletal anomalies consist of hypoplasias of the thumbs. The 1st metacarpals as well as the phalanges of the thumb are hypoplastic. There may also be hypoplasia of the middle phalanges of the 5th digits. The first metatarsal is usually normal. The phalanges of the great toes are normal, and there may be lateral deviation of the distal phalanges of the great toe.

EFFECT OF RADIATION ON GROWING BONE[10,163,201]

Irradiation in sufficient dosages causes an arrest of bone growth. This effect assumes great practical importance in the radiation therapy of infants and children with Wilms' tumor, neuroblastoma, and medulloblastoma, in whom long-term survival can be expected. The sequelae are postirradiation scoliosis and undergrowth of the hemipelvis and ribs included in the treatment field. Scoliosis is not as severe as in advanced forms of idiopathic scoliosis. There are 2 types, a lateral flexion curve and a rotary scoliosis. The latter originates from changes in the lamina and pedicles. The changes are related to dose, size of treatment field, and age of the patient. Radiographic changes may be detected as early as 6 months following treatment. The earliest changes are osteoporosis and interference with enchondral bone formation. The vertebral body changes depend on dose levels and can be divided into three types. At less than 1,000 rads, no changes are found. Between 1,000 and 2,000 rads, horizontal lines give a "bone-within-a-bone" appearance. This can be present as a normal variant. Between 2,000 and 3,000 rads, irregularity and scalloping of the vertebral end-plates are present, associated with loss of height and accentuated trabeculation (Fig. 5–100). The pedicles may be involved. The intervertebral spaces remain normal. At higher dosages the vertebral bodies show gross abnormalities of contour similar to those seen in osteochondrodystrophy or achondroplasia. There may be flattening or anterior beaking of the involved vertebral bodies, with a residual small size (Figs. 5–101, 5–102). The small

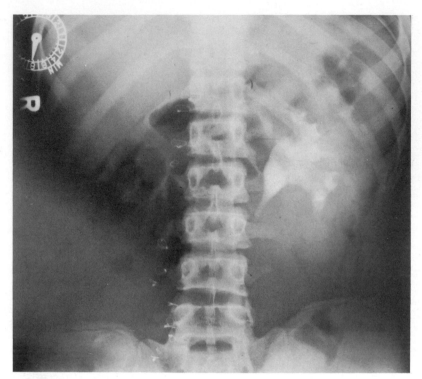

FIG. 5–100. Postradiation change, minimal (lumbar spine and ilia) — excretory urogram; male, age 18 years. The right kidney had been removed 6 years earlier for Wilms' tumor, and 4,500 rads were delivered to the renal area. There is minimal irregularity of the vertebral end-plates and minimal lack of growth of the right side of the vertebral bodies, as is best seen in the body of L-4. Undergrowth of the right iliac crest is also apparent. The pedicles are intact. Compensatory hypertrophy of the left kidney may be noted.

joints show irregularities and there may be loss of height of disk spaces. Also, the size of the spinal canal may be reduced with narrow lumbar interpediculate spaces, similar to achondroplasia. The vertebral body is not usually triangulated at the apex of the curvature as it is in idiopathic scoliosis. The pelvis, if included in the treatment field, shows undergrowth of the iliac crest, widening of the sacroiliac joint, and reduction in the size of the sacrum. A pelvic tilt is present. Reduction in soft tissue and muscle mass also occurs.

ACROMEGALY AND GIANTISM

Excess of pituitary somatotrophic growth hormone from the eosinophilic cells of the anterior pituitary gland results in acromegaly after epiphyseal closure and giantism prior to epiphyseal closure. The excess secretion may result from:

1. Eosinophilic adenoma of the pituitary gland
2. Hyperplasia of eosinophilic cells
3. Diffuse multiplication of eosinophilic cells
4. Excessive secretion of a normal number of eosinophilic cells
5. Adenocarcinoma of the anterior pituitary lobe

Giantism represents a rapid bony growth over a prolonged period. Skeletal maturation may be normal or delayed. There is retardation of sexual development. Large stature is attained. The long bones are also increased in their transverse diameter. This condition is to be differentiated from cerebral giantism, which includes mental retardation, rapid growth during the first 4 years of life, accelerated skeletal maturation, and early pubescence.

Acromegaly[123] clinically shows a typical facies of large mandible, thick lips, large tongue, large nose, prominent supraciliary ridge, and thick, coarse skin. There is an enlarged chest and dorsal kyphosis. The hands and feet are enlarged and there is clubbing of the digits. Dysfunction of other endocrine glands occurs. Diabetes mellitus and hyperthyroidism are common. Testicular atrophy in men and amenorrhea in women develop.

Radiologically, acromegaly is characterized by abnormal growth of cartilage, bone, and fibrous tissue after normal enchondral growth has ceased. Chondroblastic activity resumes at articular and other cartilage sites with enchondral bone formation. The hands and feet show the greatest enlargement because of the large number of articulations. The terminal tufts of the distal phalanges show a "spadelike" configuration and clubbing (Fig. 5–103). A tuft

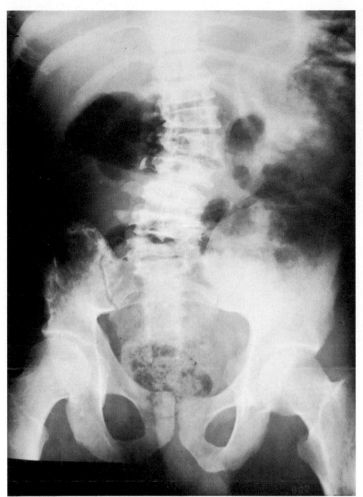

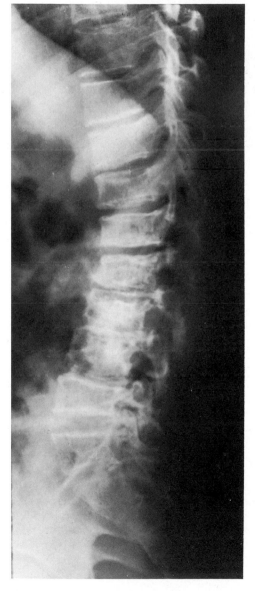

FIG. 5–101. Radiation effect (lumbar spine and pelvis), moderately severe—male, age 25 years, who received a full course of radiation therapy for Wilms' tumor on the right at age 4 years. Note rotary scoliosis of the lumbar spine, with flattening of the vertebral bodies due to involvement of both bodies and pedicles. There is loss of bone density with trabecular accentuation, and marked undergrowth of the right iliac wing. The intervertebral spaces are preserved. Vascular calcification to the right of the spine is also visible.

FIG. 5–102. Radiation effect (lumbar spine)—same patient as Fig. 5–101. Note flattening of the lumbar vertebral bodies, irregularities of the end-plates, loss of bone density, accentuated trabecular pattern, and inferior beaking, particularly of L-1.

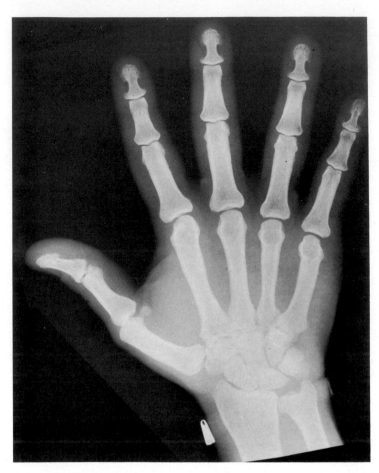

FIG. 5–103. Acromegaly (hand). The hand is markedly enlarged. Note prominence of the terminal phalangeal tufts—the "spadelike" configuration. There is no osteoarthritis.

breadth of over 12 mm in men and over 10 mm in women is said to be virtually diagnostic of acromegaly. The long bones are thickened by periosteal new bone formation. The ribs are increased in caliber and length, increasing the anteroposterior diameter of the chest. If there is erosion by an adenoma, the skull shows enlargement of the sella turcica (Fig. 5–104). There is enlargement of the paranasal sinuses and mastoid air spaces. The frontal bone is thickened to form a supraciliary ridge, and the occipital bone is thickened to form a large protuberance (Figs. 5–105, 5–106). The tongue is enlarged, with resultant depression of the hyoid bone and narrowing of the pharyngeal airway.[9] The mandible becomes markedly enlarged and thickened—one of the most characteristic features of this disease (Fig. 5–107). The vertebral bodies become enlarged by a collar of appositional bone at the anterior and lateral aspects (Fig. 5–108). Osteoporosis may be superimposed. Scalloping of the posterior aspects of the vertebral bodies, particularly in the

lumbar area, may also occur.[230] The joint spaces become widened owing to cartilage hypertrophy. Osteoarthritis, a frequent concomitant condition, is not accompanied by marked joint space narrowing (Fig. 5–109). The soft tissue of the heel is thickened, and a positive "heel pad" sign of acromegaly may be inferred if the soft tissue is thicker than 23 mm (Fig. 5–110). This sign may, however, occur in other conditions and is normally thicker in black men and in Nigerians[31] (see Chapter 8). Another auxiliary roentgen sign of acromegaly is the sesamoid index.[113] There is enlargement of the medial sesamoid bone at the first metacarpophalangeal joint that increases with duration of the disease. The sesamoid index is calculated by multiplying the greatest diameter in mm of the medial sesamoid by the greatest diameter perpendicular to the first one. This index did not prove to have the high discriminatory value originally claimed.[56] The upper limit in normal controls is 40 for men and 32 for women. In acromegalics it ranges from 30 to 63 in men and

FIG. 5–104. Acromegaly (sella turcica) — tomogram. Marked enlargement of the sella turcica, with thinning of the clinoid processes due to a pituitary eosinophilic adenoma, is seen.

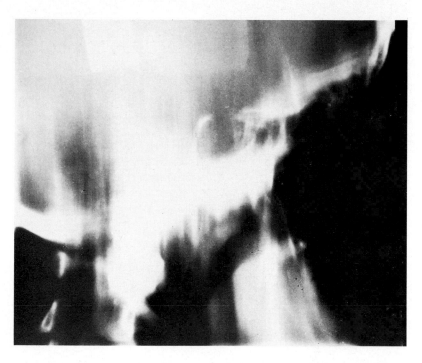

FIG. 5–105. Acromegaly (skull). There is erosion of the posterior floor of the sella turcica due to a pituitary eosinophilic adenoma. Note thickening of the calvarium, particularly in the frontal region and at the external occipital protuberance.

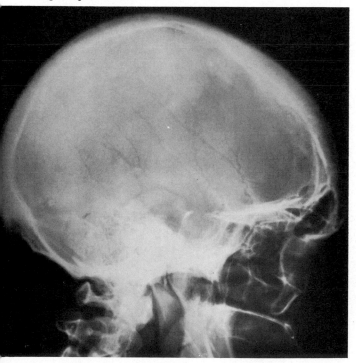

from 31 to 55 in women (Fig. 5–111). Calcification of the pinna of the ear may also be seen (Fig. 5–112).

HOMOCYSTINURIA

Homocystinuria[20,36,222] is an inborn error of metabolism caused by lack of activity of the enzyme cystathionine synthetase, which catalyzes the condensation of homocystine and serine to form cystathionine. Two other enzymatic deficiencies have been discovered: methyltetrahydrofolate homocysteine methyltransferase, and methylenetetrahydrofolate reductase. Elevated serum levels of homocystine and homocystinuria result. Plasma methionine levels may also be elevated. There is evidence that there are at least two genetically heterogenous diseases, pyridoxine-responsive and pyridoxine-resistant cystathionine synthase deficiencies.

The condition is inherited as a mendelian recessive. Males and females are equally affected.

(Text continued on p. 320)

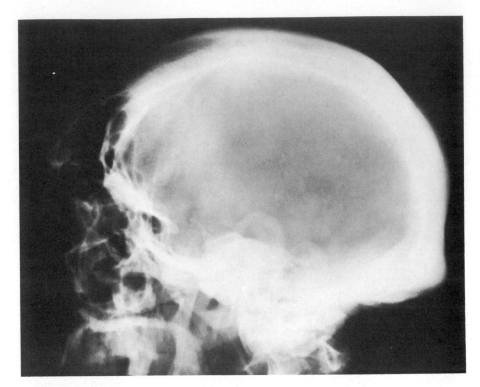

FIG. 5–106. Acromegaly (skull). There is marked thickening of the entire calvarium and of the external occipital protuberance. Note marked enlargement of the sella turcica with thinning of the clinoid processes, and marked prominence of the paranasal sinuses.

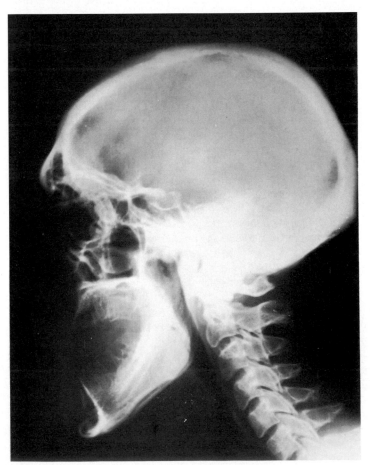

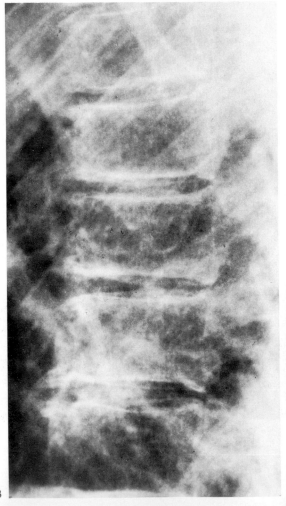

FIG. 5–107

FIG. 5–108

FIG. 5–109. Acromegaly (hands). Note widening of the joint spaces due to cartilage hypertrophy. Osteoarthritic changes, not accompanied by joint space narrowing, may be seen. Also note "spadelike" configuration of the terminal tufts and increased size of the hands.

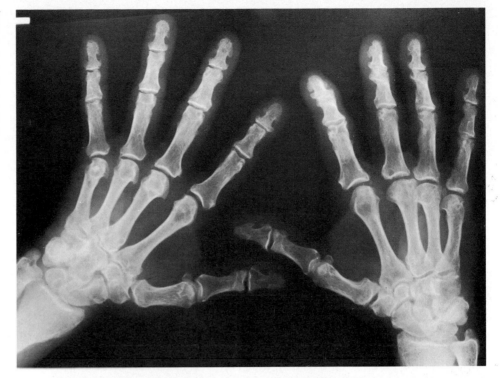

FIG. 5–107. Acromegaly (skull). The mandible is markedly enlarged. The skull shows thickening of the calvarium and prominence of the frontal sinuses. The sella turcica is normal.

FIG. 5–108. Acromegaly (dorsal spine). Enlargement of the anterior aspects of the vertebral bodies due to appositional bone is noted.

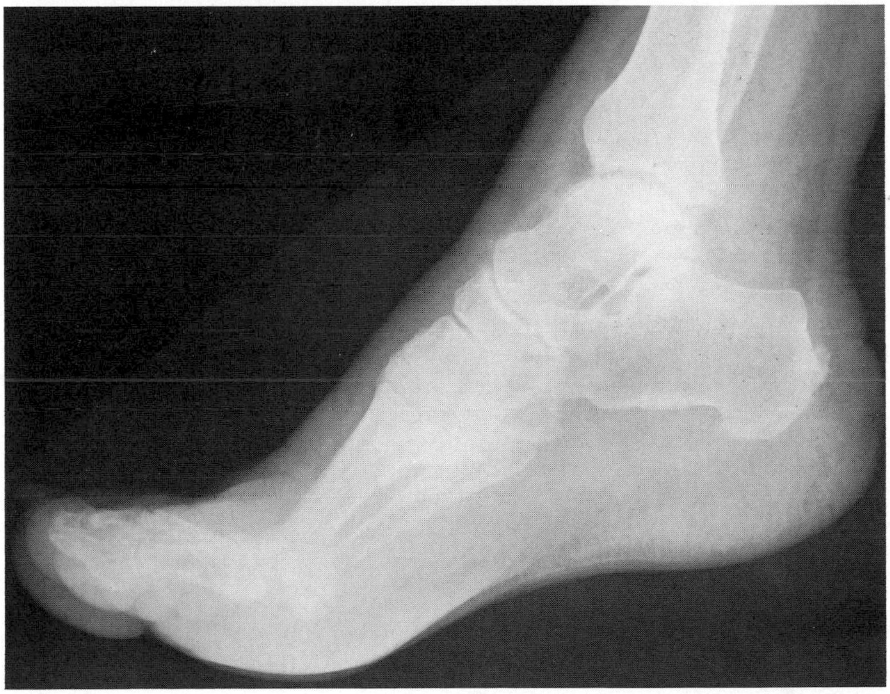

FIG. 5–110. Acromegaly (foot). Positive "heel pad" sign is present; the soft tissue inferior to the calcaneus measures 30 mm. Calcaneal spurs are also visible.

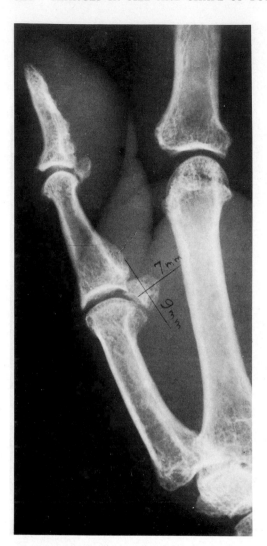

FIG. 5–111. Acromegaly (sesamoid index). The long axis is 9 mm and the perpendicular axis is 7 mm, giving a sesamoid index of 63. This high figure is said to have a high discriminatory value for acromegaly. Note also widening of the metacarpophalangeal joint spaces with mild osteoarthritic spurring.

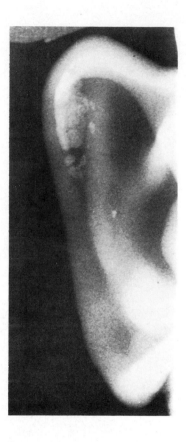

FIG. 5–112. Acromegaly (ear) —same patient as in Fig. 5–111. Calcification of the pinna of the ear is present.

Clinically, the patients are normal at birth. About one-half of patients are mentally retarded. About one-third of patients show changes similar to those seen in Marfan's syndrome, including lens luxations, high palate, scoliosis, dolichostenomelia, arachnodactyly, pectus carinatum or excavatum, and pes planus or cavus. The principal cause of death is vascular thromboembolism. Surgery and angiography are to be avoided wherever possible because of this danger. Convulsions and fractures are not uncommon.

Radiologically, the features are a combination of osteoporosis, metaphyseal and physeal changes, maturation disturbances, and Marfan-like changes. Osteoporosis is noted as a general loss of bone density with biconcavity (Fig. 5–113) or flattening of the vertebral bodies. This finding is present in most cases. The biconcavity may be on the basis of central vascular thrombosis, as in sickle-cell disease. Metaphyseal irregularities and cupping, as well as longitudinal densities, are present. Metaphyseal widening, best seen at the knees, may also be present, as well as enlargement of the epiphyseal ossification centers (Fig. 5–114). The epiphyseal cartilage plate contains calcified spicules and dots, larger than those seen in phenylketonuria, and it may be widened. Enlargement and malformation of the carpal bones frequently occur. The femoral heads may be enlarged, and coxa valga is not uncommon. Widening of the ilium in the supra-acetabular region is sometimes seen. Pathological fractures may occur. Prominent growth lines may be seen. Foot deformities with flat feet or pes cavus are common. Skeletal maturation may be accelerated or delayed. Selective retardation of the lunate has been reported, but this may be due to skeletal imbalance. The Marfan-like changes include arachnodactyly (Figs. 5–115, 5–116), dolichostenomelia, kyphoscoliosis, humerus varus, pectus carinatum or excavatum. Microcephaly may also be present, with large paranasal sinuses. Vascular calcifications and medullary sponge kidney have also been observed.

MARFAN'S SYNDROME (ARACHNODACTYLY)

Marfan's syndrome[34] is a congenital multisystem growth disturbance caused by failure to produce normal collagen. It is transmitted as an autosomal dominant. Most commonly involved are the bones, the cardiovascular system, and the eyes. Mentation is normal. Thromboses do not occur.

Clinically, the patients are tall, usually over 6 feet in height. The long bones are elongated and

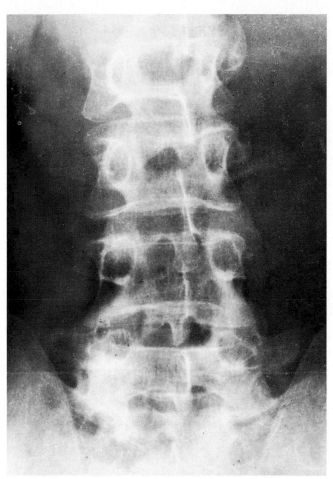

FIG. 5–113. Homocystinuria (spine). Osteoporosis of the spine is seen, with biconcavity of the vertebral bodies.

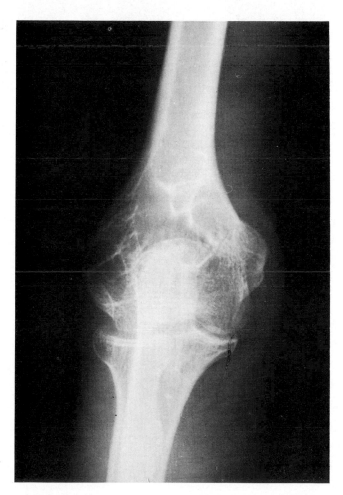

FIG. 5–114. Homocystinuria (elbow). Widening of the metaphysis and epiphysis of the distal humerus, with loss of bone density and mild trabeculation, is noted.

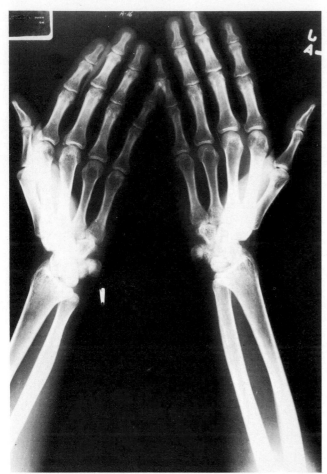

FIG. 5–115. Homocystinuria (hands). Arachnodactyly with elongation of the fingers is seen, as well as osteoporosis. The latter finding distinguishes this condition from Marfan's syndrome.

thinned. There is a high arched palate and a double row of teeth. There may be a funneled thorax with slender ribs. Poor muscular development and tonus, associated with hypermotility of the joints, are present. One-half of patients have bilateral lens luxations and contracted pupils that do not respond to mydriatics. Congenital heart anomalies, most frequently atrial septal defect, occur in about one-third of patients. The most serious cardiovascular complication is dissecting aneurysm, which often kills the patient in early adult life.

Radiologically, in the skeletal system, elongation and thinning of the tubular bones is present, most pronounced in the hands and feet (Figs. 5–117, 5–118). The characteristic feature is arachnodactyly, with long, slender metatarsals, metacarpals, and phalanges. The long bones are slender and gracile. The spine may show severe scoliosis. Abnormally tall lumbar vertebrae may be seen, in contrast to the flattening in homocystinuria. Osteoporosis does not occur. Sternal deformities may be present, and the ribs may be slender with a downward pitch

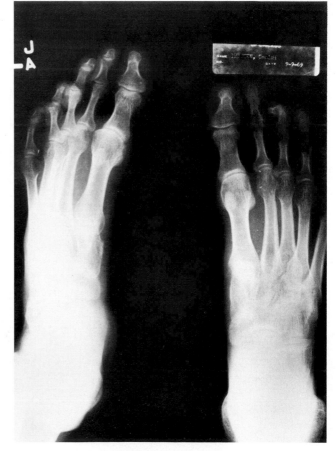

FIG. 5–116. Homocystinuria (feet). Arachnodactyly of the feet is noted.

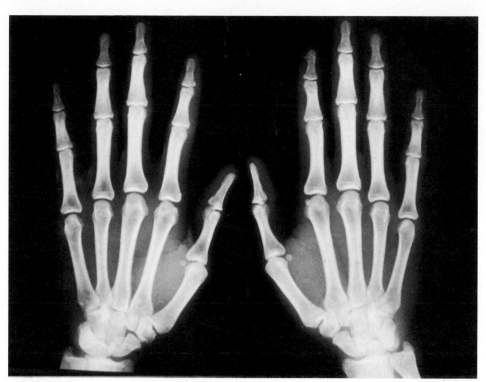

FIG. 5–117. Marfan's syndrome (hands). Note marked elongation of the metacarpals and phalanges. There are no joint changes, and the bone density is maintained.

FIG. 5–118. Marfan's syndrome (foot) showing long, thin bones of the feet.

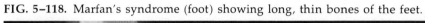

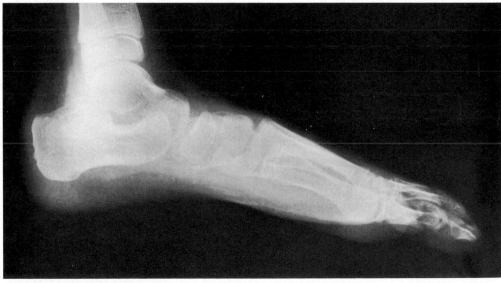

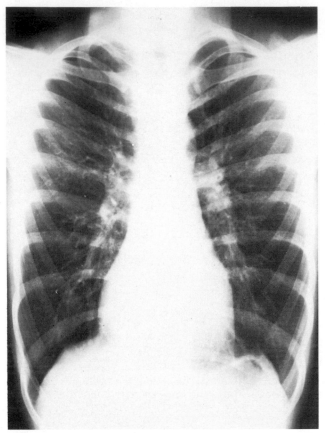

FIG. 5–119. Marfan's syndrome (chest). The ribs are thin, and there is an upward pitch to the posterior ribs and a downward pitch to the anterior ribs.

(Fig. 5–119). A vertical ilium with a wide pelvic cavity may be seen. Coxa valga is frequent. Widening of the spinal canal and posterior scalloping of the vertebral bodies, possibly due to a defective dura, is an associated condition. An anterior sacral meningocele has been reported in this condition.[229]

A marfanoid habitus has been described in multiple endocrine adenomatosis type IIb, which comprises medullary thyroid carcinoma, parathyroid disorders, pheochromocytoma, and associated abnormalities.[30]

MACRODACTYLY

Macrodactyly[17, 23] is a rare idiopathic localized enlargement of digits. True macrodactyly is not to be confused with secondary overgrowth from causes such as hemangioma. There are two forms of true macrodactyly: congenital and noncongenital. Congenital or static macrodactyly is seen at birth and does not increase disproportionately in size. The second or noncongenital type is very rare. There is a disproportionate growth of the involved radials. This is complicated by overgrowth of fatty tissue in the palm, dorsum of the hand, and forearm. Soft-tissue thickening may predominate on only one side of the involved finger (Fig. 5–120).

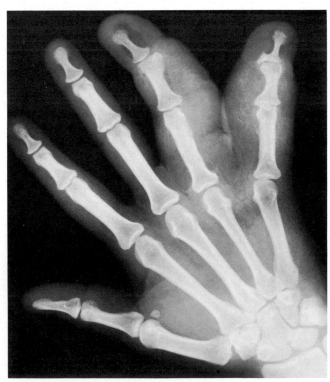

FIG. 5–120. Macrodactyly (hand) — enlargement of the fourth and fifth fingers. Note soft-tissue swelling, predominantly at the ulnar side of the fourth finger and at the radial side of the fifth finger. Biopsy showed fatty tissue to be present. This condition was not present at birth and represents the noncongenital type of idiopathic macrodactyly often complicated by the presence of fatty tissue.

IDIOPATHIC HEMIHYPERTROPHY

Idiopathic hemihypertrophy[241] is a congenital malformation causing enlargement of an entire side of the body, including all tissue components. It is present at birth and may diminish with advancing age. Maturation on the involved side may be accelerated. Elevation of urinary gonadotropins has been reported in this condition. These patients are at risk of developing malignant tumors of the adrenal, kidney, and liver.[176] Hamartomas and genitourinary anomalies also are associated. Medullary sponge kidney is rarely an associated condition.[60] A case has been reported of associated lipomatosis, arthropathy, and psoriasis in a 74-year-old woman.[147] A related condition is macrodystrophia lipomatosa. The *Klippel–Trenaunay syndrome*[138] is composed of bone hypertrophy confined to one lower extremity, associated with varicose veins and port-wine cutaneous hemangiomas. If arteriovenous malformations are also present, it is known as the *Parkes–Weber syndrome*.

NEUROFIBROMATOSIS
(VON RECKLINGHAUSEN'S DISEASE)

Neurofibromatosis,[48,84,86,87,91,181] is a hereditary disturbance of mesodermal and neuroectodermal tissues. The extent may range from minimal to extensive generalized involvement. The prime lesions are neurofibromas of the peripheral and cranial nerves. Frequently associated findings are café-au-lait spots (smooth marginated or "coast of California" type), skin neurofibromas, plexiform neurofibromas, bone deformities, angular kyphoscoliosis which is severe and may lead to paraplegia, localized giantism, elephantoid hypertrophy, intrathoracic meningocele, glial tumors, hypertrophied sebaceous glands, and lipomas. Neurofibrosarcoma may rarely complicate the picture. Repeated biopsies predispose to malignant change. Skeletal deformities are due to mesodermal dysplasia and erosions from neurofibromata.

Radiologically, skin neurofibromas can be seen as multiple soft-tissue densities (Fig. 5–121). Approximately 50% of patients with this disease have bone changes. The spine may show a sharp angular kyphoscoliosis with dysplasia of the vertebral bodies (Fig. 5–122). Erosions, particularly in the intervertebral foramina, may occur from "dumbbell" neurofibromas (Fig. 5–123). Posterior scalloping[206] of the vertebral bodies may occur, but this is not limited to this condition (Fig. 5–124; also see Table 5–8). A meningocele may be present at this site, but not in all instances. Intrathoracic meningocele may occur, and is not to be mistaken for a paravertebral mass due to neurofibromata. Anterior and lateral scalloping of the vertebral bodies have also been described.[42] Vertebral body collapse may also occur. In this disease, the skull shows a characteristic defect involving the posterior superior wall of the orbit[27] (Fig. 5–125), caused by a developmental defect of the wings of the sphenoid and the orbital plate of the frontal bone. The temporal lobe is in contact with the orbital soft tissues, leading to a pulsating exophthalmos. The orbit becomes enlarged. Other cranial changes include defects of the calvarium, absent or deformed clinoid processes,

(Text continued on p. 329)

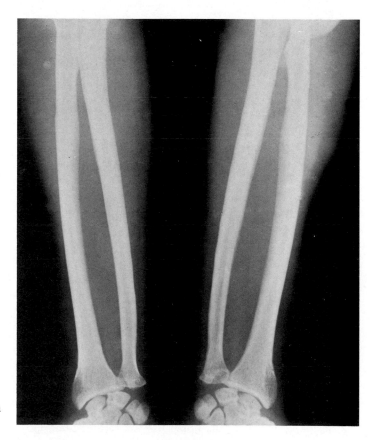

FIG. 5–121. Neurofibromatosis (forearms). Multiple skin nodules (neurofibromas) are apparent.

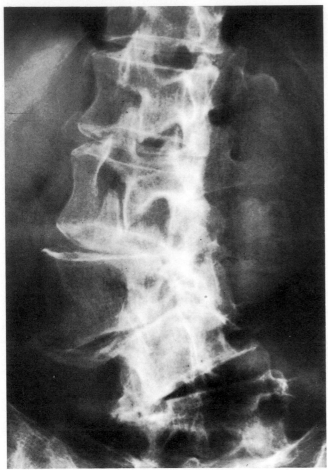

FIG. 5–122. Neurofibromatosis (lumbar spine). Note sharp rotary lumber scoliosis with an appearance of near-extrusion of the third lumbar vertebral body.

FIG. 5–124. Neurofibromatosis (lumbar vertebrae) — myelogram showing posterior scalloping of the lumbar vertebrae and dural ectasia.

FIG. 5–125. Neurofibromatosis (skull). There is agenesis of the greater wing of the right sphenoid, with absence of the superior orbital fissure, and marked elevation of the sphenoid ridge. Erosion or lack of development of the tip of the right petrous pyramid is apparent. The right orbit is enlarged, with encroachment on the lacrimal canal and maxillary antrum. (Courtesy of Dr. Jack Melamed, Chicago, IL)

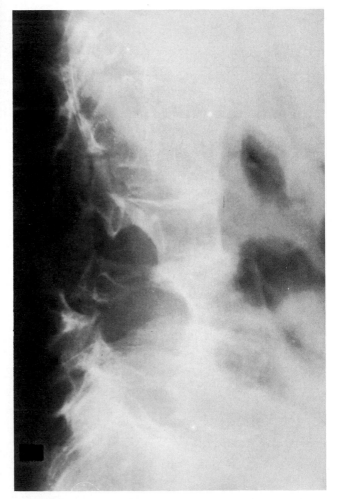

FIG. 5–123. Neurofibromatosis (lumbar spine) — lateral view of Fig. 5–122. Note marked erosions of the intervertebral foramina due to "dumbbell" neurofibromas, and posterior scalloping of the upper lumbar vertebral bodies.

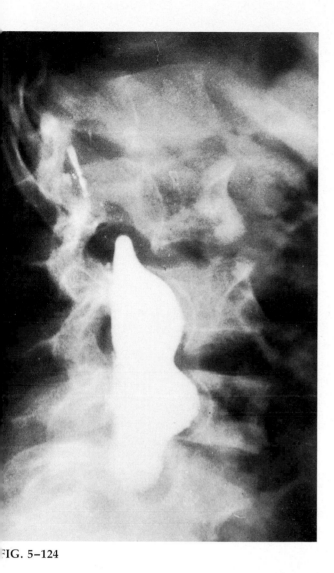

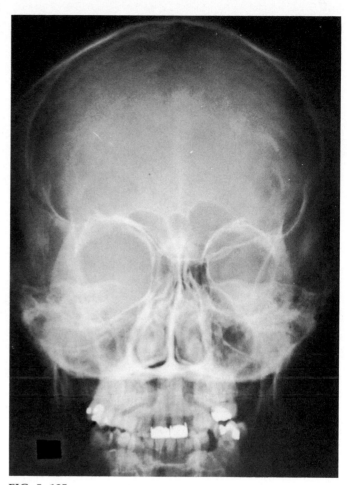

FIG. 5–125

FIG. 5–124

FIG. 5–126. Neurofibromatosis (ribs). Note multiple rib erosions bilaterally due to intercostal neurofibromas and rounded neurofibromas in the apices.

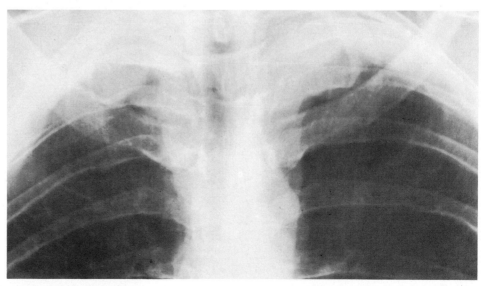

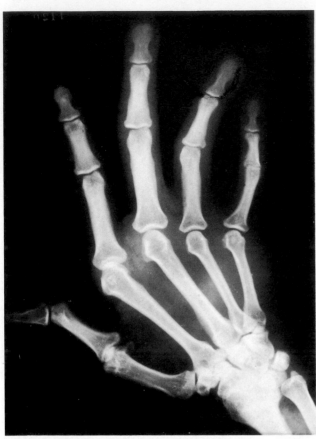

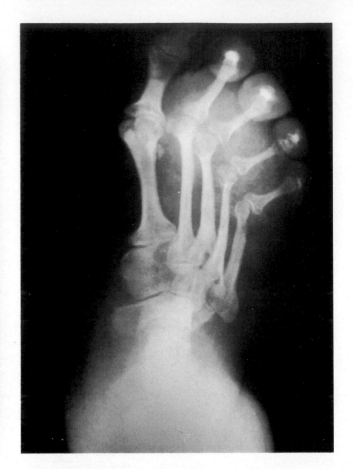

FIG. 5–127. Neurofibromatosis (right hand). Marked overgrowth of the hand may be noted, with ulnar deviation of the fingers. There is also thickening of the cortices and prominence of the terminal phalangeal tufts.

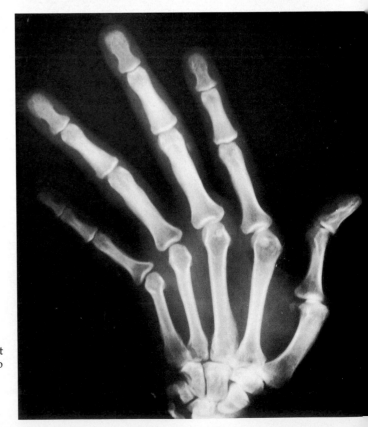

FIG. 5–128. Neurofibromatosis (left hand)—same patient as in Fig. 5–127. Note changes similar and symmetrical to those of the right hand.

FIG. 5–129. Neurofibromatosis (foot)—same patient as in Figs. 5–127 and 5–128. Enlargement of the foot with elongation of the metatarsals and phalanges, and lack of development of the tarsals at the lateral aspect. Marked soft-tissue enlargement due to plexiform neurofibroma is also present.

FIG. 5–130. Neurofibromatosis (leg). Note overconstriction resulting in a thin fibula, and pseudoarthrosis formation at the distal fibula. Bowing of the shaft of the tibia with cortical thickening, and regional osteoporosis of the ankle are also present.

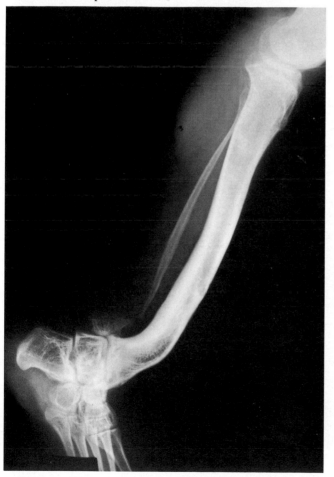

and enlargement of the middle cranial fossa. Macrocranium is frequently present in children.[243] The ribs show superior and inferior erosions from intercostal neurofibromas (Fig. 5–126). There may be attenuation and deformity with a "twisted ribbon" appearance, owing to hypoplasia.

The long bones may show localized overgrowth associated with plexiform neurofibromas (Figs. 5–127, 5–128, 5–129), or overtubulation of the shafts with a long, slender, bowed appearance (Fig. 5–130). Rarely, the long bones may be smaller. Pseudarthroses commonly occur (Fig. 5–131). Although not all congenital pseudarthroses are associated with neurofibromatosis, a large percentage are. There is usually no neurofibromatous tissue at the pseudarthrotic site. Intraosseous neurofibromas may be seen, presenting as a subperiosteal or cortical cystlike structure with a smooth expanded outer margin.[207] A subperiosteal hematoma with exuberant periosteal new bone formation is a rare complication.[120] There may be cortical thickening and increased density of bone (Figs. 5–132, 5–133). Osteomalacia has been reported as associated with neurofibromatosis, said to result from renal artery stenosis leading to renal failure. There is a high incidence of associated congenital anomalies that are not specific for this disease, such as segmentation errors of the spine, spina bifida occulta, and pes cavus.

OSTEOGENESIS IMPERFECTA (OSTEOPSATHYROSIS, FRAGILITUS OSSIUM, MOLLITIES OSSIUM, LOBSTEIN'S DISEASE)

Osteogenesis imperfecta[112] is an inherited generalized disorder of connective tissue, transmitted as an autosomal dominant. The basic bone defect is an deficiency of osteoblasts, which leads to a form of congenital osteoporosis.

Clinically, there are two types, the congenital and the tarda form. The congenital form (Vrolik) is most severe and is present at birth, with multiple fractures. The tarda form (Lobstein) may not become manifest until puberty or adulthood. These patients have osteoporosis, and develop multiple fractures and milder deformities of the long bones at varying times following birth.

Blue sclera are often found in this disease, associated with a white ring surrounding the cornea ("Saturn's ring"). Deafness may develop later in life. The prime symptom of this disease is marked susceptibility to fractures from light trauma, lead-

(Text continued on p. 331)

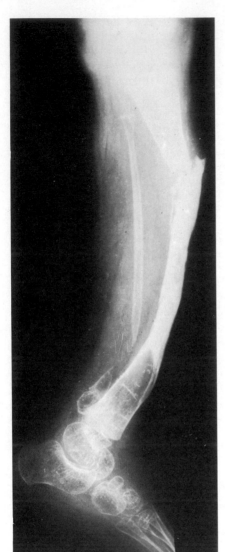

FIG. 5–131. Neurofibromatosis (leg) — male, age 5 years, with café-au-lait spots and skin neurofibromas. Note bowing of the tibia and fibula anteriorly, with pseudarthrosis in the proximal third of the shaft of the tibia, and pseudarthrosis in the distal portion of the shaft of the fibula with a sharp, smooth margin at the latter site. Sclerosis of the midshaft of the tibia and osteoporosis at other areas are visible. Pseudarthrosis is not limited to neurofibromatosis (see pp. 344–348).

FIG. 5–132. Neurofibromatosis (legs). There is bowing of all leg bones, with marked cortical thickening.

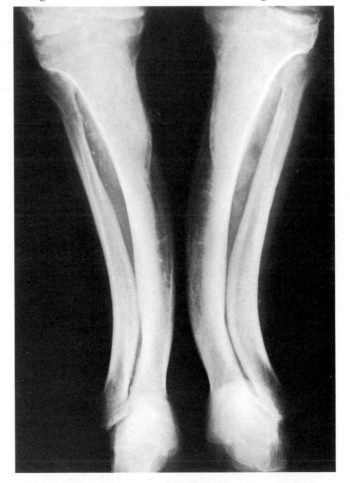

FIG. 5–133. Neurofibromatosis (pelvis). There is enlargement of the left hemipelvis, with cortical thickening in the pelvis as well as cortical thickening of the right upper femur. A beaklike projection of the anterior superior iliac spine is noted. Enlargement and irregularity of the ischiopubic synchondrosis as well as the junction between the superior ramus of the pubis and the ilium are present, with irregular calcification. Elongation and detachment of the left lesser trochanter is seen, as well as flattening of the left femoral head.

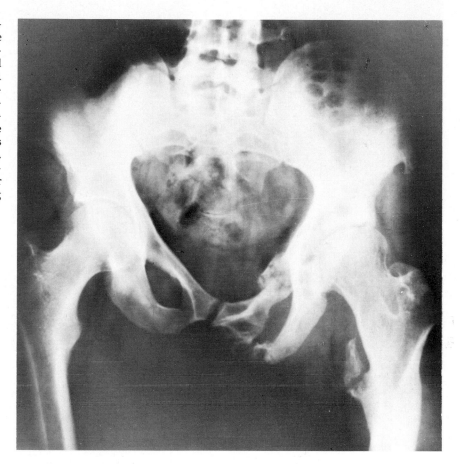

ing to deformities. The severity often diminishes after skeletal maturation. Hemorrhagic disease has been reported associated with this condition.

Radiologically the long bones are long, slender, and overconstricted, with deformities from previous fractures (Fig. 5–134, 5–135). Enchondral bone formation continues, while periosteal bone apposition is diminished, leading to a thin cortex and osteoporosis. Bowing deformities are present, and osteogenesis imperfecta is the only form of osteoporosis with this finding. There is marked fragility and tendency to fracture. The femur, humerus, tibia, and forearm, in that order of frequency, are most likely to fracture. An apparent shortening and thickening of bone may be caused by "telescoping" fractures, or deformity with cortical thickening secondary to fracture (Figs. 5–136, 5–137, 5–138), characterizing the severe form of this disease. Dislocations of the radial heads may be seen. Pseudarthroses may also be present (Fig. 5–139). Excessive callus formation is a characteristic finding

in this disease and is not to be confused with a tumor (Fig. 5–140). The callus may be massive and exuberant, enveloping the entire length of a long bone.[15] The alkaline phosphatase may be elevated. Persistent enlargement of the bone and functional loss may ensure.[197] Multiple cystic lesions owing to accentuated trabeculae may also be seen at bone ends. The skull shows thinning of the calvarium and wormian bone formation (Fig. 5–141). The vertebral bodies are osteoporotic and have a nonuniform biconcave configuration. Scoliosis is common. The pelvis shows protrusio acetabuli. Coxa vara is present. Odontogenesis imperfecta with defective enamel formation, separation of enamel, and obliteration of the root canals is a characteristic associated condition. The deciduous teeth are more severely affected. Well-circumscribed bony rarefactions distributed throughout the skeleton may be seen in both congenita and tarda forms.[107] Osteosarcoma has been reported in this condition.[114]

(Text continued on p. 335)

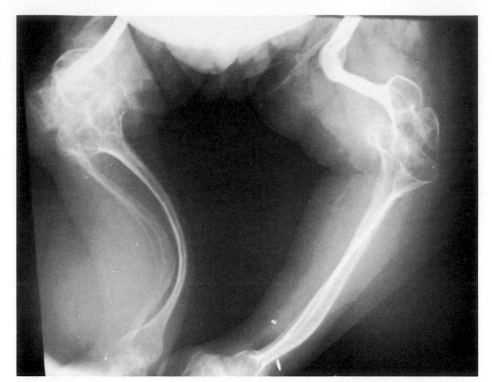

FIG. 5–134. Osteogenesis imperfecta (lower extremities). Note overconstriction of the long bones with very severe deformities of the femora, and bowing, particularly in the right tibia and fibula. Severe osteoporosis is also present.

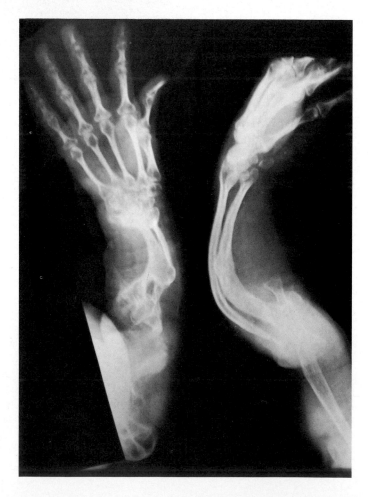

FIG. 5–135. Osteogenesis imperfecta (upper extremities) — same patient as in Fig. 5–134. Note thinning and bowing of the tubular bones, with shortening of the right radius and ulna. Cystic rarefactions at the proximal right ulna are also present.

FIG. 5–136. Osteogenesis imperfecta. Note multiple fractures involving the long bones and the ribs, with callus formation at fracture sites. Thickening of bones in the lower extremities, due to telescoping fractures with associated shortening, is also visible.

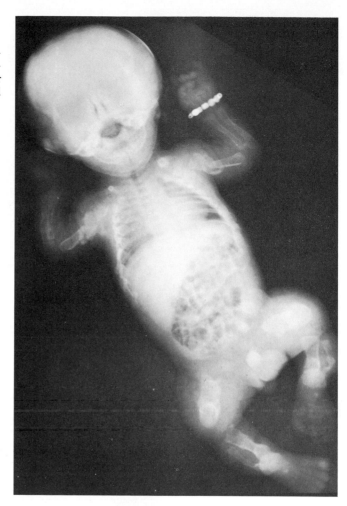

FIG. 5–137. Osteogenesis imperfecta (right upper extremity) — same patient as in Fig. 5–136 after 8 months. There has been healing of the fracture of the humerus, with shortening and thickening of the humeral shaft. Incomplete and healed fractures of the radius and ulna are also present.

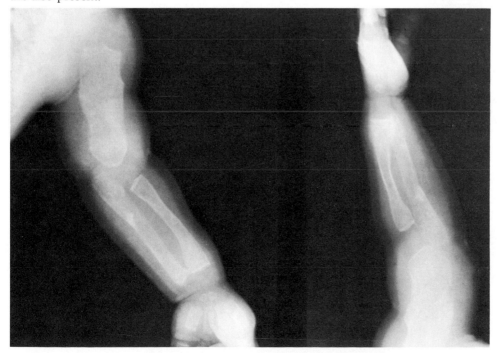

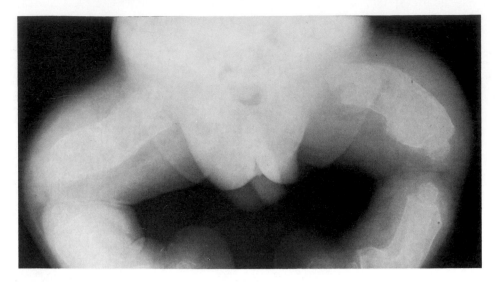

FIG. 5–138. Osteogenesis imperfecta (lower extremities)—same patient as in Figs. 5–136 and 137, 8 months after last picture was taken. Shortening and thickening of both femora, and severe deformities of the tibiae and fibulae, are apparent.

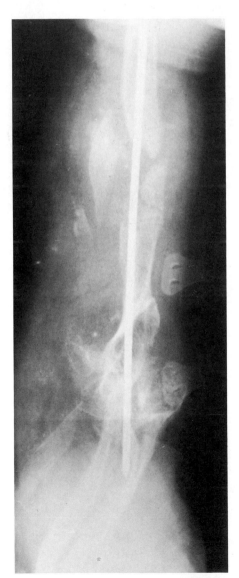

FIG. 5–139. Osteogenesis imperfecta (femur)—pseudarthrosis. Fragments are transfixed by intramedullary rod. Marked deformity of the tibia and fibula may also be seen.

FIG. 5–140. Osteogenesis imperfecta (femur). Note excessive callus formation of the right femoral shaft.

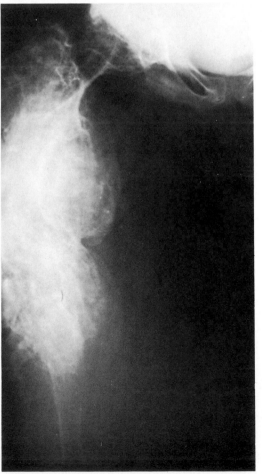

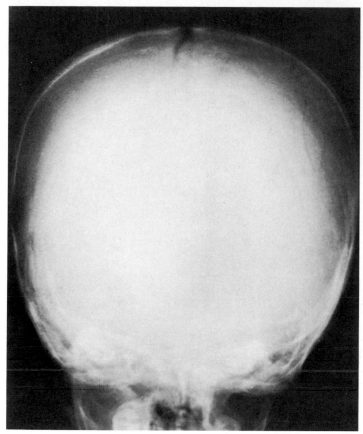

FIG. 5–141. Osteogenesis imperfecta (skull). There is wormian bone formation. Thinning of the calvarium and a granular osteoporosis may also be noted.

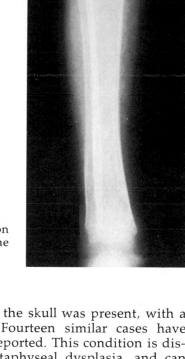

FIG. 5–142. Pyle's disease (lower extremity). Note lack of tubulation of the long bones, resulting in an "Erlenmeyer flask" deformity. The skull appeared normal in this case.

PYLE'S DISEASE
(FAMILIAL METAPHYSEAL DYSPLASIA)[74]

The disease originally described by Pyle, and followed in the same patient and family by Bakwin and Krida, had the following changes: tall stature with prominence of the frontal region, genu valgum, and massive ends of the long bones. *Radiologically*, symmetrical enlargement of the proximal portions of the clavicles, thickening of the ribs, "paddle-shaped" enlargement of the metaphyses of the long bones (Fig. 5–142), and unusually long femora and tibiae were seen. Cortical thinning and osteoporosis were also present. Only mild involvement of the skull was present, with a supraorbital bulge. Fourteen similar cases have subsequently been reported. This condition is distinct from craniometaphyseal dysplasia, and can easily be differentiated from it by lack of significant skull changes. The inheritance of Pyle's disease is probably autosomal recessive.

CRANIOMETAPHYSEAL DYSPLASIA

Craniometaphyseal dysplasia[41, 212] is a rare bone dysplasia characterized by failure of normal tubulation

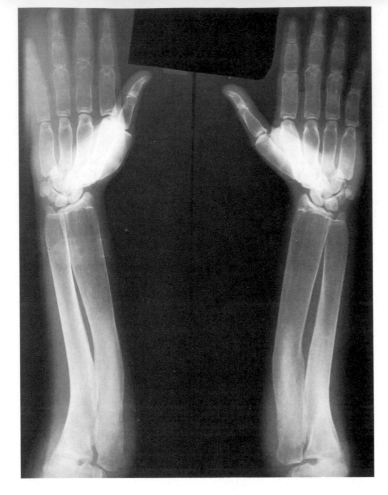

FIG. 5–143. Craniometaphyseal dysplasia (forearms and hands). There is underconstriction of the shafts of the tubular bones of the forearm and hand, with thinning of the cortex and loss of bone density.

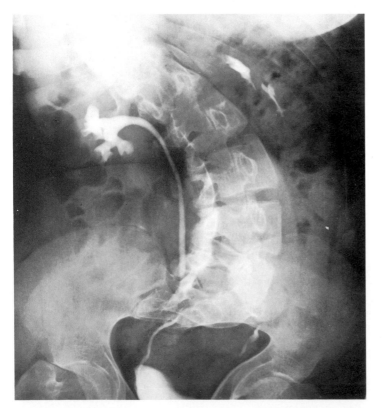

FIG. 5–144. Craniometaphyseal dysplasia. Severe scoliosis of the lumbar spine, pelvic deformity, and marked widening of the entire shafts of the ribs are present. Excretory urogram shows the renal collecting systems to be normal.

FIG. 5–145. Craniometaphyseal dysplasia (skull). Thickening of the vault, lack of development of the paranasal sinuses, lack of mastoid aeration, and sclerosis of the mandible are present. Defective dentition is also visible.

of bone, coupled with skull abnormalities. It is congenital and familial.

Clinically, the patients have a typical facies, with hypertelorism, a broad, flat nose, and defective dentition. Progressive hearing loss may occur. Significant cranial nerve deficits also affecting vision have been reported, as well as facial paralysis.

Radiologically, the most characteristic feature is lack of tubulation of the tubular bones resulting in an "Erlenmeyer flask" deformity. This also occurs in other conditions (see pp 344–348). Diaphyseal widening may also occur. The cortex is thin at the widened areas and osteoporosis may be present. These changes are most pronounced at the distal femur, radius, and ulna, but the short bones are also involved (Fig. 5–143).

The ribs are widened to the ends, and unlike in Hurler's syndrome, do not have a spatulate configuration. The vertebrae, although sometimes normal, may show flattening and sclerosis of the bodies as well as severe scoliosis (Fig. 5–144). The clavicles show splaying similar to that seen in the long bones.

The skull may show sclerosis of the base and calvarium. Lack of aeration of the paranasal sinuses and mastoids is also present. Sclerosis of the petrous and sphenoid ridges, and hypertelorism are seen (Fig. 5–145). The mandible is markedly thickened and sclerotic, with defective dentition. Fractures may occur.

WEISMANN–NETTER SYNDROME (TOXOPACHYOSTÉOSE DIAPHYSAIRE TIBIO–PÉRONIÈRE)[2,106]

The Weismann–Netter syndrome is a congenital condition with nonprogressive anterior bowing of the tibiae and fibulae, clinically manifest as a "sabre shin." Bilateral symmetric changes are combined with shortness of stature. This condition has been reported in elderly individuals. The stigmata of congenital lues or healed rickets are not present. Other skeletal changes are minor and inconstant (Fig. 5–146).

Another cause of bowing is acute traumatic plastic bowing of the forearm in children.[32] Congenital pseudoarthrosis of the radius and ulna may also be associated with bowing.[45]

APLASIA, HYPOPLASIA, AND MALSEGMENTATION[168]

The cause of congenital malformations of the extremities is incompletely understood. Thalidomide has been shown to cause phocomelia, with absence of the shaft segment but presence of the hand or foot (Figs. 5–147, 5–148), and maternal virus infection is suspected in other cases. The deformities may range from complete amelia to complete, radial (Fig. 5–149), or ulnar (Fig. 5–150) paraxial hemimelia, to oligodactylia (Fig. 5–151) or adactylia (Fig. 5–152). Apparent extra distal phalanges have been observed in fetal dilantin syndrome. Other congenital anomalies also occur with maternal anticonvulsive treatment. The most commonly involved aplastic or hypoplastic long bones are the fibula, radius, femur, ulna, and humerus. Short stature may result from femoral maldevelopment. The classification is summarized below.

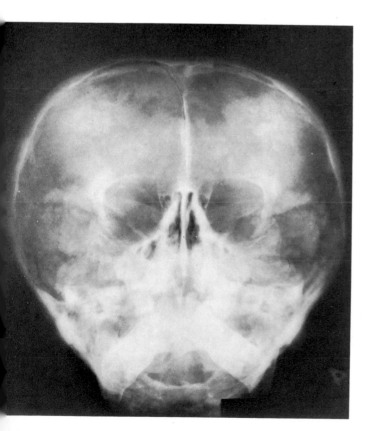

SHORT STATURE FROM FEMORAL MALDEVELOPMENT*

Partial deficiency of the femur

1. Coxa vara
2. Proximal focal femoral deficiency (PFFD)
3. Middle focal femoral deficiency (MFFD)
4. Distal focal femoral deficiency (DFFD)

Complete absence of the femur

* Modified from Bailey JA: Disproportionate Short Stature. Diagnosis and Management. Philadelphia, WB Saunders, 1973

(Text continued on p. 341)

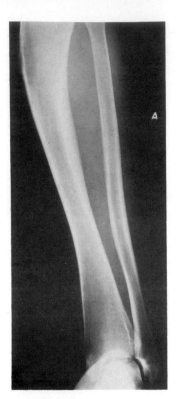

FIG. 5–146

FIG. 5–147

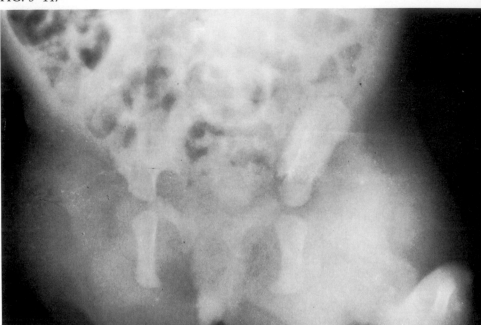

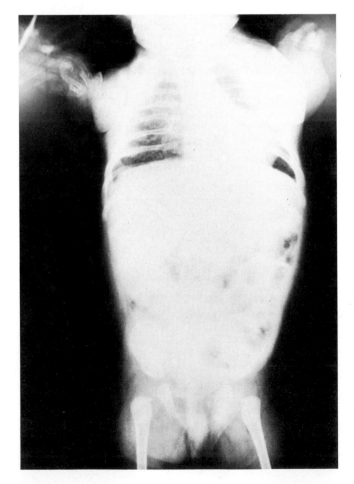

FIG. 5–146. Weisman-Netter syndrome. Bowing of the tibia, and to a lesser extent the fibula, is noted.

FIG. 5–147. Phocomelia. Left lower extremity with absence of thigh and leg bones, but with rudimentary bones of the foot, is seen. Amelia of the right lower extremity is noted.

FIG. 5–148. Phocomelia. Rudimentary long bones of the upper extremities are present with the hands attached close to the trunk. The lower extremities are normal.

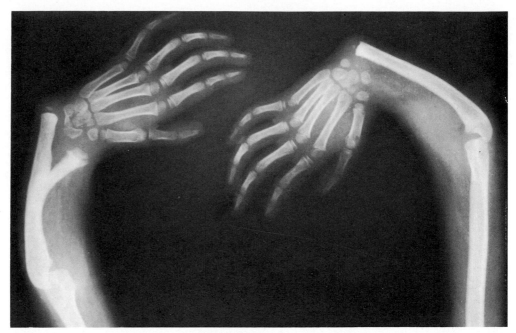

FIG. 5–149. Radial paraxial hemimelia—complete type on the left and partial type on the right.

FIG. 5–150. Ulnar paraxial hemimelia. Distal portion of the ulna and of radials 3, 4, and 5, and the carpal bones at their ulnar aspects, failed to develop.

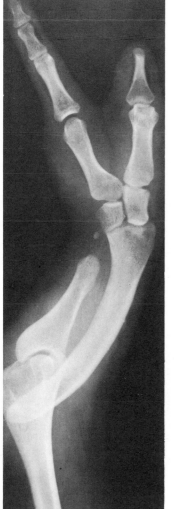

FIG. 5–151. Oligodactylia. Failure of development of middle two radials bilaterally is noted.

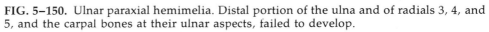

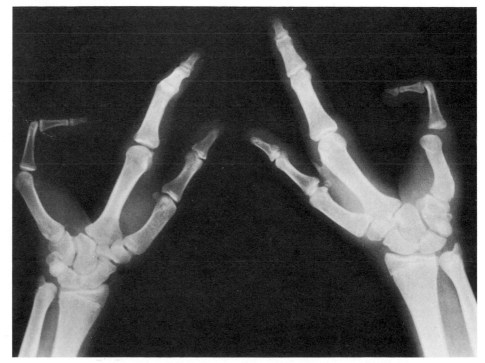

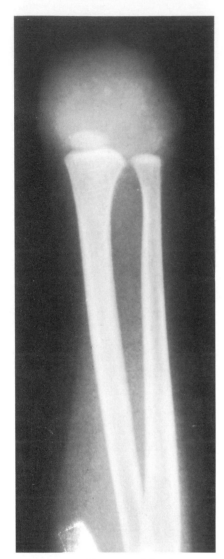

FIG. 5–152. Absence of the bones of the hands.

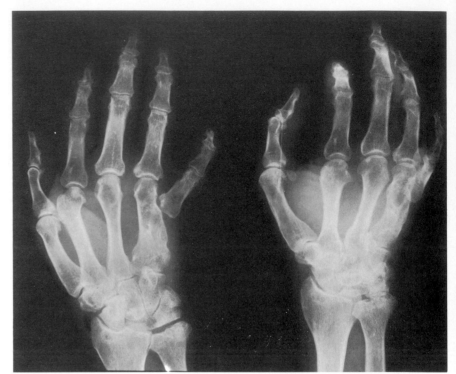

FIG. 5–153. Segmentation anomaly involving the fourth and fifth metacarpals.

FIG. 5–154. Absence of the distal interphalangeal joints of several fingers bilaterally, or symphalangism.

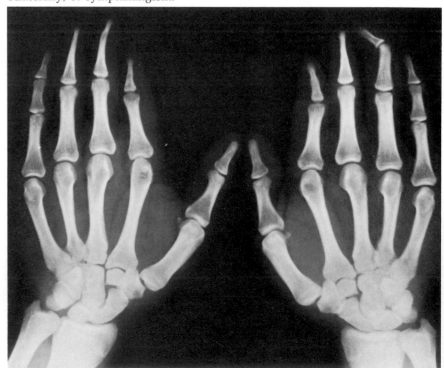

PROXIMAL FEMORAL FOCAL DEFICIENCY[134,208]

Proximal femoral focal deficiency is a distinct clinicoradiologic entity. It is characterized by lower limb length discrepancy due to defective development of the proximal femur. Its severity has been classified on a scale of A to D—D being the most severe—with the acetabulum and femoral head both absent. Other bony anomalies may be associated, most commonly with ipsilateral absence of the fibula. This picture may also be part of the caudal regression syndrome.[199]

The most common error of segmentation is proximal radioulnar synostosis in the long bones, also seen in Klinefelter's XXXXY variant. There may be longitudinal undersegmentation of the short bones resulting in syndactylism (Fig. 5–153). Absence of the articular spaces, or symphalangism, may be seen (Fig. 5–154). This finding is particularly common in the distal interphalangeal joint of the little toe, where it may be regarded as a normal variant. Oversegmentation of the short bones results in polydactyly (Fig. 5–155). Undersegmentation or fusion of the tarsal bone is called coalition and is often associated with pes planus. Carpal fusion may also occur (Fig. 5–156). Three phalanges of the thumbs may rarely be seen[79] (Fig. 5–157). This has been reported as a familial condition, and may represent an arrested attempt to form another thumb. Pelvic and coccygeal ribs have been reported.[171, 231] Bizarre

teratoid malformations may be seen (Fig. 5–158).

DIFFERENTIAL DIAGNOSIS OF CONGENITAL MALFORMATION SYNDROMES WITH RESPECT TO THE CARPALS, METACARPALS, AND PHALANGES

The carpal anomalies that may occur in the congenital malformation syndromes include extra carpals, abnormal carpals, carpal angle abnormalities, and carpal fusion. The two supernumerary ossicles of greatest interest are the os centrale and the os triangulare. The os centrale phylogenetically is a remnant of the central row of carpals present in lower animals. It normally fuses with the scaphoid, but may persist in some conditions. The os triangulare is a small ossicle near the ulna, which may occasionally be present also in some congenital conditions, or may be an infrequent variant in normal individuals. Carpal anomalies have been summarized by Poznanski and Holt,[188] and are presented in Table 5–3.

Precise statistical methods for mensuration and evaluation of metacarpal and phalangeal lengths by row and ray are described by Garn *et al*[72] as useful in the diagnosis of syndromes of chromosomal, genetic, and endocrine origin. Tables of standards for bone length have been developed.

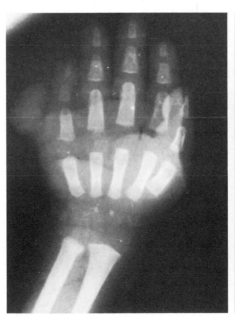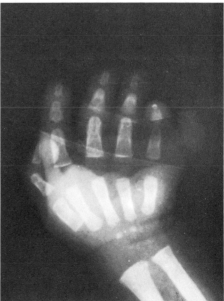

FIG. 5–155. Oversegmentation resulting in polydactyly with a supernumerary digit budding off the lateral aspects of the fifth digits bilaterally.

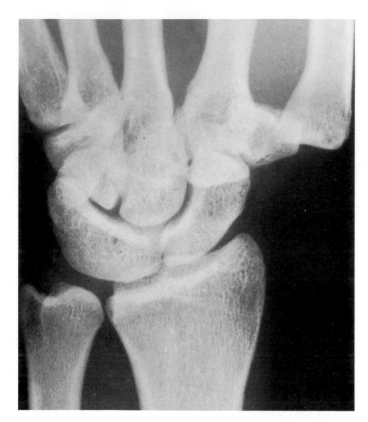

FIG. 5–156. Carpal fusion (wrist). The proximal carpal row is fused into two masses.

FIG. 5–157. Bilateral congenital anomaly of the thumbs with formation of proximal, middle, and distal phalanges. The middle phalanges assume a peculiar "cup and saucer" shape. No other abnormalities are present.

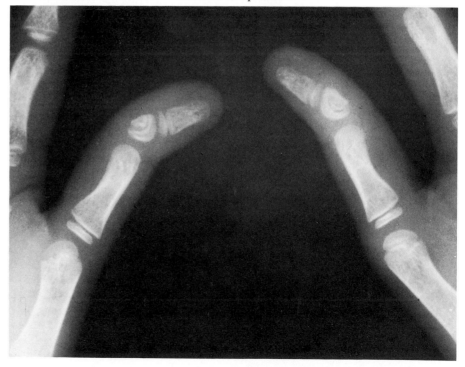

TABLE 5–3. Carpal Anomalies*

	Os Centrale (one or more)	Extra Distal Carpals	Os Triangulare	Irregular Carpal Margins	Abnormally Shaped Scaphoid	Absent or Hypoplastic Scaphoid	Scaphoid Fused to Other Carpals	Abnormally Shaped Capitate	Absent or Hypoplastic Capitate	Some Carpal Fusion	Decreased Carpal Angle	Increased Carpal Angle	Diminution in Size of the Carpus
Arthrogryposis			O		O		O	O		X		X	X
Diastrophic dwarfism		X		X	O		O	O		O		O	X
Dyschondrosteosis										O	X		
Ellis-van Creveld syndrome										X			
Epiphyseal dysplasia					X	O		X	X			X	X
Fanconi's anemia					X	X							
Hand-foot-uterus syndrome	X				X		X			X			
Holt-Oram syndrome	X		O		X	O	X	O		O			
Homocystinuria							X						
Otopalatodigital syndrome	O	O			O			O	X	O			O
Symphalangism								O		X			
Turner's syndrome										O	X		

X = Commonly present
O = Occasionally present

* Modified from Poznanski AK, Holt JF: Am J Roentgen 112:443–459, 1971

A graphic method, called the "metacarpophalangeal pattern profile," has been developed by Poznanski et al,[187] and depicts lengthening and shortening of the tubular bones of the hand, and their relationship to one another. Many congenital malformations have characteristic metacarpophalangeal pattern profiles. This method can be useful for individual diagnosis, as well as for inter-syndrome comparison.

Abnormalities of the thumb may occur as isolated anomalies or associated with congenital malformation syndromes. The changes may consist of enlargement, duplication, hypoplasia, absence, abnormal ossification centers, or abnormality in position. Tables of the relative proportions of the bones of the thumb have been developed by Poznanski et al.[186] The appearance of the thumb in various congenital malformation syndromes is presented in Table 5–4.

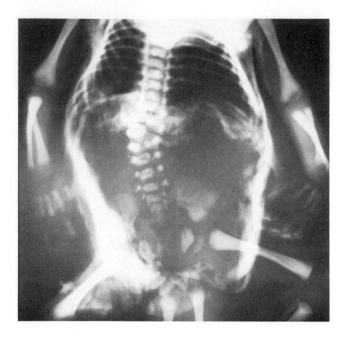

FIG. 5–158. Teratoid malformation (four-legged monster).

DIFFERENTIAL DIAGNOSIS OF SPECIFIC ROENTGEN SIGNS RELATED TO ALTERATION OF BONE SIZE AND SHAPE

1. Brachydactyly or Shortening of Metacarpals
   Pseudohypoparathyroidism (PH)
   Pseudopseudohypoparathyroidism (PPH)
   Turner's syndrome
   Sickle-cell anemia
   Basal-cell nevus syndrome (Gorlin's syndrome
   Injury to epiphyseal cartilage
   Enchondromatosis
   Marchesani's syndrome
   Epiphyseal dysostosis
   Neonatal hyperthyroidism
   Idiopathic causes
2. Shortening of Hands and Feet
   Peripheral dysostosis (cupping of metaphysis)
   Chondroectodermal dysplasis (cupping of metaphysis)
   Rheumatoid arthritis
   Hurler's syndrome
   Morquio's syndrome
   Metaphyseal dysostosis
   Achondroplasia
   Acrodysplasia
   Cephaloskeletal dysplasia
   Cockayne's syndrome
   Fibrous dysplasia with skin pigmentation and precocious puberty (McCune–Albright)

   Noonan's syndrome
   Orodigitofacial syndrome
   Prader–Willi syndrome
   Progeria
   Pseudohypoparathyroidism (PH)
   Rhinotrichophalangeal syndrome (Giedion)
   Shawl scrotum syndrome (Aarskog–Scott)
   Smith–Lemli–Opitz syndrome
   Spherophakia–brachymorphia syndrome (Weil–Marchesani)
3. Hypoplasia or Absence of First Radials or Radius
   Fanconi's anemia
   Myositis ossificans progressiva
   Holt–Oram syndrome (upper limb)
   Cornelia de Lange syndrome
   Congenital hypoplastic thrombocytopenic purpura
   Otopalatodigital syndrome
   Trisomy 18
   Basal-cell nevus syndrome (Gorlin's syndrome)
   Sporadic
4. Clinodactyly of fifth digit
   Mongolism
   Cornelia de Lange syndrome
   Otopalatodigital syndrome
   Cretinism
   Achondroplasia
   Fanconi's anemia
   Erythrogenesis imperfecta
   Myositis ossificans progressiva
   Kirner's deformity (distal phalanx)[29]
   Normal variant
5. Epiphyseal or Metaphyseal Injury Resulting in Shortening of Bone
   Trauma
   Infection[47]
   Infarction[47]
   Thermal
   Neoplasm
   Vitamin A intoxication
   Radiation
6. Generalized Overgrowth of Bone
   Hyperpituitarism
   Marfan's syndrome
   Homocystinuria

TABLE 5–4. Thumb Appearance in Various Syndromes*

	Distal Phalanx				Proximal Phalanx				Metacarpal						
	Cone Epiphysis	Short $\frac{Met.2}{D1}$	Broad	Triphalangeal Thumb	Short $\frac{Met.2}{P1}$	Long $\frac{Met.2}{P1}$	Triangular	Thin Short	Wide $\frac{Met.2}{Met.1}$	Long $\frac{Met.2}{Met.1}$	Pseudo-epiphysis	Clasped Thumb	"Hitchhiker" Thumb	Duplication	Absent Thumb
Apert's and other acrocephalosyndactyly		X	X		X		X							O	O
Arthrogryposis												X			
Cardiomelic (Holt-Oram)		X		X				X		X					X
Cornelia de Lange		X							X						
Diastrophic dwarfism		O			O				X				X		
Hand-foot-uterus	X	O			O				X		X				
Myositis ossificans		X			O	O			X		O				
Otopalatodigital	X	X													
Pancytopenia-dysmelia (Fanconi's anemia)		X						X						O	X
Rubinstein-Taybi		X	X		X	X							X		
Thalidomide embryopathy				X											O
Trisomy 18		O			O										O

O = Occasional   P 1 = Proximal phalanx of thumb
X = Frequent   D 1 = Distal phalanx of thumb

* Modified from Poznanski AK, Garn SM, Holt JF: Radiology 100:115–129, 1971

Klinefelter's syndrome
Hemihypertrophy
Total lipodystrophy (absence of fat)
Cerebral giantism (hypothalamic)
7. Localized Overgrowth of Bone
   Hyperemia
   Neurofibromatosis
   Hemangiomatosis
   Lymphangiomatosis
   Chronic osteitis
   Tuberculosis
   Chronic arthritis
   Arteriovenous fistula
   Neoplasm
   Healing fracture

Hemophilic hemarthrosis
Infantile cortical hyperostosis
Ollier's disease
Trevor's disease
Congenital macrodactyly
Infiltrating angiolipoma
Idiopathic causes
8. Overtubulation
   Neurofibromatosis
   Congenital pseudoarthrosis
   Fibrous dysplasia
   Rheumatoid arthritis
   Progeria
   Atrophy of disuse
   Enchondromatosis

Neuromuscular and paralytic states
Marfan's syndrome
Homocystinuria
Osteogenesis imperfecta

9. Undertubulation
Pyle's disease
Craniometaphyseal dysplasia
Metaphyseal injury
Cartilaginous dystrophies
Osteopetrosis
Hypervitaminosis D
Lead poisoning (late)
Neoplasm
Diaphyseal aclasia
Enchondromatosis
Healing rickets
Healing scurvy
Healing fracture
Fibrocystic disease of pancreas
Cooley's anemia (thalassemia)
Gaucher's disease
Infantile cortical hyperostosis
Adult hypophosphatasia
Cleidocranial dysostosis (atypical)
Hurler's disease
Rubella embryopathy
Peripheral dysostosis
Total lipodystrophy
Engelmann's disease
Hyperphosphatasia

10. Proximal Tapering of Tubular Bones
Hurler's syndrome
Hurler-like syndromes
Cornelia de Lange syndrome

11. Distal Tapering of Short Bones
Neurotrophic
Diabetes mellitus
Leprosy
Epidermolysis bullosa
Thermal injury

12. Pseudarthroses
Congenital pseudarthrosis
Neurofibromatosis
Fibrous dysplasia
Nonunion of fractures

13. Exostoses
Osteochondroma (metaphyseal)
Trevor's disease (epiphyseal)
Intracapsular chondroma (joint)
Supracondylar spur (humerus)
Chondroectodermal dysplasia (tibial)
Turner's syndrome (medial tibial condyle)
Pseudohypoparathyroidism (PH)
Dyschondrosteosis (tibial)

Traumatic
Myositis ossificans
Turret exostosis
Subungual exostosis
Following radiation
Hypertrophic spur
Expansion of cortex by central chondroma

14. Tibiotalar slant
Multiple epiphyseal dysplasia
Hemophilia
Juvenile rheumatoid arthritis

15. Decrease in Carpal Angle or Radioulnar Angle
Turner's syndrome
Hurler's syndrome
Diaphyseal aclasia

16. Accessory Epiphyseal Ossification Centers (Fig. 5–159)
Peripheral dysostosis
Cleidocranial dysostosis
Otopalatodigital syndrome
Mongoloidism
Hypothyroidism
Idiopathic

17. Slipped Epiphyses
Idiopathic (ages 9–17)
Traumatic
Rickets
Renal rickets
Scurvy
Lues
Metaphyseal dysostosis
Hyperparathyroidism (primary and secondary)
Congenital coxa vara
Pseudohypoparathyroidism (PH)
Pseudopseudohypoparathyroidism (PPH)

18. Metaphyseal Cupping
Normal variant triangular shape
Rachitiform diseases
Metaphyseal dysostosis
Scurvy with crumpling fracture
Phenylketonuria
Homocystinuria
Achondroplasia
Hypophosphatasia
Peripheral dysostosis
Chondroectodermal dysplasia
Sickle-cell anemia
Infarction
Infection
Lues
Trauma
Thermal injuries
Vitamin A intoxication

Congenital hyperthyroidism
19. Proximal Radioulnar Synostosis
    Klinefelter variant
    Trisomy 18
    Idiopathic
20. Radioulnar Dislocation (proximal)
    Hereditary onycho-osteodysplasia
    Cornelia de Lange syndrome
    Otopalatodigital syndrome
    Fanconi's anemia
    Madelung's deformity (distal)
    Dyschondrosteosis (distal)
21. Shortened Ribs
    Achondroplasia
    Asphyxiating thoracic dysplasia (Jeune syndrome)
    Chondroectodermal dysplasia
22. Widened Ribs
    Pyle's disease (entire length)
    Thalassemia (proximal)
    Hurler's syndrome (spatula configuration
    Rickets (end)
    Scurvy (end)
    Paget's disease
23. "Sail" Upper Lumbar Vertebra
    Hurler's syndrome (inferior peg)
    Hurler-like syndromes
    Hypothyroidism
    Morquio's syndrome (central peg)
    Achondroplasia
24. Increase in Size of Vertebra
    Paget's disease
    Hemangioma
    Congenital
    Compensatory increase from nonweight-bearing
    Fibrous dysplasia
    Acromegaly
25. "Squaring" of the Vertebral Bodies
    Ankylosing spondylitis
    Paget's disease
26. Generalized Scalloping of the Posterior Aspects
    of the Vertebral Bodies
    Achondroplasia
    Hurler's syndrome
    Hurler-like syndromes
    Morquio's syndrome
    Neurofibromatosis
    Marfan's syndrome
    Ehler's–Danlos syndrome
    Communicating hydrocephalus
    Acromegaly
    Idiopathic
27. Wormian Bones

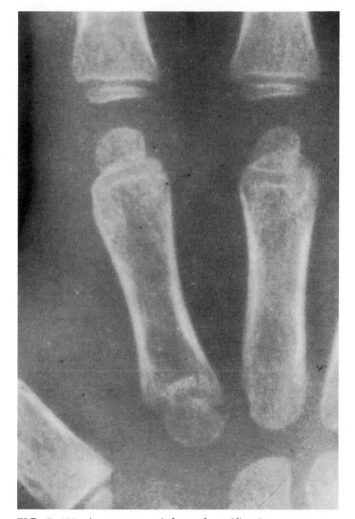

FIG. 5–159. Accessory epiphyseal ossification center at the proximal aspect of the second metacarpal.

Osteogenesis imperfecta
Cleidocranial dysostosis
Progeria
Hypothyroidism
Otopalatodigital syndrome
Chondrodystrophia calcificans congenita
Cerebrohepatorenal syndrome
Pycnodysostosis
Idiopathic osteolysis
Prader–Willi syndrome
28. Increased Thickness or Density of Skull in Children
    Anemias
    Fibrous dysplasia
    Osteopetrosis

Craniometaphyseal dysplasia
Idiopathic hypercalcemia
Idiopathic hyperphosphatasia
Otopalatodigital syndrome
Leontiasis ossea
Myotonia dystrophica
Following dilantin medication[102]
Treated hydrocephalus[7]
Ex-vacuo
Adrenogenital syndrome
Pseudohypoparathyroidism (PH)
Pseudopseudohypoparathyroidism (PPH)
Treated hyperparathyroidism
Progressive diaphyseal dysplasia (Engelmann's disease)

29. Excess Callus Formation
Osteogenesis imperfecta
Cushing's disease
Familial excess callus formation

30. Delayed and/or Defective Dentition
Cretinism
Osteopetrosis
Chondroectodermal dysplasia
Hurler's syndrome
Pseudohypoparathyroidism (PH)
Mongoloidism
Craniometaphyseal dysplasia
Fluoride intoxication
Osteogenesis imperfecta
Cleidocranial dysostosis
Hypophosphatasia
Fibrous dysplasia with skin pigmentation and precocious puberty (McCune–Albright)
Oculodento-osseous dysplasia
Prader–Willi syndrome

Progeria
Stanesco's dysplasia

31. Polydactyly
Asphyxiating thoracic dysplasia (Jeune)
Bloom's syndrome
Chondroectodermal dysplasia (Ellis–van Creveld)
Mesomelic dwarfism
Smith–Lemli–Opitz syndrome
Trisomy 13 sydrome
Carpenter's syndrome

32. Syndactyly, Other Fusions
Apert's syndrome
Chondroectodermal dysplasia (Ellis–van Creveld)
Cornelia de Lange syndrome
Oculodento-osseous dysplasia
Orodigitofacial syndrome
Otopalatodigital syndrome
Smith–Lemli–Opitz syndrome

33. Bowing of limbs at birth[221]
Prenatal bowing
Congenital pseudarthrosis
Osteogenesis imperfecta
Hypophosphatasia
Thanatophoric dwarfism
Campomelic dwarfism

34. Changes in carpal length[184]
Shortening of the carpus
Multiple epiphyseal dysplasia
Otopalatodigital syndromes
Turner's syndrome
Arthrogryposis
Juvenile rheumatoid arthritis
Large carpus
Achondroplasia

(Continued on p. 357)

TABLE 5–5. Minor Syndromes of Osteochondrodysplasia or Dwarfism

Syndrome Paris Classification*	Inheritance Sex Predilection	Clinical Features	Salient Radiological Features
Mesomelic dwarfism: type Langer[126]	Autosomal recessive	Recognized at birth. Normal mentation. No significant physical disability. Short extremities with relatively normal trunk.	Skull, spine, and pelvis normal. Hypoplasia of mandible. Shortening of radius and ulna, with curvature of radius. Shortening of tibia and fibula, with ossification of only distal fibula early. Lesser shortening of humerus and femur with metaphyseal flaring.
Osteochond. 1–A–17b			No Madelung's deformity.

* Established by the European Society for Pediatric Radiology (Paris), revised 1977[92]

TABLE 5–5. Minor Syndromes of Osteochondrodysplasia or Dwarfism (Continued)

Syndrome Paris Classification*	Inheritance Sex Predilection	Clinical Features	Salient Radiological Features
Mesomelic dwarfism: type Nievergelt Osteochond. 1–A–17a	Autosomal dominant	Recognizable at birth. Flexion deformities of elbows and fingers. Forearms and legs about one-third the length of arms and thighs. Gross disturbances in walking and standing.	Humerus longer than normal. Shortened, thickened, and curved radius and ulna. Rhomboid-shaped tibia and fibula.
Hypochondroplasia Osteochond. 1–B–1	Autosomal dominant	Usually recognized in childhood. Mild mental retardation. Mild dwarfism of extremities. "Atypical achondroplastic dwarfism."	Skull, hands, and feet normal. Lumbar interpediculate distances narrowed, but less so than in achondroplasia. Posterior scalloping. Mild mesomelic or rhizomelic dwarfism. Elongation of fibula and radius. Shortening of tibia and ulna. Flaring of metaphyses.
Spondylometaphyseal dysplasia (Kozlowski)[66,196] (Kozlowski's spondylo-metaphyseal dysostosis) Osteochond. 1–B–7a	Autosomal dominant	Recognized in childhood. Mild growth retardation between ages 1 and 4. Short neck and short trunk. Normal length extremities. Kyphoscoliosis. Limited motion (mild) of elbow, hip and knee. Normal facies. Laboratory values normal. Variable odontoid dysgenesis.	At age of 2 years—generalized platyspondyly with anterior "tongue deformity." "Sail" vertebra of D–12 or L–1. Horizontal acetabular roof. Short femoral neck. Irregularities of all metaphyses. Similar to metaphyseal dysostosis. Retarded bone age.
Hereditary arthro-opthalmopathy (Sticker syndrome) (Variant: Cervenka syndrome) Osteochond. 1–B–9	Autosomal dominant	Recognizable at birth. Myopia, retinal detachment, cataract, glaucoma. Cleft palate, flattened midface. Enlargement and hypermobility of joints. Dislocated patella.	Disturbances of epiphyseal ossification. Irregularity of articular surfaces. Joint spaces intact. Thin shafts of long bones. Dislocation of patella. Flaring of metacarpal heads.
Acrodysplasia: Rhinotricho-phalangeal (Giedion)[21,65]	Autosomal dominant or recessive	Thin, scanty hair. Bulbous nose, pear-shaped. (Facies may be normal.) Short hands (some with deformities of fingers). Fairly short stature.	Shortening of metacarpals and phalanges with cone-shaped phalangeal epiphyses (peripheral dysostosis). Bone age may be retarded. Small epiphyses at hips and possible coxa plana.
Acrodysplasia: Epiphyso-metaphyseal (peripheral dysostosis, Brailsford) (Variant: acrodysostosis)	Autosomal dominant	Recognizable at birth. Small, short hands and feet. Short stature. Otherwise normal. (Variant acrodysostosis associated with mental retardation and minor axial skeletal abnormalities.)	Shortening of metacarpals, metatarsals, and phalanges. Cone-shaped epiphyses of phalanges.

* Established by the European Society for Pediatric Radiology (Paris), revised 1977[92]

TABLE 5–5. Minor Syndromes of Osteochondrodysplasia or Dwarfism (Continued)

Syndrome Paris Classification*	Inheritance Sex Predilection	Clinical Features	Salient Radiological Features
Acrodysplasia: Epiphyseal (Thiemann)		Multiple epiphyseal dysplasia tarda with selective involvement of hands and feet. Short hands and feet.	Hands and feet only have changes of multiple epiphyseal dysplasia
Tubular stenosis (Kenny–Caffey)[37, 71] 3–14		Proportionate dwarfism. Tetany in early infancy, from hypocalcemia. Myopia. Delayed closure of anterior fontanelle. Hyperphosphatemia.	Tubular bones show symmetric endosteal thickening with narrowing of medulla. Outer diameter overconstricted. Sclerosis of calvarium, with thinning and lack of differentiation into outer and inner tables. Coxa valga.
Osteodysplasia (Melnick-Needles,[155] familial osteodysplasia) 3–16	Autosomal dominant Possible female predominance	Peculiar physiognomy with prominent brows, flattening of nasal bridge, and micrognathia. Scoliosis. Possible elevated serum phosphorus.	Sclerosis of base of skull and mastoids. Delay in closure of anterior fontanelle and general delay of ossification. Increased vertebral body height, anterior concavity, decreased lumbar disk spaces, coxa valga. Cortical irregularity of tubular bones with mild bowing and metaphyseal flaring. Thin and irregular ribs.
Frontometaphyseal dysplasia[85] 3–17		Recognizable in childhood. Normal mentation. Prominent supraorbital ridges, high arched palate, micrognathia with defective dentition. Defective vision and hearing. Limited motion of joints. Poorly developed musculature.	Skull shows internal hyperostosis, perisutural sclerosis, supraorbital exostoses with absence of frontal sinuses, and basilar invagination. Scoliosis and irregular contours of vertebral bodies. Irregular rib contours. Protrusio acetabuli and coxa valga. "Erlenmeyer flash" deformities of long bones. Widened, elongated middle phalanges and elongation of metacarpals and metatarsals.
Oculodento-osseous dysplasia (oculodentodigital dysplasia, Meyer–Schwickerath syndrome)	Autosomal dominant	Recognizable at birth. Small eyes, microcornea, glaucoma, and iris anomalies. Thin nose. Soft-tissue syndactyly of fourth and fifth digits.	Broad mandible, small orbits, broad tubular bones. Hypoplasia of one or more middle phalanges. Absence of one or more middle phalanges of the toes. "Erlenmeyer flask" deformity of distal femora.

* Established by the European Society for Pediatric Radiology (Paris), revised 1977[92]

TABLE 5–5. Minor Syndromes of Osteochondrodysplasia or Dwarfism (Continued)

Syndrome Paris Classification*	Inheritance Sex Predilection	Clinical Features	Salient Radiological Features
Craniofacial dysostosis[110] (Crouzon)[172] Dys. 1–2		Variable short stature. Exophthalmos with divergent strabismus. Prognathism. Beaked nose. Convulsions. Mental retardation. Progressive loss of vision.	Generalized craniostenosis. Digital impressions. Hypoplasia of the facial bones. Hypertelorism, scaphocephaly, trigonocephaly. Small maxilla, oversized mandible.
Mandibulofacial dysostosis (Treacher–Collins–Franceschetti) Dys. 1–5		Characteristic facies due to absent zygoma and small mandible. Over 35% of patients are deaf.	Absence of zygomatic bones and zygomatic processes of temporal bones, or hypoplasia. Small maxillary sinuses and mandible.
Oculomandibulofacial syndrome (Hallermann-Streiff–François)[121] Dys. 1–6		Proportionate dwarfism. Microphthalmia with congenital cataracts. Hypoplastic mandible. Small face with beaked nose. Hypotrichosis.	Hypoplasia of mandibular rami with anterior displacement of the temporomandibular joints. Thin bones of calvaria with poor marginal ossification. Thin gracile ribs and slender tubular bones.
Cervico-oculoacoustic syndrome (Wildervanck) Dys. 2–2	Sex-linked dominant Females	Short stature. Short neck. Deafness. Abducens paralysis.	Cervical spine resembles that in Klippel–Feil syndrome (shortening, block vertebrae, hemivertebrae). Abnormalities of petrous temporal bone.
Spondylocostal dysostosis[70] (spondylocostal dysplasia) Dys. 2–4	Dominant form and recessive form	Congenital or developmental kyphoscoliosis. Short stature owing to reduced height of the trunk. Genitourinary anomalies. Recessive form results in early death.	Deformities of spine, with block vertebrae, hemivertebrae, butterfly vertebrae, coronal cleft vertebrae, and open neural arches. Rib fusion anomalies and lateral protrusion of ribs.
Oculovertebral syndrome (Weyers syndrome) Dys. 2–5	Nonhereditable	Unilateral microphthalmia, facial asymetry.	Asymetrical hypoplasia of orbit, zygoma, and frontal bone. Hydrocephalus. Multiple variable malformations of vertebral bodies.
Pectoral–aplasia–dysdactylia syndrome[93, 177] (Poland's syndrome) Dys. 3–13		Recognizable at birth. Partial absence of pectoralis major muscle. Ipsilateral syndactyly.	Unilateral hypoplasia or asplasia of pectoralis major muscle simulating appearance of radical mastectomy. Associated rib deformities. Soft-tissue syndactyly. Microdactyly or brachydactyly. Hypoplastic forearm

* Established by the European Society for Pediatric Radiology (Paris), revised 1977[92]

TABLE 5–5. Minor Syndromes of Osteochondrodysplasia or Dwarfism (Continued)

Syndrome Paris Classification*	Inheritance Sex Predilection	Clinical Features	Salient Radiological Features
Rubinstein–Taybi syndrome Dys. 3–14		Dwarfism. Microcephaly. Mental retardation Ocular and motor disturbances. Characteristic facies with small head, beaked nose anti-monogoloid slant, hypertelorism, strabismus. Broad, curved thumbs and great toes.	Microcephaly. Short and wide distal phalanx of thumbs and great toes. Possible duplication. Tufted terminal phalanges of fingers. Flaring of ilia.
Laurence–Moon–Biedl (Bardet)[135]	Autosomal recessive	Retinitis pigmentosa. Polydactyly. Obesity (Frölich type). Genital hypoplasia. Mental retardation. Incomplete forms possible. Dwarfism. Mongoloid facies. Microphthalmos and cataracts. Deafness. Diabetes insipidus. Congenital heart disease. Renal anomalies.	Polydactyly of hands and feet. Syndactyly. Subluxation of hips. Coxa valga. Valgus deformities of knees.
Primordial dwarfism (panhypopituitarism) Prim. 1	Autosomal recessive or X-linked	Process begins in early infancy. "Elfin facies." Truncal obesity. Sexual infantilism. Craniofacial disproportion. Hypoglycemia.	Small sella turcica and craniofacial disproportion. Proportional dwarfism. Marked retardation of skeletal maturation. Narrow delicate tubular bones.
Bird-headed dwarfism (Virchow, Seckel) Prim. 3	Autosomal recessive	Recognizable at birth. Low birth weight. Small head circumference. Short trunk. Beaklike protrusion of nose. Antimongoloid slant. Genitourinary anomalies. Mental retardation.	Hypoplasia of zygoma and mandible. Joint dislocations. Kyphoscoliosis. Clinodactyly. Clubbing of fingers. Absence of patella. Retardation of bone maturation.
Leprechaunism Prim. 4	Autosomal recessive	Coarse features. Hypertrichosis. Enlarged nipples, breast, clitoris, kidneys, and ovaries. Hyperplasia of islands of Langerhans. Nodules in the liver. Dwarfism.	No diagnostic roentgen features.
Russell–Silver syndrome Prim. 5	Sporadic	Recognizable at birth. Hemihypertrophy. Small triangular face with downturned corners of the mouth. Precocious puberty. Café-au-lait spots.	Hemihypertrophy. Clinodactyly of fifth finger. Retarded and asymmetrical maturation of bone.

* Established by the European Society for Pediatric Radiology (Paris), revised 1977[92]

TABLE 5–5. Minor Syndromes of Osteochondrodysplasia or Dwarfism (Continued)

Syndrome Paris Classification*	Inheritance Sex Predilection	Clinical Features	Salient Radiological Features
Cockayne's syndrome[4, 195] Prim. 7	Autosomal recessive	Truncal dwarfism with onset within first 2 years of life. Small head. Prognathism. Deafness. Retinal abnormalities. Mental retardation.	Microcephaly. Intracranial calcification. Posterior tapering of thoracic vertebral bodies. Small pelvis. Steep iliac angle. Slender ribs and clavicles Long extremities. Large tarsal and carpal bones. Osteoporosis. Sclerosis of ossification centers. Hands and feet variable.
Bloom's syndrome (Bloom–German syndrome) Prim. 8	Autosomal recessive—chromosomal breaks	Intrauterine dwarfism. Telangiectatic erythema sensitive to the sun, with facial lesions resembling those of lupus erythematosus. Molar hypoplasia. Hypogammaglobulinemia. Increased incidence of leukemia and other neoplasms.	Supernumerary digits. Absent digits. Clinodactyly. Short lower extremities.
Geroderma osteodysplastica Prim. 9	X-linked, less severe in females	Hyperlaxity, atrophy, and aging of skin. Hyperlaxity of joints. Fractures. Growth retardation. Dislocated hips. Muscular hypotonia. Flat feet. Characteristic facies of "Walt Disney" dwarf.	Biconcavity of vertebral bodies. Generalized osteoporosis. Growth retardation.
Spherophakia–Brachymorphia syndrome (Weil–Marchesani), (congenital mesodermal dysmorphodystrophy) Prim. 10	Autosomal recessive	Short trunk with disproportionately shortened extremities. Ectopia lentis, or spherical shape of lens.	Brachycephaly or scaphocephaly. Brachydactyly.
Larsen's syndrome		Flat facies. Multiple joint dislocations. Clubfoot. Micrognathia. Cleft palate. Congenital heart disease. Hypertelorism.	Dislocations of large joints. Supernumerary carpal and tarsal bones. Broad thumbs, shortening of metacarpals and distal phalanges. Multiple vertebral anomalies.

* Established by the European Society for Pediatric Radiology (Paris), revised 1977[92]

Syndrome Paris Classification*	Inheritance Sex Predilection	Clinical Features	Salient Radiological Features
Hand–foot–uterus syndrome[189]	Autosomal dominant Males and females	Females have duplication anomalies of the genital tract. Small feet with unusually short great toes. Shortening of radials of hands with abnormal thumbs. Normal mentation.	Short metacarpals and phalanges of thumb. Clinodactyly of little fingers with shortening of middle phalanx, and pseudoepiphysis. Abnormal scaphoid. Trapezium–scaphoid fusion. Os centrale. Long ulnar styloid. Pointed distal phalanx of great toe. Short first metatarsal. Tarsal fusions involving cuneiforms. Delay in appearance of cuneiforms.
Parastremmatic dwarfism[129]	Autosomal or X-linked dominance	Recognizable in first year of life. Skeletal deformities, spinal deformities. Severe twisted dwarfism with kyphoscoliosis, bowing of extremities, contractures. Long arms, short hands. No mucopolysacchariduria.	Uniform platyspondyly with biconcave deformity. Decrease in bone density. Metaphyseal flaring with coarse trabeculation, dense stippling and streaking, and irregularity of articular surfaces. Small iliac wings and dysplastic acetabula. Short femoral necks. Thin and bowed tubular bones. Short hands.
Orodigitofacial syndrome (Papillon–Léage syndrome) (Psaume)[214] Dys. 3–17a	X-linked dominant Females	Lobulated tongue bound to floor of the mouth by a thick frenulum. Cleft palate, harelip, dental dysplasia. Malformed hands and feet. Mental retardation.	Skull shows a steep anterior fossa, a "J-shaped" sella turcica, and depression of posterior fossa. Hypoplastic mandible. Hands show brachydactyly, clinodactyly, syndactyly, or supernumerary digits. Possible irregularity of outline and reticular architectural pattern. Bone maturation is normal.
Otopalotodigital syndrome (Taybi's syndrome)	X-linked or autosomal dominant	Recognizable at birth. Characteristic facies with frontal bossing, broad nasal bridge, flat face, "battered prize-fighter's appearance." Cleft palate and small mandible. Hearing loss or deafness. Mild dwarfism. Mental retardation. Deformities of hands and feet. Pectus excavatum.	Skull shows vertical clivus, supraorbital thickening, and wormian bones. Lack of development of paranasal sinuses and mastoid air cells. Hands show clinodactyly of fifth finger, short thumb with cone-shaped metaphysis of distal phalanx. Shortening of other distal phalanges. Carpal and tarsal malformation and fusions. Incomplete ossification of neural arches.

* Established by the European Society for Pediatric Radiology (Paris), revised 1977[92]

Syndrome Paris Classification*	Inheritance Sex Predilection	Clinical Features	Salient Radiological Features
Oculoauriculo- vertebral dysplasia (Goldenhar's syndrome)[51]	Not hereditary	Epibulbar dermoids and/or lipodermoids. Coloboma, anophthalmia or microphthalmia, cataract. Preauricular appendices, fistulae, deformities of external ear. Possible deafness. Micrognathia. Vertebral anomalies.	Mandibular ramus hypoplasia. Zygomatic hypoplasia. Temporal bone hypoplasia. Hypoplasia of maxillary sinus, depression of orbit. Block vertebrae, hemivertebrae, incomplete fusion of neural arches. Elongation of odontoid process.
Oculocerebrorenal syndrome (Lowe's syndrome)	X-linked recessive Males	Severe mental retardation. Hyporeflexia. Hypotonia. Congenital bilateral glaucoma and cataracts. Decreased ability of renal tubules to secrete hydrogen ions and to produce ammonia. Hyperaminoaciduria and proteinuria. Retarded growth.	Rachitic changes secondary to renal dysfunction. Osteoporosis. Retarded growth.
Prader–Willi syndrome[178]	Not hereditable Male preponderance	Neonatal hypotonia. Obesity. Sexual infantilism. Severe mental retardation. Poor dentition. Decreased muscle mass. Increased adipose tissue.	Skull shows wormian bones, increased suture serrations, persistent metopic suture, small sella turcica, absent frontal sinuses. Small hands with overtubulation of phalanges and metacarpals. Clinodactyly. Scoliosis, irregularites of vertebral end-plates. Overtubulation of long bones.
Smith–Lemli– Opitz syndrome		Dwarfism. Low birth weight. Ptosis and low-set ears. Microcephaly. Genital hypoplasia. Swallowing mechanism dysfunction. Congenital heart disease, pyloric stenosis. Clubfeet. Mental retardation.	Polydactyly, brachydactyly, or syndactyly. Microcephaly. Micrognathia. Stippled epiphyses.
Kniest's dwarfism (Kniest's disease)[35]	Heredity uncertain	Shortened arms, legs at birth. Fusiform swelling of joints. Abnormal skull with large head. Round face, depressed nasal bridge. Short neck. Lordosis and kyphoscoliosis. Progressive stiffness of joints. Altered gait. Myopia, cataract, retinal detachment. Deafness. Cleft palate. Normal mentation.	Craniofacial disproportion. Severe platyspondyly. Narrow lumbar interpediculate distances. Shortening of long bones with metaphyseal flaring and large irregular punctate epiphyses. Small pelvic bones, large dislocated femoral heads and necks. Hypoplasia of odontoid process.

* Established by the European Society for Pediatric Radiology (Paris), revised 1977[92]

Syndrome Paris Classification*	Inheritance Sex Predilection	Clinical Features	Salient Radiological Features
Campomelic dwarfism	Sporadic	Multiple skeletal abnormalities. Bowing of legs. Death in early infancy. Small face. Cleft palate. Renal anomalies. Maldevelopment of trachea.	Medial bowing of tibia. Short and bowed fibula. Femoral bowing. Hypoplastic scapula. Wide space between ischia.

Beckwith–Wiedemann
syndrome
(Exomphalus–
macroglossia gigantism
syndrome, EMG
syndrome)
		Recognizable at birth.
		Hypoglycemia, spontaneously
		  subsiding at 4 months of age.
		Increased birth weight.
		Flame nevus of face.
		Omphalocele.
		Macroglossia.
		Hepatomegaly.
		Some patients with mental
		  retardation.
			Renal enlargement.
			Microcephaly.
			Visceromegaly with large
			  umbilical hernia.
			Broad metaphyses.
			Thickened cortex of long bones.
			Periosteal new bone formation.
			Advanced bone age.
			Hemihypertrophy.

Dyggve–Melchior–
Clausen dysplasia[225]
 	
Osteochond. 1–B–13
	Autosomal
	recessive
		Mental retardation.
		Short trunk.
		Sternal protrusion.
		Abnormal spinal
		  curvature.
		Waddling gait.
		Recognizable between
		  1 and 18 months.
			Platyspondyly.
			Notched vertebral end plates.
			Small ilia with lacy crests.
			Lateral displacement of
			  femoral capital epiphyses.
			Accessory ossification centers.

Dysosteosclerosis[89]
 	
Osteochond. 3–21
	Autosomal
	recessive
		Possible blindness.
		Dental hypoplasia.
		Cutaneous and
		  neurological mani-
		  festations.
			Thickening and sclerosis
			  of the base of the skull.
			Dense ribs and vertebral
			  bodies.
			Erlenmeyer-flask
			  deformities with lucency.
			Flattening of vertebral bodies.

Aglossia–Adactylia[100]
 	
Dys. 3–4
	Probable
	extrinsic
	insult
		Recognizable at
		  birth.
		Normal intelligence.
		Hypoplastic tongue
		  or Aglossia.
		Cleft lip and/or
		  palate.
			Asymmetrical distribution.
			Guillotine-like amputation
			  varying from loss of a few
			  digits to major amputations
			  of all four limbs.
			Micrognathia

Facio–digital–
genital syndrome
(Aarskog syndrome)[62]
	X-linked
	recessive
	(males)
		Short stature.
		Peculiar facies.
		Saddle deformity of
		  the scrotum.
		Antimongoloid slant.
		Genital hypoplasia.
		Inguinal hernia.
			Short fifth fingers.
			Hypertelorism.
			Maxillary hypoplasia.
			Spinal anomalies,
			  pectus excavatum,
			  syndactyly.

Aicardi's[179]
syndrome
		Recognizable at
		  birth.
		Spasms and tonic
		  seizures.
		Mental retardation.
		Chorioretinopathy.
			Multiple vertebral
			  anomalies, including
			  hemivertebrae and
			  fusions.
			Agenesis of the corpus
			  callosum.

* Established by the European Society for Pediatric Radiology (Paris), revised 1977[92]

Syndrome Paris Classification*	Inheritance Sex Predilection	Clinical Features	Salient Radiological Features
Cranio–carpo-tarsal dysplasia[166]		Microstomia. Prominent forehead. Hypertelorism. Recognizable at birth. Muscle wasting.	Bilateral hip dislocations. Bilateral vertical talus. Tall vertebral bodies. Ulnar deviation of fingers. Brachycephaly. "Helmet" skull.
The VATER[16] Association		Ventricular septal defect. Anorectal malformation. Tracheoesophageal fistula. Renal anomalies.	Hemivertebrae. Hypoplasia of vertebral bodies. Small or absent pedicles. Scoliosis. Radial aplasia or hypoplasia. Polydactyly. Proximal focal femoral deficiency.

* Established by the European Society for Pediatric Radiology (Paris), revised 1977[92]

INTERNATIONAL NOMENCLATURE OF CONSTITUTIONAL DISEASES OF BONE

Osteochondrodysplasias

(Abnormalities of cartilage and/or bone growth and development)

Defects of growth of tubular bones and/or spine

A. Identifiable at birth
1. Achondrogenesis type I, Parenti–Fraccaro
2. Achondrogenesis type II, Langer–Saldino
3. Thanatophoric dysplasia
4. Thanatophoric dysplasia with cloverleaf skull
5. Short rib-polydactyly syndrome type I, Saldino-Noonan (perhaps several forms)
6. Short rib-polydactyly syndrome type II, Majewski
7. Chondrodysplasia punctata.
   a. Rhizomelic form
   b. Dominant form
   c. Other forms, excluding symptomatic stippling in other disorders (e.g., Zellweger syndrome, Warfarin embryopathy)
8. Campomelic dysplasia
9. Other dysplasias with congenital bowing of long bones (several forms)
10. Achondroplasia
11. Diastrophic dysplasia
12. Metatropic dysplasia (several forms)
13. Chondroectodermal dysplasia, Ellis Van Creveld
14. Asphyxiating thoracic dysplasia, Jeune
15. Spondyloepiphyseal dysplasia congenita
    a. Type Spranger–Wiedemann
    b. Other forms (see B, 11–12)
16. Kniest dysplasia
17. Mesomelic dysplasia
    a. Type Nievergelt
    b. Type Langer (probable homozygous dyschondrosteosis)
    c. Type Robinow
    d. Type Rheinhardt
    e. Other forms
18. Acromesomelic dysplasia
19. Cleidocranial dysplasia
20. Larsen syndrome
21. Otopalatodigital syndrome
B. Identifiable in later life
1. Hypochondroplasia
2. Dyschondrosteosis
3. Metaphyseal chondrodysplasia type Jansen
4. Metaphyseal chondrodysplasia type Schmid
5. Metaphyseal chondrosyplasia type McKusick
6. Metaphyseal chondrodysplasia with exocrine pancreatic insufficiency and cyclic neutropenia
7. Spondylometaphyseal dysplasia

      a. Type Kozlowski
      b. Other forms
  8. Multiple epiphyseal dysplasia
      a. Type Fairbanks
      b. Other forms
  9. Arthroophthalmopathy, Stickler
10. Pseudoachondroplasia
      a. Dominant
      b. Recessive
11. Spondyloepiphyseal dysplasia tarda
12. Spondyloepiphyseal dysplasia, other forms (see A, 15–16)
13. Dyggve–Melchior–Clausen dysplasia
14. Spondyloepimetaphyseal dysplasia (several forms)
15. Myotonic chondrodysplasia, Catel–Schwartz–Jampel
16. Parastremmatic dysplasia
17. Trichorhinophalangeal dysplasia
18. Acrodysplasia with retinitis pigmentosa and nephropathy Saldino–Mainzer

Disorganized development of cartilage and fibrous components of skeleton
1. Dysplasia epiphyseal hemimelica
2. Multiple cartilagenous exostoses
3. Acrodysplasia with exostoses, Giedion-Langer
4. Enchondromatosis, Ollier
5. Enchondromatosis with hemangioma, Maffucci
6. Metachondromatosis
7. Fibrous dysplasia, Jaffe–Lichtenstein
8. Fibrous dysplasia with skin pigmentation and precocious puberty, McCune–Albright
9. Cherubism (familial fibrous dysplasia of the jaws)
10. Neurofibromatosis

Abnormalities of density of cortical diaphyseal structure and/or metaphyseal modeling
1. Osteogenesis imperfecta congenita (several forms)
2. Osteogenesis imperfecta tarda (several forms)
3. Juvenile idiopathic osteoporosis
4. Osteoporosis with pseudoglioma
5. Osteopetrosis with precocious manifestations
6. Osteopetrosis with delayed manifestations (several forms)
7. Pycnodysostosis
8. Osteopoikilosis
9. Osteopathia striata
10. Melorheostosis
11. Diaphyseal dysplasia. Camurati–Engelmann
12. Craniodiaphyseal dysplasia
13. Endosteal hyperostosis

      a. Autosomal dominant, Worth
      b. Autosomal recessive, Van Buchem
14. Tubular stenosis, Kenny-Caffey
15. Pachydermoperiostosis
16. Osteodysplasty, Melnick–Needles
17. Frontometaphyseal dysplasia
18. Craniometaphyseal dysplasia (several forms)
19. Metaphyseal dysplasia, Pyle
20. Sclerosteosis
21. Dysosteosclerosis
22. Osteoectasia with hyperphosphatasia

Dysostoses

(Malformation of individual bones singly or in combination)

Dysostoses with cranial and facial involvement
1. Craniosynostosis (several forms)
2. Craniofacial dysostosis, Crouzon
3. Acrocephalosyndactyly, Apert (and others)
4. Acrocephalopolysyndactyly, Carpenter (and others)
5. Mandibulofacial dysostosis
      a. Type Treacher–Collins, Franceschetti
      b. Other forms
6. Oculomandibulofacial syndrome, Hallermann–Streiff–Francois
7. Nevoid basal-cell carcinoma syndrome

Dysostoses with predominant axial involvement
1. Vertebral segmentation defects, including Klippel–Feil
2. Cervicooculoacoustic syndrome, Wildervanck
3. Sprengel anomaly
4. Spondylocostal dysostosis
      a. Dominant form
      b. Recessive forms
5. Oculovertebral syndrome, Weyers
6. Osteoonychodysostosis
7. Cerebrocostomandibular syndrome

Dysostoses with predominant involvement of extremities
1. Acheiria
2. Apodia
3. Ectrodactyly syndrome
4. Aglossia–adactyly syndrome
5. Congenital bowing of long bones (several forms) (see also osteochodrodysplasias)
6. Familial radioulnar synostosis
7. Brachydactyly (several forms)
8. Symphalangism
9. Polydactyly (several forms)
10. Syndactyly (several forms)

11. Polysyndactyly (several forms)
12. Camptodactyly
13. Poland syndrome
14. Rubinstein–Taybi syndrome
15. Pancytopenia-dysmelia syndrome, Fanconi
16. Thrombocytopenia–radial–aplasia syndrome
17. Orodigitofacial syndrome
    a. Type Papillon–Leage
    b. Type Mohr
18. Cardiomelic syndrome, Holt–Oram (and others)
19. Femoral facial syndrome
20. Multiple synostoses (includes some forms of symphalangism)
21. Scapuloiliac dysostosis, Kosenow–Sinios
22. Hand–foot–genital syndrome
23. Focal dermal hypoplasia, Goltz

Idiopathic Osteolyses

1. Phalangeal (several forms)
2. Tarsocarpal
   a. Including Francois form (and others)
   b. With nephropathy
3. Multicentric
   a. Hajdu–Cheney form
   b. Winchester form
   c. Other forms

Chromosomal Aberrations

Specific entities not listed.

Primary Metabolic Abnormalities

Calcium and/or phosphorus
1. Hypophosphatemic rickets
2. Pseudodeficiency rickets, Prader, Royer
3. Late rickets, McCance
4. Idiopathic hypercalcuria
5. Hypophosphatasia (several forms)
6. Pseudohypoparathyroidism (normo- and hypocalemic forms, include acrodysostosis)

Complex carbohydrates
1. Mucopolysaccharidosis, type I (alpha-L-iduronidase deficiency)
   a. Hurler form
   b. Scheie form
   c. Other forms
2. Mucopolysaccharidosis, type II, Hunter (sulfoiduronate sulfatase deficiency)
3. Mucopolysaccharidosis, type III San Filippo
   a. Type A (heparin sulfamidase deficiency)
   b. Type B (N-acetyl-alpha-glucosaminidase deficiency)
4. Mucopolysaccharidosis, type IV, Morquio (N-acetylgalactosamine-6-sulfate-sulfatase deficiency)
5. Mucopolysaccharidosis, type VI, Maroteaux–Lamy (aryl sulfatase B deficiency)
6. Mucopolysaccharidosis, type VII (beta-glucuronidase deficiency)
7. Aspartylglucosaminuria (aspartylglucosaminidase deficiency)
8. Mannosidosis (alpha-mannosidase deficiency)
9. Fucosidosis (alpha-fucosidase deficiency)
10. GM1-gangliosidosis (beta-galactosidase deficiency)
11. Multiple sulfatase deficiency, Austin, Thieffry
12. Neuraminidase deficiency (formerly mucolipidosis I)
13. Mucolipidosis II
14. Mucolipidosis III

Lipids
1. Niemann–Pick disease
2. Gaucher disease

Nucleic acids
1. Adenosine-deaminase deficiency and others

Amino acids
1. Homocystinuria and others

Metals
1. Menkes kinky hair syndromes and others

REFERENCES

1. Aegerter E, Kirkpatrick J A: Orthopedic Diseases, 3rd ed. Philadelphia, W B Saunders, 1968

2. Alavi S M, Keats T E: Toxopachyostéose diaphysaire tibio-péronière: Weismann–Netter syndrome. Am J Roentgen 118:314–317, 1973

3. Altman K I, Miller G: Disturbance of tryptophan metabolism in congenital hypoplastic anemia. Nature 172:868, 1953

4. Alton D J, McDonald P, Reilly B J: Cockayne's syndrome. A report of 3 cases. Radiology 102:403–406, 1972

5. Amin R: Basal cell nevus syndrome. Brit J Radiol 48:402–407, 1975

6. Amuso S J: Diastrophic dwarfism. J Bone Joint Surg 50–A:113–122, 1968

7. Anderson R et al: Thickening of the skull in surgically treated hydrocephalus. Am J Roentgen 110:96–101, 1970

8. Anton H C: Hand measurements in acromegaly. Clin Radiol 23:445–450, 1972

9. Ardyan G M, Kemp F H: The tongue and mouth in acromegaly. Clin Radiol 23:434–444, 1972

10. Arkin A M, Pack G T, Ransohoff N S, Simon N: Radiation-induced scoliosis. J Bone Joint Surg 32–A:401–404, 1950.

11. Austin J H M, Preger L, Siris E, Taybi H: Short hard palate in newborn: Roentgen sign of mongolism. Radiology 92:775–776, 1969

12. Aviad I, Stein H, Zilberman Y: Roentgen findings of pseudo-Hurler polydstrophy in the adult, with a note on cephalometric changes. Am J Roentgen 122:56–66, 1974

13. Bailey J A: Disproportionate Short Stature. Diagnosis and Management. Philadelphia, W B Saunders, 1973

14. Baker D H, Berdon W E, Morishima A, Conte F: Turner's syndrome and pseudo-Turner's syndrome. Am J Roentgen 100:40–47, 1967

15. Banta J V, Schreiber R R, Kulik W J: Hyperplastic callus formation in osteogenesis imperfecta simulating osteosarcoma. J Bone Joint Surg 53–A:115–122, 1971

16. Barnes J C, Smith W L: The Vater Association. Radiology 126:445–449, 1978

17. Barsky A J: Macrodactyly. J Bone Joint Surg 49–A:1255–1266, 1967

18. Bartalos M, Baramski T A: Medical Cytogenetics. Baltimore, Williams & Wilkins, 1967

19. Beals R K: Hypochondroplasia. A report of 5 kindreds. J Bone Joint Surg 51–A:728–736, 1969

20. Beals R K: Homocystinuria. A report of 2 cases and review of the literature. J Bone Joint Surg 51–A:1564–1572, 1969

21. Beals R K: Tricho-rhino-phalangeal dysplasia. Report of a kindred. J Bone Joint Surg 55–A:821–826, 1973

22. Beals R K, Eckhart A L: Hereditary onycho-osteodysplasia (nail-patella syndrome). A report of 9 kindreds. J Bone Joint Surg 51–A:505–516, 1969

23. Ben-Bassat M, Casper J, Kaplan I, Laron Z: Congenital macrodactyly. A case report with a 3-year follow-up. J Bone Joint Surg 48–B:359–364, 1966

24. Berkshire S B, Maxwell E N, Sams B F: Bilateral symmetrical pseudarthrosis in a newborn. Radiology 97:389–390, 1970

25. Bernhang A M, Levine S A: Familial absence of the patella. J Bone Joint Surg 55–A: 1088–1090, 1973

26. Bigongiari L R: Pseudotibiotalar slant: A positioning artifact. Radiology 122:669–670, 1977

27. Binet E F, Kieffer S A, Martin S H, Peterson H O: Orbital dysplasia in neurofibromatosis. Radiology 93:829–833, 1969

28. Bitter T, Muir H, Mittwoch V, Scott J D: A contribution to the differential diagnosis of Hurler's disease and forms of Morquio's syndrome. J Bone Joint Surg 48–B:637–645, 1966

29. Blank E, Girdany B R: Symmetric bowing of the terminal phalanges of 5th fingers in a family (Kirner's deformity). Am J Roentgen 93:367–373, 1965

30. Block M B et al: Multiple endocrine adenomatosis type IIb. JAMA 234:710–714, 1975

31. Bohner S P, Ude A C: Heel pad thickness in Nigerians. Skel Rad 3:108–112, 1978

32. Borden S: Roentgen recognition of acute plastic bowing of the forearm in children. Am J Roentgen 125:524–530, 1975

33. Borov Von Z, Mielecki T, Czernik J, Wronecki K: Klippel-Trenaunayches syndrome. Fortschr Roentgenstr 123:355–358, 1975

34. Brenton D P et al: Homocystinuria and Marfan's syndrome. J Bone Joint Surg 54–B:277–298, 1972

35. Brill P W, Kim H J, Beratis N G, Hirschhorn K: Skeletal abnormalities in the Kniest syndrome with mucopolysacchariduria. Am J Roentgen 125:731–738, 1975

36. Brill P W, Mitty H A, Gaull G E: Homocystinuria due to cystathionine synthase deficiency: Clinical-roentgenologic correlations. Am J Roentgen 121:45–54, 1974

37. Caffey J: Congenital stenosis of medullary spaces in tubular bones and calvaria in 2 proportionate dwarfs—mother and son—coupled with transitory hypocalcemic tetany. Am J Roentgen 100:1–11, 1967

38. Caffey J, Silverman F N: Pediatric X-ray Diagnosis, 5th ed. Chicago, Year Book Publishers, 1967

39. Campbell R E: Thanatophoric dwarfism in utero. Am J Roentgen 112:198–200, 1971

40. Carbonara P: Hereditary osteo-onycho-dysplasia (HOOD). Am J Med Sci 248:139–151, 1964

41. Carlson D H, Harris G B C: Craniometaphyseal dysplasia. A family with 3 documented cases. Radiology 103:147–152, 1972

42. Casselman E S, Mandell G A: Vertebral scalloping in neurofibromatosis. Radiology 131:89–94, 1979

43. Chawla S: Cranioskeletal dysplasia with acroosteolysis. Brit J Radiol 37:702–705, 1964

44. Clawson D K, Loop J W: Progressive diaphyseal dysplasia (Engelmann's disease). J Bone Joint Surg 46–A:143–150, 1964

45. Cleveland R H, Gilsanz V, Wilkinson R H: Congenital pseudarthrosis of the radius. Am J Roentgen 130:955–957, 1978

46. Clinical Chromosomology, 1967. New Eng J Med 277:825–826, 1967

47. Cockshott P W: Dactylitis and growth disorders. Brit J Radiol 36:19–26, 1963

48. Curtis B H, Fisher R L, Butterfield W L, Saunders F P: Neurofibromatosis with paraplegia. Report of 8 cases. J Bone Joint Surg 51–A:843–861, 1969

49. Curtis J A, O'Hara A E, Carpenter G G: Spurs of the mandible and supracondylar process of the humerus in Cornelia de Lange syndrome. Am J Roentgen 129:156–158, 1977

50. Danziger J, Bloch S: The widened cervical intervertebral foramen. Radiology 116:671–674, 1975

51. Darling D B, Feingold M, Berkman M: The roentgenological aspects of Goldenhar's syndrome (Oculoauriculovertebral dysplasia). Radiology 91:254–260, 1968

52. Darlington D, Hawkins C F: Nail-patella syndrome with iliac horns and hereditary nephropathy. J Bone Joint Surg 49–B:164–174, 1967

53. Dorst J P, Scott C I, Hall J G: The radiological assessment of short stature – dwarfism. Radiol Clin N Amer 10:393–414, 1972

54. Dunbar R D, Toomey F B, Centerwall W R: Radiological signs of the 4P-(Wolf) syndrome. Radiology 117:395–396, 1975

55. Duncan J G, Souter W A: Hereditary onychoosteodysplasia: Nail-patella syndrome. J Bone Joint Surg 45–B:242–258, 1963

56. Duncan T R: Validity of the sesamoid index in the diagnosis of acromegaly. Radiology 115:617–619, 1975

57. Duthie R B, Townes P L: The genetics of orthopaedic conditions. J Bone Joint Surg 49–B:229–248, 1967

58. Edeiken J, Hodes P J: Roentgen Diagnosis of Diseases of Bone, 2nd ed. Baltimore, Williams & Wilkins, 1973

59. Eisenberg K S, Potter D E, Bovill E G: Osteoonychodystrophy with nephropathy and renal osteodystrophy. A case report. J Bone Joint Surg 54–A:1301–1305, 1972

60. Eisenberg R L, Pfister R C: Medullary sponge kidney associated with congenital hemihypertrophy (asymmetry): A case report and survey of the literature. Am J Roentgen 116:773–777, 1972

61. Ellis R W B, Andrew J B: Chondroectodermal dysplasia. J Bone Joint Surg 44–B:626–636, 1962

62. Escobar V, Weaver D D: Aarskog syndrome. JAMA 240:2638–2641, 1978

63. Evans C A, Christiansen R L: Cephalic malformations in Saethre–Chotzen syndrome: acrocephalosyndactyly type III. Radiology 121:399–403, 1976

64. Fairbank H A T: Myositis ossificans progressiva. J Bone Joint Surg 32–B:108–116, 1950

65. Felman A H, Frias J L: The trichorhinophalangeal syndrome: Study of 16 patients in one family. Am J Roentgen 129:631–638, 1977

66. Felman A H, Frias J L, Rennert O M: Spondylometaphyseal dysplasia: A variant form. Radiology 113:409–415, 1974

67. Felman A H, Kirkpatrick J A: Madelung's deformity: Observations in 17 patients. Radiology 93:1037–1042, 1969

68. Felson B (ed): Dwarfs and other little people. Seminars Roentgen, Vol VIII(2), April 1973

69. Ford N, Silverman F C, Kozlowski K: Spondyloepiphyseal dysplasia (pseudoachondroplastic type). Am J Roentgen 86:462–472, 1961

70. Francheschini P et al: The autosomal recessive form of spondylocostal dysostosis. Radiology 112:673–675, 1974

71. Fresch R S, McAlister W H: Medullary stenosis of the tubular bones associated with hypocalcemic convulsions and short stature. Radiology 91:457–461, 1968

72. Garn S M, Hertzog K P, Poznanski A K, Nagy J M: Metacarpophalangeal length in the evaluation of skeletal malformation. Radiology 105:375–381, 1972

73. Goidanich I F, Lenzi L: Morquio–Ullrich disease. A new mucopolysaccharidosis. J Bone Joint Surg 46–A:734–746, 1964

74. Gorlin R J, Koszalka M F, Spranger J: Pyle's disease (familial metaphyseal dysplasia). A presentation of 2 cases and argument for its separation from craniometaphyseal dysplasia. J Bone Joint Surg 52–A:347–354, 1970

75. Greenberg S R, Karabell S, Saade G A: Pseudohypoparathyroidism. A disease of the 2nd messenger (3', 5'-cyclic AMP). Arch Intern Med 129:633–637, 1972

76. Greulich W W: A comparison of the dysplastic middle phalanx of the 5th finger in mentally normal Caucasians, Mongoloids, and Negroes with that of individuals of the same racial groups who have Down's syndrome. Am J Roentgen 118:259–281, 1973

77. Groover R V, Burke E C, Gordon H, Berdon W E: The genetic mucopolysaccharidoses. Seminars Hemat 9:371–402, 1972

78. Grossman H, Danes B S: Neurovisceral storage disease. Roentgenographic features and mode of inheritance. Am J Roentgen 103:149–153, 1968

79. Haas S L: Three-phalangeal thumbs. Am J Roentgen 42:677–682, 1939

80. Harper H A: Review of Physiological Chemistry, 11th ed. Los Altos, CA, Lange Medical Publications, 1967

81. Harper H A S, Poznanski A K, Garn S M: The carpal angle in American populations. Invest Rad 9:217–221, 1974

82. Hawkins, H B, Shapiro R, Petrillo C J: The association of cleidocranial dysostosis with hearing loss. Am J Roentgen 125:944–947, 1975

83. Heselson N G, Cremin B J, Beighton P: The radiographic manifestations of hypochondroplasia. Clin Rad 30:79–85, 1979

84. Holt J F, Wright S M: Radiologic features of neurofibromatosis. Radiology 51:647–664, 1948

85. Holt J F, Thompson G R, Arenberg I K: Frontometaphyseal dysplasia. Radiol Clin N Amer 10:225–243, 1972

86. Holt J F: Neurofibromatosis in children. Am J Roentgen 130:615–639, 1978

87. Holt J F, Kuhns L R: Macrocranium and macrencephaly in neurofibromatosis. Skel Rad 1:25–28, 1976

88. Horrigan D W, Baker D H: Gargoylism: Review of roentgen skull changes with description of new findings. Am J Roentgen 86:473–477, 1961

89. Houston C S, Gerrard J W, Ives E J: Dysosteosclerosis. Am J Roentgen 130:988–991, 1978

90. Houston C S, Zaleski W A: The shape of vertebral bodies and femoral necks in relation to activity. Radiology 89:59–66, 1967

91. Hunt J C, Pugh D G: Skeletal lesions in neurofibromatosis. Radiology 76:1–20, 1961

92. International nomenclature of constitutional diseases of bone. Am J Roentgen 131:352–354, 1978

93. Ireland D C R, Takyama N, Flatt A E: Poland's syndrome. A review of 43 cases. J Bone Joint Surg 58:52–58, 1976

94. James A E, Atkins L, Feingold M, Janower M L: The cri-du-chat syndrome. Radiology 92:50–52, 1969

95. James A E, Belcourt C L, Atkins L, Janower M L: Trisomy 18. Radiology 92:37–43, 1969

96. James A E, Belcourt C L, Atkins L, Janower M L: Trisomy 13–15. Radiology 92:44–49, 1969

97. James A E, Metz T, Janower M L, Dorst J P: Radiological features of the most common autosomal disorders: Trisomy 21–22 (mongolism or Down's syndrome), trisomy 18, trisomy 13–15, and the cri-du-chat syndrome. Clin Radiol 22:417–433, 1971

98. Jarvis J L, Keats T E: Cleidocranial dysostosis: A review of 40 new cases. Am J Roentgen 121:5–16, 1979

99. Jeune M, Beraud C, Carron R: Dystrophic thoracique asphyxiante de caractère familial. Arch Franc Pédiat 12:886, 1955

100. Johnson G F, Robinson M: Aglossia-adactylia. Radiology 128:127–132, 1978

101. Juhl H, Wesenberg R L, Gwinn J L: Roentgenographic findings in Fanconi's anemia. Radiology 89:646–653, 1967

102. Kattan K R: Calvarial thickening after Dilantin medication. Am J Roentgen 101:102–105, 1970

103. Kattan K R: Thickening of the heel-pad associated with long-term Dilantin therapy. Am J Roentgen 124:52–56, 1975

104. Kaufman J M, O'Brien W M: Hyperuricemia in mongolism. New Eng J Med 276:953–956, 1967

105. Keats T E: Cleidocranial dysostosis. Some atypical roentgen manifestations. Am J Roentgen 100:71–74, 1967

106. Keats T E, Alavi M S: Toxopachyostéose diaphysaire tibio-péroniére (Weismann–Netter syndrome). Am J Roentgen 109:568–574, 1970

107. Keats T E, Anast C S: Circumscribed skeletal rarefactions in osteogenesis imperfecta. Am J Roentgen 84:492–498, 1960

108. Keats T E, Burns T W: The radiographic manifestations of gonadal dysgenesis. Radiol Clin N Amer 2:297–313, 1964

109. Keats T E, Riddervold H O, Michaelis L L: Thanatophoric dwarfism. Am J Roentgen 108:473–480, 1970

110. Keats T E, Smith T H, Sweet D E: Craniofacial dysostosis with fibrous metaphyseal defects. Am J Roentgen 124:271–275, 1975

111. Kemperdick H, Janssen F, Lenz W: Mesomelic dwarfism. Fortschr Roentgenstr 123:450–454, 1975

112. King J D, Bobechko W P: Osteogenesis imperfecta. J Bone Joint Surg 53–B:72–89, 1971

113. Kleinberg D L, Young I S, Kupperman H S: The sesamoid index. An aid in the diagnosis of acromegaly. Ann Intern Med 64:1075–1078, 1966

114. Klenerman L, Okenden B G, Townsend A C: Osteosarcoma occurring in osteogenesis imperfecta. J Bone Joint Surg 49–B:314–323, 1967

115. Kohler E, Babbit D P: Dystrophic thoraces and infantile asphyxia. Radiology 94:55–62, 1970

116. Korn D: Congenital hypoplastic thrombocytopenia. Report of a case and review of the literature. Am J Clin Pathol 37:405–413, 1962

117. Kosowica J: Roentgen appearance of the hand and wrist in gonadal dysgenesis. Am J Roentgen 93:354–361, 1965

118. Kozlowski R et al: Neonatal death dwarfism. Fortschr Roentgenstr 129:626–633, 1978

119. Kozlowski K, Zychowiczc D: Dyschondrosteosis. Acta Radiol (Diagn) 11:459–466, 1971

120. Kullmann L, Wouters H W: Neurofibromatosis, gigantism, and subperiosteal hematoma. J Bone Joint Surg 54–B:130–138, 1972

121. Kurlander G J, Lavy N W, Campbell J A: Roentgen differentiation of the oculodentodigital syndrome and the Hallerman–Streiff syndrome in infancy. Radiology 86:77–86, 1966

122. Lamy M, Maroteaux P: Le nanisme diastrophique. Press Méd 68:1977–1980, 1960

123. Lange E K, Bessler W T: Roentgenologic features of acromegaly. Am J Roentgen 86:321–328, 1961

124. Langer L O: Diastrophic dwarfism in early infancy. Am J Roentgen 93:399–404, 1965

125. Langer L O: Dyschondrosteosis, a hereditable bone dysplasia with characteristic roentgenographic features. Am J Roentgen 95:178–188, 1965

126. Langer L O: Mesomelic dwarfism of the hypoplastic ulna, fibula, mandible type. Radiology 89:654–660, 1967

127. Langer L O: The roentgenographic features of the oto-palato-digital (OPD) syndrome. Am J Roentgen 100:63–70, 1967

128. Langer L O, Carey L S: The roentgenographic features of the K S mucopolysaccharidosis of Morquio (Morquio–Brailsford's disease). Am J Roentgen 97:1–20, 1966

129. Langer L O, Peterson D, Spranger J: An unusual bone dysplasia: Parastremmatic dwarfism. Am J Roentgen 110:550–560, 1970

130. Langer L O, Spranger J W, Greinacher I, Herdman R C: Thanatophoric dwarfism. A condition confused with achondroplasia in the neonate, with brief comments on achondrogenesis and homozygous achondroplasia. Radiology 92:285–294, 1969

131. LaRose J G, Gay B B: Metatrophic dwarfism. Am J Roentgen 106:156–161, 1969

132. Lee F A, Kenny F M: Skeletal changes in the Cornelia de Lange syndrome. Am J Roentgen 100:27–39, 1967

133. Leeds N E, Jacobson H G: Spinal neurofibromatosis. Am J Roentgen 126:617–623, 1976

134. Levinson E D, Ozonoff M B, Rogan P M: Proximal femoral focal deficiency (PFFD). Radiology 125:197–203, 1977

135. Levy M, Lotem M, Fried A: The Laurence–Moon–Beidl–Bardet syndrome. J Bone Joint Surg 52–B:318–324, 1970

136. Lewis K B, Bruce R A, Baum D, Motulsky A G: The upper limb cardiovascular syndrome: An autosomal dominant genetic effect on embryogenesis. JAMA 193:1080–1086, 1965

137. Lile H A, Rogers J F, Gerald B: The basal-cell nevus syndrome. Am J Roentgen 103:214–217, 1968

138. Lindenauer S M: The Klippel–Trenaunay syndrome. Ann Surg 162:303–314, 1965

139. Lipson S J: Dysplasia of the odontoid process in Morquio's syndrome causing quadriparesis. J Bone Joint Surg 59–A:340–344, 1977

140. Macpherson R I: Craniodiaphyseal dysplasia. A disease or group of diseases? J Canad Assn Rad 25:22–33, 1974

141. Mainzer F, Minagi H, Steinbach H L: The variable manifestations of multiple enchondromatosis. Radiology 99:377–388, 1971

142. Mandell G A: The pedicle in neurofibromatosis. Am J Roentgen 130:675–678, 1978

143. Margolin F R, Steinbach H L: Progeria–Hutchinson–Gilford syndrome. Am J Roentgen 103:173–178, 1968

144. Maroteaux P, Lamy M: Les formes pseudoachondroplatiques des dysplasies spondyloépiphysaires. Presse Med 67:383–386, 1959

145. Maroteaux P, Lamy M, Robert J M: Thanatophoric dwarfism. Presse Méd 75:2519–2524, 1967

146. Martel W, Upham R, Stimson C W: Subluxation of the atlas causing spinal cord compression in a case of Down's syndrome with a "manifestation of an occipital vertebra." Radiology 93:839–840, 1969

147. McCarthy D M, Dorr C A, Mackintosh C E: Unilateral localised gigantism of the extremities with lipomatosis arthropathy and psoriasis. J Bone Joint Surg 51–B:348–353, 1969

148. McCracken J S, Gordon R R: "Cri-du-chat" syndrome. Lancet 1:23–25, 1965

149. McCredie J: Congenital fusion of bones: Radiology, embryology, and pathogenesis. Clin Radiol 26:47–51, 1975

150. McKusick V A: Heritable Disorders of Connective Tissue, 4th ed. St. Louis, C V Mosby, 1972

151. McKusick V A et al: Dwarfism in the Amish. II. Cartilage-hair hypoplasia. Bull Johns Hopkins Hosp 116:285–326, 1965

152. McKusick V A, Ruddle F H: The status of the gene map of the human chromosomes. Science 196:390–405, 1977

153. McKusick V A, Scott C I: A nomenclature for constitutional disorders of bone. J Bone Joint Surg 53–A:978–986, 1971

154. Melham R, Dorst J P, Scott C I, McKusick V A: Roentgen findings in mucolipoidosis III (Pseudo-Hurler polydystrophy). Radiology 106:153–160, 1973

155. Melnick J C, Needles C F: An undiagnosed bone dysplasia. A 2-family study of 4 generations and 3 generations. Am J Roentgen 97:39–48, 1966

156. Mills J, Foulkes J: Gorlin's syndrome: A radiological and cytogenic study of 9 cases. Brit J Radiol 40:366–371, 1967

157. Minagi H, Steinbach H L: Roentgen appearance of anomalies associated with hypoplastic anemias of childhood: Fanconi's anemia and congenital hypoplastic anemia (erythrogenesis imperfecta). Am J Roentgen 97:100–109, 1966

158. Mitchell G E, Lourie H, Berne A S: The various causes of scalloped vertebrae with notes on their pathogenesis. Radiology 89:67–74, 1967

159. Morreels C, Fletcher B D, Weilbaecher R G, Dorst J P: The roentgenographic features of homocystinuria. Radiology 90:1150–1158, 1968

160. Mortensson W, Hall B: Abnormal pelvis in newborn infants with Down's syndrome. Acta Radiol (Diagn) 12:847–855, 1972

161. Moseley J E, Wolf B S, Gottlieb M K: The trisomy 17–18 syndrome, roentgen features. Am J Roentgen 89:905–913, 1963

162. Nagel D A: Urinary excretion of acid mucopolysaccharides. A study of 64 patients with abnormal enchondral bone formation and other skeletal abnormality. J Bone Joint Surg 47–A:1176–1184, 1965

163. Neuhauser E B D, Wittenborg M H, Berman C Z, Cohen J: Irradiation effects of roentgen therapy on the growing spine. Radiology 59:637–650, 1952

164. Newcombe D S, Keats T: Roentgenographic manifestations of hereditary peripheral dysostosis. Am J Roentgen 106:178–189, 1969

165. Novak D, Bloss W: Radiological aspects of the basal-cell naevus syndrome (Gorlin–Goltz syndrome). Fortschr Roentgenstr 124:11–16, 1976

166. O'Connell D J, Hall C M: Cranio-carpo-tarsal dysplasia: A report of 7 cases. Radiology 123:719–722, 1977

167. Ohsawa T et al: Roentgenographic manifestations of Klinefelter's syndrome. Am J Roentgen 112:178–184, 1971

168. O'Rahilly R: Morphological patterns in limb deficiencies and duplications. Am J Anat 89:135–187, 1951

169. Ozonoff M B, Clemett A R: Progressive osteolysis in progeria. Am J Roentgen 100:75–79, 1967

170. Ozonoff M B, Ogden J A: Sjogren–Larsson syndrome with epiphyseal-metaphyseal dysplasia. Am J Roentgen 118:187–192, 1973

171. Pais M J, Levine A, Pais S O: Coccygeal ribs: Development and appearance in 2 cases. Am J Roentgen 131:164–166, 1978

172. Palacios E, Schimke R N: Craniostenosis-syndactylism. Am J Roentgen 106:144–155, 1969

173. Patel D V, Ferguson L, Schey W L: Enlargement of the intervertebral foramina: An unusual cause. Am J Roentgen 131:911–913, 1978

174. Patriguin H B, Kaplan P, Kind H P, Giedion A: Neonatal mucolipidosis II (I-cell disease: Clinical and radiological features in 3 cases. Am J Roentgen 129:37–43, 1977

175. Pfeiffer R A: Acromesomelic dwarfism. Fortschr Roentgenstr 125:171–173, 1976

176. Pfister R C, Weber A L, Smith E H, Wilkinson R H, May D A: Congenital asymmetry (hemihypertrophy) and ab-

dominal disease. Radiological features in 9 cases. Radiology 116:685–691, 1975

177. Pearl M, Chow T F, Friedman E: Poland's syndrome. Radiology 101:619–623, 1971

178. Pearson K D, Steinbach H L, Bier D M: Roentgenographic manifestations of the Prader–Willi syndrome. Radiology 100:369–377, 1971

179. Phillips H E et al: Aicardi's syndrome: Radiologic manifestations. Radiology 127:453–455, 1978

180. Pirnar T, Neuhauser E B D: Asphyxiating thoracic dystrophy of the newborn. Am J Roentgen 98:358–364, 1966

181. Pitt M J, Mosher J F, Edeiken J: Abnormal periosteum and bone in neurofibromatosis. Radiology 103:143–146, 1972

182. Ponseti I V: Skeletal growth in achondroplasia. J Bone Joint Surg 52–A:701–716, 1970

183. Poznanski A K: The Hand in Radiological Diagnosis. Philadelphia, W B Saunders, 1974

184. Poznanski A K et al: Carpal lengths in children: A useful measurement in the diagnosis of rheumatoid arthritis and some congenital malformation syndromes. Radiology 129:661–668, 1978

185. Poznanski A K, Gall J C, Stern A M: Skeletal manifestations of the Holt–Oram syndrome. Radiology 94:45–53, 1970

186. Poznanski A K, Garn S M, Holt J F: The thumb in congenital malformation syndromes. Radiology 100:115–129, 1971

187. Poznanski A K, Garn S M, Nagy J M, Gall J C: Metacarpophalangeal pattern profiles in the evaluation of skeletal malformations. Radiology 104:1–11, 1972

188. Poznanski A K, Holt J F: The carpals in congenital malformation syndromes. Am J Roentgen 112:443–459, 1971

189. Poznanski A K, Stern A M, Gall J C: Radiographic findings in the hand-foot-uterus syndrome (HFUS). Radiology 95:129–134, 1970

190. Poznanski A K, Werder E A, Gledjon A: The pattern of shortening of the bones of the hand in PHP and PPHP. A comparison with brachydactyly E, Turner syndrome, and acrodysostosis. Radiology 123:707–718, 1977

191. Preger L, Miller E H, Winfield J S, Choy S H: Hereditary onycho-osteo arthrodysplasia. Am J Roentgen 100:546–549, 1967

192. Preger L et al: Roentgenographic abnormalities in phenotypic females with gonadal dysgenesis. A comparison of chromatin positive patients with chromatin negative patients. Am J Roentgen 104:899–910, 1968

193. Rabinowitz J G, Sacher M: Gangliosidosis (GM₁). A reevaluation of the vertebral deformity. Am J Roentgen 121:155–158, 1974

194. Riggs W: Roentgen findings in Noonan's syndrome. Radiology 96:393–395, 1970

195. Riggs W, Seibert J: Cockayne's syndrome: Roentgen findings. Am J Roentgen 116:623–633, 1972

196. Riggs W, Summitt R L: Spondylometaphyseal dysplasia (Kozlowski). Radiology 101:375–381, 1971

197. Roberts J B: Bilateral hyperplastic callus formation in osteogenesis imperfecta: A case report. J Bone Joint Surg 58–A:1164–1166, 1976

198. Robinson A E, Parry W H, Blizard E B: Mosaic trisomy 18. A case report with some unusual radiographic features. Radiology 100:379–380, 1971

199. Rubenstein M A, Bicy J G: Caudal regression syndrome: The urological implications. J Urology 114:934–937, 1975

200. Rubin P: Dynamic Classification of Bone Dysplasias. Chicago, Year Book Publishers, 1964

201. Rubin P, Duthie R B, Young L W: The significance of scoliosis in postirradiated Wilm's tumor and neuroblastoma. Radiology 79:539–559, 1962

202. Rukavina J G, Falls H F, Holt J F, Block W D: Leri's plenosteosis. A study of a family with a review of the literature. J Bone Joint Surg 41–A:397–408, 1959

203. Russell J G B, Chouksey S K: Asphyxiating thoracic dystrophy. Brit J Radiol 43:814–815, 1970

204. Saldino R M: Lethal short-limbed dwarfism: Achondrogenesis and thanatophoric dwarfism. Am J Roentgen 112:185–197, 1971

205. Saldino R M, Steinbach H L, Epstein C J: Familial acrocephalosyndactyly (Pfeiffer syndrome). Am J Roentgen 116:609–622, 1972

206. Salerno N R, Edeiken J: Vertebral scalloping in neurofibromatosis. Radiology 97:509–510, 1970

207. Sane S, Yunis E, Greer R: Subperiosteal or cortical cyst and intramedullary neurofibromatosis—uncommon manifestation of neurofibromatosis. A case report. J Bone Joint Surg 53–A:1194–1200, 1971

208. Schatz S L, Kopits S E: Proximal femoral focal deficiency. Am J Roentgen 131:289–295, 1978

209. Schinzel A: Trisomy 9ₚ. A chromosome aberration with distinct radiologic findings. Radiology 130:125–133, 1979

210. Schauerte E W, St Aubin P M: Progressive synosteosis in Apert's syndrome (acrocephalosyndactyly). Am J Roentgen 97:67–73, 1966

211. Schenk E A, Haggerty J: Morquio's disease. A radiologic and morphologic study. Pediatrics 34:839–850, 1964

212. Schwartz E: Craniometaphyseal dysplasia. Am J Roentgen 84:461–466, 1960

213. Schwartz E: Roentgen findings in progeria. Radiology 79:411–414, 1962

214. Schwartz E, Fish A: Roentgenographic features of a new congenital dysplasia. Am J Roentgen 84:511–517, 1960

215. Semine A A et al: Cervical spine instability in children with Down syndrome (trisomy 21). J Bone Joint Surg 60–A:649–652, 1978

216. Silver H K, Kempe C H, Bruyn H B: Handbook of Pediatrics, 7th ed. Los Altos, CA, Lange Medical Publications, 1967

217. Silverman F N: Differential diagnosis of achondroplasia. Radiol Clin N Amer 6:233–237, 1968

218. Silverman F N: Nomenclature for constitutional intrinsic diseases of bones. Pediatrics 47:431–434, 1971

219. Singleton E B, Daeschner C W, Teng C T: Peripheral dysostosis. Am J Roentgen 84:499–505, 1960

220. Singleton E B, Rosenberg H S, Yang S J: The radiographic manifestations of chromosomal abnormalities. Radiol Clin N Amer 2:281–295, 1964

221. Six R R, Thompson W M, Grossman H L: Bowed Limbs at Birth: A Differential Diagnosis. Scientific Exhibit, Chicago, RSNA, 1973

222. Smith S W: Roentgen findings in homocystinuria. Am J Roentgen 100:147–154, 1967

223. Spranger J, Gebler J, Cantz M: The radiographic features of mannosidosis. Radiology 119:402–407, 1976

224. Spranger J W, Langer L O: Spondyloepiphyseal dysplasia congenita. Radiology 94:313–322, 1970

225. Spranger J, Maroteaux P, Kaloustian V M D: The Dyggve–Melchior–Clausen syndrome. Radiology 114:415–421, 1975

226. Steinbach H L, Preger L, Williams H E, Cohen P: The Hurler syndrome without abnormal mucopolysacchariduria. Radiology 90:472–478, 1968

227. Steinbach H L, Rudhe U, Jonsson M, Young D A: Evolution of skeletal lesions in pseudohypoparathyroidism. Radiology 85:670–676, 1965

228. Steinbach H L, Young D A: The roentgen appearance of pseudohypoparathyroidism (PH) and pseudopseudohypoparathyroidism (PPH). Differentiation from other syndromes associated with short metacarpals, metatarsals, and phalanges. Am J Roentgen 97:49–66, 1966

229. Strand R D, Eisenberg H M: Anterior sacral meningocele in association with Marfan's syndrome. Radiology 99:653–654, 1971

230. Stuber J L, Palacios E: Vertebral scalloping in acromegaly. Am J Roentgen 112:397–400, 1971

231. Sullivan D, Cornwell W S: Pelvic rib. Report of a case. Radiology 110:355–357, 1974

232. Taber P, Gyepes M T, Philippart M, Ling S: Roentgenographic manifestations of Leroy's I-cell disease. Am J Roentgen 118:213–221, 1973

233. Taybi H: Diastrophic dwarfism. Radiology 80:1–10, 1963

234. Taybi H: Generalized skeletal dysplasia with multiple anomalies; note on Pyle's disease. Am J Roentgen 88:450–457, 1962

235. Taybi H, Linder D: Congenital familial dwarfism with cephaloskeletal dysplasia. Radiology 89:275–281, 1967

236. Tishler J, Martel W: Dislocation of the atlas in mongolism. Radiology 84:904–906, 1965

237. Tjio J H, Levan H: The chromosome number of man. Hereditas (Lund) 42:1, 1956

238. Valdeuza A F: The nail-patella syndrome. A report of 3 families. J Bone Joint Surg 55–B:145–162, 1973

239. Villaverde M M, DaSilva J A: Turner-monogolism polysyndrome. JAMA 234:844–847, 1975

240. Voorhess M L, Aspillaga M J, Gardner L I: Trisomy 18 syndrome with absent radius, varus deformity of the hand, and rudimentary thumb: Report of a case. J Pediat 65:130–133, 1964

241. Ward J, Lerner H H: A review of the subject of congenital hemihypertrophy and a complete case report. J Pediat 31:403–414, 1947

242. Wasserman D: Radiographic exhibit: Unilateral iliac horn (central posterior iliac process). Case report. Radiology 120:562, 1976

243. Weichert K A, Drive M S, Benton C, Silverman F N: Macrocranium and neurofibromatosis. Radiology 107:163–166, 1973

244. Williams H J, Hoyer J R: Radiographic diagnosis of osteoonychodysostosis in infancy. Radiology 109:151–154, 1973

245. Winchester P, Grossman H, Lim W N, Danes B S: A new acid mucopolysaccharidosis with skeletal deformities simulating rheumatoid arthritis. Am J Roentgen 106:121–128, 1969

246. Wood B P, Young L W: Pseudohyperphalangism in fetal dilantin syndrome. Radiology 131:371–372, 1979

247. Yoon I L et al: Mixed gonadal dysgenesis. JAMA 235:524–526, 1976

248. Young R S et al: Thanatophoric dwarfism and cloverleaf skull (Kleeblattschaedel). Radiology 106:401–405, 1973

DISEASES WITH ALTERED
IMMUNOGLOBULINS
OSTEOMYELITIS
  Acute Hematogenous Osteomyelitis
  Chronic Osteomyelitis
  Secondary Osteomyelitis
  Tuberculous Osteomyelitis
  Atypical Acid-Fast Bacilli
  BCG Osteomyelitis
  Chronic Granulomatous Disease of
  Childhood
  Virus Osteomyelitis
  Luetic Osteomyelitis
LEUKEMIA
  Childhood Leukemia
  Adult Leukemia
BURKITT'S TUMOR
MYCOSIS FUNGOIDES
HISTIOCYTOSIS X
  Acute or Subacute Disseminated
  Histiocytosis X
  Chronic Disseminated Histiocytosis X
  Eosinophilic Granuloma of Bone
  Radiographic Findings in
  Histiocytosis X
MASSIVE OSTEOLYSIS
MISCELLANEOUS RARE BENIGN
SYNDROMES CAUSING WIDESPREAD
LYTIC LESIONS OF BONE
BONE RESORPTION
  LEPROSY
  BURNS
  EPIDERMOLYSIS BULLOSA
THE PERIOSTEUM
  PULMONARY HYPERTROPHIC
  OSTEOARTHROPATHY
  THYROID ACROPACHY
  PACHYDERMOPERIOSTOSIS
  INFANTILE CORTICAL HYPEROSTOSIS
  HYPERVITAMINOSIS A
  PERIOSTEAL TUMORS
THE CORTEX
  CORTICAL THICKENING
    Progressive Diaphyseal Dysplasia
  HEREDITARY MULTIPLE DIAPHYSEAL
  SCLEROSIS
    Hyperphosphatasemia
    Van Buchem's Disease
    Melorheostosis
    Halliday's Hyperostosis
  "SPLITTING" OF THE CORTEX
  EROSION OF THE CORTEX
  EXPANSION OF THE CORTEX

DISEASES CHARACTERIZED BY
WIDESPREAD INCREASE IN BONE
DENSITY
  OSTEOPETROSIS
  PYCNODYSOSTOSIS
  OSTEOPOIKILOSIS
  BONE ISLANDS
  OSTEOPATHIA STRIATA
  OSTEOBLASTIC METASTASES
  MYELOFIBROSIS
  URTICARIA PIGMENTOSA
  TUBEROUS SCLEROSIS
  HYPERVITAMINOSIS D AND IDIOPATHIC
  HYPERCALCEMIA
  FLUOROSIS
  TERMINAL PHALANGEAL
  OSTEOSCLEROSIS
DESTRUCTION OF BONE
  OSTEOLYTIC METASTASES
  MULTIPLE MYELOMA AND OTHER

DISEASES CHARACTERIZED BY WIDESPREAD INCREASE IN BONE DENSITY

Increase in bone density can be due to several different etiologies. One mechanism is the failure of primary spongiosa to be absorbed in the metaphysis during the process of enchondral bone formation. There may also be errors of internal modeling of compacta and spongiosa. Certain lesional tissues can stimulate normal osteoblasts to form excessive new bone, at times as a reparative process. The periosteum, cortex, or endosteum may each respond singly or in combination. Periosteal new bone formation assumes a variety of patterns that are of great diagnostic significance. The osteoblastic response of the compacta is somewhat limited, as space for the addition of new bone is sparse. The major response causing bone sclerosis is that of endosteal osteoblasts depositing new bone on the surface of trabeculae in the spongiosa. New bone in the intertrabecular spaces is also formed. Why certain lesions consistently evoke an osteoblastic reaction while others do not is unknown; however, these tendencies can be utilized for roentgen diagnostic purposes.

An increase in bone density can also be caused by neoplastic new bone formation in the osteogenic and cartilaginous types of tumors. This is more often seen in solitary lesions. Another mechanism of new bone formation is by metaplasia to osteoblasts, the best example of which is myositis ossificans. New bone formation, both intra- and extraosseous, must be differentiated from calcification. Mature bone shows organization into cortex and trabeculae, in contrast to the amorphous clumps of varying size seen in calcification. Immature and early bone formation can be seen as an ill-defined cloud of increased density with few, if any, dense conglomerations. Diseases characterized by widespread increase in density of the spongiosa are summarized below.

DISEASES CHARACTERIZED BY WIDESPREAD INCREASE IN BONE DENSITY

Paget's disease (sclerotic stage)
Osteopetrosis
Pycnodysostosis
Osteopoikilosis
Bone islands
Osteopathia striata
Osteoblastic metastases
Hodgkin's disease
Leukemia
Myelofibrosis
Urticaria pigmentosa
Tuberous sclerosis
Vitamin D intoxication
Idiopathic hypercalcemia
Fluorosis
Phosphorus intoxication
Heavy metal intoxication
Renal osteodystrophy
Cretinism
Terminal phalangeal osteosclerosis
Charcot's joints
Healed brown tumors of hyperparathyroidism
Osteitis condensans illii[149]

Rare Causes of Bone Sclerosis

Leprosy
Gaucher's disease
Pseudohypoparathyroidism
Multiple myeloma with osteosclerosis
Craniometaphyseal dysplasia
Sclerosis associated with pheochromocytoma (infarcts)
Long-standing cyanotic congenital heart disease
Hereditary multiple diaphyseal sclerosis
Diffuse familial osteoplastic disease[207] (Falchi–Vallebona)
Congenital stenosis of medullary spaces with dwarfism[41]
Multiple osteosarcomata[63]
Hypoparathyroidism

Cleidocranial dysostosis[304]
Idiopathic osteosclerosis[265]

OSTEOPETROSIS (ALBERS–SCHÖNBERG DISEASE, OSTEOSCLEROSIS FRAGILIS, OSTEOPETROSIS GENERALISATA, MARBLE BONES, CHALK BONES)

Osteopetrosis[244] is a rare hereditary bone abnormality characterized radiologically by symmetrical generalized increase in bone density, failure of tubulation, and a "bone-within-a-bone" appearance. The primary defect is failure of absorption of primary spongiosa in the process of enchondral bone formation. Vascular mesenchyme, which would erode this tissue, is absent, leading to increase in bone density. An enzyme deficiency may be the basis for this condition.

The epiphyses, metaphyses, and diaphyses are all involved. The distinction between cortex and medulla is lost. All other stages of enchondral bone formation proceed normally. The process in some cases is undoubtedly intermittent, as periods of abnormal bone production alternate with normal phases to produce the "bone-within-a-bone" appearance that is so characteristic of this condition.

Laboratory studies have shown normal serum calcium, phosphorus, and alkaline phosphatase values in the majority of patients. There are, however, reports of an associated metabolic condition resembling hyperparathyroidism with hypercalcemia. Blood studies may range from normal to marked depression of all elements, most commonly normocytic, normochromic anemia. Abnormal cells may also be present, as well as hematopoiesis in spleen, lymph nodes, and liver. There is no correlation between the severity of anemia and the degree of bone disease.

Clinically, the disease varies in severity and time of recognition, with a range in age from prenatal to 75 years. Congenita and tarda (benign) forms are recognized. The congenital form is inherited as an autosomal recessive and is known as the clinically malignant form. The tarda form is dominantly inherited and is the clinically benign form. Hepatosplenomegaly and anemia do not occur in the latter, and approximately 50% of patients are asymptomatic. The number of reported cases of each type is almost equal.

In the congenital form, stillbirths may occur. If born alive, the neonate shows jaundice, adenopathy, hepatosplenomegaly, and failure to thrive. Growth and maturation may be retarded. Increased bone fragility causes multiple fractures. Skull defor-

mities may lead to optic atrophy. Symptoms of anemia are evident.

In the tarda form, pathological fractures are a prominent part of the clinical picture. Dentition is defective with carious teeth, leading to osteomyelitis of the mandible and maxilla. Symptoms of anemia and thrombocytopenia may be prominent. Bone deformities are rare, and joints are not involved.

Radiologically, the most characteristic feature is marked, uniform, symmetrical increase in bone density with loss of distinction between cortex and medulla. The condition may be recognized *in utero*. All bones and all components of the bone may be involved. The mandible shows the lowest incidence

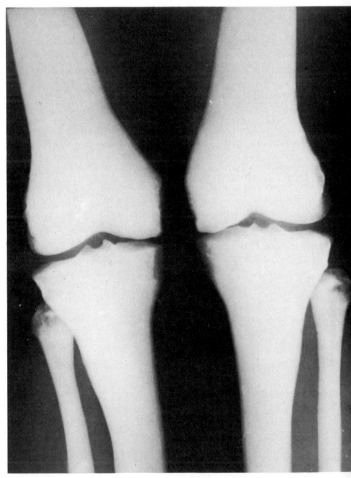

FIG. 6–1. Osteopetrosis (knees). Note marked uniform and symmetrical increase in bone density with loss of distinction between the cortex and the medulla. Underconstriction or an "Erlenmeyer flask" deformity of the distal femora and proximal tibiae may be seen.

of involvement. There is invariably an underconstriction of the tubular bones, resulting in "Erlenmeyer flask" deformities and widening of the diaphyses (Fig. 6–1). The feature that, when present, distinguishes osteopetrosis from other causes of bone sclerosis is a miniature inset of an earlier bone within the confines of a tubular, flat, or cuboid bone, giving the "bone-within-a-bone" appearance; this is due to the intermittency of the process.

The tubular bones may be of normal length or show proportional shortening. There may be multiple transverse or longitudinal metaphyseal striations. Pathological fractures are common and sometimes can be recognized only by callus formation.

The skull shows increased density and thickening of both base and calvarium, with loss of the diploic space. The density of the skull may equal or exceed that of the teeth. There is a small pituitary fossa and clubbing of the posterior clinoid process. The facial bones show thickening and poor aeration of the paranasal sinuses and mastoid air cells. The mandible is not often involved (Figs. 6–2, 6–3). The clavicle and ribs show changes similar to those of the long bones (Fig. 6–4).

The vertebrae may show uniform increased density, or there may be a "bone-within-a-bone" appearance of the bodies (Fig. 6–5). A somewhat similar appearance of "ghost" infantile vertebrae within the adult skeleton following Thorotrast administration in childhood may be seen. The pelvis also may show changes.[301] There may also be increased density at the end-plates, giving rise to "sandwich vertebrae" (Fig. 6–6). The vertebral bodies have a normal size and shape, and the intervertebral spaces are preserved. The carpal and tarsal bones also show increased density (Fig. 6–7). Their time of appearance is usually normal. The pelvis shows alternating bands of increased and decreased density paralleling the iliac crest, in addition to sclerosis

(Text continued on p. 374)

FIG. 6–2. Osteopetrosis (skull)—male, age 8 years. Note marked sclerotic changes of the calvarium and facial bones, and marked widening of the cranial sutures. There is lack of development of the paranasal sinuses. The mandible appears relatively normal.

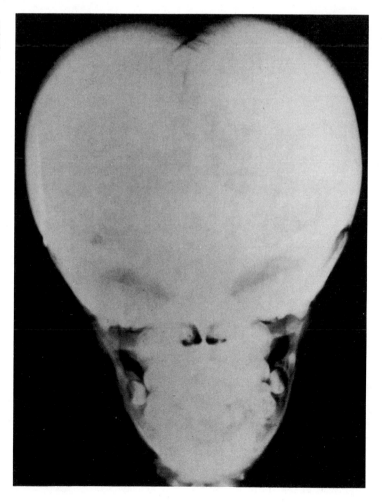

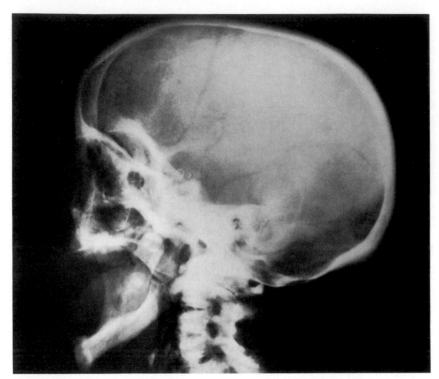

FIG. 6–3. Osteopetrosis tarda (skull) — female, age 19 years. Note thickening of the base of the skull, a small pituitary fossa with sclerosis and clubbing of the posterior clinoid processes. The patient is edentulous. There is thickening of the end-plates of the cervical vertebral bodies to give a "sandwich vertebra" appearance.

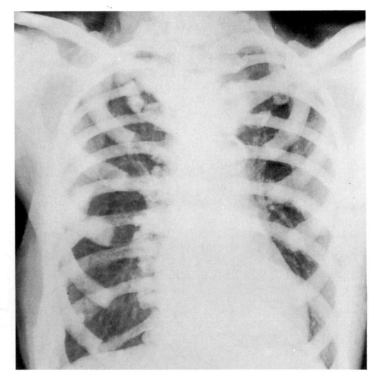

FIG. 6–4. Osteopetrosis tarda (chest) — female, age 19 years. Uniform sclerosis of the clavicles and ribs, with flaring of the sternal ends of several ribs, is noted. The scapulae are also involved. The presence of cervical ribs is an incidental finding. Marked calcification of the transverse aorta may also be seen.

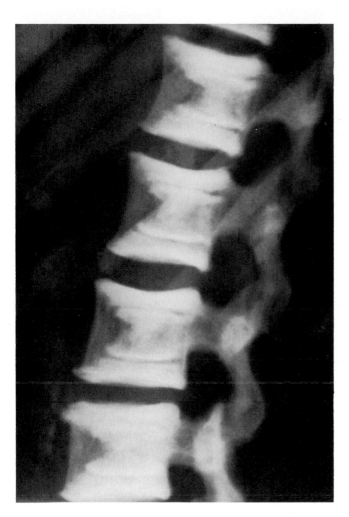

FIG. 6–5. Osteopetrosis tarda (lumbar spine)—female, age 33 years. A miniature inset may be seen in each vertebral body, giving a "bone-within-a-bone" appearance. Sclerosis at the end-plates is also present. Calcification in the abdominal aorta may also be noted.

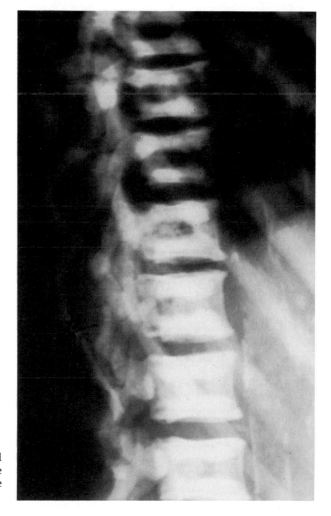

FIG. 6–6. Osteopetrosis tarda (spine), showing increased density at the end-plates or "sandwich vertebra." The spine appears otherwise normal. Note marked calcification of the abdominal vasculature.

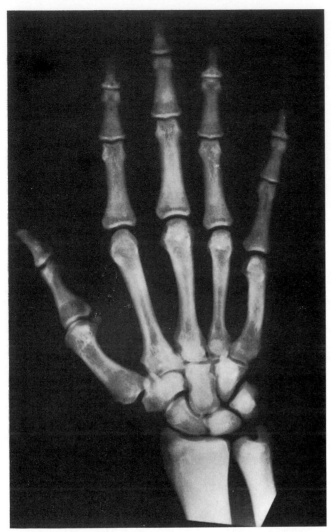

FIG. 6–7. Osteopetrosis tarda (hand), showing increase in density of the tubular bones and increase in density of several carpal bones.

(Fig. 6–8). There may be marked calcification in the soft tissues and of the arteries that is associated with hypercalcemia.

Caffey cites a case of limited involvement with regional asymmetrical osteopetrotic-like changes.[42] Palmer reports a case of osteopetrosis associated with multiple epiphyseal dysplasia.[232] Dension *et al* report a case of portal hypertension associated with osteopetrosis owing to extramedullary hematopoiesis with increased splenic blood flow.[65] Moss *et al*[208] report a case of erosion of the terminal phalanges of both feet in benign osteopetrosis.

PYCNODYSOSTOSIS

Pycnodysostosis[80,214,284] is a rare hereditary bone abnormality characterized by increased bone density, short stature, hypoplasia of the mandible, dysplasia of skull bones, partial aplasia of the terminal phalanges, and an increased tendency toward pathological fractures. Thirty-six cases have been reported to date. It is transmitted as an autosomal recessive. Sex distribution is equal. Blood chemistries are characteristically normal. There is no anemia, in contrast to osteopetrosis. The patients are of normal mentation, and no cranial nerve compression is present. Cytogenic abnormalities with short-arm deletion, probably of a G–22 chromosome, have been reported in association with this condition.[78]

Radiologically, the most characteristic feature is generalized osteosclerosis. In contrast to osteopetrosis, the long bones do not show an "Erlenmeyer flask" deformity, nor is there a "bone-within-a-bone" appearance (Fig. 6–9). The tubular bones are thin and gracile, except when fracture has occurred. The fractures are usually transverse, and heal slowly. There may be overgrowth and bowing of the radius, resulting in an abnormal radiocarpal joint. The hands are shortened, with aplasia of the tufts of the distal phalanges or tapering (Fig. 6–10).

The skull shows characteristic findings of hypoplasia of the mandible with flattening of the mandibular angles. The calvarium is sclerotic with widening of the sutures and fontanelles. Platybasia may be present. There is hypoplasia of the facial bones with lack of aeration of the paranasal sinuses (Fig. 6–11). Defective dentition is also present. Rudimentary clavicles have been reported, particularly at the distal ends. The pelvis may show shallow acetabular fossae with an increase in acetabular angles (Fig. 6–12). Coxa valga may also be present. The spine may show sclerosis, but no "bone-within-a-bone" appearance is present (Fig. 6–13). Persistent infantile notching of the anterior vertebral bodies is present. Stature is proportionately shortened.

OSTEOPOIKILOSIS (SPOTTED BONES, OSTEOPATHIA CONDENSANS DISSEMINATA, OSTEOPECILIA, OSTEODERMATOPOIKILOSIS, OSTEOSCLEROSIS GENERALISATA)

Osteopoikilosis[117] is a rare hereditary bone disorder characterized by the presence of multiple, small, circumscribed round or ovoid areas of increased bone density, widely distributed, caused by local

(*Text continued on p. 378*)

FIG. 6–8. Osteopetrosis tarda (pelvis)—female, age 33 years. There are alternating bands of sclerosis of the ilia, cortical thickening and increased density of the remainder of the bones. The sclerosis is distributed symmetrically.

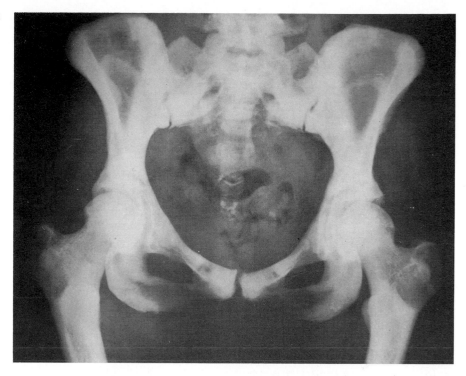

FIG. 6–9. Pycnodysostosis (lower extremity). Note uniform bone sclerosis, with no evidence of a "bone-within-a-bone" appearance nor of "Erlenmeyer flask" deformity. An incomplete fracture at the anterior aspect of the lower tibia is present.

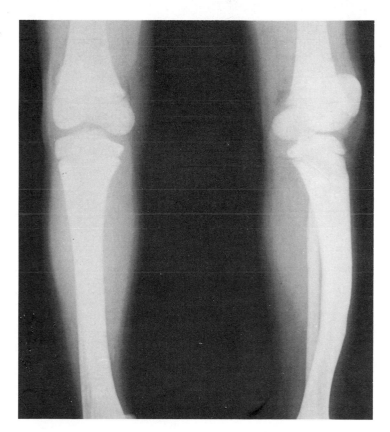

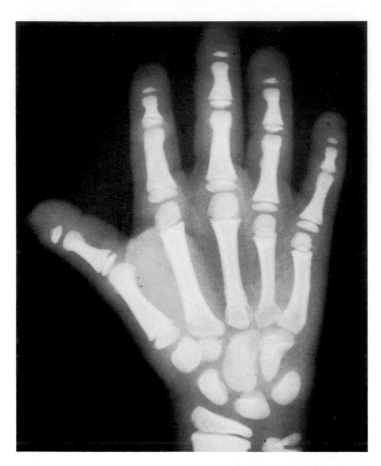

FIG. 6–10. Pycnodysostosis (hand)—same case as in Fig. 6–9. Hypoplasia of the distal phalanges of all of the fingers with a conical tapering is present.

FIG. 6–11. Pycnodysostosis (skull)—same case as Figs. 6–9 and 6–10. Note widening of the sutures, particularly the prominent posterior fontanelle, hypoplasia of the mandible, with flattening of the mandibular angle, and long, thin condylar processes. The sella turcica and posterior clinoid processes are prominent. There is prominent sphenooccipital synchondrosis. Platybasia (but not basilar invagination) is present. There is lack of development of the paranasal sinuses and the mastoid air cells.

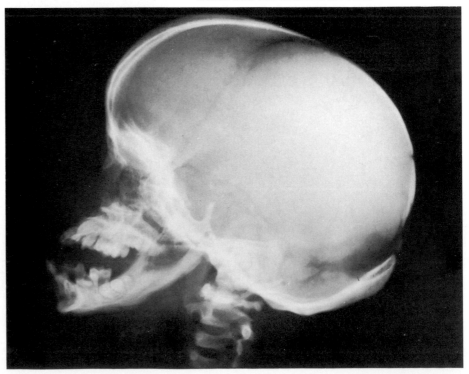

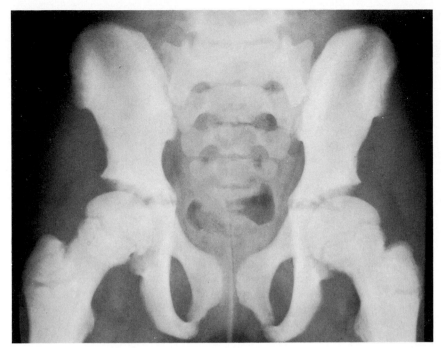

FIG. 6–12. Pycnodysostosis (pelvis)—same case as in Figs. 6–9 to 6–11. Note increased uniform bone sclerosis, without concentric stripes in the iliac wings. There is also some widening of the acetabular cartilage. The acetabular angles are increased slightly. Coxa valga is present bilaterally.

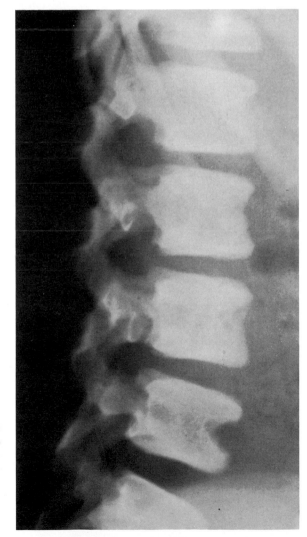

FIG. 6–13. Pycnodysostosis (spine)—same case as in Figs. 6–9 to 6–12. There is slight sclerosis of the vertebral bodies, but no evidence of the "bone-within-a-bone" appearance seen in osteopetrosis. Note residual infantile notching of the anterior vertebrae.

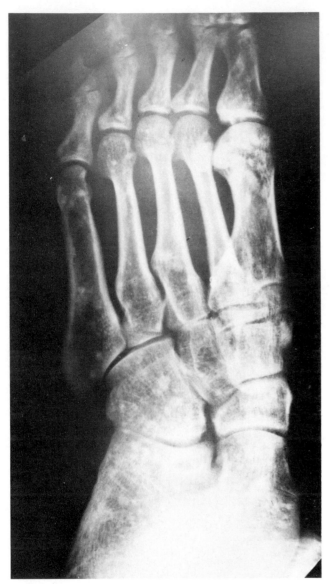

FIG. 6–14. Osteopoikilosis (foot). Small foci of bone sclerosis in the tarsal bones and at the metaphyseal aspects of the metatarsals and the phalanges are seen.

condensations of the spongiosa. The etiology is unknown. Familial occurrence has been reported. The condition is believed to be transmitted as an autosomal dominant. Laboratory studies show no abnormalities.

Clinically, there are no symptoms, and the disease is accidentally discovered on roentgenograms taken for other reasons. The age of discovery is usually between 15 and 60 years, although prenatal and geriatric cases have been reported. Many associated conditions have been reported, including dermatofibrosis lenticularis disseminata, scleroderma, syndactyly, dwarfism, endocrine abnormalities, melorrheostosis, and cleft palate.

Radiologically, there are small foci of bone sclerosis ranging in size from a few millimeters to several centimeters. These are round or ovoid and contain radiolucent centers. They are said not to progress; however, disappearance and reappearance have been reported.

In the long bones, the lesions are seen in the metaphyses and epiphyses but not the shaft. The small bones and cuboid bones can all be involved (Fig. 6–14). The pelvis is often involved, with the chief distribution about the acetabula (Fig. 6–15). The scapula may show involvement about the glenoid. The skull, mandible, ribs, sternum, and vertebrae are only rarely involved.

BONE ISLANDS (INSULA COMPACTA)

Bone Islands[25, 177] are solitary small areas of dense bone similar histologically to the lesions of osteopoikilosis. They are asymptomatic and should be considered as normal variants. They have the capacity to increase slowly in size until they are many times the size they were when originally discovered.

Radiologically, they present as well-circumscribed areas of increased density that may be present in tubular or flat bones (Fig. 6–16), occurring most commonly in the pelvis and upper femora. The skull is not involved. The lesions are small, rarely exceeding 1 cm in size. The margins are characterized by thorny radiations or a "brush" border. Giant bone islands, up to 4 cm in diameter, have been reported.[291]

Differentiation from an osteoblastic metastasis may be made by this lesion's sharper margination or "brush" border. An osteoma usually involves the skull or protrudes from the surface of the bone.

FIG. 6–15. Osteopoikilosis (pelvis). Note multiple small areas of bone sclerosis bilaterally in the pelvis, as well as in the femoral heads, necks, and metaphyseal regions. The shafts are not involved.

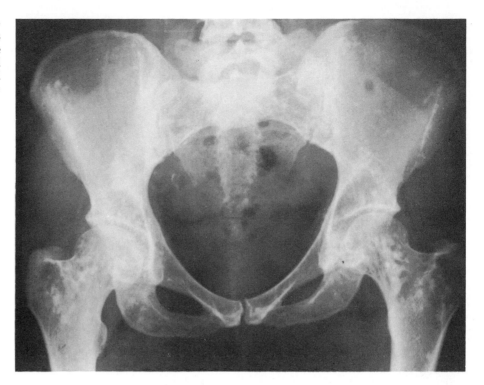

FIG. 6–16. Bone island. A small, well-circumscribed area of increased density is present in the ilium. This is similar to lesions seen in osteopoikilosis, but is solitary.

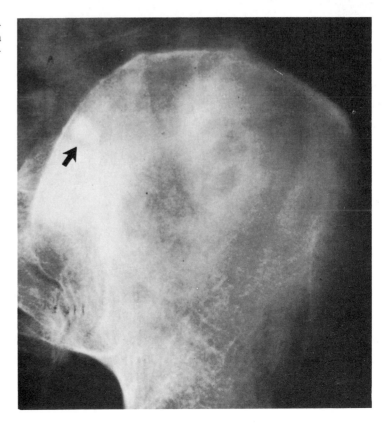

OSTEOPATHIA STRIATA (VOORHOEVE'S DISEASE)

Osteopathia striata[46, 88] is a rare bone disorder involving an error in internal bone modeling and characterized by dense longitudinal bone striations. Laboratory values are normal. The etiology is unknown. The patient is asymptomatic.

Radiologically, dense longitudinal streaking at the metaphyses of the tubular bones is seen. The lengths of the striations are proportional to the rate of growth in different bones, so that they are longest at the distal femora (Figs. 6–17, 6–18). Occasionally, there may be epiphyseal involvement. The ilium may be affected, in which case the striations fan out centrifugally from the acetabulum. Striations in the vertebral bodies may also be seen. The base of the skull has been reported to show sclerosis and thickening. Unilateral involvement has been reported. A case of osteopathia striata associated with craniometaphyseal dysplasia has been reported.[60]

OSTEOBLASTIC METASTASES

Osteoblastic metastases may result from a large variety of tumors. All carcinomas (except, most rarely, adenocarcinoma of the thyroid and hypernephroma),[254] as well as lymphomas and leukemias, may cause sclerotic response.[156,239,275,311] Mucinous carcinomas are prone to do so.

The most frequently seen osteoblastic metastases are from carcinoma of the prostate. Elevated serum acid phosphatase level and elevated serum alkaline phosphatase level are then present. Early metastases from carcinoma of the prostate are difficult to detect. In a series of 219 patients with adenocarcinoma of the prostate, classification into positive and negative bone scans was made. Of those with proven metastases, 43% had no bone pain, 39% had normal acid phosphatase levels, 23% had normal alkaline phosphatase levels, and 19% had normal levels of both enzymes. Of the patients with normal enzyme levels and unsuspected bone metastases, 24% had positive bone scans and 62% of these had normal radiographs. The ^{99m}Tc-diphosphonate bone scan is claimed to be most sensitive for the detection of early prostate metastases.[280] Serum acid phosphatase is also elevated in Gaucher's disease. Also, osteosclerotic lesions may not uncommonly be secondary to (in order of frequency): carcinoma of the lung[215] (particularly small-cell and adenocarcinoma), breast (particularly following treatment), and pancreas; malignant carcinoid; and carcinoma

of the urinary bladder and colon. In children, osteoblastic metastases secondary to cerebellar and medulloblastoma or cerebellar sarcoma, particularly following surgery, have been reported,[36, 64] with a leukoerythroblastic anemia and a resultant diffuse osteosclerosis owing to metastatic invasion of the bone marrow.[10] The tumor cells stimulate osteoblasts to form osteoid in an unknown manner. Osteoblastic response is said to be related to a slow rate of growth, but this is not necessarily a true as-

FIG. 6–17. Osteopathia striata (knee) — infant, age 5 months. Note longitudinal metaphyseal streaking of alternating dense and radiolucent bands involving the distal femur and proximal tibia. Finding of osteopathia striata was incidental to examination for a needle in the soft tissues.

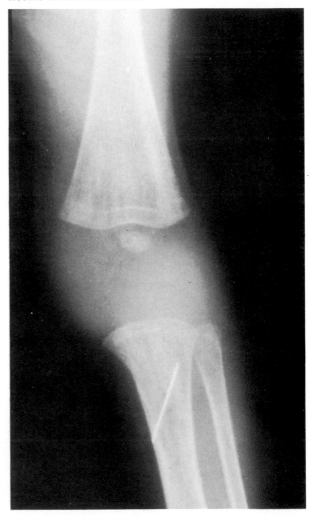

sumption. Osteoblastic response to treatment of metastatic prostate carcinoma has been reported.[246] Hypocalcemia, with serum calcium values of less than 8.6 mg%, has been reported in a series of patients with osteoblastic metastases from prostatic carcinoma.

Radiologically, ill-defined areas of increased density are seen initially (Figs. 6–19, 6–20), and may progress to complete loss of architectural landmarks. The lesions occur as discrete foci of variable sizes with ill-defined margins (Fig. 6–21), or as a diffuse sclerosis (Figs. 6–22, 6–23). Rarely, all bones are involved with a dense uniform sclerosis (Fig. 6–24). Periosteal reaction may be evoked, causing an increase in bone size (Fig. 6–25), or more rarely, a spiculated type of periosteal new bone response (Figs. 6–26, 6–27, 6–28, 6–29). The latter occurs most frequently in the pelvis. The vertebrae may show sclerosis of a pedicle (Fig. 6–30). Sclerosis or hypertrophy of a pedicle may also result from stress due

(Text continued on p. 389)

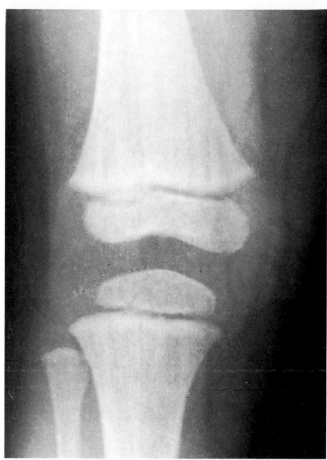

FIG. 6–18. Osteopathia striata (knee). Note alternating radiolucent and sclerotic metaphyseal bands oriented vertically.

FIG. 6–19. Osteoblastic metastases (knees) from carcinoma of the prostate. Ill-defined, patchy, sclerotic areas are present.

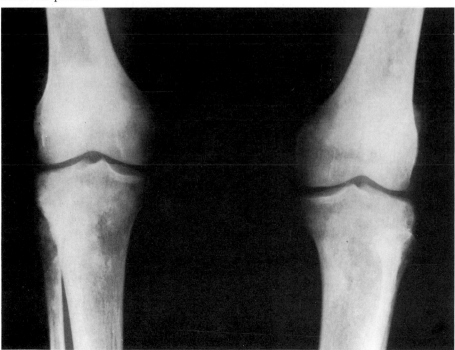

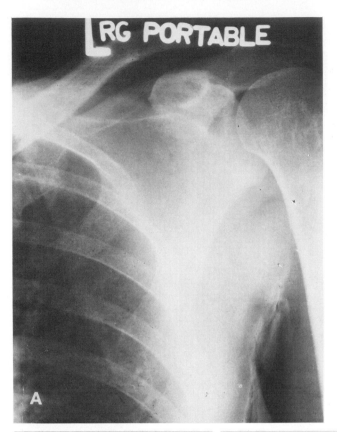

FIG. 6–20. Osteoblastic metastases from carcinoma of the breast. **A.** Left shoulder. Diffuse sclerosis of the scapula is seen about the glenoid region. **B.** Radionuclide Scan. Area of increased activity in the left scapula is seen. **C.** CT scan. Dense sclerosis of the left scapula is noted.

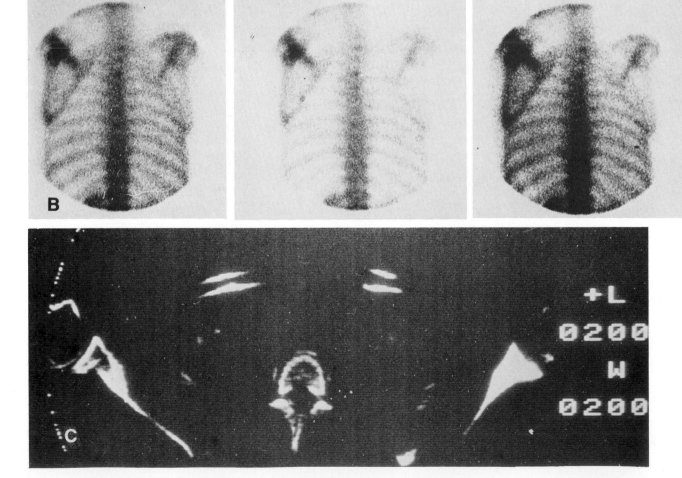

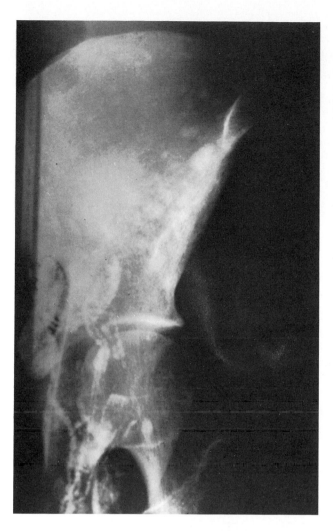

FIG. 6–21. Hodgkin's disease (ilium). Well-circumscribed, discrete foci of bone sclerosis of varying sizes are present in the ilium and in the proximal femur. These lesions are similar to those of osteopoikilosis except for greater variability in size. Lymphangiogram shows lymph node enlargement.

FIG. 6–22. Osteoblastic metastases (pelvis) from carcinoma of the prostate. There is a diffuse sclerosis of the pelvis, vertebrae, and upper femora with loss of distinction between cortex and medulla in some areas. The fifth lumbar vertebral body is densely sclerotic. However, the caliber of the bone is not enlarged, in contrast to what one may expect to find in Paget's disease.

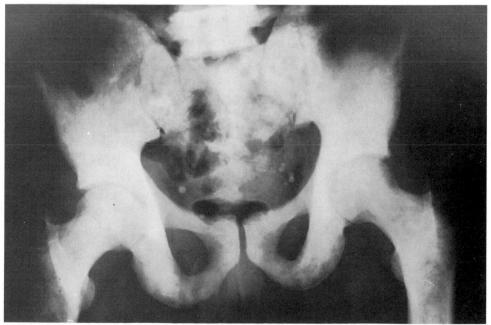

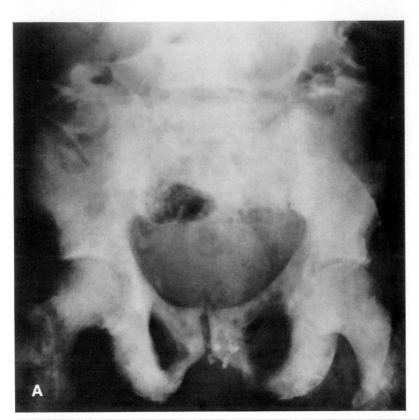

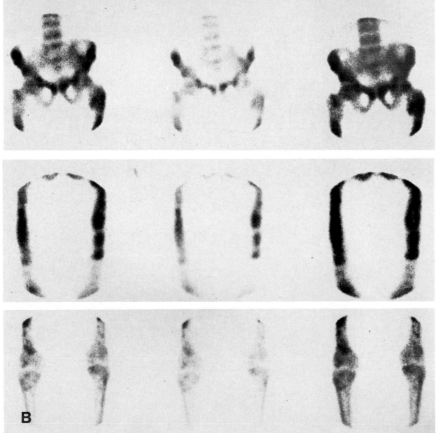

FIG. 6–23. Osteoblastic metastases to the pelvis. **A.** Extensive patchy sclerotic areas throughout the entire pelvis and proximal femora are noted. **B.** Radionuclide scan showing increased activity in the pelvis and femora. **C.** CT scan. Dense sclerosis of the femoral heads is seen. **D.** CT scan. Dense sclerosis of the sacrum and iliac wings is noted.

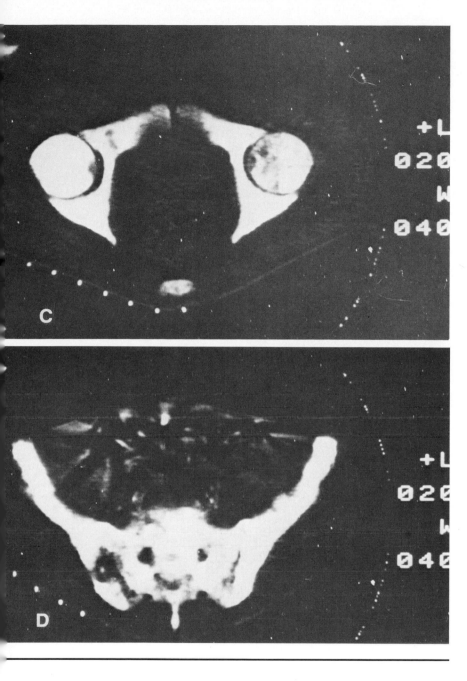

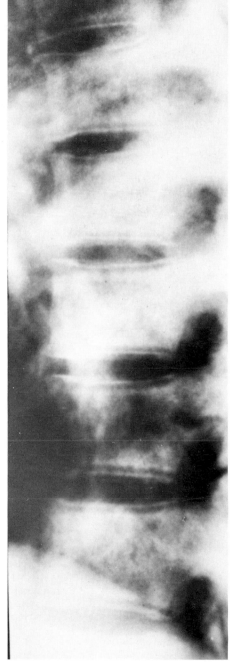

FIG. 6–24. Osteoblastic metastasis (spine) from large-cell, undifferentiated carcinoma of the lung. Dense sclerosis of the vertebral bodies is present, as well as subchondral radiolucent lines. The latter is a rare finding.

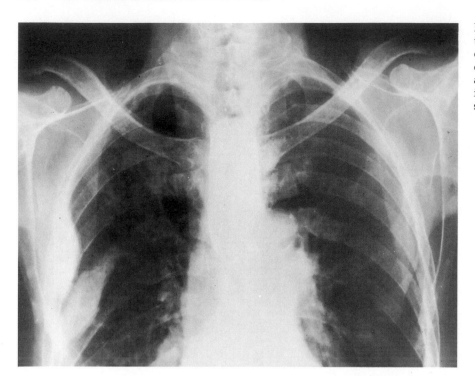

FIG. 6–25. Osteoblastic metastases to the ribs and scapulae from carcinoma of the esophagus. Dense expanding lesions of the right ribs are due to osteoblastic metastatic involvement. Sclerotic foci in both scapulae are also present.

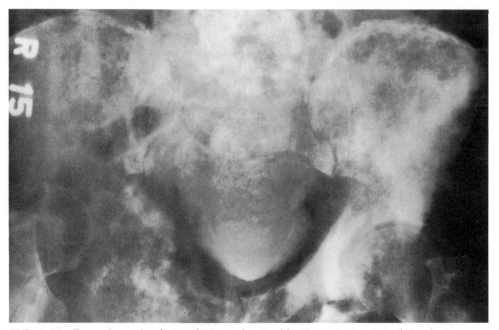

FIG. 6–26. Extensive mixed osteolytic and osteoblastic metastases (pelvis) from carcinoma of the prostate. There is destruction of the right side of the pelvis with the right femoral head "floating free" in a destroyed acetabulum. Osteoblastic areas are present. The lesions in the left side of the pelvis are predominantly osteoblastic with a spiculated margin of new bone formation along the left ilium and the pelvic rim.

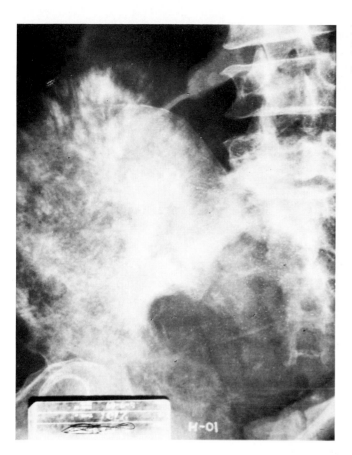

FIG. 6–27. Osteoblastic metastasis (ilium) from carcinoma of the prostate. A marked spiculated type of periosteal new bone formation is noted, as well as bone sclerosis and destructive areas.

FIG. 6–28. Metastases from carcinoma of the prostate to the right ischium. Patchy sclerosis is noted as well as enlargement of the bone and invasion of the soft tissues with spiculated periosteal new bone formation, best seen in the obturator foramen. Patchy sclerotic changes in the left ischium are also noted.

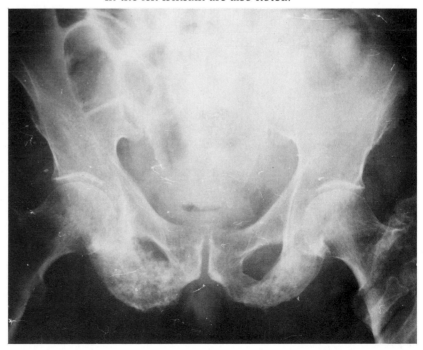

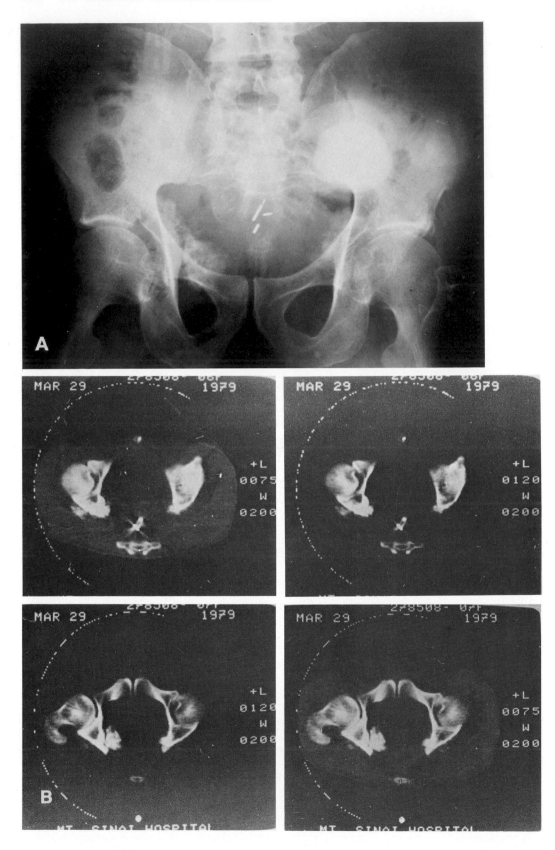

FIG. 6–29. Patient with carcinoma of the rectum with osteoblastic exophytic metastases to bone. **A.** Film of the pelvis shows invasion of the soft tissues bilaterally with new bone formation. **B.** CT scan shows exophytic metastatic bone protruding into the pelvis posterior to the acetabuli, more marked on the right.

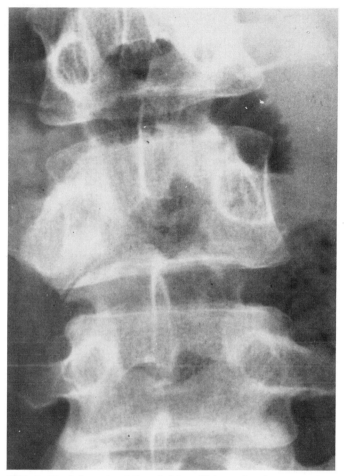

FIG. 6–30. Osteoblastic metastases (spine) from carcinoma of the prostate. Note osteosclerotic metastases to the left pedicle of the involved vertebra.

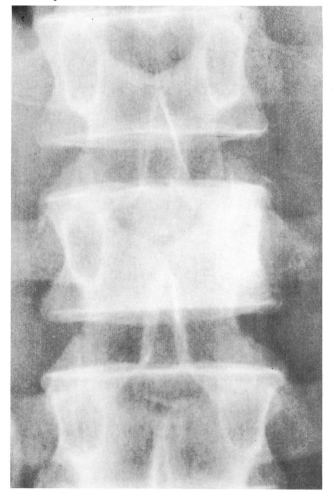

FIG. 6–31. Sclerosis of the right pedicle and enlargement associated with an ipsilateral neural arch defect.

to a neural arch defect on either side (Fig. 6–31), or it may be idiopathic.[133,191,281] Metastases may result in uniform increase in density of a body (Fig. 6–32). A dense body or "ivory" vertebra[66] is most likely to be caused by osteoblastic metastases, Hodgkin's disease (Fig. 6–33), or the sclerotic stage of Paget's disease. Hodgkin's disease may show an erosion or scalloping of the anterior margin of the vertebral body from the lymphadenopathy that is frequently present, a feature not found in osteoblastic metastases. Reduction in density and restoration of the trabecular pattern has been reported following radiation therapy.[141] Paget's disease causes enlargement of the vertebral body and cortical thickening to give a "picture frame" appearance in the combined phase of the disease.

Osteoblastic metastases to the calvarium are exceptionally rare, even in carcinoma of the prostate with its widespread sclerotic lesions in other skeletal parts (Fig. 6–34). Prostatic metastases to the sphenoid and zygomatic bones simulating meningeoma en plaque have been reported.[169] The optic canals were normal. Osteoblastic metastases from carcinoid tumors showing the unusual features of expansion and long filiform spiculation have been reported.[238] An associated soft-tissue mass is a very rare finding, but may occur. Lesions distal to the knees and elbows are rare (Figs. 6–35, 6–36). Diffuse osteosclerosis with lymphocytic lymphoma has been reported.[94]

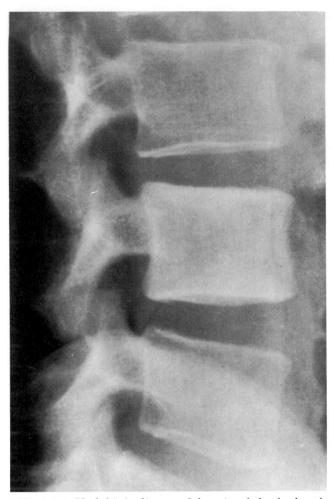

FIG. 6–33. Hodgkin's disease. Sclerosis of the body of the fourth lumbar vertebra without changes in contour is seen. This was the only bony lesion.

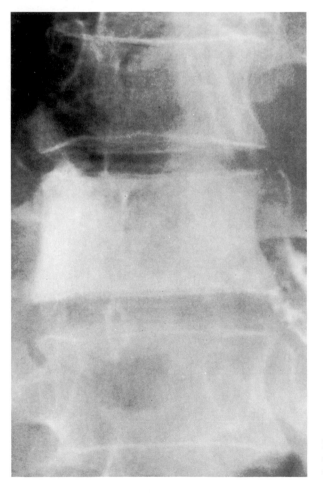

FIG. 6–32. Osteoblastic metastases (spine) from carcinoma of the prostate to a vertebral body. There is diffuse sclerosis of the entire vertebral body without increase in size.

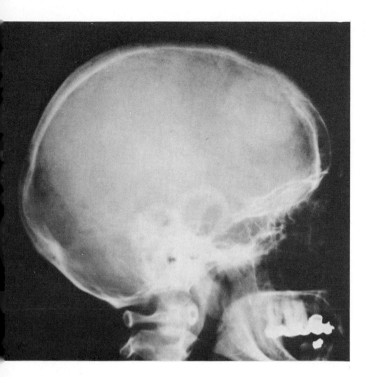

FIG. 6–34. An area of patchy sclerosis is seen in the frontal bone due to invasion by a meningioma.

FIG. 6–35. Osteoblastic metastases from carcinoma of the prostate, causing diffuse sclerosis of the calcaneus without change in contour. This is an unusual site.

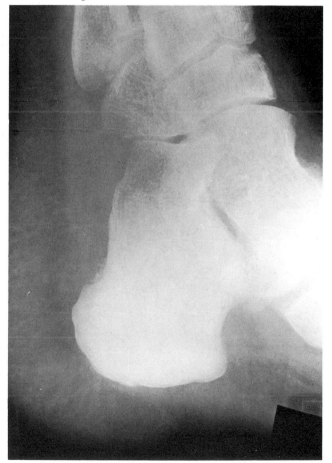

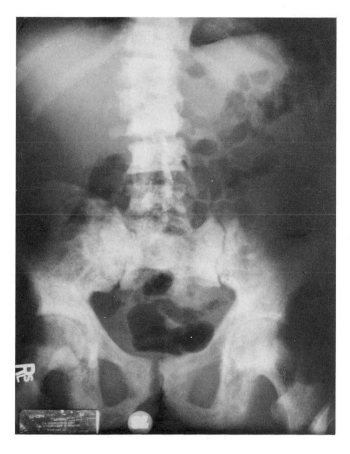

FIG. 6–36. Lumbar spine and pelvis. Typical changes of Paget's disease with coarsening of the trabecular pattern and cortical thickening are noted. In addition, osteoblastic metastases are seen in the lumbar spine.

MYELOFIBROSIS (MYELOSCLEROSIS, AGNOGENIC MYELOID METAPLASIA, OSTEOSCLEROTIC ANEMIA, MYELOPHTHISIC SPLENOMEGALY, ALEUKEMIC MEGAKARYOCYTIC MYELOSIS)

Myelofibrosis[151,197,242] is a hematological disorder characterized by anemia, a leukemoid blood picture, progressive fibrosis of the bone marrow, marked splenomegaly, and osteosclerotic changes.

The etiology is unknown. Fibrosis of the bone marrow may be associated with leukemia or polycythemia vera, but current opinion is that myelofibrosis is a separate and distinct entity.

Clinically, the majority of patients are over 50 years old, with an age range of 34 to 85 years. The sex distribution is equal. There is an insidious onset of vague symptoms related to anemia, bleeding tendency, bone pain, and secondary gout. Splenomegaly, which may be massive, is consistently present. There is often elevation of the basal metabolic rate. The blood picture shows a normochromic normocytic anemia with circulating immature red cells and immature leukocytes. The leukocyte count and platelet count are variable. A large percentage of patients have antecedent polycythemia vera.

Radiologically, the basic types of lesions are:

1. Osteosclerosis
2. Destructive
3. Splenomegaly
4. Extramedullary hematopoiesis
5. Secondary gout

Approximately 50% of all patients develop osteosclerosis, which may vary in degree from mild to severe. There may be thickening of bone trabeculae or a "ground glass" appearance.

The increase in density may be uniform or patchy (Figs. 6–37, 6–38). A uniform sclerosis is the most frequent finding. Periosteal new bone formation, irregular and thick, is most frequently seen at the medial margins of the distal femora, the lateral margins of the proximal tibiae, and the ankles (Fig. 6–39). The changes at the knees and ankles are characteristic. Endosteal thickening of the inner aspect of the cortices of long bones, causing narrowing of the medullary spaces, also occurs. The ribs, spine, pelvis, humeri, and femora are the bones most frequently involved in the osteosclerotic process. Skull changes also occur, which may be sclerotic, lucent, or mixed. The hands and feet may rarely be involved.

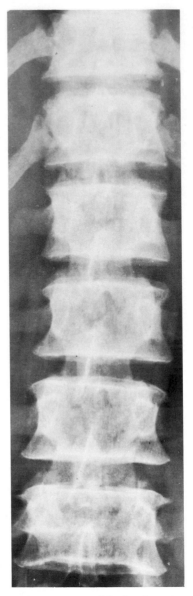

FIG. 6–37. Myelosclerosis (spine). Increase in density of vertebral bodies is seen.

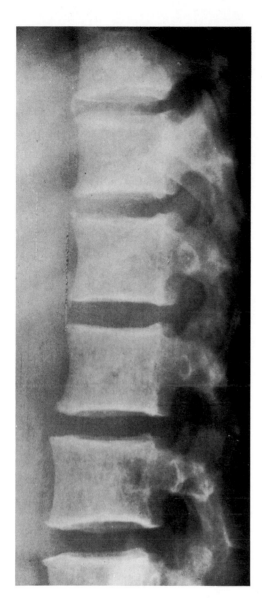

FIG. 6–38. Myelosclerosis (spine, lateral view) — same patient as in Fig. 6–37. Uniform sclerotic changes in vertebral bodies are better noted in this view.

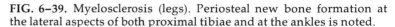

FIG. 6–39. Myelosclerosis (legs). Periosteal new bone formation at the lateral aspects of both proximal tibiae and at the ankles is noted.

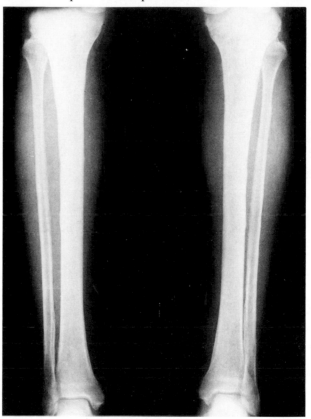

Osteolytic changes are sometimes seen.[249] There may be discrete ovoid radiolucencies with the long axis of the lesion parallel to the long axis of the shaft, or a "moth-eaten," ill-defined, destructive process may be evident. This may be mixed with sclerosis, or (rarely) it may be purely lytic (Figs. 6–40, 6–41). Splenomegaly, usually marked, is most often present, although not in all cases. Soft-tissue masses of extramedullary hematopoiesis may be seen (Fig. 6–42). These foci have been described in liver, spleen, skin, paraspinal region, adrenals, lungs, choroid plexus, lymph nodes, and as an ex-

trapleural mass adjacent to an area of rib destruction. Hyperuricemia may be present, resulting in secondary gout. The destructive bony lesions are indistinguishable from those of primary gout; however, progression is more rapid. An aggressive, rapidly progressive form, termed *malignant myelosclerosis* has been described which may simulate metastatic bone disease.[240] Myelofibrosis has also been reported as being associated with multiple myeloma,[59] and developing in treated histiocytosis-X.

(Text continued on p. 396)

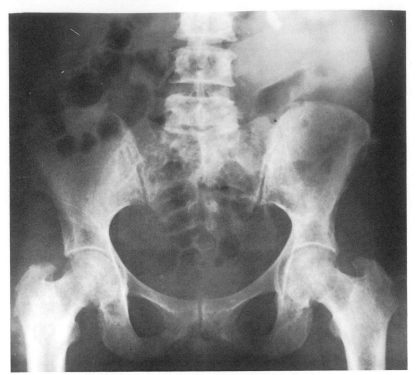

FIG. 6–40. Myelosclerosis (pelvis). Areas of increased density in the ilia, and multiple small radiolucent foci in the ischia may be seen. Also note sclerotic changes in the femora. There is a left renal calculus.

FIG. 6–41. A patient with myeloproliferative disease with leukemia, polycythemia, and myelosclerosis. A. Left shoulder. A pathological fracture of the humeral neck is noted. B. Right forearm. Permeative destruction of both radius and ulna is seen with tiny radiolucencies oriented with their long axes along the long axis of the bone.

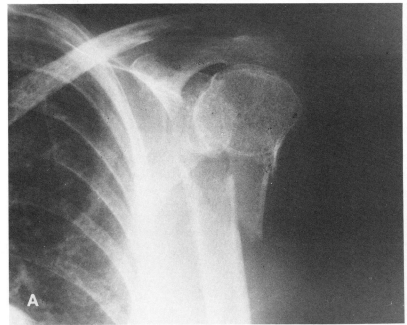

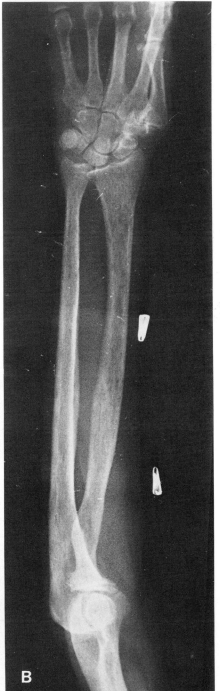

FIG. 6–42. Myelosclerosis (chest). Widening of the paramediastinal stripe is best seen as an increased density limited laterally by a sharp line medial to the aorta on the left. This is due to extramedullary hematopoiesis. Enlargement of the spleen may also be seen.

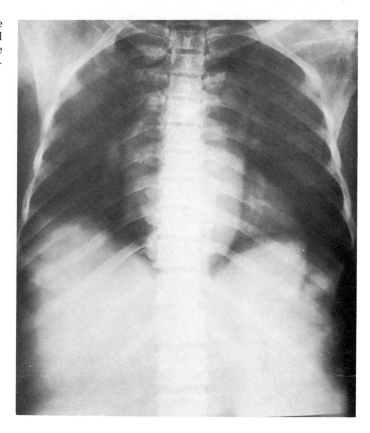

FIG. 6–43. Mastocytosis (pelvis). Diffuse osteosclerosis is present with trabecular accentuation. There is cortical thickening in the upper femora. (Courtesy of Dr. Malvin Barer, Mayo Clinic)

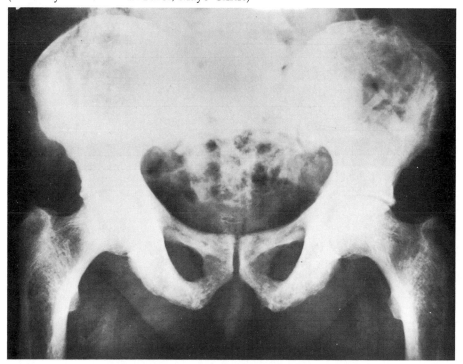

URTICARIA PIGMENTOSA (MASTOCYTOSIS)

Urticaria pigmentosa[15,19,154] is a condition in which an abnormal number of tissue mast cells are present in the skin. In some patients, generalized visceral mast cell proliferation occurs, including bone marrow, liver, spleen, lungs, lymph nodes, and peripheral blood. Bone marrow involvement results in osteosclerosis.

Clinically, the majority of patients develop skin lesions during the first year of life. These appear as umbilicated papules, discrete and coalescent. There may be hepatosplenomegaly and lymphadenopathy. The blood picture shows anemia, leukocytosis or leukopenia, and may show thrombocytopenia.

Radiologically, two types of bone changes have been described — generalized and focal — with a mixture of osteosclerosis and osteoporosis. There may be trabecular thickening or diffuse sclerosis alternating with areas of cystic rarefaction (Fig. 6–43). The lesions are confined almost entirely to cancellous bone, with sclerosis obliterating the architectural landmarks. There may also be scattered, well-defined sclerotic foci (Fig. 6–44). The areas most often involved are the spine, ribs, pelvis, humeri, and femora. The skull may also be involved, showing stippling of the calvarium and thickening of the tables.

Mastocytosis with skeletal involvement has also been reported in infancy. The frequency of bone involvement in children is claimed to be 15%, with findings of sclerotic and lytic lesions, coarse trabeculation, undertubulation, Scheuermann-like changes, and thickening of selected bones.[187]

TUBEROUS SCLEROSIS

Tuberous sclerosis[173, 188] is a rare familial disease with a basic defect of development of ectodermal structures, and a classic clinical triad of adenoma sebaceum of the face, epilepsy, and mental deficiency. Many systems, particularly the central nervous system, show involvement. Widespread hamartomas, particularly in the kidney, are common, and malignant change may occur. There is an increased incidence of associated congenital anomalies, including harelip, polydactyly, spina bifida, and congenital heart disease. Small nodules of gliosis, up to 3 cm in diameter, are scattered throughout the cerebral cortex and are detectable radiologically as small scattered foci of intracranial calcification,

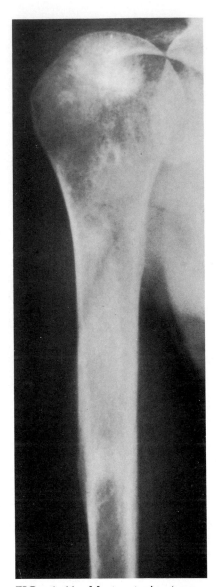

FIG. 6–44. Mastocytosis (upper humerus) — same patient as Fig. 6–43. Several well-defined, circular, sclerotic patches are seen in the humeral head and shaft. (Courtesy of Dr. Malvin Barer, Mayo Clinic)

rarely unilateral. Malignant degeneration may occur. Congenital tumors of the retina, called phakomas, also may be present. The skin in areas other than the face shows thickened plaques, café-au-lait spots, and subungual fibromas. The lungs may show a reticular and honeycomb pattern.

Radiologically, the characteristic changes in the skeletal system are patches of osteosclerosis. These may be round, ovoid, flame-shaped, or of irregular outline, and vary in size from several millimeters to several centimeters (Fig. 6–45). There is no coarsened trabecular pattern and no enlargement of the bone. The lesions involving the ilium are centrally located. All bones may be involved with osteoblastic lesions, with 40% involvement of the pelvis and lumbar spine, and 40% involvement of the cranial vault. The hands and feet may show cystlike areas, particularly in the distal phalanges. Periosteal new bone formation of the large and small tubular bones may be seen. Sclerotic and cystlike areas may be mixed. Sclerosis and widening of a rib have also been reported.[217] The spine may be involved, with sclerosis of the pedicles. Scattered intracranial calcifications, ovoid or curvilinear, ranging up to several centimeters in size and usually in close relationship to the walls of the lateral ventricles or the cerebellum, may also be seen. The roentgen findings may occur without the usual clinical picture.[299]

HYPERVITAMINOSIS D AND IDIOPATHIC HYPERCALCEMIA

Hypervitaminosis D results from excessive intake, usually of vitamin D_2. The intake can range from 50,000 to 1,000,000 IU daily, over a period ranging from a few days to several years. *Idiopathic hypercalcemia* is considered to be the result of excessive vitamin D intake, hypersensitivity to vitamin D, or inborn errors of cholesterol metabolism with resultant sterol intermediates possessing vitamin D-like properties in children. The serum calcium level is elevated even in the presence of a low calcium intake.

Clinically, the most damaging effects are due to renal calcifications, leading to renal failure. The symptoms are nausea, vomiting, polyuria, polydipsia, and abdominal cramps. The blood-urea-nitrogen and serum creatinine levels become elevated. In severe cases, convulsions and coma occur.

Radiologically, the long bones show increase in depth of the provisional zones of calcification, leading to dense metaphyseal bands (Fig. 6–46). Cortical thickening and bone sclerosis occur (Fig. 6–47). In the adult, and in cases of prolonged intake in children, loss of bone density develops. There may be thickening of the calvarium. The vertebral bodies show dense end-plates and a subcortical radio-

FIG. 6–45. Tuberous sclerosis (pelvis). Multiple discrete osteosclerotic patches, rounded and ovoid in shape, are centrally located in both ilia. (Courtesy of Dr. P. Elian, Chicago, IL and Dr. J. F. Holt, Ann Arbor, MI)

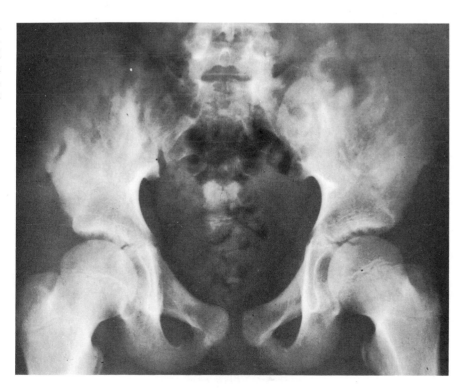

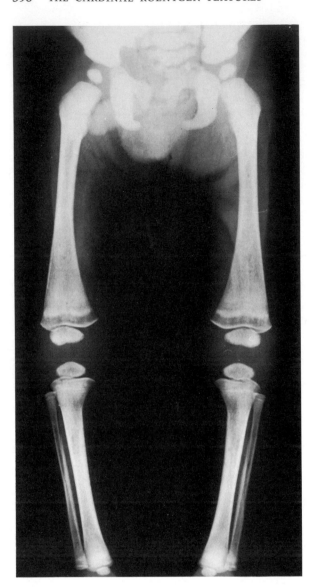

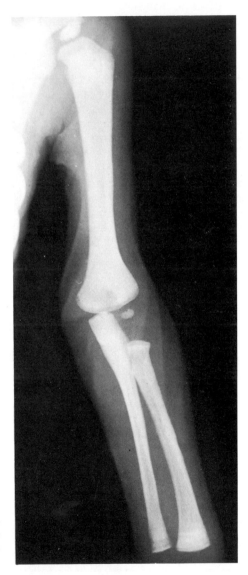

FIG. 6–46. Idiopathic hypercalcemia (lower extremities). Note multiple dense transverse metaphyseal bands, and a wide zone of radiolucency at the distal femora. (Courtesy of Dr. Harvey White, Children's Memorial Hospital, Chicago, IL)

FIG. 6–47. Idiopathic hypercalcemia (upper extremity). Note generalized bone sclerosis, multiple transverse bands at the distal radius, and radiolucent bands at the distal ulna. (Courtesy of Dr. Harvey White, Children's Memorial Hospital, Chicago, IL)

FIG. 6–48. Fluorosis (spine), showing uniform sclerosis of the vertebral bodies. ▶

lucency. Metastatic calcifications are common and have been reported in widespread areas, including the skin, cornea, gastric wall, joints, bursa, thyroid, adrenals, and pancreas. Calcification of the falx cerebri is consistently seen, and tentorial calcification may also be present. Premature vascular calcification is often noted. Marked puttylike periarticular calcification occurs when excessive vitamin D is administered as a treatment for rheumatoid arthritis or gout. Calcium is then deposited in tophi of gout, a circumstance that does not always occur in gout because the tophi are composed of sodium urate. Premature closure of the cranial sutures may occur in severe cases.

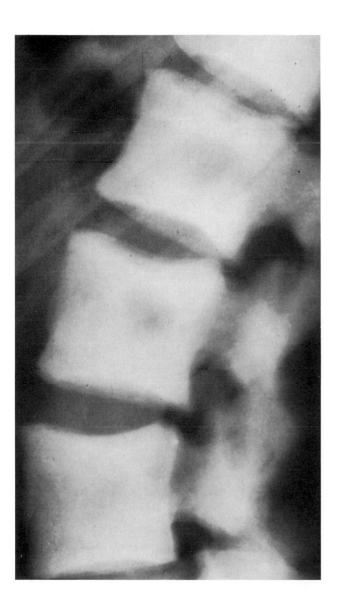

Idiopathic hypercalcemia[90] is clinically divided into two forms. A mild form (Syndrome I) is transient and no radiologic abnormalities of bone or soft tissue are seen. The severe chronic form (Syndrome II) is characterized by hypercalcemia associated with a triad of azotemia, osteosclerosis, and physical and mental retardation. *Roentgen findings* are unstable, being dependent on the metabolic state. Sclerosis of the orbital rim and sphenoids, giving a "spectacle" appearance to the skull, is the most striking feature. The mandible may also be sclerotic, as well as the vertebral bodies, with a characteristic peripheral cortical sclerosis. Widespread metaphyseal sclerosis, including the acetabular roofs, is seen. "Erlenmeyer flask" deformities of the distal femora also may be present. Craniostenosis may occasionally occur. Sclerotic rings about the epiphyseal ossification centers and the carpal and sternal centers are seen. Metastatic soft-tissue calcification occurs. The muscle cylinder ratio is diminished.[49]

FLUOROSIS

Osteosclerosis due to *fluorosis*[205] may occur from drinking water with a fluoride concentration in excess of 8 parts per million, or from agricultural or industrial fluoride contamination. Sporadic cases occur in the southwestern United States, in Arizona and Texas. Several cases have been reported in Spain from drinking wine containing fluorine.

Clinically, there is marked variation in individual responses. The most pronounced feature is "mottling" of the enamel of the teeth. The bone changes produce few symptoms. Anemia may be present. The fluoride inhibits bone resorption either by inhibiting osteoclastic activity or by reducing the solubility of bone salts. The synthesis of normal collagen is also disturbed.

Radiologically, there is initially a thickening of the bony trabecular pattern best seen in the vertebral bodies, but also involving the clavicles, ribs, and pelvis. This then progresses to a dense uniform symmetrical sclerosis that obliterates the bony architectural landmarks (Fig. 6–48). All bones may be involved, with most pronounced changes in the axial skeleton. The calvarium rarely shows changes, but the base of the skull and the posterior clinoids may be sclerosed (Fig. 6–49). Marked osteophytosis, which projects deeply into the soft tissues, develops at the areas of muscle, ligament, and tendon attachments. The osteophytes characteristically show sclerosis. The bones may be widened. The ribs occasionally show needlelike calcifications projecting

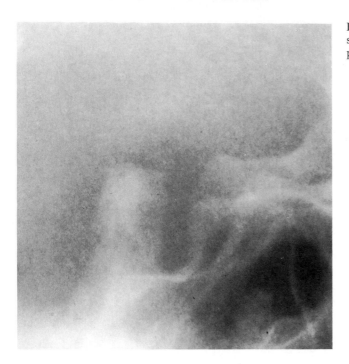

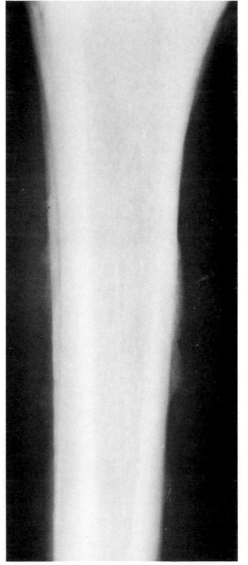

FIG. 6–49. Fluorosis (skull). Detail of sella turcica. The only significant change is sclerosis of the posterior clinoid process.

FIG. 6–50. Fluorosis (leg). Periosteal elevation along the diaphysis of the tibia and fibula may be seen.

out at the attachments of the intercostal muscles. A rarefying osteitis and a mixed form have been described. Marked periosteal proliferation (Fig. 6–50), with an unusually thick, solid, undulating periosteal cloaking, has been described as a variant form termed "periostitis deformans."[294] Joint changes or fluoric arthroses also develop, particularly in the hips, knees, and elbows. This is caused by marked osteophytosis limiting joint movement and calcification of the periarticular ligaments. Another characteristic roentgen feature is ligamentous calcification, particularly of the sacrospinous and sacrotuberous ligaments. Calcified sacral ligaments in the presence of bone sclerosis are common in fluorosis but may also be seen in renal osteodystrophy.

TERMINAL PHALANGEAL OSTEOSCLEROSIS

Osteosclerosis of the terminal phalanges[116] is a relatively common finding and has been observed as a benign entity in women older than 40 years. Sclerosis has also been observed in the terminal phalanges associated with collagen diseases such as scleroderma, rheumatoid arthritis, systemic lupus erythematosus, and to a lesser degree in osteoarthritis, trauma, gout, and periarteritis nodosa. The sclerosis may be localized or diffuse. It is claimed

FIG. 6–51. Terminal phalangeal osteosclerosis. Note sclerotic changes in the terminal phalanges ranging from almost complete medullary sclerosis to minimal involvement. There is no periostitis nor change in the contour of the bone. The predominant picture is that of localized sclerosis, which is not specific.

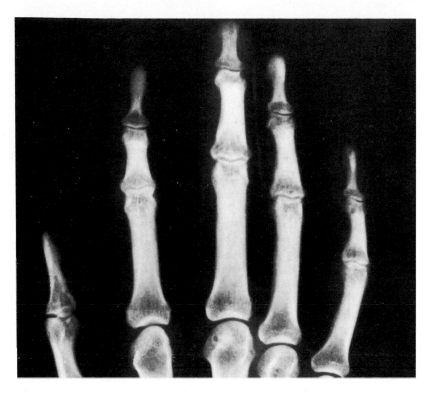

that the diffuse form of terminal sclerodactylia is most often associated with collagen disease (Fig. 6–51).

DESTRUCTION OF BONE

A basic response of bone to injury is destruction. Loss of bone substance may occur by resorption through the action of osteoclasts or, as is claimed by Jaffe,[153] direct destruction of trabeculae by metastatic tumor cells. Tissue culture studies with time-lapse motion pictures have shown dissolution of bone before an advancing osteoclastic front. Osteoclasts, by virtue of their secretory activity, lyse both mineral and organic matrix of bone. Halisteresis, or the concept of decalcification of bone with a residual normal matrix, is no longer considered valid, except on a minor scale. Hyperemia is said to facilitate osteolysis.

Early bone destruction may be recognized radiologically as a subtle alteration of bone texture or a barely perceptible decrease in bone density. There is a latent period between histological destruction and roentgen demonstrability of about 10 days under the most favorable of circumstances, and may be much longer in the case of a slow process in rarefied bone. At this stage, a radioisotope-uptake bone scan is a much more sensitive indicator of increased bone turnover than conventional radiographs.

Several factors are involved in the radiographic visibility of a destructive focal lesion other than sheer size. The ratio of volume of bone destroyed to the density of adjacent uninvolved bone is of prime importance. A destructive focus is more apparent in the cortex than in the medulla, and more readily seen in bone of normal density than in osteoporotic bone. The margination of the lesion is significant. A sharply circumscribed lesion has much greater visibility than one in which the edges fade off into imperceptibility. Radiographic technique is important. Attention should be paid to obtaining the exposure that will give proper density (MAS) and contrast (KV), as well as maximum sharpness (small focal spot, nonscreen films) and limitation of scattered radiation (collimation or grid).

Bone destruction has a wide spectrum of appearance, and several patterns along this spectrum can be discerned. The simplest and the most benign in appearance are cystlike dissolutions. These represent small areas of well-marginated radiolucencies, most commonly see in the arthritides, that may contain synovial fluid or fibrous or granulation tissue.

The radiological term "cyst" does not necessarily connote a fluid-filled cavity. A larger solitary focus may be seen, representing a lesion that grows slowly enough to destroy all of the bone in the involved area before progressing. This circumscribed lysis has been termed "geographic" by Lodwick.[186] Another pattern, the result of multiple smaller endosteal excavations, appears as many moderate-sized radiolucencies that tend to become confluent and represent a more active lesion. This regional invasive pattern has been termed "moth-eaten." A larger endosteal destructive area appears as a "punched-out" lesion. The most aggressive and infiltrative lesions tunnel in the cortex and cause a myriad of tiny radiolucencies with no definite border between the involved area and normal bone. This diffuse invasive pattern is termed *permeative*.

The margination of a destructive lesion is an indication of its aggressiveness and of the reparative response that is evoked. The margins may be ill-defined or sharply defined, partially or completely. There may be irregular or smooth edges. There may be no wall, a fine thin wall, or a thick sclerotic wall surrounding the lesion. A sharp margin or abrupt transition indicates a slowly growing or expanding lesion, while a wide zone of transition indicates an aggressive lesion. Trabeculation within the lesion may be light or heavy. If the rate of growth of the lesion is slower than the reparative potential of the bone, expansion will occur. Expansion is an indicator of the rate of growth of a lesion and not a valid differential point between malignant and benign tumors.

Loss of bone substance can also be caused by pressure erosion from a process extrinsic to bone. This has a typical smooth appearance descriptively termed "saucerization." Bone can also be invaded from a soft-tissue malignant tumor.

Another cause of bone deficit is resorption. This process may take the form of an ill-defined fading away of terminal bony segments, or a "pencil-like" or "candlestick-like" contour with sharp, well-defined borders.

The diseases characterized by generalized bone destruction are summarized below.

DISEASES CHARACTERIZED BY WIDESPREAD AREAS OF BONE DESTRUCTION

Osteolytic metastases (carcinomas, sarcomas and lymphomas)
Multiple myeloma
Osteomyelitis (of various etiologies)
Leukemia
Burkitt's tumor
Reticuloses
Gout

Rare Causes of Widespread Bone Destruction

Massive osteolysis
Intraosseous hemangiomatosis
Cystic lymphangiomatosis of bone
Congenital scattered fibromatosis
Weber-Christian disease
Primary systemic amyloidosis
Electrical injury

OSTEOLYTIC METASTASES[95,227]

All malignant tumors, with few exceptions if any, may metastasize to bone, and the skeleton is one of the most common sites of metastases. The usual route of tumor cell emboli to the osseous system is by way of the bloodstream. Metastases may lodge in the spine, bypassing the lungs by way of the vertebral vein system as described by Batson. Lymphatic spread to bone is rare. Direct extension and invasion of bone may occur, and this is seen not uncommonly in carcinoma of the cervix extending to the pelvic wall (Figs. 6–52, 6–53). The area of greatest predilection is the red-marrow-containing central skeleton: the skull, spine, ribs, pelvis, humeri, and femora. Metastatic lesions distal to the knees and elbows, although rare, do occur.[210]

The distribution pattern of metastatic bone disease from various primaries is presented below.[174]

DISTRIBUTION OF METASTATIC BONE DISEASE[174]

Axial skeleton		60%
Dorso-lumbar spine		32%
Skull		10%
Sacroiliac joint		5%
Upper ⎫		
Lower ⎬ Extremities		11%
Forearm ⎫		
Hand ⎪		
Leg ⎬		4%
Foot ⎭		

The most probable cause of osteolytic metastases in a child is neuroblastoma; in an adult man, carcinoma of the lung; and in an adult woman, carcinoma of the breast. Carcinoma of the kidney and thyroid also commonly cause osteolytic lesions and have distinctive roentgen features. The rate of frequency of metastases to bone from various primary carcinomas is as follows: breast, 35%; prostate (including osteoblastic), 30%; lung, 10%; kidney, 5%;

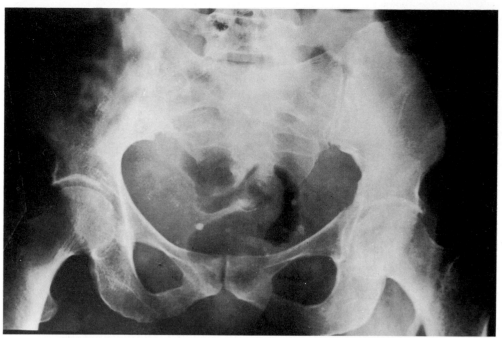

FIG. 6–52. Destruction (pelvis) by direct extension from carcinoma of the cervix. The left pelvic rim shows a destructive area.

FIG. 6–53. Destruction (pelvic wall) by direct extension from carcinoma of the cervix. A soft-tissue mass may be seen in the pelvis, along with opaque surgical sutures and clips. There is ragged destruction of the left pelvic rim with mottled destruction of the ilium.

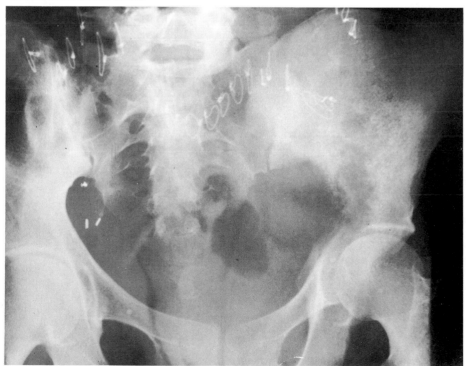

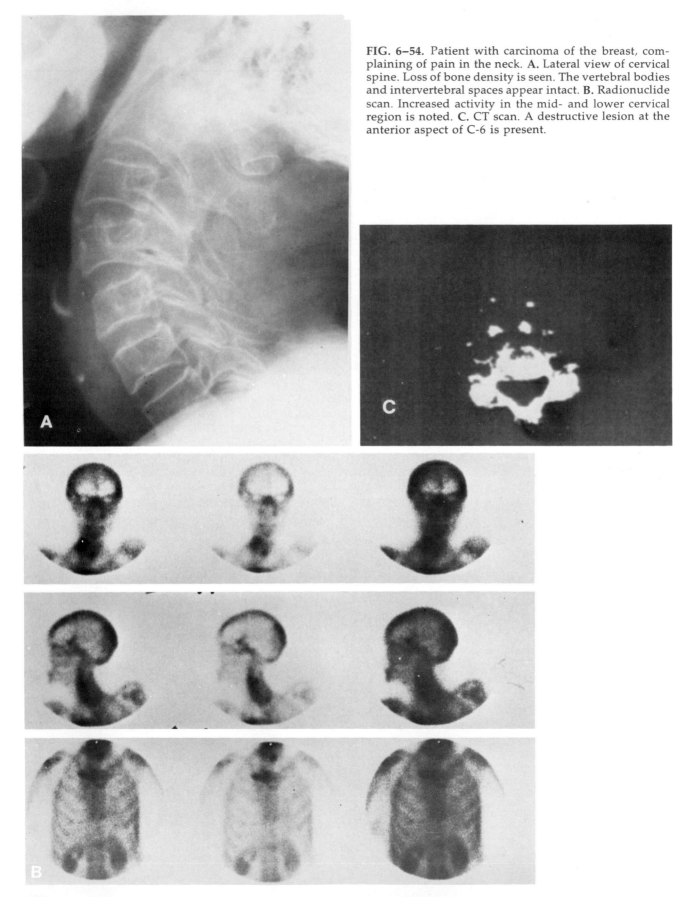

FIG. 6–54. Patient with carcinoma of the breast, complaining of pain in the neck. A. Lateral view of cervical spine. Loss of bone density is seen. The vertebral bodies and intervertebral spaces appear intact. B. Radionuclide scan. Increased activity in the mid- and lower cervical region is noted. C. CT scan. A destructive lesion at the anterior aspect of C-6 is present.

uterus, 2%; thyroid, 2%; stomach, 2%; colon, 1%; other organs, 13%.

Clinically, the metastatic focus may first call attention to the presence of disease with pain, edema, and inflammatory signs. Pathological fracture is not uncommon. Solitary or multiple lesions may be present, causing general disability. Neurological signs or paraplegia may result from spinal involvement. Hypercalcemia and an elevated serum alkaline phosphatase level occur. Associated toxic manifestations of hypercalcemia may complicate the clinical picture.

In the interests of efficiency and cost containment, a logical order of work-up for osseous metastases should be adopted. This includes an understanding of the limitations and capabilities of all available modalities. It should be understood that false-positive and false-negative radionuclide bone scans may occur.[164] CT scans are of value for the detection of central skeletal lesions. (Figs. 6–54, 6–55).

Some of these may not be visualized in any other way. Percutaneous needle biopsy under radiological control is another satisfactory method.[67]

The methods available for the diagnosis of bone metastases, in logical order, are presented below.

METHODS AVAILABLE FOR DIAGNOSIS OF BONE METASTASES

1. Radionuclide scan
2. Bone survey
3. Directed radiologic examination
4. Tomography
5. Computed tomography
6. Needle or open biopsy

Radiologically, a pure osteolytic metastasis does not evoke reactive bone proliferation (Fig. 6–56). If this is an accompanying factor, then the process is referred to as mixed metastases (Fig. 6–57). The lesions may be single or multiple, and develop from tumor embolic deposits in the spongiosa. They are usually ill-defined and poorly marginated, progress to destroy the compacta, and cause pathological fractures (Fig. 6–58). They can also present as sharply circumscribed destructive lesions. "Button sequestra" within osteolytic lesions are a rare finding (Fig. 6–59). Cartilage is resistant to tumor, the intervertebral spaces are preserved, and joint spaces are spared. Resultant hyperemia from a lesion at the end of a bone may cause osteoporosis of the adjacent bone, giving a false impression of extension across a joint (Fig. 6–60). Periosteal reaction is rare. The skull may show solitary or scattered foci in the calvarium (Fig. 6–61), or mottled destruction

(Fig. 6–62). Metastases to the nasal bones from breast carcinoma have been reported at a site of previous fractures.[226] This demonstrates the concept of *locus minoris resistentiae.* The spine shows involvement of the bodies and pedicles (Fig. 6–63), progressing to wedge or waferlike compression of the bodies (Fig. 6–64). Involvement of the pedicles usually differentiates this process from multiple myeloma, and the preservation of the intervertebral spaces effectively excludes an infective process. Pathological fractures of the odontoid process have been described resulting from metastases from breast carcinoma.[178]

In peripheral bone lesions, the feet are involved more often than the hands (Figs. 6–65, 6–66), and there may be multiple foci. The incidence of metastases to the periphery is estimated at 2% to 4%.[245] They are usually seen in the terminal phalanges, and have been reported in tarsal bones but not in carpal bones. The primary tumor is usually carcinoma of the lung. These are symptomatic, destructive lesions with no periosteal reaction. There may be destruction of the major portion of the terminal phalanx with a thin layer of intact bone adjacent to the articular surface[118] (Figs. 6–67, 6–68). The *clinical* presentation may simulate gout.[313] Many different primary sites have been reported as metastasizing to the hand. These are summarized below.

METASTASES TO THE HAND[314]

Lung
Breast
Kidney
Parotid
Prostate
Colon
Rectum
Lymphosarcoma
Oral Cavity

Very Rare

Tonsil
Nasopharynx
Esophagus
Stomach
Testicle
Bladder
Brain
Adrenal
Skin
Uterus
Larynx
Thyroid

(Text continued on p. 414)

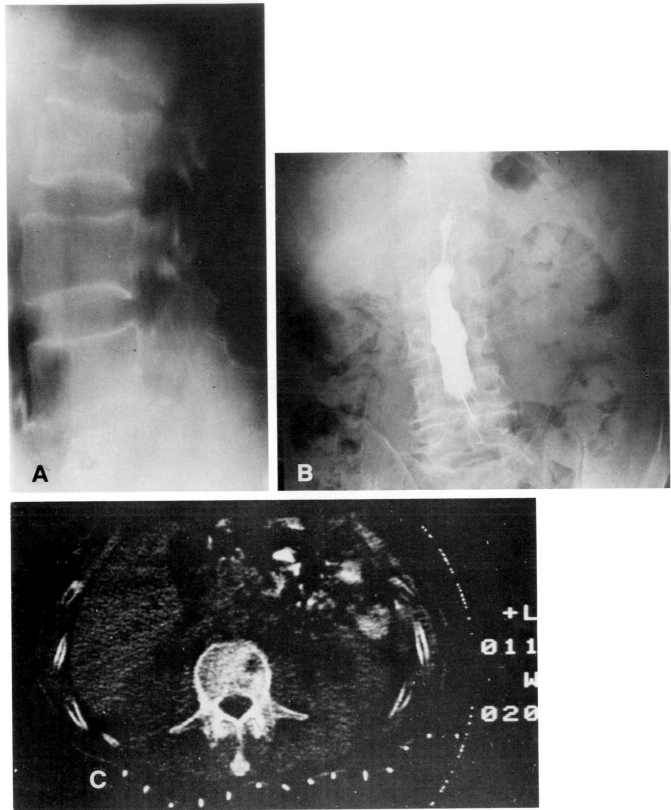

(Continued)

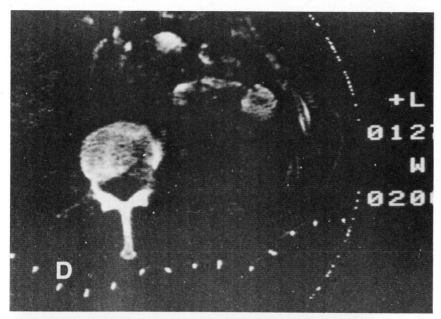

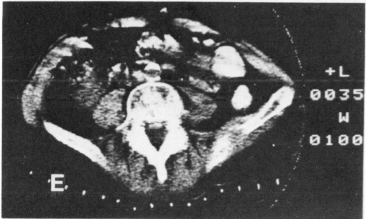

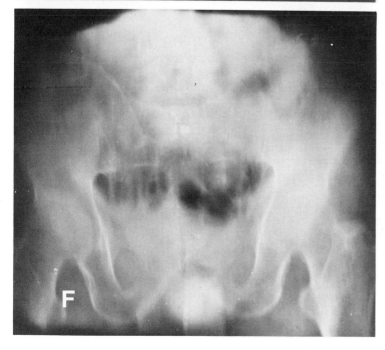

FIG. 6–55. 60-year-old male complaining of severe back pain. Further workup was negative. The patient had an old fracture of the first lumbar vertebra. **A.** Lateral tomogram of the lumbar spine. The second, third, and fourth lumbar vertebral bodies appear normal. The intervertebral spaces are preserved. **B.** Myelogram showing an extradural pressure effect on the left at the level of L-2. **C, D.** CT scans of the L-2 level. Destructive lesions within the vertebral body are noted, with cortical destruction at the left posterior aspect. **E.** CT scan of the L-4 level showing a destructive lesion of the left ilium with an associated soft tissue mass. **F.** Tomogram reveals a subtle destructive lesion at the left iliac crest. A biopsy showed undifferentiated carcinoma.

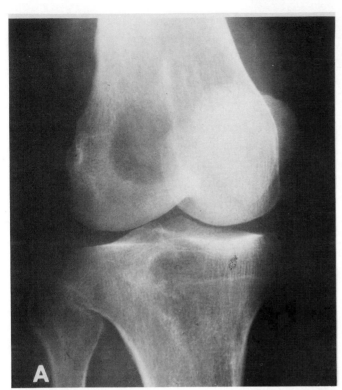

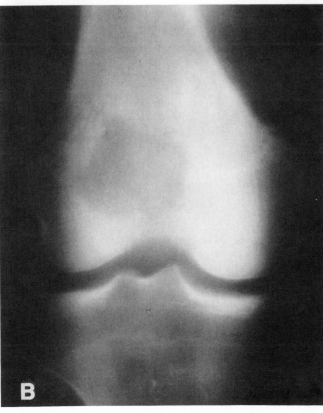

FIG. 6–56. Patient with carcinoma of the esophagus. **A.** Oblique view of the knee shows a localized radiolucent lesion in the epiphysis and metaphysis. **B.** The tomogram shows that this lesion has a wide zone of transition. Metastatic carcinoma was found.

FIG. 6–57. Mixed metastases (femur) from carcinoma of the breast. Multiple osteolytic and sclerotic areas are present with a pathological fracture of the proximal third shaft of the femur. The osteolytic areas are ill-defined.

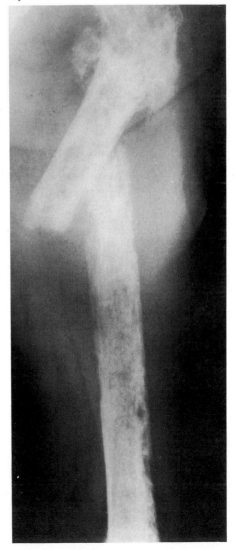

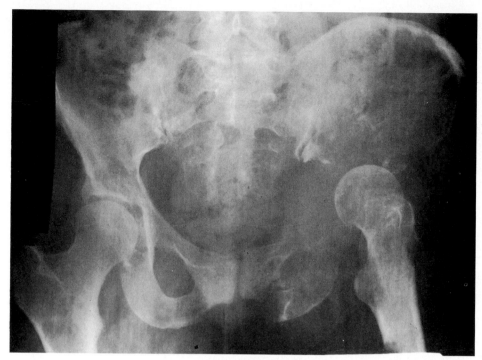

FIG. 6–58. Osteolytic metastases (pelvis) from carcinoma of the breast. Note extensive destruction of the left side of the pelvis and of the right iliac crest, with no sclerotic reaction. The articular cartilage of the hip joint serves as an effective barrier to the spread of tumor, sparing the femoral head.

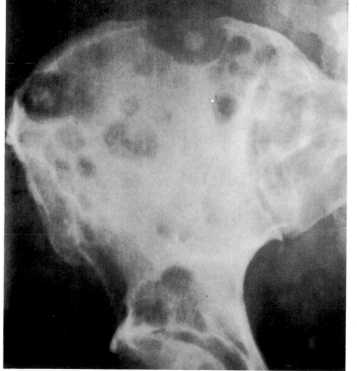

FIG. 6–59. Osteolytic metastases (pelvis) from carcinoma of the breast. Well-circumscribed, "punched-out," destructive lesions may be seen, several of which contain central round areas of residual bone or "button sequestra."

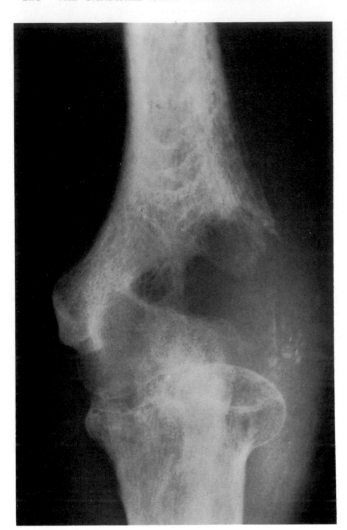

FIG. 6–60. Metastases (distal humerus) from carcinoma of the lung. A geographic area of destruction of the lateral condyle of the distal humerus is seen. Very minimal, if any, periosteal new bone formation is present. There is osteoporosis of the radial head, with a thin but intact cortical margin. The elbow joint cartilage serves as an effective barrier against the spread of the tumor, which does not involve the radius or ulna.

FIG. 6–61. Metastases (skull) from carcinoma of the breast. Several discrete, large, well-circumscribed, osteolytic lesions are present. The inferiormost occipital lesion extends to the foramen magnum.

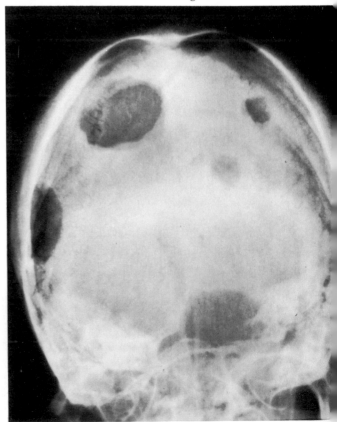

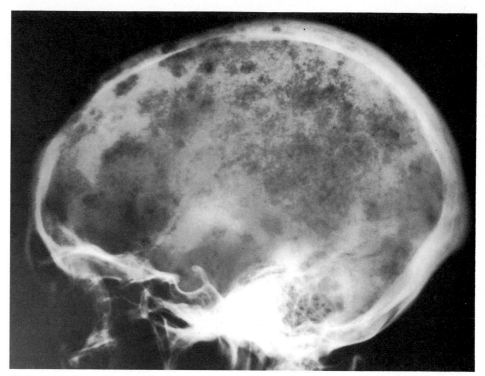

FIG. 6–62. Osteolytic metastases (skull) from carcinoma of the breast. Note extensive mottled destruction of the skull, with only several islands of bone density remaining.

FIG. 6–63. Metastases (spine) from carcinoma of the breast. The left pedicle of the fourth lumbar vertebra is destroyed, in contrast to the intact right pedicle. The vertebral body is intact. This is the "one-eyed vertebra" sign, if one considers the pedicles of the vertebrae as the eyes and the spinous process as the nose.

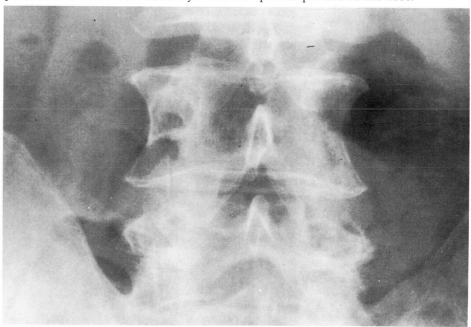

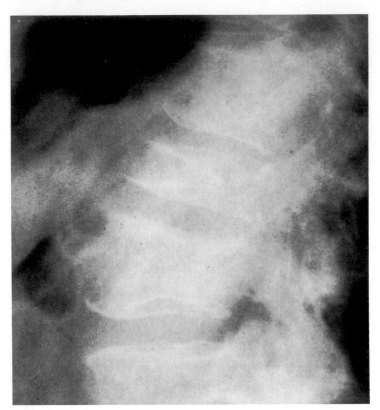

FIG. 6–64. Spine with metastases to the vertebral bodies from carcinoma of the breast. Waferlike compression of the second lumbar vertebral body is seen, with a destructive area at the anterior margin and partial collapse of the third lumbar vertebral body. The intervertebral spaces are preserved, a characteristic of metastatic tumor involving the spine.

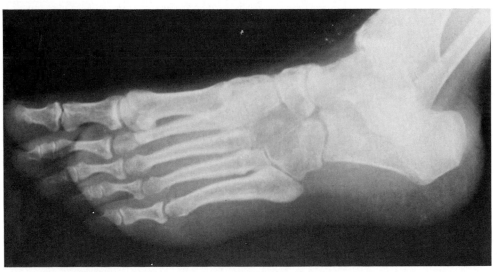

FIG. 6–65. Metastases to the tarsus from carcinoma of the cervix showing destruction of the cuneiform, cuboid, and involvement of the navicular.

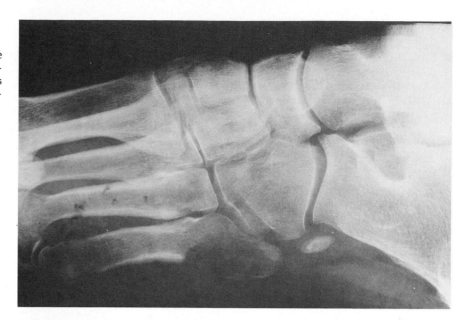

FIG. 6–66. Metastases to the base of the fifth metatarsal from a melanoma. A destructive lesion is noted with neither new bone formation nor reactive sclerosis.

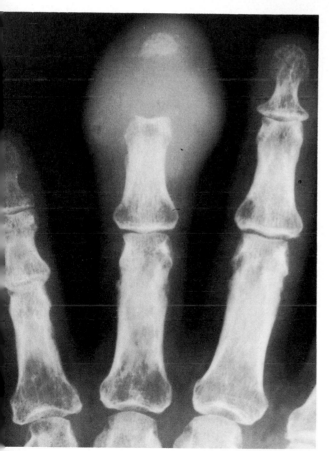

FIG. 6–67. Osteolytic metastases to the terminal phalanx of the ring finger. A large soft-tissue mass may be seen, with destruction of the major portion of the distal phalanx. The terminal tip and a small spicule at the proximal end persist. The middle phalanx is not invaded. There is spotty osteoporosis of the remaining bones.

FIG. 6–68. Metastases to the terminal phalanx from carcinoma of the lung. Soft-tissue mass and destruction of the major portion of the terminal phalanx may be seen, with a small, thin, intact sliver of bone at the base that is adjacent to the articular cartilage. (From Greenfield GB, Escamilla CH, Schorsch HA: The hand as an indicator of generalized disease. Am J Roentgen 99:736–745, 1967)

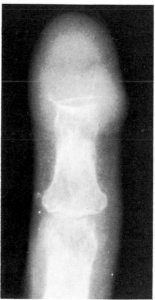

Metastases from carcinomas of the kidney (Figs. 6–69, 6–70) and thyroid (Fig. 6–71) may present as expansile, marginated, trabeculated lesions—the so-called "blowout" metastases. Other tumors, *e.g.* pheochromocytoma, melanoma (Fig. 6–72), and carcinoma of the lung and breast, may also rarely show this configuration. A renal metastasis may present as a solitary "soap bubble" septated lesion, and this may occur rarely in the presence of an apparently normal excretory urogram.

Lymphomas sometimes present as small destructive foci, elliptical in shape, with their long axes parallel to the axis of the shaft of the bone (Fig. 6–73), or as destructive areas (Figs. 6–74, 6–75). Endosteal scalloping may be an associated finding.

Metastatic neuroblastoma resembles leukemia with extensive mottled bony destruction (Fig. 6–76). A subepiphyseal band of rarefaction, as in leukemia, is also seen. The skull shows mottled destruction, "splitting" of the sutures due to increased intracranial pressure (Fig. 6–77), and perpendicular spicules of new bone formation similar to those found in the anemias (Figs. 6–78, 6–79). Destruction of a vertebral body may also occur (Fig. 6–80).

MULTIPLE MYELOMA (MYELOMATOSIS) AND OTHER DISEASES WITH ALTERED IMMUNOGLOBULINS[293]

Five distinct classes of immunoglobulins normally present in human serum have been identified. These are designated as immunoglobulins I_gG, I_gA, I_gM, I_gD, and I_gE. Their basic molecular structure consists of 4 polypeptide chains: two identical heavy chains (H-chains) and two identical light chains (L-chains), which are linked by disulfide bonds and covalent interactions.

The heavy chain has a molecular weight of about 55,000 while the light chain has a molecular weight of about 22,000. The heavy chain provides the molecular basis for the identification of the different immunoglobulin classes. The heavy chains of I_gG, I_gA, I_gM, I_gD, and I_gE have been denoted γ (gamma), α (alpha), μ (mu), δ (delta), and ϵ (epsilon), respectively. Two types of light chains termed κ (kappa) and λ (lambda) have been identified. Combinations of the above make up the various types and subtypes of human immunoglobulins.

Two main components derived from proteolytic cleavage of an I_gG molecule are the F_c (crystallizable fragment) and F_{ab} (antibody-combining fragment).

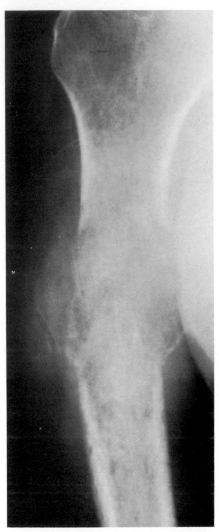

FIG. 6–69. Metastases (humeral shaft) from clear-cell carcinoma of the kidney. An expansile lesion with a pathological fracture is present, as well as permeative destruction. There is no sclerotic change. This is the "blowout" metastasis sometimes seen in renal and also thyroid carcinoma.

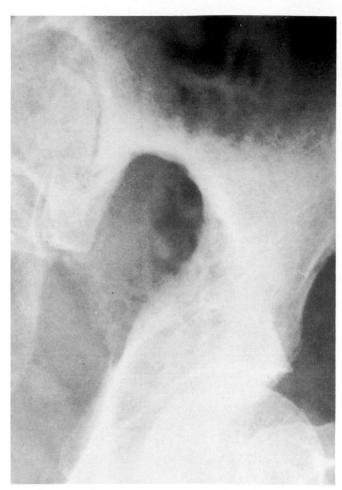

FIG. 6–70. "Blowout" metastasis (pelvis) from carcinoma of the kidney.

The F_c fragment consists of the major portions of the heavy chain, while the F_{ab} fragment consists of the light chain and the remainder of the heavy chain.

The major diseases characterized by altered immunoglobulins are heavy chain disease, macroglobulinemia, and multiple myeloma, which is by far the most common.

Heavy chain disease[100] (HCD) is a group of several clinical syndromes associated with the production of heavy chain fragments (Fig. 6–81). There are three recognized forms: α (alpha), γ (gamma), and μ (mu) chain disease.

The most common entity may be αHCD, presenting with lymphoma-like progressive intestinal involvement. It occurs in younger age groups and does not involve the marrow, liver, or spleen.

(Text continued on p. 421)

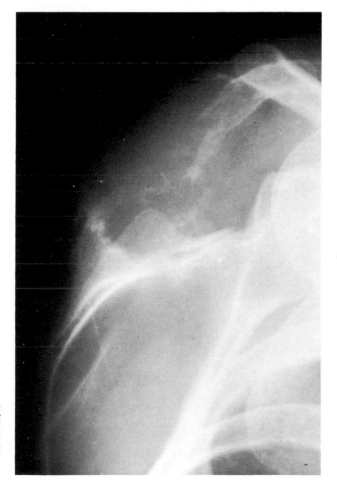

FIG. 6–71. Metastases (scapula) from carcinoma of the thyroid. Destructive expansile lesion involving the base of the acromion process of the scapula is seen, with partial destruction of the expanded margins. No reactive sclerosis is present. This also represents the so-called "blowout" metastases.

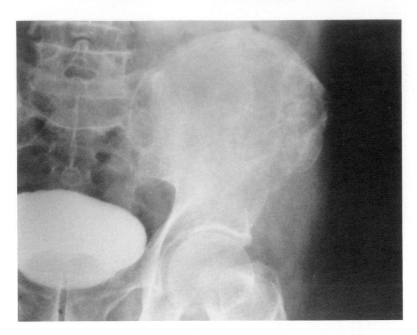

FIG. 6–72. Metastases to the ilium from melanoma. An expansile trabeculated lesion is noted involving the major portion of the left ilium.

FIG. 6–74. Hodgkin's disease (pelvis). Note extensive destruction of the ilium. The destroyed area does not cross the sacroiliac joint nor does it involve the sacral wing.

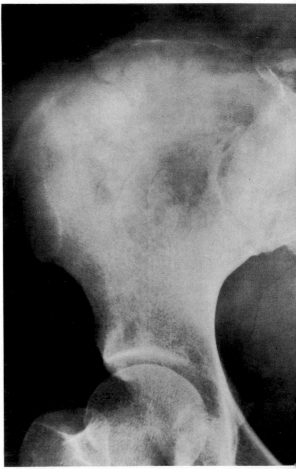

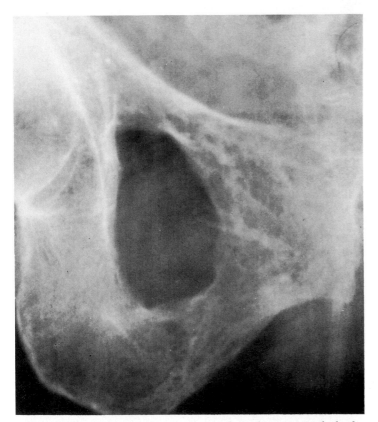

FIG. 6–73. Lymphosarcoma involving the pelvis, particularly the pubis and ischium. Small, ovoid, destructive foci are present, the majority of which parallel the axis of the pubis and ischium.

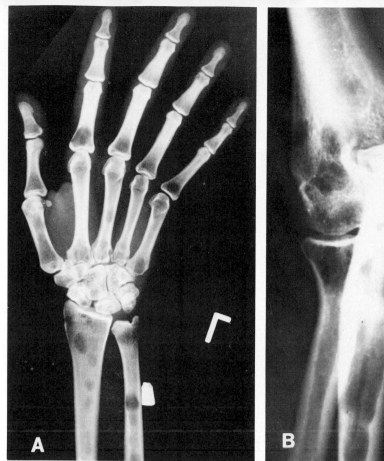

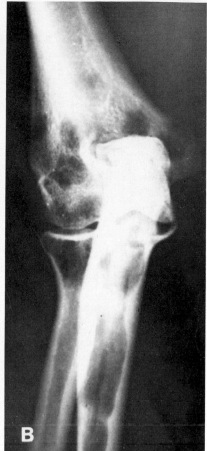

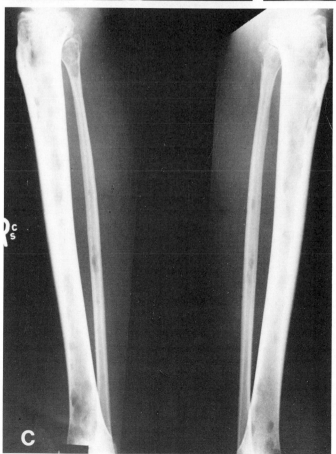

FIG. 6–75. Metastatic lymphosarcoma, primary in the breast. A. Wrist and hand. Multiple small and medium-sized well-circumscribed lesions, causing endosteal destruction with no reactive sclerosis, are seen distributed throughout the radius, ulna, carpals, metacarpals, and phalanges. B. Elbow. Similar destructive changes are seen in the distal humerus and proximal radius and ulna. C. Legs. Similar destructive changes are seen, most markedly in both tibiae.

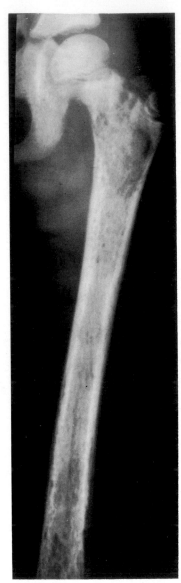

FIG. 6–76

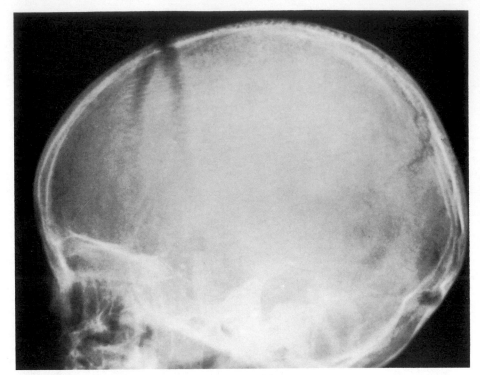

FIG. 6–77
FIG. 6–78

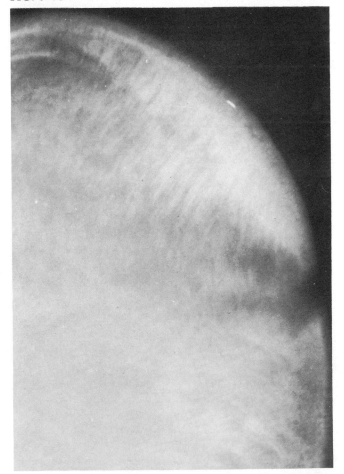

◀ FIG. 6–76. Metastatic neuroblastoma (femoral shaft)—female, age 5 years. Extensive mottled or permeative destruction of the shaft of the femur may be seen, with periosteal new bone formation.

◀ FIG. 6–77. Metastatic neuroblastoma (skull)—same patient as in Fig. 6–76. Note "splitting" of the coronal suture.

◀ FIG. 6–78. Metastatic neuroblastoma (skull). Wide separation of the coronal suture and fine long linear streaks of new bone formation are present.

FIG. 6–79. Metastatic neuroblastoma (skull). Spiculated perpendicular fine striations of new bone extending outward from the outer table are seen.

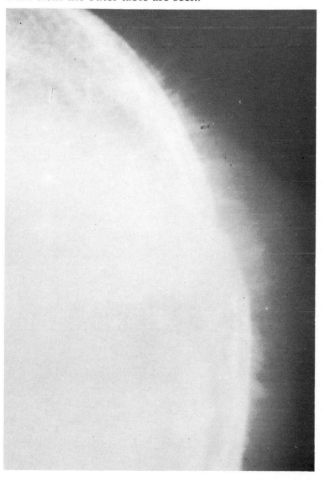

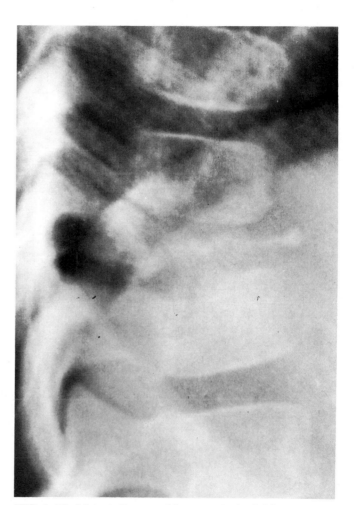

FIG. 6–80. Metastatic neuroblastoma (spine). Note extensive destruction of the twelfth vertebral body, with a "waferlike" flattening. The intervertebral spaces are preserved, as in other metastatic processes.

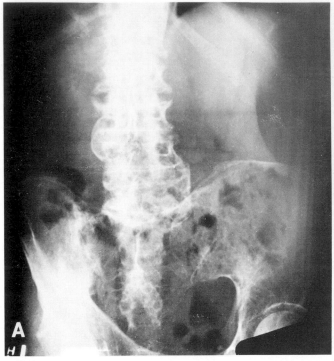

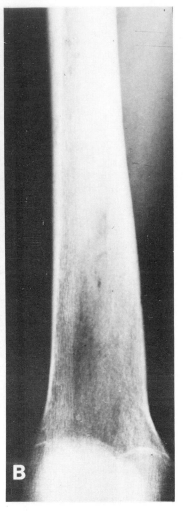

FIG. 6–81. Heavy chain disease. **A.** Spine and pelvis. Extensive destructive changes are present. The pedicles are all intact. **B.** Femur. Permeative destructive changes along the femoral shaft are noted.

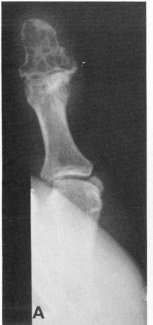

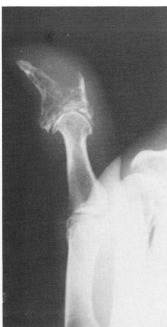

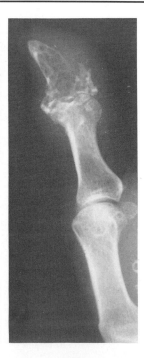

(Continued)

Clinical features of γHCD resemble those of a malignant lymphoma rather than multiple myeloma. Thirty patients have been reported to date, with an age range of 18 to 76 years, but the disease occurs most often in elderly men. Lymphadenopathy and hepatosplenomegaly are common. Bone roentgenograms have been negative in most cases, but bony lesions were visible at autopsy in one patient.

A rare abnormality associated with chronic lymphocytic leukemia is μHCD.

Primary macroglobulinemia[27,255,318,324] (Waldenström's macroglobulinemia) is a disease characterized by excessive proliferation of those plasma cell populations normally responsible for synthesis of I_gM globulins. Large quantities of monoclonal (M type) I_gM globulins are elaborated and associated with a variable clinical pattern featuring anemia, bleeding tendency, and symptoms related to large amounts of macroglobulin in the serum (hyperviscosity syndrome). Men and women are equally affected, and the disease manifests itself in the fifth to sixth decades of life. Background conditions of infections and cholecystitis are often associated. Lymphadenopathy and hepatosplenomegaly develop in some patients, producing a clinical picture of lymphoma or leukemia rather than multiple myeloma. Cold sensitivity, vascular occlusion, gangrene, and Raynaud's phenomenon are cryoglobulin-related symptoms. Bence–Jones proteinuria is present in some patients, but renal functional impairment is less common than in myeloma.

The bone marrow shows an increased number of abnormal lymphocytes and plasma cells. Osteolytic skeletal lesions, although rare in primary macroglobulinemia, do occur, and resemble those seen in multiple myeloma.

Multiple myeloma[114,139,207] is a primary malignant tumor of the bone marrow, characterized by proliferation of cells arising from primitive marrow reticulum that resemble plasma cells. This is the most common primary malignant neoplasm involving bone elements. There is a tendency of the tumor to remain confined to the osseous system, although both involvement of other systems and primary extraskeletal origin may occur. The disease is most often widespread, but may be uncommonly localized to a solitary osseous focus that is called a solitary plasmacytoma. The majority of these lesions disseminate throughout the skeletal system, or arise in multicentric sites (Fig. 6–82); however, an occasional plasmacytoma remains confined to a localized area (Fig. 6–83).

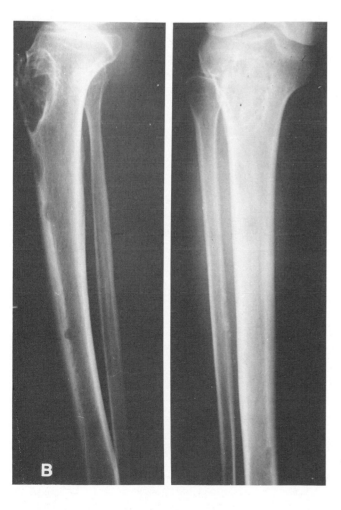

FIG. 6–82. A patient with multicentric plasmacytomas. The patient is still alive 13 years after initial diagnosis. **A.** Expansile destructive trabecular lesion involving the entire distal phalanx of the thumb is noted. **B.** An expansile lesion of the anterior tibial metaphysis is seen with trabeculations, as well as several "punched-out" lesions along the tibial shaft. (Courtesy of Dr. Dharmashi V. Bhate, VA Hospital, Hines, IL)

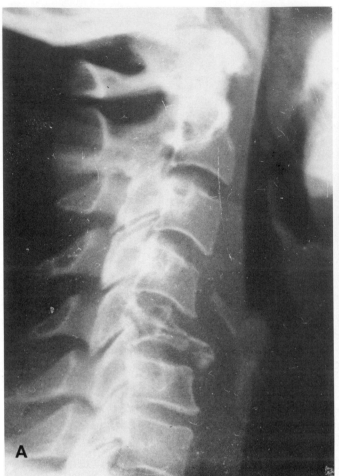

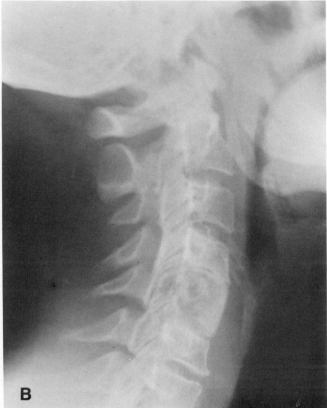

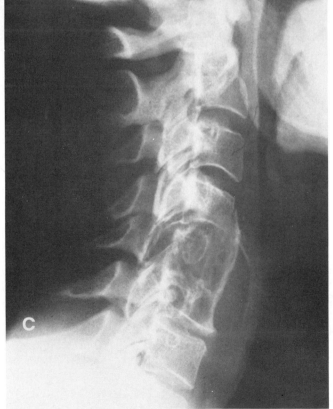

FIG. 6–83. **A.** There is a waferlike collapse of the fifth cervical vertebra. The intervertebral spaces are preserved. This lesion proved to be a solitary plasmacytoma. **B.** Lateral view of cervical spine shows postsurgical changes taken approximately 18 months after surgery. **C.** Six months later. Recurrence of lesion with destruction at the site of previous graft. **D.** CT scan of the fifth cervical vertebral region showing expansion, destruction and trabeculation of the vertebral body. Encroachment on the spinal canal has also resulted in spinal stenosis.

(Continued)

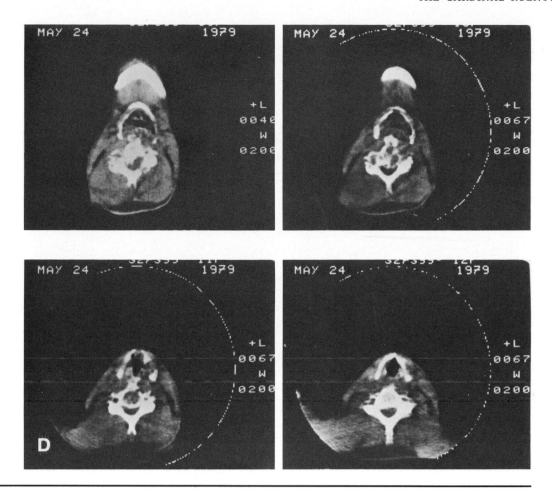

Clinically, 75% of patients are between the ages of 50 and 70 years. Multiple myeloma is definitely rare under the age of 30 years; however, it may occur in the younger age group. Jaffe cites a case with an age of onset of 13 years.[153] Males are affected twice as commonly as females. The symptoms are of insidious onset with vague complaints. Bone pain with progressive severity, usually referred to the lower back, is present in most cases. This can be complicated by pathological vertebral fracture leading to severe pain and paraplegia. Pain in other bones and soft-tissue masses from extraskeletal invasion of myeloma tissue eventually occurs, as well as fever and symptoms resulting from the severe accompanying anemia.

The role of the intravenous pyelogram in this condition has been reevaluated in recent years, and it is now felt that if dehydration is avoided, an IVP is not contraindicated[13] in the absence of renal failure. Renal failure in multiple myeloma is usually not accompanied by hypertension, and is second to

pneumonia as the most frequent cause of death. Hepatosplenomegaly and lymphadenopathy, as well as amyloid or paramyloid deposition, are common. Metastatic calcifications, particularly in the kidneys but occasionally in the lungs and other organs, not infrequently occur.

The blood picture shows a normochromic, normocytic anemia ranging from mild to severe. Marked rouleau formation may be seen in blood smears. The white cell count is usually within normal limits, although numerous plasma cells are occasionally found in the blood, a condition referred to as *plasma-cell leukemia.* Thrombocytopenia, which is partially responsible for the bleeding tendency commonly seen, is also present. The diagnosis can be established by marrow puncture smears when the proportion of plasma cells is greater than 10%. Increased numbers of plasma cells may also be found in Waldenström's macroglobulinemia and F_c fragment (heavy chain) disease.

The serum calcium level is elevated in over 50%

of patients, owing to mobilization of calcium from bones. Hypercalcemia may be present with or without hyperproteinemia. The serum phosphorus level becomes elevated only in the presence of renal insufficiency, which is a frequent concomitant condition. The serum alkaline phosphatase level is within normal limits, except in advanced disease with pathological fractures. The serum uric acid level is elevated, leading to secondary gout.[33]

The serum proteins show characteristic changes. The majority of patients show hyperglobulinemia with reversal of the A/G ratio. In the presence of proteinuria, the serum proteins need not be elevated. The albumin fraction is normal or slightly lowered.

Multiple myeloma is typically associated with a monoclonal increase of immunoglobulins arising from a single clone of antibody-forming cells. This finding is present in certain lymphoproliferative diseases, and has also been found in the serum of patients with nonreticular neoplasms, inflammatory diseases, and in normal-aged individuals. The monoclonal proteins, designated M components, are thought to be normal immunoglobulins present in abnormal quantities. Two distinct M components have been found in some patients.

Bence–Jones protein is the light chain of an immunoglobulin. It is a complete polypeptide chain. It has a peculiar thermal behavior in that it first coagulates and then dissolves at temperatures above 60° C. About 40% of myeloma patients show detectable Bence–Jones proteinuria by the heating method, and a higher percentage may be detected by electrophoresis. A 5% incidence of Bence–Jones proteinuria is said to be observed in such conditions as malignant lymphomas, metastatic bone tumors, idiopathic hemolytic disease, and essential cryoglobulinemia. The protein abnormalities may precede visible bony lesions by several years.

Histologically, multiple myeloma is cellular with no supporting stroma between tumor cells. The cells are plasma cells that vary in size from small to large.

Radiologically, the findings in the skeletal system in myeloma vary widely in extent and pattern, ranging from a solitary focus to overall involvement. The patterns may take the following forms, alone or in combination:

1. Loss of bone density
2. Alteration of bone texture
3. "Punched-out" lesions
4. Diffuse bone destruction
5. Expanding lesions
6. Osteosclerosis[81, 89] (very rarely)
7. Soft-tissue masses.

Loss of bone density results from diffuse marrow involvement with myeloma tissue, causing reduction of the bone trabeculae and thinning of the cortices. It is a roentgen picture similar to that of osteoporosis, and can be most severe (Fig. 6–84). The spine is markedly involved, and a case has been reported in which the vertebral bodies assumed a greater radiolucency than the intervertebral spaces.[309] The trabecular pattern can be accentuated by a similar mechanism, and in the absence of destructive lesions the roentgen appearance may be similar to that of other diseases in which there is a proliferation of marrow elements (Fig. 6–85). The central skeleton is most often affected because of the primary involvement of red marrow. The vertebral bodies, pelvis, ribs, skull, and mandible are most often involved. The vertebral pedicles are involved much less frequently than the bodies because of the lack of red marrow in the pedicles. This has been referred to by Jacobson *et al* as the "pedicle sign," and is a valid differential point between myeloma and osteolytic metastases[152] (Fig. 6–86). However, destruction of an entire posterior vertebral arch may occur.

Loss of bone density in the spine may be the only roentgen sign of multiple myeloma. The radiological hallmark of this disease, however, is the sharply circumscribed "punched-out" lesion. These lesions are multiple, round, sharply marginated, and purely lytic: they may involve the inner surface of the cortex, causing scalloping; and they vary in size and tend to coalesce, destroying large segments of bone. These lesions are widely distributed, and the areas most commonly involved are the skull (Figs. 6–87, 6–88) and the long bones (Fig. 6–89). "Punched-out" vertebral lesions are rare. The outer end of the clavicle and the acromion are frequently involved (Fig. 6–90), as are the ribs. Subglenoid erosion may be seen. Pathological fractures are common, and may also occur in the sternum. The skull base[306] may be involved with a destructive lesion, and a solitary myeloma involving the petrous bone and occiput has been reported.

Severe diffuse bone destruction, particularly of the pelvis (Fig. 6–91) and sacrum, is common, as well as widely scattered, poorly circumscribed destructive lesions. Such bone lesions can resemble osteolytic metastases in every way, and differentiation on the roentgen picture alone is not always possible. The terminal phalanges may also rarely be involved.

Expansion of bone is not uncommon, and there may be a "soap bubble" expansile lesion showing trabeculations, most often in the ribs, long bones,

(*Text continued on p. 427*)

FIG. 6–84. Multiple myeloma (spine). Marked loss of bone density with relative increase of density of the vertebral end-plates. Severe compression of the vertebral bodies is present. In several areas the vertebral bodies actually appear more radiolucent than the intervertebral spaces.

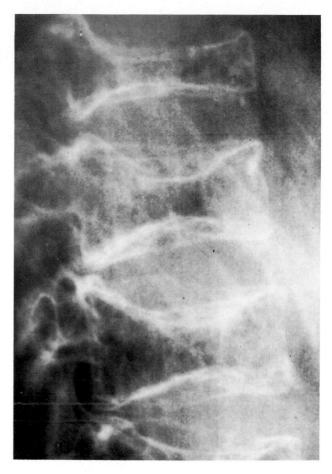

FIG. 6–85. Multiple myeloma (pelvis)—diffuse type. There is loss of bone density and accentuation of the trabecular pattern without frank destructive areas.

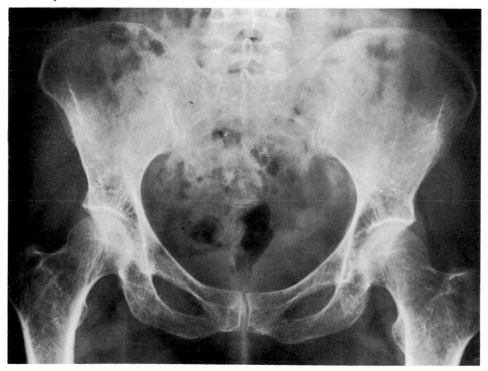

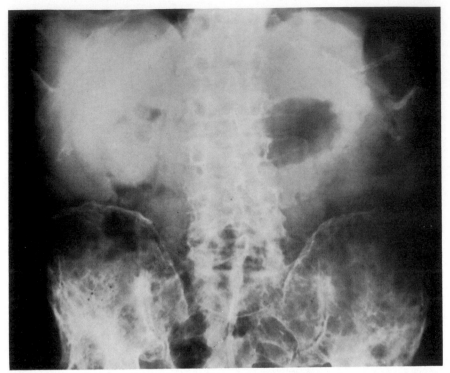

FIG. 6–86. Multiple myeloma (spine and pelvis). Extensive destructive changes in the vertebral bodies with partial collapse of all of the vertebral bodies may be seen, as well as extensive destructive changes in the ilia. The pedicles are all intact. The roentgen pattern is indistinguishable from that of severe osteolytic metastases, however, with this amount of involvement in carcinoma metastases, the pedicles would be expected to show involvement.

FIG. 6–87. Multiple myeloma (skull). Note multiple small, ''punched-out'' radiolucencies.

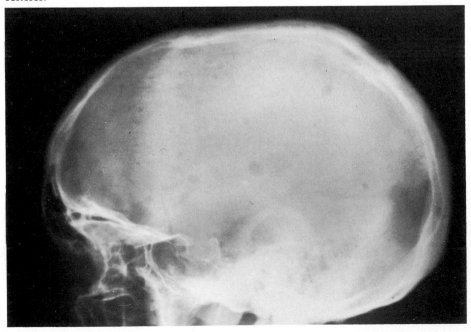

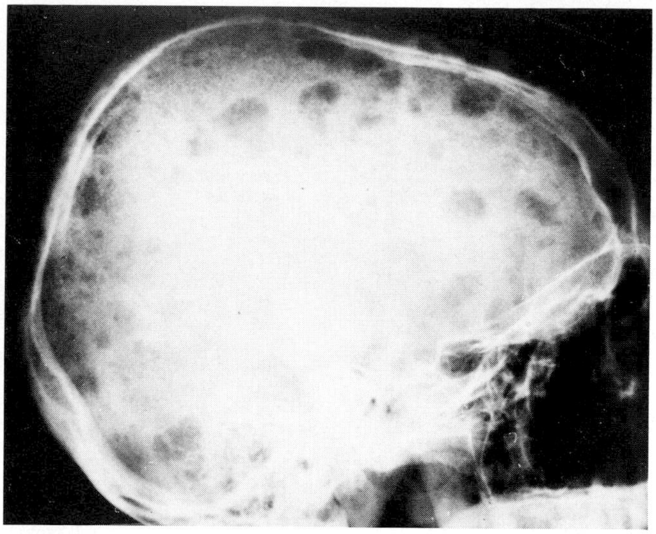

FIG. 6–88. Multiple myeloma (skull). Extensive destruction may be seen, showing multiple well-circumscribed radiolucencies without any reactive sclerotic margin.

FIG. 6–89. Multiple myeloma (hip). Multiple "punched-out" discrete lesions of the proximal femoral shaft are present, along with endosteal scalloping. Note also the extensive destruction in the pelvis.

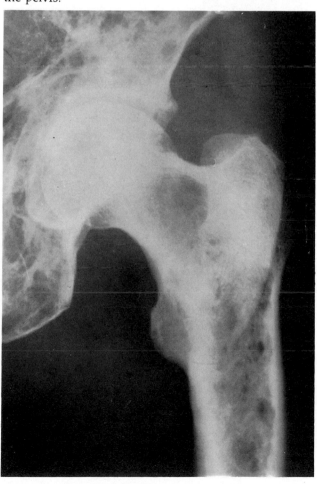

or pelvis. Endosteal scalloping may be present. A solitary myeloma may present with expansion.

Several patterns of bone sclerosis have been described as very rare occurrences. There may be a fine sclerotic margin completely or partially surrounding a "punched-out" lesion. Perpendicular spicules of periosteal new bone formation may be associated with a lesion similar to that seen in osteosarcoma. Focal sclerosis with "ivory vertebrae," or generalized patchy (Fig. 6–92) or uniform bone sclerosis (Fig. 6–93), has been reported, possibly preceding destructive lesions, or in the absence of such lesions. A solitary "ivory vertebra" in the dorsal spine has been reported.[261] Amyloid lesions of bone may exist coexistently with myeloma and may be seen as lytic or expansile. These do not respond to radiation therapy, as does myeloma.[142]

Invasion of soft tissues by myelomatous tumor commonly occurs (Fig. 6–94), and can often be seen as a paraspinal or extrapleural mass (Fig. 6–95). The most common sites of palpable tumor are the ribs, ilium, clavicle, and sternum.

Rarely, the radiological findings and usual criteria for multiple myeloma may be present, but the disease is definitively absent. Metastases or osteoporosis may be responsible. Such a condition has been termed *pseudomyeloma*.[38] Scattered osteoblastic lesions with dense plasmacytic infiltrates, with slow growth and normal laboratory findings, have been reported as *plasma-cell granuloma* rather than myeloma.[303]

(Text continued on p. 431)

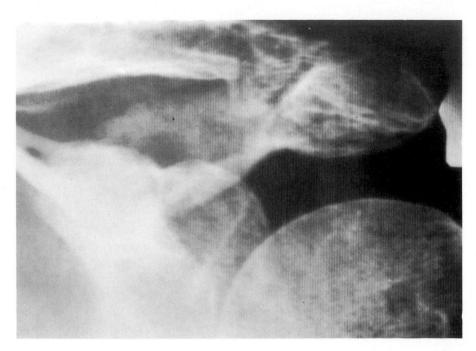

FIG. 9–90. Multiple myeloma (shoulder). A destructive process in the distal clavicle and a destructive and expansile process at the base of the acromion process of the scapula may be seen. A small "punched-out" lesion in the humeral head may also be noted.

FIG. 6–91. Multiple myeloma (pelvis). Marked diffuse destructive changes are present in the ilia, pubis, and ischia, and in the proximal femur.

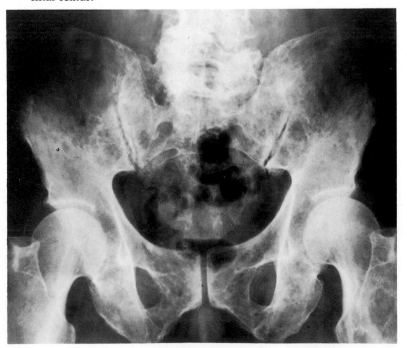

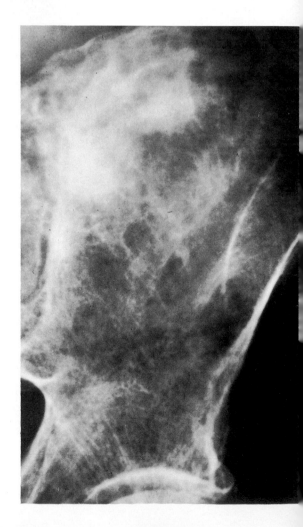

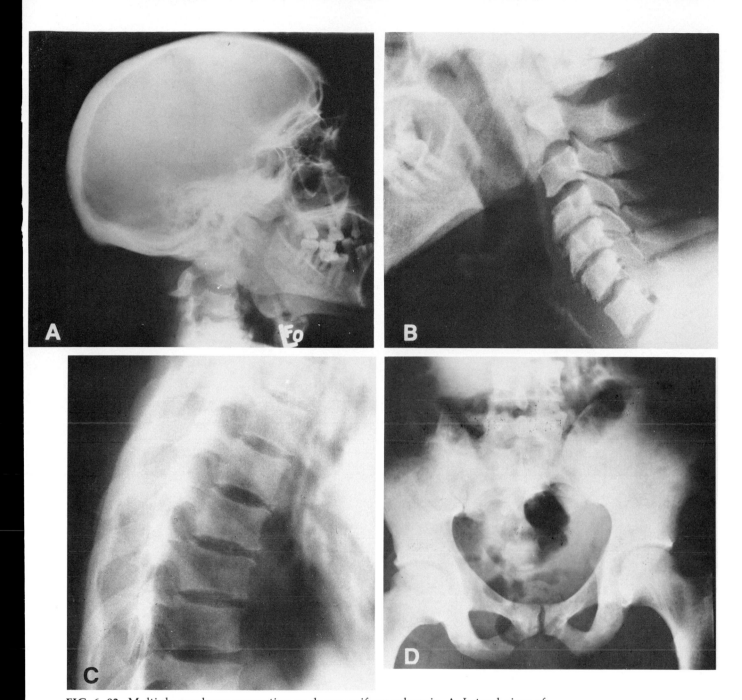

FIG. 6–93. Multiple myeloma presenting as dense uniform sclerosis. A. Lateral view of the skull showing sclerosis about the base of the skull. B. Lateral view of the cervical spine showing marked sclerosis of the bodies of the mid- and lower cervical region. C. Lateral view of the dorsal spine showing uniform sclerosis of the bodies. D. Pelvis. Uniform bony sclerosis is seen.

◀ FIG. 6–92. Osteosclerosis in multiple myeloma (ilium). Patchy sclerotic areas of the ilium are present alongside widespread diffuse destruction. This is a very rare finding in multiple myeloma.

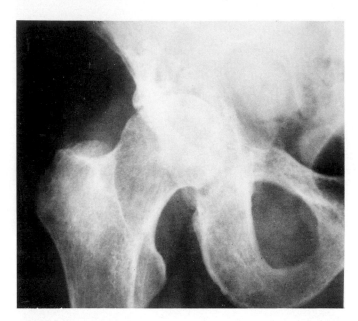

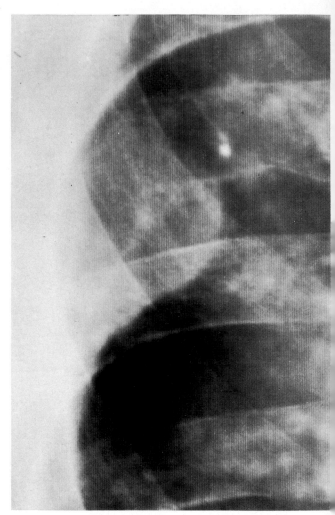

FIG. 6–94. Multiple myeloma (hip). A geographic destructive lesion in the acetabular area is noted, with a large soft-tissue mass extending into the pelvis.

FIG. 6–96. Pseudomonas osteomyelitis (spine) in a drug addict—tomogram. There is narrowing of the intervertebral space with destructive changes at the contiguous vertebral margins.

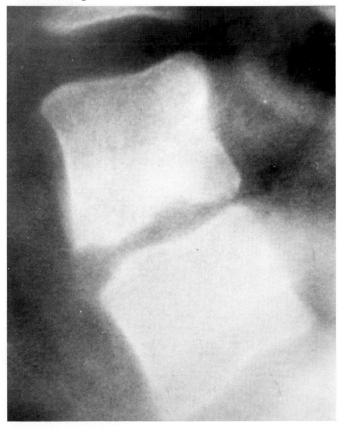

FIG. 6–95. Multiple myeloma (ribs)—rib destruction with extrapleural sign. This is a common finding of multiple myeloma, but may be seen in other conditions as well (see p. 562).

OSTEOMYELITIS

Osteomyelitis is most often caused by *Staphylococcus aureus.* Tuberculous, luetic, and streptococcal osteomyelitis are not infrequent. Salmonella osteomyelitis frequently occurs in children with sickle-cell anemia. There has been a sharp rise in recent years in the incidence of osteomyelitis as a complication of intravenous drug abuse.[168] The most frequent causative organisms are *Pseudomonas aeruginosa*[268] and *Klebsiella aerobacter.* The most frequent site of involvement is the spine (Fig. 6–96), with the sacroiliac joints, symphysis pubis, bony protuberances, and sternoclavicular joints also being affected. Pneumococci, meningococci, brucella, fungi,[37] parasites, and viruses occasionally invade bone. The usual route to bone is through the bloodstream. Osteomyelitis secondary to diabetes mellitus and diabetic gangrene is common. Compound fractures, penetrating wounds, and direct extension from soft-tissue infection are other mechanisms of bone involvement. Osteomyelitis of the ilium complicating Crohn's disease has also been reported.[106] The process may be acute or chronic, localized or diffuse.

ACUTE HEMATOGENOUS OSTEOMYELITIS[45, 108]

Acute hematogenous osteomyelitis is a frequently occurring form of bone infection. It usually affects infants and children, but adults are not immune. There is a latent period of about 10 days between the onset of symptoms and evidence of bony roentgen change. Soft-tissue changes may be seen after 3 days. The invading bacteria settle in the terminal capillary loops of the metaphysis and epiphysis, causing multiple abscesses and bone destruction. This initial focus may follow several pathways. It may penetrate the articular cartilage into the joint, an event which is more common in adults than children. The process may extend to involve a part or all of the medullary canal. Most commonly, pus spreads through the haversian system to the subperiosteal space. The periosteum is stripped from the cortex and elevated as the pressure from the pyogenic process increases. The cortex has two sources of blood supply, the nutrient vessels and the periosteal vessels. The nutrient branches are occluded by bacterial emboli. The periosteal vessels are ruptured by the process of elevation. Thus, deprived of its blood supply, the bone dies. The periosteum retains its osteogenic properties and forms new bone at its elevated site, enclosing the dead shaft. The dead bone is called the sequestrum

and the new shell of bone is called the involucrum. New bone also forms from cortex and endosteum. The regional uninvolved bone becomes osteoporotic, due to disuse and possibly the action of toxins. Associated soft-tissue inflammation occurs more commonly in infants than in children or adults. Defects in the involucrum called cloaca are usually present, and permit the discharge of pus and debris. On healing, the involucrum remodels and gradually assumes a normal contour. The process may become chronic and continue indefinitely. The infection may localize to form an abscess, or a low-grade sclerosing osteitis may occur without suppuration.

Radiologically, no osseous findings are present in the initial stages of the disease. The first sign is localized, deep soft-tissue swelling adjacent to the metaphysis of a growing bone with displacement of the lucent deep muscle plane away from the bone, followed by obliteration of the lucent planes between the muscles. In infants or children, the earliest osseous roentgen sign is a metaphyseal area of bone destruction (Figs. 6–97, 6–98, 6–99). Destructive changes may also be present in the epiphyseal ossification center (Fig. 6–100) and extend down the shaft (Figs. 6–101, 6–102). Periosteal new bone formation occurs as a solid or cloaking pattern, forming the involucrum in the involved area. The cortex becomes sequestered (Fig. 6–103) and multiple defects are seen. The periosteum may also show a laminated (Fig. 6–104) or spiculated appearance (Fig. 6–105). Regional osteoporosis occurs, and as the sequestrum becomes separated by granulation tissue, it stands out as chalky white. This relative radio-density is a requisite for designation of a fragment of bone as a sequestrum. Sequestra vary widely in size and may be situated within the involucrum or be extruded through a cloaca (Fig. 6–106). The cloaca leaves areas of intact cortex between destroyed segments, in contrast to a malignant tumor, which usually destroys the involved area uniformly (Fig. 6–107). An exception to this rule is Ewing's sarcoma. Antibiotic treatment diminishes the destructive phase and accentuates the involucrum. Residual epiphyseal damage may cause shortening of the bone or a "ball-and-socket" metaphyseal deformity. Destruction of the epiphysis[259] and metaphysis may lead to bizarre residual deformities with malalignment. Part of the etiology is ischemia following occlusion of the blood supply. Increase in bone length may be caused by chronic hyperemia.

In infants, the infection is usually caused by a streptococcus. Soft-tissue and joint involvement

(Text continued on p. 437)

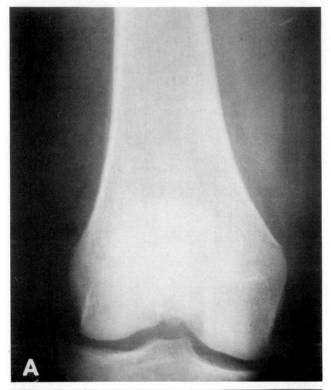

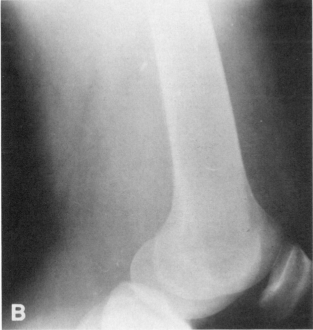

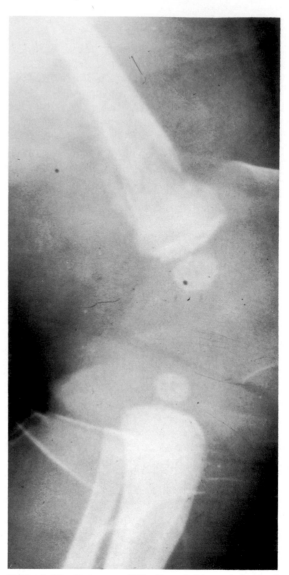

FIG. 6–98. Osteomyelitis (knee) in an infant. A large metaphyseal destructive area in the distal femur is present.

FIG. 6–97. Distal femur—osteomyelitis—anteroposterior view. **A.** Thin line of periosteal new bone formation at the distal medial femur is noted. **B.** Lateral view of the distal femur shows periosteal new bone formation posteriorly, as well as deep soft-tissue swelling.

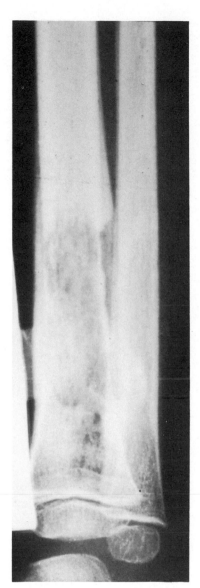

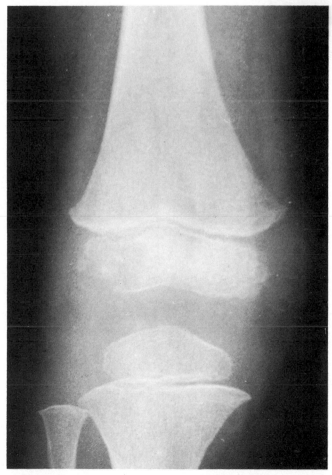

FIG. 6–99. Acute hematogenous osteomyelitis (leg). There is a large area of destruction involving the metaphysis and the distal tibial shaft, associated with solid periosteal new bone formation.

FIG. 6–100. Pyogenic epiphysitis. A destructive area at the lateral aspect of the distal femoral epiphysis is present. (Courtesy of Dr. Harvey White, Children's Memorial Hospital, Chicago, IL)

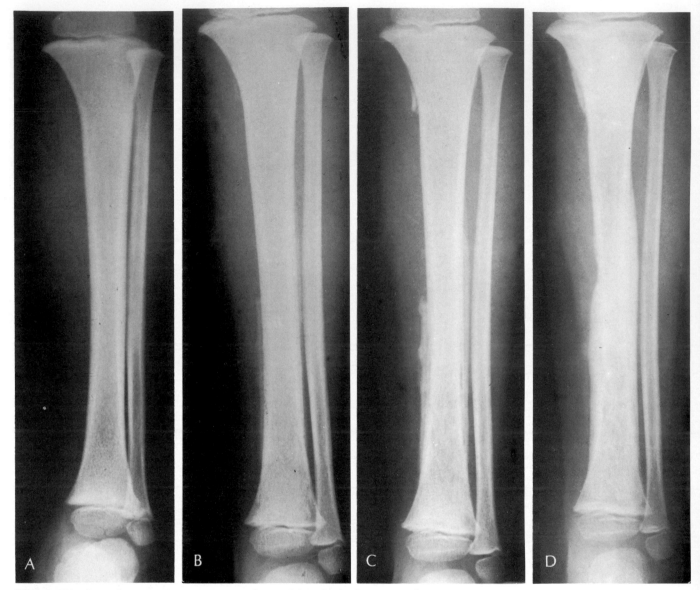

FIG. 6–101. Acute hematogenous osteomyelitis (tibia). **A.** At the onset of symptoms no visible bone changes are present. **B.** Two-week interval after. **A.** Note extensive periosteal new bone formation of the solid type along the tibial shaft, associated with light metaphyseal destructive changes at the distal end. **C.** One-week interval after **B.** Note thickening of the periosteal new bone, and permeative destructive change along the distal tibial shaft. A small area of periosteal new bone formation along the proximal medial tibial shaft may also be seen. **D.** Five-week interval after **C.** Note extensive thickened solid periosteal new bone formation with small scattered areas of radiolucency in the distal tibial shaft (see Fig. 6–102).

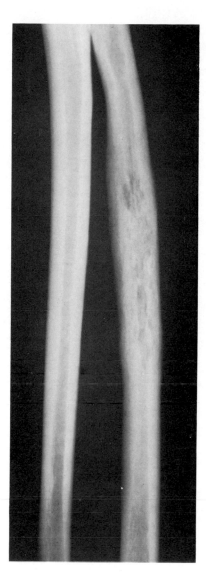

FIG. 6–102. Osteomyelitis in a patient with sickle-cell anemia. Note permeative destructive changes in the midshaft of the radius. The midshaft is more frequently involved in sickle-cell disease with osteomyelitis, because a diaphyseal infarct forms a locus for deposition of circulating bacteria.

FIG. 6–103. Osteomyelitis (tibia). There is sequestration of the cortex with an involucrum peripherally, separated by cortical bone which shows several small white areas. The roentgen criteria for sequestrum are separation of bone and a chalky white appearance. Air in the soft tissues may also be noted.

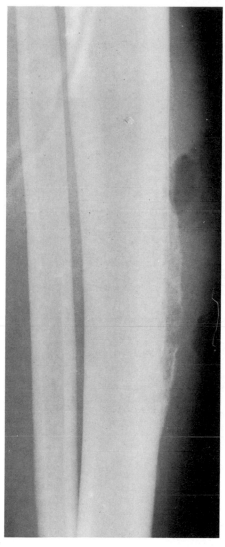

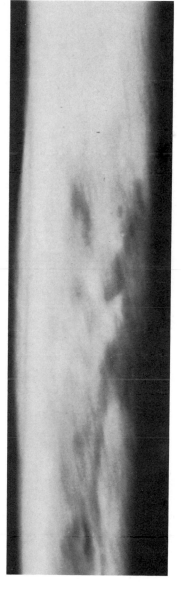

FIG. 6–104. Osteomyelitis—tomogram. Note laminated periosteal new bone formation and chalky white sequestra within destructive areas. The periosteal laminations are thick and solid.

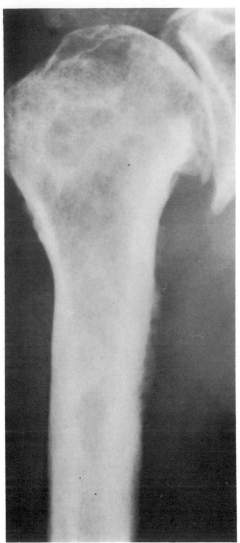

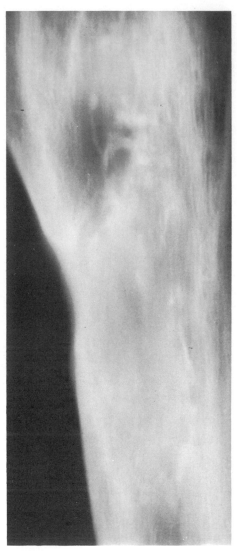

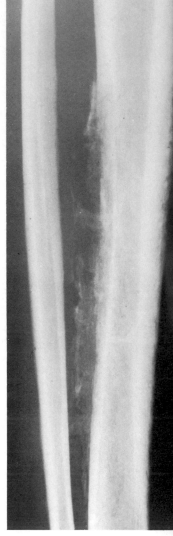

FIG. 6–105   FIG. 6–106   FIG. 6–107

FIG. 6–105. Osteomyelitis (humerus) showing spiculated type of periosteal elevation along the upper medial shaft of the humerus. The spiculations are short and thick in contrast to the fine long spiculations commonly seen in osteosarcoma.

FIG. 6–106. Osteomyelitis—tomogram. Multiple small chalky white sequestra may be seen. There is a loss of cortex, indicating a cloaca through which pus and sequestra may extrude.

FIG. 6–107. Cortical destruction and involucrum formation by osteomyelitis. The destroyed segment of cortex has areas of normal cortex interspersed through it, which helps to differentiate this process from a malignant tumor. A Codman's triangle is formed at the superior aspect of the process.

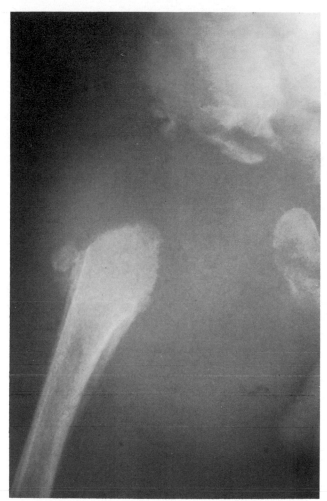

FIG. 6–108. Osteomyelitis and septic arthritis (hip joint) in an infant, with marked widening of the hip joint space. There are destructive changes about the acetabulum and periosteal elevation of the femoral shaft.

(Fig. 6–108) are more common than in older children. There is less tendency to form sequestra and healing is more rapid. The epiphyseal cartilage plate forms a barrier against spread after the age of 8 months. Adults also show a somewhat different picture. There is a greater tendency toward involvement of a joint in adults than in children. The infection may be localized to the metaphysis or the shaft. Adult osteomyelitis shows a greater tendency to chronicity.

In children, nontubular bones may also be involved, particularly if multiple sites are affected. The most common flat bone to be involved is the pelvis, with a predilection for the sacroiliac area. This site is followed in frequency by the clavicle and the calcaneus.[203]

The flat and irregular bones can be considered to have anatomic subdivisions analogous to long bones. Prior to skeletal maturation, areas adjacent to joints and apophyses are claimed to have metaphyseal-type vascular anatomy.[223] These metaphyseal equivalent sites, such as the areas adjacent to the sacroiliac joint or triradiate cartilage, and so forth, are said to harbor 30% of hematogenous osteomyelitis to nontubular bones.

CHRONIC OSTEOMYELITIS

Chronic osteomyelitis appears as a thickened, irregular, sclerotic bone, containing several radiolucent areas, with elevated periosteum (Figs. 6–109, 6–110, 6–111, 6–112). A destructive area may uncommonly develop rapidly at the site of a chronic draining sinus (Fig. 6–113). This is usually due to a squamous cell carcinoma,[160] although the development of a fibrosarcoma has also been reported at this site.[161, 204] Squamous cell carcinomas at this site can metastasize.[93] Chronic sclerosing osteitis (Garré) is a low-grade chronic infection causing sclerotic reaction without destruction or sequestration (Fig. 6–114). It is a rare condition. In the spine, osteomyelitis causes vertebral destruction and collapse. Earliest changes may only be detected on the radionuclide scan. A subtle destruction of a portion of the cortex of a vertebral body may initially occur. This may progress to total destruction of the vertebral body associated with a soft-tissue abscess.[213] The intervertebral space is usually involved (Fig. 6–115), while it is not in neoplasm. Intervertebral-diskspace inflammation in children is a not uncommon clinical entity, usually due to *Staphylococcus aureus*.[295] Involvement of the atlantoaxial region with complete disappearance of the odontoid

(Text continued on p. 441)

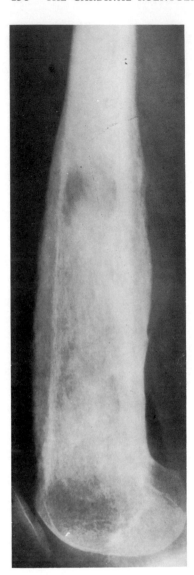

FIG. 6–109. Chronic osteomyelitis (femur). Note marked thickening of the diaphysis in the involved area, along with scattered radiolucent destructive areas and solid periosteal new bone formation. Also note bone sclerosis.

FIG. 6–110. Chronic osteomyelitis (femur). Note very marked thickening of the femoral shaft with bone sclerosis and a "lacelike" periosteal new bone formation. The sequestered cortex lies centrally, giving a "bone-within-a-bone" appearance. Fracture of the femoral neck with destructive changes in the femoral head may also be seen.

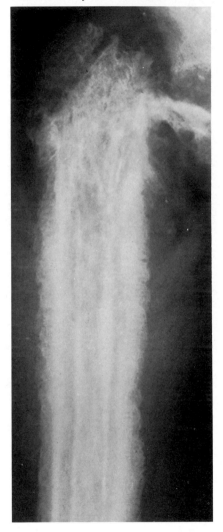

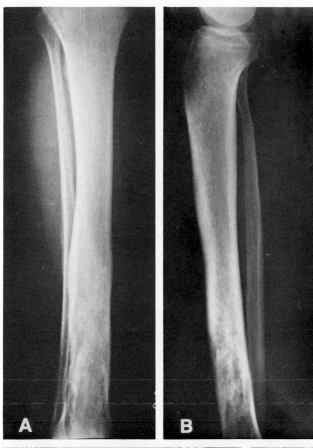

FIG. 6–111. Chronic osteomyelitis of the tibia. A, B. Anteroposterior and lateral views showing expansion and patchy radiolucency and sclerosis as well as sequestration. C. CT scan showing enlargement of the bone with thickening of the cortex and central sequestration on the left. Compare to normal right tibia.

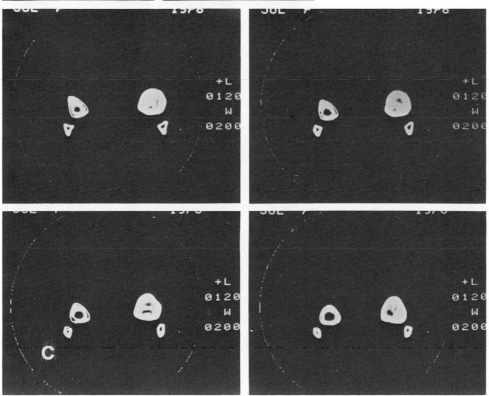

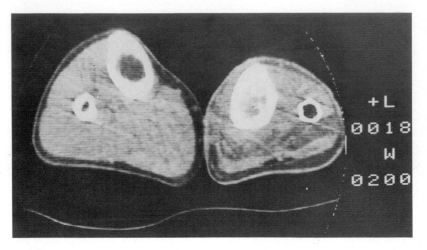

FIG. 6–112. Osteomyelitis of the tibia in an amputation stump. The left tibia shows cortical thickening and sequestration in the medulla. Comparison of the density of the marrow cavity with the fibula and the normal right tibia shows that the central density has been elevated to that of soft tissue by the infectious process. Atrophy of the left leg, secondary to more distal amputation, is also noted.

FIG. 6–113

FIG. 6–114

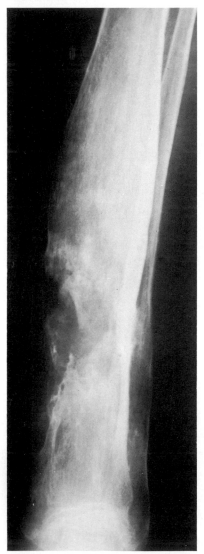

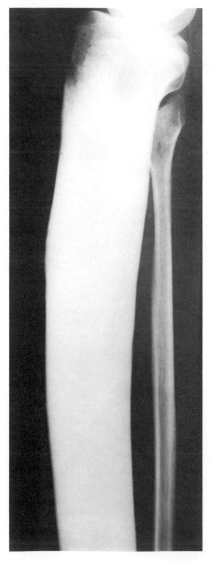

FIG. 6–113. Chronic osteomyelitis (leg) with the development of a large destructive area at drainage site. There is marked widening of the shaft of the tibia and, to a lesser extent, of the fibula. An irregular area of bone destruction at the distal medial aspect of the tibia is associated with soft tissue irregularity. Note localized cortical destruction. This appearance was due to the development of a squamous cell carcinoma at a chronic draining site.

FIG. 6–114. Chronic sclerosing osteitis Garré (leg). Diffuse sclerosis of the tibia without marked destruction or periosteal reaction is present, in contrast to the normal architecture of the fibula.

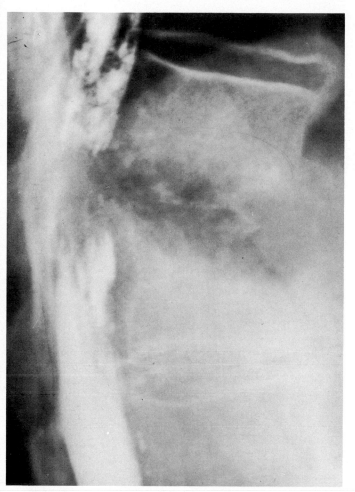

FIG. 6–115. Osteomyelitis (spine) causing spinal cord compression. There is involvement of the intervertebral space and destruction of the contiguous vertebral margins. Note irregularity of the margins of the process, and pressure from the abscess into the spinal canal on the myelogram.

process has been reported.[4] The process in bone may be localized to form an abscess. This usually occurs at the end of a bone, and characteristically appears as a radiolucent area with a sclerotic margin or a central sequestrum (Fig. 6–116).

An irregular, marginated tract to the cartilage plate and epiphyseal ossification center may sometimes by seen. Occasionally, a chronic abscess that has never had an acute stage is seen. This is a painful lesion surrounded by marked sclerosis, and is known as Brodie's abscess (Figs. 6–117, 6–118, 6–119, 6–120). It is usually in the metaphysis, but presents in a spectrum of radiological appearances. One-third of the lesions are in the diaphysis, half show cortical thickening, 40% show periosteal new bone formation, and 20% contain sequestra.[200] An amorphous calcification in the adjacent soft tissues may rarely be seen. Brodie's abscess is similar in appearance to osteoid osteoma but can be differentiated by lack of vascular flush in a nidus or an arteriogram and lack of enhancement on postinfusion CT scan.[184] Osteomyelitis in flat bones appears as a mixture of patchy destruction and sclerosis. It may not be possible radiologically to differentiate osteomyelitis from Ewing's sarcoma, particularly in the pelvis or calcaneus. Involvement of the metatarsal sesamoid bones has been reported secondary to neuropathy, or as the site of hematogenous osteomyelitis.

SECONDARY OSTEOMYELITIS

Secondary osteomyelitis results from spread of infection to bone from the contiguous soft tissues. This most commonly occurs in the feet and hands of diabetic patients, as well as in patients with other types of vascular insufficiency. The infection may spread from a skin abscess or a decubitus ulcer to cause destruction of adjacent bones and joints. Gram-negative osteomyelitis has been reported following puncture wounds of the foot.[199] There may be purely destructive changes, or more rarely a marked degree of osteosclerosis and periosteal new bone formation (Figs. 6–121 to 6–125).

A remarkable degree of reconstitution of bone in the toes of patients with diabetic osteomyelitis has been reported. This seems to indicate that lack of visibility of bone in these instances is partly caused by osteoporosis rather than frank destruction.

(Text continued on p. 447)

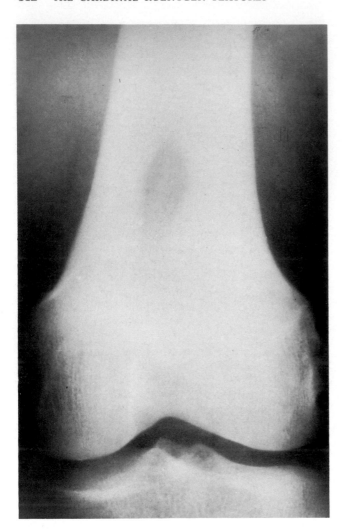

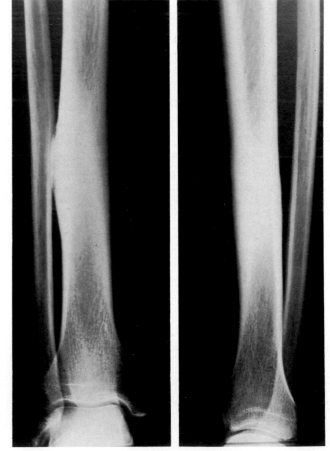

FIG. 6–116. Brodie's abscess (distal femur). Radiolucent area with surrounding reactive diffuse sclerosis is noted.

FIG. 6–117. Chronic cortical abscess (leg)—anteroposterior and lateral views. Localized thickening of the cortex of the tibial shaft may be seen. On lateral view a small radiolucent area may be noted, which proved surgically to be an abscess. It is not possible to differentiate this process from an osteoid osteoma on conventional roentgen film.

FIG. 6–118. Brodie's abscess (distal tibia). Radiolucent lesion with slight surrounding reactive sclerosis is noted.

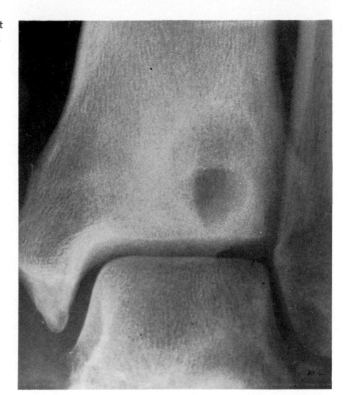

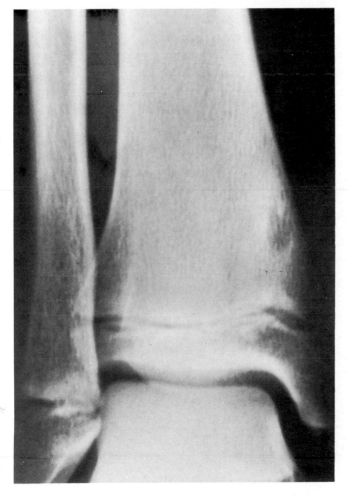

FIG. 6–119. Brodie's abscess (ankle). Small cortical radiolucency with minimal surrounding sclerosis is noted.

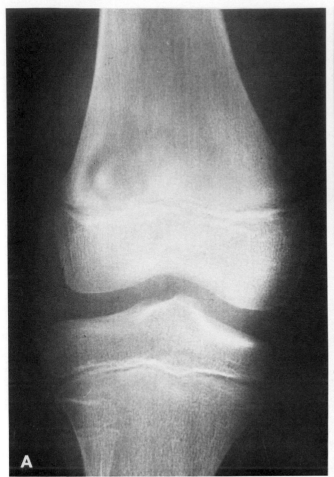

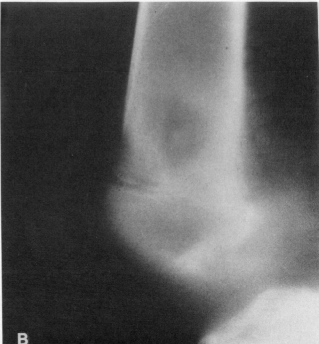

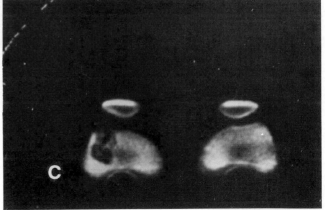

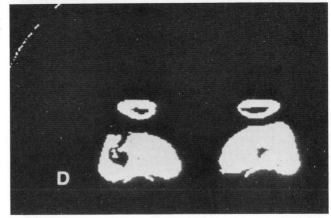

FIG. 6–120. Adolescent with metaphyseal osteomyelitis containing a sequestrum. **A.** A radiolucency of the lateral aspect of the distal femoral metaphysis is noted which contains a dense sequestrum. **B.** Lateral tomogram confirming the presence of radiolucency with a sequestrum. In addition, cortical breakthrough at the anterior aspect is seen. **C, D.** CT scans at two different windows and levels. A destructive lesion at the lateral aspect of the right femoral metaphysis is seen which contains a sequestrum and is seen to open into the anterior cortex. There is an increase in the patello-femoral distance on the right as well.

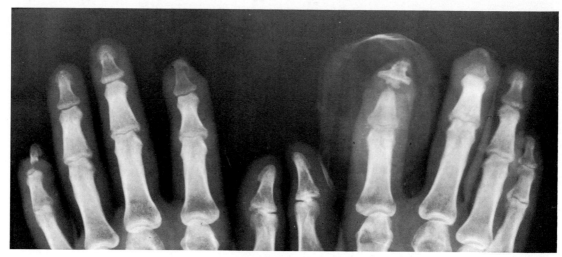

FIG. 6–121. Secondary osteomyelitis (hands) due to diabetes. Bony destructive areas of several of the phalanges without sclerosis of periosteal reaction may be noted bilaterally.

FIG. 6–122. Osteomyelitis and septic arthritis (hip joint) from a decubitus ulcer in a paraplegic. Note destruction of the femoral neck with bony debris, and soft-tissue air in a decubitus ulcer.

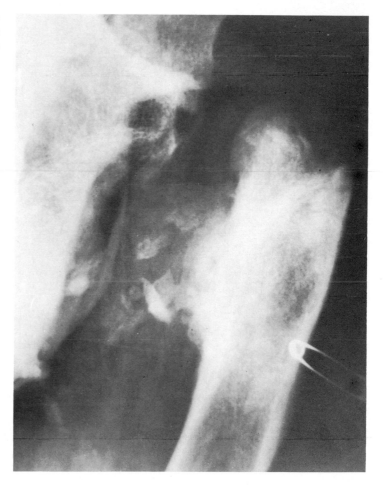

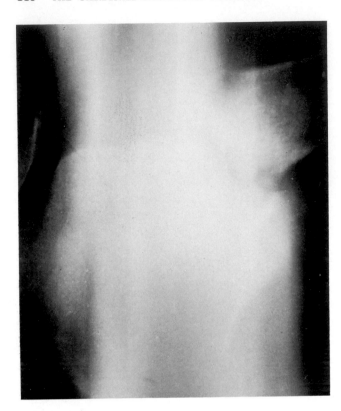

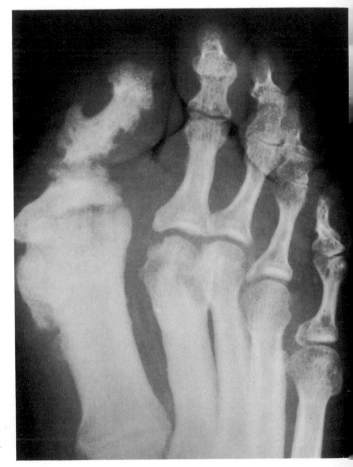

FIG. 6–123. Osteomyelitis and septic arthritis of the left sternoclavicular joint secondary to a pin prick—tomogram. Note narrowing of the joint space and marginal irregularity, and the destructive area at the clavicle.

FIG. 6–124. Osteomyelitis (foot) secondary to diabetes. Destructive changes are associated with marked sclerotic changes of the great toe and metatarsal and with cortical thickening in the adjacent metatarsals.

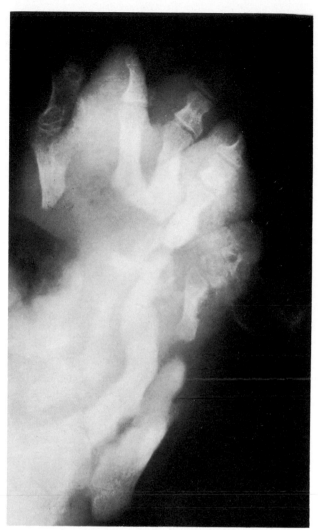

FIG. 6–125. Diabetic osteomyelitis (foot). Extreme destruction of the metatarsals with osteosclerotic reaction, marked soft-tissue swelling, and a large soft-tissue ulcer medially.

TUBERCULOUS OSTEOMYELITIS[176, 247]

Tuberculous osteomyelitis is much less common than tuberculous arthritis. Bone involvement may occur in the presence or absence of pulmonary tuberculosis. It is most common in patients under 30 years of age. Usually the acute symptoms of osteomyelitis are lacking, although in some cases inflammatory signs may be prominent.

Radiologically, the findings are similar to those of pyogenic osteomyelitis, except that osteoporosis is usually seen earlier and is more pronounced, while sclerotic and periosteal reaction is less, and there is less tendency toward sequestration. The sites of involvement are generally the same as in pyogenic infection, and definitive differentiation on a roentgen basis alone usually cannot be made.

The long bones may show involvement with a destructive lesion in the epiphyses, metaphyses, or diaphyses (Figs. 6–126, 6–127). In the short tubular bones, particularly phalanges, a characteristic expansile lesion may occasionally be seen, with trabecular destruction, cortical destruction, and a ballooned-out appearance. This is the "spina ventosa tuberculosa," which can be differentiated from a somewhat similar dactylitis of lues by the lack of cortical thickening and the lack of a dense shell (Figs. 6–128, 6–129). Spina ventosa usually occurs in children, but may occur in adults.[91] It has also been reported in the metacarpals, metatarsals, ulnae, and humeri. Twenty-five percent of cases have multiple peripheral lesions. Initially, soft-tissue swelling may be present. In addition to spina ventosa, a lesion composed of deossification, periosteal reaction, destruction, and pathological fracture may be seen in adults. Diffuse sclerosis of a short tubular bone with scattered areas of destruction and marked periostitis is another picture that may be seen, as well as honeycombing of bone with or without a pathological fracture. Chronic draining sinuses are common. If a joint is involved, severe osteoporosis of the extremity distal to the joint is characteristic.

In the flat bones, "punched-out" cystlike lesions with little or no reactive sclerosis are typical (Figs. 6–130, 6–131). There may be secondary infection of chronic draining sinuses, causing a mixed infection that is indistinguishable from pyogenic osteomyelitis.

Disseminated bone tuberculosis with multiple cystlike, scattered lesions is a rare form that may be seen in both children and adults. Hypercalcemia may be associated.[228]

One of the most common sites of involvement is the spine. The usual locus of infection is the centrum of a body, leading to destruction of vertebrae and intervertebral spaces, and causing collapse (Fig. 6–132), gibbus formation, reactive sclerosis (Fig. 6–133), and a calcified (Fig. 6–134) or noncalcified paraspinal soft-tissue mass and psoas abscess. This

(Text continued on p. 453)

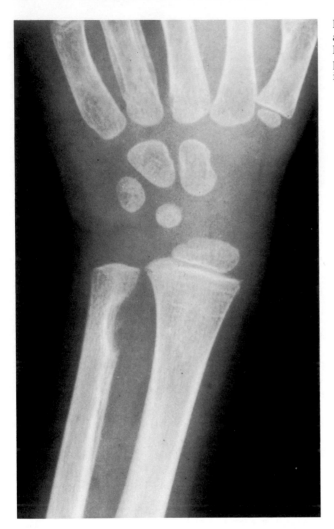

FIG. 6–126. Tuberculosis. Destructive metaphyseal lesion at the distal ulna is seen. There is regional osteoporosis. Note the slight degree of periosteal new bone formation proximal to the lesion, and periosteal new bone formation in the fourth metacarpal.

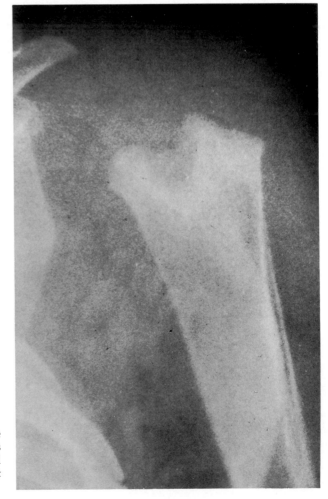

FIG. 6–127. Tuberculosis (humerus). Metaphyseal destructive lesion in the center of the proximal humeral metaphysis is noted. There is no marked degree of osteoporosis. A small amount of periosteal new bone formation at the lateral aspect of the humeral shaft is present.

FIG. 6–128. Tuberculosis (fingers). Expansion of the third proximal phalanx with a thin cortex and lack of sclerotic reaction is noted. This is called the "spina ventosa tuberculosa."

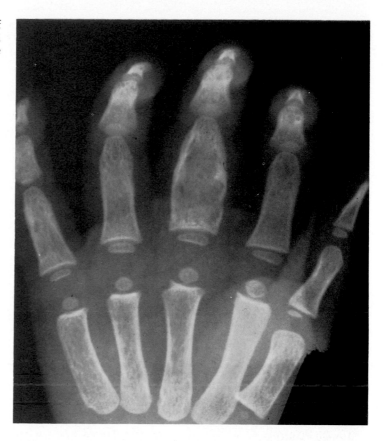

FIG. 6–129. Tuberculosis (hand). Expansion of the third proximal phalanx with a thin cortex is seen—spina ventosa tuberculosa. Soft-tissue swelling is also present.

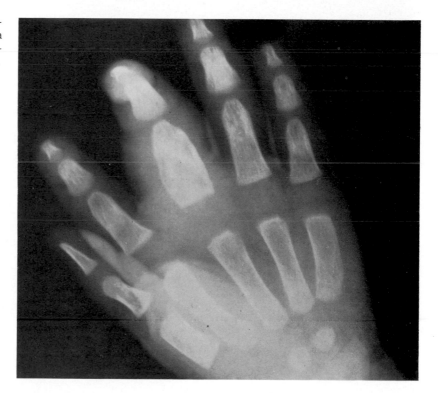

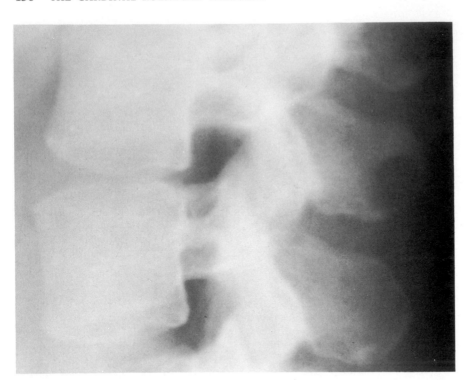

FIG. 6–130. Tuberculosis (spine). "Punched-out" lytic lesion in the spinous process with no reactive sclerotic change is noted.

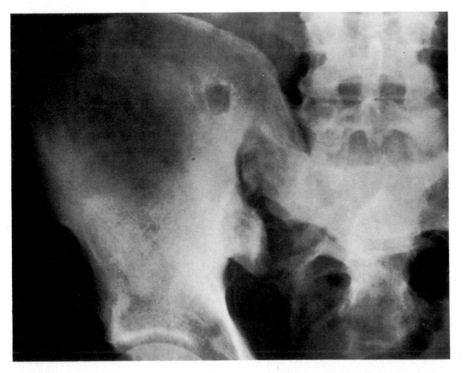

FIG. 6–131. Tuberculosis (flat bones). There is a destructive process of the right sacroiliac joint with no reactive sclerosis. Also note the small "punched-out" lesion in the ilium.

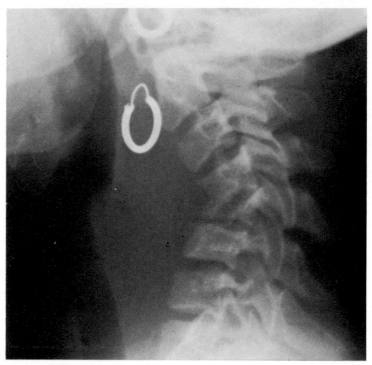

FIG. 6-132. Tuberculosis (cervical spine). There is collapse of the body of the fifth cervical vertebra with destruction of the adjacent intervertebral space. A large retrolaryngeal mass with calcifications is present.

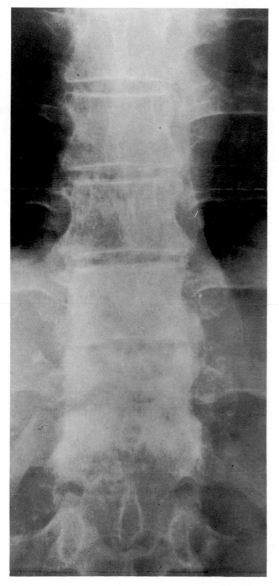

FIG. 6-133. Tuberculosis with involvement of the lower dorsal vertebrae and intervertebral spaces. Note a paraspinal soft-tissue mass, and reactive sclerosis in the lower dorsal vertebral bodies.

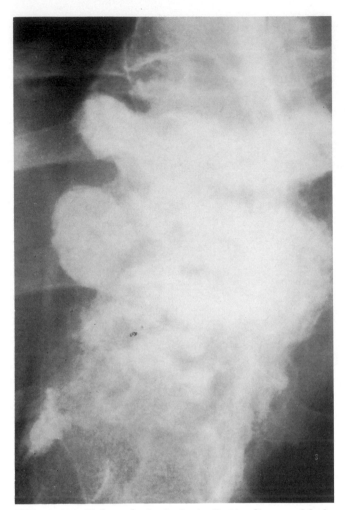

FIG. 6–134. Tuberculosis (spine)—Pott's disease. Markedly calcified soft-tissue paraspinal mass in the involved area.

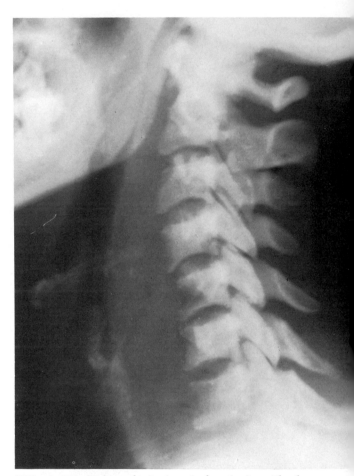

FIG. 6–135. Tuberculosis (cervical spine), with destruction of the anterior aspects of the vertebral bodies. There is no vertebral collapse and the intervertebral spaces are preserved. A retrolaryngeal and retrotracheal abscess is present. This represents the rare form of spinal tuberculosis with anterior involvement.

FIG. 6–136. Elbow. *Mycobacterium kansasii.* Multiple ▶ destructive, well-marginated, radiolucent areas are seen. On anteroposterior view the lesion in the proximal ulna has an overhanging margin. (Courtesy of Dr. Dharmashi V. Bhate, VA Hospital, Hines, IL)

is the picture of Pott's disease. More rarely, the anterior aspects of the vertebral bodies may be involved with anterior destruction, associated with an anterior cold abscess but without vertebral collapse (Fig. 6–135). This may occur in the retropharyngeal and retrotracheal regions. Tuberculosis of the vertebral pedicles[17] occurs in about 2% of spinal cases. The pedicles may be destroyed unilaterally or bilaterally, isolated or at multiple levels. Large paravertebral abscesses are present, which may lead to paraplegia. Healing may show restoration of the pedicles. Tuberculosis of the ribs[331] and of the sphenoid bone[328] has also been reported.

ATYPICAL ACID-FAST BACILLI[61,77,140]

Atypical acid-fast bacilli may also cause osteomyelitis. The classification comprises photochromogens (including *Mycobacterium kanasii, Mycobacterium marinum*),[325] scotochromogens, nonchromogens (Battey type), and rapid-growers. The bony lesions may be similar to those of tuberculous osteomyelitis or arthritis. Scattered central radiolucent defects with variable margins of sclerosis (Fig. 6–136), or bone sclerosis with periostitis, have been described.

BCG OSTEOMYELITIS[20,84,206]

BCG osteomyelitis is an infrequent complication. Osteolytic lesions similar to those seen in tuberculosis have been reported. A metaphyseal destructive or cystic lesion that sometimes extends into the epiphysis may be seen. The clinical picture is that of a low-grade osteomyelitis.

CHRONIC GRANULOMATOUS DISEASE OF CHILDHOOD[330]

Chronic granulomatous disease of childhood is a usually fatal, genetically transmitted syndrome affecting males, based on inability of leukocytes to kill certain organisms after phagocytosis. A granulomatous response is manifested in many organs and in the skeleton. The causative organisms include *Serratia marcescens, Aerobacter aerogenes, Staphylococcus aureus,* and *Aspergillus fumigatus.* The roentgen picture is that of osteomyelitis with a predilection for the small bones of the hands and feet. Expansion, similar to that seen in tuberculous spina ventosa, may be seen, probably due to granulomatous changes.

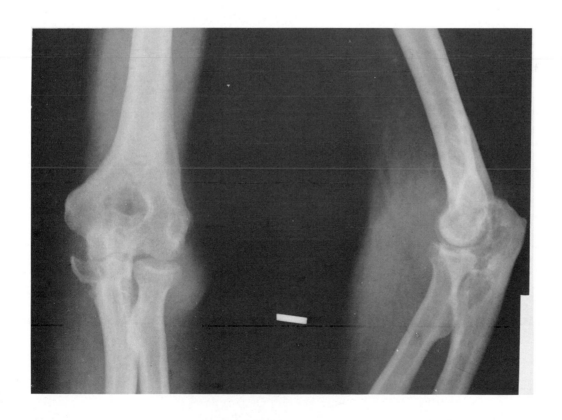

VIRUS OSTEOMYELITIS[288]

Osteomyelitis may also be caused by fungi, echinococcus and viruses,[62] particularly smallpox[216] and rubella viruses.

Smallpox is claimed by the WHO to be eradicated, but time will tell if this is true. *Osteomyelitis variolosa* is a complication of smallpox that results in deformities with shortening, tapering, and resorption of bone. Rubella is discussed elsewhere.

Vaccinia osteomyelitis is a very rare complication of vaccination, which may be related to infantile cortical hyperostosis.[288] Bone destruction, sequestration, and periostitis may occur. Cytomegalic inclusion disease may cause bone changes similar to rubella with loss of density and streaking of the metaphysis.

LUETIC OSTEOMYELITIS

Luetic osteomyelitis may be present in congenital syphilis (Chap. 4) or in the acquired form. In acquired syphilis, bone lesions are usually seen in the tertiary stage, however they have been reported in the primary and secondary stages,[68] and may present as dense periostitis, bone sclerosis, gummatous destruction, luetic osteomyelitis (Figs. 6–137, 6–138), or neurotrophic changes. Irregular cortical thickening may be present, and at the anterior tibia this produces the characteristic "sabre shin." Periosteal reaction may be irregular or lacelike, or may show spiculation perpendicular to the shaft of the bone. The latter change is usually associated with a gumma. Gumma formation is often seen as an area of destruction within sclerotic and thickened bone, with permeative destruction in the flat bones or calvarium (Fig. 6–139). Isolated gummas with little or no surrounding changes may also be seen. The lesions tend to be anterior.

Neurotrophic manifestations may appear as resorption of bone or as the classical Charcot's joint with dense bony sclerosis, fragmentation, and marked soft-tissue debris. The atrophic form of Charcot's joint is most commonly seen in the shoulder. There is resorption of the head of the humerus with soft-tissue debris and possibly sclerotic changes. This is similar in appearance to the neurotrophic joint found in syringomyelia, other neurological conditions, and diabetes mellitus (Fig. 6–140). The dense productive type of Charcot's joint is most often seen in the knees and the spine[157] (Figs. 6–141, 6–142).

LEUKEMIA

Radiologically detectable skeletal involvement in *leukemia*[35,207] occurs in 50% to 70% of cases of childhood leukemia and up to 10% of cases in adults. It is not correct to state that these lesions represent metastases, but rather primary bone involvement from neoplastic proliferation of marrow elements.

The chief clinical complaint is pain in the bones and joints in patients with bone involvement. There may be bone pain without demonstrable lesions, and demonstrable lesions without pain. Arthralgia may be due to referred pain from nearby bone lesions or leukemic synovial infiltrates. The roentgen appearance of the osseous system in leukemia is somewhat different in children and adults.

CHILDHOOD LEUKEMIA[21,224,289,326]

Childhood leukemia has a wide range of age incidence, from congenital leukemia upward. Congenital leukemia may present with metaphyseal lucent bands.[285] These are nonspecific findings in infancy and may be seen with prematurity and malnutrition. There maybe widening of the medullary cavity and thinning of the cortex. Occasionally sclerotic bands occur adjacent to the radiolucent bands. It is rarely associated with bilateral agenesis of the radii. The peak incidence is between 2 and 5 years of age. Three to 5% of cases occur during the first year of life. The clinical picture is usually acute and the cell type is most commonly lymphatic. Males are affected more often than females. There may be no circulating lymphocytes—the "aleukemic" type—and the roentgen picture is then important for diagnosis.

Four types of roentgenographically observable lesions of bones were found by Silverman:[287] transverse bands of diminished density, osteolysis, osteosclerosis, and subperiosteal new bone formation. Generalized bony demineralization may also be present. Osteolysis was present most often in Silverman's series. The lesions are most prominent about the knees, ankles, and wrists. A transverse radiolucent metaphyseal band is usually the earliest sign (Fig. 6–143). This finding may also be seen in severe illness of any type and in other specific diseases, if the patient is under 2 years of age (see Chap. 4). This band is formed by nonspecific depression of enchondral bone formation combined with a pressure effect of leukemic tissue on labile

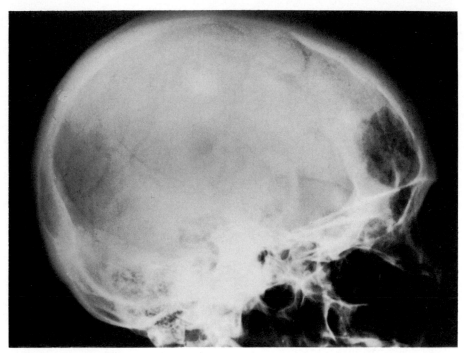

FIG. 6–137. Lues (skull). Note a large destructive area in the frontal bone and several sclerotic patches. Patient is a 60-year-old woman with tertiary syphilis, who had an associated soft-tissue swelling in the frontal region.

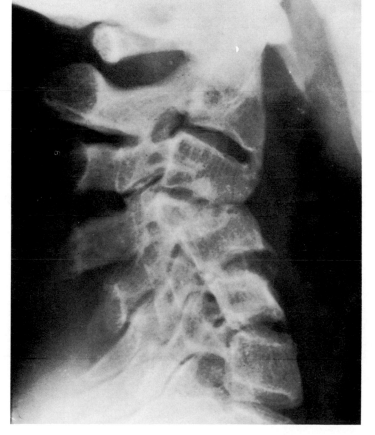

FIG. 6–138. Tertiary acquired syphilis (cervical spine) — same patient as in Fig. 6–137. Gummatous destruction of the body of the fourth cervical vertebra with anterior wedging and gibbus formation.

osseous trabeculae. These bands may be deeply situated and assume wide dimensions (Fig. 6–144). Analogous horizontal radiolucent bands in the vertebral bodies adjacent to the end-plates may rarely be seen. They may regress on therapy (Fig. 6–145). A residual dense metaphysis simulating the appearance of lead poisoning has been reported in a large percentage of those patients undergoing chemotherapy.[262] The bone abnormalities may persist for many months after the initiation of treatment. Occasionally, sclerotic zones may border the radiolucent bands on both sides. The zone of provisional calcification and the cortex remain intact. There is a transition from a wide band to a frank osteolytic lesion (Fig. 6–146). A large zone of metaphyseal rarefaction occurs, with cortical erosion. Generalized loss of bone density may also occur (Fig. 6–147). Small radiolucencies occur at the metaphyseal ends of the long bones in a "moth-eaten" pattern, and later extend along the diaphysis and also in other bones. These appear as ill-defined lytic lesions or "punched-out" radiolucencies (Fig. 6–148). Osteosclerosis may rarely occur, and can be seen in patches alternating with destructive areas, or as a uniform sclerosis (Fig. 6–149). Jaffe states that the latter may represent osteopetrosis complicated by leukemia.[153] Periosteal new bone formation of the long bones and ribs not uncommonly occurs as a result of subperiosteal proliferation of leukemic cells (Fig. 6–150). This may be the presenting roentgen sign, with no evidence of destruction or metaphyseal bands. Meningeal involvement yields increased intracranial pressure with resultant splitting of the cranial sutures. All of the findings of leukemia may be mimicked by neuroblastoma metastatic to bone. The age incidence is the same and the clinical picture may not be clear. Laboratory differentiation can be made by the presence, in neuroblastoma, of urinary vanillylmandelic acid (VMA) and vanilphenylethylamine, which are metabolic intermediary products.

ADULT LEUKEMIA

Adult leukemia shows bone changes much less often than childhood leukemia. Osseous lesions are said not to occur in the acute form, but very rarely they do so. The majority of adults with bone lesions have chronic lymphatic leukemia, or more rarely chloroma.

(*Text continued on p. 464*)

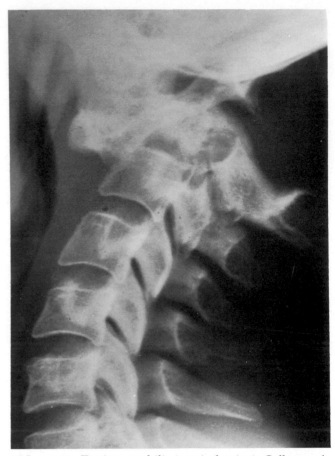

FIG. 6–139. Tertiary syphilis (cervical spine). Collapse of the second cervical vertebral body with destruction, sclerosis, and marked anterior displacement are noted.

FIG. 6–140. Diabetic patient with syringomyelia who sustained a fracture to the left shoulder. **A.** Fracture of the humeral head with rotation of the head fragment. **B.** Six-month interval film after **A.** There is marked soft-tissue debris with new bone formation at the lateral aspect of the humerus. Smoothening of the fracture line and severe hypertrophic changes at the glenoid may be seen. **C.** Two-year interval film after **B.** There has been organization of the new bone that was formed along the lateral aspect of the humerus. Severe hypertrophic changes with organization at the inferior aspect of the glenoid, and soft-tissue debris may be noted. The humeral head has not reconstituted. (Courtesy of Dr. Miriam Liberson, West Side VA Hospital, Chicago, IL)

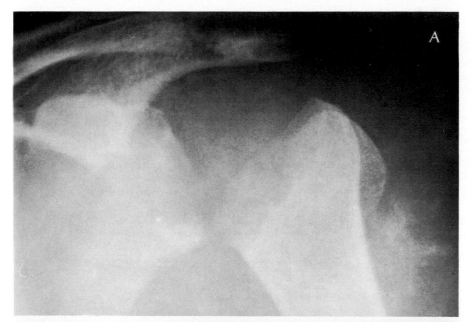

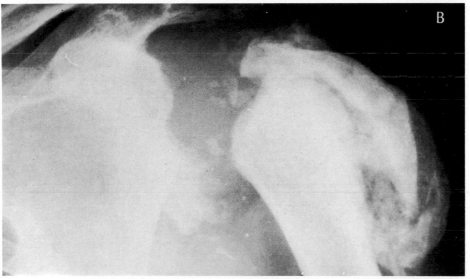

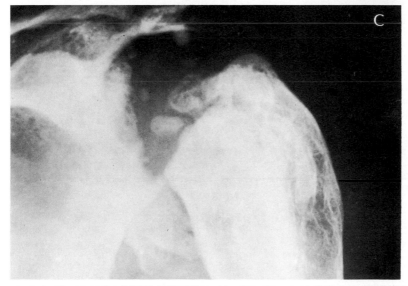

457

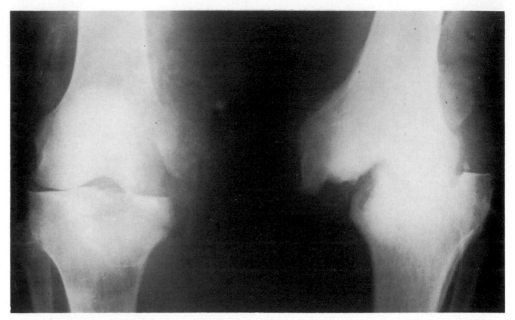

FIG. 6–141. Tertiary syphilis (Charcot's knees). Note articular destruction and disorganization, reactive sclerosis, and soft-tissue debris. Subluxation on left.

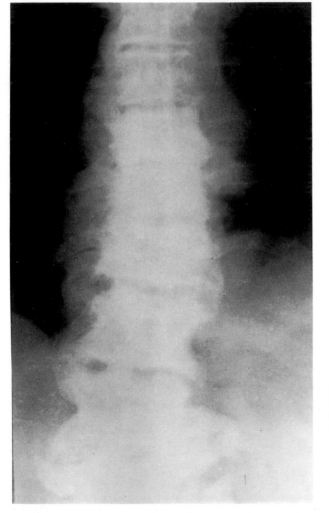

FIG. 6–142. Acquired tertiary syphilis (Charcot spine). There is marked sclerosis, disk space degeneration, and hypertrophic change in the spine associated with paraspinal soft-tissue mass.

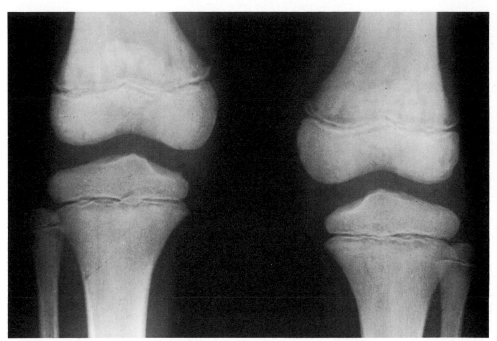

FIG. 6-143. Leukemia (knees). Note submetaphyseal radiolucent bands. The zone of provisional calcification is intact and there is no cortical destruction. All visible metaphyses are involved.

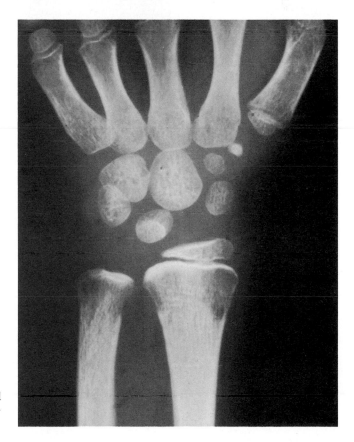

FIG. 6-144. Leukemia (wrist). Deep, wide metaphyseal band is noted. The cortex and the zone of provisional calcification remain intact.

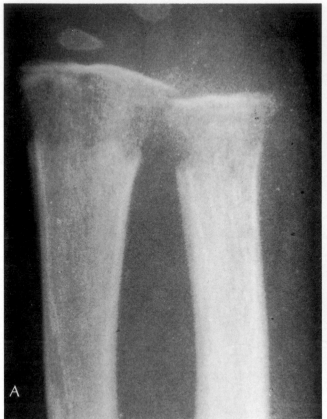

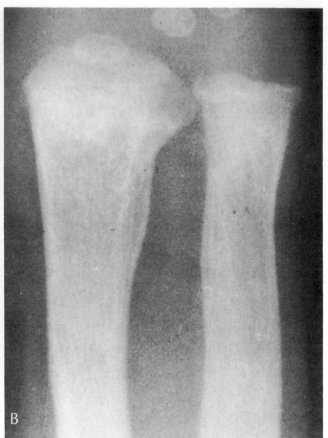

FIG. 6–145. Leukemia (wrist). A. Deep transverse metaphyseal bands at the distal radius and ulna with beginning areas of cortical destruction. B. Fourteen-month interval film after A. The radiolucent bands have regressed following therapy.

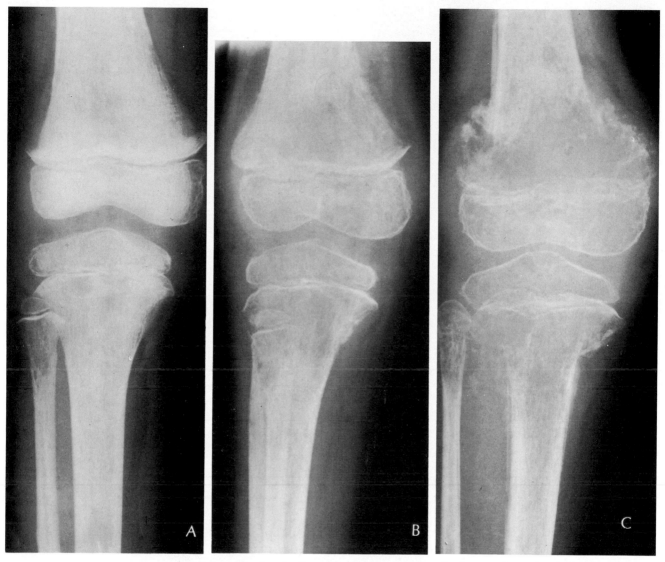

FIG. 6–146. Leukemia (knees). A. Wide bands of submetaphyseal radiolucency in the proximal tibial and fibular metaphyses. There is a rounded, ill-defined radiolucent lesion at the central metaphyseal aspect of the distal femur. Relative sclerosis at the distal femoral metaphyses may also be seen. B. Three-month interval film after A. Marked progression of destructive changes and loss of bone density. Soft-tissue atrophy may also be noted. However, the cortex is still intact in the major portion of the involved areas. C. Six-week interval film after B. Progression of lesions to severe destruction and periosteal new bone formation. Note the "moth-eaten" appearance in the distal femur proximal to the major destructive lesion and the permeative destructive pattern in the proximal tibial shaft.

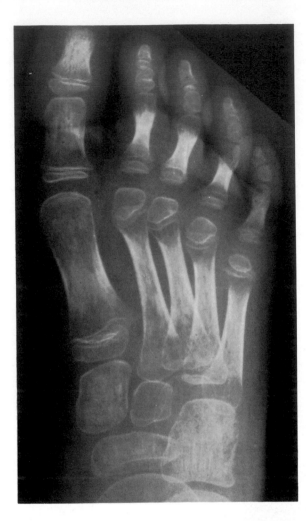

FIG. 6–147. Leukemia (foot). Generalized loss of bone density of the foot with a periarticular distribution is seen.

FIG. 6–148. Leukemia (skull). Multiple focal destructive lesions in the calvarium are noted. Some appear ill-defined and some appear as well-marginated or "punched-out" lesions.

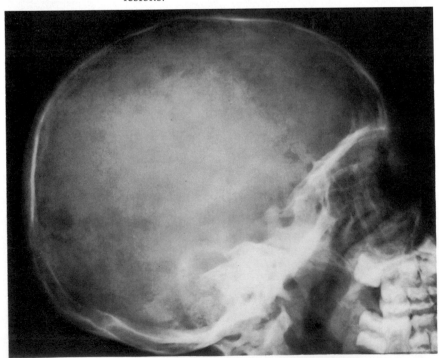

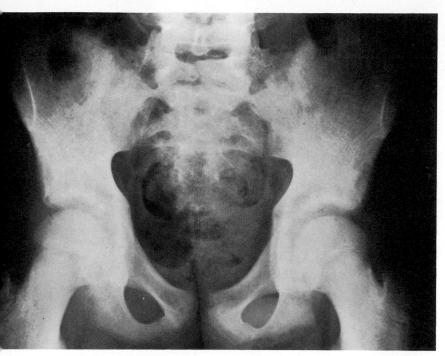

FIG. 6–149. Leukemia (pelvis). Osteosclerosis with coarsening of the trabecular pattern is noted.

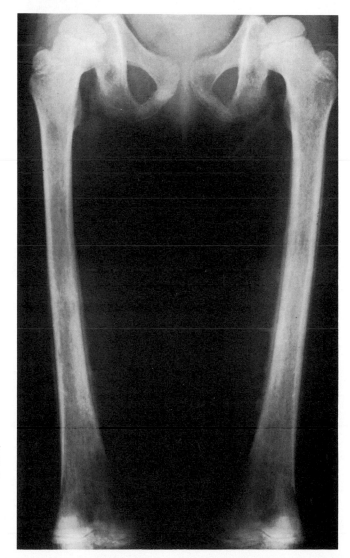

FIG. 6–150. Leukemia (femora). Marked periosteal new bone formation along the shaft of the femora, associated with metaphyseal destructive changes and destructive changes in the ischia, is seen.

Radiologically, there is a generalized loss of bone density. Metaphyseal bands are seen only very rarely. The rarefaction is most marked in the vertebrae, ribs, skull, and pelvis. Vertebral collapse may follow. There is thinning of the cortex and resorption of bony trabeculae. Fractures, particularly of the ribs, may occur. Scattered lytic destructive areas occur in all bones (Fig. 6–151), including the small bones of the hands and feet, and circumscribed lytic areas occur in the calvarium. The long axes of the lytic lesions may parallel the axis of the shaft of a long bone. Periosteal new bone formation and cortical erosion may occur. Patchy sclerosis, alternating with destructive areas, is a rare finding (Fig. 6–152). Generalized osteosclerosis is only very rarely seen and more likely represents myelofibrosis with a leukemoid picture than leukemia. A very rare manifestation is leukemic acropachy, with clubbing of the fingers and bilateral symmetrical destruction of the terminal phalanges.[112]

BURKITT'S TUMOR

Burkitt's tumor[6,18,57,92] is an uncommon, distinctive, malignant reticuloendothelial tumor, reported from Africa, South America, and the United States. It arises from B-lymphocytes, and is a disease of children with a peak age incidence of 6 to 7 years, but adults also may be involved. An association with the Ebstein–Barr virus is postulated. Multifocal lesions involving the bones and the viscera are present. The gastrointestinal and genitourinary tracts are usually involved, but the lungs are spared. Americans with Burkitt's lymphoma have a lower incidence of jaw tumors, but a higher incidence of abdominal tumors, pleural effusions, and peripheral lymph node involvement.[73]

Radiologically, destructive lesions are seen with a permeative pattern involving the metaphyses and diaphyses of the long bones. Usually the humerus, femur, and tibia show lesions. Interrupted periosteal new bone formation of the spiculated or laminated types may be present. The mandible is frequently involved, with destruction and loss of the lamina dura (Fig. 6–153).

MYCOSIS FUNGOIDES

Mycosis fungoides is an unusual form of malignant lymphoma with primary origin in the skin.[229] Over 1,000 new patients are affected each year. Its peak onset is in the fourth or fifth decade, affecting males predominantly. The disease progresses to involve the lymph nodes and the internal organs. Bone involvement is rare. Permeative or discrete areas of medullary destruction, progressing to cortical destruction, may be seen. Multiple areas may be involved, without expansion or periosteal new bone formation. The peripheral skeleton may also be involved.

HISTIOCYTOSIS X

Histiocytosis X[9,83,144,183] is generally considered to consist of three clinical syndromes of varying severity, with identical pathogenesis. The basic defect is probably cellular, with the deposition of lipids, chiefly cholesterol and its esters, within histiocytes. The etiology is unknown. No association with any

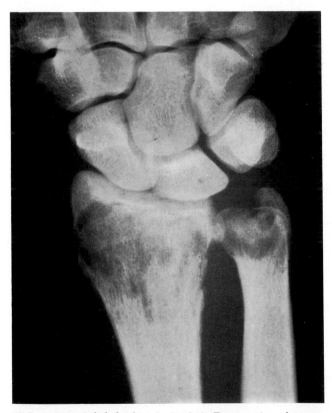

FIG. 6–151. Adult leukemia (wrist). Destructive changes in the metaphyses of the distal radius and ulna occurred after fusion of the epiphyseal growth center. This is an unusual finding. The bone density in adjacent areas is normal. The patient is a 50-year-old male with lymphocytic leukemia. (Courtesy of Dr. Miriam Liberson, West Side VA Hospital, Chicago, IL)

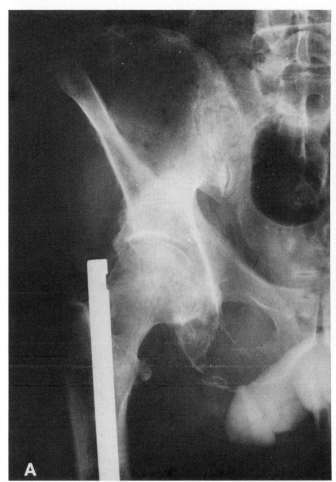

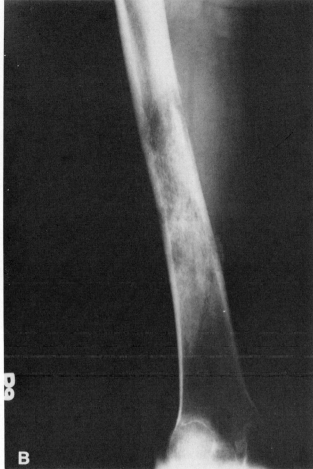

FIG. 6–152. Patient with granulocytic sarcoma. **A.** Destructive lesion involving the right ischium is seen. An intramedullary rod in the right femur for pathological fracture is present. **B.** The right femur prior to fracture showed permeative destructive lesions in the midshaft, with cortical destruction and periosteal new bone formation. (Courtesy of Dr. Dharmashi V. Bhate, VA Hospital, Hines, IL)

known infectious agent or abnormality of lipid metabolism has been found. The syndromes are:

1. Acute or subacute disseminated histiocytosis X (Letterer–Siwe disease)
2. Chronic disseminated histiocytosis X (Hand–Schueller–Christian disease)
3. Eosinophilic granuloma of bone

The fundamental lesions are proliferations of reticulum cells containing a variable amount of lipids, which is generalized in Letterer–Siwe's disease. In Hand–Schueller–Christian disease and eosinophilic granuloma, there are focal granulomas containing lipidized and nonlipidized histiocytes and eosinophils. Hyperlipemia, hypercholesterolemia, and eosinophilia are rare and not characteristic.

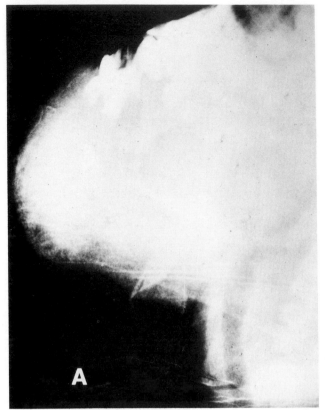

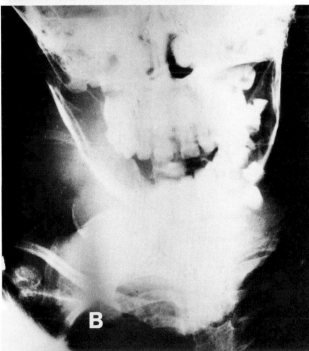

FIG. 6–153. Burkitt's tumor (mandible). **A.** Lateral view. Note extensive soft-tissue swelling, mandibular destruction, and appearance of "floating teeth." **B.** Anteroposterior view showing similar findings.

ACUTE OR SUBACUTE DISSEMINATED HISTIOCYTOSIS X (LETTERER–SIWE'S DISEASE)

Clinically, the disease is usually seen in patients under the age of 2 years, although older individuals may be affected. Hand–Schueller–Christian disease terminally may show a transition to this form. It is characterized by a sudden onset and a rapidly progressive malignant course with fever, hemorrhagic tendency, anemia, hepatosplenomegaly, and lymphadenopathy. Characteristic maculopapular skin lesions and petechiae are seen. Pulmonary nodular densities due to histiocytic infiltration are noted on chest radiographs; these are followed by bronchopneumonia. Bone lesions may be absent, particularly if there is a rapid course, but the cranium is most often involved. The bone lesions are similar to those seen in the chronic forms in roentgen appearance, but the incidence of bone lesion is less than in Hand–Schueller–Christian disease.

CHRONIC DISSEMINATED HISTIOCYTOSIS X (HAND–SCHUELLER–CHRISTIAN DISEASE)

Clinically, the disease most commonly occurs in children under the age of 5 years, but may be seen up to adulthood. Classically, a triad of exophthalmos, diabetes insipidus, and skull lesions have been considered a hallmark of this process. However, the concurrent presence of these signs is found in under 10% of cases. The chief clinical symptomatology in the various phases of this disease is related to the organ system involved. The most common findings in various combinations are: diabetes insipidus (in one-half of patients), skin and mucous membrane lesions similar to those in Letterer–Siwe's disease, hepatosplenomegaly, bone pain, unilateral or bilateral exophthalmos (in one-third of patients), loose teeth, chronic otitis media, weakness, weight loss, anorexia and signs of chronic debilitating disease. The course is chronic, with remissions and exacerbations. The mortality rate is 13%.

EOSINOPHILIC GRANULOMA OF BONE[99, 225]

Clinically, this form of histiocytosis X usually occurs in patients under the age of 10 years, but may rarely affect even the elderly. The most common form is monostotic; however, disseminated bony lesions may also be seen. The patients consistently complain of bone pain and limitation of motion of the involved area. Local inflammatory signs and fever may also be present. This is the most benign phase of this disease. The skull, ribs, mandible, spine, pelvis, and extremities are most often involved. The epiphysis is not usually involved.

RADIOGRAPHIC FINDINGS IN HISTIOCYTOSIS X

Radiologically, bone lesions may not be seen in either Hand–Schueller–Christian or Letterer–Siwe disease. When present, they are due to bone destruction by granulation tissue and are similar in all three forms of histiocytosis X. The basic lesion is an area of osteolysis that may involve any portion of any bone. Initially, small radiolucencies are seen that may be ill-defined or sharply marginated (Fig. 6–154). As the lesions enlarge, they may show endosteal scalloping (Fig. 6–155), a multilocular appearance, or bone expansion. There is a peculiar beveling with multiple undulating contours of the margin, or a "hole-within-a-hole" overlap giving a three-dimensional effect to the lesion in some cases (Figs. 6–156, 6–157). In contrast, other cases show poorly defined, patchy destructive areas or a coarsened trabecular pattern. The cortex may be destroyed, and some lesions may originate in the cortex (Fig. 6–158). Periosteal reaction of the solid or laminated type may be locally or extensively present (Fig. 6–159). Osteoporosis occurs in the debilitating stages. In the long bones, the epiphyses, diaphyses, or metaphyses may be involved. True expansion and pathological fractures are rare. Reactive sclerosis (Fig. 6–160), particularly following therapy, may also occur. Sequestration within destructive areas may rarely be seen.

The skull is more commonly involved than other areas. The lesions typically begin as small "punched-out" areas originating in the diploë; they expand (Fig. 6–161) and perforate both inner and outer tables unevenly, leading to the appearance of a double contour. More often, there is an ill-defined

(Text continued on p. 472)

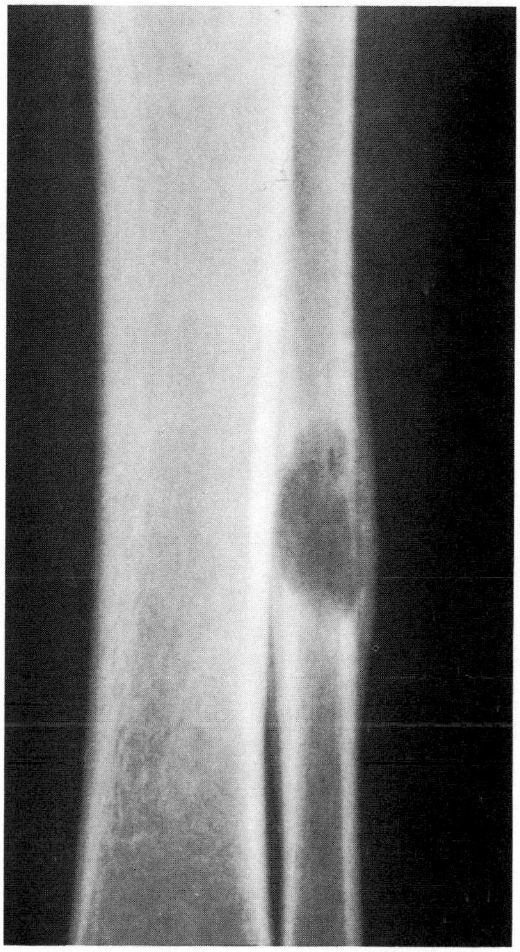

FIG. 6–154. Eosinophilic granuloma. Note the small, well-defined lesion in the fibular diaphysis and surrounding periosteal new bone formation.

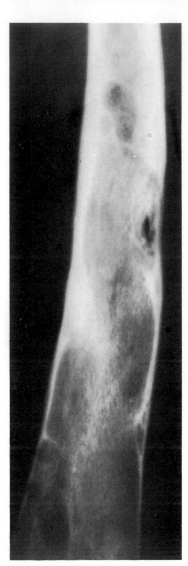

FIG. 6–155. Hand-Schueller-Christian disease (femur). Osteolytic lesion in the femoral shaft with endosteal scalloping is noted.

FIG. 6–156. Hand-Schueller-Christian disease. There are multiple radiolucent lesions in the proximal humerus. The most proximal metaphyseal lesion has a double contour, giving a "hole-within-a-hole" or three-dimensional effect.

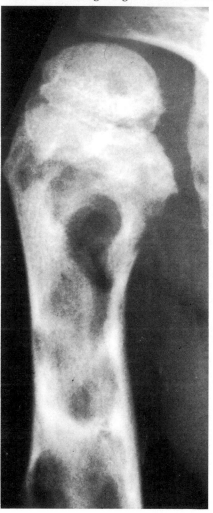

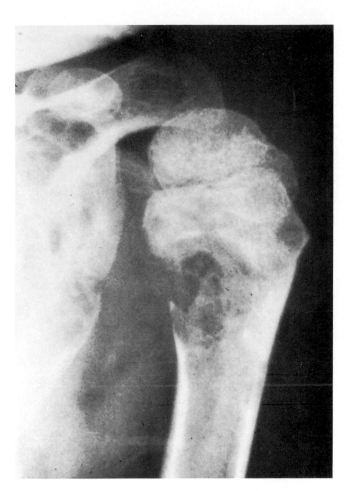

FIG. 6–157. Hand-Schueller-Christian disease—same patient as in Fig. 6–156. Beveled contour of metaphyseal lesion gives a three-dimensional "hole-within-a-hole" effect. Destructive changes in the scapula may also be seen.

FIG. 6–158. Eosinophilic granuloma originating in the cortex. Note extensive eccentric cortical destruction with a scalloped margin in the lower femoral shaft medially. A soft-tissue component is also present.

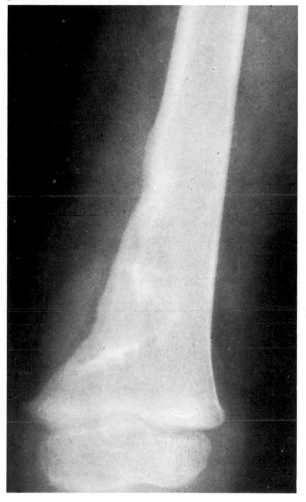

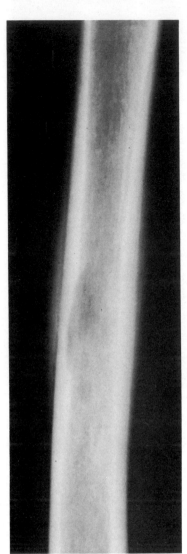

FIG. 6–159. Eosinophilic granuloma (femoral shaft). Ill-defined area of bone destruction in the midfemoral shaft causing endosteal scalloping and laminated periosteal new bone formation is noted.

FIG. 6–160. Eosinophilic granuloma (proximal femur) simulating osteoid osteoma. Reactive bone sclerosis at the outer aspect of the proximal femur is present, and the small radiolucent area represents the eosinophilic granuloma. (Courtesy of Dr. Marion Magalotti)

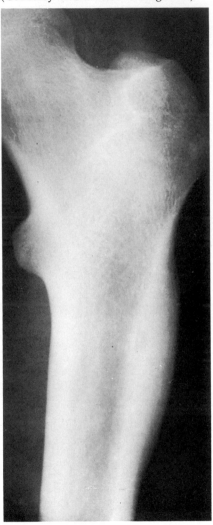

FIG. 6–162. Hand-Schueller-Christian disease (skull). Extensive multiple destructive lesions are seen in the skull. Most lesions are sharply marginated, but several have beveled edges.

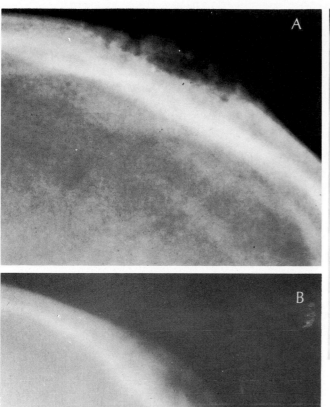

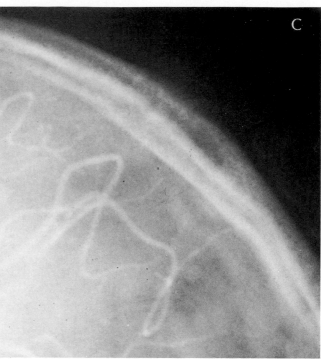

FIG. 6–161. Eosinophilic granuloma (skull—parietal bone). **A.** A radiolucent lesion expanding the outer table with an intact cortex may be seen. **B.** Tomogram showing radiolucent area with expansion of the diploic space and intact inner and outer tables. **C.** Cerebral arteriogram showing vascular fill of both internal and external carotid branches with no vascular flush in the radiolucent lesion.

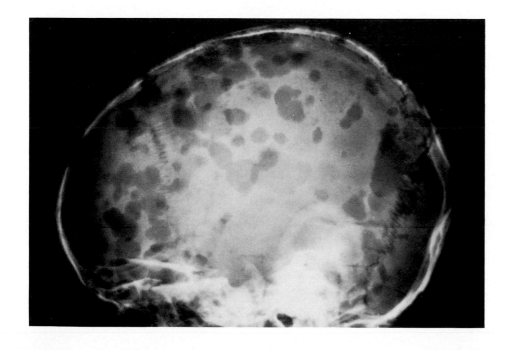

margin, or there may be sharply marginated extensive lesions (Fig. 6–162). Palpable soft-tissue tumors may be present in the involved areas. Extensive confluence of lesions later develops to give the "maplike" or "geographic skull" (Fig. 6–163) in the disseminated forms of the disease. A "button sequestrum" within the lesions may rarely be seen. Destruction of the sella turcica, petrous bone, mastoids, base of the skull, and orbits occurs; there is also involvement of the paranasal sinuses. Orbital osteolytic lesions are common, involving the orbital roof, lateral wall, and sphenoid wings. Healing results in a dense orbital sclerosis which should be differentiated from fibrous dysplasia.[218] Mandibular lesions begin about the apices of the teeth, destroying periodontal bone and giving the characteristic appearance of "floating teeth" (Fig. 6–164).

Pelvic manifestations are common and are usually situated in the supra-acetabular area. Reactive sclerosis, particularly along the superior margin of the destructive lesion, is said to be a characteristic finding (Fig. 6–165). The ribs may show expansile lesions with pathological fractures (Fig. 6–166).

The spine may be affected, with involvement of the vertebral body or partial destruction of the pedicles in all three forms of the disease. Three phases of vertebral body involvement are recognized. The destructive phase shows spotty radiolucencies in the centrum (Fig. 6–167), then proceeds to the phase of collapse in which the vertebral body assumes the shape of a flat thin disk (Fig. 6–168). The regenerative phase follows with a residual vertebra plana. The intervertebral spaces are preserved. A wedge-like collapse may also be seen. It is now considered that Calvé's disease is due to eosinophilic granuloma rather than ischemic necrosis. Widening of the paravertebral shadow may also be seen.

MASSIVE OSTEOLYSIS (DISAPPEARING BONE DISEASE)

Massive osteolysis[26,39,127,167,234,266,267], is a rare condition of unknown etiology characterized by the progressive resorption of large areas of bone. Microscopically it is associated with hemangioma or lymphangioma, without the presence of pathologically malignant tissue.

Clinically, the age of the patient is usually under 30 years, with a reported range of 1½ to 58 years. The onset sometimes follows trauma. There is no evidence of heredity, nor of metabolic or endocrine disturbances. There is an insidious onset of pain

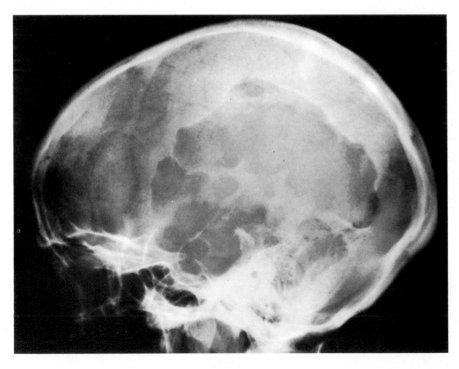

FIG. 6–163. Hand-Schueller-Christian disease (skull). Confluence of destructive lesions gives the "geographic skull" appearance. The major portion of the destroyed area has a beveled margin, indicating that the inner and outer tables are perforated unevenly.

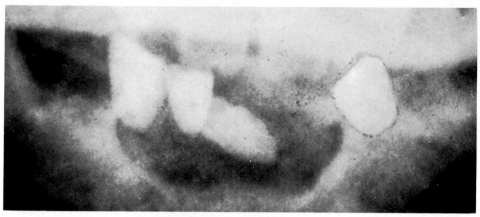

FIG. 6–164. Hand-Schueller-Christian disease (mandible). Periodontal destruction about the incisors gives the "floating teeth" appearance.

FIG. 6–165. Eosinophilic granuloma (pelvis). There is a large destructive lesion in the iliac wing with a smaller satellite lesion at its inferior aspect. A fine margin of reactive sclerosis at its superior margin is present.

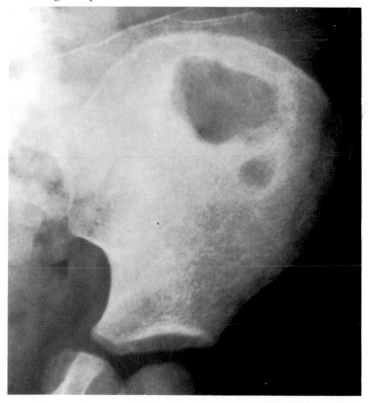

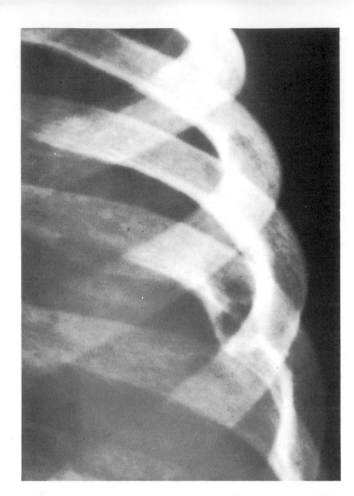

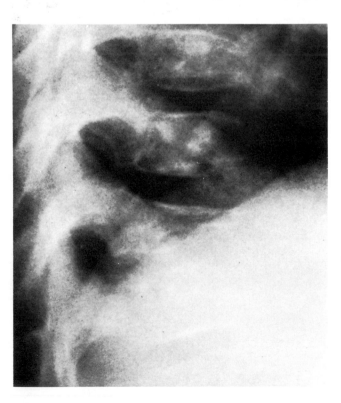

FIG. 6–166. Hand-Schueller-Christian disease (ribs). Destructive and expansile lesions in the ribs are noted.

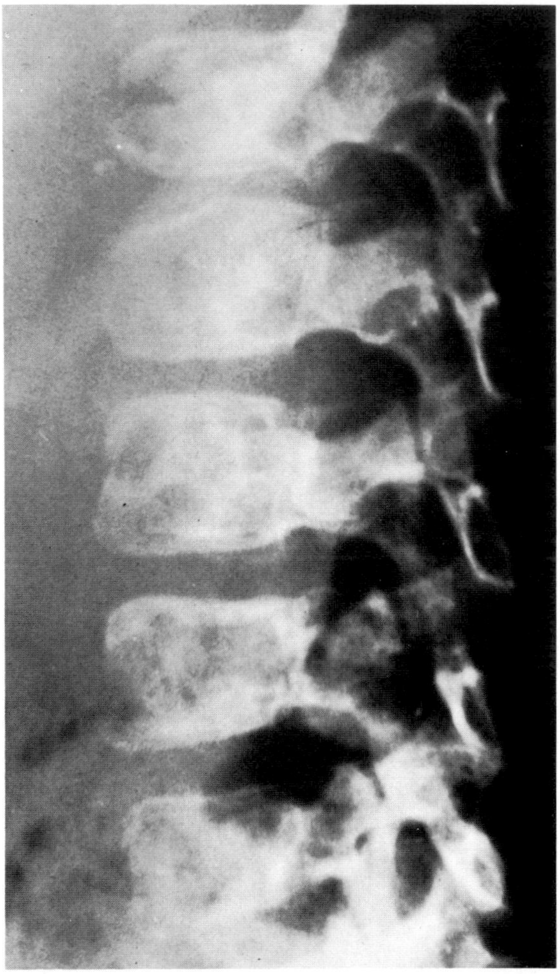

FIG. 6–167. Hand-Schueller-Christian disease (spine). There are multiple destructive lesions in the bodies of the lumbar vertebrae. Vertebral collapse has not yet occurred.

FIG. 6–168. Eosinophilic granuloma (spine). The body of the eleventh dorsal vertebra has collapsed.

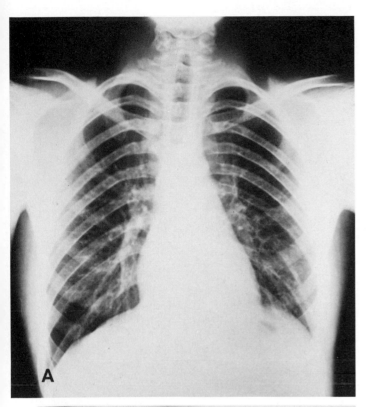

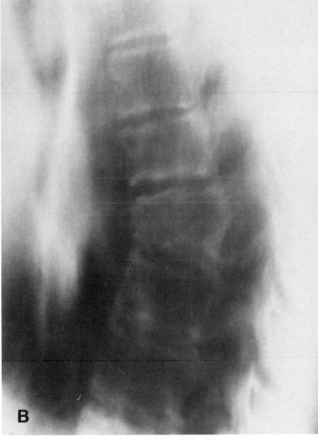

followed by severe deformity and occasionally pathological fracture. The progress of the disease may spontaneously be arrested, or continue inexorably to cause death, particularly in cases with rib cage involvement. Laboratory studies show no characteristic changes except for a rise in alkaline phosphatase in the event of a pathological fracture. At surgery, simply no bone is found at the involved site. Bone grafts also become resorbed. A single case has been reported with spontaneous reossification.[44] This occurred in an elderly patient following a fracture of the humerus. Massive osteolysis of the ribs and cervical spine has been reported in a single case of scleroderma.[135]

Radiologically, massive resorption of bone is seen. All bones in the body may be affected, most frequently the pelvis, ribs, spine, and long bones (Fig. 6–169). The process spreads with ease across joints and intervertebral spaces to involve adjacent bones, causing massive areas of vanished bone. The characteristic finding in tubular bone is tapering of the margin of the lesion to a conelike contour. This is due to simultaneous intra- and extraosseous involvement. There is no coarsening of the trabecular pattern nor is there osteosclerotic reaction. No periosteal reaction is seen. Soft-tissue debris or phleboliths are not present. Occasionally cutaneous hemangiomas are present.

Hereditary osteolysis of the carpal, tarsal, and adjacent bones with arthropathy has been described as a distinct syndrome. The appearance of the patients is similar to that seen in Marfan's syndrome. This disease is inherited as an autosomal dominant.[16, 172]

Several syndromes of acroosteolysis have been described including a dominant and a recessive.[312] *Hajdu–Cheney syndrome* has its onset in the second decade with digital clubbing and lysis in the distal phalanges.[316] Other forms include series reported by Schinz and Joseph.[16] Other causes are neurogenic disease, lipodermatoarthritic, and *Farber's disease*, which is an inborn error of lipid metabolism or mucopolysaccharide metabolism of the fibroblast. It is characterized by periarticular swelling, joint contractures, and bone destruction. The condition is usually fatal within 2 years.

FIG. 6–169. Massive osteolysis, or vanishing bone disease. **A.** PA chest film. Destruction of the left eighth and ninth ribs are seen. **B.** Tomogram of dorsal spine. Partial collapse of the middorsal vertebrae is noted with sharp gibbus formation. (Courtesy of Dr. Tom Hinckle, Beaumont, TX)

MISCELLANEOUS RARE BENIGN SYNDROMES CAUSING WIDESPREAD LYTIC LESIONS OF BONE

Multiple widespread bone defects may be caused by *intraosseous hemangiomatosis,* without the characteristic appearance seen in other forms of this disease, such as massive osteolysis, vertebral hemangioma, hemangioma of the skull, or soft-tissue hemangiomatosis. Association with hereditary hemorrhagic telangiectasia has been reported as a very rare finding.[201] *Cystic lymphangiomatosis*[28, 34,136,274] may involve all bones with erosive or "soap bubble" lesions, or ill-defined radiolucencies. Although the symptoms are mild, there is a relentless progression of osteolysis. Pathological fractures may ensue. Children are usually affected. Mixed lymphangiomas and hemangiomas may be present (cystic angiomatosis).

Congenital scattered fibromatosis[11, 138] is characterized by the presence of multiple fibromas in the subcutaneous tissues and viscera. At times, these may be calcified. The flat and long bones show widespread osteolytic defects and expansion. The disease is usually fatal in those patients who have visceral involvement.

Weber–Christian disease[71] is a diffuse panniculitis characterized by painful subcutaneous nodules. The condition results from a disturbance in fat metabolism. There are multiple "punched-out" or "moth-eaten" lesions involving the calvarium, pelvis, and medullary bone. The appearance is similar to that of myelomatosis. The spine is said not to be involved. *Primary systemic amyloidosis*[103,121,320] rarely shows bone involvement. When bones are involved, multiple osteolytic areas may be seen, owing to replacement of bone tissue by amyloid. There is a predilection for the proximal humeral and femoral heads. Also, there is soft-tissue swelling about the joints, due to synovial amyloidosis. Diffuse infiltration of the bone marrow may cause loss of bone density and collapse of vertebrae (Fig. 6–170). Ischemic necrosis of the femoral head has also been reported. *Membranous lipodystrophy*[5] is a recently described rare condition in which multiple radiolucencies are found symmetrically distributed

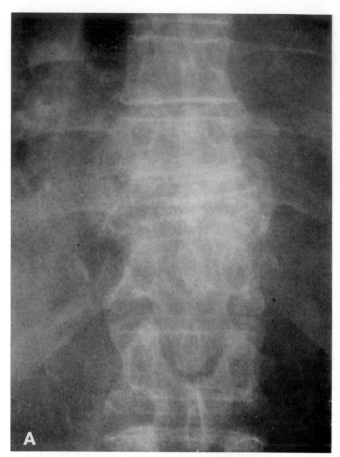

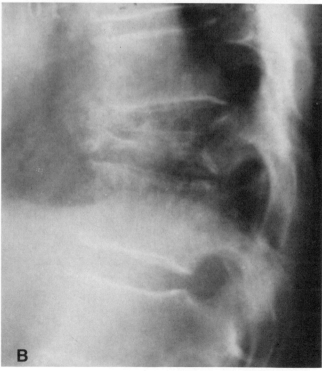

FIG. 6–170. Primary amyloidosis. **A, B.** Anteroposterior and lateral views of the lower dorsal spine reveal a wafer-like collapse of the 11th dorsal vertebra with preservation of the intervertebral spaces. (Courtesy of Dr. Dharmashi V. Bhate, VA Hospital, Hines, IL)

476

in the peripheral skeleton. The long bones in the vicinity of the joints, and the hands and the feet are chiefly involved. The lesions are cystic and expansile, with irregular margins and light trabeculation. The lesions contain a yellow lipidlike substance with a membranocystic structure. Pathologic fractures may occur.

The differential diagnosis of nonmalignant multiple skeletal radiolucencies includes:

Histiocytosis X
Fibrous dysplasia
Intraosseous hemangiomatosis
Cystic lymphangiomatosis
Cystic angiomatosis
Familial multiple nonosteogenic fibromas
Congenital scattered fibromatosis
Aggressive fibromatosis
Weber–Christian disease
Primary systemic amyloidosis
Hydatidosis
Familial hypercholesterolemia[24]
Membranous lipodystrophy

Electrical injury[32] may leave persistent discrete areas of rarefaction in bones, as well as periostitis, resorption of the phalangeal tufts, fracture dislocations, or fine fractures. Small rounded densities, or "bone pearls," may be seen, which may result from the actual melting of bone by intense heat. Delayed effects[14] may be manifested as extensive ischemic necrosis.

Frostbite injuries may show soft-tissue swelling or interstitial gas. Soft-tissue atrophy may follow. Bone changes include delayed appearance of sclerosis, "punched-out" areas, tuft resorption, epiphyseal fragmentation, and premature fusion of the epiphysis. Joint changes may include marginal spurs or fusion.

BONE RESORPTION

Resorption of bone may be due to a vast variety of causes. The basic mechanisms have vascular, neuropathic, inflammatory, or metabolic etiologies. Local factors, such as trauma or thermal injuries, may be causative, or a widespread, generalized disease may have a resorptive component.

Radiologically, the most significant sites of resorption are the terminal phalanges, distal clavicles, superior aspects of the ribs (not to be confused with rib notching of the inferior surfaces through vascular erosion, Fig. 6–171), and the calcanei at tendinous insertions. The many causes of bone resorption at these sites are summarized below.

CONDITIONS ASSOCIATED WITH BONE RESORPTION AT SPECIFIC SITES

I. Distal Clavicles

1. Hyperparathyroidism
2. Rheumatoid arthritis (Fig. 6–172)
3. Scleroderma
4. Posttraumatic osteolysis[126,150,290] (Fig. 6–173)
5. Progeria
6. Pycnodysostosis
7. Reticulohistiocytoma (lipoid dermatoarthritis)
8. Hurler's syndrome

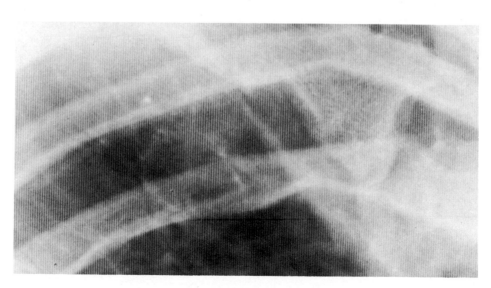

FIG. 6–171. Notching of the inferior surfaces of the ribs due to coarctation of the aorta. This is caused by bone erosion from dilated intercostal arteries. Many other conditions can give a similar picture.

II. Terminal Phalangeal Tufts (May Show Sharply Marginated Conical Tapering, a "Candlestick Effect" with a Central Depression, or Ill-Defined Regional Loss of Bone Density)

1. Scleroderma[118] (may be associated with calcification, Fig. 6–174)
2. Raynaud's disease and allied conditions
3. Occlusive vascular disease (Fig. 6–175)
4. Traumatic vascular disease
5. Thromboangiitis obliterans
6. Diabetes mellitus (Fig. 6–176)
7. Tabes dorsalis
8. Syringomyelia
9. Leprosy
10. Psoriasis (Fig. 6–177)
11. Epidermolysis bullosa[31, 125] (may be associated with calcification)
12. Pityriasis rubra
13. Hyperparathyroidism
14. Osteomalacia
15. Malabsorption syndrome
16. Hunger osteopathy
17. Burns[86] (Fig. 6–178)
18. Frostbite injuries (Fig. 6–179)
19. Electrical injuries[32]
20. Osteolysis in polyvinyl chloride workers[101]
21. Acro-osteolysis[51]
22. Progeria[231]
23. Pycnodysostosis
24. Reticulohistiocytoma (lipoid dermatoarthritis)
25. Benign proliferative lesions
26. Disseminated lipogranulomatosis
27. Rothmund's syndrome[193] (may be associated with calcification)
28. Sarcoidosis[118] (rare)
29. Sjögren's syndrome[286]
30. Gout

III. Superior Aspects of the Ribs[269]

1. Hyperparathyroidism
2. Rheumatoid arthritis (Fig. 6–180)
3. Scleroderma[165] (Fig. 6–181)
4. Lupus erythematosus
5. Sjögren's syndrome
6. Neurofibromatosis
7. Poliomyelitis[22]
8. Progeria
9. Localized pressure (Fig. 6–182)
10. Osteogenesis imperfecta
11. Marfan's syndrome
12. Radiation damage
13. Restrictive lung disease[166]

IV. Calcanei

1. Rheumatoid arthritis
2. Hyperparathyroidism
3. Reiter's syndrome (Figs. 9–106, 9–107)
4. Localized osteomyelitis (Fig. 6–183)
5. Reticulohistiocytoma (Fig. 9–133)

V. Generalized Bone Resorption May also be Seen in:

1. Paraplegia
2. Myositis ossificans[137] (Fig. 6–184)

(Text continued on p. 483)

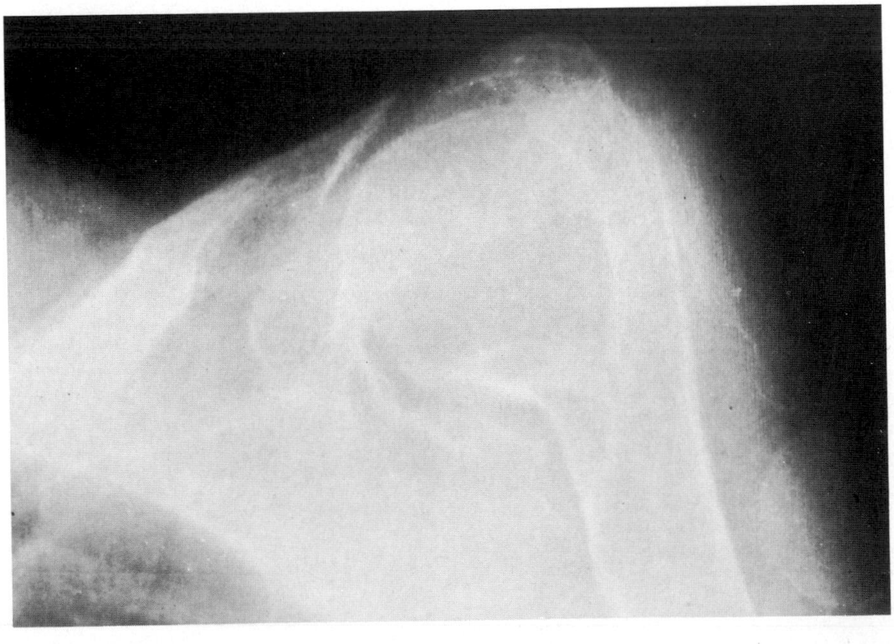

FIG. 6–172. Rheumatoid arthritis (shoulder). Resorption of the distal clavicle with a sharply defined pencillike configuration is noted. The well-demarcated margin differentiates this condition from hyperparathyroidism, in which the margins are usually ill-defined. Resorption of the glenoid and erosion at the humeral neck may also be seen.

FIG. 6–173. Posttraumatic osteolysis. Resorption of the distal clavicle following trauma is noted.

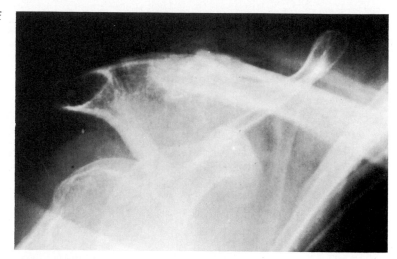

FIG. 6–174. Scleroderma (hand). Marked resorption of all of the distal phalanges. Calcification in the soft tissues is not present in this case. The bone density and texture are not severely affected.

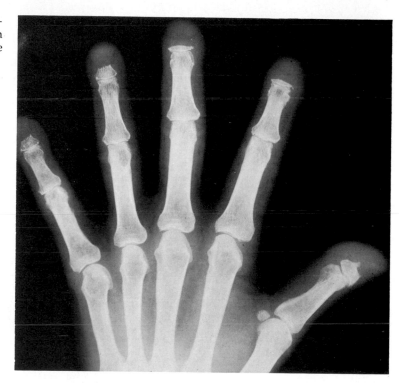

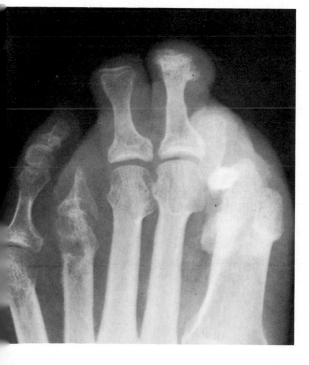

FIG. 6–175. Occlusive arteriosclerosis (foot). Resorption of the distal phalanges is noted down to the proximal phalanx of the fourth toe, forming a pencillike deformity. Also note the focus of osteomyelitis at the distal fourth metatarsal.

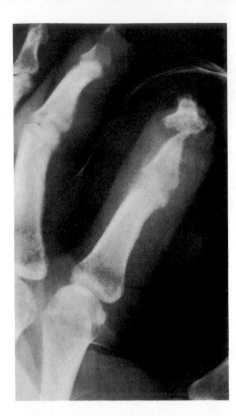

FIG. 6–176. Diabetes mellitus (hand). Note resorption of the terminal tuft of the distal phalanx of the index finger, and of the distal aspect of the middle phalanx to give a pencillike effect. A focus of osteomyelitis in the distal phalanx of the middle finger is also present.

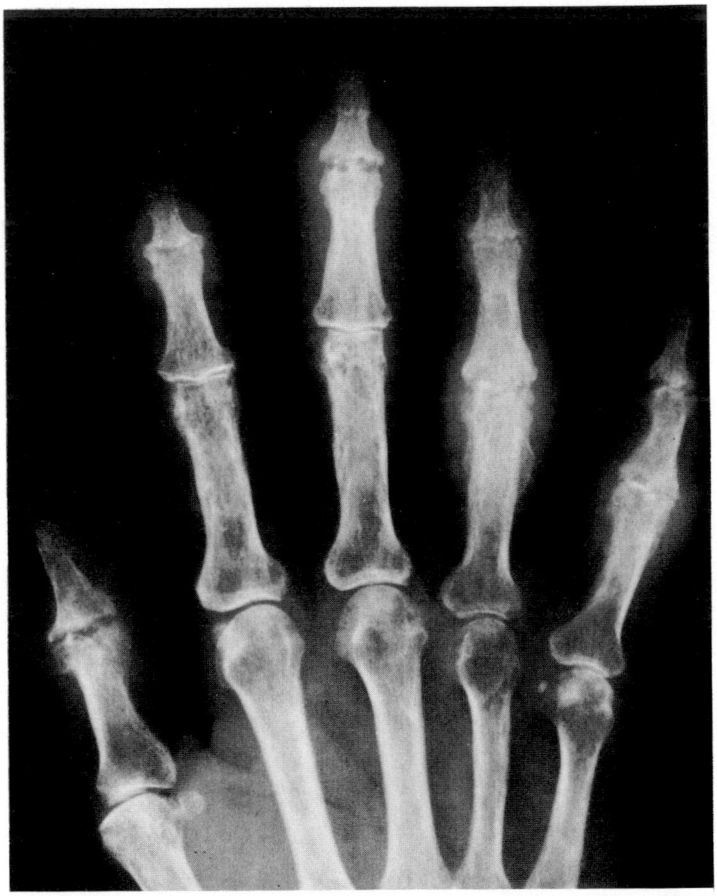

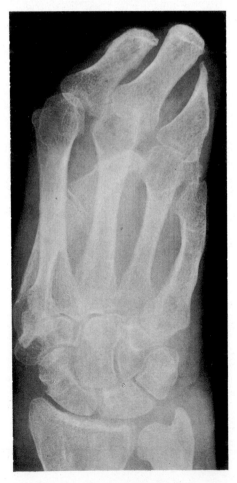

FIG. 6–177. Psoriasis (hand). Note ill-defined resorption at the terminal phalangeal tufts. Typical changes of psoriatic arthritis, including resorption and widening of the distal interphalangeal joints, and, to a lesser degree, the proximal interphalangeal joints are noted.

FIG. 6–178. Hand following burn. Severe resorption of the phalanges with a pencillike deformity of the proximal phalanx of the ring finger can be seen. Soft-tissue contracture may also be seen.

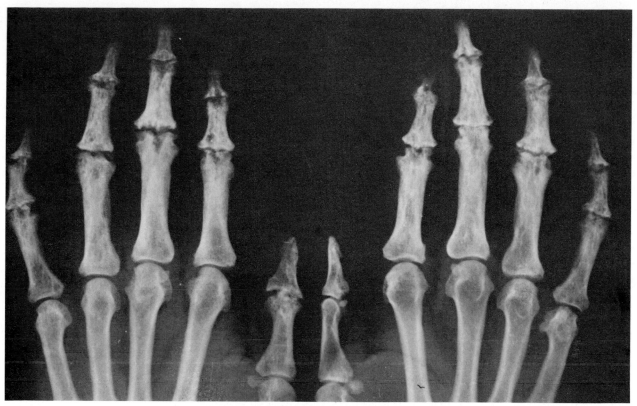

FIG. 6–179. Frostbite (hands). Destructive changes of the proximal and distal interphalangeal joints are noted, as well as bony sclerosis. (Courtesy of Dr. Dharmashi V. Bhate, VA Hospital, Hines, IL)

FIG. 6–180. Rheumatoid arthritis (ribs). Resorption at the superior aspect of the posterior third rib is noted.

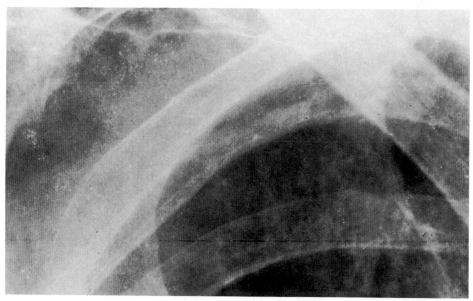

FIG. 6–181. Scleroderma (ribs). Resorption with loss of cortical sharpness at the superior aspect of the sixth rib is noted.

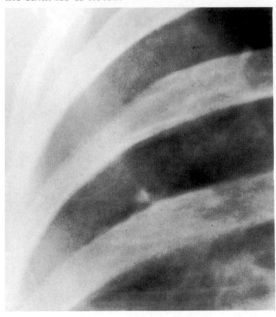

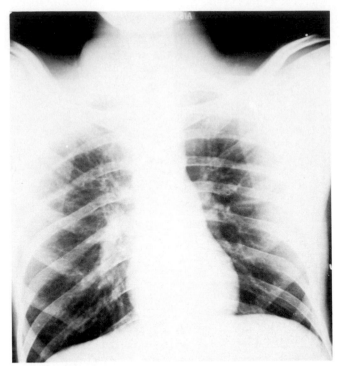

FIG. 6–182. Paraplegia (ribs). Resorption of the superior aspects of the third, fourth, fifth, and sixth ribs bilaterally, due to pressure from scapulae secondary to use of crutches, is noted.

FIG. 6–183. Localized osteomyelitis (calcaneus) from decubitus ulcer. Resorptive and destructive changes at the posterior aspect of the calcaneus are seen.

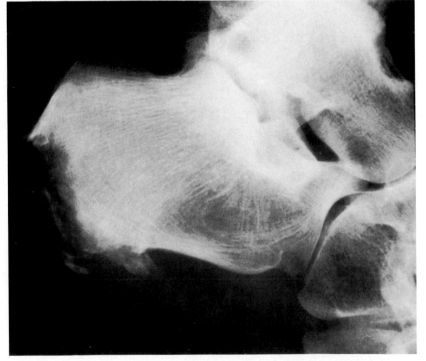

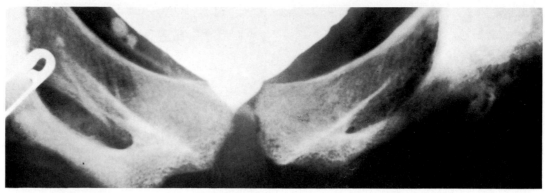

FIG. 6–184. Paraplegia. Resorption at the inferior aspects of both ischia and small foci of myositis ossificans may be seen.

LEPROSY

Leprosy[82, 220] is caused by infection with *Mycobacterium leprae.* There are two types of involvement, lepromatous and neural. Bone changes are seen most often in the neural form, but may also be present in the lepromatous type, in which case the bone is directly involved with granulomatous tissue.

In neural leprosy, severe neurotrophic changes and atrophy result. The hands and the feet are chiefly affected. There is marked resorption and tapering deformity of the phalanges, similar to, but much more severe than, other neurotrophic changes. In severe cases, all of the phalanges of the hands may be completely resorbed (Fig. 6–185), and tapering of the distal metacarpals may be seen. In the feet, the changes usually begin at the metatarsophalangeal joints, and destruction and resorption proceed in both directions (Fig. 6–186). There is resorption of the midportion of the shafts of the phalanges, leading to fracture and destruction. Neurotrophic changes of the Charcot type may also be present (Fig. 6–187). Tarsal bone disintegration may occur.[134, 319] Flexion deformities may be present, as well as enlargement of the nutrient foramina in the hands.

In the lepromatous type, periosteal and endosteal thickening may be seen, most often involving the ulna and fibula. Cystic changes in the hands and feet may also be seen, as well as expansion. Absorption of the facial bones may occur.

Angiography[158, 159] of the lower limb in leprosy showed decreased circulation through narrow and constricted vessels in the distal third of the lower limb. These findings may precede clinical symptoms. Arteriovenous shunting was also seen.

BURNS[277]

The following changes have been described in areas involved with *burns:* heat necrosis of bone with sequestrum formation and secondary osteomyelitis, osteoporosis, periosteal reaction, bone resorption, soft-tissue contractures and webbing, soft-tissue and periarticular calcification particularly about the elbow, myositis ossificans, articular destruction, arthropathy, and ankylosis (Fig. 6–178).

EPIDERMOLYSIS BULLOSA

Epidermolysis bullosa[145] is a rare hereditary skin disease characterized by the formation of vesicles and bullae spontaneously or following slight trauma. *Radiological changes* include resorption and thinning of the terminal phalanges. The shafts of the long bones are overconstricted. Flexion contractures and subluxations may occur, and a cocoon of epidermis may envelop the entire hand or foot. Dental abnormalities are also present.

THE PERIOSTEUM

Elevation of the periosteum from the cortex followed by new bone formation is a fundamental response of bone to disease processes. The periosteum may be lifted by any agent, be it blood, pus, neoplasm, granulomatous tissue, or edema. The cambium layer of the periosteum retains its osteogenic properties, and if not destroyed, will form new bone. The presence of periosteal elevation is of

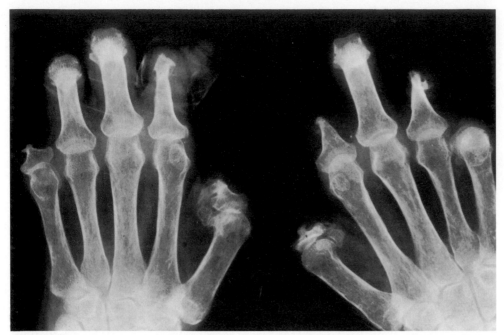

FIG. 6–185. Leprosy, neural form (hands)—severe phalangeal resorption. Several digits have the major portion of all phalanges resorbed. Typical pencillike configurations are present.

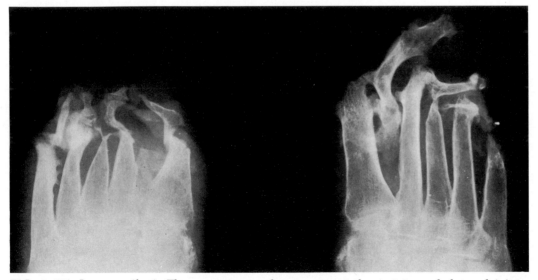

FIG. 6–186. Leprosy (feet). The most severe changes are at the metatarsophalangeal joints, where marked pencillike resorption is present with subluxations. The process proceeds both proximally and distally from this point.

FIG. 6–187. Leprosy (shoulder)—neurotrophic joint. Note flattening and eburnation of the humeral head and the glenoid fossa, and soft-tissue calcific debris.

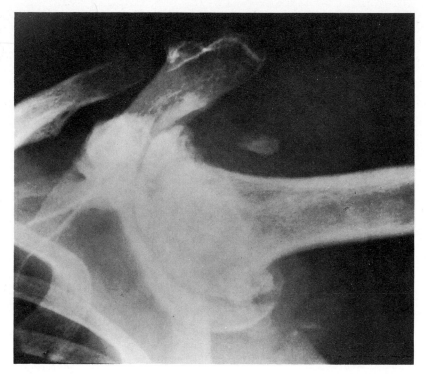

lesser diagnostic significance than the pattern that is assumed.

Three basic forms of periosteal reaction can be discriminated: the solid, the laminated, and the spiculated. Each of these forms can be present in either malignant or benign processes; however, the presence of their specific subtypes indicates the probability of malignancy or benignity.

The solid periosteal type may be thin or dense, straight or undulating. A thin, solid periosteal reaction is not useful as a diagnostic indicator, because both malignant (*e.g.*, leukemia) and benign (*e.g.*, pulmonary hypertrophic osteoarthropathy) conditions cause this finding. Edeiken *et al*[75, 76] state that solid periosteal reaction greater than 1 mm in thickness indicates a benign process. Thick, undulating periosteal reaction, commonly seen in venous stasis, also is an indication of benignity.

Rapidly developing osteoporosis with longitudinal loss of mineral from the cortices may simulate periosteal new bone formation.[97]

Laminated or "onionskin" periosteal reaction occurs in malignant tumors and in benign conditions such as pulmonary hypertrophic osteoarthropathy and osteomyelitis. It is an indicator of an intermittent or cyclic process and deserves no special mystique. It is, however, most commonly associated with Ewing's sarcoma. Lodwick[186] states that the laminations are delicate with side spacing in Ewing's sarcoma, in contrast to the coarse laminations of osteosarcoma.

Spiculated periosteal reaction[122, 180] is due to a disturbance in the reparative stage that follows periosteal elevation. The spicules are not tumor bone. Tumors or other agents prevent the filling in of the subperiosteal space with bone. Spicules then form along the stretched periosteal vessels and the extensions of Sharpey's fibers. Electrical fields due to piezoelectrical effects of deformed bone crystal may also contribute to this picture, which represents a rapid, aggressive process that can be either malignant or benign. Angiography may show blood vessels running parallel to the spicules. Several localized primary malignant tumors of bone, metastases, osteomyelitis and lues, thyroid acropachy, hemangiomas, and anemias may cause a spiculated appearance. Lodwick[186] has divided spiculation into three roentgen patterns: the "sunburst," or radiating from a central point (osteosarcoma); the "hair-on-end" or parallel, involving a long segment (Ewing's); and "velvet," or low and slanting (chondrosarcoma). Malignant spicules tend to be long and slender, while benign spicules tend to be short and squat.

When periosteum is locally elevated and destruction of the apex of the formed triangle occurs at a rate that exceeds the osteogenic potential, a periosteal cuff called *Codman's triangle* is seen at the margin of the lesion. This may be formed in both malignant and benign processes. The absence of periosteal new bone formation is also of diagnostic significance, particularly in localized lesions. The so-called "fibrocystic" lesions of bone are characterized by this absence.

The benign conditions associated with generalized periosteal elevation are summarized below.

PERIOSTEAL ELEVATION

Benign Conditions Characterized by Generalized Periosteal Elevation

Pulmonary hypertrophic osteoarthropathy
Thyroid acropachy
Pachydermoperiostosis
Infantile cortical hyperostosis
Hypervitaminosis A

Other Benign Conditions Commonly Associated with Generalized Periosteal Elevation

Prematurity
Venous stasis
Subacute lupus erythematosus (arteritis)[12]
Polyarteritis nodosa
Rheumatoid arthritis
Reiter's syndrome
Psoriatic arthritis
Battered child syndrome
Thermal injuries
Widespread osteomyelitis
Widespread infarcts of bone (especially hand–foot syndrome in sickle-cell anemia)
Congenital lues
Rubella
Scurvy[155]
Healing rickets
Infantile Hurler's syndrome
Gaucher's disease
Histiocytosis X
Myelosclerosis
Fluorosis
Cornelia de Lange syndrome II (pseudomuscular hypertrophy)
Idiopathic

PULMONARY HYPERTROPHIC OSTEOARTHROPATHY

Pulmonary hypertrophic osteoarthropathy[7,119,332] is composed of the triad of periosteal new bone formation, clubbing of the fingers and toes, and synovitis. It is associated with a wide variety of pulmonary and pleural conditions, which may be inflammatory, suppurative, neoplastic, benign, malignant, primary, or metastatic. When seen in adults, the condition is most commonly caused by carcinoma of the lung. In infants and children, it not uncommonly results from fibrocystic disease or pulmonary metastases. Hilar metastases secondary to nasopharyngeal carcinoma, without peripheral pulmonary metastases, has also been reported to cause this condition.[143] This entity is different from simple clubbing of the fingers without periostitis or arthritis, which has a much broader range of etiologies (Chap. 8).

A neurogenic mechanism produces the changes. The afferent pathway is the vagus nerve, but the efferent pathway is unknown. Vagotomy reduces blood flow to the affected areas. Osteoarthropathy regresses following removal of the primary lung lesion, unilateral vagotomy, or even exploratory thoracotomy (Fig. 6–188).

Clinically, the triad of clubbing, periostitis, and arthralgia may be entirely present, or may be manifest in various combinations and in various orders of appearance. Clubbing of the fingers due to intrathoracic neoplasms is somewhat different from that due to chronic pulmonary insufficiency. The former is often painful, appears acute with a red rim surrounding the base of the nail, and develops rapidly. The periostitis is painful, and the arthritis shows some similarity to the rheumatoid type. This condition may be the first sign of an intrathoracic lesion. An increase in estrogen excretion in pulmonary hypertrophic osteoarthropathy has been reported.

Pathologically, the tubular bones show periosteal new bone apposition and cortical thickening, most marked at the diaphysis. The bone ends and epicondyles are not involved. At first, the osteoperiostitic deposit is sharply demarcated from the original cortex, and is composed of meshing trabecular primitive bone. As the deposit thickens, the deeper part undergoes lamellar reconstruction and can merge with the cortex. There is no endosteal deposition of bone. The joints show synovial inflammatory changes and occasionally intra-articular effusion. The articular cartilages may show subcapsular vascularization.

Radiologically, the soft-tissue signs are clubbing of the fingers with soft-tissue prominence at the terminal tufts (Fig. 6–189). There are no bone changes in the distal phalanges; specifically, there is no periosteal new bone formation nor a spadelike configuration as in acromegaly.

Periosteal changes are evident in the diaphyses of the tubular bones, sparing the ends. In decreasing order, the following structures are most frequently involved: the radius and ulna, the tibia and fibula, the humerus and femur, the metacarpals and meta-

tarsals, and the proximal and middle phalanges. Five types of periosteal changes have been seen:

1. Simple or solid elevation of the periosteum, in which a radiolucent area is seen between the periosteum and the cortex (Figs. 6–190, 6–191)
2. Laminated or "onionskin" effect (Fig. 6–192)
3. Irregular "bursts" of periosteal new bone sporadically distributed (Fig. 6–193)
4. Solid periosteal cloaking with a wavy contour (Fig. 6–194)
5. Cortical thickening, in which the periosteal new bone has merged with the cortex and no separating radiolucent line is evident (Fig. 6–195)

(Text continued on p. 490)

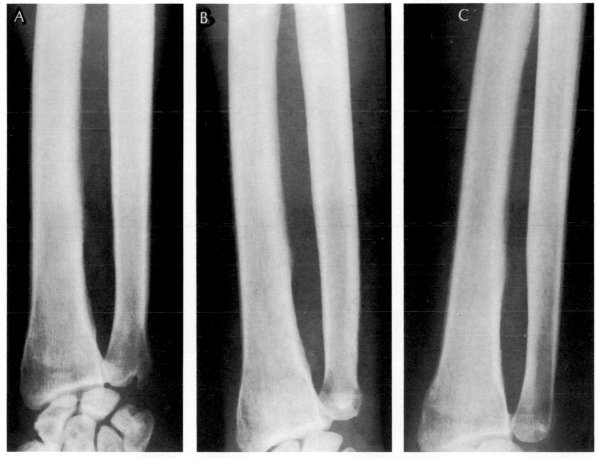

FIG. 6–188. Pulmonary hypertrophic osteoarthropathy (forearm). This series shows regression of simple periosteal new bone formation, secondary to carcinoma of the lung following surgery. **A.** Simple periosteal elevation of the radius and ulna. The bone ends are spared (presurgical film). **B.** One-year interval film following surgery and **A.** Considerable diminution in the amount of periosteal elevation is noted. **C.** Three-month interval film following **B**, showing progressive diminution of periosteal new bone.

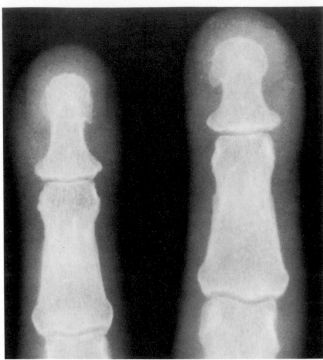

FIG. 6–189. Pulmonary hypertrophic osteoarthropathy (hand) secondary to carcinoma of the lung. Clubbing with soft-tissue prominence of the distal phalanges, but without periosteal new bone formation, may be seen. There is no "spadelike" configuration of the terminal tufts.

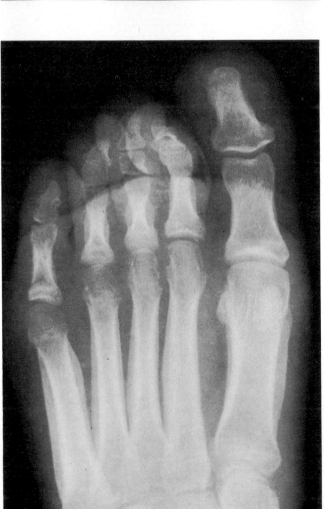

FIG. 6–190. Pulmonary hypertrophic osteoarthropathy (hand) secondary to carcinoma of the lung. Simple periosteal elevation may be seen involving the metacarpals and the proximal and middle phalanges. The distal phalanges are spared. Soft-tissue clubbing may also be noted.

FIG. 6–191. Pulmonary hypertrophic osteoarthropathy (foot). Note solid periosteal new bone formation involving the metatarsals, proximal phalanges, and the medial aspect of the distal phalanx of the great toe. The latter finding is unusual.

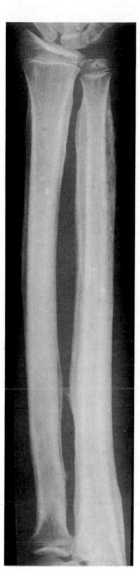

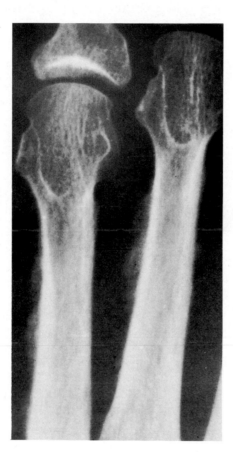

FIG. 6–192. Pulmonary hypertrophic osteoarthropathy (forearm)—male, age 14 years, with pulmonary metastases from osteosarcoma. Note extensive laminated periosteal new bone formation of the radius and ulna. The new bone characteristically does not involve the epiphyses or metaphyses.

FIG. 6–193. Pulmonary hypertrophic osteoarthropathy (metatarsals), secondary to carcinoma of the lung. Irregular "bursts" of periosteal new bone formation may be seen.

FIG. 6–194. Pulmonary hypertrophic osteoarthropathy (leg). Solid periosteal cloaking with a wavy and lacelike contour is noted.

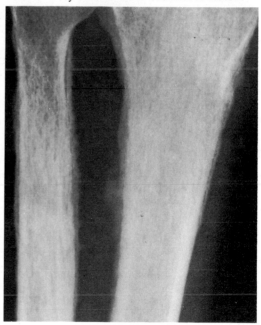

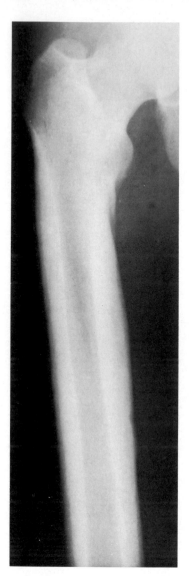

FIG. 6–195. Pulmonary hypertrophic osteoarthropathy (femur) secondary to pulmonary metastases from mixed tumor of the parotid gland. Marked cortical thickening of the femur is present, which characteristically does not involve the ends of the bones.

FIG. 6–196. Thyroid acropachy (hands). Spiculated periosteal new bone formation is present bilaterally and symmetrically. The first and second radials show most pronounced changes at the radial side while the fifth radial shows most pronounced changes at the ulnar side. Soft-tissue masses are associated with the periosteal new bone formation. The spicules are short and squat, characteristic of a benign spiculative process. (From Greenfield GB, Escamilla CH, Schorsch HA: The hand as an indicator of generalized disease. Am J Roentgen 99:736–745, 1967)

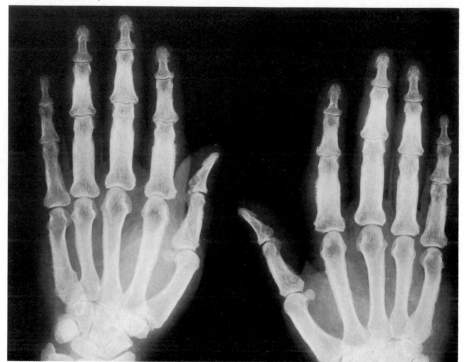

No recognizable roentgen manifestations of joint erosions or cartilage destruction occur; however, occasionally massive distention of the knee joint may be seen.

Other conditions associated with clubbing of the fingers and periosteal new bone formation are thyroid acropachy and pachydermoperiostosis.

THYROID ACROPACHY

Thyroid acropachy[79,118,194,209,272,310] is a rare complication of hyperthyroid disease characterized by progressive exophthalmos, relatively asymptomatic swelling of the hands and feet, clubbing of the digits, pretibial myxedema, and periosteal new formation. The onset is insidious and usually follows ablation of the thyroid after a period from several weeks to many years. Ninety-five percent of cases developed following therapy for the primary disease. The overall incidence is less than 1% in hyperthyroid patients.[321] The patients are euthyroid or hypothyroid, and range in age from young adults to the elderly. Men and women are equally affected. The etiology may be related to TSH (thyroid-stimulating hormone), LATS (long-acting thyroid stimulator), EPS (exophthalmos-producing substance), or calcitonin, but this has not been proven.

Radiological findings are present in over 90% of cases.

Radiologically, the periosteal proliferations characteristically involve the midportions of the diaphyses, causing a fusiform contour, usually with asymmetrical involvement. The periosteal new bone may be irregular with multiple small radiolucencies, causing a "bubbly" appearance, or short squat spiculations may be present. This is in contrast to pulmonary osteoarthropathy. The periostitis is usually associated with soft-tissue swellings. The hands and feet are most often involved, and rarely the forearms and legs show periosteal new bone.

In the hands, the bones at the radial aspect show most pronounced changes at their radial sides, while if the fifth metacarpal is involved, the periostitis is more marked at the ulnar side (Fig. 6–196). Changes were observed most frequently in the first, second, and fifth metacarpals, the first metatarsals, and their proximal phalanges.

PACHYDERMOPERIOSTOSIS (CHRONIC IDIOPATHIC HYPERTROPHIC OSTEOARTHROPATHY WITH PACHYDERMIA)

Pachydermoperiostosis[48,258,276] is an uncommon familial condition characterized by a marked thickening of the skin of the forehead and face and of the forearms and legs, clubbing of the fingers, painful swollen joints, hyperhydrosis of the hands and feet, nontender periosteal new bone formation, and cortical thickening. The onset is at puberty or adolescence, involving males almost exclusively. It is self-limiting, progressing for several years, then ceasing. It is transmitted as an autosomal dominant with variable penetrance.

Radiologically, irregular periosteal new bone formation is seen, which tends to blend with the cortex. There is symmetrical involvement. The cortex is thickened and the medulla narrowed. The midportion of the diaphysis is the site of greatest change, although the bone ends and epicondyles may also be involved (Fig. 6–197). This is in contrast to what is seen in pulmonary osteoarthropathy. The sites most frequently involved are the distal radius, ulna, tibia, and fibula. The metacarpals and proximal and midphalanges may show cortical thickening (Fig. 6–198). Rarely, there may be thickening of the skull, facial bones, and mandible. The paranasal sinuses may be enlarged. A thickened heel pad may also be present. A "forme fruste" has been reported in which periostitis is absent or minimal. Pachydermoperiostosis associated with acroosteolysis has

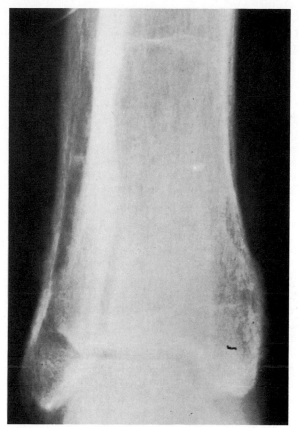

FIG. 6–197. Pachydermoperiostosis. Periosteal new bone formation of the tibia and fibula are present with involvement of the distalmost portions of bone. This is in contrast to what is seen in pulmonary hypertrophic osteoarthropathy. (Courtesy of Dr. Leon Bobrow, Weiss Memorial Hospital, Chicago, IL)

been reported[123] as well as its association with gross extramedullary hematopoiesis.[222] Cases have also been seen showing the features of this condition since childhood without pachydermia, in which case it is termed *Idiopathic hypertrophic osteoarthropathy* (Fig. 6–199).[23] Differentiation from acromegaly must be made.

INFANTILE CORTICAL HYPEROSTOSIS (CAFFEY'S SYNDROME)

Infantile cortical hyperostosis[42, 54] is a now uncommon disease characterized by hyperirritability, soft-tissue swellings, periosteal new bone formation, and cortical thickening of the underlying bones. The etiology is unknown. Familial incidence has been observed in some cases.[56] The onset very rarely, if ever, occurs past the age of 5 months, and is usually seen about the ninth week of life. The disease has been reported *in utero*. Late recurrence in older children has been reported.[298]

Clinically, there is a sudden onset of tender soft-tissue swellings without discoloration or marked warmth. Fever almost invariably accompanies the condition, and there may be pallor, pleuritis, or pseudoparalysis. In the acute phase, the erythrocyte sedimentation rate is increased and there is elevated serum phosphatase activity. Anemia may be present. Other laboratory studies have shown no consistent abnormalities. The disease may be acute, subacute, or chronic. Residual deformities may be seen very rarely up to adult life.[56] Deformities and delayed muscular development may occur in the chronic stage. The severity of the disease may range from the barely perceptible to widespread involvement. Males and females are equally affected.

Radiologically, the bone underlying the soft-tissue swellings shows periosteal new bone formation and cortical thickening. When the tubular bones are involved, only the diaphysis is affected, causing a spindle shape of the bone (Fig. 6–200). The process spares the bone ends and the metaphyses, differentiating this entity from the various diseases that involve the epiphyseal region. Massive cortical thickening, widening of bone (Fig. 6–201), bridging across the interosseous membranes and enlargement, marginal hyperostosis, and sclerosis of the flat bones occur (Fig. 6–202). During the healing phase, but not in the acute stage, laminated periosteal reaction may be seen. In chronic cases, there may be expansion of the shaft resulting in a thin cortex with a wide medulla.

The distribution of lesions is characteristic. The mandible (Fig. 6–203), clavicles, and ulnae are the bones most frequently involved. The long bones, ilia, lateral ribs (Fig. 6–204), and skull are often affected, as is the scapula, which usually shows unilateral involvement. All bones of the body have been implicated except the phalanges, vertebral bodies, and cuboidal bones. There may be asymmetrical involvement. Recovery may be complete in a period ranging from a few weeks to several months. Roentgen changes usually completely regress within a year after acute symptoms have subsided. A case originating in the first metatarsal has been reported.[132]

(Text continued on p. 496)

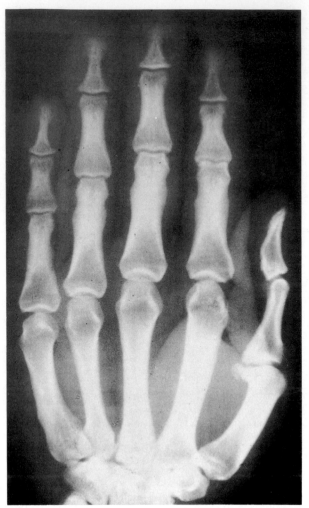

FIG. 6–198. Pachydermoperiostosis (hand). Clubbing of the phalanges and cortical thickening with narrowing of the medullary canal of the metacarpals and proximal and middle phalanges are seen. The latter finding is not present in pulmonary hypertrophic osteoarthropathy. (Courtesy of Dr. Leon Bobrow, Weiss Memorial Hospital, Chicago, IL)

FIG. 6–199. Idiopathic osteoarthropathy without pachydermia. **A.** Hands. Cortical thickening of the mid-portions of the phalanges and metacarpals is noted. **B.** Forearms. Cortical thickening with undulating borders of both radius and ulna is noted. **C.** Legs. Marked cortical thickening and periosteal new bone formation are seen. **D.** Lateral view of ankle showing cortical thickening, particularly of the distal fibula.

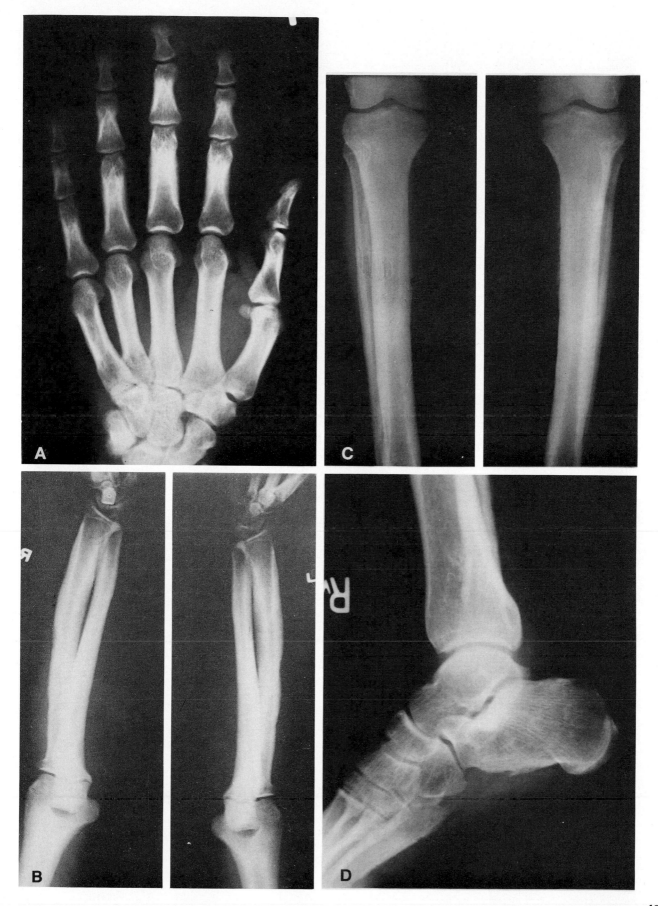

493

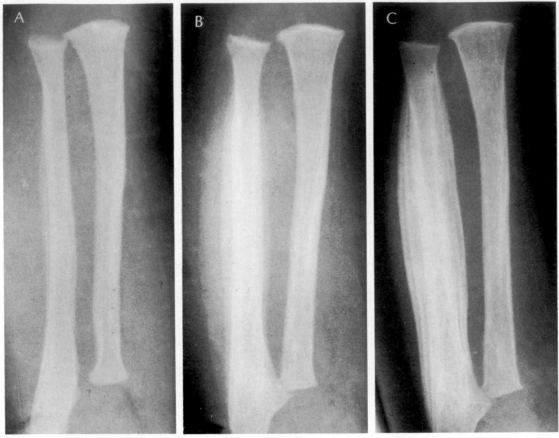

FIG. 6–200. Infantile cortical hyperostosis (forearm) — male, age 5 months. **A.** Note simple periosteal elevation along the shaft of the ulna. **B.** Ten-day interval film. Thickened periosteal new bone formation along the ulnar shaft may be seen involving the diaphysis. **C.** Three-week interval film showing marked progression of periosteal new bone formation with a laminated appearance in the ulna. There is a fusiform appearance of thickening of the bone, as the bone ends are spared.

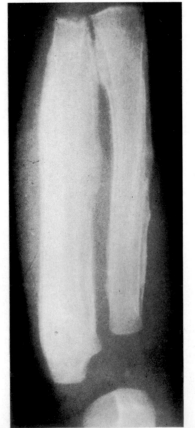

FIG. 6–201. Infantile cortical hyperostosis (forearm). Massive cortical thickening and widening of the bones with periosteal new bone formation are seen. The ends of the bone are not involved.

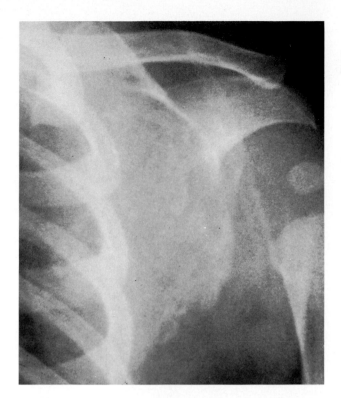

FIG. 6–202. Infantile cortical hyperostosis with enlargement and sclerosis of the scapula.

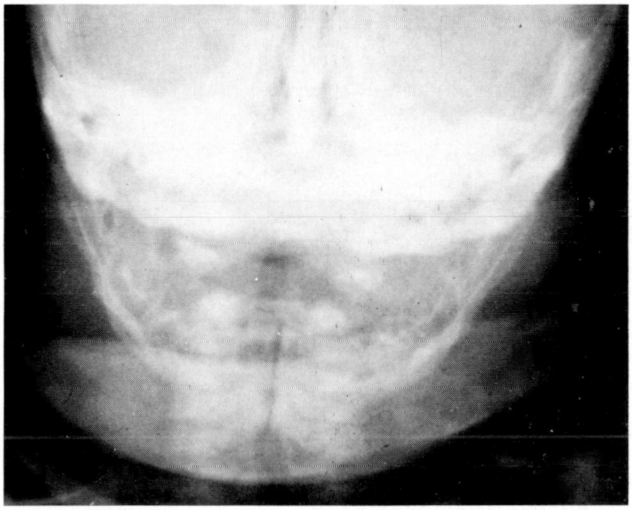

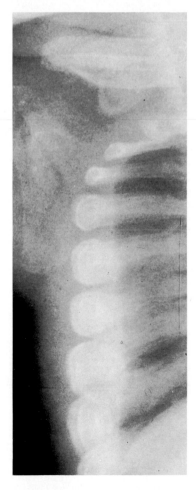

FIG. 6–203. Infantile cortical hyperostosis (mandible). Marked soft-tissue swelling and periosteal new bone formation involving the mandible are seen.

FIG. 6–204. Infantile cortical hyperostosis (ribs). Periosteal new bone formation of the ribs associated with pleural reaction and widening of the clavicle is seen.

495

HYPERVITAMINOSIS A

Excessive intake of vitamin A results in characteristic symptoms and roentgen changes.[40] Acute and chronic forms exist. Ingestion of more than 1,000,000 IU may cause acute symptoms, the most ominous of which are due to increased intracranial pressure. Chronic hypervitaminosis A usually is seen between the ages of 1 and 3 years, and has been reported at the age of 2 months in a patient who had received 70,000 IU daily since birth.

Clinically, loss of appetite and pruritis are followed by hard, tender masses in the extremities. Hepatosplenomegaly, fissures of the lips, loss of hair, and jaundice may occur. The blood vitamin A level is increased, as are the serum lipids. The serum alkaline phosphatase is elevated. A long latent period between the beginning of excessive intake and onset of symptoms usually occurs.

Radiologically, the long bones underlying the tender masses show periosteal new bone formation. The ulnae and metatarsals are the bones most commonly affected. The diaphyses are involved, while the bone ends are spared (Figs. 6–205, 6–206). The periosteal new bone initially may have the appearance of a smooth, wavy, undulating contour, later blending the cortex to cause thickening. This condition can be differentiated from infantile cortical hyperostosis by the different distribution of lesions, the older age group, and the high serum vitamin A levels. Permanent arrest of bone growth in vitamin A intoxication has been reported.[237, 264] Shortening of the shaft, splaying of the metaphysis, enlargement, and premature fusion of the ossification centers are seen. The shortenings are asymmetrical (Fig. 6–207). The presence of scoliosis in one such case has been reported.

PERIOSTEAL TUMORS

The region of the periosteum may rarely give rise to a neoplasm. The following tumors have been described (see Chap. 7):

1. Parosteal sarcoma
2. Juxtacortical chondrosarcoma[58]
3. Juxtacortical chondroma[47]
4. Periosteal osteoid osteoma
5. Periosteal benign osteoblastoma
6. Parosteal lipoma
7. Giant-cell tumor[282]
8. Periosteal desmoid.

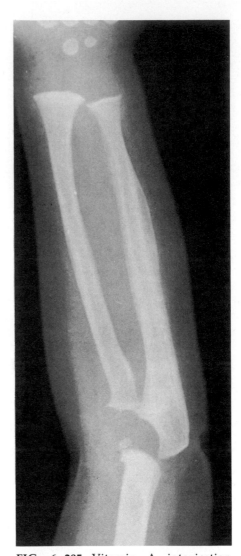

FIG. 6–205. Vitamin A intoxication (forearm). Periosteal new bone formation along the diaphysis of the ulna is seen, with partial blending with the cortex at the proximal outer aspect. The bone ends are not involved. (Courtesy of Dr. Harvey White, Children's Memorial Hospital, Chicago, IL)

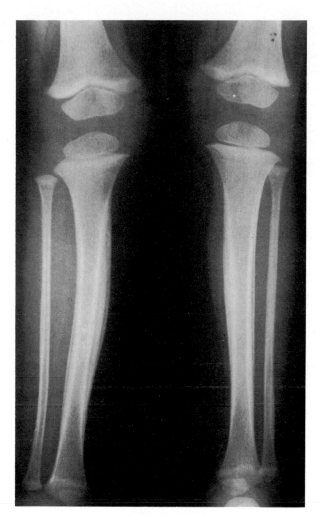

FIG. 6–206. Vitamin A intoxication (legs). Periosteal new bone formation with a laminated effect is present along the shafts of the tibiae. Note the undulating contour on the right and the slight amount of fibular periosteal new bone formation. The bone ends are not involved. (Courtesy of Dr. Harvey White, Children's Hospital, Chicago, IL)

FIG. 6–207. Vitamin A intoxication (femora). There is shortening of the shaft of the right femur with splaying of the metaphysis and enlargement of the epiphyseal ossification center. The involvement is asymmetrical. (Courtesy of Dr. Harvey White, Children's Memorial Hospital, Chicago, IL)

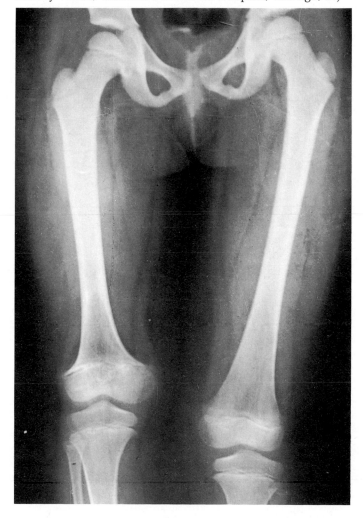

THE CORTEX

Radiologically, the cortex may show thickening, thinning, splitting, destruction, erosion, endosteal erosion, or expansion.

CORTICAL THICKENING

Cortical thickening may be due to local causes such as osteoid osteoma, or as part of a generalized process. A thickened cortex may result from blending of elevated periosteal new bone, or excess periosteal or endosteal new bone formation, without the stripping of the periosteum away from the cortex. The causes of generalized cortical thickening are summarized below.

CAUSES OF GENERALIZED CORTICAL THICKENING

1. All processes in which periosteal new bone has blended with the cortex
2. Paget's disease
3. Fibrous dysplasia
4. Progressive diaphyseal dysplasia (Engelmann–Camurati disease)
5. Hereditary multiple diaphyseal sclerosis (Ribbing's disease)
6. Hyperphosphatasemia
7. Van Buchem's disease
8. Melorheostosis

PROGRESSIVE DIAPHYSEAL DYSPLASIA (ENGELMANN'S DISEASE, ENGELMANN–CAMURATI DISEASE)

Progressive diaphyseal dysplasia[111,146,219,329] is a rare condition characterized by progressive midshaft cortical thickening associated with neuromuscular dystrophy and wasting. It is transmitted as an autosomal dominant.

Clinically, the usual age of onset is between 4 and 12 years. A waddling gait, muscular weakness, and malnutrition are constant features. There may be tenderness over the involved bones. There is no mental retardation. Laboratory values are normal except for slight elevation of the serum alkaline phosphatase level in some cases.

Radiologically, the characteristic finding is cortical thickening in the midshaft of a long bone. The process begins in the midportion and progresses peripherally. The medullary cavity is narrowed. The bone ends are spared. There may be elongation of the bone. The result is a spindle-shaped bone with an undertubulated appearance and a relatively abrupt transition to normal bone at the ends. The distribution of lesions is symmetrical. All of the long bones are involved (Fig. 6–208 *A* to *C*).

The bones of the hands and feet are less often affected. The pelvis, ribs, clavicles, and scapula rarely are involved. The vertebral bodies may rarely show diffuse sclerosis or vertical dense striations. The base of the skull is more often involved than the calvarium (Fig. 6–208 *D*). Muscular underdevelopment can be detected. Associated lamellated periosteal reaction has been reported.

HEREDITARY MULTIPLE DIAPHYSEAL SCLEROSIS (RIBBING'S DISEASE)

Ribbing's disease[257] represents a rare entity that may represent the adult form of Engelmann's disease after clinical symptoms have subsided. There is a familial incidence, and the age of occurrence is during adolescence and young adulthood. The neuromuscular symptoms seen in Engelmann's disease are not present. Bone pain may be present.

Radiologically, lesions similar to those of Engelmann's disease, with cortical thickening of the midshaft, fusiform contour of bone, and sparing of the bone ends are seen. The distribution of lesions is limited, with asymmetrical involvement of one or several bones. When several bones are involved there is a tendency toward symmetry. There is no progression of lesions.

HYPERPHOSPHATASEMIA

Hyperphosphatasemia[147, 202] is a rare condition in which there are marked cortical thickening and bowing deformities of the long bones associated with elevated serum alkaline phosphatase levels. The high alkaline phosphatase activity is thought to result from excess bone activity rather than to be the casual factor. Bowing deformities are usuallly noted from several months to years after birth. Muscle weakness is usually present, and arterial hypertension has been reported. There is no mental retardation.

Radiologically, all bones are involved with a marked cortical thickening. The long bones show diffuse cortical thickening involving the entire bone, in contrast to Engelmann's disease, which is fusiform. There is narrowing or obliteration of the medullary cavity. Lateral bowing of the femora is seen. The short tubular bones of the hands and feet also show cortical thickening. There is marked

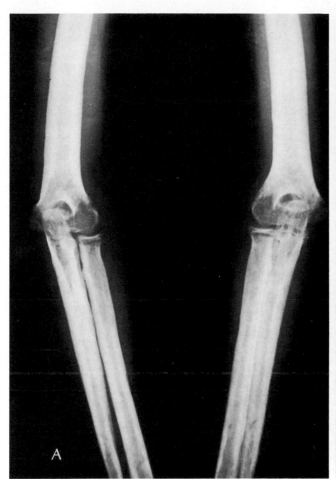
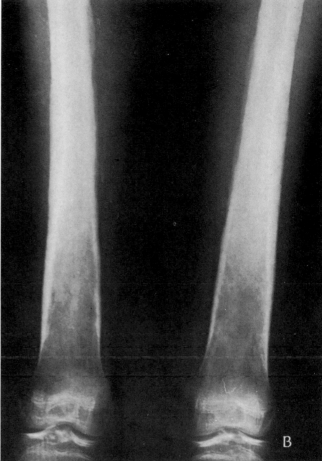

thickening of the calvarium with patchy sclerosis. Localized rarefactions and loss of lamina dura may be seen in the mandible. The ribs are thickened and may show pseudofractures. The cuboidal bones are usually uninvolved. "Splitting" of the cortex may also be seen. A report of a long-term follow-up showed, in addition, marked osteophyte formation, vertebral body sclerosis, and calcification of the spinal ligaments. Associated pseudoxanthoma elasticum has been reported.[202] Improvement of the radiological appearance following treatment with calcitonin has been reported.[323]

VAN BUCHEM'S DISEASE (HYPEROSTOSIS CORTICALIS GENERALISATA)

Van Buchem's disease[74,98,230,315,317] is a rare condition characterized by symmetrical middiaphyseal cortical thickenings associated with an elevated serum

FIG. 6–208. Engelmann's disease. The patient is a female who appeared normal at birth. A waddling gait was seen at the age of 18 months, and diagnosis was established. The patient complained of increasing progressive lumbar lordosis over the years. Urine and blood studies were normal except for a slightly elevated serum alkaline phosphatase level. **A.** Arms, showing undertubulation of the bones. Cortical thickening involves the diaphysis but spares the epiphysis. **B.** Femora, showing thickening of the cortex of the diaphysis without epiphyseal involvement, and undertubulation. **C.** Legs. Cortical thickening, involving the diaphyses of both tibiae and fibulae (greatest at the midshaft but sparing the ends of the bone) and undertubulation of both tibiae are noted. **D.** Skull. Note thickening of the base of the skull and cloudlike irregular sclerosis of the calvarium.

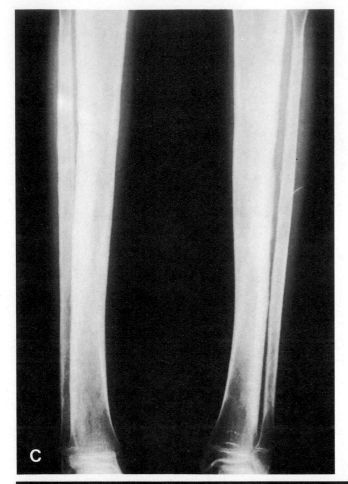

FIG. 6–208

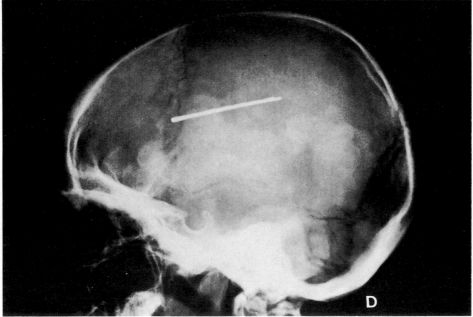

FIG. 6–208

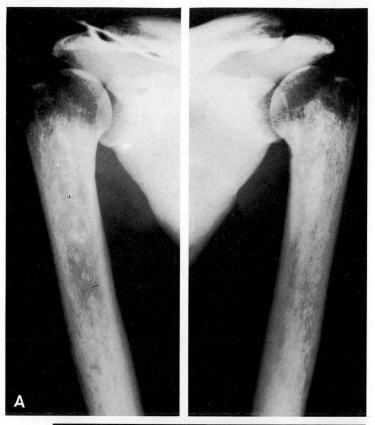

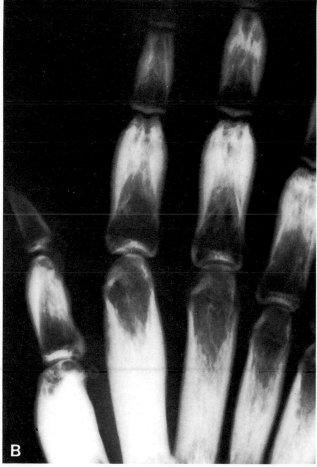

FIG. 6–209. Van Buchem's disease. A. Humeri, showing diaphyseal sclerosis. B. Hand, showing diaphyseal sclerosis, cortical thickening, and fusiform contour of the short bones. C. Skull—anteroposterior and lateral views. Extensive sclerosis of all bony structures, with obliteration of paranasal and mastoid air spaces is noted. D. Pelvis, showing patchy and diffuse sclerotic changes. (From Fosmoe RJ, Holm RS, Hildreth RC: Van Buchem's disease (hyperostosis corticalis generalizata familiaris). A case report. Radiology 90:771–774, 1968)

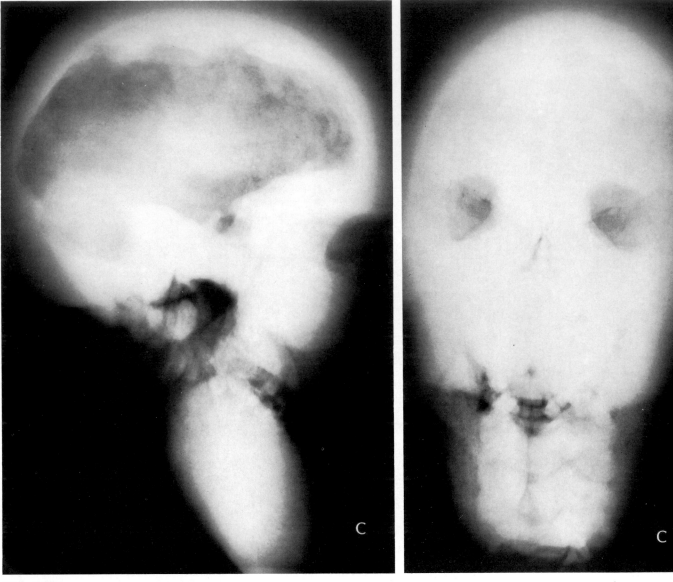

FIG. 6–209

alkaline phosphatase level, occurring in adults. Caffey[42] states that this may represent the adult form of hyperphosphatasemia, and Rubin[263] claims that it represents the tarda form of the same disease.

Clinically, the patients may range in age up to the fifth decade, with a greater incidence in males. There is a widened chin without prognathism. Neurological symptoms occur, owing to thickening of the base of the skull. There is no muscular weakness.

Radiologically, diffuse symmetrical cortical thickening of all of the long bones occurs (Fig. 6–209 *A*). Bowing has not been reported. The cortical thickening is chiefly caused by endosteal sclerosis. The midshaft appears more affected than the bone ends. Fusiform changes are seen in short tubular bones (Fig. 6–209 *B*). Thickening of the ribs and pelvic bones and marked thickening of both the base and the vault of the skull are seen (Fig. 6–209 *C* and *D*). The mandible and clavicle are also sclerotic, and the spine may be involved.

MELORHEOSTOSIS (LERI)

Melorheostosis[43, 117] is a rare condition of cortical thickening of unknown etiology. There is a wide range of age incidence, from 3 years to 59 years. The

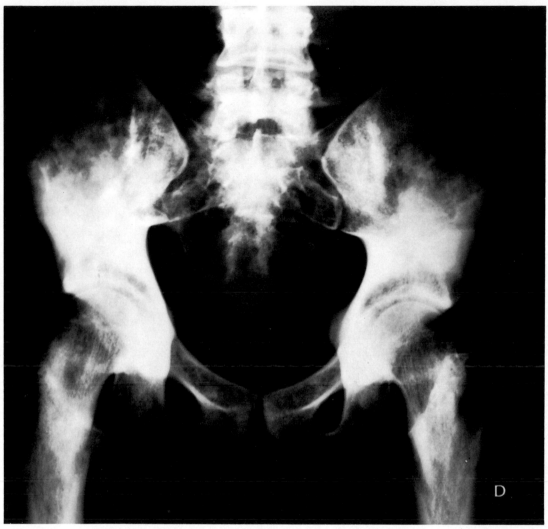

FIG. 6–209

disease may be asymptomatic, but the most common complaint is pain of varying severity. Limitation of motion, contracture, or fusion of an adjacent joint may occur. There may be decreased growth of an extremity, luxation of the patella, and muscular atrophy and contractures. There is an insidious onset and chronic course. Linear scleroderma-like changes of the overlying skin may be present.[292]

Radiologically, cortical sclerosis and thickening that may encroach on the medullary canal are seen. The process begins as a faint linear hyperostosis which progresses. Uniform cortical thickening, or involvement of only one side of a bone, may occur (Fig. 6–210). A smooth, irregular outline of hyperostosis, involving initially the end of the bone and proceeding toward the center, has been likened to the flowing of wax down a burning candle, and has inspired the name of this disease. The involved

bone may be shorter or longer than normal. Limb deformities and muscle wasting may be present. Commonly, there is monomelic involvement; however, multiple limbs may be affected. The long bones are most frequently involved. Other sites include the short tubular bones, pelvis, shoulder girdle, spine, and skull. The lesions are sharply demarcated from normal bone. Soft-tissue calcifications or ossifications in the region of joints may also be found. There is no report of regression of lesions. The distribution of lesions is reported by Murray[212] to correspond to sclerotomes, which represent the zones of the skeleton supplied by individual spinal sensory nerves. Associated arteriovenous aneurysms[233] have been reported. Cases have been described with features of melorheostosis, osteopoikilosis, and osteopathia striata, and these are referred to as *mixed sclerosing bone dystrophy.*[2]

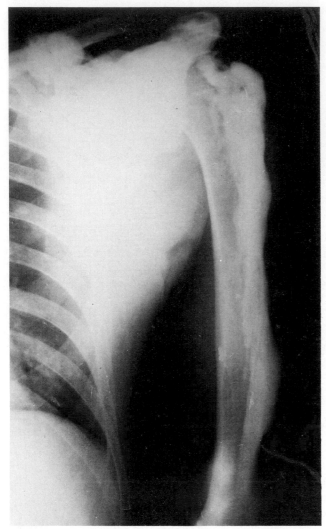

FIG. 6–210. Melorheostosis (shoulder and humerus). Note the dense sclerosis of the scapula and of the outer humeral cortex with an undulating margin. (Courtesy of Dr. Antonio Pizzaro, Hines VA Hospital, Hines, IL)

Regression of melorheostosis in this condition has been reported.[162]

HALLIDAY'S HYPEROSTOSIS

In 1949, Halliday[128] reported a case that is quoted in the literature in the differential diagnosis of bone sclerosis. The patient showed a thick skull, wide and dense ribs and clavicles, underconstricted long bones with a thin cortex, ballooning of the metacarpals, and hypertelorism. The appearance of the illustrations supplied in Halliday's report suggests that this actually represents a case of craniometaphyseal dysplasia; Moseley[207] also states this opinion. Halliday's hyperostosis should not be considered as a distinct entity.

"SPLITTING" OF THE CORTEX

"Splitting" of the cortex to form a double layer is not a rare finding. The conditions is which this sign may be encountered are summarized below.

CONDITIONS ASSOCIATED WITH "SPLITTING" OF THE CORTEX

1. Sickle-cell anemia
2. Osteomyelitis
3. Hyperphosphatasemia
4. Osteopetrosis
5. Gaucher's disease
6. Battered child syndrome
7. Scurvy
8. Bone graft (local)

EROSION OF THE CORTEX

Endosteal scalloping, or erosion or resorption of the inner margin of the cortex, is frequently encountered, chiefly in the myeloproliferative diseases. The conditions in which this finding is seen are summarized below.

CONDITIONS ASSOCIATED WITH SCALLOPING OF THE INNER CORTICAL MARGIN

1. Hodgkin's disease
2. Multiple myeloma
3. Leukemia
4. Reticulum-cell sarcoma
5. Mastocytosis
6. Histiocytosis X
7. Gaucher's disease
8. Hyperparathyroidism
9. Fibrous dysplasia
10. Osteopetrosis

Erosion or "saucerization" of the outer margin of the cortex not infrequently occurs, and is most often caused by aneurysms (Fig. 6–211), nodes, soft-tissue tumors, or pigmented villonodular synovitis.

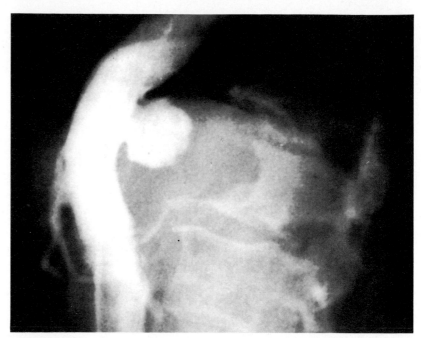

FIG. 6–211. Erosion of the anterior aspect of a vertebral body by an abdominal aortic aneurysm—aortogram.

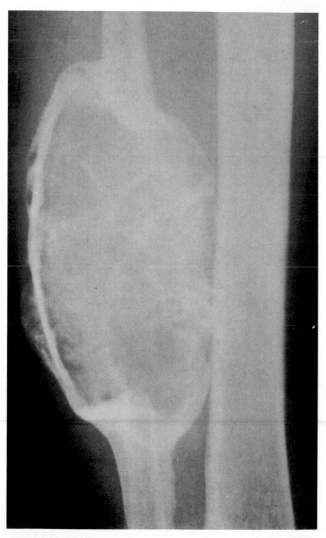

FIG. 6–212. Large expansile lesion of the fibula which shows a dense outer margin and light trabeculation. This represents a metastatic focus from endometrial carcinoma following radiation therapy.

EXPANSION OF THE CORTEX

Expansion of the cortex is related to the slow rate of growth or enlargement of a lesion with respect to the rate of bone repair. It only indicates a slowly growing lesion, and is not a valid criterion of malignancy or benignity. The expanded area may be centrally or eccentrically located. The more common causes of bone expansion are listed below.

CAUSES OF BONE EXPANSION

Primary Benign Tumors of Bone

1. Giant-cell tumor
2. Enchondroma
3. Benign chondroblastoma
4. Chondromyxoid fibroma
5. Desmoplastic fibroma
6. Lipoma of bone

Tumorlike Processes

1. Unicameral bone cyst
2. Fibrous dysplasia
3. Aneurysmal bone cyst
4. Eosinophilic granuloma
5. Dermoid inclusion cyst

Primary Malignant Tumors of Bone

1. Multiple myeloma
2. Malignant giant-cell tumor
3. Chondrosarcoma
4. Fibrosarcoma
5. Adamantinoma (long bone)
6. Osteosarcoma (rare feature)

Tumors Metastatic to Bone

1. Carcinoma of kidney
2. Carcinoma of thyroid
3. Treated metastases (Fig. 6–212)

Differential Diagnosis of an Expansile Lesion in a Rib — Most Probable Lesions

1. Fibrous dysplasia
2. Multiple myeloma or plasmocytoma
3. Histiocytosis X
4. Chondromyxoid fibroma
5. Aneurysmal bone cyst[260]
6. Chondrosarcoma
7. Gaucher's disease

REFERENCES

1. Abel M S, Smith G R: The case of the disappearing pelvis. Radiology 111:105–106, 1974

2. Abramson M N: Disseminated asymptomatic osteosclerosis with features resembling melorheosis, osteopoikilosis, and osteopathia striata. A case report. J Bone Joint Surg 50–A:991–996, 1968

3. Aegerter E, Kirkpatrick J A: Orthopedic Diseases, 3rd ed. Philadelphia, W B Saunders 1968

4. Ahlback S, Collert S: Destruction of the odontoid process due to atlanto-axial pyogenic spondylitis. Acta Radiol (Diagn) 10:394–400, 1970

5. Akal M et al: Membranous lipodystrophy—a clinicopathological study of 6 cases. J Bone Joint Surg 59–A:802–809, 1977

6. Alford B A, Coccia P F, C'Heureuz P R: Roentgenographic features of American Burkitt's lymphoma. Radiology 124:763–770, 1977

7. Ameri M R, Alebouyeh M, Donner M W: Hypertrophic osteoarthropathy in childhood malignancy. Am J Roentgen 130:992–993, 1978

8. Amin P H, Evans A N W: Essential osteolysis of carpal and tarsal bones. Brit J Radiol 51:539–541, 1978

9. Arcomano J P, Barnett J C, Wunderlich H O: Histiocytosis X. Am J Roentgen 85:663–679, 1961

10. Bach M, Simpson W J, Platts, M E: Metastatic cerebellar sarcoma (desmoplastic medulloblastoma) with diffuse osteosclerosis and leukoerythroblastic anemia. A case report and review of the literature. Am J Roentgen 103:38–43, 1968

11. Baer J W, Radkowski M.A: Congenital multiple fibromatosis: A case report with a review of the world literature. Am J Roentgen 118:200–205, 1973

12. Ball J, Grayzell A I: Arteritis and localized periosteal new bone formation. J Bone Joint Surg 46–B:244–250, 1964

13. Baltzer G, Jacob H, Esselborn H: Contrast media and renal function in multiple myeloma. Fortschr Roentgenstr 129:208–211, 1978

14. Barber J W: Delayed bone and joint changes following electrical injury. Radiology 99:49–53, 1971

15. Barer M et al: Mastocytosis with osseous lesions resembling metastatic malignant lesions in bone. J Bone Joint Surg 50–A:142–152, 1968

16. Beals R K, Bird C B: Carpal and tarsal osteolysis. J Bone Joint Surg 57–A:681–686, 1975

17. Bell D, Cockshott W P: Tuberculosis of the vertebral pedicles. Radiology 99:43–48, 1971

18. Beltran G, Baez A, Correa P: Burkitt's lymphoma in Colombia. Am J Med 40:211–216, 1966

19. Bendel W L, Race G J: Urticaria pigmentosa with bone involvement. Case report and analysis of 21 cases from the literature. J Bone Joint Surg 45–A:1043–1056, 1963

20. Bergdahl S, Fellander M, Robertson B: BCG osteomyelitis. J Bone Joint Surg 58–B:212–216, 1976

21. Bernhard W G, Gore I, Kilby R A: Congenital leukemia. Blood 6:990–1001, 1951

22. Bernstein C, Loeser W D, Manning L E: Erosive rib lesions in paralytic poliomyelitis. Radiology 70:368–372, 1958

23. Bhate D V, Pizarro A J, Greenfield G B: Idiopathic hypertrophic osteoarthropathy without pachyderma. Radiology 129:379–382, 1978

24. Bjersand A J: Bone changes in hypercholesterolemia. Radiology 130:101–102, 1979

25. Blank N, Lieber A: The significance of growing bone islands. Radiology 85:508–511, 1965

26. Blundell G, Midgley R L, Smith G S: Massive osteolysis — disappearing bones. J Bone Joint Surg 40–B:494–501, 1958

27. Bottomly J P, Bradley J, Whitehouse G H: Waldenstrom's macroglobulinemia and amyloidosis with subcutaneous calcification and lymphographic appearances. Brit J Radiol 47:232–235, 1974

28. Boyle W J: Cystic angiomatosis of bone. J Bone Joint Surg 54–B:626–636, 1972

29. Brailsford J F: The radiology of gout. Brit J Radiol 32:472–478, 1959

30. Branan R, Wilson C B: Arachnoid granulations simulating osteolytic lesions of the calvarium. Am J Roentgen 127:523–525, 1976

31. Brinn L B, Khiliani M T: Epidermolysis bullosa with characteristic hand deformities. Radiology 89:272–274, 1967

32. Brinn L B, Moseley J E: Bone changes following electrical injury. Am J Roentgen 97:682–686, 1966

33. Bronsky D, Bernstein A: Acute gout secondary to multiple myeloma. A case report. Ann Intern Med 41:820–822, 1954

34. Brower A C, Culver J E, Keats T E: Diffuse cystic angiomatosis of bone: Report of 2 cases. Am J Roentgen 118:456–463, 1973

35. Brünner S, Gudbjerg C E, Iverson T: Skeletal lesions in leukemia in children. Acta Radiol 49:419–424, 1958

36. Brutschin P, Culver G J: Extracranial metastases from medulloblastomas. Radiology 107:359–362, 1973

37. Bryan C S: Vertebral osteomyelitis due to cryptococcus neoformans. A case report. J Bone Joint Surg 59–A:275–276, 1977

38. Buonocore E, Salomon A, Kerley H E: Pseudomyeloma. Radiology 95:41–46, 1970

39. Cadenat H, Combelles R, Fabert G, Clovet M: Ostéolyse cryptogénétique de la mandibule. J Radiol Electrol 59:509–512, 1978

40. Caffey J: Chronic poisoning due to excess of vitamin A. Pediatrics 5:672–688, 1950

41. Caffey J: Congenital stenosis of medullary spaces in tubular bones and calvaria in 2 proportionate dwarfs — mother and son — coupled with transitory hypocalcemic tetany. Am J Roentgen 100:1–11, 1967

42. Caffey J, Silverman F N: Pediatric X-ray diagnosis, 5th ed. Chicago, Year Book Publishers, 1967

43. Campbell C J, Papademetriou T, Bonfiglio M: Melorheostosis. A report of the clinical, roentgenographic, and pathological findings in 14 cases. J Bone Joint Surg 50–A:1281–1304, 1968

44. Campbell J, Almond H G A, Johnson R: Massive osteolysis of the humerus with spontaneous recovery. J Bone Joint Surg 57–B:238–240, 1975

45. Capitanio M A, Kirkpatrick J A: Early roentgen observations in acute osteomyelitis. Am J Roentgen 108:488–496, 1970

46. Carlson D H: Osteopathia striata revisited. J Canad Assn Rad 28:190–192, 1977

47. Cary G R: Juxtacortical chondroma. A case resport. J Bone Joint Surg 47–A:1405–1407, 1965

48. Chamberlain D S, Whitaker J, Silverman F N: Idiopathic osteoarthropathy and cranial defects in children. Am J Roentgen 93:408–415, 1965

49. Chang C H, Gaskell J R, Chun C S: Abnormal muscle cylinder ratio in idiopathic infantile hypercalcemia: A new roentgen sign. Am J Roentgen 108:533–536, 1970

50. Chawla S: Cranioskeletal dysplasia with acroosteolysis. Brit J Radiol 37:702–705, 1964

51. Cheney W D: Acroosteolysis. Am J Roentgen 94:595–607, 1965

52. Chevrot A, Pallardy G, Ledoux P, Lebard G: Skeletal manifestations of hyperthyroidism. J Radiol Electrol 59:167–173, 1978

53. Cheyne C: Histiocytosis X. J Bone Joint Surg 53–B:366–382, 1971

54. Claesson I: Infantile cortical hyperostosis: Report of a case with late manifestation. Acta Rad 17:594–600, 1976

55. Clarisse P D T, Staple T W: Diffuse bone sclerosis in multiple myeloma. Radiology 99:327–328, 1971

56. Clemett A R, Williams J G: The familial occurrence of infantile cortical hyperostosis. Radiology 80:409–416, 1963

57. Cockshott W P: Radiological aspects of Burkitt's tumour. Brit J Radiol 38:172–180, 1965

58. Cooper R R: Juxtacortical chondrosarcoma. A case report. J Bone Joint Surg 47–A:524–528, 1965

59. Coughlin C, Greenwald E S, Schraft W C, Grossman S: Myelofibrosis associated with multiple myeloma. Arch Int Med 138:590–592, 1978

60. Culver G J, Thumasathit C: Osseous changes of osteopathia striata and Pyle's disease occurring in a patient with an 11-year follow-up. A case report. Am J Roentgen 116:640–643, 1972

61. Danigelis J A, Long R E: Anonymous mycobacterial osteomyelitis. A case report of a 6-year-old child. Radiology 93:353–354, 1969

62. Davidson J C, Palmer P E S: Osteomyelitis variolosa. J Joint Surg 45–B:687–693, 1963

63. Davidson J W, Chacha P B, James W: Multiple osteosarcomata. Report of a case. J Bone Joint Surg 47–B:537–541, 1965

64. Debnam J W, Staple T W: Osseous metastases from cerebellar medulloblastoma. Radiology 107:363–365, 1973

65. Denison E K, Peters R L, Reynolds T B: Portal hypertension in a patient with osteopetrosis. A case report with discussion of the mechanism of portal hypertension. Arch Intern Med 128:279–283, 1971

66. Dennis J M: The solitary dense vertebral body. Radiology 77:618–621, 1961

67. de Santos L E et al: Percutaneous needle biopsy of bone in the cancer patient. Am J Roentgen 130:641–650, 1978

68. Dismukes W E et al: Destructive bone disease in early syphilis. JAMA 236:2646–2648, 1976

69. Dodds W J, Steinbach H L: Gout associated with calcification of cartilage. New Eng J Med 275:745–749, 1966

70. Doe W F, Henry K, Doyle F H: Radiological and histological findings in 6 patients with alpha-chain disease. Brit J Radiol 49:3–11, 1976

71. Doel G: Bone involvement in Weber–Christian disease. Brit J Radiol 36:140–142, 1963

72. DuBois P J, Orr D P, Meyersen E N, Barnes L E: Undifferentiated parotid carcinoma with osteoblastic metastases. Am J Roentgen 129:744–746, 1977

73. Dunnick N R: Radiographic manifestations of Burkitt's lymphoma in American patients. Am J Roentgen 132:1–6, 1979

74. Eastman J R, Bixler D: Generalized cortical hyperostosis (Van Buchem Disease): Nosologic considerations. Radiology 125:297–304, 1977

75. Edeiken J, Hodes P J: Roentgen Diagnosis of Diseases of Bone, 2nd ed. Baltimore, Williams & Wilkins, 1973

76. Edeiken J, Hodes P J, Caplan L H: New bone production and periosteal reaction. Am J Roentgen 97:708–718, 1966

77. Ellis W: Multiple bone lesions caused by Avian–Battey mycobacteria. J Bone Joint Surg 56–B:323–326, 1974

78. Elmore S M et al: Pycnodysostosis with a familial chromosome anomaly. Am J Med 40:273–282, 1966

79. Elson M W: The syndrome of exophthalmos, hypertrophic osteoarthropathy, and pretibial myxedema. Am J Roentgen 85:114–118, 1961

80. Emami–Ahari Z, Zarabi M, Javid B: Pycnodysostosis. J Bone Joint Surg 51–B:307–312, 1969

81. Engels E P, Smith R C, Krantz S: Bone sclerosis in multiple myeloma. Radiology 75:242–247, 1960

82. Enna C D, Jacobson R R, Rausch R O: Bone changes in leprosy: A correlation of clinical and radiographic features. Radiology 100:295–306, 1971

83. Ennis J T, Whitehouse G, Ross F G M, Middlemiss J H: The radiology of bone changes in histiocytosis. Clin Radiol 24:212–220, 1973

84. Erikson V, Hjelmstedt A: Roentgenologic aspects of BCG osteomyelitis. Radiology 101:575–578, 1971

85. Evans G A, Park W M: Familial multiple nonosteogenic fibromata. J Bone Joint Surg 60–B:416–419, 1978

86. Evans E B, Smith J R: Bone and joint changes following burns. A roentgenographic study — preliminary report. J Bone Joint Surg 41–A:785–799, 1959

87. Ewald F C: Unilateral mixed sclerosing bone dystrophy associated with unilateral lymphangiectasis and capillary hemangioma. A case report. J Bone Joint Surg 54–A:878–880, 1972

88. Fairbank H A T: Osteopathia striata. J Bone Joint Surg 32–B:117–125, 1950

89. Fairley G H, Jackson D C, McDonald P: Osteosclerosis in myelomatosis. Brit J Radiol 37:852–855, 1964

90. Feinberg S, Margulis A R: Severe idiopathic hypercalcemia of infancy. Am J Roentgen 80:468–474, 1958

91. Feldman F, Auerbach R, Johnston A: Tuberculous dactylitis in the adult. Am J Roentgen 112:460–479, 1971

92. Ferris R A, Hakkal H G, Cigtay O S: Radiologic manifestations of North American Burkitt's lymphoma. Am J Roentgen 123:614–620, 1975

93. Fitzgerald R H, Brewer N S, Dahlin D C: Squamous-cell carcinoma complicating chronic osteomyelitis. J Bone Joint Surg 58–A:1146–1148, 1976

94. Foley W D, Baum J K, Wheeler R H: Diffuse osteosclerosis with lymphocytic lymphoma. A case report. Radiology 117:553–554, 1975

95. Forbes G S, McLeod R A, Hattery R R: Radiographic manifestations of bone metastases from renal carcinoma. Am J Roentgen 129:61–66, 1977

96. Fornasier V L: Hemangiomatosis with massive osteolysis. J Bone Joint Surg 52–B:444–451, 1970

97. Forrester D M, Kirkpatrick J: Periostitis and pseudoperiostitis. Radiology 118:597–601, 1976

98. Fosmoe R J, Holm R S, Hildreth R C: Van Buchem's disease (hyperostosis corticalis generalizata familiaris). A case report. Radiology 90:771–774, 1968

99. Fowles J V, Bobechko W P: Solitary eosinophilic granuloma in bone. J Bone Joint Surg 52–B:238–243, 1970

100. Frangione B, Franklin E C: Heavy chain diseases: Clinical features and molecular significance of the disordered immunoglobulin structure. Seminars Hemat 10:53–64, 1973

101. Gama C, Meira J B B: Occupational acroosteolysis. J Bone Joint Surg 60–A:86–90, 1978

102. Gantz N M: Gonococcal osteomyelitis. An unusual complication of gonococcal arthritis. JAMA 236:2431–2432, 1976

103. Gardner H: Bone lesions in primary systemic amyloidosis. Brit J Radiol 34:778–783, 1961

104. Gehweiler J A, Bland W R, Carden T S, Daffner R H: Osteopathia striata — Voorhoeve's disease. A review of the roentgen manifestations. Am J Roentgen 118:450–455, 1973

105. Geoffroy J et al: Les lesions osteoarticulaires du pied chez le diabetique. J Radiol Electrol 59:557–562, 1978

106. Ghahremani G G: Osteomyelitis of the ilium in patients with Crohn's disease. Am J Roentgen 118:364–370, 1973

107. Gillison E W, Grainger R G, Fernandez D: Osteoblastic metastases in carcinoma of the pancreas. Brit J Radiol 43:818–820, 1970

108. Gilmour W N: Acute haematogenous osteomyelitis. J Bone Joint Surg 44–B:841–853, 1962

109. Gilsantz V, Grunebaum M: Radiographic appearance of iliac marrow biopsy sites. Am J Roentgen 128:597–598, 1977

110. Gilula L A, Bliznak J, Staple T W: Idiopathic nonfamilial acroosteolysis with cortical defects and mandibular ramus osteolysis. Radiology 121:63–68, 1976

111. Girdany B R: Engelmann's disease (progressive diaphyseal dysplasia), a nonprogressive familial form of muscular dystrophy with characteristic bone changes. Clin Orthop 14:102–109, 1959

112. Glatt W, Weinstein A: Acropachy in lymphatic leukemia. Radiology 92:125–126, 1969

113. Golding F C: Radiology and orthopedic surgery. Sixth Watson–Jones Lecture, Royal College of Surgeons, England, September 1964. J Bone Joint Surg 48–B:320–335, 1966

114. Gompels B M, Vataw M L, Martel W: Correlation of radiological manifestations of multiple myeloma with immunoglobulin abnormalities and prognosis. Radiology 104:509–514, 1972

115. Gondos B: The pointed tubular bone. Its significance and pathogenesis. Radiology 105:541–546, 1972

116. Goodman N: The significance of terminal phalangeal osteosclerosis. Radiology 89:709–712, 1967

117. Green A E, Ellswood W II, Collins J R: Melorheostosis and osteopoikilosis. Am J Roentgen 87:1096–1111, 1962

118. Greenfield G B, Escamilla C H, Schorsch H A: The hand as an indicator of generalized disease. Am J Roentgen 99:736–745, 1967

119. Greenfield G B, Schorsch H A, Shkolnik A: The various roentgen appearances of pulmonary hypertrophic osteoarthropathy. Am J Roentgen 101:927–931, 1967

120. Griffiths D L: Orthopaedic aspects of myelomatosis. J Bone Joint Surg 48–B:703–728, 1966

121. Grossman R E, Hensley G T: Bone lesions in primary amyloidosis. Am J Roentgen 101:872–875, 1967

122. Grunow O H: Radiating spicules, a nonspecific sign of bone disease. Radiology 65:200–205, 1955

123. Guyer P B, Brunton F J, Wren M W G: Pachydermoperiostosis with acroosteolysis. J Bone Joint Surg 60–B:219–223, 1978

124. Gyepes M T, D'Angio G J: Extracranial metastases from CNS tumors in children and adolescents. Radiology 87:55–63, 1966

125. Hadley M, MacDonald A F: Epidermolysis bullosa. Brit J Radiol 33:646–649, 1960

126. Halaby F A, DiSalvo E I: Osteolysis: A complication of trauma: Report of 2 cases. Am J Roentgen 94:591–594, 1965

127. Halliday D R, Dahlin D C, Pugh D G, Young H H: Massive osteolysis and angiomatosis. Radiology 82:637–644, 1964

128. Halliday J: A rare case of bone dystrophy. Brit J Surg 37:52–63, 1949

129. Harbison J B, Nice C M: Familial pachydermoperiostosis presenting as an acromegalylike syndrome. Am J Roentgen 112:532–536, 1971

130. Harper H A: Review of Physiological Chemistry, 14th ed. Los Altos CA, Lange Medical Publications 1973

131. Harris J R, Brand P W: Patterns of disintegration of the tarsus in the anaesthetic foot. J Bone Joint Surg 48–B:4–16, 1966

132. Harris V J, Ramilo J: Caffey's disease: A case originating in the 1st metatarsal and review of a 12-year experience. Am J Roentgen 130:335–337, 1978

133. Hart K Z, Brower A C: Unilateral hypertrophy of multiple pedicles. Am J Roentgen 129:739–740, 1977

134. Harverson G, Warren A G: Tarsal bone disintegration in leprosy. Clin Rad 30:317–322, 1979

135. Haverbush T J, Wilde A H, Hawk W A, Scherbel A L: Osteolysis of the ribs and cervical spine in progressive systemic sclerosis (scleroderma). J Bone Joint Surg 56–A:637–640, 1974

136. Hayes J T, Brody G L: Cystic lymphangiectasis of bone. A case report. J Bone Joint Surg 43–A:107–117, 1961

137. Heilbrun N, Kuhn W G: Erosive bone lesions and soft-tissue ossification associated with spinal cord injuries (paraplegia). Radiology 48:579–593, 1947

138. Heiple K G, Perrin E, Masamichi A: Congenital generalized fibromatosis. A case limited to osseous lesions. J Bone Joint Surg 54–A:663–669, 1972

139. Heiser S, Schwartzmann J J: Variations in the roentgen appearance of the skeletal system in myeloma. Radiology 58:179–191, 1952

140. Heitzman E R, Bornhurst R A, Russell J P: Disease due to anonymous mycobacteria. Am J Roentgen 103:533–539, 1968

141. Hertz M, Solomon A, Aghai E: "Ivory vertebra" in Hodgkin's disease. Restoration of trabecular pattern after therapy. JAMA 238:2402, 1977

142. Himmelfarb E, Sebes J, Raninowitz J: Unusual roentgenographic presentations of multiple myeloma. Report of 3 cases. J Bone Joint Surg 56–A:1723–1728, 1974

143. Hock T B: Nasopharyngeal carcinoma with hypertrophic pulmonary osteoarthropathy. Singapore Med J 9:103–107, 1968

144. Hodgson J R, Kennedy R L J, Camp J D: Reticuloendotheliosis. Radiology 57:642–652, 1951

145. Horner R L, Wiedel J D, Bralliar F: Involvement of the hand in epidermolysis bullosa. J Bone Joint Surg 53–A:1347–1356, 1971

146. Hundley J D, Wilson F C: Progressive diaphyseal dysplasia. Review of the literature and report of 7 cases in one family. J Bone Joint Surg 55–A:461–474, 1973

147. Iancu T C et al: Chronic familial hyperphosphatemia. Radiology 129:669–676, 1978

148. Inoue Y: A new finding in bone scintigram. Three cases of defect findings. Fortschr Roentgenstr 128:258–261, 1978

149. Isley J K: Prognosis in osteitis condensans illii. Radiology 72:234–237, 1959

150. Jacobs P: Posttraumatic osteolysis of the outer end of the clavicle. J Bone Joint Surg 46–B:705–707, 1964

151. Jacobson H G et al: Agnogenic myeloid metaplasia. Radiology 72:716–725, 1959

152. Jacobson H G, Poppel M H, Shapiro J H, Grossberger S: The vertebral pedicle sign. A roentgen finding to differentiate metastatic carcinoma from multiple myeloma. Am J Roentgen 80:817–821, 1958

153. Jaffe H L: Tumors and Tumorous Conditions of the Bones and Joints. Philadelphia, Lea & Febiger, 1958

154. Jensen W N, Lasser E C: Urticaria pigmentosa associated with widespread sclerosis of the spongiosa of bone. Radiology 71:826–832, 1958

155. Joffe N: Some radiological aspects of scurvy in the adult. Brit J Radiol 34:429–437, 1961

156. Joffe N, Antonioli D A: Osteoblastic bone metastases secondary to adenocarcinoma of the pancreas. Clin Rad 29:41–46, 1978

157. Johns D: Syphilitic disorders of the spine. J Bone Joint Surg 52–B:724–731, 1970

158. Johnson A et al: Lower limb angiography in leprosy. Radiology 126:327–332, 1978

159. Johnson A C, James A E, Reddy E R, Johnson S: Relation of vascular and osseous changes in leprosy. Skel Rad 3:36–41, 1978

160. Johnson L L, Kempson R L: Epidermoid carcinoma in chronic osteomyelitis. Diagnostic problems and management, report of 10 cases. J Bone Joint Surg 47–A:133–145, 1965

161. Johnston R M, Miles J S: Sarcomas arising from chronic osteomyelitic sinuses. J Bone Joint Surg 55–A:162–168, 1973

162. Kanis J A, Thomson J G: Mixed sclerosing bone dystrophy with regression of melorheostosis. Brit J Radiol 48:400–402, 1975

163. Kattan K R, Babcock D S, Felson B: Solitary phalangeal defect in the hand. Report of 2 rare cases. Am J Roentgen 124:29–31, 1975

164. Kaufman R A et al: False negative bone scans in neuroblastoma metastatic to the ends of long bones. Am J Roentgen 130:131–135, 1978

165. Keats T E: Rib erosions in scleroderma. Am J Roentgen 100:530–532, 1967

166. Keats T E: Superior marginal rib defects in restrictive lung disease. Amer J Roentgen 124:449–450, 1975

167. Kery L, Wouters H W: Massive osteolysis. A report of 2 cases. J Bone Joint Surg 52–B:452–459, 1970

168. Kido D, Bryan D, Halpern M: Hematogenous osteomyelitis in drug addicts. Am J Roentgen 118:356–363, 1973

169. Kirkwood J R, Margolis T, Newton T H: Prostatic metastasis to the base of the skull simulating meningioma en plaque. Am J Roentgen 112:774–778, 1971

170. Kittredge R D, Finby N: The many facets of lymphangioma. Am J Roentgen 95:56–66, 1965

171. Klumper A: Congenital diaphyseal venous dysplasia. Fortschr Roentgenstr 125:396–399, 1976

172. Kohler E, Babbitt D, Huizenga B, Good T A: Hereditary osteolysis. A clinical, radiological, and chemical study. Radiology 108:99–105, 1973

173. Komar N N, Gabrielsen T O, Holt J F: Roentgenographic appearance of lumbosacral spine and pelvis in tuberous sclerosis. Radiology 89:701–705, 1967

174. Krishnamurthy G T et al: Distribution pattern of metastatic bone disease. JAMA 237:2504–2506, 1977

175. Kutzner J, Kohler H, Vehlinger E: Sternocostoclavicular hyperostosis. Fortschr Roentgenstr 123:446–449, 1975

176. La Fond E M: An anlysis of adult skeletal tuberculosis. J Bone Joint Surg 40–A:346–364, 1958

177. Lagier R, Nussle D: Anatomy and radiology of a bone island. Fortschr Roentgenstr 128:261–264, 1978

178. Lally J F, Cossrow J L, Dalinka M K: Odontoid fractures in metastatic breast carcinoma. Am J Roentgen 128:817–820, 1977

179. Lazarus J H, Galloway J K: Pachydermoperiostosis: An unusual cause of finger clubbing. Am J Roentgen 118:308–313, 1973

180. Lehrer H Z, Maxfield W S, Nice C M: The periosteal "sunburst" pattern in metastatic bone tumors. Am J Roentgen 108:154–161, 1970

181. Leonhardt W, Taenzer V: The acroosteolysis syndrome. Fortschr Roentgenstr 123:179–181, 1975

182. Leucutia T: Multiple myeloma and intravenous pyelography. Am J Roentgen 85:187–189, 1961

183. Lichtenstein L: Histiocytosis X (eosinophilic granuloma of bone, Letterer–Siwe disease, and Schuller–Christian disease). Further observations of pathological and clinical importance. J Bone Joint Surg 46–A:76–90, 1964

184. Lindbom A, Lindvall N, Soderberg G, Spjut H: Angiography in osteoid osteoma. Acta Radiol 53:377–384, 1960

185. Lodge T: Development defects in the cranial vault. Brit J Radiol 48:421–434, 1975

186. Lodwick G S: Solitary malignant tumors of bone: The application of predictor variables in diagnosis. Seminars Roentgen 1:293–313, 1966

187. Lucaya J et al: Mastocytosis with skeletal and gastrointestinal involvement in infancy. Radiology 131:363–366, 1979

188. MacCarty W C, Russel D G: Tuberous sclerosis. Radiology 71:833–839, 1958

189. Macpherson R I, Letts R M: Skeletal diseases associated with angiomatosis. J Canad Assn Rad 29:90–100, 1978

190. Madsen B: Osteolysis of acromial end of clavicle following trauma. Brit J Radiol 36:822–828, 1963

191. Maldague B E, Malghem J J: Unilateral arch hypertrophy with spinous process tilt: A sign of arch deficiency. Radiology 121:567–574, 1976

192. Martel W, Abell M R, Duff I F: Cervical spine involvement in lipoid dermatoarthritis. Radiology 77:613–617, 1961

193. Maurer R M, Langford O L: Rothmund's syndrome. A cause of resorption of phalangeal tufts and dystrophic calcification. Radiology 89:706–708, 1967

194. McCarthy J, Twersley J, Lion M: Thyroid acropachy. J Canad Assn Rad 26:199–202, 1976

195. McLean F C, Urist M R: Bone. An Introduction to the Physiology of Skeletal Tissue, 2nd ed. Chicago, University of Chicago Press, 1961

196. McNulty J G, Pim P: Hyperphosphatasia: A report of a case with a 30-year follow-up. Am J Roentgen 115:614–618, 1972

197. Meszaros W T, Sisson M: Myelofibrosis. Radiology 77:958–967, 1961

198. Middlemiss J H, Braband H: Juvenile gout. Clin Radiol 13:149–152, 1962

199. Miller E H, Semian D W: Gram-negative osteomyelitis following puncture wounds of the foot. J Bone Joint Surg 57–A:535–537, 1975

200. Miller W B, Murphy W A, Gilula L A: Brodie abscess: Reappraisal. Radiology 132:15–23, 1979

201. Mirra J M, Arnold W D: Skeletal hemangiomatosis in association with hereditary hemorrhagic telangiectasia. A case report. J Bone Joint Surg 55–A:850–854, 1973

202. Mitsudo S M: Chronic idiopathic hyperphosphatasia associated with pseudoxanthoma elasticum. J Bone Joint Surg 53–A:303–314, 1971

203. Morrey B F, Bianco A J, Rhodes K H: Hematogenous osteomyelitis at uncommon sites in children. Mayo Clin Proc 53:707–713, 1978

204. Morris J M, Lucas D B: Fibrosarcoma within a sinus tract of chronic draining osteomyelitis. Case report and review of the literature. J Bone Joint Surg 46–A:853–857, 1964

205. Morris J W: Skeletal fluorosis among Indians of the American Southwest. Am J Roentgen 94:608–615, 1965

206. Mortensson W, Eklof O, Jorulf H: Radiologic aspects of BCG osteomyelitis in infants and children. Acta Radiol Diag 17 Fasc 6:845–855, 1976

207. Moseley J E: Bone Changes in Hematologic Disorders (Roentgen Aspects). New York, Grune & Stratton, 1963

208. Moss A A, Mainzer F: Osteopetrosis: An unusual cause of terminal-tuft erosion. Radiology 97:631–632, 1970

209. Moule B, Grant M C, Boyle I T, May H: Thyroid acropachy. Clin Radiol 21:329–333, 1970

210. Mulvey R B: Peripheral bone metastases. Am J Roentgen 91:155–160, 1964

211. Murray R O: Iatrogenic lesions of the skeleton. Caldwell Lecture, 1975, Am J Roentgen 126:5–22, 1976

212. Murray R O, McCredie J: Melorheostosis and the sclerotomes: A radiological correlation. Skel Rad 4:57–71, 1979

213. Musher D M et al: Vertebral osteomyelitis. Arch Intern Med 136:105–110, 1976

214. Muthukrishnan N, Shetty M U K: Pycnodysostosis. Report of a case. Am J Roentgen 114:247–252, 1972

215. Napoli L D, Hansen H H, Muggia F M, Twigg H L: The incidence of osseous involvement in lung cancer, with special reference to the development of osteoblastic changes. Radiology 108:17–21, 1973

216. Nathan P A, Trung N B: Osteomyelitis variolosa. Report of a case. J Bone Joint Surg 56–A:1525–1528, 1974

217. Nathanson N, Anvet N L: An unusual X-ray finding in tuberous sclerosis. Brit J Radiol 39:786–787, 1966

218. Nesbit M E, Wolfson J J, Kieffer S A, Peterson H O: Orbital sclerosis in histiocytosis X. Am J Roentgen 110:123–128, 1970

219. Neuhauser E B D, Shwachman H, Wittenborg M, Cohn J: Progressive diaphyseal dysplasia. Radiology 51:11–22, 1948

220. Newman H, Casey B, DuBois J J, Gallagher T: Roentgen features of leprosy in children. Am J Roentgen 114:402–410, 1972

221. Ngan H, Preston B J: Non-Hodgkin's lymphoma presenting with osseous lesions. Clin Rad 26:351–356, 1975

222. Neiman H L, Gompels B M, Martel W: Pachydermoperiostosis with bone marrow failure and gross extramedullary hematopoiesis. Report of a case. Radiology 110:553–554, 1974

223. Nixon G W: Hematogenous osteomyelitis of metaphyseal-equivalent locations. Am J Roentgen 130:123–129, 1978

224. Nixon G W, Gwinn J L: The roentgen manifestations of leukemia in infancy. Radiology 107:603–609, 1973

225. Ochsner S F: Eosinophilic granuloma of bone: Experience with 20 cases. Am J Roentgen 97:719–726, 1966

226. O'Connell D: Metastasis in the nasal bones. Clin Radiol 9:97–98, 1958

227. O'Connell D J, Frank P H, Riddel R H: The metastases of meningioma-radiologic and pathologic features. Skel Rad 3:30–35, 1978

228. O'Connor B T, Steel W M, Sanders R: Disseminated bone tuberculosis. J Bone Joint Surg 52–A:537–542, 1970

229. O'Reilly G V, Clark T M, Crum C P: Skeletal involvement in mycosis fungoides. Am J Roentgen 129:741–743, 1977

230. Owen R H: Van Buchem's disease. Brit J Radiol 49:126–132, 1976

231. Ozonoff M B, Clemett A R: Progressive osteolysis in progeria. Am J Roentgen 100:75–79, 1967

232. Palmer P E S: Case report: Osteopetrosis with multiple epiphyseal dysplasia. Brit J Radiol 33:455–457, 1960

233. Patrick J H: Melorheostosis associated with arteriovenous aneurysm of the left arm and trunk. J Bone Joint Surg 51–B:126–129, 1969

234. Patrick J H: Massive osteolysis complicated by chylothorax successfully treated by pleurodesis. J Bone Joint Surg 58–B:347–349, 1976

235. Paul L W, Juhl J H: Essentials of Roentgen Diagnosis of the Skeletal System. New York, Hoeber Medical Division (Harper and Row), 1967

236. Pear B L: The plasma cell in radiology. Am J Roentgen 102:908–915, 1968

237. Pease C N: Focal retardation and arrestments of growth of bones due to vitamin A intoxication. JAMA 182:980–985, 1962

238. Peavy P W, Rogers J V, Clements J L, Burns J B: Unusual osteoblastic metastases from carcinoid tumors. Radiology 107:327–330, 1973

239. Peterson R T, Haidak D J, Ferris R A, MacDonald J S, Schein P S: Osteoblastic bone metastases in Zollinger–Ellison syndrome. Radiology 118:63–64, 1976

240. Peison B, Benisch B: Malignant myelosclerosis simulating metastatic bone disease. Radiology 125:62, 1977

241. Peterson C C, Silbiger M L: Reiter's syndrome and psoriatic arthritis: Their roentgen spectra and some interesting similarities. Am J Roentgen 101:860–871, 1967

242. Pettigrew J D, Ward H P: Correlation of radiologic, histologic, and clinical findings in agnogenic myeloid metaplasia. Radiology 93:541–548, 1969

243. Pinckney L, Parker B R: Myelosclerosis and myelofibrosis in treated histiocytosis X. Am J Roentgen 129:521–523, 1977

244. Pincus J B, Gittleman I F, Kramer B: Juvenile osteopetrosis. Am J Dis Child 73:458–472, 1947

245. Pirschel J, Metzger H O F J, Wismann C: Malignant metastases to the periphery of the skeleton. Fortschr Roentgenstr 129:621–626, 1978

246. Pollen J J, Schlaer W J: Osteoblastic response to successful treatment of metastatic cancer of the prostate. Am J Roentgen 132:927–931, 1979

247. Poppel M H, Lawrence L R, Jacobson H G, Stein J: Skeletal tuberculosis. A roentgenographic survey with reconsideration of diagnostic criteria. Am J Roentgen 70:936–963, 1953

248. Probst F P: Chronic multifocal cleidometaphyseal osteomyelitis of childhood. Acta Rad 17:531–537, 1976

249. Raia T J, Hentz E C, Theros E G: Case of the month from AFIP. An exercise in radiologic pathologic correlation. Radiology 89:941–946, 1967

250. Ramin D: Tertiary yaws: Skeletal changes in the spine and ribs. Fortschr Roentgenstr 125:185–186, 1976

251. Raskin P, McClain C J, Medsger T A: Hypocalcemia associated with metastatic bone disease. A retrospective study. Arch Intern Med 132:539–543, 1973

252. Reed M H, Shokeir M H K, Macpherson R I: Skeletal metastases from retinoblastoma. J Canad Assn Rad 26:249–254, 1975

253. Reese E J, Baker H L, Scanlon P W: The roentgenologic aspects of metastatic pheochromocytoma. Am J Roentgen 115:783–793, 1972

254. Reidy J F: Osteoblastic metastases from a hypernephroma. Brit J Radiol 48:225–227, 1975

255. Renner R R, Nelson D A, Lozner E L: Roentgenological manifestations of primary macroglobulinemia (Waldenström). Am J Roentgen 113:499–508, 1971

256. Reynolds D G, Csonka G W: Radiological aspects of Reiter's syndrome ("Venereal" arthritis). Clin Radiol 9:44–49, 1958

257. Ribbing S: Hereditary multiple diaphyseal sclerosis. Acta Radiol 31:522–536, 1949

258. Rimoin D L: Pachydermoperiostosis. New Eng J Med 272:923–931, 1965

259. Roberts P H: Disturbed epiphyseal growth at the knee after osteomyelitis in infancy. J Bone Joint Surg 52–B:692–703, 1970

260. Robinson A E, Thomas R L, Monson D M: Aneurysmal bone cyst of the rib. A report of 2 unusual cases. Am J Roentgen 100:526–529, 1967

261. Rodriguez A R, Lutcher C L, Coleman F W: Osteosclerotic myeloma. JAMA 236:1872–1874, 1976

262. Rosenfeld N S, McIntosh S: Prospective analysis of bone changes in treated childhood leukemia. Radiology 123:413–415, 1977

263. Rubin P: Dynamic Classification of Bone Dysplasias. Chicago, Year Book Publishers, 1964

264. Ruby L K, Mital M A: Skeletal deformities following chronic hypervitaminosis A. A case report. J Bone Joint Surg 56–A:1283–1287, 1974

265. Russell W J, Bizzozero O J, Omori Y: Idiopathic osteosclerosis. Radiology 90:70–76, 1968

266. Sacristan H D, Portal L F, Castresana F G, Pena D R: Massive osteolysis of the scapula and ribs. A case report. J Bone Joint Surg 59–A:405–406, 1977

267. Sage M R, Allen P W: Massive osteolysis, J Bone Joint Surg 56–B:130–135, 1974

268. Salahuddin J I, Madhavan T, Fisher E J, Cox F, Quinn E L, Eyler W R: Pseudomonas osteomyelitis: Radiologic features. Radiology 109:41–47, 1973

269. Sargent E N, Turner A F, Jacobson G: Superior marginal rib defects. An etiologic classification. Am J Roentgen 106:491–505, 1969

270. Satin R, Usher M S, Goldenberg M: More causes of button sequestrum. J Canad Assn Rad 27:288–289, 1976

271. Scalley J R, Collins J: Thymoma metastatic to bone. Report of a case. Diagnosed by percutaneous biopsy. Radiology 96:423–424, 1970

272. Scanlon G T, Clemett A R: Thyroid acropachy. Radiology 83:1039–1042, 1964

273. Schaffzin E A, Chung S M K, Kaye R: Congenital generalized fibromatosis with complete spontaneous regression. A case report. J Bone Joint Surg 54–A:657–662, 1972

274. Schajowicz F et al: Cystic angiomatosis (hamartous haemolymphangiomatosis) of bone. J Bone Joint Surg 60–B:100–106, 1978

275. Schatzki S C, McIlmoyle S, Lowis S: Diffuse osteoblastic metastases from an intracranial glioma. Am J Roentgen 128:321–323, 1977

276. Schawarby K, Ibrahim M S: Pachydermoperiostosis. A review of the literature and report on 4 cases. Brit Med J 1:763–766, 1962

277. Schiele H P, Hubbard R B, Bruck H M: Radiographic changes in burns of the upper extremity. Radiology 104:13–18, 1972

278. Schwarz E, Fish A: Reticulohistiocytoma: A rare dermatologic disease with roentgen manifestations. Am J Roentgen 83:692–697, 1960

279. Scott W C, Gautby T H T: Hyperostosis corticalis generalizata familiaris. Brit J Radiol 47:500–503, 1974

280. Shaffer D L, Pendergrass H P: Comparison of enzyme, clinical, radiographic, and radionuclide methods of detecting bone metastases from carcinoma of the prostate. Radiology 121:431–434, 1976

281. Sherman F C, Wilkinson R H, Hall J E: Reactive sclerosis of a pedicle and spondylosis in the lumbar spine. J Bone Joint Surg 59–A:49–54, 1977

282. Seth H N, Majid M A, Rao B D P: Giant-cell tumor arising from the periosteum. Report of a case occurring in the femur. J Bone Joint Surg 46–A:844–847, 1964

283. Shopfner C E, Allen R P: Lymphangioma of bone. Radiology 76:449–453, 1961

284. Shuler S E: Pycnodysostosis. Arch Dis Child 38:620–625, 1963

285. Silberstain M J et al: Bone changes in a neonate with congenital leukemia. Radiology 131:370, 1979

286. Silbiger M L, Peterson C C: Sjogren's syndrome: Its roentgenographic features. Am J Roentgen 100:554–558, 1967

287. Silverman F N: The skeletal lesions in leukemia, clinical and roentgenographic observations in 103 infants and children, with a review of the literature. Am J Roentgen 59:819–844, 1948

288. Silverman F N: Virus diseases of bone. Do they exist? Am J Roentgen 126:677–703, 1976

289. Simmons C R, Harle T S, Singleton E B: The osseous manifestations of leukemia in children. Radiol Clin N Amer 6:115–130, 1968

290. Smart M J: Traumatic osteolysis of the distal ends of the clavicles. J Canad Assn Radiol 23:264–266, 1972

291. Smith J: Giant bone islands. Radiology 107:35–36, 1973

292. Soffa D J, Sire D J, Dodson J R: Melorheostosis with linear sclerodermatous skin changes. Radiology 114:577–578, 1975

293. Solomon A, McLaughlin C L: Immunoglobulin structure determined from products of plasma cell neoplasms. Seminars Hemat 10:3–17, 1973

294. Soriano M, Manchon F: Radiological aspects of a new type of bone fluorosis, periostitis deformans. Radiology 87:1089–1095, 1966

295. Spiegel P G, Kengla K W, Isaacson A S, Wilson J C: Intervertebral disc-space inflammation in children. J Bone Joint Surg 54–A:284–296, 1972

296. Stetten D W: Basic sciences in medicine: The example of gout. New Eng J Med 278:1333–1336, 1968

297. Stewart W R et al: Skeletal metastases of melanoma. J Bone Joint Surg 60–A:645–649, 1978

298. Swerdloff B A, Ozonoff M B, Gyepes M T: Late recurrence of infantile cortical hyperostosis (Caffey's disease). Am J Roentgen 108:461–467, 1970

299. Teplick G J: Tuberous sclerosis. Extensive roentgen findings without the usual clinical picture. A case report. Radiology 93:53–55, 1969

300. Teplick G J, Haskin M E, Schimert A P: Roentgenologic Diagnosis, vol 1. Philadelphia, W B Saunders, 1967

301. Teplick J G et al: Ghost infantile vertebrae and hemipelves within adult skeleton from thorotrast administration in childhood. Radiology 129:657–660, 1978

302. Terry D W, Isitman A T, Holnes R A: Radionuclide bone images in hypertrophic pulmonary osteoarthropathy. Am J Roentgen 124:571–576, 1975

303. Theros E: Plasma cell granuloma of pelvis and femora. RPC case of the month from AFIP. Radiology 95:679–686, 1970

304. Thoms J: Cleidocranial dysostosis. Acta Radiol 50:514–520, 1958

305. Tishler J M: The soft-tissue and bone changes in frostbite injuries. Radiology 102:511–513, 1972

306. Toland J, Phelps P D D: Plasmacytoma of the skull base. Clin Radiol 22:93–96, 1971

307. Tonge K: Periosteal reaction in polyarteritis nodosa. Brit J Radiol 45:698–701, 1972

308. Torgerson W R, Hammond G: Osteomyelitis of the sesamoid bones of the 1st metatarsophalangeal joint. J Bone Joint Surg 51–A:1420–1422, 1969

309. Torrance D J: "Negative" bone density in a case of multiple myeloma. Radiology 70:864–865, 1958

310. Torres–Reyes E, Staple T W: Roentgenographic appearance of thyroid acropachy. Clin Radiol 21:95–100, 1970

311. Tsai F Y, Lisella R S, Lee K F, Roach J F: Osteosclerosis of base of skull as a manifestation of tumor invasion. Am J Roentgen 124:256–264, 1975

312. Tyler T, Rosenbaum H D: Idiopathic multicentric osteolysis. Am J Roentgen 126:23–31, 1976

313. Vaezy A, Budson D C: Phalangeal metastases from bronchogenic carcinoma. JAMA 239:226–227, 1978

314. Uriboro I M F, Morchio F J, Marin J C: Metastases of carcinoma of the larynx and thyroid gland to the phalanges of the hand. Report of 2 cases. J Bone Joint Surg 58–A:134–135, 1976

315. Van Buchem F S P, Hadders H N, Hansen J F, Woldring M G: Hyperostosis corticalis generalizata: Report of 7 cases. Am J Med 33:387–397, 1962

316. Vanek J: Idiopathic osteolysis of Hadju–Cheney. Fortschr Roentgenstr 128:75–79, 1978

317. Vayssairat M et al: New cases of familial generalized cortical hyperostosis with dominant transmission (Worth's type). J Radiol Electrol (Paris) 57:719–724, 1976

318. Vermess M, Pearson K D, Einstein A B, Fahey J L: Osseous manifestations of Waldenstrom's macroglobulinemia. Radiology 102:497–504, 1972

319. Warren G: Tarsal bone disintegration in leprosy. J Bone Joint Surg 53–B:688–695, 1971

320. Weinfeld A, Stern M H, Marx L H: Amyloid lesions of bone. Am J Roentgen 108:799–805, 1970

321. Werner S C, Ingbar S H: The Thyroid, 3rd ed, p 519. New York, Hoeber Medical Division (Harper & Row), 1971

322. Whalen J P: The resorption of bone and its control: Its roentgen significance. Radiology 113:257–266, 1974

323. Whalen J P et al: Calcitonin treatment in hereditary bone dysplasia with hyperphosphatasemia: A radiographic and histologic study of bone. Am J Roentgen 129:29–35, 1977

324. Whitehouse G H, Bottomley J P, Bradley J: Lymphangiographic appearances in Waldenstrom's macroglobulinemia. Brit J Radiol 47:226–229, 1974

325. Williams C S, Riordan D C: Mycobacterium marinum (atypical acid-fast bacillus). Infections of the hand. A report of 6 cases. J Bone Joint Surg 55–A:1042–1050, 1973

326. Willson J K V: The bone lesions in childhood leukemia: A survey of 140 cases. Radiology 72:672–681, 1959

327. Winterberger A R: Radiographic diagnosis of lymphangiomatosis of bone. Radiology 102:321–324, 1972

328. Witcombe J B, Gremin B J: Tuberculous erosion of the sphenoid bone. Brit J Radiol 51:347–350, 1978

329. Wolf B H, Ford H W: An unusual radiographic manifestation of Engelmann's disease in a young Negro child. Radiology 99:401–402, 1971

330. Wolfson J J, Kane W J, Laxdal S D, Good R A, Quie P G: Bone findings in chronic granulomatous disease of childhood. A genetic abnormality of leukocyte function. J Bone Joint Surg 51–A:1572–1583, 1969

331. Wolstein D, Rabinowitz J G, Twersky J: Tuberculosis of the rib. J Canad Assn Rad 25:307–309, 1974

332. Zornosa J, Cangir A, Green B: Hypertrophic osteoarthropathy associated with nasopharyngeal carcinoma. Am J Roentgen 128:679–681, 1977

A solitary lesion of bone may be etiologically:

1. Neoplastic
2. Hammartomatous
3. Inflammatory
4. Traumatic
5. Neurogenic
6. Histiocytic
7. Metabolic
8. Ischemic
9. Vascular
10. Congenital
11. Developmental
12. Miscellaneous

It is in the area of the solitary bone lesion, more than any other, that the limitations of the roentgen examination must be understood in order to allow the correct emphasis on the radiographic interpretation within the total information picture. The roentgenogram alone often does not permit an etiologic diagnosis. An example of this is Ewing's tumor vs osteomyelitis, which can have similar appearances in both long and flat bones. It is in the evaluation of solitary lesions that the close cooperation among the radiologist, the clinician, and the pathologist is imperative. Each must understand the basis of the other's discipline in order to be able to arrive at a meaningful diagnosis.

If the roentgen picture fits a typical pattern (*e.g.*, nonossifying fibroma), or it is known that a malignant tumor is present (as in the presence of pulmonary metastases), diagnosis from the radiographic pattern is relatively easy. In the absence of these conditions, however, the purpose of the roentgen examination is to provide a picture of the gross pathology to supplement the biopsy. It does not constitute diagnostic nihilism when a specific diagnosis is not hazarded on an atypical radiological picture. Indeed, such a statement would serve no useful purpose. Rather, a list of differential diagnostic possibilities should be prepared, based on careful analysis of the roentgen pattern. This should be compared to the clinical picture, particularly in regard to the age group, and the list should be narrowed down to the most probable entities. Histo-logical study, when correlated with the above information, will most often, but not always, yield a correct diagnosis. The final judge of a correct or incorrect diagnosis is not the consultant pathologist, but rather the patient and his subsequent survival or demise.

TUMORS PRIMARY TO BONE

It is of little advantage to the radiologist to be partisan to the discussions of the histogenesis and classification of bone tumors that concern the research pathologist. Within the vast spectrum of possible histological types and subtypes of neoplasms, there are condensations of a finite number of definite clinicopathological entities.

The WHO classification of bone tumors is presented below.

HISTOLOGICAL TYPING OF PRIMARY BONE TUMORS AND TUMORLIKE LESIONS (WHO)

   I. Bone-Forming Tumors
      A. Benign
         1. Osteoma
         2. Osteoid osteoma and osteoblastoma (benign osteoblastoma)
      B. Malignant
         1. Osteosarcoma (osteogenic sarcoma)
         2. Juxtacortical osteosarcoma (parosteal osteosarcarcoma)
  II. Cartilage-Forming Tumors
      A. Benign
         1. Chondroma
         2. Osteochondroma (osteocartilaginous exostosis)
         3. Chondroblastoma (benign chondroblastoma, epiphyseal chondroblastoma)
         4. Chondromyxoid fibroma
      B. Malignant
         1. Chondrosarcoma
         2. Juxtacortical chondrosarcoma
         3. Mesenchymal chondrosarcoma

517

III. Giant-Cell Tumor (Osteoclastoma)
IV. Marrow Tumors
    1. Ewing's sarcoma
    2. Reticulosarcoma of bone
    3. Lymphosarcoma of bone
    4. Myeloma
V. Vascular Tumors
   A. Benign
    1. Hemangioma
    2. Lymphangioma
    3. Glomus tumor (glomangioma)
   B. Intermediate or Indeterminate
    1. Hemangioendothelioma
    2. Hemangiopericytoma
   C. Malignant
    1. Angiosarcoma
VI. Other Connective Tissue Tumors
   A. Benign
    1. Desmoplastic fibroma
    2. Lipoma
   B. Malignant
    1. Fibrosarcoma
    2. Liposarcoma
    3. Malignant mesenchymoma
    4. Undifferentiated sarcoma
VII. Other Tumors
    1. Chordoma
    2. "Adamantinoma" of long bones
    3. Neurilemmoma (schwannoma, neurinoma)
    4. Neurofibroma
VIII. Unclassified Tumors
IX. Tumorlike Lesions
    1. Solitary bone cyst (simple or unicameral bone cyst)
    2. Aneurysmal bone cyst
    3. Juxta-articular bone cyst (intraosseous ganglion)
    4. Metaphyseal fibrous defect (nonossifying fibroma)
    5. Eosinophilic granuloma
    6. Fibrous dysplasia
    7. "Myositis ossificans"
    8. "Brown tumor" of hyperparathyroidism

THE ORIGIN OF THE LESION

L. C. Johnson,[130] in his general theory of bone tumors, stresses that bone is an organ with varying functions in different parts of the skeleton. He states that there is a metabolic gradient within each individual bone that is minimal in the midshaft, low in the epiphysis, high in the metaphysis, and maximal in the metaphysis of a rapidly growing end. This gradient can be correlated with fields of cell activity. A tumor of a specific cell type tends to originate in the field of maximal activity of homologous normal cells. The preferential sites and times of origin of the various tumors are thus determined and are of the greatest diagnostic significance, along with the roentgen pattern. The preferential sites of origin of various tumors are summarized below.

PREFERENTIAL SITE OF ORIGIN OF VARIOUS TUMORS OF BONE

EPIPHYSIS
   Chondroblastoma
   Giant-cell tumor after fusion of growth plate

METAPHYSIS
   Osteosarcoma
   Parosteal sarcoma
   Chondrosarcoma
   Fibrosarcoma
   Nonossifying fibroma
   Giant-cell tumor prior to fusion of growth plate
   Unicameral bone cyst (non-neoplastic)

DIAPHYSIS
   Myeloma
   Ewing's tumor
   Reticulum-cell sarcoma

Although a wide span of age in most tumors is possible, a large number of bone tumors develop at the time of the last growth spurt in late adolescence. Other tumors develop in childhood and in adult life. The preferential time of origin of the various tumors is summarized in Table 7–1.

In very young patients, malignant bone tumors are likely to be metastases from neuroblastoma or leukemia. In the first decade, the most likely primary bone tumors are Ewing's tumor and, later, osteosarcoma. In adolescence and adult life, the various primary bone tumors are probable. In the older age groups, the vast majority of bone tumors are metastatic carcinomas. Multiple myeloma also occurs in this age group.

Biochemical studies in the evaluation of solitary tumors have limited diagnostic value. All benign tumors of bone show normal serum values. Osteosarcoma is usually associated with an elevated serum alkaline phosphatase level. Other malignant tumors and giant-cell tumors may show slight elevation of

TABLE 7–1. Preferential Time of Origin of Various
Tumors of Bone

Tumor	Age of Maximum Incidence (Decades)
Osteosarcoma	2,3 (smaller peak at 7)
Parosteal sarcoma	4,5
Chondrosarcoma	4,5,6
Fibrosarcoma	4
Giant-cell tumor	3,4
Ewing's tumor	2
Reticulum-cell sarcoma of bone	3,4
Multiple myeloma	5,6,7
Benign chondroblastoma	2
Chondromyxoid fibroma	2,3
Nonossifying fibroma	2
Osteoid osteoma	2,3
Non-Neoplastic Lesions	
Solitary bone cyst	1,2
Aneurysmal bone cyst	2,3

serum alkaline phosphatase values. The chief value of serum calcium and phosphorus determinations in solitary lesions is to exclude a brown tumor of hyperparathyroidism.

ROENTGEN PATTERNS OF SOLITARY BONE LESIONS

Lodwick[156, 158] has pointed out the basic patterns of tumor behavior and bone response, and has assigned the probability values of a specific diagnosis to various combinations of features. In addition to the basic features of destruction, expansion, periosteal response, cortex, origin, and bone production, which have been discussed in previous sections, the location, size, margination, trabeculation, shape, and pattern of matrix calcification or ossification are important factors.

The location of a lesion is of diagnostic significance with respect to which bone is involved, which portion (epiphysis, metaphysis, diaphysis), whether the lesion is central or eccentric, or involves the medulla, cortex, or periosteum. The size of a lesion is also of significance, because malignant tumors are not often small when first seen. Margination and trabeculation are important considerations. Malignant tumors tend to have an indistinct margin or "wide zone of transition," and the entire circumference of any lesion must be carefully inspected so as not to overlook a segmental wide zone. Some lesions are characteristically lightly trabeculated (giant-cell tumor), but others often have

heavy trabeculation. A round shape favors a rapidly growing neoplasm, and an elongated shape usually favors a bone cyst or a benign tumor. Calcification or ossification within the tumor matrix (as opposed to reactive bone sclerosis) indicates the osteogenic or chondrogenic series of tumors, if calcification is not in necrotic tissue.

In recent years, computed tomography has become important in the evaluation of primary bone tumors, particularly in the axial skeleton. Important information concerning the size, location, definition, anatomic relations to neural, vascular, and osseous structures as well as determination of vascularity on post-infusion study may be gained with great accuracy.[109] Visualization of the soft-tissue component is accomplished with ease,[14] as is follow-up after therapy. A radionuclide skeletal survey for metastases from primary bone tumors, particularly in the pediatric age group, is significantly more sensitive than conventional radiographic examination alone.[89] Angiography in primary bone tumors is of proven value in determining the extent and vascularity of a tumor. Ultrasonography is useful in delineating the extent of soft-tissue components of pelvic and abdominal primary bone tumors.[61]

It is no longer sufficient to use the radiological examination only to predict the histology of a primary bone tumor. The newer modalities have the capability of supplying much valuable information that can be used in treatment planning.

PRIMARY MALIGNANT TUMORS OF BONE

OSTEOSARCOMA (CENTRAL OSTEOSARCOMA)

Osteosarcoma[59,150,168] is a primary malignant tumor of bone in which osteoid is formed directly from sarcomatous tissue. Osteoid may also be formed from cartilaginous tissue, which can be present in abundance. This is an entity distinct from fibrosarcoma of bone, which does not give rise to osteogenesis, and chondrosarcoma, which is a malignant tumor of cartilage.

Osteosarcoma may be grouped by location as central, parosteal (juxtacortical) sarcoma, multiple osteogenic sarcomatosis, and soft-tissue osteosarcoma (see Chap. 8). The clinical picture and prognosis are different for each.

Microscopically, the typical appearance consists of osteoid arising directly from neoplastic cells. The amount and calcification of this osteoid may vary greatly, along with the amount of cartilage that may be present. The lesion may be highly vascular. Tumor cells of great variability in degree of anaplasia are present, as well as giant cells.

Recently, there has been a tendency to subclassify osteosarcomas on the basis of different clinical and histological features.[51] About 75% of the tumors are still considered conventional osteosarcomas. The remainder fall into small subgroups that are distinctive. There is a group that arises from abnormal bone. Another variety arises in the jaws; this group has a better prognosis than ordinary osteosarcomas. A small group of tumors results from the dedifferentiation of chondrosarcomas. These have the distribution of the latter tumor, but a poor prognosis. Some tumors have histologies similar to malignant fibrous histiocytoma, but osteoid is produced by malignant cells. Another group is called *telangiectatic osteosarcoma*. It is lytic throughout and radiographically may simulate Ewing's sarcoma. These tumors are bloody and necrotic, and the prognosis is poor.

Low-grade intraosseous osteosarcoma is another small group. It may be mistaken for fibrous dysplasia. *Periosteal osteosarcoma* is another distinctive type of lesion. It characteristically is seen on the surface of the tibial shaft, and is a small tumor with periosteal spiculation without medullary involvement. The prognosis is better than that of ordinary osteosarcoma.

Clinically, osteosarcoma is the second most common primary sarcoma of bone component tissue. (Multiple myeloma is the most common.) The ratio of involvement of males and females is about 2:1. The majority of these tumors arise in the 10- to 25-year age bracket. A smaller peak incidence occurs in the older age groups. Osteosarcomas in the older age groups may be associated with Paget's disease, postirradiated bone or osteochondromas, or they may arise *de novo*, with features and distribution similar to these tumors in younger age groups. It is probable that the incidence in association with fibrous dysplasia is not very high, although cases have been reported. Association with osteogenesis imperfecta has been reported,[140] although often a spurious picture is present, owing to hyperplastic callus formation.[11] Radiation-induced osteosarcomas can be due to teletherapy, or ingested radium and mesothorium, or Thorotrast administration. Common instances in which radium was ingested in the past are watch dial painters and those patients who were given radium water as a treatment for arthritis.

In the younger patient, osteosarcoma most often involves the tubular bones. When it occurs in an

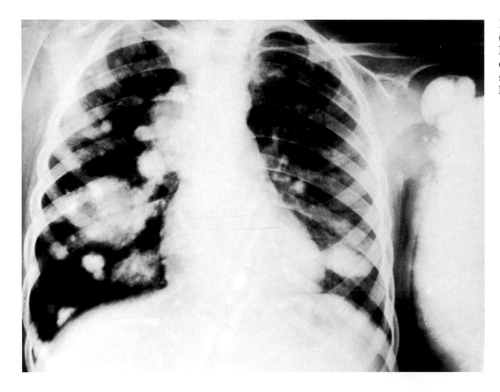

FIG. 7–1. Multiple metastases (chest) from osteosarcoma. Note calcific density of several of the metastases, and extensive osteosarcoma of the left humerus.

older individual, the flat bones are most often involved.

In the vast majority of instances, the tumor metastasizes by way of the bloodstream, and will probably have done so by the time the diagnosis is established, even though metastases cannot be demonstrated. The most common site of metastasis is the lungs, where osseous parenchymal densities (Fig. 7–1), or, rarely, cavitating metastases (Fig. 7–2) are visible on the chest radiograph. Occasionally, visceral or skeletal metastases may be seen, the latter usually involving the skull, spine, or pelvis (Figs. 7–3, 7–4, 7–5). Calcified renal metastases have been reported.[180] In very rare instances, metastases may spread by way of the lymphatics,[274] in which case a cloud of ossification is seen radiographically in a regional lymph node (Fig. 7–6). In centrally located lesions of the shoulder and pelvic girdles, lymphatic involvement is more common than in peripheral osteosarcomas. The mediastinal or para-aortic lymph nodes may be involved (Fig. 7–7).[25] Lymphangiography would be of value.

The chief clinical symptom prior to metastasis is pain at the tumor site. The pain begins insidiously and intermittently, and progresses to severe constancy. A palpable mass develops, with associated inflammatory signs and local venous dilatation. Effusion in a contiguous joint is common. Pathological fracture may occur. Systemic symptoms then follow. The duration of symptoms prior to diagnosis averages several months. The serum alkaline phosphatase is usually slightly elevated in the presence of a large lesion.

The prognosis is poor, with a mortality rate in some series of 95%. In a few cases, so rare as to be a medical curiosity, osseous pulmonary metastases have inexplicably stabilized and permitted long-term survival of the patient.

Radiologically, the areas most commonly involved in central osteosarcoma are the distal femur and the proximal tibia. This is seen in about 75% of the cases in which tubular bones are affected. The proximal humerus, the distal radius, and the pelvis are not uncommon sites of tumor, and there may be involvement of the femoral shaft, maxilla, sternum, ribs, cervical spine,[81] and skull, or rarely almost any bone in the body, including the patella.[95] The computed relative distribution of tumors is presented in Table 7–2.

(Text continued on p. 525)

TABLE 7–2. Osteosarcoma

Skull	********	8
Mandible	*****	5
Cerv. spine	*	1
Dors. spine	*	1
Lumb. spine	*	1
Ribs	**	2
Clavicle	*	1
Scapula	**	2
Sternum	*	1
Humerus	****************	16
Radius & Ulna	**	2
Hand & Carpus	*	1
Pelvis	*************	13
Sacrum	**	2
Femur	********************************	
Femur	********************************	63
Tibia	****************************	28
Foot & Tarsus	*	1
Other	****	4

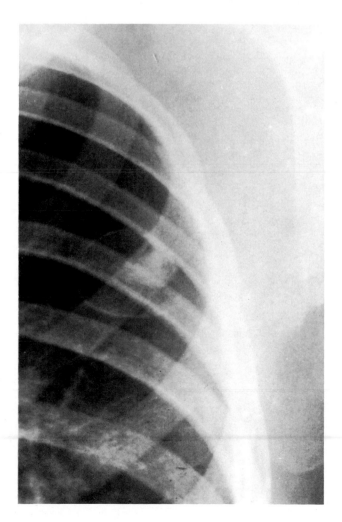

FIG. 7–2. Thin-walled cavitating metastases from osteosarcoma. These lesions eventually progressed to spontaneous pneumothorax.

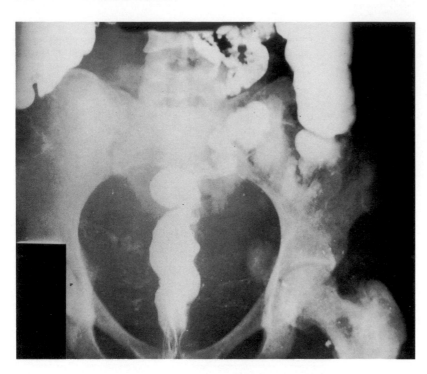

FIG. 7–3. Osteosarcoma primary in the greater trochanter of the left femur which has involved the soft tissues of the pelvis. Note large soft-tissue mass with streaky tumor new bone formation. The tumor has metastasized to the bony pelvis as well. The soft-tissue mass displaces the barium-filled colon.

FIG. 7–4. Metastases to the ilium, following disarticulation for osteosarcoma. An ovoid osteosclerotic lesion is seen near the iliac crest.

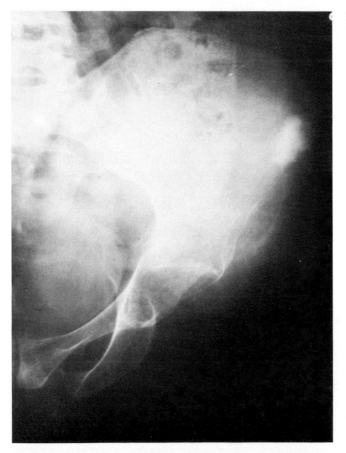

FIG. 7–6. Osteosarcoma of the distal radius metastatic to a supratrochlear lymph node. A. Note soft-tissue swelling containing streaky calcific densities. B. Note area of sclerosis at the distal radius, involving the metaphysis and the diaphysis but not the epiphysis. The radiolucency is secondary to biopsy. A large soft-tissue mass, perpendicular streaks of periosteal new bone formation, and Codman's triangle are also visible.

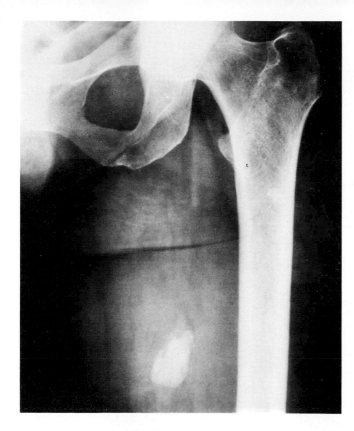

FIG. 7–5. Osteosarcoma with skeletal and soft-tissue metastases. Osteoblastic lesions in the proximal left femur are noted, as well as a large ovoid, calcified, metastatic deposit in the soft tissues of the thigh.

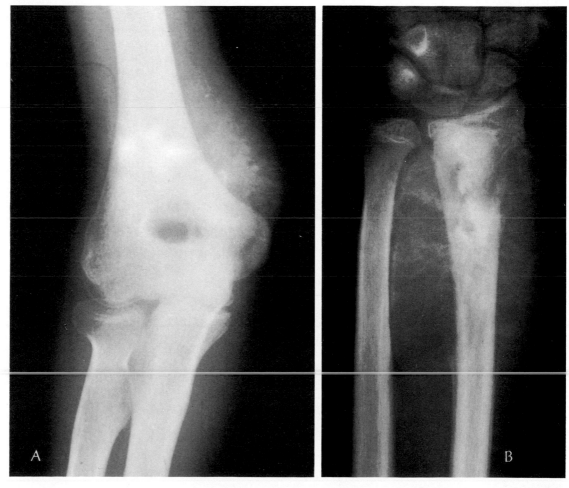

A

B

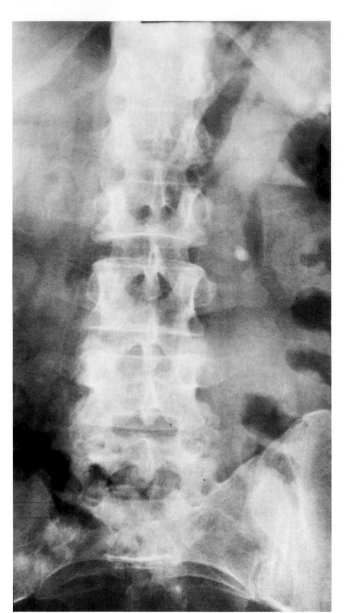

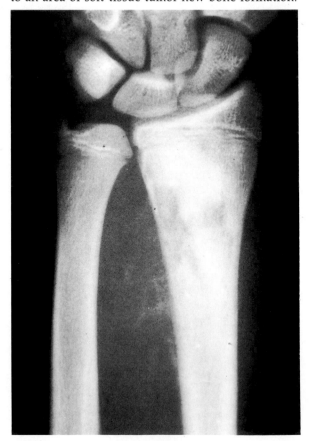

FIG. 7–7. Metastases from osteosarcoma—same case as Fig. 7–5. Osteoblastic lesions at the level of the right sacroiliac joint are noted, as well as metastatic abdominal calcification representing a left para-aortic lymph node and a node at the hilum of the spleen.

FIG. 7–8. Osteosarcoma (distal radius). Note area of sclerosis in the metaphysis; the epiphyseal ossification center is not involved. Radiolucency represents site of biopsy. A small amount of periosteal new bone formation at the ulnar aspect of the distal radius may be seen, forming a Codman's triangle adjacent to an area of soft-tissue tumor new bone formation.

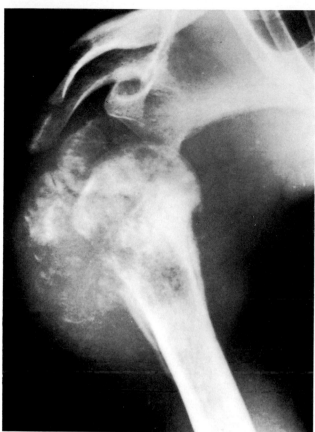

FIG. 7–9. Osteosarcoma (proximal humerus). The epiphyseal end of the bone is involved in a mixed sclerotic and lytic type of lesion. There is a large soft-tissue mass following breakthrough of the cortex at the outer aspect of the upper humerus. Note marked tumor new bone formation within the mass, and periosteal elevation at the distal aspect of the tumor. Also note the solid nature of this periosteal new bone formation, particularly at the medial side.

FIG. 7–10. Osteosarcoma (femur), diaphyseal origin. Long, spiculated, periosteal new bone formation may be seen in the involved area, associated with a more solid type of periosteal new bone.

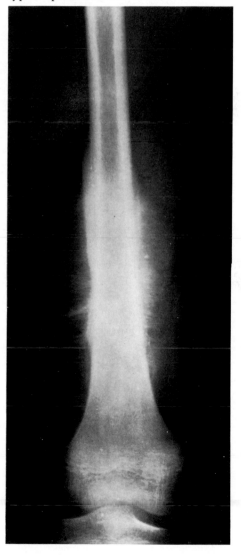

In the tubular bones, the tumor usually originates in the metaphysis (Fig. 7–8). If the epiphyseal cartilage is present, it usually forms an effective barrier against epiphyseal spread. After epiphyseal fusion has taken place, the end of the bone is commonly involved (Fig. 7–9). The joint forms an effective barrier against transarticular spread. Rarely, the tumor may originate in the diaphysis (Fig. 7–10). Transepiphyseal (Fig. 7–11) and transarticular spread (Fig. 7–12) may occur in advanced cases. A large area of involvement, usually greater than 6 cm, extending from the metaphysis down the shaft, is frequently seen.

It must be understood that the term *osteosarcoma* refers to the histological production of osteoid and not the roentgen appearance of sclerosis. The tumor may show a dense sclerosing roentgen picture[174] in about 50% of cases (Figs. 7–13, 7–14, 7–15), or a moderately ossifying appearance, a mixed productive and destructive appearance (Fig. 7–16), or rarely a pure osteolytic lesion (Figs. 7–17, 7–18).

(Text continued on p. 530)

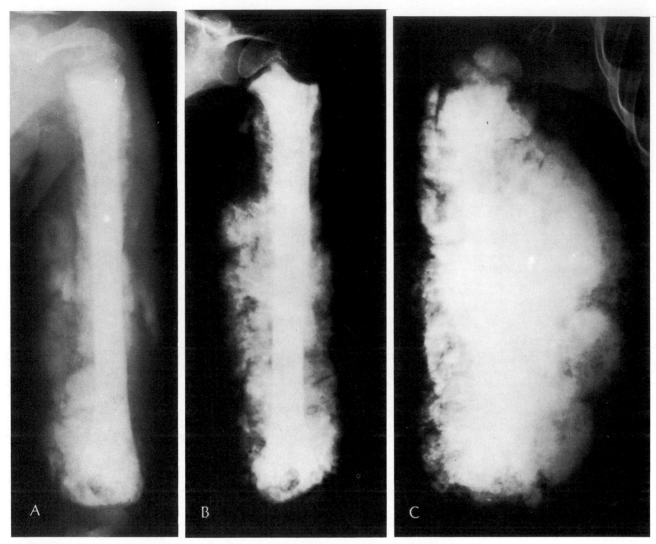

FIG. 7–11. Osteosarcoma (humerus). **A.** Involvement of the entire diaphysis. The epiphyses at both ends of the humerus are spared. Note soft-tissue involvement, with extensive tumor bone formation and spiculated periosteal new bone formation. **B.** One-month interval film after **A**. Involvement of the humerus and soft tissues has progressed, and the bases of the epiphyseal ossification centers are starting to be invaded. **C.** Four-month interval film after **B**. There is now extreme soft-tissue ossification and complete involvement of the epiphyseal ossification centers. Sarcoma has not spread across the joints. (Chest film of this patient is shown in Fig. 7–1.)

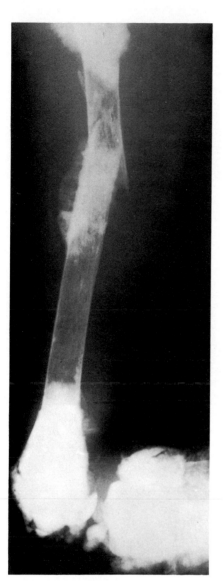

FIG. 7–12. Advanced osteosarcoma. Note involvement of the knee with sclerosis of all bones, a pathological fracture of the femoral shaft, and sclerosis at the proximal femur.

FIG. 7–13. Osteosarcoma (proximal tibia). Dense, sclerotic appearance of the epiphysis and upper shaft may be seen. Epiphyseal fusion has already occurred. Area of radiolucency at the medial aspect of the tibia is biopsy site. There is no evidence of periosteal reaction or new bone formation, and no destructive areas are visible. This is a purely sclerotic osteosarcoma.

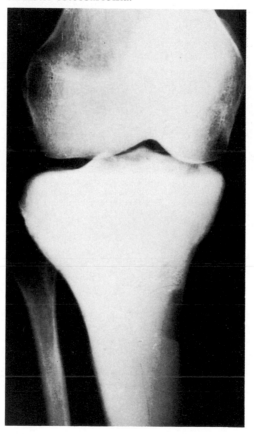

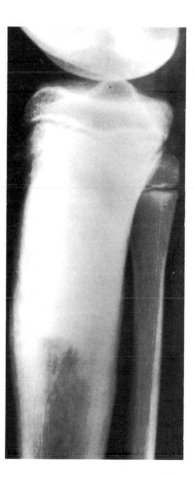

FIG. 7–14. Osteosarcoma, sclerosing type (proximal tibial metaphysis). Note dense sclerotic area involving the metaphysis, limited by the epiphyseal cartilage plate and showing a fairly well circumscribed distal margin.

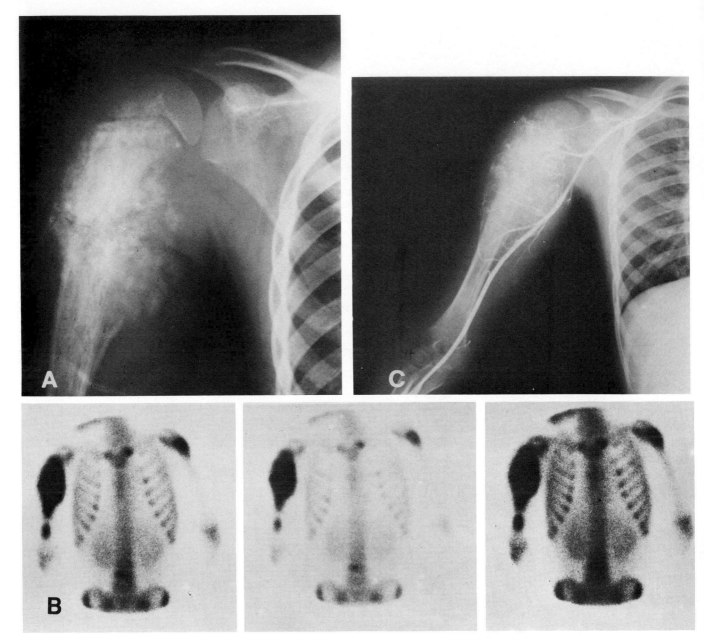

FIG. 7–15. Osteosarcoma (humerus). **A.** Anteroposterior view showing an extensive sclerotic and destructive lesion of the proximal humeral metaphysis and shaft. There has been invasion of the medial soft tissue with soft-tissue ossification. There is a large Codman's triangle. Permeative destruction along the shaft is also seen. A small area of involvement of the epiphyseal ossification center is also noted. **B.** Radionuclide scan showing increased activity of the humerus. **C.** Angiogram showing increased vascularity in the tumor area with small vessels running parallel to the periosteal bone spicules.

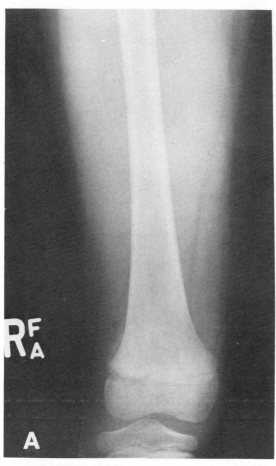

FIG. 7–16. Osteosarcoma (distal femoral metaphysis). **A.** Small area of increased sclerosis and periosteal new bone formation is seen at the lateral aspect of the distal femoral metaphysis. **B.** The radionuclide scan showing almost symmetrical activity bilaterally, however a definite asymmetry is seen with the lateral aspect on the right of the active area extending to a lower level than the normal side.

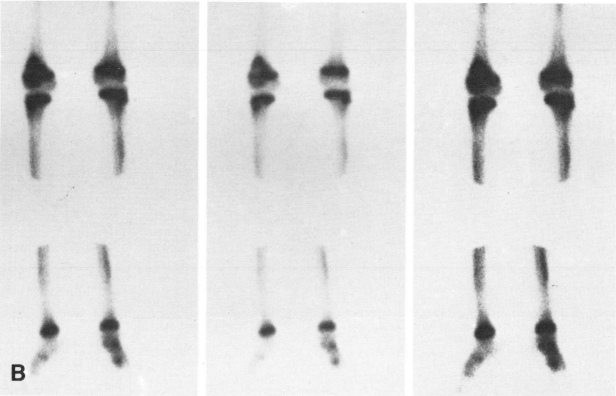

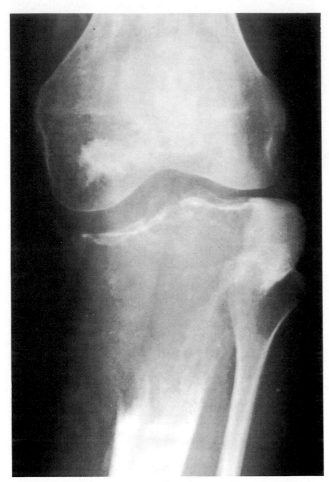

FIG. 7–17. Osteosarcoma—female, age 17 years. This is a purely destructive lesion of the proximal tibia. The margin of the destroyed area is irregular, and several "moth-eaten" areas of destruction may be seen extending down the shaft. There is no expansion of bone. The latter two findings differentiate this from a giant-cell tumor. Osteoporosis of the distal femur is present, causing a radiolucent appearance not due to invasion by tumor.

These variations in density depend upon the amount of calcified osteoid and vascularity present and do not represent basic differences in type of tumor. Bone sclerosis may be of extreme density, but extreme bone density is not pathognomonic of this condition, because other conditions such as Charcot's joint, osteoid osteoma, or sclerosing osteomyelitis may also induce bone densities as osteosclerotic as osteosarcoma. When the lesion is lytic, the pattern is "moth-eaten" or permeative with ill-defined margins blending imperceptibly with normal uninvolved bone and a characteristic wide zone of transition. A "geographic" area may rarely be seen.

The appearance of the periosteum is the best known feature of this lesion. In the classic case, the typical filiform radiating spiculation or "sunburst" pattern is seen (Figs. 7–19, 7–20). A long segment pattern of spiculation may also be present (Fig. 7–10). Spiculated periosteal reaction may also be seen in metastatic tumors, particularly carcinoma of the prostate, as well as benign conditions such as osteomyelitis and thyroid acropachy. Malignant spicules tend to be long and thin, while benign spicules are short and squat. Rarely, other cases may show lamellated periosteal response. Lodwick[156] claims that these laminations are coarser in osteosarcoma than in Ewing's tumor. A Codman's triangle is often present (Fig. 7–21). This triangle may, however, also be found in benign conditions. Rarely, an expansile lesion in a flat bone is seen (Fig. 7–22).

Another characteristic finding in osteosarcoma is destruction of the cortex and invasion of the soft tissues. The soft-tissue mass may at times by very

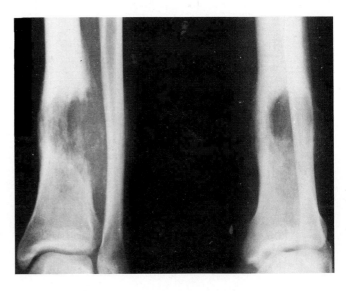

FIG. 7–18. Osteosarcoma. A large geographic area of bone destruction is present in the distal tibia, with a very wide zone of transition. Soft-tissue calcification is present, as well as a proximal Codman's triangle. Local osteoporosis distal to the lesion is also noted. No bone sclerosis is seen. (Courtesy of Drs. A. Pizarro and J. F. Kurtz, VA Hospital, Hines, IL)

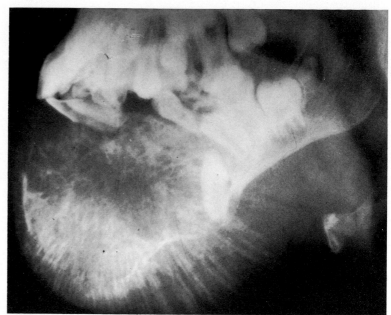

FIG. 7–20. Osteosarcoma involving the mandible, with long, slender, spiculated, periosteal new bone formation, or the "sunburst" pattern. Destructive and sclerotic changes in the mandible are also present, representing a mixed type of osteosarcoma.

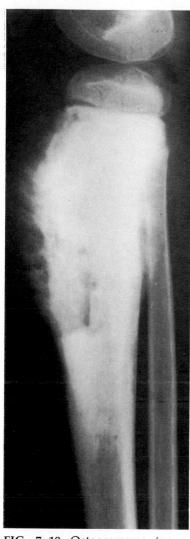

FIG. 7–19. Osteosarcoma (proximal tibia). Note perpendicular, spiculated, periosteal new bone formation, or "sunburst" pattern. There is dense sclerosis of the metaphysis extending down toward the shaft; the epiphysis is not involved. A biopsy site is also visible, and soft-tissue swelling is present.

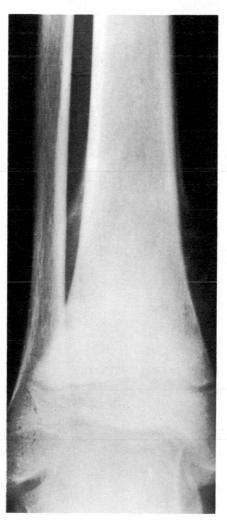

FIG. 7–21. Osteosarcoma (distal tibial metaphysis). Codman's triangles may be seen at the proximal aspect of the lesion.

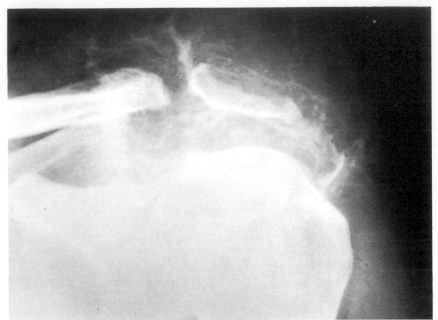

FIG. 7–22. Male, age 49 years, with no evidence of antecedent bone disease. There is an expansile, trabeculated destructive lesion of the scapula at the base of the acromion process. Soft-tissue invasion has occurred. Light streaky densities simulating trabeculations may be seen within the tumor mass. A majority of prominent consulting pathologists concurred with the diagnosis of osteosarcoma. This represents an unusual roentgen picture. (Courtesy of Dr. Miriam Liberson, West Side VA Hospital, Chicago, IL)

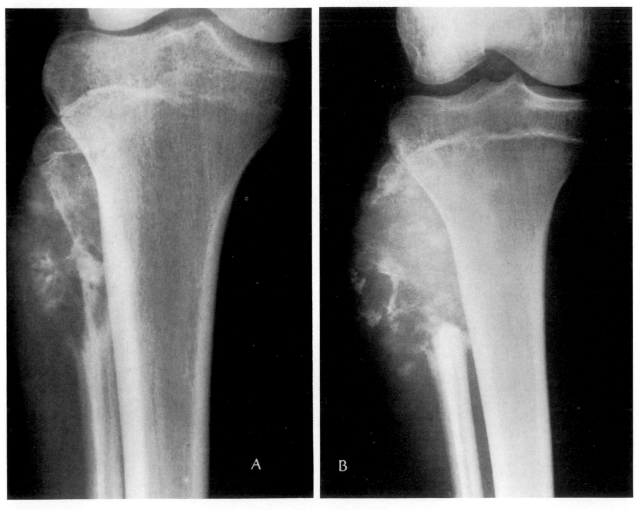

large, particularly following biopsy (Fig. 7–23, 7–24). Areas of ossification or amorphous calcification may be present in the soft-tissue mass (Fig. 7–25), and there may be an apparent alignment of calcific densities radiating outward from the central tumor. The amount of new bone formation in the soft-tissue component may exceed that in the intraosseous component. Pathological fractures are common.

Angiography of osteosarcoma is of value for determining the intra- and extraosseous extent of the tumor, as well as the selection of a biopsy site.[285] Osteosarcomas are vascular tumors, with fibroblastic and chondroblastic subtypes less vascular than conventional osteosarcoma. This technique also aids in differentiation from other lesions, such as healing fractures, myositis ossificans, and osteomyelitis. The vascular supply of an osteosarcoma arises from the surrounding tissues. A typical angiographic appearance of an osteosarcoma is a "sunburst" effect of many vessels running along and between the periosteal perpendicular spicules (Fig. 7–15 C).[210]

OSTEOSARCOMA DEVELOPING IN ABNORMAL BONE

Although osteosarcoma may develop *de novo* in the older age groups, the possibility of an underlying bone abnormality as a precursor must be considered. One possibility is the malignant transformation of a previously benign tumor, such as osteochondroma. Other than local transformation of a benign tumor, the development of osteosarcoma in bone involved with Paget's disease, or in bone that has been previously radiated, is not uncommon. Osteosarcoma rarely develops in fibrous dysplasia. In an area of chronic osteomyelitis with long-standing discharge of a sinus, the skin may be involved with a squamous-cell carcinoma. This causes a destructive pattern in bone, and is to be differentiated from sarcomatous degeneration, which may also occur, most commonly as a fibrosarcoma.

OSTEOSARCOMA AS A COMPLICATION OF PAGET'S DISEASE

Paget's disease is common in the northern sections of the United States, in England, and in the Western European Plain. It is a disease of unproven etiology characterized by destructive and reparative changes in bone. Malignant transformation has been estimated to occur in from 3% to 14% of patients. The Paget's disease may be quite limited and still be a site of sarcoma. Paget's sarcoma originates only in involved bone.

Clinically, the alkaline phosphatase is usually elevated in Paget's disease. With the development of an osteosarcoma, the alkaline phosphatase value tends to become yet higher.

The type of sarcoma developing in Paget's disease, in approximately 50% of cases, is osteosarcoma; in another 25% fibrosarcoma occurs, with anaplastic sarcoma, giant-cell sarcoma and reticulosarcoma accounting for the remainder of cases in which tumors arise. Giant-cell tumor has also been described in association with Paget's disease.

The mean age of discovery of this sarcoma (according to Price)[203] is 67.6 years in England. In the United States, the mean age is 55 years. The age range is from 46 to 91 years. The ratio of men to women is 2:1. There is a high incidence of pathological fractures.

Radiologically, the areas involved are not limited. The pelvis, humerus, and femur are frequently involved. The calvarium, scapula, mandible,[216] calcaneus, vertebral column, and other long bones may also be involved. An area of bone destruction with ill-defined margins and a wide zone of transition is usually seen (Fig. 7–26). Areas of increased density resembling ordinary osteosarcoma may rarely be seen (Fig. 7–27). Spiculated periosteal new bone response may be present, and increased density in the soft tissues may also be seen due to soft-tissue invasion. The osteolytic form tends to predominate. The lesions may be multiple, suggesting multifocal origin. The tumor usually spreads by the

(Text continued on p. 536)

FIG. 7–23. Osteosarcoma (proximal fibula). **A.** Note destructive and sclerotic changes of the proximal fibula, with an associated soft-tissue mass, periosteal and tumor new bone formation, and a Codman's triangle. This is the prebiopsy picture. **B.** One-month interval film following **A** and biopsy. Note marked increase in the soft-tissue mass, and increase in tumor new bone formation within the mass. **C.** One-month interval film after **B.** Note very marked increase in size of the soft-tissue mass.

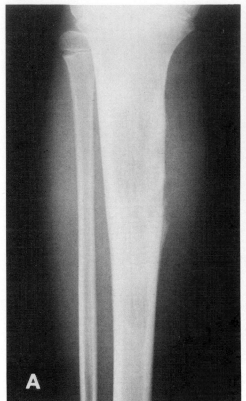

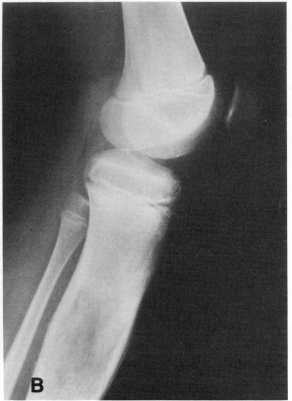

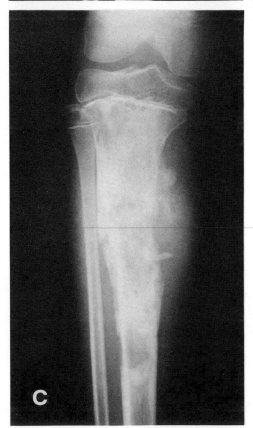

FIG. 7–24. Osteosarcoma—fibrous type. **A.** Anteroposterior view of the leg. An expansile area in the upper tibial diaphysis is noted with patchy destructive and sclerotic regions. Periosteal new bone formation is seen as well as a Codman's triangle at the medial aspect. **B.** Lateral view shows expansion and periosteal new bone formation. **C.** AP view of the leg taken 6 months after patient had refused surgery. There has been extensive soft-tissue invasion, soft-tissue ossification, and bony destruction.

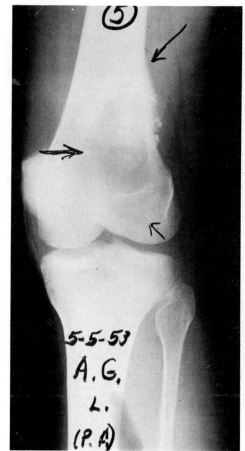
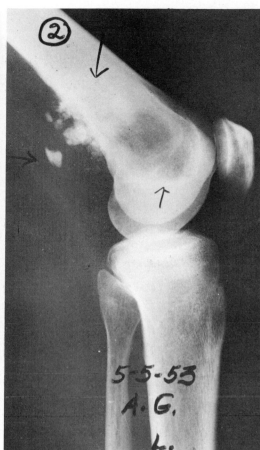

FIG. 7–25. Osteosarcoma of the distal femoral metaphysis. An osteolytic lesion is noted in the distal femur. The lesion has broken through the cortex and invaded the soft tissues. Multiple amorphous clumps of calcification in the soft-tissue mass are present. (Courtesy of Drs. A. Pizarro and J. F. Kurtz, VA Hospital, Hines, IL)

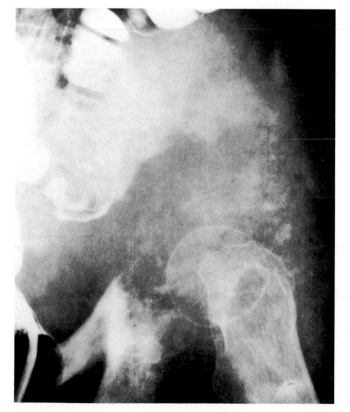

FIG. 7–26. Osteosarcoma of the pelvis associated with Paget's disease. Note extensive destructive area in the acetabulum and ilium. New bone formation in the tumor mass is apparent. The tumor does not cross the articular surface, and the femoral head is spared. Changes of Paget's disease in the ischium and pubis are also visible. The associated soft-tissue mass may be seen to cause displacement of the barium-filled colon. This represents the radiologically osteolytic picture of osteosarcoma.

535

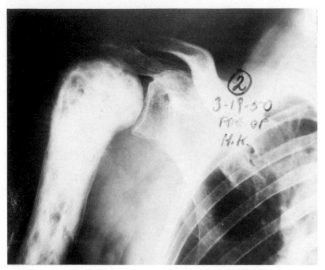

FIG. 7–27. Osteosarcoma (proximal humerus) in Paget's disease. The classical changes of Paget's disease are present with cortical thickening and accentuation of the trabecular pattern. In addition, a dense area of osteosclerosis involving the humeral head and neck and a portion of the shaft is seen, which proved to be osteosarcoma. Slight periosteal reaction suggesting spiculation at the medial aspect is noted. (Courtesy of Drs. A. Pizarro and J. F. Kurtz, VA Hospital, Hines, IL)

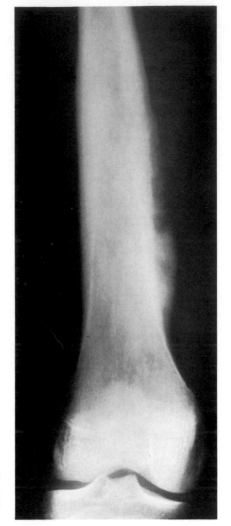

FIG. 7–28. Periosteal osteosarcoma. Note area of new bone formation at the distal femur, with ossified matrix and periosteal elevation. The cortex is intact. Irregularity at the proximal aspect of the lesion is present.

hematogenous route, but lymphogenous metastases may also occur.

OSTEOSARCOMA DEVELOPING IN PREVIOUSLY IRRADIATED BONE

Ionizing radiation may lead to the formation of malignant tumors. These changes may result from either internal[9,31] or external[288] radiation sources. Internal radiation effects on humans are well documented by Martland,[9] in his account of watch dial painters who had ingested radium and mesothorium during the course of their work. These individuals developed anemia, bone necrosis, osteomyelitis, pathological fractures, carcinomas of the paranasal sinuses and mastoids, and bone sarcomas. The ingested radioactive substances were metabolized in the body in the same manner as calcium, and were deposited in bone. Other "bone-seeking" radioactive isotopes, particularly radiostrontium, may have the same effect.

External sources, when a skeletal part is in a radiation treatment field, can cause radiation osteitis of bone, destructive areas, pathological fractures, sclerosis, and local inhibition of bone growth.

The incidence of postradiation sarcoma in long-term survivors of breast cancer has been reported as being between 0.07% and 0.22%. Approximately 200 cases of sarcoma developing in bone following external irradiation have been reported in English language literature to date.

The latent period ranges from 3 to 42 years. Sarcoma may develop either in normal bone that has been in the radiation treatment field, or at the site of a preexisting irradiated lesion. Osteosarcoma and fibrosarcoma are the usual types seen. Chondrosarcoma and Ewing's tumor may also occur, while other tumors may show a complex histological picture. The age range is from 8½ to 77 years, with an average of 47 years.

Preexisting lesions that show sarcomatous development after radiation include giant-cell tumor (which represents the largest group), aneurysmal bone cyst, osteoblastoma, and fibrous dysplasia.

FIBROUS DYSPLASIA WITH SARCOMATOUS CHANGE

While *fibrous dysplasia* is a relatively common lesion of the skeleton, the development of sarcoma in fibrous dysplasia is a rare event, following or without prior irradiation. Albright's syndrome may rarely be present. The fibrous dysplasia may be polyostotic or monostotic. The sex incidence is approximately equal.

The age range at the onset or discovery of the sarcoma is from 11 to 54 years. The sites involved, in approximate order, are the mandible, femur, pelvis, scapula, humerus, tibia, maxilla, and fibula. The cell types seen are osteosarcoma, fibrosarcoma, spindle cell, giant cell, or chondrosarcoma. The sarcomas arise in bone affected with fibrous dysplasia.

Radiologically, the changes of fibrous dysplasia are apparent. The sarcoma usually manifests itself as an area of destruction. Areas of rarefaction and cortical destruction may be present. There may be an expansile or trabeculated lesion. Marked bone sclerosis and a "sunburst" type of periosteal reaction may be present, manifesting an osteosarcoma.

OSTEOSARCOMA IN OSTEOGENESIS IMPERFECTA

Osteogenesis imperfecta may rarely show a large soft-tissue mass containing dense ossification. This is usually due to hyperplastic callus formation, which has been described as simulating sarcoma. Very rarely the simulator is simulated, and a true osteosarcoma is found.

A single case has been reported of osteosarcoma associated with osteopoikilosis.[169]

PERIOSTEAL OSTEOSARCOMA

Periosteal osteosarcoma[60,270] is an entity distinct from the conventional medullary and parosteal

types. The average age of patients is in the late 20s, with a 2:1 male preponderance. It usually occurs in the diaphysis, with the most common location being the proximal third of the femur. The cortex is always involved, but the medulla is spared. The typical radiographic appearance is that of a nonhomogenous spiculated mass attached to the cortex for a variable length. It does not outgrow the base and the lesion is denser at its cortical base (Fig. 7–28). The character of the spicules varies from coarse to fine. They are not as dense as in parosteal sarcoma, and may resemble the amorphous calcification of cartilage. Periosteal new bone formation may be seen as well as a Codman's triangle. An accompanying uncalcified soft-tissue mass is common. Cortical thickening may be present, but the medullary cavity is spared. Features of the three types of osteosarcomas are compared in Table 7–3.

PAROSTEAL SARCOMA (JUXTACORTICAL OSTEOSARCOMA)

Parosteal sarcoma[5,69,205,222,254] is an entity separate from osteosarcoma, with different clinical, pathological, and radiological features. The tumor originates about the periosteum or immediate parosteal connective tissue.

Microscopically, there is wide variation in appearance and wide range in grade of malignancy; fibrous, cartilaginous, and osseous elements are present with fibrosarcomatous areas, zones of calcified and uncalcified osteoid, and chondrosarcomatous areas. Deceptive areas of benignity are also seen. About one-half of the tumors are encapsulated.

Clinically, parosteal sarcoma is a rare tumor. The age range is from childhood to the sixth decade, with the majority of cases occurring in patients over 30 years of age. Males and females are equally affected.

The chief complaint is a slowly growing mass, which interferes with articular motion when located near a joint. Pain is not an early or constant feature of this lesion. The tumor may invade the bone or metastasize by way of the bloodstream to the lungs, particularly after attempts at local excision. The prognosis is better than in central osteosarcoma. Two distinct behavior patterns of this tumor have been described: slow growth with eventual cure after major ablative surgery, and rapid growth with recurrences and metastases leading to death.

TABLE 7–3. Features of Osteosarcomas

	Age Range/ Peak	Sex	Peak Location	Matrix	Cortex	Marrow Cavity
Central Osteo-sarcoma	1–80	Men	Central metaphysis	Lytic to very dense. In general some amount of osteoid present	Destroyed	Always Involved
		Women	1) Distal femur 2) Proximal tibia			
	15	3/2				
Parosteal Osteo-sarcoma	12–58	Men	Cortical	A. Dense homogeneous lesion	Thickened at base	Occasionally Involved
		Women	1) Distal posterior femur metaphysis 2) Proximal humeral metaphysis	B. Daughter masses adjacent to principal mass C. Wraps D. Outgrows base		
	39	2/3				
Periosteal Osteo-sarcoma	13–70	Men	Cortical	A. Spiculated nonhomogeneous	Thickened under lesion	Not In-volved
		Women	1) Anterior proximal medial shaft of femur	B. Single mass		
	20	2/1	2) Anterior proximal tibial shaft	C. Does not outgrow base in length		

(Modified from deSantos LA et al. Radiology 127:123, 1978)[60]

Radiologically, the tumor originates in the parosteal region of the metaphyseal end of a tubular bone. Fifty percent of the cases are in the lower femur, with the proximal femur, proximal humerus, and tibia as other sites. Even involvement of a metacarpal has been reported. The computed relative distribution of parosteal sarcoma is presented in Table 7–4. The size of the lesion varies from a small juxtacortical mass to a huge bulky tumor completely surrounding the entire shaft of the bone. The tumor may have a homogeneous ivory density due to tumor new bone formation, or more rarely, it may show lobulated areas of calcification densely scattered (Fig. 7–29). In early stages, there is a characteristic radiolucent line of demarcation between the dense tumor and the cortex of bone that may disappear as the lesion progresses. This line represents the periosteum or fibrous capsule. The density of the tumor is usually greatest near the cortex of bone. In about 10% of cases, the tumor invades the bone, causing a radiolucent area of destruction. Round, large, dense masses in the soft tissue, separate from the bulk of the tumor, sometimes form. The tumor may grow completely around the bone without invasion (Fig. 7–30). A nonossified soft-tissue component surrounding dense neoplastic bone may also be present. A "sunburst" periosteal pattern as an atypical finding has been reported.

TABLE 7–4. Parosteal Sarcoma

Skull	*	0
Mandible	*	0
Cerv. spine	*	0
Dors. spine	*	0
Lumb. Spine	*	0
Ribs	*	0
Clavicle	*	0
Scapula	*	0
Sternum	*	
Humerus	*****	5
Radius & Ulna	**	2
Hand & Carpus	*	0
Pelvis	*	0
Sacrum	*	0
Femur	*****************************	
Femur	******	36
Tibia	*****	5
Foot & Tarsus	**	2
Other	**	2

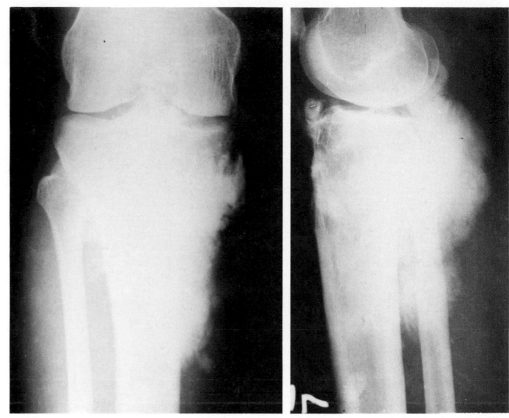

FIG. 7–29. Parosteal sarcoma. A large densely and uniformly calcific lobulated soft-tissue mass in relation to the dorsal and lateral aspect of the proximal tibia is seen. The margins are lobulated. (Courtesy of Drs. A. Pizarro and J. F. Kurtz, VA Hospital, Hines, IL)

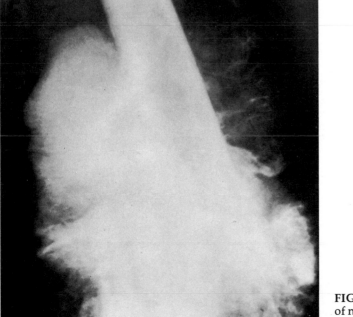

FIG. 7–30. Juxtacortical osteosarcoma. Note dense mass of new bone—due to calcified tumor matrix—which completely surrounds the distal femur and has a solid, lobulated appearance at the posterior aspect. The femur is not invaded.

MULTIPLE OSTEOGENIC SARCOMATOSIS (SCLEROSING OSTEOGENIC SARCOMATOSIS)

Multiple sclerosing osteogenic sarcomatosis[44,56,100] is a distinct clinical entity considered to represent osteosarcomas of simultaneous multicentric origin at many skeletal sites.

Clinically, this rare disease almost always occurs in childhood. It may very rarely occur in young adults, and has been reported in a 50-year-old man. Bone pain is a constant feature, followed by general debility. Metastasis to the lungs occurs early in the course of the disease. The serum alkaline phosphatase level is elevated and the serum calcium and phosphorus values are normal. This is a rapidly progressive condition with an invariably fatal outcome.

Radiologically, the characteristic lesions are dense osteosclerotic areas that may assume all of the features of an individual osteosarcoma. The lesions are all approximately the same size, suggesting multicentric origin; the presence of a single lesion much larger than the others probably indicates conventional osteosarcoma with multiple bony metastases. The lesions are distributed bilaterally and symmetrically. They chiefly involve the metaphyseal regions of the long bones, and also the pelvis, spine, sternum, ribs, and clavicles. Osseous pulmonary metastases occur early. The lesions in the tubular bones invade the epiphyses, or multiple round sclerotic areas in the epiphyseal ossification centers may develop independently. In early stages the lesions may appear as multiple, well-circumscribed metaphyseal bone islands, or may somewhat resemble the metaphyseal densities seen in heavy metal intoxication.

CHONDROSARCOMA

Chondrosarcoma[49,111,193,206,211] is a malignant tumor of cartilaginous origin that remains essentially cartilaginous in its development. The tumor may be primary, or it may develop in a preexisting cartilaginous lesion, such as osteocartilaginous exostoses or enchondromas, more commonly multiple disease than solitary lesions. Rarely, chondrosarcomas may develop in association with Paget's disease or in postirradiated bone. A chondrosarcoma has been reported to have arisen in a unicameral bone cyst.[96] Chondrosarcomas reportedly can secrete high levels of chorionic gonadotropin.[159] Low levels have been reported as being associated with osteosarcomas as well as carcinomas of the lung, liver, and kidney.

The computed relative distribution of all types of chondrosarcoma is presented in Table 7–5.

Chondrosarcomata show wide variations in their clinical, histological, and behavioral features, and several variants may be observed. They may be primary or secondary to some preexistent benign cartilage lesion. They have been classified in the following manner by Schajowicz:

PRIMARY CHONDROSARCOMAS

1. Central
2. Juxtacortical (periosteal)
3. Mesenchymal
4. Dedifferentiated
5. Clear-Cell
6. Malignant chondroblastoma?

SECONDARY CHONDROSARCOMAS

Central Chondrosarcoma

1. Chondroma (enchondroma)
2. Multiple enchondromatosis (with or without Ollier's syndrome)

Peripheral Chondrosarcoma

1. Osteochondroma (osteocartilaginous exostosis)
2. Multiple Hereditary Exostoses ("hereditary-deforming chondrodysplasia")
3. Juxtacortical (periosteal chondroma)

A chondrosarcoma that originates within a bone is termed a central chondrosarcoma, while one that originates outside the confines of the cortex is a peripheral or juxtacortical chondrosarcoma. A central chondrosarcoma may be primary or secondary. Peripheral chondrosarcoma is a term used by Jaffe for a secondary lesion.[124]

Juxtacortical chondrosarcoma, according to the WHO classification, is a rare malignant cartilage-forming tumor arising from the external surface of bone, characterized by well-differentiated cartilage with extensive areas of enchondral ossification. It is different from the chondrosarcoma arising from the cartilage cap of an osteochondroma. It may be thought of as the malignant counterpart juxtacortical chondroma.[224] Most commonly, this occurs in young adults. The shaft of a long bone, usually the femur, is involved. The prognosis is relatively favorable.

Central chondrosarcoma is more common than peripheral chondrosarcoma, and primary chondrosarcomas are considered to be much more common than secondary tumors. Any bone preformed in cartilage may be involved.

Mesenchymal chondrosarcoma is a rare variant that may originate from primitive cartilage-forming mesenchymal cells. It often arises from soft tissues and may sometimes be multicentric. This is a highly lethal tumor with a predilection for young patients.[196, 198]

Clear-cell chondrosarcoma is another rare variant that is often not recognizable as being cartilaginous on gross specimen observation.[271] It is a slow-growing tumor with a wide range of age distribution. A lytic expansile lesion, usually without calcification, may be seen. It may involve the epiphysis, with an appearance similar to a chondroblastoma.

As a group, chondrosarcomas are the third most common primary malignant tumors of bone components, following multiple myeloma and osteosarcoma.

Microscopically, the tumor tissue is cartilaginous. While it may be poorly differentiated, it can very often resemble a benign lesion. Jaffe lists the following criteria for chondrosarcoma: hypercellularity, plumpness of nuclei, irregularity in size of cells and nuclei, numerous cells with multiple nuclei, hyperchromatism of nuclei, and large or giant cartilage cells with single or multiple nuclei.[124] If osteoid is directly formed from tumor cells, the tumor must be considered an osteosarcoma. The histological changes indicative of malignancy can be so subtle as to be untrustworthy.

CENTRAL CHONDROSARCOMA

Clinically, there is a wide range of age distribution, with more than 50% of the patients older than 40 years. Males and females are about equally affected. Dull pain is the most frequent complaint, with an average duration of several years prior to the discovery of the lesion. Local swelling without inflammatory signs and disability of a contiguous joint may also be present. The tumor grows slowly and usually metastasizes late by way of the bloodstream. There is a tendency to invade the veins, and cases have been reported in which tumor had propagated through the venous channels to the heart and lungs. Lymph node metastases are very rare but may occur, with chondrosarcomatous tissue within a regional node. A small percentage of chondrosarcomas follows a fulminant course, leading to early death. In the average case, the prognosis is much better than that for osteosarcoma. The closer a cartilaginous lesion is to the central skeleton, the greater its malignant potential.

Radiologically, cartilage tissue is readily recognized by amorphous, punctate, small, flocculent, dense, irregular calcifications, the distribution of which ranges from sparse to heavy. Approximately two-thirds of central chondrosarcomas exhibit this finding. The most common site is the femur, most often at the ends, but also involving the midshaft. The proximal humerus is also commonly involved. The tibia, ribs (Figs. 7–31, 7–32), ilium (Fig. 7–33, 7–34), scapula, spine (Fig. 7–35), or sternum, as well as other sites, are occasionally involved. A large segment of the shaft of a long bone may be affected.

The tumor may present as an osteolytic expansile ragged-looking lesion, well-marginated, with either endosteal cortical thickening or thinning (Fig. 7–36). At this stage it may not be possible to differentiate this lesion from an enchondroma; however, a location in the proximal skeleton should arouse a suspicion of malignancy. There may be simple periosteal elevation or, rarely, fine spiculation or lamination.

When the rate of tumor growth exceeds the rate of bone repair, margination of the lesion is not present. The destructive area blends imperceptibly with normal bone (Fig. 7–37), and the entire shaft of a long bone may be involved. The lesion may progress to cortical destruction and invasion of the soft tissues where calcifications in the tumor mass are seen. Juxtacortical chondrosarcoma shows long-segment involvement of the diaphysis with a soft-tissue mass containing striated calcifications[224] (Fig. 7–38). Osteosarcomas with cartilage components also show this type of calcification.

TABLE 7–5. Chondrosarcoma

Skull	********	8
Mandible	*	1
Cerv. spine	****	4
Dors. Spine	******	6
Lumb. spine	****	4
Ribs	*************************	26
Clavicle	*	1
Scapula	**********	10
Sternum	****	4
Humerus	*****************	17
Radius & Ulna	*	1
Hand & Carpus	***	3
Pelvis	***************************	
Pelvis	*********************	54
Sacrum	****	4
Femur	***********************	
Femur	***************	40
Tibia	********	8
Foot & Tarsus	**	2
Other	***	3

(Text continued on p. 547)

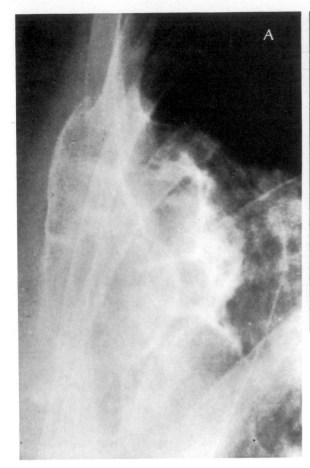

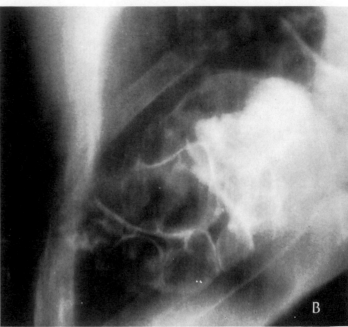

FIG. 7–31. Chondrosarcoma (rib). **A.** An expanding lesion with linear calcifications may be seen in the sixth rib. **B.** Tomogram of lesion in **A**. Details of expansile lesion with destruction and linear and circular calcifications are visible. (Courtesy of Dr. Miguel Garces, Chicago, IL)

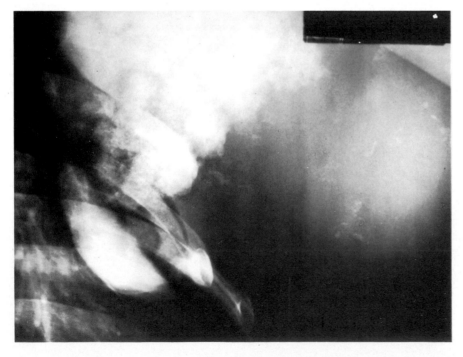

FIG. 7–32. Chondrosarcoma involving the ribs, advanced. A very large soft-tissue mass may be seen, containing dense amorphous, flocculent calcifications centrally and a more sparse calcific pattern peripherally.

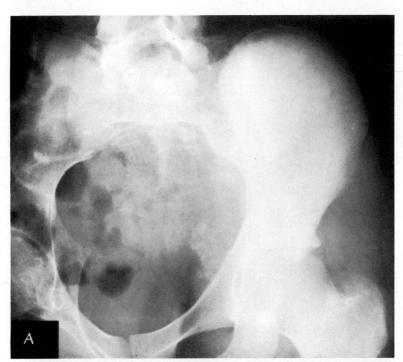

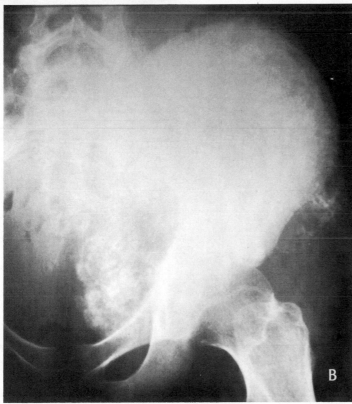

FIG. 7–33. Chondrosarcoma involving the left ilium. **A.** There is an increase in bone density, associated with a soft-tissue intrapelvic mass that contains flocculent calcifications. **B.** Four-month interval film. There has been marked increase in the size of the chondrosarcoma and increase in the soft-tissue calcifications, which have a linear and flocculent character. Destructive and sclerotic changes in the left ilium are also apparent.

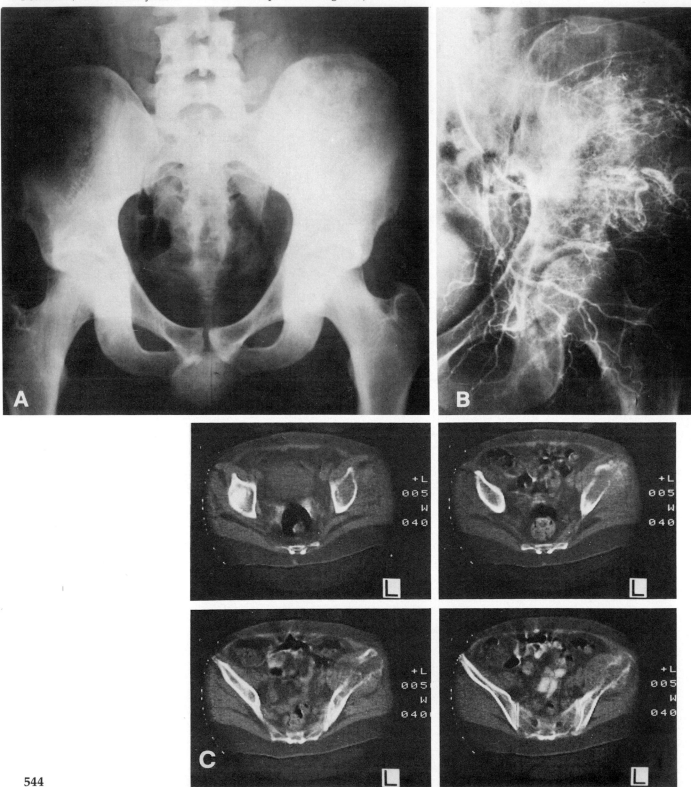

FIG. 7–34. Chondrosarcoma in 59-year-old female who presented with a mass in the left flank. **A.** Anteroposterior view of pelvis shows a destructive lesion involving the outer aspect of the ilium. **B.** Angiogram — multiple tumor vessels and puddling of contrast material. **C.** Computed tomographic examination of pelvis shows expansion and destruction of the left ilium as well as a large associated soft-tissue mass. (Courtesy of Dr. J. P. Petasnick, Rush–Presbyterian St. Luke's Hospital, Chicago, IL)

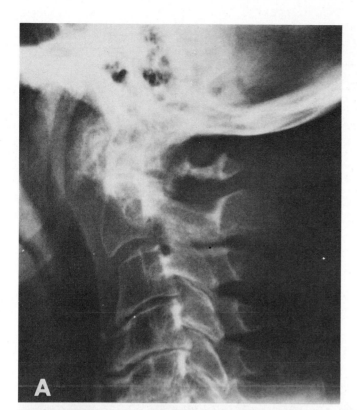

FIG. 7–35. Chondrosarcoma of the first cervical vertebra. **A.** Lateral view of spine shows destruction at the C-1 level associated with a large calcified soft-tissue mass. Degenerative changes in the lower spine are incidentally present. **B.** CT scan. The odontoid process is easily identified. Expansile, destructive, and calcific changes of the ring of C-1 are noted. (Courtesy of Dr. J. P. Petasnick, Rush–Presbyterian St. Luke's Hospital, Chicago, IL)

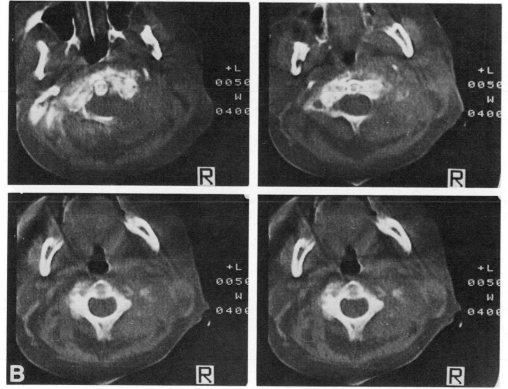

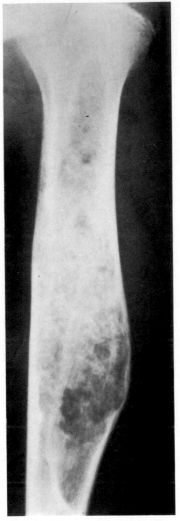

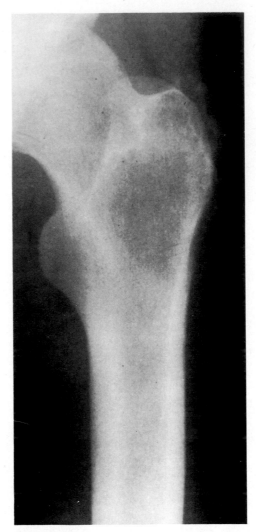

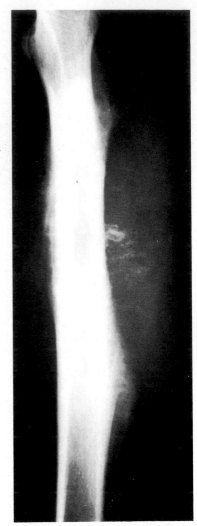

FIG. 7–36   FIG. 7–37   FIG. 7–38

FIG. 7–36. Chondrosarcoma (humerus). Note expansile lesion involving the proximal and middle third of the humeral shaft. Endosteal scalloping and thickening of the cortex at the medial margin of the lesion are apparent. The lesion is fairly well demarcated. The characteristic streaky and amorphous calcification within the matrix may be noted.

FIG. 7–37. Chondrosarcoma (femur). There is an ill defined, poorly marginated area of radiolucency in the intertrochanteric region of the femur. The outer cortex has been destroyed regionally, and a minimal amount of amorphous soft-tissue calcification may be seen. (Courtesy of Dr. Marion Magalotti)

FIG. 7–38. Chondrosarcoma (femur). There is involvement of a long segment of the femoral shaft. Cortical destruction has occurred, with breakthrough and a large soft-tissue mass. Fine, long, spiculated calcifications may be seen perpendicular to the shaft of the bone in the central portions and at the periphery. Laminated periosteal new bone formation, and a large Codman's triangle formed at the distal outer aspect, are also visible.

In femoral lesions, endosteal thickening of the medial neck and intertrochanteric area remote from the tumor is sometimes seen.

In an enchondroma that is well encapsulated, incurring malignant change may be recognized initially by irregularity and subsequent loss of the peripheral margination, followed by cortical breakthrough.

Chondrosarcoma rarely occurs in the small bones of the foot, but it has been reported,[189] with an average age of 38 years for such cases. Males apparently are more often affected than females. In the short bones, this lesion must be differentiated from osteosarcoma and tuberculosis.

PERIPHERAL CHONDROSARCOMA

Peripheral chondrosarcoma is a term reserved by Jaffe[124] for those tumors that develop from malignant degeneration of hereditary multiple exostoses or of a solitary osteocartilaginous exostosis. The frequency of this occurrence is about 25% in multiple exostoses and 1% in solitary exostosis. Peripheral chondrosarcoma is about one-fifth as common as central chondrosarcoma.

Clinically, the average age of patients with peripheral chondrosarcoma is somewhat lower than in those having the central type, with the majority of cases occurring in middle life. The chief complaint is a slowly growing painless tumor mass in a patient who usually has multiple exostoses. The mass may have reached a large size by the time the patient presents himself. The duration of symptoms may be many years. A hard, firm, nontender mass is noted, without inflammatory signs. Nerve compression may produce corresponding symptoms.

Radiologically, the most frequent areas of involvement are the pelvic and shoulder girdles, upper femur, and humerus. Occasionally other sites are affected, even the hand. The prime roentgen characteristic is flocculent or streaky radiation of calcific densities from an osteochondroma into the adjacent soft tissues. (Fig. 7–39). The lesion is not marginated. The tumor may attain large size; however, a benign osteochondroma may also attain large size. In later stages, the underlying bone may be invaded, with extensive destruction. A juxtacortical chondrosarcoma presents as flocculent soft-tissue calcifications within a soft-tissue mass, attached to bone without a preexisting osteochondroma. Pressure effects and sclerosis of underlying bone have been reported.

A chondrosarcoma may dedifferentiate to either a fibrosarcoma[170] or an osteosarcoma.

The angiographic appearance of chondrosarcomas varies from normal to increased vascularity with pathological vessels.[284] A close relationship is claimed between the number of vessels in a tumor and its degree of clinical and histopathologic malignancy.

FIBROSARCOMA OF BONE

Fibrosarcoma[74, 147] of bone is a primary malignant tumor of fibroblastic tissue that does not form neoplastic osteoid or cartilage. This entity represents a rare bone tumor. The majority of lesions arise *de novo,* but fibrosarcoma complicating Paget's disease, bone damaged by radiation, desmoplastic fibroma, ameloblastic fibroma, pre- and postirradiated giant-cell tumor, chronic osteomyelitis[6] and rarely fibrous dysplasia, bone infarcts[66] and multicentric fibrosarcomatosis has been reported. A type arising from the periosteum also rarely occurs.

Microscopically, the tumor tissue may be well differentiated, poorly differentiated, or anaplastic. The differentiated forms show spindle-shaped fibroblasts with intercellular collagen. In the poorly differentiated form, atypism and anaplasia are present. Hemosiderin, macrophages, and occasional multinucleated giant cells may also be seen. There is no tumor osteoid or cartilage.

Clinically, the course of the disease usually correlates with the histological degree of differentiation. Age distribution ranges widely, from 8 to 88 years, with the peak in adulthood. The tubular bones are more often affected in the younger patient, but older patients have a tendency toward flat bone involvement. The chief complaints are local pain and swelling. The pain progressively increases in severity. The tumor metastasizes via the bloodstream to the lungs, central skeleton, and viscera in a large percentage of cases.[127] This is one of the few bone tumors that shows a tendency to lymphatic metastasis, and consequently lymphangiography may be of value. The prognosis in central fibrosarcoma is now considered to be poor. Pathological fractures are common, as well as soft-tissue invasion.

Radiologically, the tumor may originate centrally, or, less often, periosteally. A periosteal fibrosarcoma is sometimes associated with a large soft-tissue mass. The most common sites of involvement are the distal femur and proximal tibia. The tumor usually occurs eccentrically in the metaphysis of a long bone, but may extend into the epiphysis. Other sites of involvement are the mandible, long

TABLE 7–6. Fibrosarcoma

Skull	**********	11
Mandible	*****************	18
Cerv. spine	**	2
Dors. spine	***	3
Lumb. spine	***	3
Ribs	****	4
Clavicle	*	1
Scapula	******	6
Sternum	*	0
Humerus	*************	13
Radius & Ulna	***	3
Hand & Carpus	*	0
Pelvis	*************************	26
Sacrum	*********	10
Femur	***************************	
Femur	***********************	57
Tibia	***************************	
Tibia	****	34
Foot & Tarsus	**	2
Other	***	3

bones of the upper limbs, rib, scapula, sacrum, and pelvis. The computed relative distribution of fibrosarcomas is given in Table 7–6. The size is usually larger than 6 cm. The chief roentgen feature is a bony destructive lesion that may assume any or all patterns (Fig. 7–40). There is no neoplastic new bone formation, nor can flocculent calcifications be seen within the radiolucent areas. A not uncommon finding is a bone sequestrum, varying in size, which may be present within the tumor (Fig. 7–41). Fibrosarcoma is the only primary malignant bone tumor in which sequestration is frequently found. (Sequestration has also been described in intracortical Ewing's tumor.) The lesion may erode the inner cortical margin or be expansile, with a thin cortical shell. The margination of this lesion is usually more ill-defined than that seen in a giant-cell tumor, and trabeculation, although possible, is not a prominent feature. There may be breakthrough of the expanded shell, or complete cortical destruction that affects only one side of the cortex in an eccentric lesion. Massive expansion simulating an aneurysmal bone cyst may be present. Reactive bone formation is sparse and periosteal reaction, when present, shows no spiculations. Pathological fractures may occur. The most difficult entity in the differential diagnosis is giant-cell tumor or the osteolytic type of osteosarcoma.

In the periosteal type there may be thickening, erosion, or invasion of the cortex. Invasion of the soft tissues is a feature in advanced cases of both forms of the tumor.

The angioarchitecture of fibrosarcomas is variable. The most vascular site is the least differentiated, and is the area that should be chosen for a biopsy.[284]

EWING'S TUMOR (EWING'S SARCOMA)

Ewing's tumor[48,62,139,239,278] is a primary malignant neoplasm of unknown origin, but considered by many to be derived from immature reticulum cells of the bone marrow. This is classed in the group of round-cell tumors of the diaphysis, together with myeloma and reticulum-cell sarcoma. The three tumors are similar in location, but differ greatly in age incidence. Ewing's tumor occurs less frequently than myeloma, osteosarcoma, or chondrosarcoma.

Microscopically, this is a highly cellular tumor with little supportive connective tissue. The tumor cells lack clear cell boundaries, and the nuclei, sometimes crowded together, are largely uniform in appearance. Vascularity is not striking. Large necrotic areas are present, which are surrounded by polymorphonuclear leukocytes. There is no neoplastic bone or cartilage formation.

Clinically, the peak age incidence is 15 years; the occurrence of the tumor is improbable below the age of 5 years and over the age of 30 years. It has been reported in a 13-month-old infant. The sex distribution has been reported as equal or slightly more prevalent in males. The chief clinical complaint is local pain, usually of several months' duration, which persistently increases in severity. The duration of the pain is of great diagnostic importance, because a patient with osteomyelitis may present with a similar clinical and radiological picture, but with a history of pain of only a few weeks' duration. Spread of the tumor causes pain and disability of the involved regions, including pleural effusion if a rib is involved. A soft-tissue mass is usually present, and is tender but not warm. Regional dilated veins are present.

The tumor tends to become necrotic, which contributes to systemic symptomatology. Malaise, fever sometimes as high as 105°F, leukocytosis, anemia, and a rapid erythrocyte sedimentation rate are usually present. The tumor spreads by direct infiltration and by early hematogenous dissemination to other bones and the lungs. The 5-year survival rate is probably less than 5%.

Radiologically, the distribution varies somewhat according to the age of the patient, owing to the differing locations of red marrow at various ages. In the younger patient, the tubular bones are most

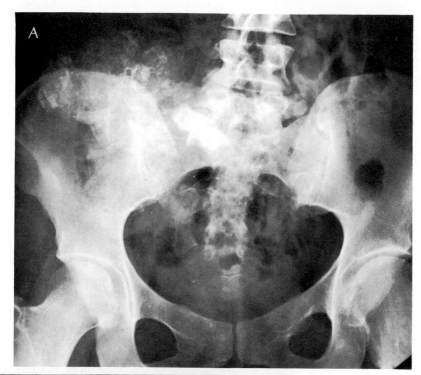

FIG. 7–39. **A.** Peripheral chondrosarcoma (pelvis). There has been malignant degeneration of an osteochondroma. A large intrapelvic mass may be seen, containing disoriented streaky and flocculent calcifications. The patient has multiple osteochondromatosis, which is visible at the left femoral neck and left pubis. **B.** Recurrent chondrosarcoma, same patient as **A**, one year after resection of tumor and iliac crest. There has been massive recurrence with formation of a large mass in the pelvis and on the right side of the abdomen, exhibiting flocculent and disorganized linear streaky calcification.

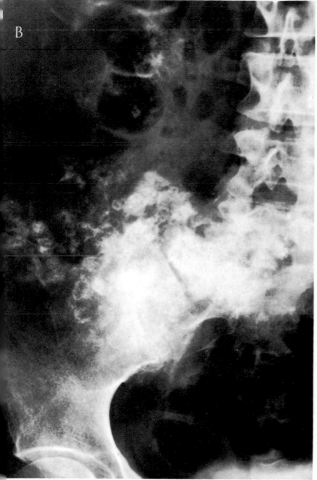

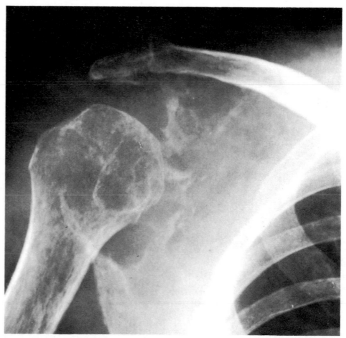

FIG. 7–40. Fibrosarcoma (scapula). There is marked destruction of the scapula, including the glenoid fossa, coracoid process, and base of the acromion. The margins are irregular. Residual bone spicules, which do not represent neoplastic new bone formation, may be seen within the destroyed area.

TABLE 7–7. Ewing's Sarcoma

Skull	**	2
Mandible	**	2
Cerv. spine	*	1
Dors. spine	*	1
Lumb. spine	***	3
Ribs	***************	15
Clavicle	****	4
Scapula	***********	11
Sternum	*	1
Humerus	**********************	22
Radius & Ulna	*****	5
Hand & Carpus	*	1
Pelvis	*****************************	
Pelvis	*****	35
Sacrum	*********	10
Femur	******************************	
Femur	*************	44
Tibia	*****************	17
Foot & Tarsus	**********	11
Other	*************	13

likely to be involved, but in the patient over 20 years of age, the flat bones are the most frequent sites. Of the long bones, the femur is most commonly affected, followed by the tibia. The os calcis is not infrequently involved, and no bone is immune. In the flat bones, the most frequent site is the innominate bone. Four cases have been reported in the hand.[64] The computed relative distribution of Ewing's tumor is presented in Table 7–7.

Ewing's tumor in the flat bones has a characteristic roentgen appearance of mottled destruction (Figs. 7–42, 7–43) and patchy reactive bone sclerosis (Figs. 7–44, 7–45). The os calcis has a similar appearance.

The "classic" appearance in the long bones is present in only about 25% to 50% of cases. This consists of an ill-defined permeative area of bone destruction involving a large central portion of the midshaft, with a fusiform configuration associated with a fine, delicate, lamellated, periosteal new bone response (Figs. 7–46, 7–47). If this picture is seen in a patient between the ages of 5 and 20 years, having the clinical symptomatology described previously, then Ewing's tumor is most probable, although osteomyelitis with an atypical diaphyseal localization must be excluded.

The tumor may atypically develop centrally in the metaphysis (Fig. 7–48), intracortically in the diaphysis or metaphysis, or involve the epiphysis before or after fusion. Typically, the tumor cells permeate the haversian canals and invade the soft tissues,

(Text continued on p. 554)

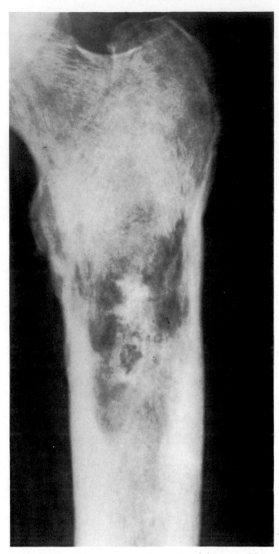

FIG. 7–41. Fibrosarcoma (proximal femur). Note localized but poorly marginated destructive area at the proximal femoral shaft, containing a small segment of increased density which represents a sequestrum. Scalloping of the endosteum at the lateral aspect of the lesion is also apparent.

FIG. 7–42. Ewing's tumor (scapula). Note ill-defined area of destruction involving the body of the scapula, the glenoid, and the acromion process, with several small areas of reactive bone sclerosis.

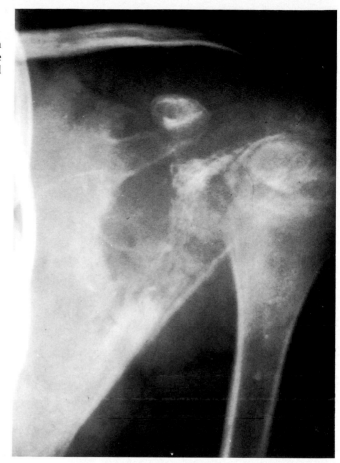

FIG. 7–43. Ewing's tumor (scapula). **A.** An area of destruction of the scapula is noted with reactive bone sclerosis. **B.** Same area 3 months after 4000 rads of roentgen therapy. Reconstitution of the bone, which now has a mottled sclerotic appearance, is seen.

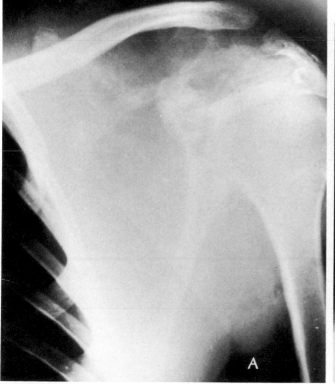

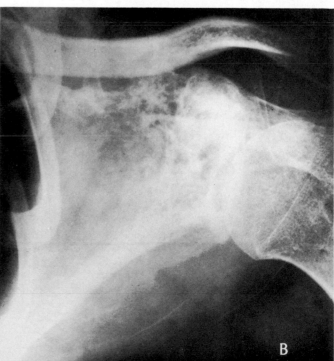

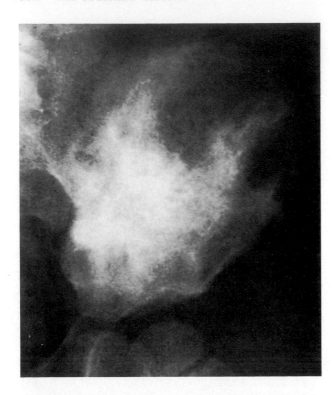

FIG. 7–44. Ewing's tumor (ilium). Mottled sclerosis of the left ilium may be noted, with several marginal destructive areas.

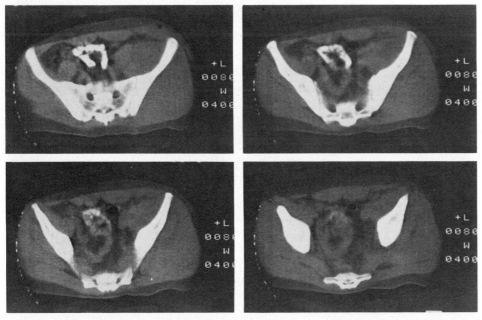

FIG. 7–45. Ewing's tumor (ilium). CT scan shows a large soft-tissue mass in the left side of the pelvis adjacent to the ilium. There is no evidence of cortical breakthrough of the ilium itself. (Courtesy of Dr. J. P. Petasnick, Rush–Presbyterian St. Luke's Hospital, Chicago, IL)

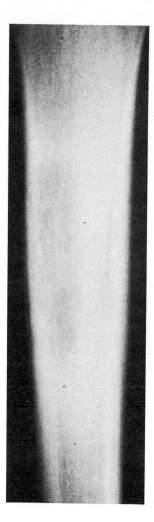

FIG. 7–46. Ewing's tumor (tibial shaft). Note ill-defined area of radiolucency with a segment of fine periosteal new bone formation at the medial aspect. (Courtesy of Dr. Edward Salinas, Chicago, IL)

FIG. 7–47. Ewing's sarcoma involving the midshaft of the femur. Laminated periosteal new bone formation and reactive cortical thickening are present.

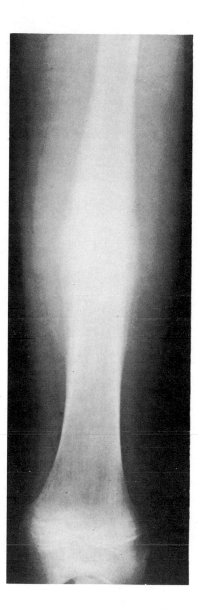

FIG. 7–48. Ewing's tumor. Note ill-defined permeative and "moth-eaten" destruction of the femoral neck, trochanteric region, and proximal shaft. The cortex is intact and there is no periosteal new bone formation.

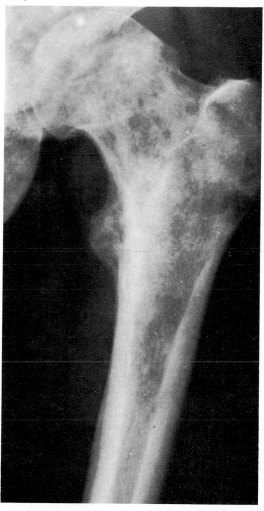

leaving an intact cortex, cortical sequestration, or a cortex only segmentally destroyed (Fig. 7–49), unlike other tumors but similar to osteomyelitis. In tumors of cortical origin, the outer surface of the cortex is destroyed with invasion of the soft tissues to form a large mass, while the inner cortical surface remains intact. These mechanisms permit the formation of a large soft-tissue component with a relatively intact cortex. Because the tumor forms no osteoid or chondroid, the soft-tissue mass is free of calcifications except for periosteal new bone formation or debris.

Variations in the "classic" destructive pattern and reactive bone sclerosis occur in the majority of instances. The rate of growth may be slower, leading to a discrete zone of destruction. An expansile lesion in the short tubular bones, with a thin and segmentally destroyed cortex, may be seen.[64] Bone sclerosis may range from minimal to prominent, and may be patchy or take the form of thickened trabeculae. No neoplastic new bone is formed. Cortical thickening may also be present.

"Onionskin" periosteal reaction is not pathognomonic of Ewing's tumor, and need not be present. Simple, delicate periosteal elevation may be present, as well as a Codman's triangle. A spiculated periosteal response may sometimes be seen, with thin delicate strands of periosteal perpendicular new bone extending parallel to each other, involving a long segment of the shaft. This differs from the periosteal pattern sometimes seen in osteosarcoma in that there is no radiation from a central point or "sunburst" effect.[158]

When the vertebrae are involved, the lesion leads to vertebral body collapse. Sclerotic reaction and a paraspinal soft-tissue mass may also be present. The ribs, when involved, usually show a lytic, fusiform, expansile lesion without periosteal reaction. An associated extrapleural soft-tissue mass is frequently present.

When skeletal metastases have occurred, extreme bone destruction may result and differentiation from other causes of widespread destruction becomes difficult. The most difficult entities in the differential diagnosis are osteomyelitis, eosinophilic granuloma of bone, and osteosarcoma.

RETICULUM-CELL SARCOMA OF BONE

Reticulum-cell sarcoma[98,121,191] primary to bone is a rare malignant tumor derived from primitive marrow mesenchyme; this is a separate clinicopathologic entity distinct from Ewing's tumor, myeloma, and generalized reticulum-cell sarcoma.

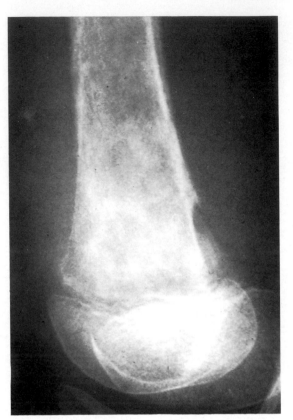

FIG. 7–49. Ewing's tumor (femur). The tumor originated in the distal femoral metaphysis, causing an ill-defined area of destruction. The anterior cortex has been invaded in several separate localities. No periosteal new bone formation is present.

TABLE 7–8. Reticulum-Cell Sarcoma

Skull	***	3
Mandilble	****	4
Cerv. spine	*	1
Dors. spine	***	3
Lumb. spine	**	2
Ribs	****	4
Clavicle	*	0
Scapula	******	6
Sternum	**	2
Humerus	*************	13
Radius & Ulna	*****	5
Hand & Carpus	*	1
Pelvis	********	9
Sacrum	**	2
Femur	*******************************	31
Tibia	**************	15
Foot & Tarsus	**	2
Other	***	3

Microscopically, the tumor is similar to reticulum-cell lymphoma and Ewing's tumor. Reticulum tumor cells are present, which may vary in appearance, with foci of lymphocytes. A variable amount of fibrous stroma is also present.

Clinically, the age (distribution) of patients is older than in Ewing's sarcoma and younger than in multiple myeloma. The majority of patients are between 20 and 40 years of age; however, wide variations are possible. Males are affected twice as often as females. Local pain and swelling with inflammatory signs of long duration are the usual chief complaints. Systemic symptoms are characteristically absent, while they are present in Ewing's tumor. Pathological fractures may occur. The tumor metastasizes late to lymph nodes and lungs, and only very rarely to other bones.

Radiologically, a large percentage of tumors are found in the lower femur and upper tibia. About 50% occur in the lower extremities, with the remainder in the humerus, scapula, vertebra, pelvis, and other bones. In the tubular bones, the lesion may occur in the shaft or in the metaphysis. The computed relative distribution of reticulum-cell sarcoma is presented in Table 7–8.

The radiologic characteristic is "moth-eaten" or permeative bone destruction in separate areas that coalesce (Figs. 7–50, 7–51). The cortex is broken through and periosteal reaction of a lamellated or amorphous type is sometimes seen. Spiculation and Codman's triangle are said to be absent. Cortical expansion may rarely be seen (Fig. 7–52). Cortical thickening and reactive bone sclerosis may also be present. Pathological fracture not infrequently occurs (Fig. 7–53). A large soft-tissue mass may be present but shows no neoplastic ossification. If the tumor is near a joint, an associated synovitis may occur. The most difficult entity in differential diagnosis is Ewing's sarcoma, which can present an identical roentgen picture. The older age group and the lack of systemic symptoms in reticulum-cell sarcoma aid in differentiating the two.

CHORDOMA

A *chordoma*[82,84,103] is a rare malignant tumor derived from notochordal remnants. The majority develop in the sacrum. They also occur in the base of the skull in the sphenoido-occipital area, with about 10% of cases occurring elsewhere along the spine. The age distribution is from 30 to 70 years. Benign notochordal rests in the sphenoido-occipital region also occur, and are not to be confused with malignant tumor. The lesions are painful, with as-

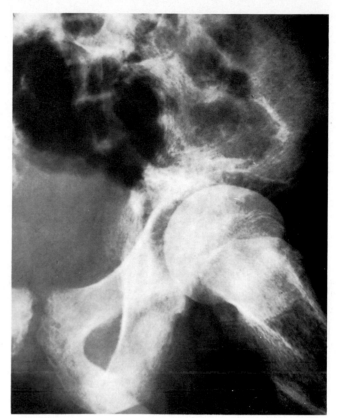

FIG. 7–50. Reticulum-cell sarcoma (pelvis). Note multiple permeative areas of bone destruction, with a large area of coalescence in the supra-acetabular region. The head of the femur is not involved.

sociated neurological symptoms and palpable mass. Prognosis is poor. Distant metastases are said to occur in less than 10% of cases, and most commonly involve lymph nodes, liver, and lungs.

Radiologically, the picture is not characteristic; however, a bulky tumor causing bone destruction and located in the midline at the base of the skull or in the caudal region suggests this condition when it occurs in a patient over 30 years of age. Ill-defined bone destruction or cortical expansion may be seen, as well as flocculent calcifications within a large soft-tissue mass. Intracranial tumors may present as sellar tumors with extensive destruction. One-half of the patients have erosion of the clivus when first seen. Over one-half show calcification, and a nasopharyngeal mass is present in one-third. Skeletal metastases may occur. Sacral tumors present as a midline destructive or expansile lesion, with or without osteosclerosis. In late stages the tumor

(Text continued on p. 558)

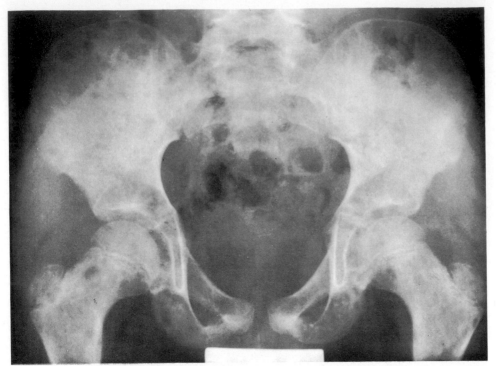

FIG. 7–51. Primary reticulum-cell sarcoma of bone (pelvis). Multiple small destructive areas in the ischia and femoral heads and necks are present. There is no reactive bone sclerosis and no periosteal new bone formation in this case. (Courtesy of Dr. Harvey White)

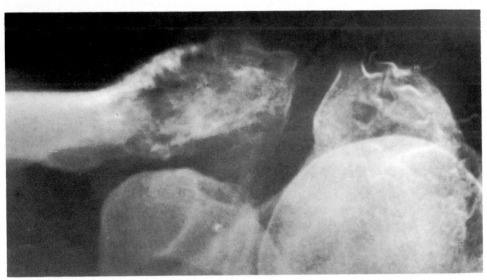

FIG. 7–52. Reticulum-cell sarcoma (distal clavicle). Small, ill-defined destructive areas are present, with expansion of the superior aspect of the distal clavicle and slight cortical thickening.

FIG. 7–53. Reticulum-cell sarcoma. **A.** Humerus. Film taken at initial complaint shows minimal permeative destructive areas in the midhumeral shaft. **B.** Humerus. Film taken after short interval now shows extensive permeative destruction of the humeral diaphysis. **C.** Xeroradiograph of the humerus shows that the destruction has progressed to a pathological fracture.

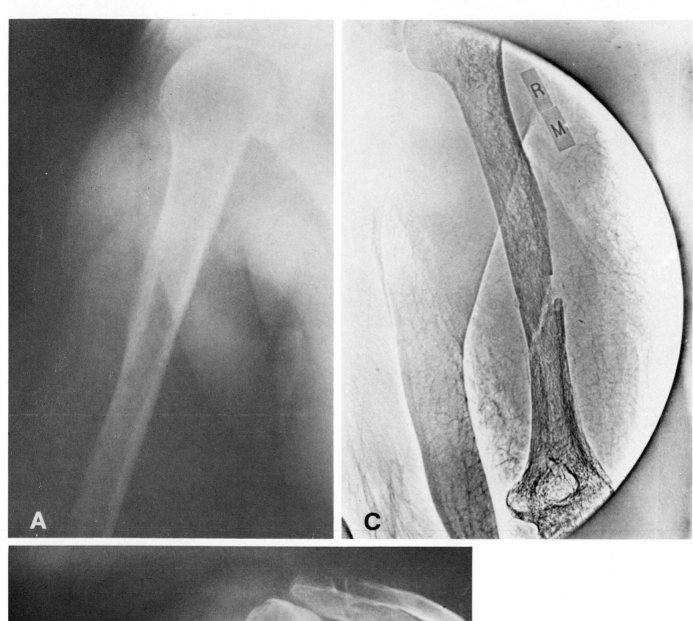

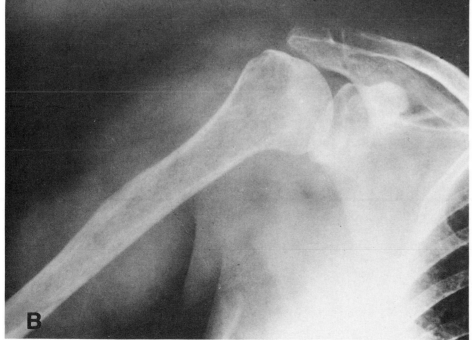

557

need not be confined to the midline (Fig. 7–54). If the tumor primarily involves the spine, the roentgen picture is not specific. Bone destruction is present with or without involvement of the intervertebral disk and 2 or more vertebrae may be involved. A paraspinal soft-tissue mass which may contain calcification is often present.[82]

GIANT-CELL TUMOR (OSTEOCLASTOMA)

Giant-cell tumor[70,122,163,171,279] is an uncommon tumor derived from skeletal connective tissue. Jaffe[124] classes this as a quasimalignant tumor. It is not possible to predict either on histological or radiological grounds the future behavior of the majority of these lesions. Nevertheless, giant-cell tumor forms a distinct clinico-pathological-radiological entity even though division into benign and malignant forms is not of great reliability. The incidence of malignancy has been estimated at about 20%.

Microscopically, ovoid or spindle-shaped cells in a vascular stroma and large multinucleated giant cells are seen. Osteoid may also be present, as well as lipid-bearing foam cells. The appearance of the stromal cells and their ratio to giant cells are considered to be an indicator of the malignant potential of the tumor.

Clinically, 75% of these lesions occur between the ages of 20 and 40 years. Rare cases have been reported in children and in patients older than 50 years. Males and females are equally affected. The chief complaint is an intermittent dull ache that may be associated with a palpable, tender mass. Symptomatology in a contiguous joint often develops, and pathological fracture may occur. The prognosis is uncertain, because the tumor may recur after excision (Fig. 7–55), or metastasize to the lungs (Fig. 7–56). Malignant change or transformation into fibrosarcoma (Fig. 7–57) or osteosarcoma following radiation therapy is a hazard of that modality of treatment. Giant-cell tumor also occurs in association with Paget's disease, in which case these tumors may be malignant or benign. Twenty-six cases have been reported to date. The most frequent sites are the skull, mandible, maxilla, innominate bone, and tibia. The average age is about 60 years. Malignant tumors are rapidly fatal.

When the diagnosis of giant-cell tumor is entertained, it is imperative to determine the serum calcium, phosphorus, and alkaline phosphatase in every case, because a brown tumor of hyperparathyroidism may simulate this lesion in every respect except metastases.

Radiologically, the classic location is in the distal femur or proximal tibia, extending to the articular surface, and off the central axis. The distal radius is another common site of lone bone involvement, and the lesion has been reported in almost all tubular bones, as well as the patella and calcaneus. The origin of the lesion is considered to be metaphyseal by Johnson, and this is confirmed by the principal metaphyseal location of the rare giant-cell tumor that arises in a young patient prior to epiphyseal fusion.[195,238] The tumor then may be limited by the cartilage plate or extend into the epiphysis. The lesion in an adult may rarely extend almost to the articular surface, or may be located in the shaft in very exceptional cases. The latter situation precludes the roentgen diagnosis of giant-cell tumor. Locations other than the long bones are en-

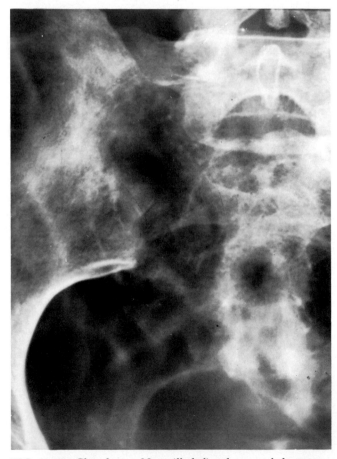

FIG. 7–54. Chordoma. Note ill-defined area of destruction, involving the sacrum and extending to the right sacral wing.

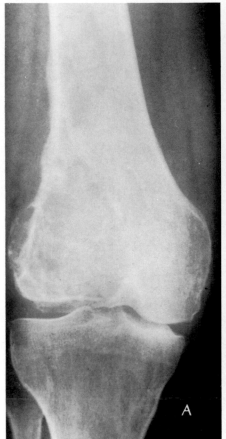
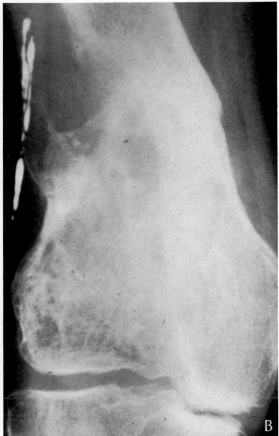

FIG. 7–55. Giant-cell tumor (distal femur) — female, age 44 years. A. There is a moderately well-circumscribed destructive area off the central axis in the distal femur that is lightly trabeculated and expands the lateral cortex to a slight degree. The lesion extends to the articular surface of the bone. B. Two-year interval film following surgery. There has been reconstitution of the major portion of the bone. Lipiodol is seen filling a draining sinus tract due to superimposed osteomyelitis. C. Two-year interval film after B. Recurrence of the giant-cell tumor is noted. Further bone destruction and expansion of the lateral cortex are also apparent. The lesion is still lightly trabeculated.

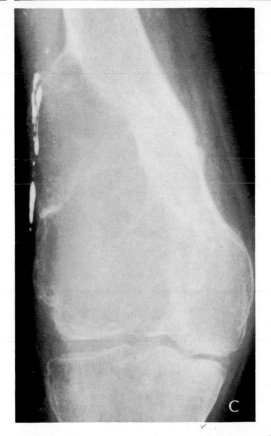

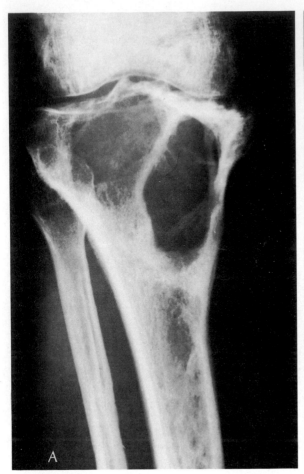

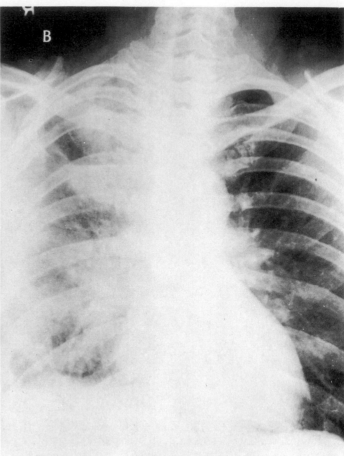

FIG. 7–56. Giant-cell tumor. **A.** Large destructive lesion at the proximal tibia, which extends to the articular surface, is well demarcated and shows light trabeculation. This tumor metastasized to the lungs following surgery. It would not be possible to predict the future behavior of this tumor with this roentgenogram. **B.** Chest film, 4-year interval after **A**. Extensive pulmonary metastases from the giant-cell tumor are present.

TABLE 7–9. Giant-Cell Tumor

Skull	***	3
Mandible	*	0
Cerv. spine	***	3
Dors. spine	*	1
Lumb. spine	**	2
Ribs	**	2
Clavicle	*	0
Scapula	*	0
Sternum	*	1
Humerus	***************	16
Radius & Ulna	***********************	25
Hand & Carpus	****	4
Pelvis	*************	13
Sacrum	***************	15
Femur	**************************	
Femur	****************************	
Femur	****	74
Tibia	**************************	26
Foot & Tarsus	***	3
Other	**********	11

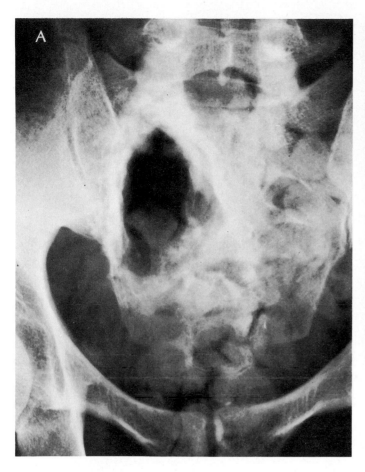

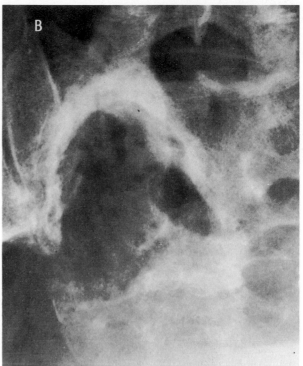

FIG. 7–57. Giant-cell tumor after radiation therapy. **A.** Note well-defined area of radiolucency, with sclerotic margins, in the right side of the sacrum. The inferior margin is sharply delimited and the lateral cortex is intact. **B.** Six-month interval film after **A**. The lesion has now recurred. Note the destruction of the lateral margin of the sacrum and the ill-defined margin of the inferior aspect of the lesion. Biopsy at this time revealed a fibrosarcoma.

countered in about 15% of cases. Mandibular involvement is rare, and brown tumors of hyperparathyroidism or giant-cell reparative granulomas have been mistaken for this lesion. Giant-cell tumors of the vertebral column are rare except in the sacrum, and may involve the body, pedicle (Figs. 7–58, 7–59), or other portions of the neural arch. The majority of radiologically similar lesions actually represent aneurysmal bone cysts. Rarely, the pelvis, ribs, or scapula may be involved (Fig. 7–60). The computed relative distribution of giant-cell tumors is presented in Table 7–9. Multiple giant-cell tumors are very rare. It is difficult to distinguish a multicentric giant-cell tumor from a primary giant-cell tumor that has metastasized. Multiple lesions tend to exhibit the same aggressive behavior as a solitary giant-cell tumor.

The classical appearance is a moderately sized expansile radiolucent lesion that may be eccentric

(Figs. 7–61, 7–62) or involve the entire diameter of the bone end (Fig. 7–63), extending to the immediate subarticular cortex. The lesion is usually round. An appearance of light trabeculation is often present, owing to uneven bone destruction. At times, no trabeculations are seen. Heavy trabeculation is not usual in an uncomplicated lesion, and its occurrence or a "soap bubble" appearance suggests postradiation change or recurrence (Fig. 7–64). The margin of the area of circumscribed osteolysis is fairly well defined, but there is usually no sclerotic rim, nor does the edge commonly fade imperceptibly into normal bone, although the latter may occur.

(Text continued on p. 565)

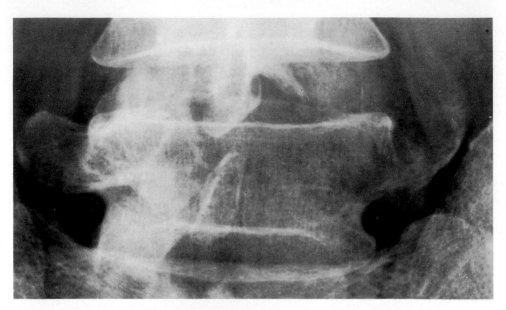

FIG. 7–58. Giant-cell tumor involving the left pedicle of the fifth lumbar vertebra, causing destruction and partial destruction of the superior aspect of the transverse process.

FIG. 7–59. Giant-cell tumor involving the left pedicle of the ninth dorsal vertebra. Tomogram shows destruction of the pedicle and of a portion of the right vertebral body.

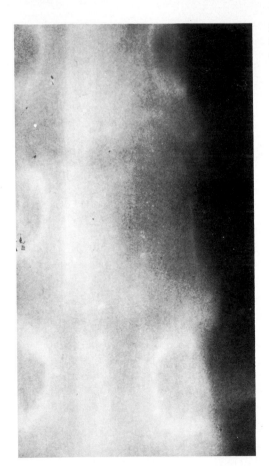

FIG. 7–60. Giant-cell tumor (scapula). Note destructive, expansile, lightly trabeculated lesion involving the scapula, the acromion, and the glenoid fossa.

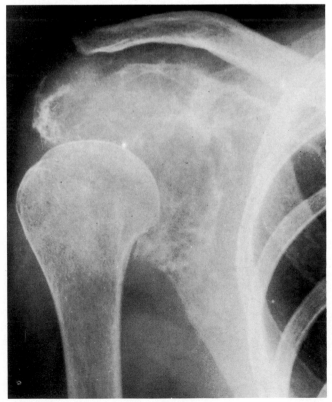

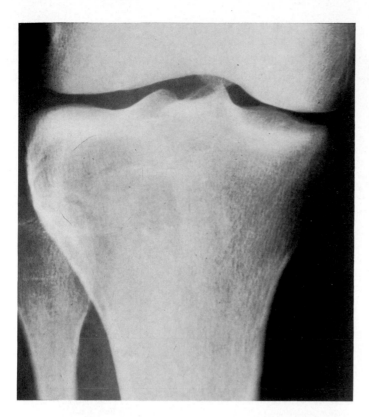

FIG. 7–61. Giant-cell tumor (proximal tibia)—early stage. Note roundish area of radiolucency at the proximal tibia off the central axis, with fairly sharply demarcated superior margins and poorly defined inferior margin. There is not periosteal reaction, and expansion of the cortex is minimal.

FIG. 7–62. Giant-cell tumor (proximal tibia)—advanced stage. Note area of radiolucency off the central axis in the proximal tibia. The lesion is slightly elongated and extends to the articular surface, with poorly defined margins and light trabeculation. A large area of cortical destruction medially may be noted, with bulging of tumor tissue into the soft tissues. It is not possible to predict malignant or benign behavior on the basis of this appearance. It is still possible for the tumor to be well encapsulated, in spite of lack of visibility of the cortex on roentgenograms.

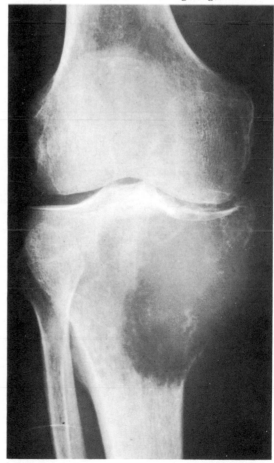

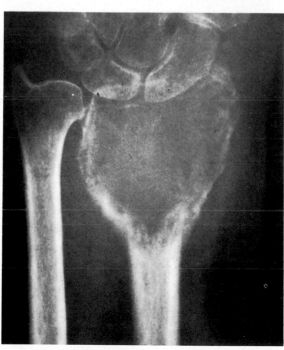

FIG. 7–63. Giant-cell tumor (distal radius). There is a central radiolucent, destructive, and expansile lesion at the distal radius, extending to the articular surface. The expanded cortex is intact. Lack of definition of the proximal margin of the lesion, and very light trabeculation may be seen. No periosteal new bone formation is present, a characteristic of this tumor.

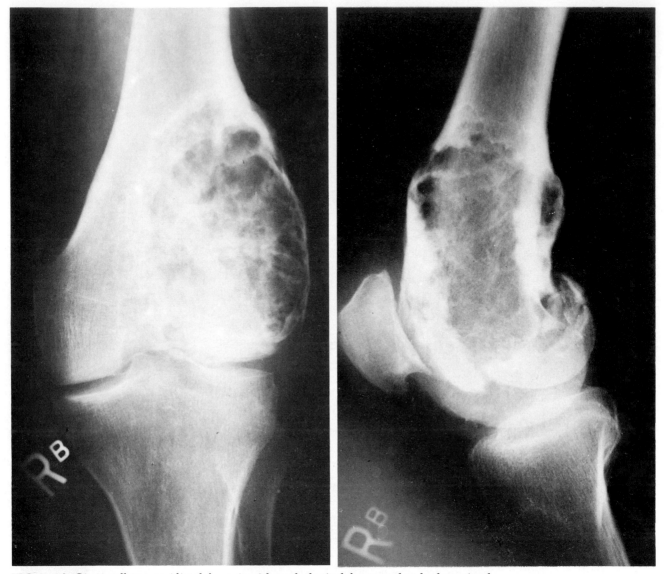

FIG. 7–64. Giant-cell tumor (distal femur) with pathological fracture that had received radiation therapy 10 years previously—anteroposterior and lateral views. A large, expansile, well-circumscribed and heavily trabeculated radiolucent lesion with a narrow zone of transition is seen in the distal femur, extending to portions of the subarticular cortex. A pathological fracture at its distal aspect is noted. This change of heavy trabeculation is consistent with prior irradiation and is not seen in an untreated giant-cell tumor.

FIG. 7–65. Giant-cell tumor (distal first metatarsal). There is an expansile radiolucent lesion extending to the articular surface of the bone, with light trabeculation. Slight thickening of the expanded cortex may be seen, indicating relatively slow growth. There is no evidence of punctate calcifications within this lesion. The sesamoid bone is visible through the radiolucent area.

The periosteum is expanded and thinned and segments may not be seen, owing to either destruction or lack of visibility. There is characteristically no periosteal elevated new bone formation over the expanded area, even when pathological fracture occurs. Very rarely, some calcification within the tumor may be seen. The cortex may be broken through and the soft tissue invaded with the formation of a soft-tissue mass. This is said to occur in both malignant and benign varieties. When a short tubular bone is involved, there is expansion of the bone end and a portion of the diaphysis (Fig. 7–65).

Computerized tomography is of value in this lesion to demonstrate the presence and extent of any soft-tissue component, to assess the intraosseous extent, (Fig. 7–66), to demonstrate the integrity of the cortex, and to evaluate the postoperative state.[63] Angiography is useful to show the vascularity and the extent of the tumor.

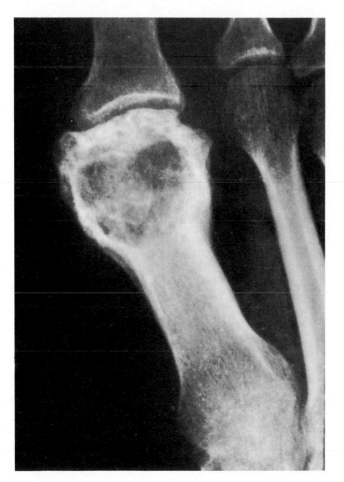

This lesion is to be differentiated from an enchondroma, which usually does not involve the end of a bone. A nonneoplastic osteolytic lesion of the base of a metacarpal, containing giant cells, has been described and termed *giant-cell reaction*.[128]

BENIGN TUMORS AND TUMORLIKE CONDITIONS OF BONE

OSTEOMA

A true *osteoma* is a benign tumor that contains only osseous tissue. These lesions may represent hamartomas. They develop only in intramembranous bone. The most common sites of origin are the inner and outer tables of the skull, the paranasal sinuses, and the mandible. Osteoma of the nasal bones may rarely occur. The lesions are asymptomatic until they block the ostia of the paranasal sinuses or cause mechanical oral disturbances. Other reported complications include reversible blindness[101] and recurrent pyogenic meningitis[241] due to frontal sinus osteomas, as well as proptosis. They are often discovered in adult life and show neither signs of progression nor malignant change.

Radiologically, they are characterized by a dense, radiopaque, structureless appearance. Round and well-circumscribed, they rarely attain a size larger than 2 cm in diameter (Figs. 7–67, 7–68), although a much greater size is possible (Figs. 7–69, 7–70). If situated in a paranasal sinus, usually the frontal or ethmoid sinuses, it may cause expansion of the sinus walls. A large tumor with the appearance of an osteoma in the periosteal region of a long bone is likely to be a parosteal sarcoma, although a parosteal osteoma may rarely occur. A round condensation of dense bone in the medulla represents an enostoma (Fig. 7–71) or bone island (see Chap. 6). Osteomalike bone response to tropical ulcer has been reported.[141]

GARDNER'S SYNDROME

Gardner's syndrome[33] is a familial disease consisting of osteomata, soft-tissue tumors, and polyposis, chiefly of the colon. It is transmitted as an autosomal dominant. The colonic polyps are premalignant, and a colonic carcinoma may be present at

(Text continued on p. 569)

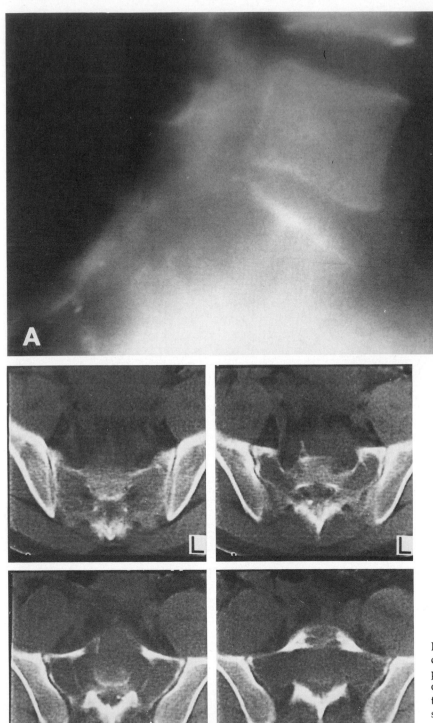

FIG. 7–66. Giant-cell tumor of the sacrum in 25-year-old male who complained of sciatica. **A.** Laterial tomogram of sacrum showing a destructive lesion at the posterior aspect of the first sacral segment with cortical destruction. **B.** CT scan showing destruction at the central aspect of the sacrum. (Courtesy of Dr. J. P. Petasnick, Rush–Presbyterian St. Luke's Hospital, Chicago, IL)

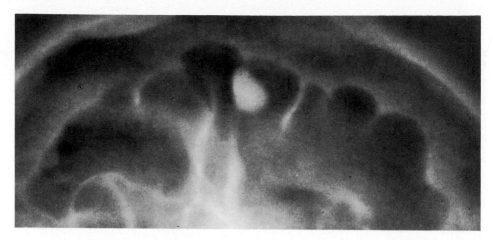

FIG. 7–67. Osteoma of the frontal sinus. Note small, dense, structureless bony condensation in the frontal sinus.

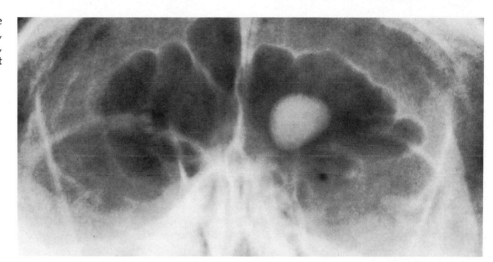

FIG. 7–68. Osteoma of the frontal sinus. Note roundish, well-circumscribed, dense, structureless lesion in the left frontal sinus.

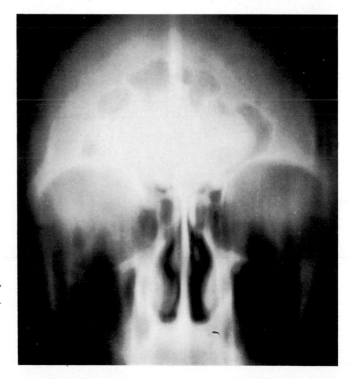

FIG. 7–69. Osteoma of the frontal sinus, measuring 4×7 cm—tomogram. A dense, structureless, irregularly outlined ossific mass is present.

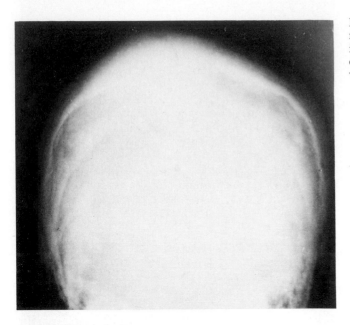

FIG. 7–70. Osteoma of the skull. A dense structureless mass involving the outer table of the calvarium, measuring 6 cm in its longest diameter, and blending with the outer table at its margins, is seen. Thickening of the calvarium and hyperostosis frontalis interna are also noted.

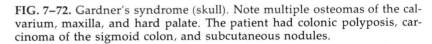

FIG. 7–71. Enostoma. A dense, structureless lesion within the medullary cavity of the proximal humerus may be seen.

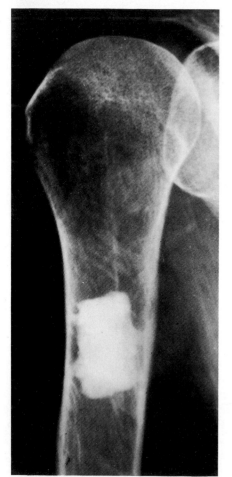

FIG. 7–72. Gardner's syndrome (skull). Note multiple osteomas of the calvarium, maxilla, and hard palate. The patient had colonic polyposis, carcinoma of the sigmoid colon, and subcutaneous nodules.

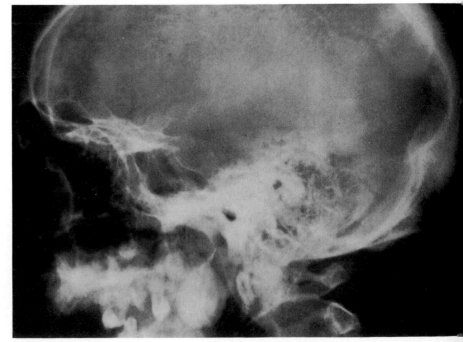

the time of diagnosis. Polyposis of the gastrointestinal tract may rarely be present outside of the colon, and adenocarcinoma of the duodenum has been reported. Approximately 150 cases of this syndrome have been reported in the literature to date. The bone lesions may precede the intestinal polyposis. Multiple dense osteomas of various sizes, from slight thickening to large masses, are distributed throughout the skeleton. Localized cortical thickening may also be present. The skull and mandible are characteristically involved. The maxilla and hard palate may also show osteomas (Fig. 7–72). In the mandible, dense, protuberant, lobulated osteomas arise from the mandibular angle. Enostoses at the roots of the teeth are also seen, as well as dental abnormalities. The tubular bones show localized or wavy cortical thickening, and may show exostoses or pedunculated osteomas. The ribs and the pelvis may show cortical thickening. Small dense osteomas of the scaphoid have also been reported.

OSTEOID OSTEOMA

Osteoid osteoma[86,149,259] is generally considered to be a benign tumor of bone. The actual lesion is 1 cm or less in size and is called the *nidus*. The nidus initially is uncalcified, but on maturity may develop calcification that may range from small flecks to calcification of its major portion (Fig. 7–73). The second component of the lesion is reactive sclerosis with cortical thickening and periosteal reaction. The degree of this reactive new bone formation varies considerably and is influenced by the location of the nidus. The nidus may be intramedullary, intracortical, or subperiosteal, and the roentgen appearances of all three are dissimilar. In addition, an intracapsular osteoid osteoma in the femoral neck provokes less reactive sclerosis because of the low-bone-producing capacity of the intracapsular periosteum.

Microscopically, the nidus consists of osteoid and osseous tissue within a highly vascular stroma. Giant cells are present. The nidus is sharply demarcated from the surrounding reactive sclerosis.

Clinically, the hallmark of this lesion is local pain that is worse at night and is ameliorated by activity. Dramatic relief is usually obtained with aspirin. The duration of symptoms ranges on the average from 6 months to 2 years before the patient seeks medical assistance. The pain is sometimes referred to a nearby joint, and later increases in severity. Regional soft-tissue swelling, point tenderness, and limitation of motion also occur, but not heat and erythema.

If the lesion is in the lower extremities, limp, weakness, and muscle atrophy are seen, as well as depressed deep tendon reflexes. When the spine is involved, osteoid osteoma produces a painful rigid scoliosis causing nerve irritation and root pain simulating a neurological lesion. Cervical radicular pain as well as torticollis may occur in a cervical spinal location.[234] There are no systemic symptoms. Rarely, a lesion may not be painful, or pain may precede a demonstrable lesion.[148] A lesion of the capitate is reported as presenting with carpal–tunnel syndrome.[114] Leg-length discrepancy in a patient with a tibial osteoid osteoma has been documented.[260]

Osteoid osteoma is not an uncommon lesion. Ninety percent of cases are seen below the age of 25 years, with the disease being very rare under 2 years and over 50 years. It has been reported in the tibia of an 8-month-old boy.[102] Males are affected twice as often as females.

Radiologically, one-half of the lesions are seen in the femur and tibia. Other common sites are the fibula, humerus, and vertebral arch. However, all bones of the body may be involved, even the skull.[55, 200] The nidus may be intracortical, intramedullary, subperiosteal, or at the articular surface. Double and triple nidi have been reported.[91] Eleven cases of such multifocal osteoid osteomas have been reported in the literature.[97] A single case of osteoid osteomas arising in adjacent bones has also been reported.[186]

The relative distribution of osteoid osteomas is presented in Table 7–10.[46] The classical roentgen appearance is that of a small, radiolucent intracortical nidus, less than 1 cm in diameter, surrounded by a large, dense, sclerotic zone of cortical thickening and solid or possibly laminated (Fig. 7–74) periosteal reaction. The dense reaction may obscure the nidus on conventional films (Fig. 7–75) and overpenetrated films or laminography may be necessary for its demonstration. The nidus may be uncalcified (Fig. 7–76), partially calcified, or have the major portion of its centrum calcified so as to present as a radiolucent halo within the sclerotic zone. The nidus need not be centrally located within the area of sclerosis, but may be eccentrically placed or even on edge. The roentgen appearance does not correlate with the duration of symptoms (Fig. 7–77). Cortical thickening at a distance from the nidus may be seen. Synovitis in an adjacent joint not involving an intracapsular lesion may be present.[237,250] An intramedullary nidus characteristically evokes little bone sclerosis (Fig. 7–78). This may cause internal cortical thickening.

(Text continued on p. 572)

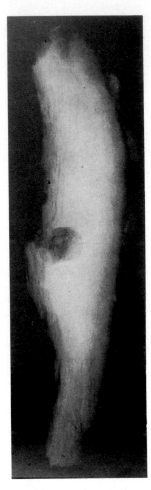

FIG. 7–73. Radiograph of resected specimen of osteoid osteoma. The actual lesion is the 7 mm round radiolucency, called the *nidus*. Surrounding reactive and sclerotic bone is present. There is a small amount of calcification within the nidus in this specimen, due to the calcification of lesional osteoid.

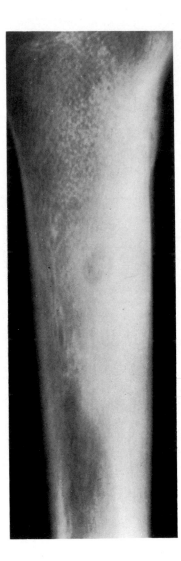

FIG. 7–74. Osteoid osteoma (femur). Note dense cortical thickening, with a radiolucent nidus.

FIG. 7–75. Osteoid osteoma. Dense cortical thickening at the proximal medial femoral shaft completely obscures the small radiolucent nidus.

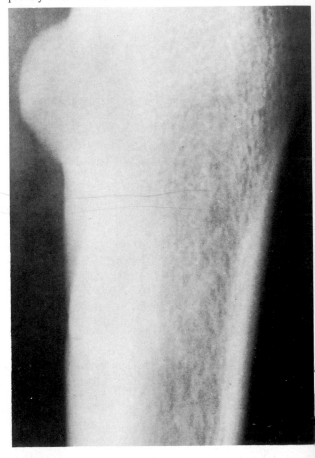

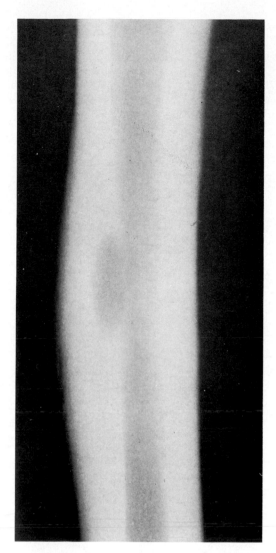

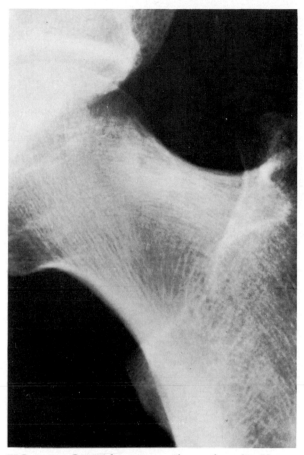

FIG. 7–76. Tomogram of osteoid osteoma with cortical location and an endosteal abutment. An ovoid radiolucent nidus with no areas of calcification is present. Note fusiform cortical thickening with periosteal new bone formation.

FIG. 7–77. Osteoid osteoma (femoral neck). Very little bone sclerosis is present. Note small radiolucent nidus at the outer aspect of the femoral neck.

TABLE 7–10. Osteoid Osteoma

Skull	*	0
Mandible	*	1
Cerv. spine	*	0
Dors. spine	***	3
Lumb. spine	******	6
Ribs	*	0
Clavicle	*	0
Scapula	****	4
Sternum	*	0
Humerus	*************	13
Radius & Ulna	******	6
Hand & Carpus	**********	10
Pelvis	*****	5
Sacrum	*	0
Femur	*****************************	
Femur	*****************************	60
Tibia	*****************************	
Tibia	**********	41
Foot & Tarsus	********	8
Other	**	2

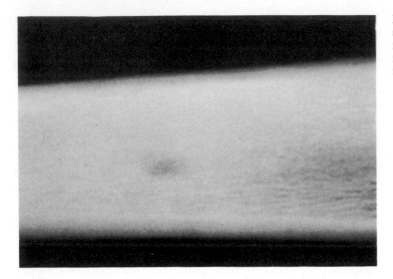

FIG. 7–78. Intramedullary osteoid osteoma. Note small radiolucent nidus with very little surrounding reactive bone sclerosis—a finding characteristic of intramedullary location of the nidus. There is no appreciable cortical thickening.

A less common site for a nidus is a subperiosteal location (Fig. 7–79). This presents as a small periosteal bulge of the contour of the bone. A radiolucency in the peripheral-most portion and a thin shell of margination, associated with some thickening of the cortex, are characteristically seen.

A not uncommon location for an intramedullary osteoid osteoma is the neck of the femur, where it sometimes may be associated with osteoporosis of the femoral head and neck (Fig. 7–80). Severe growth disturbances associated with lesions in this location have been reported. Lymphofollicular synovitis in association with intra-articular osteoid osteoma has also been described.[237,250] The roentgen findings include uniform narrowing of the interosseous space and subperiosteal bone apposition involving the affected bone as well as adjacent bones. Lymphofollicular inflammation in the adjacent soft tissues is reported to be a consistent finding in intra-articular osteoid osteoma. Differentiation must be made from rheumatoid arthritis.

In the spine, the neural arch (Fig. 7–81) and the spinous and transverse processes may be involved. If the lamina is involved, there may be enlargement of the adjacent transverse process. A rigid scoliosis occurs and the local appearance is similar to that seen in other bones. Rarely, a lesion may regress without treatment, however such a lesion may, in reality, be an abscess. As the lesion heals, the nidus becomes less radiolucent, but the sclerotic reaction does not resolve. There may also be recurrence following surgery (Fig. 7–82). Incomplete removal results in persistent or recurrent pain. Radionuclide

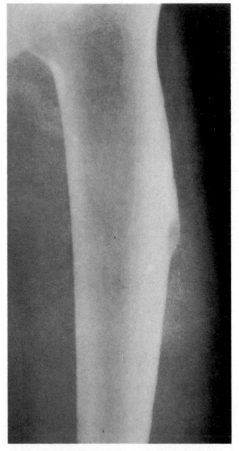

FIG. 7–79. Subperiosteal osteoid osteoma. Note bulging of the periosteum by the nidus, and cortical thickening.

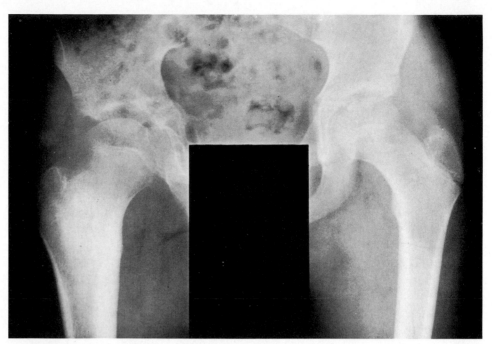

FIG. 7–80. Osteoid osteoma (right hip). Note cortical thickening at the upper medial femoral margin, with a smooth scalloped appearance, and a radiolucent area in the intertrochanteric region (which proved to be the site of the nidus). Widening of the joint space and effusion into the joint space were caused by an associated synovitis. Regional osteoporosis of the femoral head and neck may also be noted. Synovitis and effusion may occur in an intracapsular osteoid osteoma. (Courtesy of Dr. Heriberto Garcia, Chicago, IL)

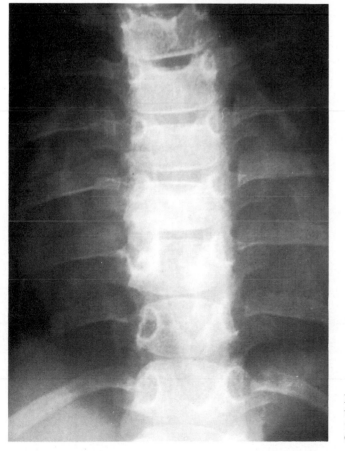

FIG. 7–81. Osteoid osteoma involving the right pedicle on the ninth dorsal vertebra. There is marked enlargement of the pedicle with sclerosis. (Courtesy of Dr. Harvey White, Children's Memorial Hospital, Chicago, IL)

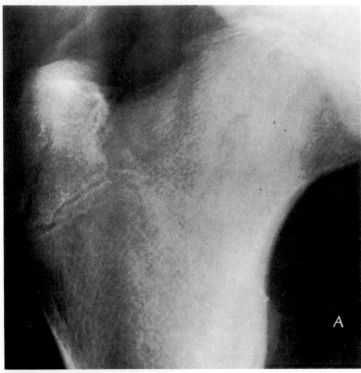

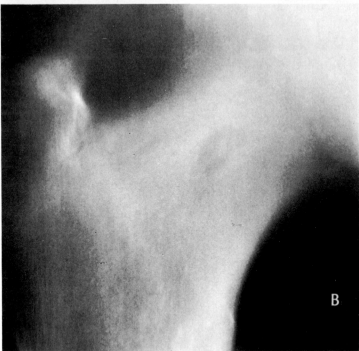

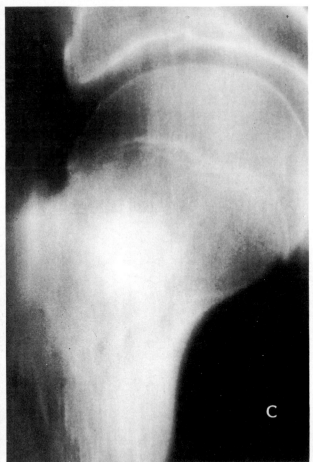

FIG. 7–82. Osteoid osteoma (femoral neck). **A.** Small radiolucent nidus in the femoral neck, without significant reactive bone sclerosis. **B.** Tomogram, taken at same time as **A**, gives a good demonstration of the nidus containing a small central calcification without reactive bone sclerosis. **C.** Eight-month interval film following surgery. Pain has recurred, and tomogram shows area of sclerosis due to recurrent tumor in the femoral neck.

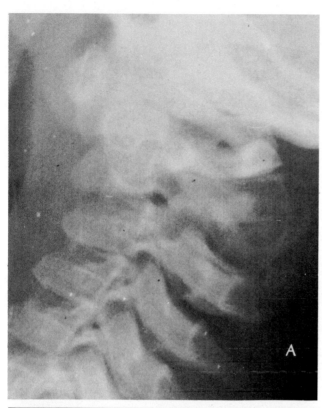

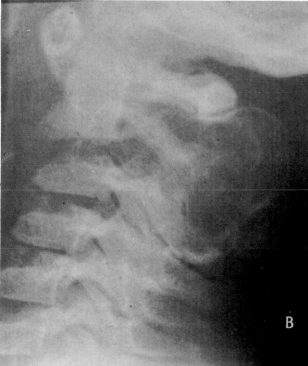

FIG. 7–83. Benign osteoblastoma (cervical spine). **A.** Well-circumscribed, expansile lesion situated *between* the spinous processes of the second and third cervical vertebrae. The bony margin is intact. Some calcification of the matrix is present. **B.** Nine-month interval film after **A.** There has been progressive growth of the lesion, with involvement of the spinous processes of both C-2 and C-3. The cortical shell of the lesion remains intact. (Courtesy of Dr. Harvey White, Children's Memorial Hospital, Chicago, IL)

imaging is of value in the event that conventional radiography fails to demonstrate the tumor.[259]

The most difficult entity in differential diagnosis is a small intracortical abscess, which may present a roentgen appearance identical to that of osteoid osteoma. An arteriogram would show a vascular flush of the nidus correlating with the histological hypervascular stroma in osteoid osteoma, but a necrotic abscess cavity demonstrates no such finding. Enhancement on post-infusion computed tomography is also said to aid in this differentiation. In the event that the nidus is not visible, differentiation from osteosarcoma or Garré's sclerosing osteomyelitis must be made.

BENIGN OSTEOBLASTOMA (GIANT OSTEOID OSTEOMA) (OSTEOBLASTOMA)

Benign osteoblastoma[50,142,153,154,166,226,267] is a rare neoplasm characterized histologically by the presence of osteoblasts and giant cells in a vascular connective tissue stroma. This lesion is similar to osteoid osteoma in microscopic appearance and in age incidence, but differs in size, location, and roentgen appearance.

Clinically, the peak age incidence is between 7 and 20 years, with a reported range of 5 to 78 years. Males are more frequently affected than females. The chief complaint is pain, which is said to be not as severe as in osteoid osteoma. A palpable mass and moderate local tenderness develop. When the spine is involved, neurological symptoms may ensue.

Radiologically, the most common location is in the vertebral arch, chiefly in the transverse and spinous processes (Fig. 7–83), but the bodies may also be affected. About 50% of the cases have vertebral involvement. An osteoblastoma of the atlas has been

TABLE 7–11. Benign Osteoblastoma

Skull	*********	9
Mandible	******************	18
Cerv. spine	*********	9
Dors. spine	***********	11
Lumb. spine	*************	13
Ribs	*****	5
Clavicle	*	0
Scapula	*	1
Sternum	*	0
Humerus	****	4
Radius & Ulna	***	3
Hand & Carpus	****	4
Pelvis	**	2
Sacrum	******	6
Femur	****************	17
Tibia	*************	13
Foot & Tarsus	*****	5
Other	***	3

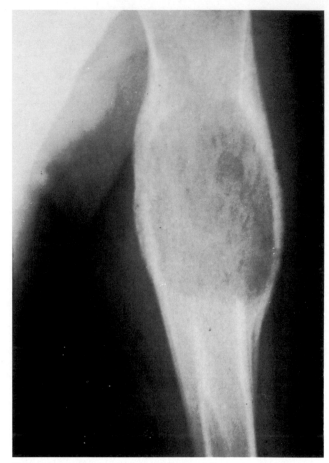

FIG. 7–84. Benign osteoblastoma (humerus). Note expansile lesion with thick cortical shell in the proximal humeral diaphysis. Extensive ossification of the matrix is present. A minimal amount of periosteal new bone formation, which has a laminated appearance, may be seen at the distal aspect of the lesion, forming a buttress. There is no periosteal new bone formation about the periphery of the lesion. (Courtesy of Dr. Harvey White, Children's Memorial Hospital, Chicago, IL)

reported.[88] The tubular bones of the hands and feet, the long bones (especially the femur and tibia), and the calvarium have been described as relatively frequent sites of involvement. The scapula, ribs, sacrum, carpals, tarsals, patella, maxilla, mandible, and pelvis may occasionally be sites of tumor. The relative distribution of benign osteoblastoma is presented in Table 7–11.[166]

In the tubular bones, the lesions are eccentrically located in the metaphysis or shaft. The epiphysis is not involved. The characteristic roentgen feature is an expansile bone lesion that is well outlined and well circumscribed (Fig. 7–84). There may be cortical breakthrough to form a soft-tissue component. The entire lesion may be surrounded by a fine calcific margin. The tumor matrix shows a variable amount of calcification and may be radiolucent, contain small spotty calcific areas, or be radiopaque, particularly following radiation therapy. The size of the tumor ranges from 2 to 12 cm, and rapid growth is possible. Pathological fracture may occur. There may be dense surrounding reactive bone sclerosis as seen in osteoid osteoma. Periosteal new bone formation may be present, and rarely may be exuberant.

In the spine, the neural arch is most commonly involved, followed by involvement of the arch and the body. The body alone is rarely involved. Two adjacent vertebrae have been reported as being involved. The tumor presents as an expansile amorphous or densely calcified mass with a diameter up to 10 cm. The margin is usually well defined, but may be poorly defined. Rarely, a cuboid bone may

be involved, with reactive sclerosis and periosteal new bone formation, which would be difficult to differentiate from an osteosarcoma. Malignant degeneration has only been reported in very few cases.[226]

In the differential diagnosis, the chief consideration is the ossifying character of the lesion. Expansion of bone with a thin marginal calcific shell and the usual lack of periosteal new bone formation would help to differentiate most lesions from an osteosarcoma. The lesion does not have the dense reactive sclerosis commonly seen in an intracortical osteoid osteoma, and the "nidus" is much larger. Differentiation from cartilaginous tumors can be made from the lack of clumps of amorphous calcification, usually seen in the latter. Differentiation from giant-cell tumor can be made by ossification of the matrix and the fact that the epiphysis is usually not involved.

OSTEOCHONDROMA (SOLITARY)

A solitary osteochondroma or *osteocartilaginous exostosis* is a projection of bone with a cartilage cap, originating from a bone preformed in cartilage, usually from the metaphysis of a tubular bone. This is the most common benign growth involving the skeleton. The mechanism of formation is thought to be similar to that seen in hereditary multiple exostoses; however, instead of a constantly present inherited abnormality, solitary osteochondroma represents a sporadic accident.

Not all exostoses are formed in the manner of solitary osteochondromas, nor represent this condition. Several different mechanisms are involved. A *supracondylar process*[57] is a small exostotic spur projected medially and distally at the distal humerus 5 to 7 cm above the medial epicondyle, and is joined to it by a band of fibrous tissue. It (Fig. 7–85) is an atavism to species of apes. It may also be associated with Cornelia de Lange syndrome. The median nerve and the brachial artery or its branches pass through the formed arch. A fracture of the spur may result in median nerve compression.[182] A *subungual exostosis*[72] is a painful spur under a fingernail or toenail (Fig. 7–86). Similar bone protrusions originate as a small focus of myositis ossifications and later blend with the cortex (Fig 7–87). An exostosis may follow irradiation[176] or trauma (Fig. 7–88). The conditions associated with these findings are listed in Chapter 5.

Microscopically, the osteochondroma is a miniature model of the epiphyseal region, except for lack of the ossification center. There is a cartilaginous cap representing the epiphysis, and a metaphysis. The cortex blends with the cortex of the parent bone, and the periosteum extends over the base to cover the exostosis. Enchondral ossification continues during the active growth period and ceases at maturity. There may be zones of cellularity in the cartilaginous cap.

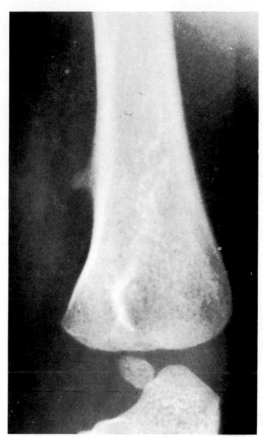

FIG. 7–85. Supracondylar process of the distal humerus. A narrow-necked, bony process may be seen projecting medially and distally. The cortex does not blend with this anomaly.

Clinically, the majority of patients are in the second decade of life at the time of discovery of the lesion, although childhood involvement is not uncommon. The most frequent complaint is a painless mass. Symptoms may be produced by pressure on contiguous vessels and nerves. Trauma may result in a fracture of the pedicle of the lesion. Malignant degeneration to chondrosarcoma is estimated to occur in less than 1% of cases. This transformation most often occurs in later life. Two cases of degeneration to osteosarcoma and one to fibrosarcoma have been reported.[7] Rapid growth of a stable lesion indicates this change. A single case report of spontaneous resolution of an osteochondroma that was of the sessile type in the midhumeral shaft has been published.[27]

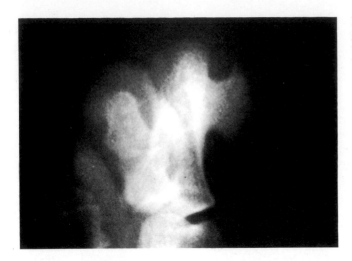

FIG. 7–86. Subungual exostosis (distal phalanx of the great toe). Note bony protrusion at the dorsal aspect of the distal phalanx. The cortex of the toe does not blend with the lesion.

FIG. 7–87

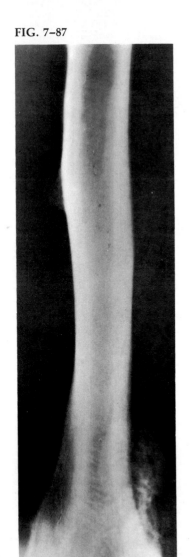

FIG. 7–88

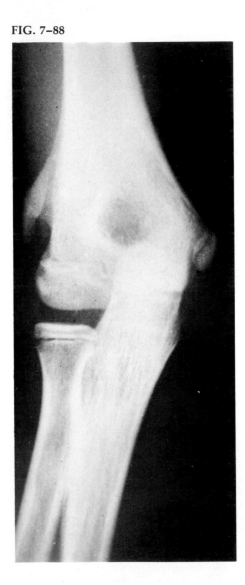

FIG. 7–89

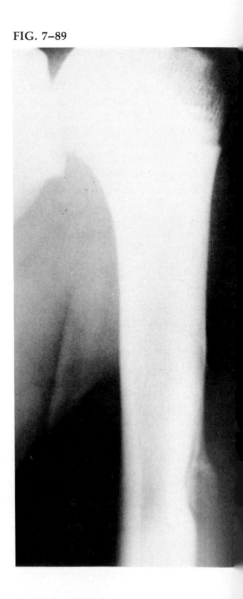

Radiologically, the most common locations are the lower femur and the upper tibia, near the metaphyseal regions. Rarely, they may originate away from the metaphysis (Fig. 7–89). The vast majority of solitary osteochondromas occur in the long bones of the extremities, with more than half in the lower extremities. Any bone preformed in cartilage may be involved. The scapula, pelvis, ribs, vertebrae, and sacrum are less common sites. The computed relative distribution of osteochondroma is presented in Table 7–12.

There are three forms of the lesion: the pedunculated, the sessile, and the calcific. The pedunculated form is an osteocartilaginous cap on a long, narrow base (Fig. 7–90). The sessile form is broad-based without an elongated projection, forming a local widening of the shaft of the bone (Fig. 7–91). The radiological hallmark of both lesions is the blending of the cortex of the exostosis with the cortex of normal bone so as to form a continuity of contour with no cortex interposed between the two. The cap shows irregularity of ossification and the cartilage may calcify when mature, sometimes extensively with an amorphous spotty appearance. Lack of modeling of the shaft, or aclasia, locally occurs. The direction of the pedunculated type is characteristically slanted away from the adjacent joint, owing to muscle pull; hence, the common term "coat hanger exostosis." The lesion may be visualized *en*

TABLE 7–12. Osteochondroma

Skull	*	0
Mandible	*	0
Cerv. spine	*	1
Dors. spine	**	2
Lumb. spine	**	2
Ribs	******	6
Clavicle	*	1
Scapula	**********	10
Sternum	*	0
Humerus	****************************	
Humerus	**********	40
Radius & Ulna	****	4
Hand & Carpus	***	3
Pelvis	***************	15
Sacrum	*	1
Femur	******************************	
Femur	******************************	
Femur	************	72
Tibia	******************************	32
Foot & Tarsus	**	2
Other	*********	9

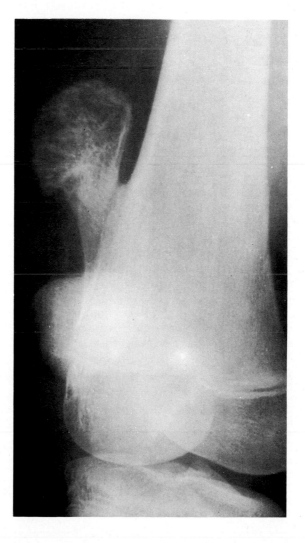

FIG. 7–87. Bony spur in the midhumeral shaft, secondary to myositis ossificans. Myositis ossificans may be seen at the distal humerus. The cortex of the bone does not blend with the spur.

FIG. 7–88. Posttraumatic exostosis (distal humerus).

FIG. 7–89. Osteochondroma of midhumeral shaft.

FIG. 7–90. Solitary osteochondroma (distal femur), pedunculated form. There is a narrow base with blending of the cortex of the parent bone with the lesion. A calcified cartilaginous cap containing several streaks of calcification is visible. The orientation of the lesion is away from the joint, due to muscle pull, hence the term "coat hanger exostosis."

face, in which case a dense ring of cortex surrounding the base is seen superimposed on the cartilage cap (Fig. 7–92). This is not to be confused with an enchondroma.

The common appearance in flat bones is a dense, amorphous, localized area of spotty calcification (Fig. 7–93). The site of attachment to bone may not be apparent. In the pelvis this form may simulate a calcified uterine fibroid, and in the thoracic inlet, thyroid calcification (Fig. 7–94).

Malignant transformation may be inferred if growth resumes in a previously stable lesion. Very extensive calcification may be present in a benign lesion (Fig. 7–95); however, a large associated soft-tissue mass that contains streaky calcification should be regarded as an indicator of malignancy. Invasion and destruction of the osteochondroma is another sign of chondrosarcoma.

HEREDITARY MULTIPLE EXOSTOSES (DIAPHYSEAL ACLASIS)

Hereditary multiple exostoses[255] is an inherited metaphyseal hyperplasia characterized by the presence of multiple osteochondromata. The current pathogenetic explanation combines two older theories, that of Keith and that of Mueller. There are defects in cortical bone formation at the juxta-epiphyseal regions of the periosteal ring, combined with disturbed function of the periosteum in forming small islets of cartilage. These factors permit enchondral bone growth perpendicular to the shaft. The exostoses are similar to those found in solitary osteochondroma.

Clinically, this is not an uncommon condition. The disease very rarely shows clinical manifestations at birth or under the age of 2 years. It is most commonly discovered between the ages of 2 and 10 years. Males are twice as often affected as females. The mode of transmission may be a mendelian dominant. Any affected person can transmit the disease. An unaffected female may be a carrier, but an unaffected male usually does not transmit this disorder. The chief complaint is the discovery of single or multiple hard, painless masses near joints. The lesions form and enlarge only during the growth period. Deformities and dwarfing may occur. The distribution is usually bilateral and may be symmetrical, but there may be a predilection for one side. About one-third of patients show a characteristic "bayonet hand" owing to shortening of the ulna. Shortening of the fingers may also occur, as well as of other long bones. Shortening of the lower extremities results in compensatory scoliosis.

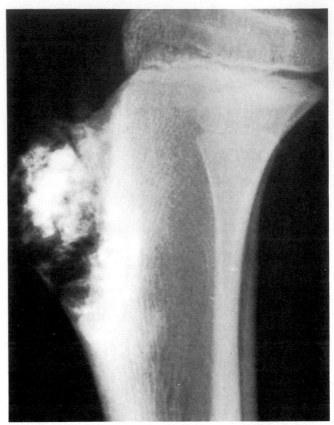

FIG. 7–91. Solitary osteochondroma — sessile type. There is a broad-based exostosis with blending of the cortex of the parent bone with the lesion. Note amorphous stippled calcification characteristic of cartilage.

Eventually the exostoses interfere with joint function. Symptoms from pressure on vessels, nerves, and the spinal cord develop.[269] Bursa form at the cartilaginous margins and may lead to inflammatory changes. Perforation of the popliteal artery with false aneurysm formation in the popliteal fossa has been reported.[115] Perforation of the lung has also been reported.[231]

The most ominous complication is transformation to chondrosarcoma, which may occur in as many as 20% of cases, according to Jaffe.[124]

Radiologically, the individual lesions are similar to those seen in solitary osteochondrodroma, but there is a tendency to form smaller protuberances. They may range in number from a few lesions to a thousand. The exostoses in the long bones are clustered about the metaphyseal region (Fig. 7–96). Epiphyseal exostosis does not represent this entity,

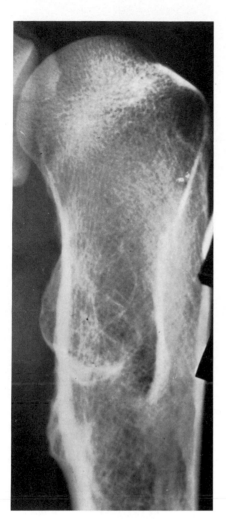

FIG. 7–92. Osteochondroma visualized *en face*. Note lack of modeling of the upper humeral shaft. Rounded density represents the osteochondroma extending perpendicular to the plane of the film.

FIG. 7–93. Osteochondroma (iliac crest), calcific type. An amorpous area of spotty calcification, well circumscribed, may be seen at the iliac crest. The precise site of attachment to the iliac bone cannot be discerned.

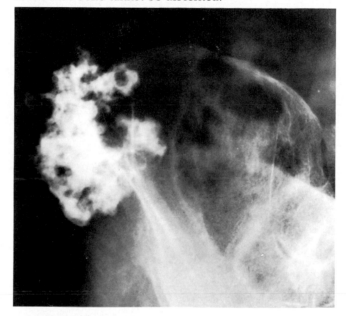

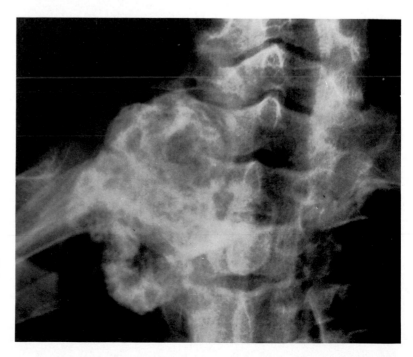

FIG. 7–94. Osteochondroma (thoracic inlet) —calcific type simulating a thyroid calcification. There is no deviation of the trachea.

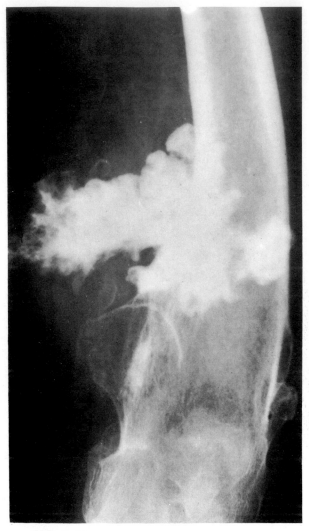

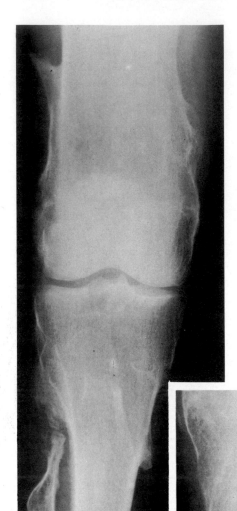

FIG. 7–95

FIG. 7–96

FIG. 7–97

FIG. 7–95. Benign osteochondroma (femur) with very extensive amorphous calcification. The margins are well defined and there is very little streaky calcification. Multiple osteochondromas are present.

FIG. 7–96. Multiple exostoses (knee). Multiple exostotic projections may be seen, directed away from the joint owing to muscle pull. There is lack of modeling of the distal femur and shortening of the fibula. The exostoses are generally smaller than those seen in solitary osteochondromas.

FIG. 7–97. Multiple exostoses (knee). Marked lack of tubulation of both distal femur and proximal tibia, hence the term "diaphyseal aclasis."

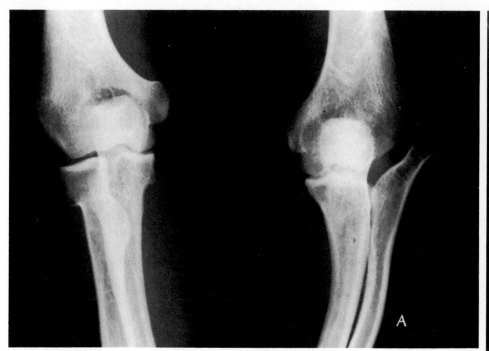
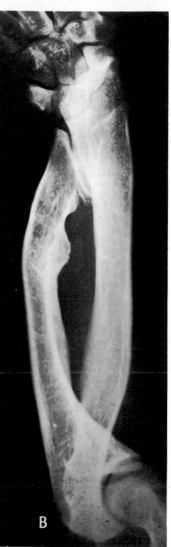

FIG. 7–98. **A.** Multiple exostoses (elbows)—congenital luxation of the head of the left radius, associated with curvature of both radius and ulna. Small exostoses of the right proximal radius and ulna may be seen. Involvement of the elbows is unusual in this condition. **B.** Multiple exostoses (forearm) (same patient). There is shortening of the ulna, with curvature. A false articulation has formed between the radius and the ulna. Also note ulnar deviation of the carpus and posterior curvature of the distal radius.

but rather represents Trevor's disease (Chap. 4). There is interference with the modeling of the shaft, hence the term *diaphyseal aclasis* (Fig. 7–97).

The most common sites of involvement are the long bones, particularly in the lower extremities, where the knees are most severely affected. In the lower extremities, both ends of all bones show lesions, whereas in the upper extremities, the elbow tends to be spared (Fig. 7–98 A). There is a characteristic shortening of the ulna and fibula. Ulnar shortening causes curvature of the radius and a false articulation between the two (Fig. 7–98 B). There may be ulnar deviation of the carpus and subluxation of the radius (Fig. 7–99). This results in a "bayonet hand" deformity.

A large exostosis of a forearm or leg bone may cause pressure erosion or deformity of the adjacent bone (Fig. 7–100). There may be interlocking exostoses (Fig. 7–101) or synostoses of varying lengths in these bones. Occasionally, shortening or deformity of the metacarpals (Fig. 7–102) and phalanges (Fig. 7–103) occurs. Although the base of the skull may be involved, the calvarium and mandible are spared. The scapula is frequently involved with multiple protrusions at the vertebral margin and inferior angle, owing to the presence of epiphysis at these sites (Fig. 7–104). Pelvic lesions are seen at the iliac crest and at the ischiopubic synchondroses. The ribs are most frequently involved at the costochondral junctions (Figs. 7–105, 7–106), and the

(Text continued on p. 586)

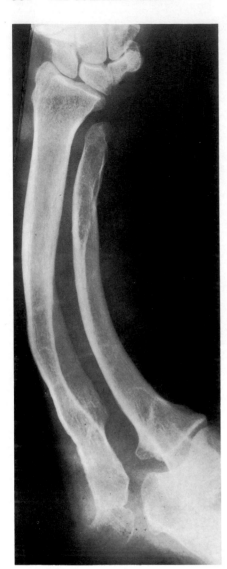

FIG. 7–99. Multiple exostoses. Note curvature of both radius and ulna, shortened ulna, and congenital dislocation of the head of the radius. Two small exostoses at the proximal ulna and a small exostosis at the distal humerus are also visible.

FIG. 7–100. Osteochondroma (distal tibia), causing pressure erosion of the distal fibula and deformity.

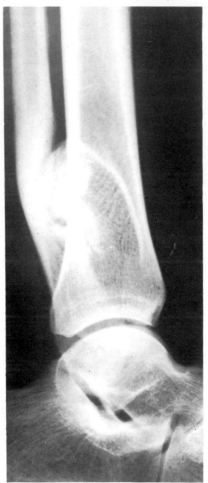

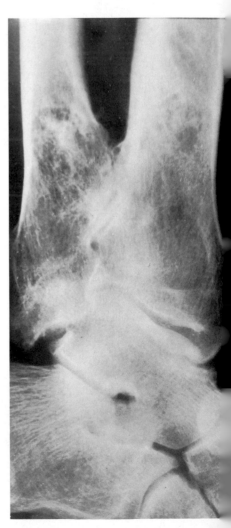

FIG. 7–101. Multiple osteochondromatosis with interlocking exostoses of the distal tibia and fibula.

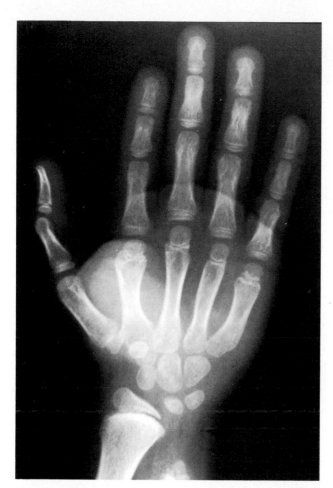

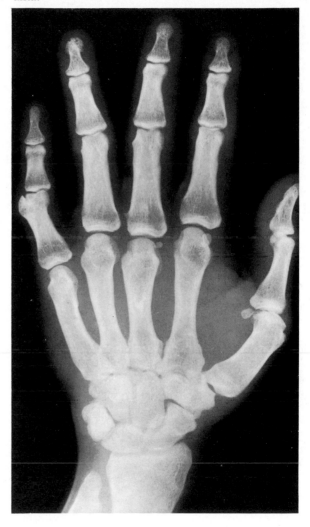

FIG. 7–102. Multiple exostoses (hand). Note shortening of the second metacarpal and of the ulna, and curvature of the radius.

FIG. 7–103. Multiple exostoses (hand). Note exostosis at the distal fifth proximal phalanx, causing shortening and deformity, and shortening of the ulna.

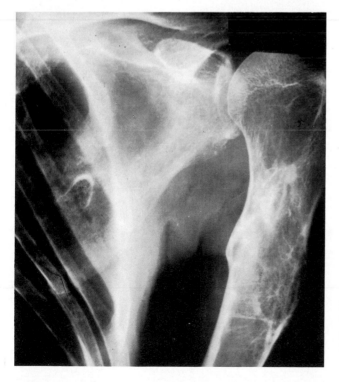

FIG. 7–104. Multiple exostoses. Note exostosis near the vertebral margin of the scapula, seen as a ringlike density *en face*. Exostoses of the humeral shaft are also apparent.

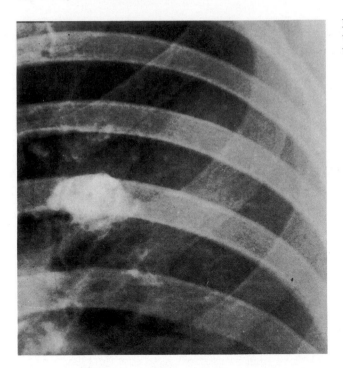

FIG. 7–105. Multiple exostoses (ribs). A calcific osteochrondroma of the third anterior rib may be seen, attached by a pedicle to the costochondral region.

FIG. 7–106. Multiple exostoses. Note deformities of several ribs due to a large osteochondroma with an area of calcification, and an osteochondroma involving the axillary margin of the scapula.

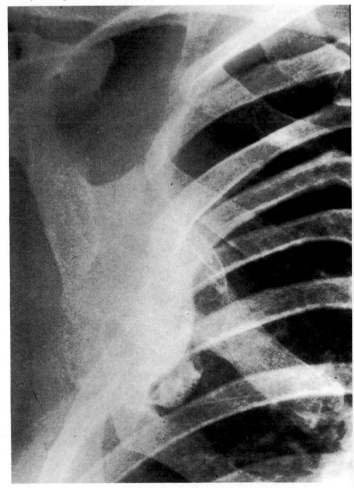

sternum and clavicles are not immune. The vertebrae are rarely involved and are most likely to show lesions near the tips of the spinous processes. The os calcis may be involved, but other cuboid bones are usually spared. A bursa occasionally forms about an exostosis, and this may rarely contain calcific loose bodies. In the event of sarcomatous degeneration, the roentgen appearance is similar to the same process in solitary exostosis. Osteochondromatosis and enchondromatosis do not coexist.

SOLITARY (EN)CHONDROMA

A *solitary enchondroma* is a benign cartilaginous tumor situated in the medullary cavity of a bone. It is thought to originate from a cartilage rest displaced from the physis. Enchondromas may be single or multiple.

Microscopically, the cellularity varies. A lesion of multiple enchondromatosis is more cellular than a solitary enchondroma. The cellularity does not approach that of a chondrosarcoma, although differentiation can be difficult at times. The cartilage cells are regularly small and uninuclear. The major tissue is mature hyaline cartilage. The malignant potential of these tumors increases the closer the lesion is to the axial skeleton.

Clinically, the entity is one of the most common benign tumors of bone. The age incidence is distributed from the second to the fifth decades. Males and females are equally affected. When the short tubular bones are involved, the lesions are usually asymptomatic and discovered either as incidental findings or when pathological fracture occurs. An occasional expansile lesion may cause visible swelling; slight pain may at times be present.

When a long bone is involved, pain of recent onset or pathological fracture may be the presenting complaint.

Radiologically, in 50% of patients with enchondroma, the short tubular bones of the hand are affected. This is the most common tumor of the bones of the hand. Any bone preformed in cartilage may be involved, and the humerus, femur, toes, metatarsals, tibia, fibula, and ulna are not uncommon sites. Rarely, the ribs (Fig. 7–107), sternum, pelvis, patella,[145] carpal bones,[263] and vertebrae may be affected. The relative distribution of enchondromas is presented in Table 7–13.[46] The site of origin in a tubular bone is usually in the metaphysis, extending down the shaft, or into the epiphysis after fusion of the growth plate. The lesion usually involves the distal and mid aspects of the metacarpals (Fig. 7–108) and the proximal aspects of the phalanges (Fig. 7–109). Prior to epiphyseal closure, the epiphysis is not involved. Initially, the lesion is off-axis but grows to a central location. The size varies from a small round or ovoid lesion in the short bones to extensive involvement of the shaft of a long bone. The lesions may attain to enormous size — up to 11.5 kg has been reported.[190] These tumors are then termed *giant chondromas,* and have been reported in the ribs, upper jaw, and patella. They may remain benign in spite of their size, although huge chondrosarcomas of the ribs have been reported. Occasionally, there may be subperiosteal origin (see Juxtacortical Chondroma).

The lesion may begin as a well-marginated radiolucency (Fig. 7–110), or it may be seen as an expansile, well-demarcated lesion with a thin cortical margin, or with a thickened cortex with endosteal scalloping. A subperiosteal chondroma shows external cortical erosion and an expanded shell of periosteal new bone surrounding the outer margin of the lesion. There is no cortical breakthrough or periostitis. The appearance of the matrix varies from radiolucent with a few flecks of calcification to extensive amorphous or spotty calcification (Fig. 7–111). At times, an enchondroma may present merely as a dense intramedullary collection of stippled calcifications without a radiolucent component or

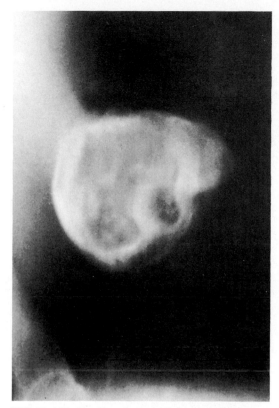

FIG. 7–107. Enchondroma of the anterior rib— tomogram. An expansile anterior rib lesion is visible, containing multiple flecks of amorphous calcification and having a dense sclerotic margin.

TABLE 7–13. Enchondroma

Skull	*	0
Mandible	*	0
Cerv. spine	**	2
Dors. spine	**	2
Lumb. spine	*	1
Ribs	****	4
Clavicle	*	0
Scapula	**	2
Sternum	*	1
Humerus	******************	18
Radius & Ulna	***	3
Hand & Carpus	******************************	
Hand & Carpus	**************************	56
Pelvis	***	3
Sacrum	*	1
Femur	***************************	27
Tibia	**	2
Foot & Tarsus	*********	9
Other	*****	5

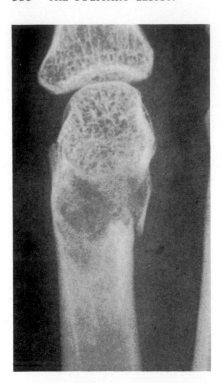

FIG. 7–108. Enchondroma of the distal fifth metacarpal. Note radiolucent area with minimal calcific densities at the outer aspect. A pathological fracture has occurred through the lesion. The end of the bone is not involved.

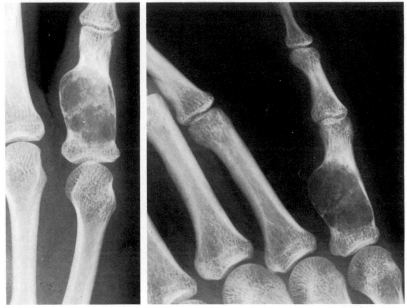

FIG. 7–109. Enchondroma involving the proximal and midaspects of the proximal fifth phalanx. The end of the bone is not involved. There is an expansile lesion with a thin but intact cortex. Several amorphous flecks and streaks of calcification are present.

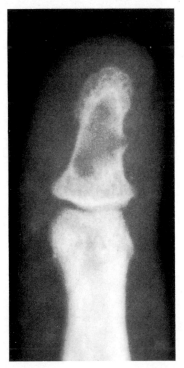

FIG. 7–110. Enchondroma (distal phalanx). Note well-marginated radiolucency with no calcific matrix. A pathological fracture at the margin has occurred.

FIG. 7–111. Enchondroma (first metacarpal). An expansile lesion at the base of the first metacarpal is visible, containing several dense, amorphous areas of calcification. The lesion extends to the proximal end of the bone.

without cortical changes (Fig. 7–112). The lesion must then be differentiated from a medullary bone infarct, which has a characteristic dense limiting outer margin and a serpiginous distribution of calcifications, neither of which occurs in enchondroma. Rarely, a completely radiolucent appearance is present, in which case a roentgen diagnosis of the presence of cartilage may be inferred from other features but cannot be established. In an extensive tumor of a long bone it may not be possible to radiologically differentiate a benign enchondroma from a chondrosarcoma. Malignant transformation to a secondary central chondrosarcoma may occur.[105, 212]

An *epidermoid inclusion cyst* of a distal phalanx may cause confusion with an enchondroma, but the lack of stippled calcification and a history of penetrating trauma would clarify the diagnosis (Fig. 7–113).

JUXTACORTICAL CHONDROMA

A *juxtacortical chondroma*[29, 213] is a rare benign cartilaginous tumor that develops in relation to the periosteum or parosteal connective tissue. Jaffe includes a periosteal chondroma in this classification.[124] It usually presents as a solitary lesion, but occasionally may be multiple. The age and sex incidence is similar to that seen in enchondroma. The usual clinical complaint is a small, firm, painless mass.

Radiologically, the lesion consists of a soft-tissue mass adjacent to the cortex of a tubular bone. It has been reported at the anterior tibial tubercle.[138] It is rarely larger than 4 cm in diameter. Uncommonly, there may be only a soft-tissue mass, in which case a radiological diagnosis cannot be established. The mass usually contains amorphous spotty calcifications to indicate its cartilaginous nature (Fig. 7–114), or is outlined by a thin calcific rim. The cortex

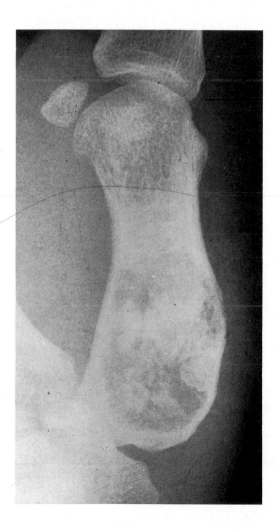

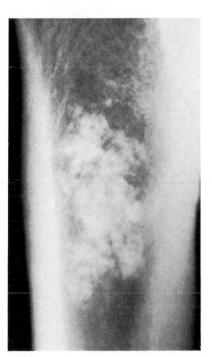

FIG. 7–112. Enchondroma. Note dense, amorphous, intramedullary calcifications localized to a limited region. There is neither radiolucency nor an expansile lesion. Minimal endosteal scalloping is present. No limiting outer margin may be seen, and the calcifications do not show a serpiginous pattern.

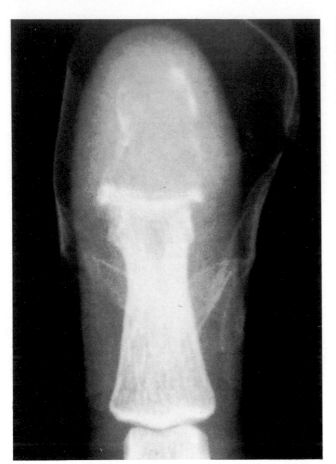

FIG. 7–113. Epidermoid inclusion cyst of the distal phalanx. An expansile lesion involving the entire distal phalanx may be seen, with loss of cortex at the terminal tuft and along the margins. There is no calcification within the lesion. In considering differential diagnosis, loss of cortical definition would be an unusual finding in an enchondroma.

FIG. 7–114. Juxtacortical chondroma. **A.** There is a 2-cm ovoid soft-tissue mass at the anterior aspect of the tibia, which contains amorphous spotty calcifications. Pressure erosion of the anterior tibial cortex has occurred. **B.** Nine-month interval film following surgery for removal of juxtacortical chondroma. Cortical thickening at the site of erosion has occurred, progressing toward a normal contour.

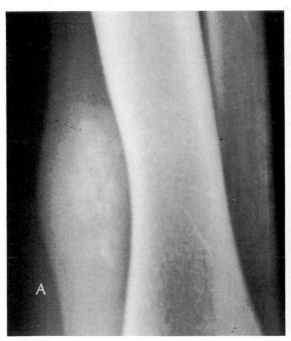

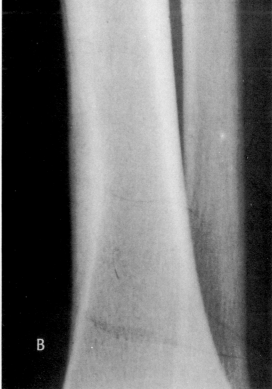

adjacent to the mass shows pressure erosion, which may be shallow or deep. Reactive cortical sclerosis can be present, and a buttress of periosteal new bone at the margins is sometimes visible. There is no invasion of the medulla. A periosteal desmoid or neurofibroma can cause difficulty in differential diagnosis. The characteristic spotty calcification serves to exclude most other entities. Synovioma should also be considered.

BENIGN CHONDROBLASTOMA (CODMAN'S TUMOR)

Benign chondroblastoma[165,183,199,225,258] is a tumor of bone developing from cells that may be chondroblasts. This represents a separate entity with distinct roentgen and microscopic appearances. The tumor is generally considered to be benign; however, Geschickter and Copeland[41] claim that a malignant chondroblastoma not uncommonly exists, and that the ratio of chondroblastomas is two benign to three malignant. This view does not appear to be widely accepted.

Microscopically, the basic cells are moderately sized polyhedral cells with little intercellular connective tissue. Focal areas of calcification of stroma and necrotic cells are present. Giant cells are also seen.

Clinically, this entity represents an uncommon primary tumor of bone. The peak age distribution is between 10 and 25 years, with a reported range between 8 and 59 years. The chief complaint is pain referred to a joint. Tenderness, swelling, limitation of joint motion, weakness, numbness, muscle atrophy, and local heat may also occur. Symptoms are said to be of shorter duration in younger patients. The tumor may be quiescent for many years and then begin to enlarge.[282]

Radiologically, this tumor in the long bones characteristically involves the epiphysis. It has its origin in the epiphyseal cartilage plate and extends into the epiphysis, and may involve the adjacent metaphysis with lesser involvement (Fig. 7–115). Rarely, it may be confined to the metaphysis,[76] abutting the epiphyseal plate. The sites of most frequent involvement according to Jaffe[124] are, in descending order of frequency: lower femur, upper tibia, upper humerus, lower tibia, upper femur (including head and greater trochanter), calcaneus,[144] astragalus, ilium, and ischium. It has also been reported in the patella,[36] finger,[181] rib, scapula, proximal fibula, distal radius, and more unusual locations including the manubrium, capitate, metatarsal, vertebra, mandibular condyle, calvarium, and mastoid.

Fifty percent of all cases have involvement about the knee joint. In the proximal humerus and femur,

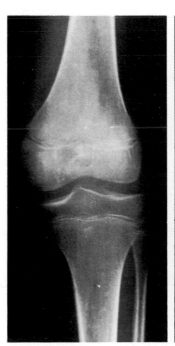
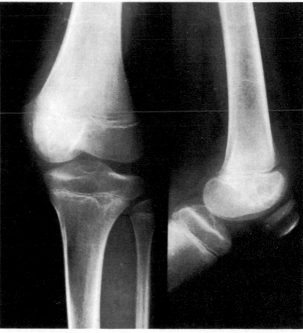

FIG. 7–115. Benign chondroblastoma (distal femoral epiphysis). Note radiolucent areas in the epiphyseal ossification center with a fine sclerotic margin and several stippled calcifications. (Courtesy of Dr. Heriberto Garcia, Chicago, IL)

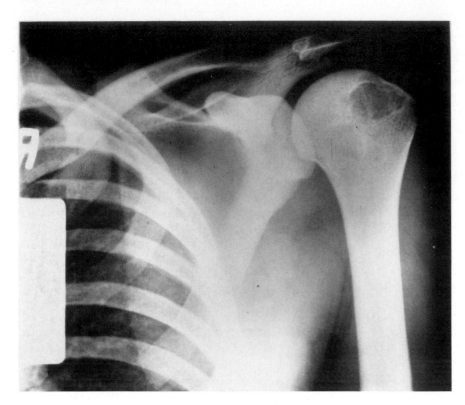

FIG. 7–116. Benign chondroblastoma. Radiolucent area in the outer aspect of the proximal humeral epiphysis is noted with a thin, sharp, sclerotic margin and containing light trabeculae.

the lesion has a tendency to develop at the greater tuberosity and the greater trochanter, respectively. Ninety percent of lesions are found in the medulla and 10% in the cortex.

Characteristically, the presenting appearance is a well-demarcated oval or round radiolucency (Fig. 7–116). The size is usually between 3 and 6 cm, but a size of 8 by 19 cm has been reported. There may be eccentric expansion of the cortex and periosteal reaction is not unknown. Rarely, a ballooned cortex may be seen. A thin, sharply demarcated sclerotic bony margin is usually present, separating the lesion from adjacent normal bone. The metaphyseal portion of the tumor may not show this sclerotic rim. At times surrounding reactive bone sclerosis of nonuniform distribution and at a slight distance from the tumor is present. A scalloped margin may also be seen. A fuzzy margin does not exclude this lesion. Cortical destruction and an associated soft-tissue mass may rarely be seen, and destruction of the articular cortex has been reported.

In a minority of cases there is a varying amount of amorphous spotty calcification to identify the lesion as being of cartilaginous origin. This has been described as a "fluffy cotton wool appearance." Rarely, light trabeculation as seen in giant-cell tumor may be present. Pathologic fracture is rare. An associated synovitis of the adjacent joint may occur.

Any flat bone preformed in cartilage may also be involved. The characteristic finding is an expanding lesion with the features described previously.

The most difficult entity in the differential diagnosis of benign chondroblastoma in the long bones is giant-cell tumor, because both lesions are commonly located in the epiphysis. The lack of matrix calcification and lack of sharp margination, the greater radiolucency, larger average size, light trabeculation, and older age group all serve to distinguish giant-cell tumor from benign chondroblastoma. A lesion in the femoral head must be distinguished from ischemic necrosis, which has a more angular configuration.[93] Malignant chondroblastomas of bone have been reported.[164] These may represent a variant of chondrosarcoma.

CHONDROMYXOID FIBROMA

Chondromyxoid fibroma[52,77,177,268,276] is an uncommon benign bone neoplasm that originates from cartilage-forming connective tissue, characterized by chondroid tissue and an intercellular mucinlike substance. Histologically, the lesion is apt to be mistaken for a chondrosarcoma. Jaffe[123] states that "there is an almost paradoxical incongruity between its ominous cytologic appearance and its generally benign clinical course."

Clinically, the peak age incidence is in the second and third decades of life, with a reported range of between 5 and 79 years. Males are more often affected than females. The chief complaint is pain, usually of several months' duration. Swelling may be present at times. Pathological fracture is rare.

Radiologically, about 50% of cases have tibial involvement. The next most frequent sites are the femur, pelvis, humerus, fibula, calcaneus, metatarsals and tarsals, ribs, and phalanges. Vertebral, radial, ulnar, mastoid, and scapular involvement have also been reported. The tibial tuberosity is not infrequently affected.

In the tubular bones, the origin of the lesion is most often metaphyseal. It may extend into the epiphysis, but the epiphysis alone is not involved. Epiphyseal extension rarely may occur prior to closure of the growth plate. A small or large portion of the epiphysis may be involved.

The characteristic appearance is an ovoid, eccentric, radiolucent lesion that causes cortical expansion. In a narrow bone, the lesion may involve the full width of the shaft. A cortical origin may also rarely be seen without medullary involvement (Fig. 7–117).

The size of the lesion is usually about 3 cm, but it may reach the size of 10 cm in its long axis. There is expansion of the cortex, and the limiting periosteal shell may be thick, thin, or not visible. The latter finding should not be interpreted as cortical destruction. No elevated periosteal new bone formation is visible. The inner margin of the lesion may be thin, dense bone or thickened, sclerotic bone on the medullary side. Scalloping of the margin is usually present. Cortical thickening may be seen at a short distance beyond the lesion. Stippled calcification—so common in chondroblastoma—is very rarely seen in this lesion. The matrix density may range from radiolucent to a heavily trabeculated appearance caused by scalloped margins. Pathological fracture may rarely occur. Satellite defects rarely may be seen in a recurrent lesion. A chondromyxoid fibroma in the femoral neck with a dense rim of sclerosis has been reported.

In the short tubular bones, the lesion typically presents as a centrally located, expansile, radiolucent lesion. In the flat and cuboid (Fig. 7–118) bones, a noncharacteristic expansile lesion is seen.

In a long bone, the differential diagnosis takes into consideration benign-appearing, expansile, radiolucent or trabeculated metaphyseal lesions, which occur in a younger individual. This list should include unicameral bone cyst, aneurysmal bone cyst, and nonossifying fibroma. A unicameral bone cyst is centrally located, only under the most unusual of circumstances involves the epiphysis, and ordinarily does not expand the contour of the bone beyond the width of the epiphyseal plate. An aneurysmal bone cyst has a typical "soap bubble" appearance, wide cortical expansion, and an ill-defined medullary margin. A nonossifying fibroma is a small eccentric lesion in the shaft that does not have a great tendency to expansion as does chondromyxoid fibroma. Periosteal elevation in an aggressive form of this tumor has been reported. Rare cases of recurrence of tumor as chondrosarcoma have been reported.

NONOSSIFYING FIBROMA (NONOSTEOGENIC FIBROMA)

A *nonossifying fibroma* is a benign lesion of bone derived from fibrous tissue. It is thought to result from proliferative activity of a fibrous cortical defect.

Microscopically, whorled bundles of spindle-shaped connective-tissue cells are seen. Cytoplasmic hemosiderin granules are present. Large nests of lipid-containing foam cells may also be present. There is no new bone formation.

Clinically, the age incidence is between 8 and 20 years in the majority of cases, in contrast to a fibrous cortical defect, which usually has spontaneously regressed in this age group. Some patients may complain of local pain, but many lesions are discovered as incidental findings. The lesion may regress spontaneously. Malignant change has not been reported.

Radiologically, the most common sites are the long bones of the lower extremities, although the upper extremities and short bones may also be affected. Characteristically, nonossifying fibromas are situated several centimeters shaftward from the metaphysis. The epiphysis is not involved. The lesion is usually off-axis, developing in the cortex (Fig. 7–119); however, a large tumor may extend entirely across the shaft.

The typical lesion is represented by an ovoid radiolucency that varies in size from 2 to 7 cm in its long axis. The margins are scalloped and there may be a multilocular appearance (Fig. 7–120). The cortex is thinned and expanded (Fig. 7–121). The med-

(Text continued on p. 596)

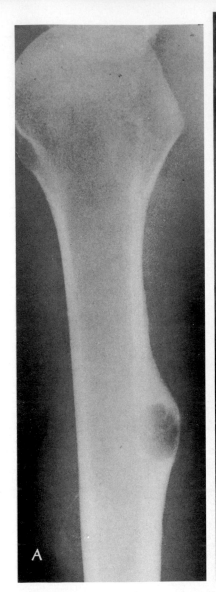
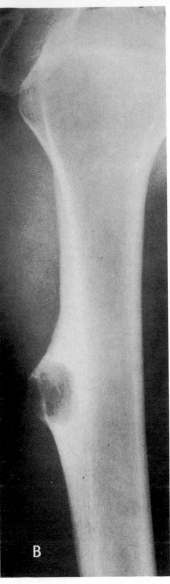

FIG. 7–117. Chondromyxoid fibroma (proximal humeral shaft). **A.** There is an ovoid, radiolucent, expansile lesion that originated in the cortex and has ballooned out the outer cortical margin without involving the endosteum. Cortical thickening, extending a small distance on either side of the lesion, is also visible. The lesion is very lightly trabeculated but contains no calcific stippling. There is no periosteal new bone formation. **B.** Same lesion, showing loss of cortical definition of the outer margin of the lesion; this is caused by lack of visibility rather than destruction and breakthrough. Light trabeculation without stippled amorphous calcification may again be noted.

FIG. 7–118. **A, B.** Chondromyxoid fibroma of the talus. An expansile, lightly trabeculated lesion with a sharp sclerotic margin is seen.

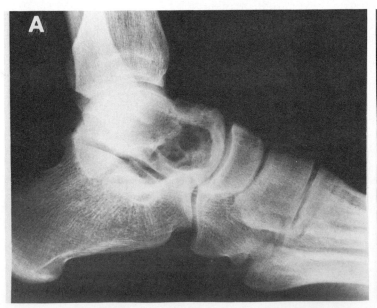
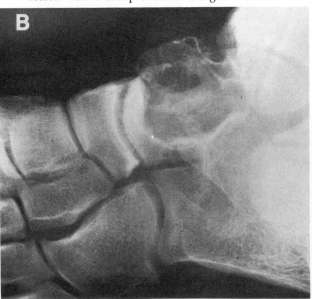

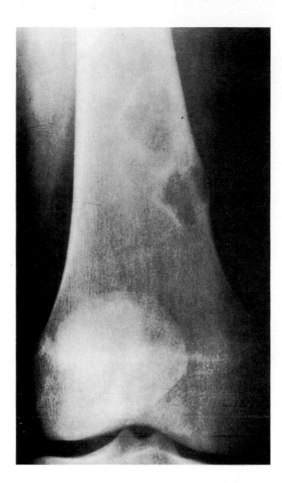

FIG. 7–119. Nonossifying fibroma (femur). Note multilocular lesion measuring 6 cm in its long axis, situated off-center and bulging the cortex. Sclerotic bone reaction at the medial margins is present. There is no calcification of the matrix.

FIG. 7–120. Nonossifying fibroma (humerus) involving the entire diameter of the shaft of the bone, 2 cm below the metaphysis and measuring 4 cm in its long axis. Note scalloped margins, multilocular appearance, and endosteal scalloping. There is no true cortical expansion.

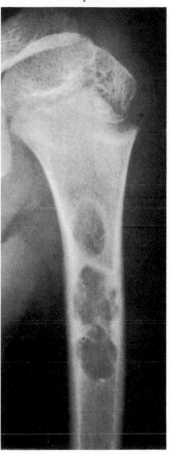

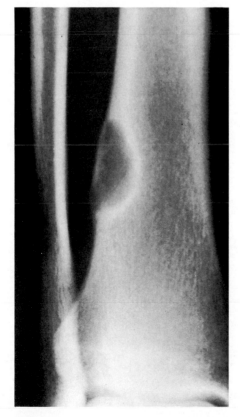

FIG. 7–121. Nonossifying fibroma. Note cortical origin with thinning and expansion of the cortex, and sclerosis of the endosteal margin. There is no calcification of the matrix. The lesion is 5 cm proximal to the metaphysis.

ullary margin has a dense, sclerotic appearance (Fig. 7–122). The long axis of the lesion is parallel to the axis of the bone. Periosteal new bone formation is not a feature. Pathological fractures may occur (Fig. 7–123). These tumors may coexist with several fibrous cortical defects or, rarely, they may be multiple.

DESMOPLASTIC FIBROMA OF BONE

Desmoplastic fibroma[37,257] of bone is a very rare benign fibrous tumor characterized by the presence of collagen fibers and small fibroblasts, with no new bone formation. Less than 20 cases in total have been reported to date. The age range is from 8 to 40 years. Local pain and swelling are common complaints.

Radiologically, the tibia appears to be a common site of involvement. The humerus, femur, and other long bones, as well as the scapula, vertebra, os calcis and mandible, have been involved. It has been reported as an expansile trabeculated lesion in the pubis.[257] The lesion is most likely to be located near the metaphysis, although it may uncommonly extend into the epiphysis (Fig. 7–124). The majority of lesions are central, although an eccentric position occurs in about one-third of cases. Tibial tubercle involvement has been reported.

The characteristic finding is a large radiolucent area, usually well demarcated. Jaffe, however, describes a case with an ill-defined patchy area of radiolucency with slight cortical expansion.[124] The lesion may be trabeculated or present as a radiolucency with a sclerotic margin. Little reactive bone formation is present. Expansion of bone is a feature in both central and eccentric lesions. The matrix does not calcify.

The differential diagnosis is difficult. Fibrosarcoma, unicameral bone cyst, and chondromyxoid fibroma may show similar roentgen appearances, and histological study is necessary for diagnosis.

PERIOSTEAL DESMOID

A *periosteal desmoid*[20,32,135] is a rare fibrous lesion associated with the periosteum. Microscopically, adult fibroblasts and intercellular collagen are characteristically present. Osteoclastic activity associated with bone erosion may also be seen. The reported age range is from 8 to 20 years.

Radiologically, the site is not uncommonly the distal femur and may be metaphyseal. The lesion originates subperiosteally and causes destruction of

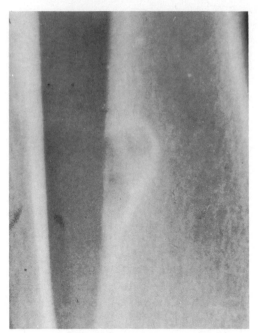

FIG. 7–122. Small nonossifying fibroma. Cortical origin is apparent. There is thinning of the cortex without expansion. Relatively dense sclerosis of the medullary margin is present.

the outer margin of the cortex. The inner margin of the lesion is usually sharply delimited. A slight amount of periosteal new bone formation is usually present (Fig. 7–125). An associated soft-tissue mass may also be seen.

An awareness of this entity, although it is rare, is of importance in order to avoid confusion with a malignant tumor.

Normal irregularity of the surface of the distal medial tibial metaphysis is not to be confused with the above conditions.[12]

FIBROUS CORTICAL DEFECT

Fibrous cortical defect[202,230] is a small metaphyseal focus of cellular fibrous tissue that erodes the cortex. The origin of the fibrous tissue is the local periosteum. A large percentage of normal children show one or more of these lesions, and the most frequent age incidence is between 4 and 8 years. They are rarely seen under 2 years of age. Spontaneous regression is the rule. Males are more often involved than females. The lesions are asymptomatic.

Radiologically, the most common location is the posterior medial aspect of the distal femoral metaphysis. The proximal tibia and the fibula are other common sites, and other tubular bones may be involved. The defects are extremely rarely found in the epiphysis (Fig. 7–126), but occur in the shaft. The typical appearance is a small round, ovoid, or flame-shaped radiolucency seen as a shallow cortical defect (Fig. 7–127). The size averages from 1 to 2 cm (Fig. 7–128). The long axis of the lesion is parallel to the axis of the bone. The margins are well defined, and may appear as a smooth or scalloped, thin, dense line. There is an appearance of lobulation in some cases. Slight bulging of the cortex may be seen in tangential views.

Occasionally, localized loss of cortex may be seen. Jaffe claims that a periosteal desmoid corresponds to a fibrous cortical defect in which collagenized connective tissue is conspicuous.[124] Upon healing, the lesions may regress to a normal appearance or persist as a sclerotic focus.

UNICAMERAL BONE CYST

A *unicameral bone cyst*[35, 157] is a true fluid-filled cyst with a wall of fibrous tissue. The mode of origin and development is subject to debate. Jaffe[124] divides these lesions into two groups, the active and the latent. Active cysts are located immediately

(Text continued on p. 600)

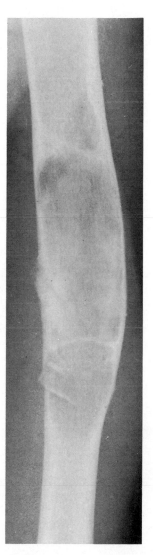

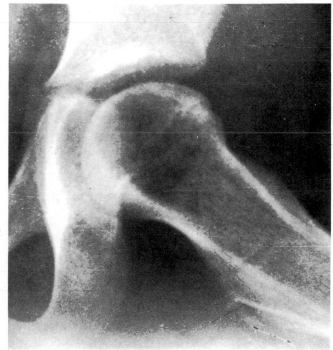

FIG. 7–123. Large nonossifying fibroma of the midshaft of the humerus with pathological fracture. Thinning and expansion of the cortex to a mild degree may be noted. There is no calcification of the matrix. Differential diagnosis from a unicameral bone cyst would be difficult.

FIG. 7–124. Desmoplastic fibroma. Note well-defined area of radiolucency in the femoral head and neck, crossing the epiphyseal cartilage plate. There is no calcification of the matrix or expansion of bone. (Courtesy of Dr. Harvey White, Children's Memorial Hospital, Chicago, IL)

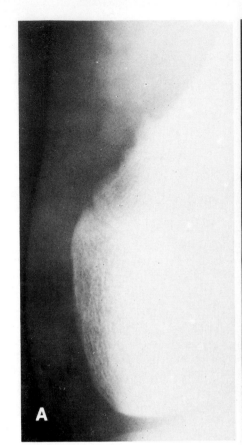
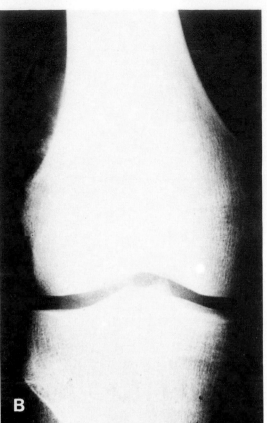

FIG. 7–125

FIG. 7–126

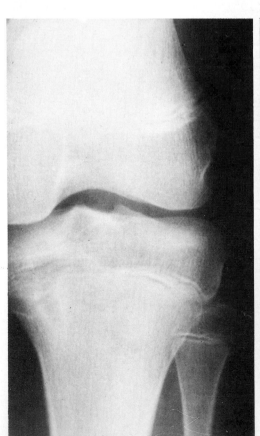
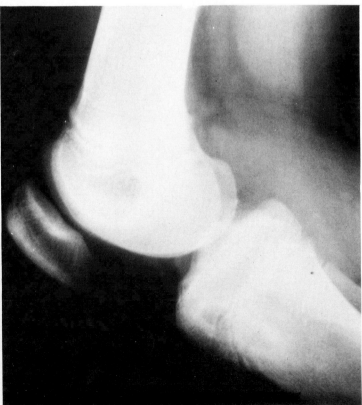

FIG. 7–125. A. Periosteal desmoid (distal femur). Bony irregularity with a thick, squat appearance is seen. **B.** Osteosarcoma in similar location for comparison. Filiform spiculated periosteal new bone formation is seen.

FIG. 7–126. Fibrous cortical defect (proximal tibia)—anteroposterior and lateral views. A portion of the lesion extends into the epiphysis.

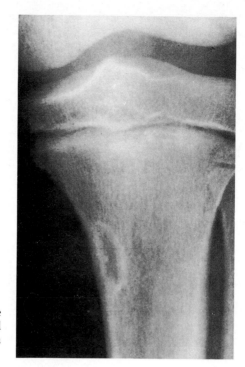

FIG. 7–127. Fibrous cortical defect (proximal tibia). Note small, ovoid-shaped radiolucency involving the medial cortex, with a thin, dense margin. There is no calcification of the matrix.

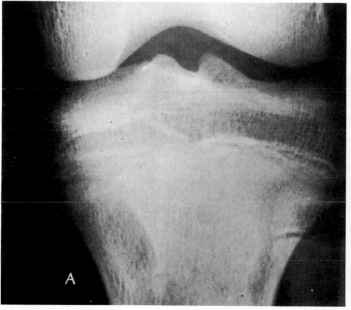
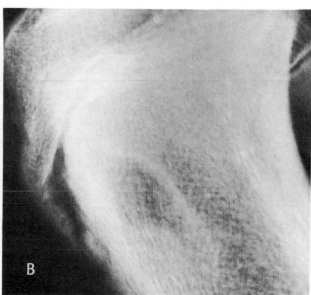

FIG. 7–128. Fibrous cortical defect (proximal tibia). **A.** Note ovoid radiolucency at the proximal tibial metaphysis, which appears slightly medially situated because of projection. The medial margin shows a thin, dense line; the outer aspect shows no such demarcation. **B.** Lateral view. The lesion measures 2 cm and seems to be in the anterior tibial cortex. The posterior margin shows a thin, dense line.

adjacent to the epiphyseal cartilage plate and retain growth potential, while latent cysts are displaced away from the growth plate by normal bone and remain as a static bone defect. However, active bone cysts in the shaft have also been described.[184] Both types may recur after surgical excision.

Microscopically, the lining is composed of fibrous and vascular tissue. Osteoid and osseous tissue are formed by metaplasia. Osteoclasts and multinuclear giant cells may also be present. Ridging of the wall may be seen, but the cavity is not divided into compartments. The fluid is clear and yellowish. If there has been a recent fracture, the fluid may be bloody.

Clinically, the age incidence in 80% of cases is between 3 and 14 years, with rare cases reported as early as 2 months and over 50 years. Males are twice as often affected as females. This represents a common lesion of bone. An active cyst grows until the time of epiphyseal fusion. The lesion is asymptomatic until pathologic fracture occurs. Spontaneous regression with reconstruction of bone to a normal appearance is said to occur very rarely, if at all.

The age of the patient has great importance in the presentation and clinical behavior of these cysts.[184] Bone cysts behave more aggressively in childhood, and the recurrence rate is 4 times greater than in the adolescent. The highest incidence of pathological fractures is under 10 years of age.

Radiologically, the proximal humerus and proximal femur are the most common sites, in contrast to most tumors that have a predilection for the knee. Seventy-five percent of bone cysts are found in the femur and humerus. The tibia, fibula, ribs, ilium, radius, ulna, phalanges,[73] and calcaneus[249] (Fig. 7–129) are other reported locations. Two cysts occurring simultaneously in the same patient have been reported.[221] In patients over 17 years of age the distribution changes. It shifts from the proximal humerus and femur to a preponderance in the pelvis and calcaneus.

The origin of the lesion is in the metaphysis. It may be immediately adjacent to the epiphyseal cartilage plate or may have migrated a considerable distance down the shaft. (More correctly, the epiphysis has migrated away from the cyst (Fig. 7–130).) Very rarely, it may extend into the base of the epiphyseal ossification center[120] (Fig. 7–131). The lesion is most often centrally located, although an off-axis position is not unknown.

The typical appearance is a fairly large radiolucent lesion that is broad at the metaphyseal end and narrower at the shaft end. The long axis is greater than the diameter to give the form of a truncated cone (Fig. 7–132). The presence of the cyst interferes

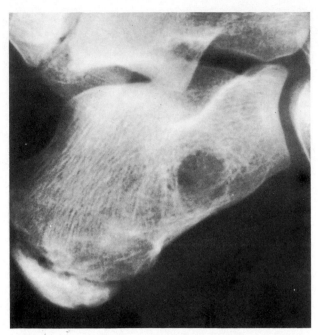

FIG. 7–129. Unicameral bone cyst (calcaneus). Note rounded area of radiolucency without expansion of bone. A radiolucent area in the calcaneus may also be seen as a normal variant. This is the typical location of a calcaneal cyst, abutting the inferior margin.

with normal modeling of the bone. The expanded cortex rarely exceeds the diameter of the epiphyseal plate, but it may do so (Fig. 7–133). At a later stage, normal bone may be interposed between the cyst and the epiphysis, and the lesion may even be located in the midshaft. An important differential point from tumors is that the cyst never penetrates the cortex to extend into the soft tissues. The lesion is sharply demarcated from normal bone, and a trabeculated appearance may be present owing to ridges and scalloping of the cortical margin. The thickness of the sclerotic rim varies. No periosteal elevated new bone formation is present, but may rarely occur after pathological fracture (Figs. 7–134, 7–135). In the event of a pathological fracture with a detached fragment, the fluid content of the cyst permits falling of the bony fragment to the most dependent portion, thus definitively differentiating a cyst from a solid tumor. This is known as the "fallen fragment sign."[208] The radiolucent lesional area usually shows no calcification. Rarely, calcification or ossification within the cyst may be seen owing to changes in old fibrin coagula.[223]

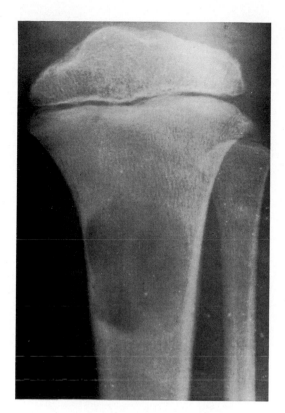

FIG. 7–130. Unicameral bone cyst. Note area of radiolucency somewhat removed from the metaphysis in the proximal tibial shaft. There is no calcification of matrix. Thinning of the cortex on the medial side is also visible.

FIG. 7–131. Unicameral bone cyst. **A.** An expansile lesion at the proximal humeral metaphysis may be noted, with light trabeculation and thinning of the cortex. The lesion has crossed the unfused epiphyseal cartilage plate and involves the epiphyseal ossification center, a very unusual finding in a unicameral bone cyst. **B.** Fourteen-month interval film following surgery. Typical roentgen appearance of postsurgical bone cyst in the proximal humerus may be seen, separated approximately 1 cm from the cartilage plate. There is a truncated appearance with lack of tubulation of the proximal humeral shaft. The epiphyseal ossification center is residually involved.

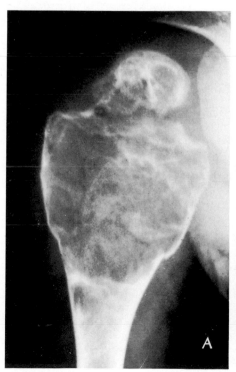

A

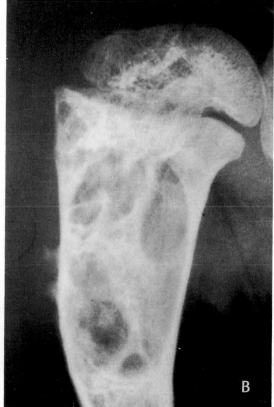

B

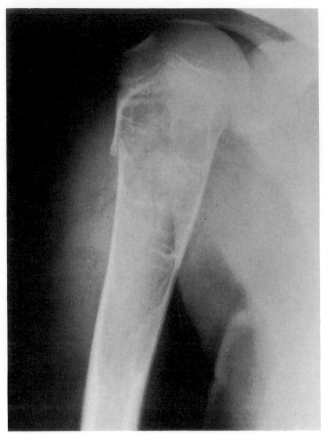

FIG. 7–132. Unicameral bone cyst (proximal humerus) — typical appearance. There is an elongated, truncated, radiolucent lesion which shows light trabeculation abutting the metaphysis but not extending into the epiphyseal ossification center. The normal modeling of bone is interfered with, but the lesion has not expanded beyond the width of the growth plate. A pathological fracture has occurred at the outer upper surface.

The differential diagnosis includes an aneurysmal bone cyst, which is eccentric and has a "blowout" cortical distension. Giant-cell tumor and benign chondroblastoma have a typical epiphyseal location. Enchondroma would be differentiated by the presence of calcific stippling. Chondromyxoid fibroma is more eccentric in location and causes more cortical expansion. Localized fibrous dysplasia may show a "ground glass" density or be heavily trabeculated with a "soap bubble" appearance (Fig. 7–136). Intrasacral cysts due to defective meningeal development also occur.

ANEURYSMAL BONE CYST

An *aneurysmal bone cyst*[17,28,47,246,274] is the only bone lesion in current terminology that derives its name from its roentgen appearance rather than from its histology. It is a bone lesion characterized by a "blown-out" cortical appearance. The name is a misnomer since it is histologically neither an

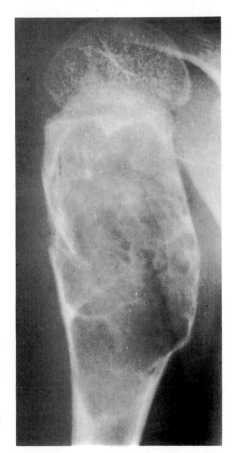

FIG. 7–133. Unicameral bone cyst. Note elongated, radiolucent, expansile lesion at the proximal humerus abutting the metaphysis. There is expansion of bone slightly beyond the width of the metaphysis, an unusual finding.

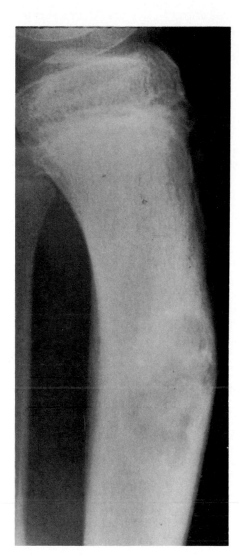

FIG. 7–134. Unicameral bone cyst. An area of radiolucency several centimeters removed from the metaphysis of the proximal tibia may be seen, causing endosteal scalloping. Note periosteal new bone formation at the posterior and anterior aspects. This is an unusual finding.

FIG. 7–135. Unicameral bone cyst (upper humerus). **A.** Pathological fracture. **B.** Healed stage, showing periosteal new bone and callus formation.

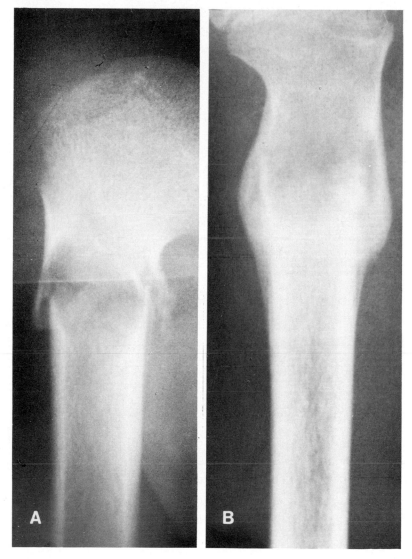

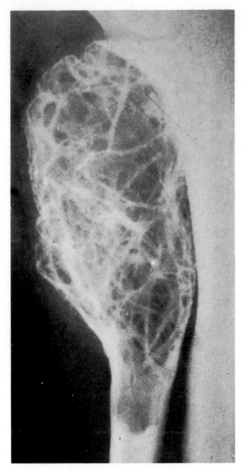

FIG. 7–136. Solitary lesion of fibrous dysplasia. There is marked expansion of the proximal radius involving the end of the bone, with very heavy trabeculation and a "soap bubble" appearance. This appearance is not consistent with a unicameral bone cyst.

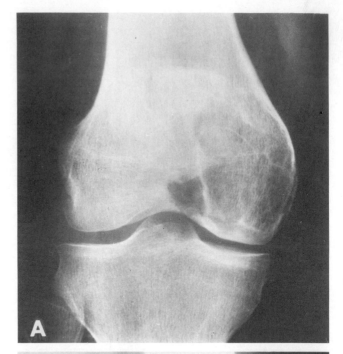

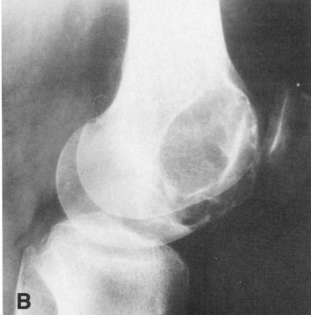

FIG. 7–137. A, B. Anteroposterior and lateral views (aneurysmal bone cyst). An expansile, lightly trabeculated lesion which does not quite extend down to the subarticular cortex is noted. It has a thin, sclerotic, sharply defined margin. **C.** Tomograph of the distal femoral metaphysis showing details of a rounded, expansile, marginated lesion.

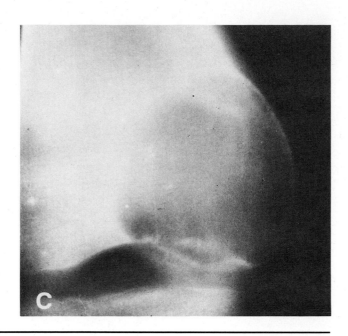

aneurysm nor a cyst. There are two types: a primary, which occurs without an associated lesion; and a secondary, which occurs in association with a bone tumor. The relationship of the two is unknown. The radiological appearance of a secondary aneurysmal bone cyst is most often that of the associated bone lesion. The bone lesions occurring with an aneurysmal bone cyst are in order of frequency:[17]

Giant-cell tumor
Osteosarcoma
Solitary bone cyst
Nonossifying fibroma
Fibrous dysplasia
Metastatic carcinoma
Chondromyxoid fibroma
Hemangioendothelioma
Osteoblastoma

Approximately two-thirds of aneurysmal bone cysts are primary, and one-third are secondary.

Microscopically, it contains interconnecting blood-filled cavernous spaces separated by fibrous septa that may show thin bone formation. The blood spaces may have an endothelial lining, and numerous multinuclear giant cells may be present. It is a nonneoplastic tumorlike lesion.

Clinically, the age distribution is in older children, adolescents, and young adults. The chief complaint is mild local pain of several months' duration. Swelling may also be present. Pain and im-

pairment of function of a contiguous joint result. When a vertebra is involved, pathological fracture often occurs with ensuing neurological symptomatology. Females are more often affected than males.

Radiologically, the most common sites of involvement are the long bones, most often the femur (Fig. 7–137). The lesion may be found in any segment of the spine in the bodies, arch, or processes.[108] In 75% of the cases, the cysts are in the long bones and spine. Any other bone may be involved, including the flat bones, (Fig. 7–138), ribs, calvarium,[23] orbit,[187] small bones, and zygoma. Multiple aneurysmal bone cysts in a 3-month-old infant have been reported.[119]

The relative distribution of aneurysmal bone cysts is given in Table 7–14.

In the tubular bones, the lesion is usually metaphyseal but may extend into the epiphysis after fusion of the ossification center (Fig. 7–139). Rarely, the lesion may encroach upon an adjacent joint. The characteristic appearance is an eccentric radiolucency that causes a marked ballooning of a thinned cortex. Light trabeculation within the lesion and elevated periosteal new bone formation near the margins of the lesion, with a periosteal buttress, are seen. The long axis of the expanded area is parallel to the axis of the bone and may reach up to 8 cm. The thin outer cortical shell may not be visible. The inner aspect of the lesion may or may not have a thin sclerotic margin. Edeiken *et al*[71] claim that there are two types of aneurysmal bone cysts: intraosseous, which originates within the

TABLE 7–14. Aneurysmal Bone Cyst

Skull	********	8
Mandible	*	1
Cerv. spine	*********	9
Dors. spine	*********	9
Lumb. spine	****	4
Ribs	***	3
Clavicle	***	3
Scapula	****	4
Sternum	*	0
Humerus	*****	5
Radius & Ulna	********	8
Hand & Carpus	****	4
Pelvis	**************	14
Sacrum	*****	5
Femur	********************	20
Tibia	*********************	21
Foot & Tarsus	*****	5
Other	***********	11

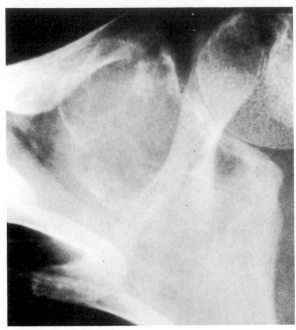

FIG. 7–138. Aneurysmal bone cyst of the scapula. There is ballooning of the body of the scapula and the coracoid process, with marked expansion of bone and thinning of the cortex. The matrix is not calcified, but light trabeculation is visible.

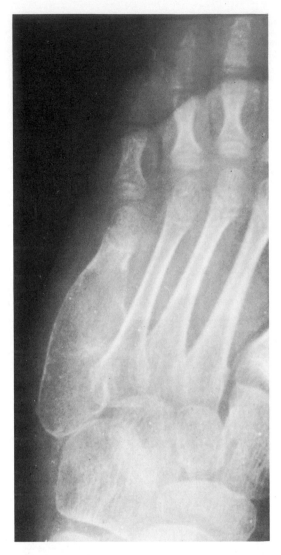

FIG. 7–139. Aneurysmal bone cyst (foot). Note expansile lesion in the fifth metatarsal with involvement of the proximal end and the major portion of the shaft. There is considerable ballooning of the cortex, but the cortical shell is intact. No periosteal new bone formation may be seen. This represents the intraosseous type of aneurysmal bone cyst. (Courtesy of Dr. Harvey White, Children's Memorial Hospital, Chicago, IL)

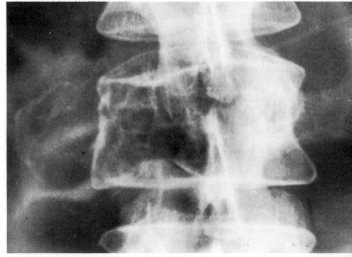

FIG. 7–140. Unbiopsied vertebral lesion. There is a radiolucent lesion in the right half of the third lumbar vertebral body, with light trabeculation. No new bone formation is present. Note expansion of the transverse process. This lesion has the radiographic appearance of an aneurysmal bone cyst. Giant-cell tumor should be considered in the differential diagnosis, as well as myeloma.

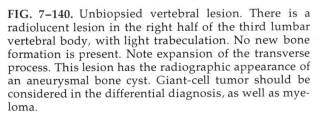

bone and balloons the cortex; and extraosseous, which begins as a soft-tissue tumor and erodes the external surface of bone. An early lytic phase has been described, which is superseded later by a mature-cystlike appearance. Pathological fractures may occur.

Vertebral involvement presents as an expanding trabeculated lesion that may attain large size. The body, arch, transverse, and spinous processes are affected alone or in combination (Fig. 7–140). Trabeculation may be absent. Collapse of the body sometimes occurs. The lesion may extend along the spine and several adjacent vertebrae may be destroyed. In the flat bones, a large expansile lesion with cortical margins may be seen (Fig. 7–141). Rib lesions may present as a large intrathoracic mass,[112] and pelvic lesions may present as an intra-abdominal or pelvic mass. In the calvarium, the most frequent site is the occipital bone.

DIFFERENTIAL DIAGNOSIS OF BENIGN CONDITIONS OF BONE

In considering the differential diagnosis between benign and malignant solitary lesions, undue emphasis should not be placed on any particular roentgen sign. Indeed, any of the radiological features that we associate with malignancy may be found in a benign condition. For example, dense bone production of equal radiopacity may be found in osteosarcoma, osteoid osteoma, or Charcot's joint; spiculated or laminated periosteal response may be found in neoplastic and inflammatory conditions; bone destruction is a feature of both malignant and benign neoplasms; and cortical breakthrough may also occur in benign tumors.

One must rather, by careful analysis of all features and clinical data, decide which specific clinicopathologic entity best fits the lesion in question. If this cannot be done, then at least the possibilities of identity must be separated from the improbable diagnoses in order to permit the pathologist to come to a meaningful conclusion.

Tumors in certain locations may defy roentgen diagnosis. This is particularly true in the pelvis. Solitary lesions are very difficult if not impossible to diagnose radiologically, if they present in an atypical location or have an atypical form.

The benign tumors and tumorlike conditions that have a distinctive appearance and are common enough to consider in a differential diagnosis are:

COMMON

> Osteoid osteoma
> Localized fibrous dysplasia
> Enchondroma
> Unicameral bone cyst
> Nonossifying fibroma

UNCOMMON

> Giant-cell tumor
> Benign chondroblastoma
> Aneurysmal bone cyst

RARE

> Benign osteoblastoma
> Chondromyxoid fibroma

The age distribution of these benign lesions is most frequent in late childhood and adolescence, with the exception of giant-cell tumor, which occurs in the 20- to 40-year group; enchondroma, which is evenly distributed in the 10- to 50-year range; and unicameral bone cyst, which has its greatest frequency between 3 and 14 years. Benign bone tumors in elderly patients are rare. The roentgen appearance of a fibrous cortical defect is diagnostic.

FIG. 7–141. Aneurysmal bone cyst (pelvis). An expansile trabeculated lesion involving the ilium, ischium, and pubis is present. (Courtesy of Dr. Harold Rosenbaum, Lexington, KY)

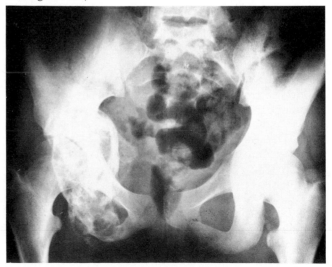

The sites of most frequent involvement for most of these lesions are the long bones, particularly in the vicinity of the knee joint. A unicameral cyst does not tend to involve the knee. Enchondroma and benign osteoblastoma also have a predilection for the short tubular bones of the hands. The spine is most commonly involved by an aneurysmal bone cyst or a benign osteoblastoma, which tends to involve the arch. Giant-cell tumor in the spine is uncommon.

In the long bones, the location may be epiphyseal, metaphyseal, or diaphyseal, and the central or eccentric position should also be considered. Most lesions are in the metaphysis when first seen, except giant-cell tumor and benign chondroblastoma, which almost always involve the epiphysis. Aneurysmal bone cysts may involve the epiphysis after fusion of the growth plate. Many metaphyseal lesions apparently migrate down the shaft. A nonossifying fibroma typically lies somewhat removed from the metaphysis.

The lesion that is most characterized by an eccentric location is an aneurysmal bone cyst. A nonossifying fibroma, chondromyxoid fibroma, and osteoid osteoma have typical eccentric locations. A giant-cell tumor also usually has an off-axis location. The lesion that is typically centrally situated is a unicameral bone cyst.

The size and shape of the lesion are also important considerations. Lesions that often attain large size are aneurysmal bone cyst, unicameral bone cyst, fibrous dysplasia, and chondromyxoid fibroma. Lesions that are typically small when seen are fibrous cortical defect, osteoid osteoma, and enchondroma in the tubular bones.

Most of the above lesions are ovoid, with the long axis parallel to the long axis of the bone. Giant-cell tumor and the nidus of osteoid osteoma are typically round. A unicameral bone cyst has the shape of a truncated pyramid with the wide base at the epiphyseal end. This lesion usually does not expand the cortex beyond the width of the epiphyseal cartilage plate. All of the above lesions, even an osteoid osteoma (subperiosteal type) expand the cortex. The most prominent expansion is found in aneurysmal bone cyst, which widely balloons out the cortex.

The margins of benign tumors and tumorlike processes are characteristically well-defined. Tumors of the cartilaginous series are likely to show dense marginal sclerosis, which may extend to a distance from the lesion. There may also be cortical thickening. The most pronounced reactive sclerosis is caused by intracortical osteoid osteoma, which

may be eccentrically located with respect to the sclerosis. The sclerosis may be severe enough to obscure the nidus. Sclerotic residua are seen in the healed stages of fibrous cortical defect and brown tumor of hyperparathyroidism. Dense sclerosis following radiation therapy for benign osteoblastoma frequently occurs.

The matrix of the tumor in enchondroma and in about 50% of the cases of benign chondroblastoma show a characteristic stippled punctate calcification, indicating the presence of cartilage. Fibrous dysplasia may show similar findings if cartilage is present, or may show a "ground glass" density if microosseous trabeculae are uniformly dispersed throughout the tissue.

Most of the other tumors are radiolucent and may show light trabeculation. Lesions that show characteristic heavy trabeculation are fibrous dysplasia, nonossifying fibroma, and chondromyxoid fibroma.

Periosteal reaction is sparse in benign tumorous lesions, even in the presence of a pathological fracture. Aneurysmal bone cyst may show solid periosteal elevation at the nonexpanded cortex near the margin of the lesion, with a periosteal buttress. Spiculated or laminated periosteal new bone formation is not seen, except possibly in subperiosteal desmoid.

In summary, a benign appearance is a combination of a well-demarcated radiolucent lesion, possibly with trabeculation or calcification, expansion of the cortex, and no periosteal reaction. This, however, is a fair description also of a solitary myeloma, "blowout" metastasis from kidney or thyroid carcinoma, fibrosarcoma, and secondary chondrosarcoma within an enchondroma prior to breakthrough. It is for this reason that any atypical or suspect malignant lesion should be biopsied in order for a definitive roentgen diagnosis of a benign lesion to be established, the specific criteria of a definite clinicopathological entity should be fulfilled.

MISCELLANEOUS, RARE, AND NONDESCRIPT BONE LESIONS

Adamantinoma of the limb bones[15, 65] *(angioblastoma)* is a rare tumor of unknown cell origin, in which the histological pattern resembles that of ameloblastoma of the jawbones. It may recur and metastasize. It is most often seen in the tibia. Adolescents and young adults tend to be affected. The typical roentgen picture is a large, loculated, expansile, radiolucent mass in the cortex of the midshaft of the tibia. It may also occur at the ends, and be of central location (Fig. 7–142). Spontaneous pneumothorax has been described as the presenting feature of metastases of adamantinoma of the tibia.[281] *Hemangiomas*[133,240,244] may occur in the long bones, but are rare in this location. When they occur, the ends of the bone are most often involved with an expansile, delicately loculated, radiolucent lesion (Fig. 7–143). A "sunburst" periosteal effect may be present, and is typical in the flat bones, particularly in the calvarium (Fig. 7–144). The vertebrae are the most common osseous location for this lesion, and have a typical appearance. *Lymphangioma* of bone

may occur.[21,143] A *glomus tumor*[264] may rarely involve bone. The most common site is the distal aspect of the terminal phalanx of a finger. Radiologically, a central circumscribed radiolucency is present in an intraosseous lesion that resembles an enchondroma. The lesion is painful, however. A subungual glomus tumor may cause pressure erosion at the same sites. *Angiosarcomas*, including hemangiosarcoma, hemangioendothelioma[22,253,260] (Fig. 7–145), hemangiopericytoma, and lymphangiosarcoma may cause solitary or multiple destructive skeletal lesions. The roentgen picture shows no distinctive features. An *arteriovenous aneurysm* may cause pressure erosion of bone, sometimes associated with local bone overgrowth. *Ossifying fibroma*

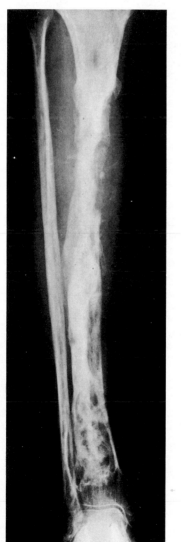

FIG. 7–142. Adamantinoma of the tibia. There is extensive involvement of the entire shaft of the tibia, with a multilocular expansile appearance at the distal aspect and a destructive appearance with periosteal new bone formation at the proximal aspect. Reactive sclerosis is also visible in the midshaft.

FIG. 7–143. Hemangioma of the fifth metacarpal. **A.** Unusual dense sclerotic cortical thickening. **B.** Arteriogram of hemangioma showing hypervascularity.

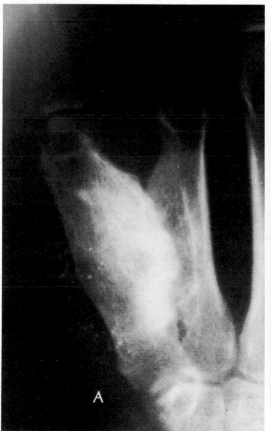

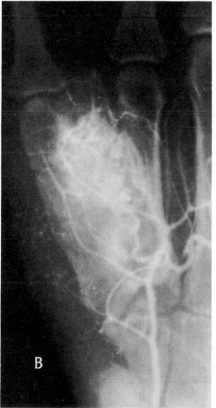

of the skull, face, and mandible[233] is a distinct lesion that is seen radiologically as a smooth roundish or expansile mass. A paranasal sinus may be expanded (Fig. 7–146). There may be reactive bone sclerosis or calcification of the tumor matrix (Fig. 7–147).

Lipoma of bone[106] is a rare tumor that may occur in the skull, ribs, or extremities. The older age groups may be affected by this tumor. Radiologically, there is an expansile lesion with a thinned cortex or there may be cortical breakthrough with a soft-tissue component. The radiolucency of fat, if visible, indicates the diagnosis. Multiple lipomas may occur in hyperlipoproteinemia.[85] Liposarcoma of bone[207,232] is a very rare malignant tumor that may show extensive destruction of both medulla and cortex in the involved area. The most common site of involvement is the tibia. Neurilemmoma[4] (Schwannoma) may rarely involve the medullary cavity of a bone. Radiologically, it is seen as a circumscribed or multilocular radiolucency with a thin sclerotic margin. It may originate subperiosteally, eroding the outer aspect of the cortex. Neurofibroma (see Chap. 5) may involve bone, either as a solitary lesion or with widespread changes. Hodgkin's disease not uncommonly involves bone. There may be destructive or productive changes. An "ivory" sclerotic vertebral body is sometimes seen, with ero-

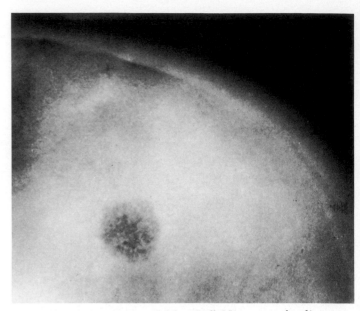

FIG. 7–144. Hemangioma of the skull. Note area of radiolucency showing small punctate stippling.

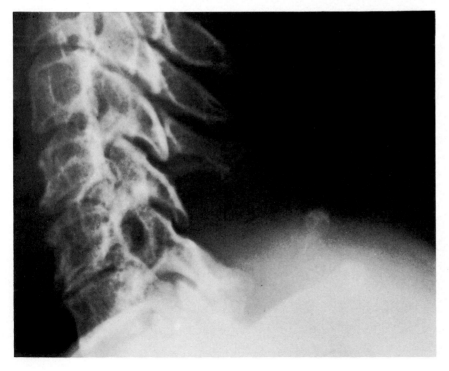

FIG. 7–145. Hemangioendothelioma of the cervical spine. Note destruction of the spinous processes of the sixth and seventh cervical vertebrae, with soft-tissue involvement. A phlebolith is present posteriorly.

FIG. 7–146. Ossifying fibroma. There is haziness of the right maxillary antrum with expansion of the superior and lateral margins.

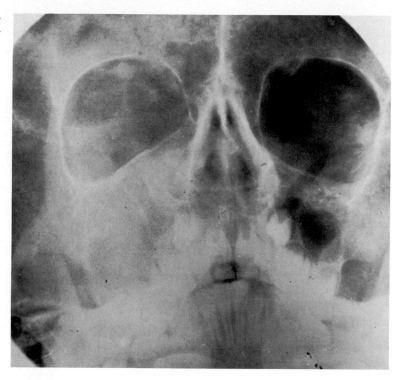

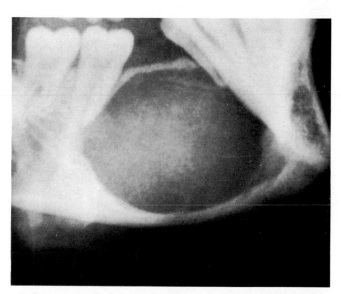

FIG. 7–147. Ossifying fibroma of the mandible. Note smooth, well-marginated, expansile lesion in the body of the mandible. Several small flecks of calcification are present within the tumor, and there is a fine, diffuse, calcific distribution.

sion of the anterior margin by an enlarged lymph node. *Pseudoplasma-cell myeloma*[2] *(plasma-cell granuloma)* is a very rare condition of bone characterized by the presence of large masses of plasma cells with a mingling of other cells. It is thought to represent a granuloma. There have been insufficient reports to formulate a typical roentgen picture; however, widespread sclerotic lesions may be present. An *anterior meningocele* may be present as a pelvic mass with deformity and erosion of the sacrum (Fig. 7–148). *Sacrococcygeal teratomas*[228] are usually benign, calcified lesions evident in the neonate. Rarely, they may be malignant. They may be extrapelvic or intrapelvic. Associated abnormalities of the spine are infrequent. The calcifications may be in any form, even representing skeletal parts.

An *epidermoid inclusion cyst*[113,151] not infrequently involves the terminal phalanx, with a well-circumscribed radiolucent lesion showing a thin cortical margin that may not be visible in its entirety (Fig. 7–113). A history of penetrating trauma is often elicited. *March fractures* or *fatigue fractures*[45,152] may first present roentgenologically as periosteal new bone formation (Fig. 7–149), and later as callus formation (Fig. 7–150). A light, irregular, linear sclerosis may traverse the diameter of the bone at the fracture site. The areas most frequently

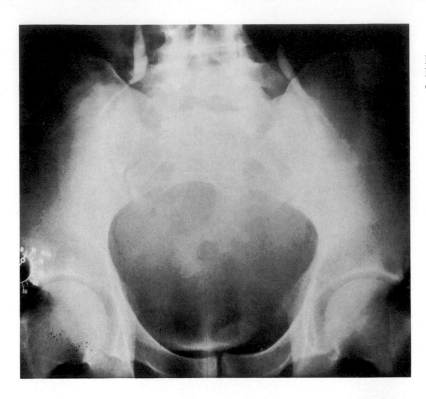

FIG. 7–148. Anterior meningocele. Note large pelvic mass and deformity and erosion of the sacrum. (Courtesy of Dr. D. Christou)

FIG. 7–149. Stress fracture (second metatarsal) — early stage. Only a slight amount of periosteal new bone formation may be noted.

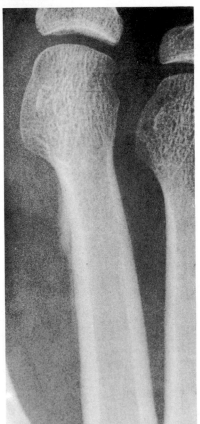

involved are the calcaneus, metatarsals, tibia, and femoral neck. Multiple stress fractures have been reported as occurring in rheumatoid arthritis.[167] Stress fractures of the ribs, usually the seventh, eighth, or ninth, but also of the first, may occur. *Thorn, and twig-induced granulomas,*[277] owing to a foreign body, produce mixed, lytic, or sclerotic lesions. An area of bone destruction with cortical thickening and periosteal reaction, sometimes laminated, may be seen. A wooden splinter-induced pseudotumor of bone has also been described.[261] An *atrophic Charcot joint*, particularly in the proximal humerus, causes para-articular bone resorption and destruction, soft-tissue swelling, and bony debris. *Posttraumatic osteolysis* is a cause of para-articular bone resorption, particularly in the distal clavicle, distal radius, and proximal humerus (Fig. 7–151). *Fibromyxoma*[24,116] of bone is a rare lesion that shows a radiolucent lesion that shows a radiolucent area with a sclerotic margin and possible calcification. *Myxofibrosarcoma*[136] has also been described. It is in the spectrum of fibrosarcoma.[46] *Intraosseous ganglion*[43,78,201,236] is a rare cause of an osteolytic lesion in bone. A well-defined radiolucency with a sclerotic margin adjacent to the articular surface is seen (Fig. 7–152). It may be in other locations. The tibia and femoral head and neck are most often involved. The lesions range in size from 2 mm to 7 cm. *Posttraumatic cysts*[265] also

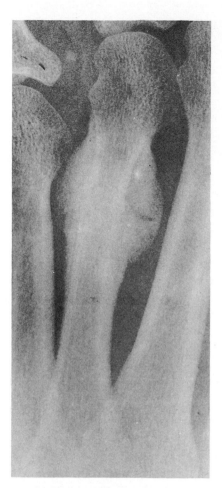

FIG. 7–150. Stress fracture (third metatarsal). Note callus formation at the fracture site.

FIG. 7–151. Posttraumatic osteolysis of the humeral head. There is absence of the humeral head in a patient who sustained trauma one year prior to this examination. Note resorption to the humeral neck, with smooth margination and soft-tissue debris. The patient had neither a neurological disease nor any other disease which could be associated with an atrophic type of Charcot joint. Biopsy showed no specific findings.

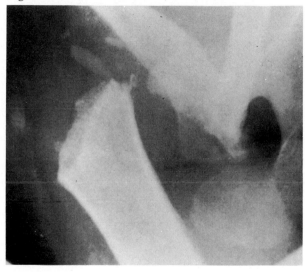

cause radiolucent changes. *Malignant fibrous histiocytoma*,[79,80,118] or *fibrous xanthoma*, may result in destructive skeletal lesions. Permeative destruction, expansion, and periosteal reaction are seen.

Areas of rarefaction in the region of the greater tuberosity, termed "pseudocysts of the humerus," but containing normal bone have been described.[110] *Intraosseous xanthomata* may be associated with hyperlipidemia and show discrete destructive foci in bone.[104,286]

Osteomyelitis albuminosa[229] is a lesion caused by staphylococci characterized by the presence of a large amount of plasma cells and serous or mucoid fluid. Radiologically, the lesion may resemble Ewing's tumor, with a localized destructive area and periosteal reaction. Schintz also cites a *tumorlike form of osteomyelitis* with localized bone destruction and replacement by chronic inflammatory tissue.[229] Amorphous, thick periosteal new bone formation may simulate a malignant tumor. *Yaws*[34] presents as

small circumscribed erosions and periosteal new bone formation. An *echinococcus cyst*[16,68,117,197] may present as a large central radiolucent area within a bone, causing endosteal scalloping and expansion. Daughter cysts may be present. The lesion is usually monostotic and the pelvis (Fig. 7–153), spine, and long bones are frequent sites. The ribs may rarely be involved. Cortical breakthrough and soft-tissue masses may occur. *Actinomycosis* most often affects the mandible and may extend to the facial bones. There is most often mixed destruction and sclerosis (Fig. 7–154). The peripheral skeleton may rarely be involved with a solitary lesion. *Blastomycosis*[132] commonly affects the skeleton in generalized disease. Osteolytic lesions are seen (Figs. 7–155, 7–156), followed by sclerosis. The vertebrae, skull, ribs, tibia, tarsus, and knees are most frequently involved. The basic patterns are focal and diffuse osteomyelitis. *Coccidioidomycosis* of bone results from hematogenous spread. A solitary oste-

(*Text continued on p. 617*)

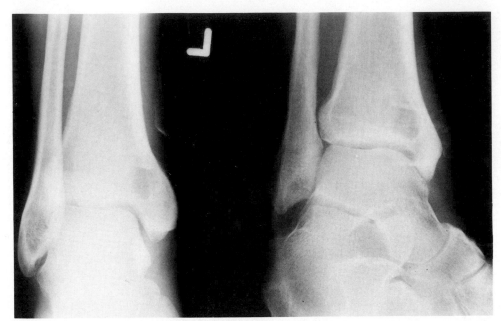

FIG. 7–152. Intraosseous ganglion (distal tibia). A small, well-marginated radiolucency is seen. (Courtesy of Dr. Harold Rosenbaum, University of Kentucky Medical Center, Lexington, KY)

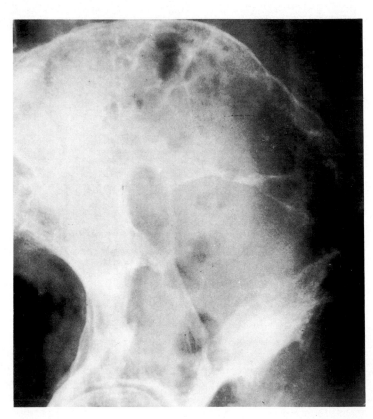

FIG. 7–153. Echinococcus cyst of the ilium. Note large area of radiolucency involving almost the entire bone, with light trabeculation.

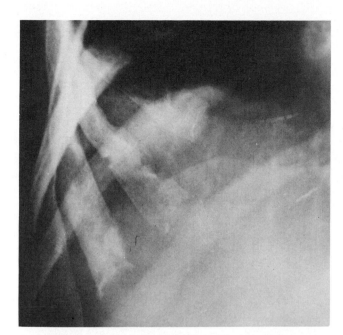

FIG. 7–154. Actinomycosis (ribs). Sclerosis and destruction of multiple lower ribs are noted. (Courtesy of Dr. Dharmashi V. Bhate, VA Hospital, Hines, IL)

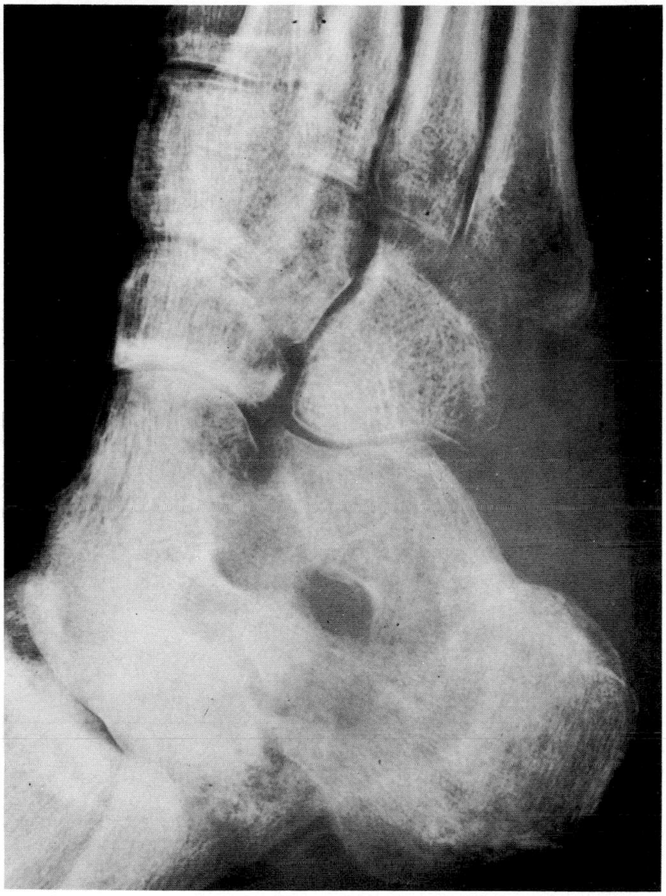

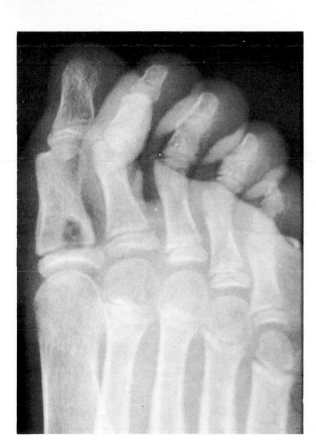

FIG. 7–155. Blastomycosis of the tarsus. Lytic lesions in the calcaneus and local osteoporosis may be seen.

FIG. 7–156. Blastomycosis. Note radiolucent lesion in the metaphysis of the proximal phalanx of the great toe. No reactive sclerosis is present. There is a minimal amount of periosteal new bone formation at the medial aspect of the shaft. (Courtesy of Dr. Harvey White, Children's Memorial Hospital, Chicago, IL)

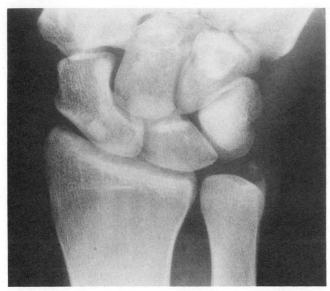

FIG. 7–157. Coccidioidomycosis (wrist). Destruction of the ulnar styloid process associated with soft-tissue swelling is noted. (Courtesy of Dr. Dharmashi V. Bhate, VA Hospital, Hines, IL)

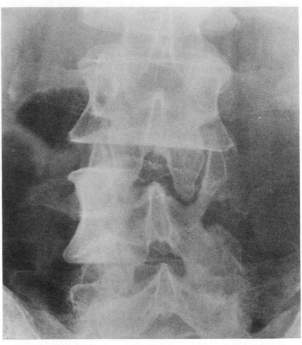

FIG. 7–158. Coccidioidomycosis. Anteroposterior view reveals destruction of the left half of the body of fifth lumbar vertebra. (Courtesy of Dr. Dharmashi V. Bhate, VA Hospital, Hines, IL)

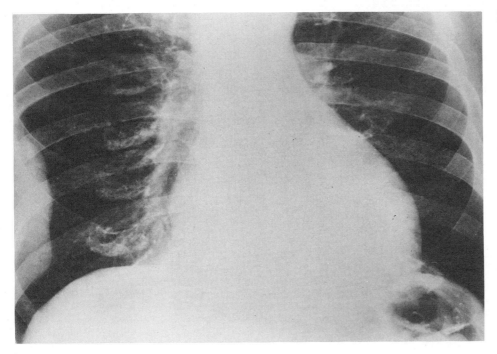

FIG. 7–159. Coccidioidomycosis (ribs). Destruction of the right seventh rib is noted in the axillary line with large, associated, soft-tissue extrapleural mass. (Courtesy of Dr. Dharmashi V. Bhate, VA Hospital, Hines, IL)

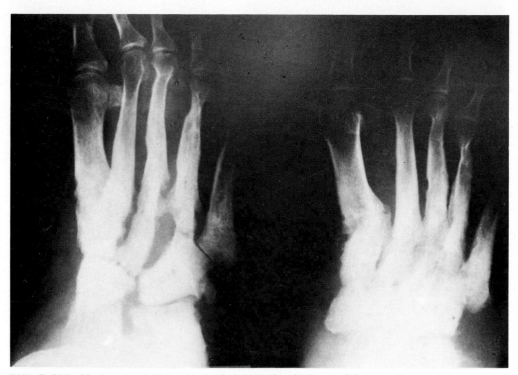

FIG. 7–160. Madura foot. Sclerotic and destructive lesions of the tarsals are seen.

olytic lesion is usually first seen without periosteal reaction (Figs. 7–157, 7–158). Multiple lesions often occur (Fig. 7–159). Spinal involvement is frequent. Chronic lesions show a variable amount of sclerosis. *Torulosis* very rarely involves bone with osteolytic lesions. *Madura foot* is a chronic infection caused by a large variety of fungi. One or all of the bones of the feet may be involved with a mixed lytic and sclerotic process that resembles chronic osteomyelitis (Fig. 7–160). *Granuloma inguinale*[137] may cause bone lesions. Multiple osteolytic areas may be seen without sclerotic reaction resembling metastases. *Sporotrichosis*[39,280] is a granulomatous disease due to infection with the fungus *Sporotrichum schenkii.* It may show osseous, synovial, or arthritic manifestations. Radiologically, in the osseous type, osteoporosis and destructive lesions may be seen. Synovial involvement may resemble villonodular synovitis, and a destructive type of arthritis may occur. The knees, elbows, wrists, and small joints of the hands are most often involved. (Figs. 7–161, 7–162, 7–163). *Aspergillosis* of bone and of the paranasal sinuses have also been described.[99,220] An *epidermoid rest* in the skull presents as a radiolucent lesion with a sclerotic margin (Fig. 7–164).

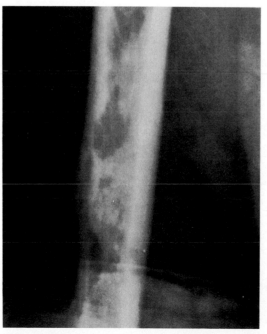

FIG. 7–161. Sporotrichosis (humerus). Note osteolytic lesions with cortical destruction and endosteal scalloping. There is no periosteal new bone formation in this case.

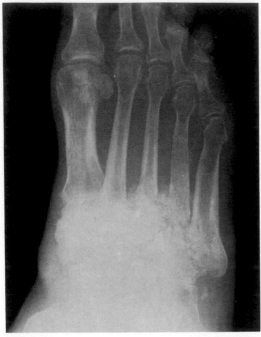

FIG. 7–162. Sporotrichosis (foot). Note expansile lesion in the fourth metatarsal with fine periosteal new bone formation. Extensive destructive changes in the tarsus are present.

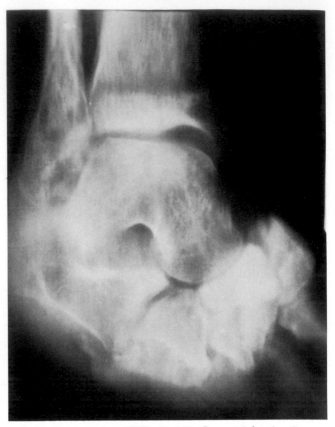

FIG. 7–163. Sporotrichosis (tomogram of tarsal bones). Same case as Fig. 7–162. Note destructive changes and reactive sclerosis.

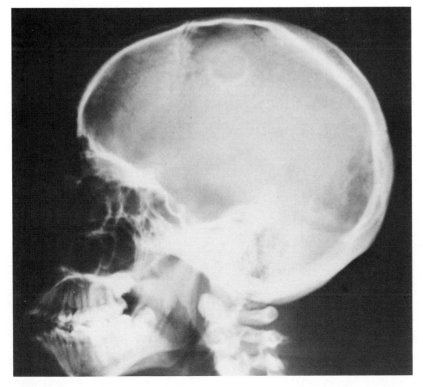

FIG. 7–164. Epidermoid rest in the skull. A radiolucency with a sclerotic margin is noted in the calvarium.

REFERENCES

1. Abell J M, Hayes J T: Charcot knee due to congenital insensitivity to pain. J Bone Joint Surg 46–A:1287–1291, 1964

2. Ackerman L V, Spjut H H: Tumors of Bone and Cartilage, Section II, Fascicle 4. Armed Forces Institute of Pathology, 1961

3. Aegerter E, Kirkpatrick J A: Orthopedic Diseases, 4th ed. Philadelphia, W B Saunders, 1975

4. Agha F P, Lilienfeld R M: Roentgen features of osseous neurilemmoma. Radiology 102:325–326, 1972

5. Ahuja S C et al: Juxtacortical (parosteal) osteogenic sarcoma. J Bone Joint Surg 59–A:632–647, 1977

6. Akbarnia B A, Wirth C K, Colman N: Fibrosarcoma arising from chronic osteomyelitis. Case report and review of the literature. J Bone Joint Surg 58–A:123–125, 1976

7. Anderson R L, Popowitz L, and Li J K H: An unusual sarcoma arising in a solitary osteochondroma. J Bone Joint Surg 51–A:1199–1204, 1969

8. Assor D: Chondroblastoma of the rib. Report of a case. J Bone Joint Surg 55–A:208–210, 1973

9. Aub J C, Evans R P, Hempelmann L H, Martland H S: The late effects of internally deposited radioactive materials in man. Medicine 31:221, 1952

10. Bahr A L, Gayler B W: Cranial chondrosarcomas. Radiology 124:151–156, 1977

11. Banta J V, Schreiber R R, Kulik W J: Hyperplastic callus formation in osteogenesis imperfecta simulating osteosarcoma. J Bone Joint Surg 53–A:115–122, 1971

12. Barnes G R, Gwinn J L: Distal irregularities of the femur simulating malignancy. Am J Roentgen 122:180–185, 1974

13. Barnes R, Catto M: Chondrosarcoma of bone. J Bone Joint Surg 48–B:729–764, 1966

14. Berger P E, Kuhn J P: Computed tomography of tumors of the musculoskeletal system in children. Radiology 127:171–175, 1978

15. Besemann E F, Perez M A: Malignant angioblastoma, so-called adamantinoma, involving the humerus. A case report. Am J Roentgen 100:538–541, 1967

16. Bonakdarpour A et al: Costal echinococcosis: Report of 6 cases and review of the literature. Am J Roentgen 118:371–377, 1973

17. Bonakdarpour A, Levy W M, Aegerter E: Primary and secondary aneurysmal bone cyst: A radiological study of 75 cases. Radiology 126:75–83, 1978

18. Braddock G T F, Hadlow V D: Osteosarcoma in enchondromatosis (Ollier's disease): Report of a case. J Bone Joint Surg 48–B:145–149, 1966

19. Broussin J, Cambuzat J M, LaCoste, F, Chabot G: Critical analysis of the arteriography of primary malignant tumors of the bones, on the occasion of 19 unedited cases. J Radiol Electrol 57:331–340, 1976

20. Brower A C, Culver J E, Keats T E: Histological nature of the cortical irregularity of the medial posterior distal femoral metaphysis in children. Radiology 99:389–392, 1971

21. Bullough P G, Goodfellow J W: Solitary lymphangioma of bone. A case report. J Bone Joint Surg 58–A:418–419, 1976

22. Bundens W D, Brighton C T: Malignant hemangioendothelioma of bone. Report of 2 cases and review of the literature. J Bone Joint Surg 47–A:762–772, 1965

23. Burns–Cox C J, Higgins A T: Aneurysmal bone cyst of the frontal bone. J Bone Joint Surg 51–B:344–345, 1969

24. Caballes R L: Fibromyxoma of bone. Radiology 130:97–99, 1979

25. Caceres E, Zaharia M, Tantalean E: Lymph node metastasis in osteogenic sarcoma. Surgery 65:421–422, 1969

26. Caffey J, Silverman F N: Pediatric X-ray Diagnosis, 5th ed. Chicago, Year Book Publishers, 1967

27. Callan J E, Wood V E: Spontaneous resolution of an osteochondroma. J Bone Joint Surg 57–A:723, 1975

28. Carlson D H, Wilkinson R H, Bhakkaviziam A: Aneurysmal bone cysts in children. Am J Roentgen 116:644–650, 1972

29. Cary G R: Juxtacortical chondroma. A case report. J Bone Joint Surg 47–A:1405–1407, 1965

30. Case records of the Massachusetts General Hospital (osteogenic sarcoma of humerus, with ossifying metastases in the regional nodes). New Eng J Med 225:953, 1941

31. Castle W B, Drinker K R, Drinker C K: Necrosis of the jaw in workers employed in applying a luminous paint containing radium. J Indust Hyg 7:371, 1925

32. Castleman B, McNeill M J: Bone and Joint Clinicopathological Conferences of the Massachusetts General Hospital. Boston, Little, Brown & Co, 1966

33. Chang C H, Piatt E D, Thomas K E, Watne A L: Bone abnormalities in Gardner's syndrome. Am J Roentgen 103:645–652, 1968

34. Cockshott W P, Davies A G M: Tumoural gummatous yaws. Two case reports. J Bone Joint Surg 42–B:785–787, 1960

35. Cohen J: Etiology of simple bone cyst. J Bone Joint Surg 52–A:1493–1497, 1970

36. Cohen J, Cahen I: Benign chondroblastoma of the patella. A case report. J Bone Joint Surg 45–A:824–826, 1963

37. Cohen P, Goldenberg R R: Desmoplastic fibroma of bone. Report of 2 cases. J Bone Joint Surg 47–A:1620–1625, 1965

38. Coleman S S: Benign chondroblastoma with recurrent soft-tissue and intra-articular lesions. J Bone Joint Surg 48–A:1554–1560, 1966

39. Comstock C, Wolson A H: Roentgenology of sporotrichosis. Am J Roentgen 125:651–655, 1975

40. Cooper R R: Juxtacortical chondrosarcoma. A case report. J Bone Joint Surg 47–A:524–528, 1965

41. Copeland M M, Geschickter C F: Cartilaginous tumors of bone. In Anderson MD Hospital and Tumor Institute: Tumors of Bone and Soft Tissue, pp 279–298. Chicago, Year Book Publishers, 1965

42. Coventry M B, Dahlin D C: Osteogenic sarcoma. J Bone Joint Surg 39–A:741–758, 1957

43. Crabbe W A: Intraosseous ganglions in bone. Brit J Surg 53:15–17, 1966

44. Cremin B J, Heselson N G, Webber B L: The multiple sclerotic osteogenic sarcoma of early childhood. Brit J Radiol 49:416–419, 1976

45. Daffner R H: Stress fractures: Current concepts. Skel Rad 2:221–229, 1978

46. Dahlin D C: Bone Tumors, 3rd ed. Springfield, Charles C Thomas, 1978

47. Dahlin D C, Besse B E, Pugh D G, Ghormley R K: Aneurysmal bone cysts. Radiology 64:56–65, 1955

48. Dahlin D C, Coventry M B, Scanlon P W: Ewing's sarcoma. A critical analysis of 165 cases. J Bone Joint Surg 43–A:185–192, 1961

49. Dahlin D C, Henderson E D: Chondrosarcoma. A surgical and pathological problem. Review of 212 cases. J Bone Joint Surg 38–A:1025–1038, 1956

50. Dahlin D C, Johnson E E: Giant osteoma. J Bone Joint Surg 36–A:559–572, 1954

51. Dahlin D C, Unni K K: Osteosarcoma of bone and its important recognizable varieties. Am J Surg Pathol 1:61, 1977

52. Dahlin D C, Wells A H: Chondromyxoid fibroma of bone. Report of 2 cases. J Bone Joint Surg 35–A:831–834, 1953

53. Dalinka M K, Chunn S P: Osteoblastoma — benign or malignant precursor? Report of a case. J Canad Assn Radiol 23:214–216, 1972

54. Dalinka M K, Dinnenberg S, Greendyke W H, Hopkins R: Roentgenographic features of osseous coccidioidomycosis and differential diagnosis. J Bone Joint Surg 53–A:1157–1164, 1971

55. Daly J G: Case report: Osteoid osteoma of the skull. Brit J Radiol 46:392–393, 1973

56. Davidson J W, Chacha P B, James W: Multiple osteosarcomata. Report of a case. J Bone Joint Surg 47–B:537–541, 1965

57. Delahaye R P, Metges P J, Lomazzi R, Capeau F: About 3 cases of sus epitrochlear process of the humerus. Radioclinical approach and review of the literature. J Radiol Electrol 57:341–345, 1976

58. deSantos L A et al: Computed tomography in the evaluation of musculoskeletal neoplasms. Radiology 128:89–94, 1978

59. deSantos L A et al: Osteogenic sarcoma after the age of 50: A radiographic evaluation. Am J Roentgen 131:481–484, 1978

60. deSantos L A et al: The radiographic spectrum of periosteal osteosarcoma. Radiology 127:123–129, 1978

61. deSantos L A, Goldstein H M: Ultrasonography in tumors arising from the spine and bony pelvis. Am J Roentgen 129:1061–1064, 1977

62. deSantos L A, Jing B S: Radiographic findings of Ewing's sarcoma of the jaws. Brit J Radiol 51:682–687, 1978

63. deSantos L A, Murray J A: Evaluation of giant-cell tumor by computerized tomography. Skel Rad 2:205–212, 1978

64. Dick H M, Francis K C, Johnston A D: Ewing's sarcoma of the hand. J Bone Joint Surg 53–A:345–348, 1971

65. Donner R, Dickland R: Adamantinoma of the tibia. A longstanding case with unusual histological features. J Bone Joint Surg 48–B:139–144, 1966

66. Dorfman H D, Norman A, Wolff H: Fibrosarcoma complicating bone infarction in a caisson worker. A case report. J Bone Joint Surg 48–A:528–532, 1966

67. Dunlop J A Y, Morton K S, Elliott G B: Recurrent osteoid osteoma. Report of a case with a review of the literature. J Bone Joint Surg 52–B:128–133, 1970

68. Duran H et al: Osseous hydatidosis. J Bone Joint Surg 60–A:685–690, 1978

69. Edeiken J, Farrel C, Ackerman L V, Spjut H J: Parosteal sarcoma. Am J Roentgen 111:579–583, 1971

70. Edeiken J, Hodes P J: Giant-cell tumors vs tumors with giant cells. Radiol Clin N Amer 1:75–100, 1963

71. Edeiken J, Hodes P J: Roentgen Diagnosis of Diseases of Bone, 2nd ed. Baltimore, Williams & Wilkins, 1973

72. Evison G, Price C H G: Subungual exostosis. Brit J Radiol 39:451–455, 1966

73. Ewald F C: Bone cyst in a phalanx of a 2½-year-old child. J Bone Joint Surg 54–A:399–401, 1972

74. Eyre–Brook A L, Price C H G: Fibrosarcoma of bone. J Bone Joint Surg 51–B:20–37, 1969

75. Farr G H, Huvos A G: Juxtacortical osteogenic sarcoma. An analysis of 14 cases. J Bone Joint Surg 54–A:1205–1261, 1972

76. Fechner R E, Wilde H D: Chondroblastoma in the metaphysis of the femoral neck. J Bone Joint Surg 56–A:413–415, 1974

77. Feldman F, Hecht H L, Johnston A D: Chondromyxoid fibroma of bone. Radiology 94–249–260, 1970

78. Feldman F, Johnston A: Intraosseous ganglion. Am J Roentgen 118:328–343, 1973

79. Feldman F, Lattes R: Primary malignant fibrous histiocytoma (fibroux xanthoma) of bone. Skel Rad 1:145–160, 1977

80. Feldman F, Norman D: Intra- and extraosseous malignant histiocytoma (malignant fibrous xanthoma). Radiology 104:497–508, 1972

81. Fielding J W et al: Primary osteogenic sarcoma of the cervical spine. J Bone Joint Surg 58–A:892–894, 1977

82. Firooznia H et al: Chordoma: Radiologic evaluation of 20 cases. Am J Roentgen 127:797–805, 1976

83. Fitzgerald R H, Dahlin D C, Sim F H: Multiple metachonous osteogenic sarcoma. Report of 12 cases with 2 long-term survivors. J Bone Joint Surg 55–A:595–605, 1973

84. Fox J E, Batsakis J G, Owano L R: Unusual manifestations of chordoma. J Bone Joint Surg 50–A:1618–1628, 1968

85. Freiberg R A, Air G W, Glueck J, Ishikawa T, Abrams N R: Multiple intraosseous lipomas with type IV hyperlipoproteinemia. A case report. J Bone Joint Surg 56–A:1729–1732, 1974

86. Freiberger R H, Loitman B S, Herpern M, Thompson T C: Osteoid osteoma. A report on 80 cases. Am J Roentgen 82:194–205, 1959

87. Gehweiler J A, Capp M P, Chick E W: Observations on the roentgen patterns in blastomycosis of bone: A review of

cases from the blastomycosis cooperative study of the Veterans Administration and Duke University Medical Center. Am J Roentgen 108:497–510, 1970

88. Gelberman R H, Olson C O: Benign osteoblastoma of the atlas. A case report. J Bone Joint Surg 56–A:808–810, 1974

89. Gilday et al: Radionuclide skeletal survey for pediatric neoplasms. Radiology 123:399–406, 1977

90. Giustra P E, Freiberger R H: Severe growth disturbance with osteoid osteoma. A report of 2 cases involving the femoral neck. Radiology 96:285–288, 1970

91. Glynn J L, Lichtestein L: Osteoid osteoma with multicentric nidus. J Bone Joint Surg 55–A:855–858, 1973

92. Goergen T G, Resnick D, Riley R R: Posttraumatic abnormalities of the pubic bone stimulating malignancy. Radiology 126:85–87, 1978

93. Gohel V K, Dalinka M K, Edeiken J: Ischemic necrosis of the femoral head simulating chondroblastoma. Radiology 107:545–546, 1973

94. Goldenberg R R, Campbell C J, Bonfiglio M: Giant-cell tumor of bone. An analysis of 218 cases. J Bone Joint Surg 52–A:619–664, 1970

95. Goodwin M A: Primary osteosarcoma of the patella. A case report. J Bone Joint Surg 43–B:338–341, 1961

96. Grabias S, Mankin H J: Chondrosarcoma arising in histologically proved unicameral bone cyst. A case report. J Bone Joint Surg 56 A:1501–1509, 1974

97. Greenspan A, Elguezbel A, Bryk D: Multifocal osteoid osteoma. A case report and review of the literature. Am J Roentgen 121:103–106, 1974

98. Griffiths H J: Marrow Tumors. In Bone Tumors, Vol V, Part 6. Berlin, Springer–Verlag, 1977

99. Grossman M: Aspergillosis of bone. Brit J Radiol 48:57–59, 1975

100. Grosswasser J R, Brunebaum M: Metaphyseal multifocal osteosarcoma. Brit J Radiol 51:671–681, 1978

101. Güttich H, Müller E S: Brosses Stirnhöhlenosteom and reversible Blindheit. HNO 15:155–158, 1967

102. Habermann E T, Stern R E: Osteoid osteoma of the tibia in an 8-month-old boy. A case report. J Bone Joint Surg 56–A:633–636, 1974

103. Hagenlocher H U, Ciba K: The radiological aspects of cervical chordomas. Fortschr Roentgenstr 125:228–232, 1976

104. Hamilton W C, Ramsey P L, Hanson S M, Schiff D C: Osseous xanthoma and multiple hand tumors as a complication of hyperlipidemia. J Bone Joint Surg 57–A:551–553, 1975

105. Hamlin J A, Adler L, Greenhaum E I: Central enchondroma —a precursor to chondrosarcoma. J Canad Assn Radiol 22:206–209, 1971

106. Hanelin L G, Sclamberg E L, Bardsley J L: Intraosseous lipoma of the coccyx. Report of a case. Radiology 114:343–344, 1975

107. Hardy R, Lehrer H: Desmoplastic fibroma vs desmoid tumor of bone. Radiology 88:899–901, 1967

108. Hay M C, Paterson D, Taylor T K F: Aneurysmal bone cysts of the spine. J Bone Joint Surg 60–B:406, 1978

109. Heelan R T, Watson R C, Smith J: Computed tomography of lower extremity tumors. Am J Roentgen 132:933–937, 1979

110. Helms C A: Pseudocysts of the humerus. Am J Roentgen 131:287–288, 1978

111. Henderson E D, Dahlin D C: Chondrosarcoma of bone. A study of 285 cases. J Bone Joint Surg 45–A:1450–1458, 1963

112. Henley F T, Richetts G L: Aneurysmal bone cyst presenting as a chest mass. A case report. Radiology 92:1103–1104, 1969

113. Hensley C D: Epidermoid cyst of the distal phalanx occurring in an 8-year-old child. A case report. J Bone Joint Surg 48–A:946–948, 1966

114. Herndon J H, Eaton R G, Littler J W: Carpal–Tunnel syndrome. An unusual presentation of osteoid-osteoma of the capitate. J Bone Joint Surg 56–A:1715–1718, 1974

115. Hershey S L, Lansden F T: Osteochondromas as a cause of false popliteal aneurysms. Review of the literature and report of 2 cases. J Bone Joint Surg 54–A:1765–1768, 1972

116. Hill J A et al: Myxoma of the toes. A case report. J Bone Joint Surg 60–A:128–130, 1978

117. Hsieh C K: Echinococcus involvement of bone with x-ray examination. Radiology 14:562–575, 1930

118. Hudson T M et al: Angiography of malignant fibrous histiocytoma of bone. Radiology 131:9–15, 1979

119. Huettig G, Rittmeyer K: Multiple aneurysmatische Knochenzysten bei 3 Monate altem Saeugling. Fortschr Roentgenstr 129:796, 1978

120. Hutter C G: Unicameral bone cyst. A report of an unusual case. J Bone Joint Surg 32–A:430–432, 1950

121. Ivins J C, Dahlin D C: Reticulum-cell sarcoma of bone. J Bone Joint Surg 35–A:835–842, 1953

122. Jacobs P: The diagnosis of osteoclastoma (giant-cell tumour): A radiological and pathological correlation. Brit J Radiol 45:121–136, 1972

123. Jaffe H L: Histogenesis of bone tumors. In Anderson MD: Hospital and Tumor Institute. Tumors of Bone and Soft Tissue, pp 41–44. Chicago, Year Book Publishers, 1965

124. Jaffe H L: Tumors and Tumorous Conditions of the Bones and Joints. Philadelphia, Lea & Febiger, 1958

125. Janecki C J, Nelson C L, Dohn D F: Intrasacral cyst. Report of a case and review of the literature. J Bone Joint Surg 54–A:423–428, 1972

126. Jeffree G M, Price C H G: Bone tumors and their enzymes. A study of the phosphatases, nonspecific esterases and beta-glucuronidase of osteogenic and cartilaginous tumours, fibroblastic and giant-cell lesions. J Bone Joint Surg 47–B:120–135, 1965

127. Jeffree G M, Price C H G: Metastatic spread of fibrosarcoma of bone. J Bone Joint Surg 58–B:418–425, 1976

128. Jernstrom P, Stark H H: Giant-cell reaction of a metacarpal. Am J Clin Path 55:77–81, 1971

129. Johnson G F: Osteoid osteoma of the femoral neck. Am J Roentgen 74:65–69, 1955

130. Johnson L C: A general theory of bone tumors. Bull NY Acad Med 29:164–171, 1953

131. Jokl P, Albright J A, Goodman A H: Juxtacortical chondrosarcoma of the hand. J Bone Joint Surg 53–A:1370–1376, 1971

132. Joyce P F et al: A rare clinical presentation of blastomycosis. Skel Rad 2:239–242, 1977

133. Karlin C A, Brower A C: Multiple primary hemangiomas of bone. Am J Roentgen 129:162–164, 1977

134. Kenin A, Levine J, Spinner M: Parosteal lipoma. A report of 2 cases with associated bone changes. J Bone Joint Surg 41–A:1122–1126, 1959

135. Kimmelstiel P, Rapp I H: Cortical defect due to periosteal desmoids. Bull Hosp Joint Dis 12:286–297, 1951

136. Kindblom L G, Merck C, Svendson P: Myxofibrosarcoma: A pathologico-anatomical, microangiographic, and angiographic correlative study of 8 cases. Brit J Radiol 50:876–887, 1977

137. Kirkpatrick D J: Donovanosis (granuloma inguinale): A rare cause of osteolytic bone lesions. Clin Radiol 21:101–105, 1970

138. Kirschner S G et al: Periosteal chondromas of the anterior-tibial tubercle — 2 cases. Am J Roentgen 131:1088–1089, 1978

139. Kittredge R D: Arteriography in Ewing's tumor. Radiology 97:609–610, 1970

140. Klenerman L, Ockenden B G, Townsend A C: Osteosarcoma occurring in osteogenesis imperfecta. Report of 2 cases. J Bone Joint Surg 49–B:314–323, 1967

141. Kolawole T M, Bohrer S P: Ulcer osteoma — bone response to tropical ulcer. Am J Roentgen 109:611–618, 1970

142. Kopp W K: Benign osteoblastoma of the coronoid process of the mandible. Report of a case. J Oral Surg 27:653–655, 1969

143. Kopperman M, Antoine J E: Primary lymphangioma of the calvarium. Am J Roentgen 121:118–120, 1974

144. Kricun M E, Kricun R, Haskin M E: Chondroblastoma of the calcaneus: Radiographic features with emphasis on location. Am J Roentgen 128:613–616, 1977

145. Lammot T R: Enchondroma of the patella. A case report. J Bone Joint Surg 50–A:1230–1232, 1968

146. Larsson S E, Lorentzon R: The incidence of primary malignant bone tumors in relation to age, sex, and site. J Bone Joint Surg 56–A:534–540, 1974

147. Larsson S E, Lorentzon R, Roquist L: Fibrosarcoma of bone. J Bone Joint Surg 58–B:412–417, 1976

148. Lawrie T R, Aterman K, Path F C, Sinclair A M: Painless osteoid osteoma. A report of 2 cases. J Bone Joint Surg 52–A:1357–1363, 1970

149. Lechner G, Knahr K, Riedl P: Das Osteoid-Osteom (osteoid osteoma). Fortschr Roentgenstr 128:511–520, 1978

150. Lee E S: Osteosarcoma: A reconnaissance. Clin Radiol 26:5–25, 1975

151. Lerner M R, Southwick W O: Keratin cysts in phalangeal bones. Report of an unusual case. J Bone Joint Surg 50–A:365–372, 1968

152. Levin D C, Blazina M E, Levine E: Fatigue fractures of the shaft of the femur: Simulation of malignant tumor. Radiology 89:883–885, 1967

153. Lichtenstein L: Bone Tumors, 3rd ed. St. Louis, CV Mosby, 1965

154. Lichtenstein L, Sawyer W R: Benign osteoblastoma. Further observations and report of 20 additional cases. J Bone Joint Surg 46–A:755–765, 1964

155. Linscheid R L, Dahlin D C: Unusual lesions of the patella. J Bone Joint Surg 48–A:1359–1365, 1966

156. Lodwick G S: The Bones and Joints. Chicago, Year Book Publishers, 1971

157. Lodwick G S: Juvenile unicameral bone cyst. Am J Roentgen 80:495–504, 1958

158. Lodwick G S: Solitary malignant tumors of bone: The application of predictor variables in diagnosis. Seminars Roentgen 1:293–313, 1966

159. Mack G R, Robey D B, Kurman R J: Chondrosarcoma secreting chorionic gonadotropin. J Bone Joint Surg 59–A:1107–1111, 1978

160. Majid M A, Mathias P F, Seth H N, Thirumalachar M J: Primary mycetoma of the patella. J Bone Joint Surg 46–A:1283–1286, 1964

161. Marcove R C et al: Osteogenic sarcoma under the age of 21. A review of 145 operative cases. J Bone Joint Surg 52–A:411–423, 1970

162. McGrath P J: Giant-cell tumour of bone. J Bone Joint Surg 54–B:216–229, 1972

163. McInerney D P, Middlemiss J H: Giant-cell tumor of bone. Skel Rad 2:195–204, 1978

164. McLaughlin R E, Sweet D E, Webster T, and Merritt W M: Chondroblastoma of the pelvis suggestive of malignancy. Report of an unusual case treated by wide pelvic excision. J Bone Surg 57–A:549–550, 1975

165. McLeod R A, Beabout J W: The roentgenographic features of chondroblastoma. Am J Roentgen 118:464–471, 1973

166. McLeod R A, Dahlin D C, Beabout J W: The spectrum of osteoblastoma. Am J Roentgen 126:321–335, 1976

167. Miller B, Markheim H R, Towbin M N: Multiple stress fractures in rheumatoid arthritis. A case report. J Bone Joint Surg 49–A:1408–1414, 1967

168. Miller C W, McLaughlin R E: Osteosarcoma in siblings. Report of 2 cases. J Bone Joint Surg 59–A:261–262, 1977

169. Mindell E R, Northrup C S, Douglass H O: Osteosarcoma associated with osteopoikilosis. J Bone Joint Surg 60–A:406–408, 1978

170. Mirra J M, Marcove R C: Fibrosarcomatous dedifferentiation of primary and secondary chondrosarcoma. Review of 5 cases. J Bone Joint Surg 56–A:285–296, 1974

171. Mnaymneh W A, Dudley H R, Mnaymneh L G: Giant-cell tumor of bone. An analysis and follow-up study of the 41 cases observed at the Massachusetts General Hospital between 1925 and 1960. J Bone Joint Surg 46–A:63–75, 1964

172. Moore T M, Row J B, Harvey J P: Chondroblastoma of the talus. J Bone Joint Surg 59–A:830–831, 1977

173. Morris E, Wolinsky E: Localized osseous cryptococcosis. A case report. J Bone Joint Surg 47–A:1027–1029, 1965

174. Morse D, Reed J O, Bernstein J: Sclerosing osteogenic sarcoma. Am J Roentgen 88:491–495, 1962

175. Morton K S, Bartlett L H: Benign osteoblastic change resembling osteoid osteoma. A report of 3 cases with unusual radiologic features. J Bone Joint Surg. 48–B:478–487, 1966

176. Murphy F D, Blount W B: Cartilaginous exostosis following irradiation. J Bone Joint Surg 44–A:662–668, 1962

177. Murphy N B, Price C H G: The radiological aspects of chondromyxoid fibroma of bone. Clin Radiol 22:261–269, 1971

178. Naji A F et al: So-called adamantinoma of long bones. Report of a case with massive pulmonary metastases. J Bone Joint Surg 46–A:151–158, 1964

179. Neer C S et al: Treatment of unicameral bone cyst. A follow-up study of 175 cases. J Bone Joint Surg 48–A:731–745, 1966

180. Nelson J A, Clark R E, Palubinskas A J: Osteogenic sarcoma with calcified renal metastases. Brit J Radiol 44:802–804, 1971

181. Neviaser R J, Wilson J N: Benign chondroblastoma of the finger. J Bone Joint Surg 54–A:389–392, 1972

182. Newman A: The supracondylar process and its fracture. Am J Roentgen 105:844–849, 1969

183. Nolan D J, Middlemiss H: Chondroblastoma of bone. Clin Rad 26:343–350, 1975

184. Norman A, Schiffman M: Simple bone cysts: Factors of age dependency. Radiology 124:779–782, 1977

185. Norman A, Ulin R: A comparative study of periosteal new-bone response in metastatic bone tumors (solitary) and primary bone sarcomas. Radiology 92:705–708, 1969

186. O'Dell C W et al: Osteoid osteomas arising in adjacent bones. Report of a case. J Canad Assn Rad 27:298–300, 1976

187. O'Gorman A M, Kirkham T H: Aneurysmal bone cyst of the orbit with unusual angiographic features. Am J Roentgen 126:896–899, 1976

188. O'Hara J M et al: An analysis of 30 patients surviving longer than 10 years after treatment for osteogenic sarcoma. J Bone Joint Surg 50–A:335–354, 1968

189. Pachter M R, Alpert M: Chondrosarcoma of the foot skeleton. J Bone Joint Surg 46–A:601–607, 1964

190. Pandey S: Giant chondromas arising from the ribs. J Bone Joint Surg 57–B:519–522, 1975

191. Parker F, Jackson H: Primary reticulum-cell sarcoma of bone. Surg Gynec Obstet 68:45–51, 1939

192. Pasquel P M, Levet S N, DeLeon B: Primary rhabdomyosarcoma of bone. A case report. J Bone Joint Surg 58–A:1176–1178, 1976

193. Patel M R, Pearlman H S, Engler J, Wollowick B S: Chondrosarcoma of the proximal phalanx of the finger. Review of the literature and report of a case. J Bone Joint Surg 59–A:401–403, 1977

194. Paul L W, Juhl J H: Roentgen Diagnosis of the Skeletal System. New York, Hoeber Medical Division (Harper and Row), 1967

195. Peison B, Feigenbaum J: Metaphyseal giant-cell tumor in a girl of 14 years. Radiology 118:145–146, 1976

196. Pepe A J, Kuhlmann R F, Miller D B: Mesenchymal chondrosarcoma. A case report. J Bone Joint Surg 59–A:256–258, 1977

197. Pintilie D C, Panoza G H, Hatman V D, Fahrer M: Echinococcosis of the humerus. Treatment by resection and bone grafting. J Bone Joint Surg 48–A:957–962, 1966

198. Pirschel J: A mesenchymal chondrosarcoma of the sternum. Fortschr Roentgenstr 124:91–93, 1976

199. Plum G E, Pugh D G: Roentgenologic aspects of benign chondroblastoma of bone. Am J Roentgen 79:584–591, 1958

200. Prabhakar B, Reddy D R, Dayananda B, Rao G R: Osteoid osteoma of the skull. J Bone Joint Surg 54–B:146–148, 1972

201. Prager P J, Menges V, DiBiase M: The intraosseous ganglion. Fortschr Roentgenstr 123:458–461, 1975

202. Prentice A I D: Variations on the fibrous cortical defect. Clin Rad 25:531–533, 1974

203. Price C H G, Goldie W: Paget's sarcoma of bone. A study of 80 cases from the Bristol and Leeds bone tumour registries. J Bone Joint Surg 51–B:205–224, 1969

204. Prichard R W, Stoy R P, Barwick J T F: Chondromyxoid fibroma of the scapula. Report of a case. J Bone Joint Surg 46–A:1759–1760, 1964

205. Ranniger K, Altner P C: Parosteal osteoid sarcoma. Radiology 86:648–651, 1966

206. Reiter F B, Ackerman L V, Staple T W: Central chondrosarcoma of the appendicular skeleton. Radiology 105:525–530, 1972

207. Retz L D: Primary liposarcoma of bone. Report of a case and review of the literature. J Bone Joint Surg 43–A:123–129, 1961

208. Reynolds J: The "fallen fragment sign" in the diagnosis of unicameral bone cysts. Radiology 92:949–953, 1969

209. Riddel R J, Louis C J, Bromberger N A: Pulmonary metastases from chondroblastoma of the tibia. Report of a case. J Bone Joint Surg 55–B:848–853, 1973

210. Rittenberg G M et al: The vascular "sunburst" appearance of osteosarcoma. A new angiographic finding. Skel Rad 2:243–244, 1978

211. Roberts P H, Price C H G: Chondrosarcoma of the bones of the hand. J Bone Joint Surg 59–B:213–221, 1977

212. Rockwell M A, Enneking W F: Osteosarcoma developing in solitary enchondroma of the tibia. J Bone Joint Surg 53–A:341–344, 1971

213. Rockwell M A, Saiter E T, Enneking W F: Periosteal chondroma. J Bone Joint Surg 54–A:102–108, 1972

214. Rosen R S, Jacobson G: Fungus disease of bone. Seminars Roentgen 1:370–391, 1966

215. Rosenfeld K, Bora F W, Lane J M: Osteoid osteoma of the hamate. A case report and review of the literature. J Bone Joint Surg 55–A:1085–1087, 1973

216. Rosenmertz S K, Schare H J: Osteogenic sarcoma arising in Paget's disease of the mandible. Review of the literature and report of a case. Oral Surg 28:304–309, 1969

217. Ross P: Gardner's syndrome. Am J Roentgen 96:298–301, 1966

218. Roth S I: Squamous cysts involving the skull and phalanges. J Bone Joint Surg 46–A:1442–1450, 1964

219. Rubin P: Dynamic Classification of Bone Dysplasias. Chicago, Year Book Publishers, 1964

220. Rudwan M A, Sheikh N A: Aspergilloma of paranasal sinuses. A common cause of unilateral proptosis in Sudan. Clin Rad 27:497–502, 1976

221. Sadler A H, Rosenhain F: Occurrence of 2 unicameral bone cysts in the same patient. J Bone Joint Surg 46–A:1557–1560, 1964

222. Sammons B P, Sarkisian S S, Krepela M C: Juxtacortical osteogenic sarcoma. Am J Roentgen 79:592:597, 1958

223. Sanerkin N G: Old fibrin coagula and their ossification in simple bone cysts. J Bone Joint Surg 61–B:194–199, 1979

224. Schajowicz F: Juxtacortical chondrosarcoma. J Bone Joint Surg 59–B:473–480, 1977

225. Schajowicz F, Gallardo H: Epiphyseal chondroblastoma of bone. J Bone Joint Surg 52–B:205–226, 1970

226. Schajowicz F, Lemos C: Osteoid osteoma and osteoblastoma. Acta Orthop Scand 41:272–291, 1970

227. Schajowicz F, Lemos C: Malignant osteoblastoma. J Bone Joint Surg 58–B:202–211, 1976

228. Schey W L, Shkolnik A, White H: Clinical and radiographic considerations of sacrococcygeal teratomas. An analysis of 26 new cases and review of the literature. Radiology 125:189–195, 1977

229. Schintz H R, Baensch W E, Friedl E, Uehlinger E: Roentgen Diagnostics. New York, Grune & Stratton, 1952

230. Schmidt M, Thiel H J, Spitz J: Der Fibroese Kortikalisdefekt. Fortschr Roentgenstr 128:521–524, 1978

231. Schmoller H, Suwandschieff N: Eine aussergewöhnliche Komplication bei Multiplen Kartilaginären Exostosen. Fortschr Roentgenstr 123:273–275, 1975

232. Schwartz A, Shuster M, Becker S M: Liposarcoma of bone. Report of a case and review of the literature. J Bone Joint Surg 52–A:171–177, 1970

233. Schwarz E: Ossifying fibroma of the face and skull. Am J Roentgen 91:1012–1015, 1964

234. Scott M, Lignelli G J, Shea F J: Cervical radicular pain secondary to osteoid osteoma of spine. JAMA 217:964–965, 1971

235. Scranton P E et al: Investigation of carbohydrate metabolism and somatomedin in osteosarcoma patients. J Surg Oncol 7:403–409, 1975

236. Seymour N: Intraosseous ganglia. Report of 2 cases. J Bone Joint Surg 50–B:134–137, 1968

237. Sherman F S: Osteoid osteoma associated with changes in the adjacent joint. Report of 2 cases. J Bone Joint Surg 29:483–490, 1947

238. Sherman M, Fabricus R: Giant-cell tumor in the metaphysis of a child. Report of an unusual case. J Bone Joint Surg 43–A:1225–1229, 1961

239. Sherman R S, Soong K Y: Ewing's sarcoma: Its roentgen classification and diagnosis. Radiology 66:529–539, 1956

240. Sherman R S, Wilner D: Roentgen diagnosis of hemangioma of bone. Am J Roentgen 86:1146–1159, 1961

241. Siegler J: Recurrent pyogenic meningitis due to an osteoma of the frontal sinus. J Laryng 78:226–228, 1964

242. Sim F H, Danlin D C, Beaubout J W: Multicentric giant-cell tumor of bone. J Bone Joint Surg 59–A:1052–1060, 1977

243. Simon G: Principles of Bone X-ray Diagnosis, 2nd ed. London, Butterworth & Company, 1965

244. Singh R, Grewal D S, Bannerjee A K, Bansal V P: Haemangiomatosis of the skeleton. J Bone Joint Surg 56–B:136–138, 1974

245. Singleton E B, Rosenberg H S, Dodd G D, Dolan P A: Sclerosing osteogenic sarcomatosis. Am J Roentgen 88:483–490, 1962

246. Slowick F A, Campbell C J, Kettelkamp D B: Aneurysmal bone cyst. An analysis of 13 cases. J Bone Joint Surg 50–A:1142–1151, 1968

247. Smith J, Ahuja S C, Huvos A G, Bullough P: Parosteal (juxtacortical) osteogenic sarcoma. A roentgenological study of 30 patients. J Canad Assn Rad 29:167–174, 1978

248. Smith J, McLachlan D L, Huvos A G, Higinbotham N L: Primary tumors of the clavicle and scapula. Am J Roentgen 124:113–123, 1975

249. Smith R W, Smith C F: Solitary unicameral bone cyst of the calcaneus. A review of 20 cases. J Bone Joint Surg 56–A:49–56, 1974

250. Snarr J W, Abell M R, Martel W: Lymphofollicular synovitis with osteoid osteoma. Radiology 106:557–560, 1973

251. Spence A J, Lloyd–Roberts G C: Regional osteoporosis in osteoid osteoma. J Bone Joint Surg 43–B:501–507, 1961

252. Spiers F W, King S D, Beddoe A H: Measurements of endosteal surface area in human long bones. Relationship of sites of occurrence of osteosarcoma. Brit J Radiol 50:769–776, 1977

253. Srinivasan C K et al: Malignant hemangioendothelioma of bone. J Bone Joint Surg 60–A:696–700, 1978

254. Stark H H, Jones F E, Jernstrom P: Parosteal osteogenic sarcoma of a metacarpal bone. A case report. J Bone Joint Surg 53–A:147–153, 1971

255. Stark J D, Adler N N, Robinson W H: Hereditary multiple exostoses. Radiology 59:212–215, 1952

256. Stewart J R, Dahlin D C, Pugh D G: Pathology and radiology of solitary bone tumors. Seminars Roentgen 1:268–292, 1966

257. Sugiura I: Desmoplastic fibroma. A case report and review of the literature. J Bone Joint Surg 58–A:126–129, 1976

258. Sundaram T K S: Benign chondroblastoma. J Bone Joint Surg 48–B:92–104, 1966

259. Swee R G, McLeod R A, Beabout J W: Osteoid osteoma. Radiology 130:117–123, 1979

260. Sweterlitsch P R, Torg J S, Watts H: Malignant hemangioendothelioma of the cervical spine. J Bone Joint Surg 52–A:805–808, 1970

261. Swischuk L E, Jorgenson F, Caden D: Wooden splinter induced "pseudotumors" and "osteomyelitis-like" lesions of bone and soft tissue. Roent 122:176–179, 1974

262. Sybrandy S, de la Fuente A A: Multiple giant-cell tumour of bone. J Bone Joint Surg 55–B:350–356, 1973

263. Takigawa K: Chondroma of the bones of the hand. A review of 110 cases. J Bone Joint Surg 53–A:1591–1600, 1971

264. Tang T T et al: Angioglomoid tumor of bone. J Bone Joint Surg 58–A:873–876, 1976

265. Taxin R N, Feldman F: The tumbling bullet sign in a post-traumatic bone cyst. Am J Roentgen 123:140–143, 1975

266. Tiedjen K U: Ewing–Sarkom bei einem 13 Monate alten Jungen. Fortschr Roentgenstr 129:798–800, 1978

267. Tulloh H P, Harry D: Osteoblastoma in a rib in childhood. Clin Radiol 20:337–338, 1969

268. Turcotte B, Pugh D G, Dahlin D C: The roentgenologic aspects of chondromyxoid fibroma of bone. Am J Roentgen 87:1085–1095, 1962

269. Twersky J, Kassner E G, Tenner M S, Camera A: Vertebral and costal osteochondromas causing spinal cord compression. Am J Roentgen 124:124–128, 1975

270. Unni K K, Dahlin D C, Beabout J W: Periosteal osteogenic sarcoma. Cancer 37:2476–2485, 1976

271. Unni K K, Dahlin D C, Beabout J W, Sim F H: Chondrosarcoma: Clear-cell variant. A report of 16 cases. J Bone Joint Surg 58–A:676–683, 1976

272. Valderrama J A F, Matthews J M: The haemophilic pseudotumour or haemophilic subperiosteal haematoma. J Bone Joint Surg 47–B:256–265, 1965

273. Vandevoort P L M, Rosenbusch G: Ossifizierende Lymph Kontenmetastasen eines Osteosarcoms. Fortschr Roentgenstr 126:492–494, 1977

274. Verbiest H: Giant-cell tumours and aneurysmal bone cysts of the spine with special reference to the problems related to the removal of a vertebral body. J Bone Joint Surg 47–B:699–713, 1965

275. Vinstein A L, Franken E A: Hereditary multiple exostoses. Report of a case with spinal cord compression. Am J Roentgen 112:405–407, 1971

276. Vix V A: Unusual appearance of a chondromyxoid fibroma. Radiology 92:365–366, 1969

277. Weston W J: Thorn- and twig-induced pseudotumours of bone and soft tissues. Brit J Radiol 36:323–326, 1963

278. Whitehouse G H, Griffiths G J: Roentgenologic aspects of spinal involvement by primary and metastatic Ewing's tumor. J Canad Assn Rad 27:290–297, 1976

279. Wilkerson J A, Cracchiolo A: Giant-cell tumor of the tibial diaphysis. J Bone Joint Surg 51–A:1205–1209, 1969

280. Winter T Q, Pearson K D: Systemic sporothrixosis. Radiology 104:579–584, 1972

281. Winter W G: Spontaneous pneumothorax heralding metastases of adamantinoma of the tibia. Report of 2 cases. J Bone Joint Surg 58–A:416–417, 1976

282. Wright J L, Sherman M S: An unusual chondroblastoma. J Bone Joint Surg 46–A:597–600, 1964

283. Yaghamai I: Angiographic features of chondromas and chondrosarcomas. Skel Rad 3:91–98, 1978

284. Yaghamai I: Angiographic features of fibromas and fibrosarcomas. Radiology 124:57–64, 1977

285. Yaghamai I: Angiographic features of osteosarcoma. Am J Roentgen 129:1073–1082, 1977

286. Yaghamai I: Intra- and extraosseous xanthomata associated with hyperlipidemia. Radiology 128:49–54, 1978

287. Yaghamai I, Abdolmahmoud S Z, Shams S, Afshari R: Value of arteriography in the diagnosis of benign and malignant bone lesions. Cancer 27:1134–1147, 1971

288. Yoneyama T, Greenlaw R H: Osteogenic sarcoma following radiotherapy for retinoblastoma. Radiology 93:1185–1186, 1969

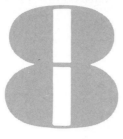

THE
SOFT
TISSUES

SOFT-TISSUE CALCIFICATION

Deposition of calcium in abnormal locations is due to a variety of causes, which can be classified as metastatic calcification, calcinosis, and dystrophic calcification.

Metastatic calcification refers to a disturbance in calcium or phosphorus metabolism leading to ectopic calcification in primarily normal tissue. This is likely to include periarticular regions.

Calcinosis refers to deposition of calcium in skin and subcutaneous and connective tissue in the presence of normal calcium metabolism.

Dystrophic calcification indicates calcium deposition in damaged tissues without a generalized metabolic derangement. Devitalized tissue, because of a lower metabolic rate, has a lower CO_2 concentration, leading to local alkalinity. Calcium and phosphorus salts are less soluble in an alkaline medium and, as a result, precipitate.

Calcification can be roentgenologically differentiated from ossification. The latter shows organization into trabeculae and a cortex. Extraskeletal ossification occurs as myositis ossificans and in other forms.

METASTATIC CALCIFICATION

Hyperparathyroidism, usually secondary to renal disease but sometimes in the primary form, leads to metastatic calcification. Renal calcification in the form of nephrolithiasis and nephrocalcinosis is common to both forms. Calcification in the pancreas, prostate, and salivary glands occasionally occurs. More commonly, the vascular system (Fig. 8–1) and cartilage are calcified. Periarticular calcinosis may also be present, as well as calcific deposits in articular cartilage, menisci, and joint capsules.

Hypoparathyroidism, both idiopathic and pseudo, can be associated with calcification of the basal ganglia (Fig. 8–2) and dentate nuclei of the cerebellum, with deposition of calcium in the colloid material that is often present in these structures.[105]

Periarticular and interstitial calcinosis have also been reported. Albright and Reifenstein state that there is an excess of interstitial ionic calcium in the presence of low serum calcium concentration occurring in this condition.[3] The causes of calcification of the basal ganglia[40] are summarized below.

CAUSES OF CALCIFICATION OF THE BASAL GANGLIA*

A. Parathyroid syndromes
   1. Idiopathic hypoparathyroidism
   2. Pseudohypoparathyroidism
   3. Postoperative hypoparathyroidism
B. Familial idiopathic basal ganglia calcification
C. Fahr's disease (idiopathic familial nonarteriosclerotic intracerebral vascular calcification)
D. Lead intoxication
E. Carbon monoxide intoxication
F. Postradiation therapy
G. Concomitant neurological disorders and basal ganglia calcification

* Modified from Harwood–Nash DCF, Reilly BJ: Am J Roentgen 108:392–395, 1970

Massive bone destructive processes, such as metastatic tumors, multiple myeloma, and leukemia, can rarely cause metastatic calcifications in the presence of hypercalcemia. *Sarcoidosis* is associated with hypercalcemia in 20% of patients. This can cause nephrocalcinosis and nephrolithiasis. Calcification, particularly in the skin, cornea, and conjunctiva can occur. Involved lymph nodes show a characteristic absence of calcification. Metastatic calcification in the soft tissues may occur in the presence of hypercalcemia in sarcoidosis which may cause confusion with hyperparathyroidism. Cortisone administration will cause a fall in serum calcium level if the hypercalcemia is due to sarcoidosis, but not if it is due to hyperparathyroidism. A similar fall in the serum calcium concentration occurs in multiple myeloma and hypervitaminosis D. Renal failure is rare in sarcoidosis.

Hypervitaminosis D results from excessive intake, usually of vitamin D_2. The intake can range from

50,000 to one million I.U. taken daily, over a period ranging from a few days to several years. *Idiopathic hypercalcemia* is considered to result from either excessive intake of vitamin D or hypersensitivity to vitamin D in children. There is a high serum calcium level even in the presence of a low calcium intake. The plasma phosphorus may be elevated, helping to differentiate idiopathic hypercalcemia from primary hyperparathyroidism. Renal calcification may occur and lead to renal failure and uremia. Metastatic calcifications are common and have been reported in widespread areas including the skin, cornea, joints, bursa, vasculature, thyroid, and pancreas. *Periarticular calcification,* particularly when excess vitamin D is given as a treatment for rheumatoid arthritis or gout, occurs. Calcium is then deposited in the tophi of gout. *Mild-alkali syndrome* may also be associated with extensive soft-tissue calcification, as well as renal calcification. Metastatic vascular calcifications in *cystic fibrosis* have been reported as a rare finding.

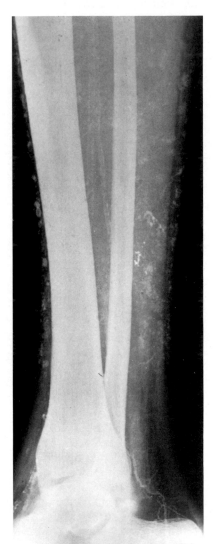

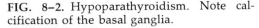

FIG. 8–1. Hyperparathyroidism. Extensive vascular and subcutaneous calcifications are present. Hyperparathyroidism was secondary to renal disease.

FIG. 8–2. Hypoparathyroidism. Note calcification of the basal ganglia.

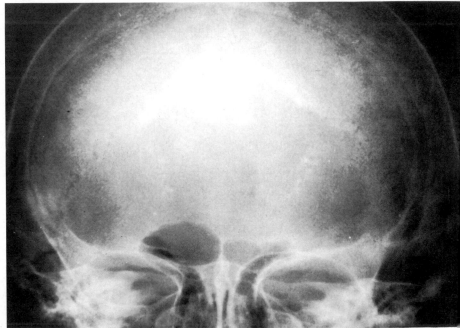

GENERALIZED CALCINOSIS

Calcinosis intersitialis universalis is a disease of unknown etiology, in which calcium is deposited subcutaneously and, later in the course of the disease, in deeper connective tissue. It occurs in younger individuals and is frequently progressive. It may lead to death. Calcium depositions occur as discrete conglomerations arranged in bands in the longitudinal direction of the limb (Fig. 8–3 *A*). Connective tissue associated with muscles, nerves, tendons, and joints becomes calcified (Fig. 8–3 *B, C*). The distal phalanges can also become calcified (Fig. 8–3 *D*). The serum calcium and phosphorus values are normal. Calcific nodules are seen in the skin. Ossification of calcified tissue does not occur.

Calcinosis circumscripta refers to localized calcific deposits in the skin and subcutaneous tissues, particularly of the hands and wrists. In about one-half of cases, it is associated with collagen disease, most often scleroderma. No underlying disease can be found in the remainder of cases.

Other diseases which may be associated with calcinosis circumscripta include rheumatoid arthritis, lupus erythematosus, and acrodermatitis atrophicans.

Scleroderma[32, 95] associated with calcinosis is known as the Thibierge–Weissenbach syndrome. Calcium deposition can occur in the fingertips (Figs. 8–4, 8–5), face, axilla, ulnar side of the arm or forearm (Fig. 8–6), subcutaneous tissues, pressure areas such as the ischial tuberosities and elbow, and muscles. Large areas of periarticular calcinosis may be present. Raynaud's phenomenon is often associated, frequently preceding calcinosis by many years. No consistent biochemical abnormality has been found. Visceral calcification may also occur. A related condition is CRST syndrome, comprising calcinosis, Raynaud's phenomenon, sclerodactyly, and telangiectasia.

Dermatomyositis[80] is associated with malignant tumors in a high percentage of adult patients. Subcutaneous calcification in the extremities, axilla (Fig. 8–7), inguinal area (Fig. 8–8), and abdominal wall (Fig. 8–9) may occur. Sometimes this calcification assumes a form more finely linear and streakier than that seen in scleroderma. It may become more globular as the disease progresses. Visceral calcification characteristically does not occur, nor does resorption of the terminal phalanges. Subcutaneous edema may be seen in early stages of the disease, and progresses to decreased muscle mass. Fibrosis leads to joint contractures and deformities. Osteoporosis results from disuse and steroid therapy. The calcification may regress.

Systemic lupus erythematosus is associated with calcinosis, although less frequently than dermatomyositis and scleroderma. Calcifications may be seen in the skin and deeper soft tissues as well as in relation to the peripheral vasculature.

Tumoral calcinosis[8,43,81,116] is a rare condition in which localized collections of calcium are found in the vicinity of joints. No other abnormality is present. The serum calcium and phosphorus levels are normal to slightly elevated. The etiology is unknown. The usual age incidence is from 6 to 25 years. Black people are most often affected. Single or multiple joints may be involved and there is a predilection for the hips, elbows, and shoulders. Although the lesions may be painless, pain, swelling, and disability are often present. Slowly growing calcific masses in the periarticular tissues of the large joints are seen. Small calcified nodules progress in size to large, solid, lobulated tumors with a linear, lacy calcific distribution (Fig. 8–10). The joint itself is not involved. In the elbow, the lower dorsal humerus is characteristically flattened. No obvious cause has been found. A case of huge symmetric lesions that showed fluid levels in the tumoral masses has been reported. These occurred in the scapular regions. The authors suggest that the etiology is chronic trauma in patients who may have an error of metabolism.[54] Similar calcific tumors may be seen in hyperparathyroidism and other causes of metastatic calcification.

DYSTROPHIC CALCIFICATION

Localized dystrophic calcification in soft tissue may occur in diseases such as Ehlers–Danlos syndrome, pseudoxanthoma elasticum and fibromatosis, or in various tumors, hematomas, in degenerative, necrotic, and postinflammatory foci, and in cartilaginous areas. The latter have a typical amorphous, flaky, mottled nodular appearance. It may also occur following physical, chemical, or thermal trauma (Fig. 8–11).

The differential diagnosis of common calcifications in specific structures is presented below.

(Text continued on p. 637)

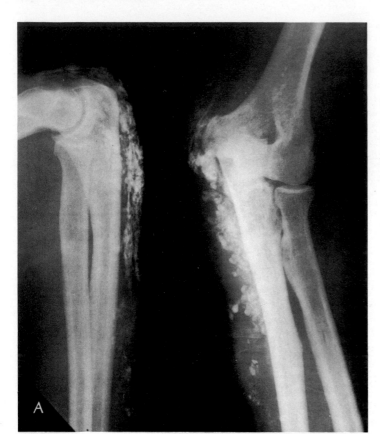

FIG. 8–3. Calcinosis universalis—female, age 24 years. **A.** Forearm. There are dense conglomerate and streaky calcifications in the soft tissues, arranged longitudinally in the direction of the long axis of the extremity. All laboratory values, including those for serum calcium, phosphorus, and alkaline phosphatase levels were normal. There was no evidence of collagen disease. **B.** Periarticular calcinosis about both knees. **C.** Periarticular calcification in the right hip, the left trochanteric region, and the left inguinal region. **D.** Calcification about the terminal tufts of several fingers and several other joints. Note that there is no evidence of resorption of the tufts, as would be expected in scleroderma.

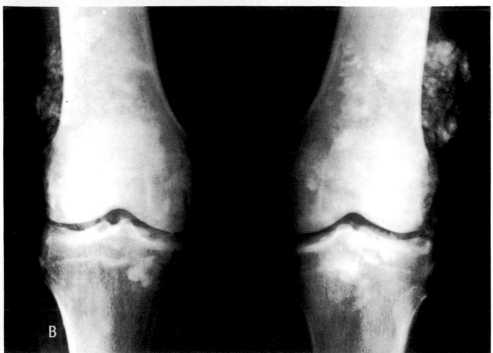

(Continued)

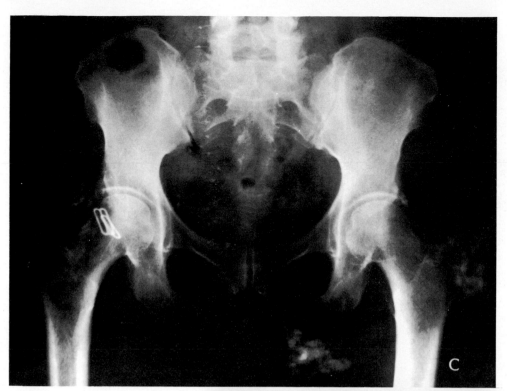

C

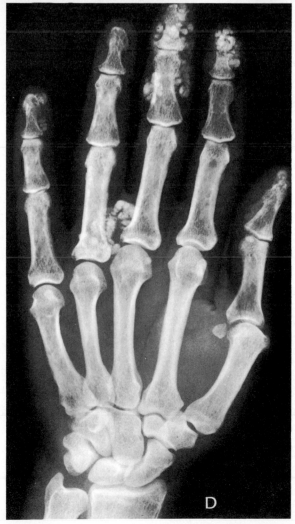

D

633

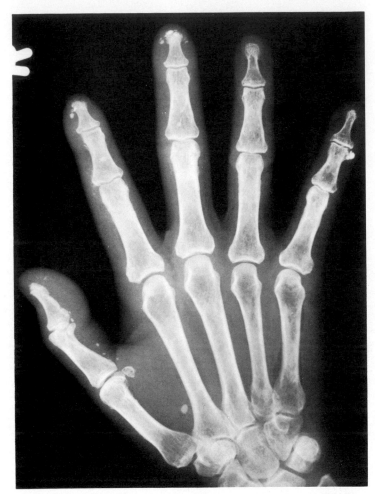

FIG. 8–4. Scleroderma (hand). There is slight resorption of the terminal phalangeal tufts, and slight calcification at several tufts and along the interphalangeal joints. This represents the Thibierge-Weissenbach syndrome.

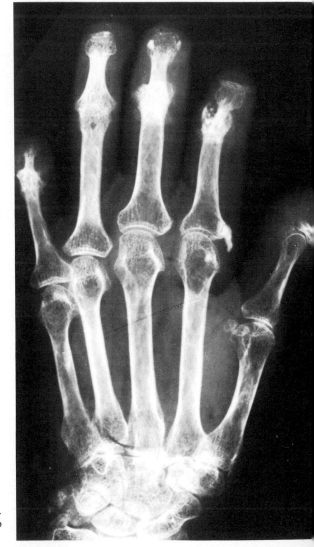

FIG. 8–5. Scleroderma. Severe resorption of the terminal phalanges. Osteoporosis and several small areas of calcification are also present.

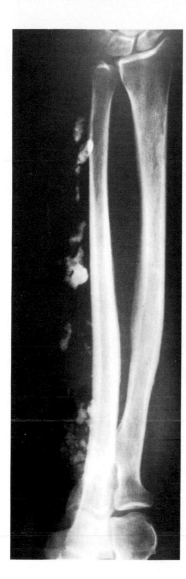

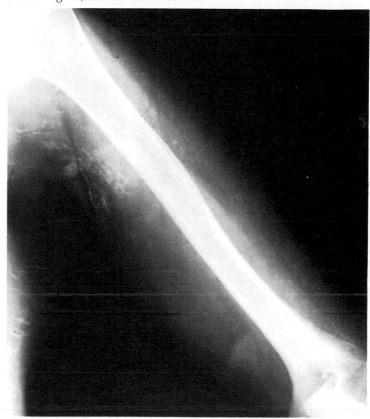

FIG. 8–6. Scleroderma (forearm). Note relatively large conglomerations of calcium in the soft tissue at the ulnar aspect of the forearm.

FIG. 8–7. Dermatomyositis. Exceptionally fine streaky calcification is visible in the axilla (extending down the arm), in the elbow region, and in the chest wall.

FIG. 8–8. Dermatomyositis. Note fine, reticular, subcutaneous calcification at the lateral aspect of the right thigh, and fine linear calcifications in both inguinal regions. This patient definitely never had a lymphangiogram.

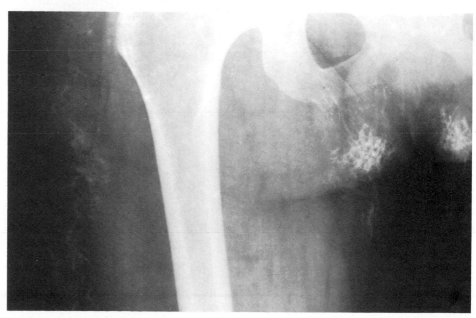

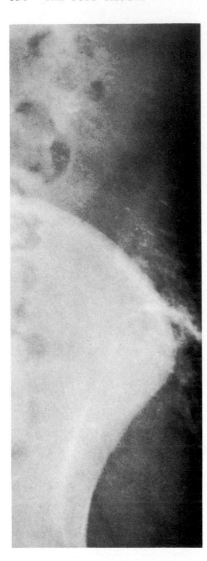

FIG. 8–9. Dermatomyositis. Note fine, streaky, linear calcification of the abdominal wall.

FIG. 8–10. Tumoral calcinosis (left thigh). Very extensive soft-tissue calcification is noted. (Courtesy of Dr. Dharmashi V. Bhate, VA Hospital, Hines, IL)

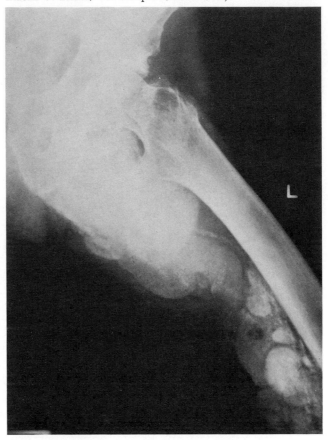

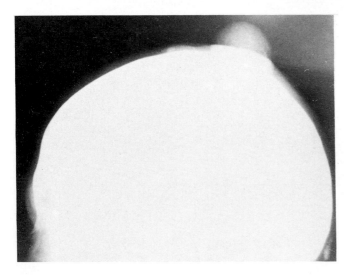

FIG. 8–11. Cutaneous metastases from carcinoma of the breast. One large and two smaller soft-tissue masses are seen in the scalp, containing amorphous dystrophic calcifications.

DIFFERENTIAL DIAGNOSIS OF CALCIFICATIONS IN SPECIFIC STRUCTURES

A. Arteries (Early or Extensive Calcification)
   1. Diabetes mellitus (Fig. 8–12)
   2. Hyperparathyroidism (primary and secondary)
   3. Renal rickets
   4. Hypervitaminosis D
   5. Atherosclerosis
   6. Homocystinuria
   7. Cushing's syndrome
   8. Nephropathies
   9. Moenckeberg's sclerosis
   10. Associated with hydramnios in infants
   11. Cystic fibrosis (rare)
B. Veins
   1. Phleboliths
   2. Phleboliths in hemangiomas (Fig. 8–13)
   3. Phleboliths following radiation therapy
   4. Calcified thrombi
C. Nerves
   1. Leprosy[107]
   2. Neurofibromatosis
D. Lymph Nodes
   1. Tuberculosis (Fig. 8–14)
   2. BCG
   3. Histoplasmosis
   4. Coccidioidomycosis
   5. Filaria bancrofti
   6. Immature metastasis from osteosarcoma (rare) (Fig. 7–6)
   7. Metastases, especially from thyroid carcinoma
   8. Malignant lymphoma, postradiation therapy
E. Tendons
   1. Peritendinitis calcaria
   2. Pellegrini–Stieda disease (can ossify) (Fig. 8–15)
   3. Calcinosis universalis
   4. Pseudogout
   5. Ochronosis
   6. De Quervain's disease (rarely, calcification in tendons of abductor pollicis longus and extensor pollicis brevis)
   7. Calcified ganglion (rare) (Fig. 8–16)
   8. Multiple tendon calcification.[11]
F. Bursa
   1. Calcific bursitis
   2. Long-standing gout
   3. Pseudogout
   4. Bursal osteochondromatosis[104]

   5. Hypervitaminosis D
   6. Calcinosis
G. Ligaments
   1. Degenerative
   2. Ankylosing spondylitis
   3. Idiopathic (Fig. 8–17)
   4. Fluorosis
   5. Renal osteodystrophy
   6. Cooper's ligament (physiologic)[102]
H. Muscle (Not Ossification)
   1. Scleroderma
   2. Postpyogenic myositis
   3. Postcarbon monoxide poisoning
   4. Calcinosis universalis
   5. Ochronosis
   6. Volkmann's contracture
   7. Parasites
      a) *Cysticercus cellulosae* (larval form of *Taenia sodium.* (Fig. 8–18)
      b) Hydatid disease (due to *Taenia echinococcus*)
      c) *Filaria bancrofti*
      d) Trichinosis (1 mm or less, too small to be detected radiologically)
      e) Schistosomiasis
      f) *Armillifer armillatus* (comma-shaped; intraperitoneal)
I. Calcified Intervertebral Discs
   1. Idiopathic (also in children)[72]
   2. Posttraumatic
   3. Ochronosis (lamellar)
   4. Pseudogout (only in annulus fibrosus, not in nucleus pulposus)
   5. Hypervitaminosis D (annulus fibrosus)
   6. Ankylosing spondylitis (Fig. 8–19)
J. Articular Cartilage
   1. Gout
   2. Hyperparathyroidism[110] (Fig. 2–51)
   3. Pseudogout (Fig. 9–181, 9–182, 9–183)
   4. Degenerative (Fig. 8–20)
   5. Ochronosis
   6. Hemochromatosis
K. Subcutaneous
   1. All above causes of generalized interstitial calcinosis
   2. Calcinosis interstitialis circumscripta
   3. Subcutaneous fat necrosis[97] (Fig. 8–21)
   4. Rheumatoid arthritis (rare)
   5. Following thermal injuries
   6. "Turtle-egg tumors" following quinine and camphor injections[101]
   7. Varicose veins
   8. Venous thrombosis
   9. Pseudogout

10. Ehlers–Danlos syndrome
11. Congenital scattered fibromatosis[24]
12. Differentiate calcification from heavy metal and Thorotrast deposits
13. Extravasation of calcium gluconate[10]

L. Periarticular
1. Hyperparathyroidism
2. Hypoparathyroidism
3. Hypervitaminosis D
   a) with gout
   b) with rheumatoid arthritis
4. Scleroderma
5. Dermatomyositis
6. Ochronosis
7. Adult diabetes
8. Tuberculosis
9. Calcinosis universalis interstitialis
10. Immature myositis ossificans
11. Synovioma
12. Pseudogout
13. Metastatic calcification
14. Tumoral calcinosis

M. Intra-articular
1. Osteochondromatosis
2. Synovioma
3. Calcific synovitis
4. Intracapsular chondroma
5. Hyperparathyroidism
6. Hypervitaminosis D
7. Posttraumatic
8. Hydroxyapatite deposition disease

N. Fingertips
1. Scleroderma (Figs. 8–4, 8–5)
2. Rothmund's syndrome[66]
3. Calcinosis interstitiasis universalis (Fig. 8–3 D)
4. Acrosclerosis
5. Raynaud's syndrome
6. Dermatomyositis
7. Lupus erythematosus
8. Epidermolysis bullosa[39]
9. CRST syndrome

O. Pinna of Ear[67,71]
1. Acromegaly (Fig. 5–112)
2. Addison's disease
3. Allergies
4. Collagen diseases
5. Diabetes mellitus
6. Familial cold hypersensitivity
7. Frostbite
8. Hypercalcemia
9. Hypertension
10. Hyperthyroidism
11. Hypopituitarism
12. Idiopathic causes
13. Inflammatory lesions
14. Luetic perichondritis
15. Ochronosis
16. Sarcoidosis
17. Trauma
18. Von Meyenburg's disease (systemic chondromalacia)

(Text continued on p. 643)

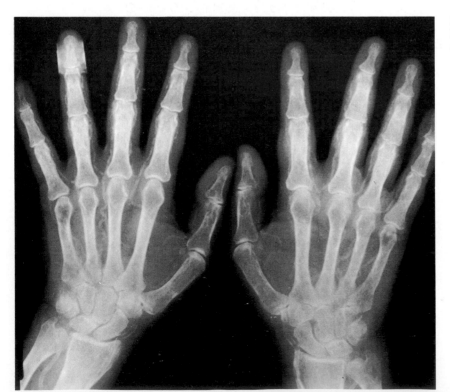

FIG. 8–12. Diabetes mellitus (hands). Note extensive vascular calcification, and osteoporosis.

FIG. 8–13. Hemangiomatosis. Large area of soft-tissue irregularity is apparent. The several small, rounded, calcific densities in the soft tissues, with dense rims, represent phleboliths.

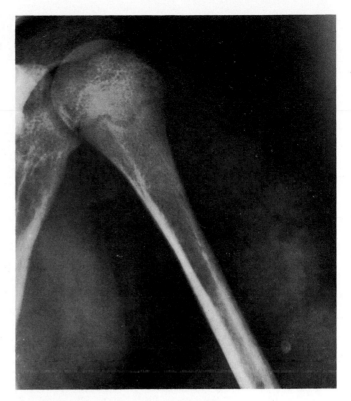

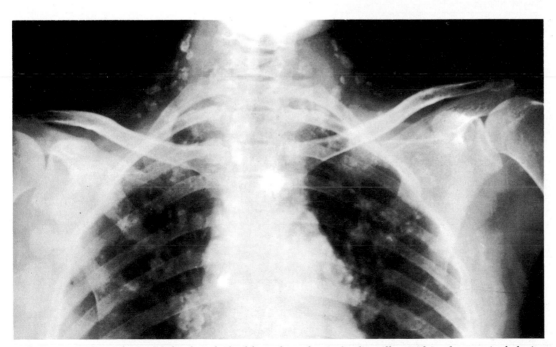

FIG. 8–14. Tuberculosis. Multiple calcified lymph nodes in both axillae and in the cervical chain may be seen. Also note hilar nodes and pulmonary calcification.

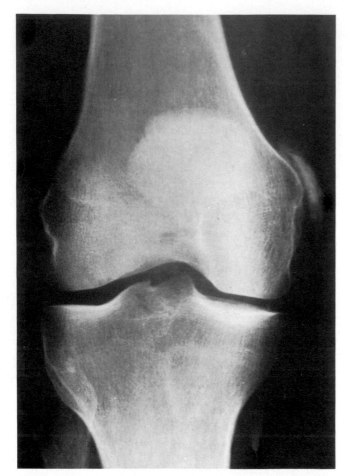

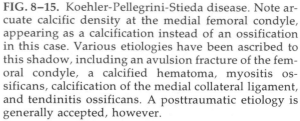

FIG. 8–15. Koehler-Pellegrini-Stieda disease. Note arcuate calcific density at the medial femoral condyle, appearing as a calcification instead of an ossification in this case. Various etiologies have been ascribed to this shadow, including an avulsion fracture of the femoral condyle, a calcified hematoma, myositis ossificans, calcification of the medial collateral ligament, and tendinitis ossificans. A posttraumatic etiology is generally accepted, however.

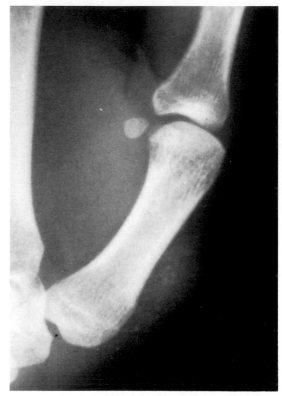

FIG. 8–16. Calcified ganglion adjacent to the first metacarpal. This represents a rare manifestation of a common finding. Small stippled calcifications are seen with a soft-tissue mass. (Courtesy of Dr. Raphael Gomez, Miami, FL)

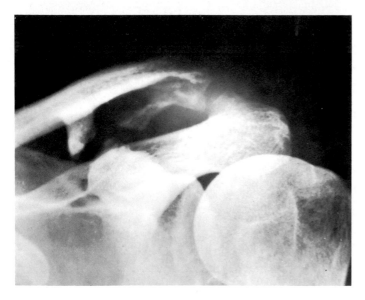

FIG. 8–17. Idiopathic calcification of the coracoclavicular ligament. The coracoacromial ligament is also calcified.

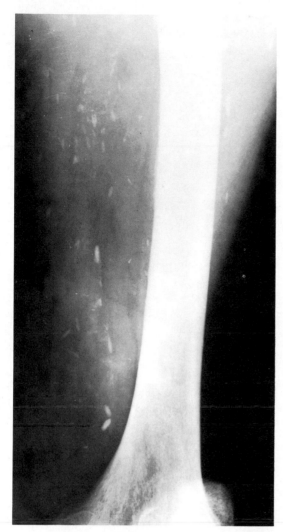

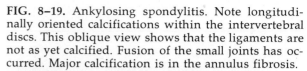

FIG. 8–18. Calcifications in the soft tissue of the thigh due to Cysticercus cellulosae. Note ovoid calcifications about 1 cm long, their long axes paralleling the long axis of the limb.

FIG. 8–19. Ankylosing spondylitis. Note longitudinally oriented calcifications within the intervertebral discs. This oblique view shows that the ligaments are not as yet calcified. Fusion of the small joints has occurred. Major calcification is in the annulus fibrosis.

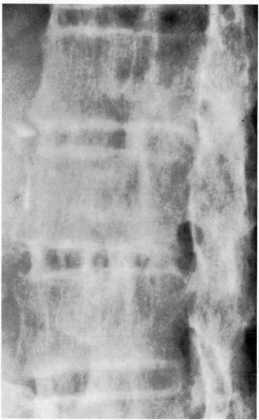

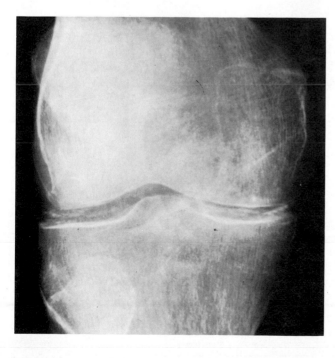

FIG. 8–20. Degenerative calcification of the articular cartilage of the knee in a male, age 87 years.

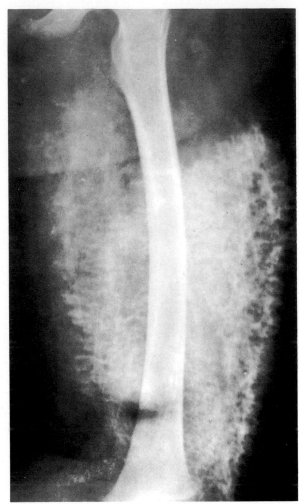

FIG. 8–21. Subcutaneous fat necrosis of the thigh. An envelope of subcutaneous calcification with a fine reticular appearance surrounds the thigh.

FIG. 8–22. Myositis ossificans. An ill-defined, cloudlike calcification at the lateral aspect of the femoral shaft may be seen.

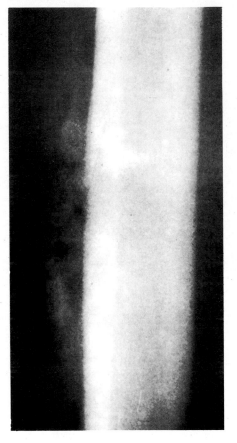

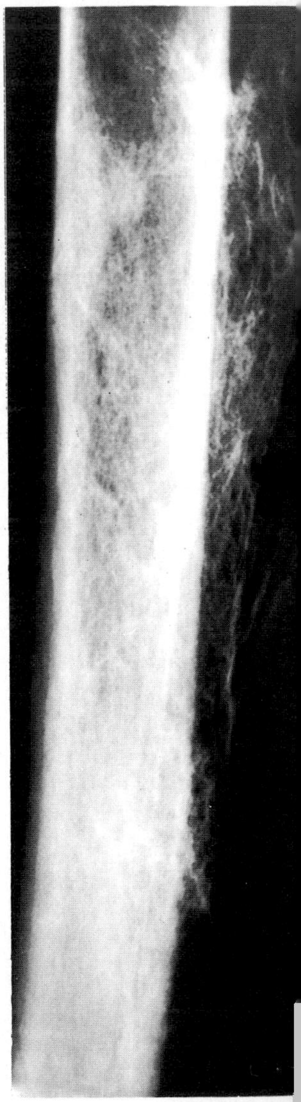

FIG. 8–23. Myositis ossificans. A veillike envelope of fine new bone may be seen surrounding a portion of the femoral shaft. The bone is organized into cortex and trabeculae and lies along the muscle axis.

OSSIFICATION IN THE SOFT TISSUES

MYOSITIS OSSIFICANS

Myositis ossificans refers to heterotopic soft-tissue ossification that can have several etiologies. It is thought not to be due to muscle inflammation, but to metaplasia of intermuscular connective tissue. The initial roentgen appearance is an ill-defined calcification (Fig. 8–22) that matures to organization into trabeculae and cortex (Fig. 8–23). The ectopic bone may lie along the axis of involved muscles, and may or may not be attached to regional bone. The periosteum adjacent to the ossification may or may not show reaction. In early stages, a radiolucent zone of soft tissue may separate the lesion from the underlying periosteal reaction and cortex. Bone erosion and blending of the new bone with the cortex can occur. Localized myositis ossificans must be differentiated from parosteal sarcoma, which in its early stages has a thin radiolucent periosteal line separating tumor from cortex. Myositis ossificans may be of three different etiologies.

Progressive myositis ossificans is a genetic dysplasia in which congenital osseous abnormalities are associated with an inexorable progressive soft-tissue ossification. There is usually hypoplasia of the phalanges of the thumbs (Fig. 5–95), the first metacarpals, and the phalanges of the great toes. Some cases have also shown hypoplasia of the middle phalanges of the little fingers. Ossification may be present at the end of the first year of life. This may be preceded by an inflammatory reaction, followed by necrosis and ossification of connective tissue and muscle. The neck and back are usually initially involved, progressing to generalized skeletal involvement and ankylosis of joints (Figs. 5–98, 5–99).

Myositis ossificans associated with neurological disease[41] may be due to a variety of conditions. These have been summarized (below) by Voss.[111]

NEUROLOGICAL CAUSES OF MYOSITIS OSSIFICANS*

I. Brain Diseases and Cerebral Hemiplegia
 1. Epidemic encephalitis
 2. Progressive paralysis
 3. Syphilis of central nervous system
 4. Arteriosclerotic bleeding and thrombosis
 5. Embolic encephalitis
 6. Posttraumatic brain lesions
 7. Brain hemorrhage with intracranial hemangioma
 8. Cerebral hemiplegia of unknown etiology
II. Diseases of the Spinal Cord
 1. Meningocele
 2. Traumatic section of cord
 3. Extramedullary tumor
 4. Myeloencephalitis
 5. Syphilitic meningomyelitis
 6. Tuberculous meningomyelitis
 7. Acute anterior poliomyelitis
 8. Funicular myelosis with circumscript thrombosis
 9. Tabes dorsalis
 10. Syringomyelia
III. Diseases of the Cauda Equina
 1. Compression of the cauda equina
IV. Diseases of the Peripheral Nerves
 1. Polyneuritis
V. Tetanus[38, 74]

Extensive soft-tissue ossifications are present, particularly in the para-articular regions, leading to ankylosis. There are no accompanying bone lesions other than disuse osteoporosis and bone erosions. The periosteum shows no reaction. The area of ossification may blend with and obscure the cortex. Erosive lesions develop at bony prominences such as the trochanters and ischia. The greater trochanter loses its outward bulge and becomes flattened (Fig. 8–24). Ossification may form rapidly. Myositis ossificans develops below the level of the neurological lesion.

Myositis ossificans posttraumatica or *circumscripta*[78, 84] is localized ossification caused by acute or chronic trauma. A soft-tissue mass is present soon after injury. After about 1 month, flocculent densities within the mass and periosteal reaction are seen. After 6 to 8 weeks a lacy pattern of bone circumscribed by a cortex appears. Myositis about the elbow joint is particularly common (Fig. 8–25). The ectopic bone may lie parallel to the bone shaft (Fig. 8–26) or along the axis of a muscle in a feathery pattern. The best known example of heterotopic bone caused by chronic trauma is "rider's bone" or ossification of the adductor longus muscle. Ossification may occur in the brachialis, the soleus, and in other locations. Similar localized changes may be

---

* Modified from Voss H: Fortschr Roentgenstr 55:423–441, 1937

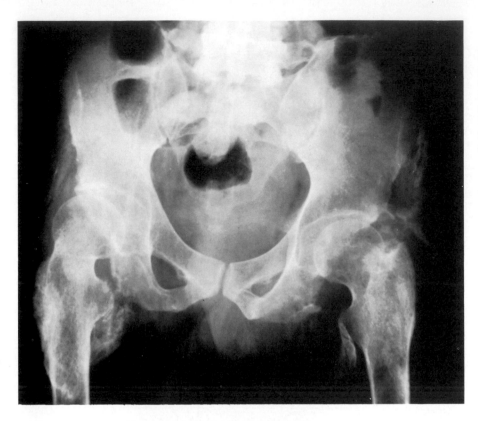

FIG. 8–24. Myositis ossificans in a paraplegic. Extensive soft-tissue ossification at the lateral aspects of the pelvis and about the hip joints may be seen. Note resorption of both greater trochanters, with flattening of their contour, and resorption at both ischia.

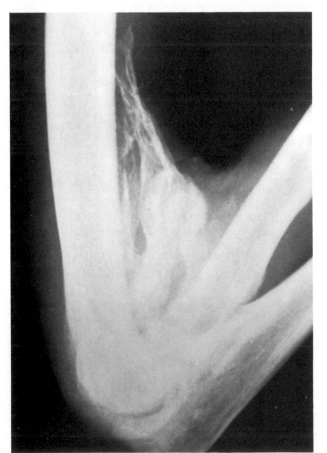

FIG. 8–25. Posttraumatic myositis ossificans of the elbow. The elbow joint is fixed in flexion and there is ectopic bone formation parallel to the muscles of the distal humerus.

FIG. 8–26. Myositis ossificans—posttraumatic. An area of ectopic bone at the anterior aspect is visible; the superior portion is beginning to blend with the cortex. The long axis of the ectopic bone lies parallel to the muscle plane. A hole from traction device may be seen at the distal femoral shaft.

FIG. 8–27. A small mature focus of myositis ossificans is noted in the foot between the third and fourth toes, showing definite organization into cortex and trabeculae, and eroding the shaft of contiguous proximal phalanges.

seen without a definitive history of trauma (Fig. 8–27). A true ossifying hematoma in the thigh has been reported[117] with a large, ovoid, ossified mass, remote from bone, with a thin cortical shell, and containing central areas of hemorrhage. Angiographic differentiation from a malignant lesion rests on absence of arteriovenous shunting, venous laking, and vessel amputations in myositis ossificans circumscripta.[44] In the active stage fine vessels cause a diffuse stain. In the healing stage the lesions are usually avascular.[115] Drug-induced myositis ossificans circumscripta due to attempts at injection of narcotics into the antecubital vein has been reported.[22] Myositis ossificans, particularly mul-

tiple areas in patients with partial clotting factor deficiencies, has been reported.[48]

TUMORAL OSSIFICATIONS OF SOFT TISSUE

Osteosarcoma developing in the soft tissues[29,51,61] is a very rare but well-documented entity. It may develop *de novo* or it may occur as a late complication of radiation therapy. It has been reported as developing in the heart, lungs, pulmonary artery, pleura, breast,[5] uterus,[50] retroperitoneum, and soft tissues of the neck, extremities, or trunk. Some of these tumors arising in organs may represent malignant growth of a single component of a teratoma.

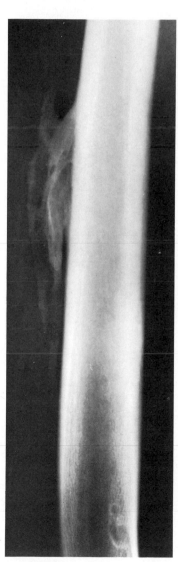

FIG. 8–26

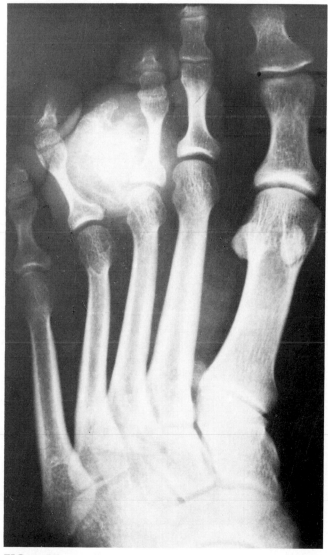

FIG. 8–27

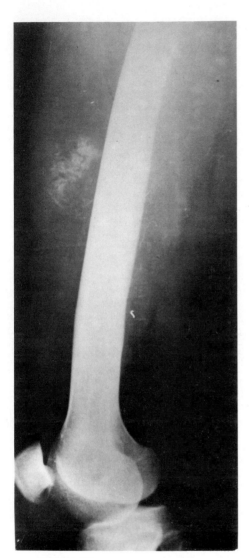

FIG. 8–28.

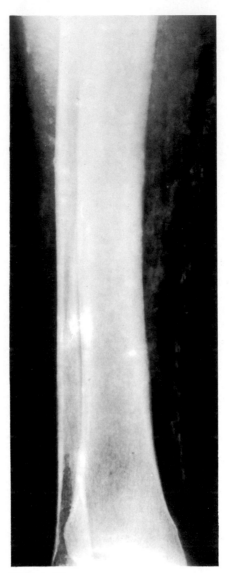

FIG. 8–29.

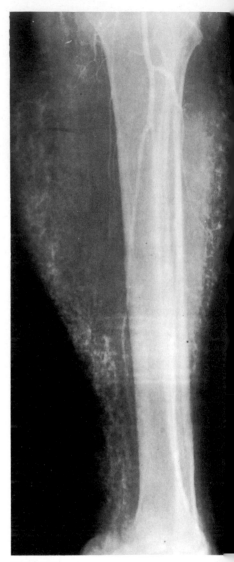

FIG. 8–30.

FIG. 8–28. Soft-tissue osteosarcoma. A soft-tissue mass in the midanterior thigh is noted, containing amorphous calcification with peripheral streaking. A thin calcific rim at its inferior margin is also noted. (Courtesy of Drs. A. Pizarro and T. F. Kurtz, VA Hospital, Hines, IL)

FIG. 8–29. Varicose veins. Note extensive subcutaneous ossification with a nodular and fibrillar pattern.

FIG. 8–30. Venous thrombosis. There is massive edema of the leg associated with a fine fibrillar pattern of subcutaneous ossification. Arteriogram shows patency of the arterial system.

The age group tends to be older than in osteosarcoma of bone, with a reported age range from 8 to 70 years, but the disease is rare in the first two decades of life. The site of involvement in 90% of cases is in the extremities, most commonly the lower extremities.

Radiologically, a soft-tissue mass that may attain a size of up to 10 cm is seen. Varying amounts of streaky radiopacity may be seen. The opacification may be fuzzy and show some spiculation at its periphery (Fig. 8–28).

The adjacent bone may be secondarily invaded. This condition can be differentiated from an osteosarcoma of bone invading the soft tissues by a saucerized cortical defect, indicating an external origin. At this stage, radiological differentiation from a parosteal sarcoma may be difficult.

In the differential diagnosis several entities must be considered. A soft-tissue density showing radiopacity should be classified into lesions showing calcification or lesions showing ossification. Ossification can be determined by the recognition of organization into cortex and trabecular pattern, although in early stages and in undifferentiated lesions this may be very difficult.

Calcifications would include metastatic calcification, calcinosis, and dystrophic calcification.

Of the lesions that show true ossification, a pseudomalignant osseous soft-tissue tumor should first be considered. Myositis ossificans circumscripta should also be considered. These two entities may be related.

Streaky opacity may also be seen in soft-tissue fibrosarcomas, liposarcomas, and lipomas[75] (see Fig. 8–35). A chondrosarcoma characteristically shows amorphous spotty or streaky calcification.

Heterotopic bone-forming metastases have been reported from carcinoma of the colon, breast, and urinary tract.[21] These lesions are associated with bone destruction and adjacent soft-tissue ossification.

Pseudomalignant osseous tumor of soft tissue[20,31,47] is a rare tumor occurring in young adults and adolescents. Females are more often affected than males. There is a predilection for the soft tissues of the lower extremities. The tumor usually attains a size of not larger than 3 cm. The lesion exhibits a zone phenomenon with a periphery of mature bone, which under favorable circumstances can be detected roentgenologically. There is no antecedent trauma, as is present with localized myositis ossificans. Posttraumatic myositis ossificans will mature and growth will stop, a situation that does not occur with pseudomalignant tumor. Fine and Stout,[29] however, consider this entity to represent an atypical form of myositis ossificans.

MISCELLANEOUS SOFT-TISSUE OSSIFICATIONS

Varicose veins can be associated with subcutaneous ossification. This is seen radiographically as ranging from small subcutaneous ossicles to a dense meshwork of fine osseous fibrils (Fig. 8–29). Periosteal elevated new bone formation of regional bones is usually present. *Thrombophlebitis* causing subcutaneous ossification of the leg in a 6-month-old infant has been cited by Caffey.[18] It is said to have been due to metaplasia and not fat necrosis. *Venous thrombosis* may also be associated with subcutaneous ossifications (Fig. 8–30). *Ossification in scars* has been reported. *Melorheostosis*, in addition to the dense bone lesions, may have soft-tissue inflammatory involvement. Calcification and ossification may also be present.

RADIOLOGY AND THE DIAGNOSIS OF SOFT-TISSUE TUMORS[2,65,86,98]

All soft-tissue tumors are of unit or water density except:

1. Tumors with fat content (more radiolucent)
2. Masses with hemosiderin content (dense)
3. Long-standing, large tophi (may rarely calcify)
4. Masses with calcification or ossification

A definitive diagnosis on the basis of roentgen features alone is not possible, therefore, in the majority of cases. The location, size, and distribution of these tumors can usually be accurately determined. The fat, hemosiderin, and calcium content can also be specified. The behavior of the tumor with respect to bone (*i.e.*, saucerization, erosion or invasion, and sclerotic reaction) can be seen. Infiltration of a fatty tumor along muscle planes can be determined. Specific characteristics, such as phleboliths and bone formation, are important clues to the identity of a tumor.

Tumor vascularity can be studied by angiography. The angiographic picture correlates with histological vascularity, and a characteristic pattern of malignancy may be seen, but it is hazardous to attempt to specify a cell type on the basis of an angiogram.

Computed tomography[112] of soft-tissue tumors in the extremities is of value both for anatomical localization and for the prediction of histology. The preoperative delineation of tumor margins, their relationship to fascial planes, the proximity to neighboring bones, muscles, nerves, and blood ves-

(Text continued on p. 650)

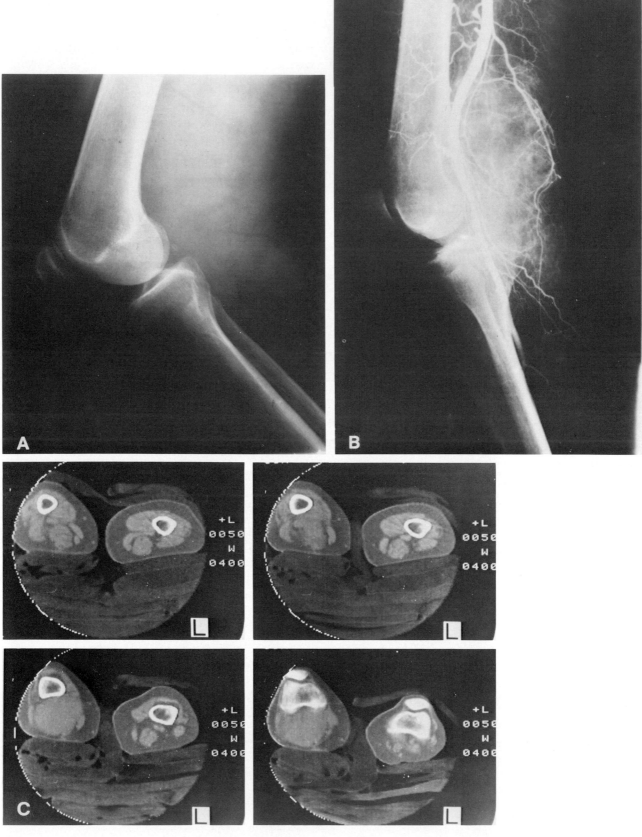

FIG. 8-31. Undifferentiated soft-tissue sarcoma in the popliteal area in a 70-year-old male. **A.** Lateral view of the knee shows soft-tissue swelling posteriorly. **B.** Angiogram shows anterior displacement of the popliteal artery, a large soft-tissue mass showing tumor vessels, and puddling of contrast material. **C.** CT scan showing a large soft-tissue mass of muscle density posterior to the knee joint. (Courtesy of Dr. J.P. Petasnick, Rush–Presbyterian St. Luke's Hospital, Chicago, IL)

FIG. 8–32. CT scan of thighs. **A.** Preinfusion. A large soft-tissue mass containing several low-density areas is seen on the right. **B.** Postinfusion. Irregular, patchy enhancement is present. On biopsy, this lesion proved to be an undifferentiated sarcoma.

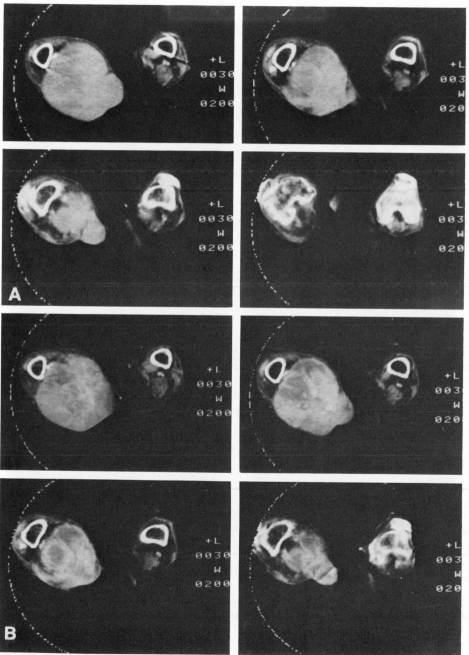

sels can best be demonstrated by the cross-sectional view that this modality permits. More sensitive definition of the density of the tumor matrix is possible by this method than by conventional tomography or xeroradiography (Figs. 8-31 *A-C*, 8-32 *A*, *B*).

The types of soft-tissue tumors are listed below.

SOFT-TISSUE PRIMARY TUMORS

I. Tumors of Muscle
   1. Leiomyoma[34]
   2. Leiomyosarcoma
   3. Rhabdomyosarcoma[26] (Fig. 8-33)
     a) Embryonal
     b) Alveolar
     c) Pleomorphic

II. Tumors of Fat
   1. Lipoma (Figs. 8-34, 8-35)
     a) Infiltrating angiolipoma[33]
     b) Lipoma arborescens[113]
   2. Hibernoma
   3. Liposarcoma[88] (Figs. 8-36, 8-37
     a) Well-differentiated myxoid
     b) Round-cell type
     c) Well-differentiated type
     d) Pleomorphic type
   4. Lipoblastoma[56]

III. Tumors of Connective Tissue
   1. Fibromatoses[27,36,49]
   2. Desmoid
   3. Quasi-neoplastic benign proliferations of connective tissue
     a) Nodular pseudosarcomatous fasciitis
     b) Juvenile xanthogranuloma
     c) Proliferative myositis
   4. Fibrosarcoma (Figs. 8-38, 8-39)
   5. Fibroxanthosarcoma[17]

IV. Tumors of Nerve and Supportive Tissue
   1. Neuroma
   2. Neurilemmoma
   3. Malignant schwannoma
   4. Neurofibroma (Figs. 8-40, 8-41)
   5. Neurofibrosarcoma (Figs. 8-42, 8-43)
   6. Ganglioneuroma (Fig. 8-44 *A, B*)

V. Tumors of Vessels
   1. Hemangioma (Figs. 8-45, 8-46)
   2. Hemangiosarcoma
   3. Hemangioendothelioma
   4. Hemangiopericytoma
   5. Lymphangioma (Fig. 8-47)

VI. Tumors of Mesothelium
   1. Synovioma (Figs. 8-48, 9-211)
     a) Pseudoglandular
     b) Fibrosarcoma
     c) Endothelioid

   2. Pigmented villonodular synovitis

VII. Tumors of Uncertain and Mixed Tissue Origin
   1. Granular cell myoblastoma (Fig. 8-49)
   2. Alveolar soft-part tumor
   3. Mesenchymoma (Fig. 8-50)
   4. Malignant fibrous histiocytoma[99]
   5. Soft-tissue Ewing's sarcoma[4]

VIII. Soft-Tissue Osteosarcoma and Chondrosarcoma.

IX. Others (Including processes that may mimic tumors)
   1. Metastases (Fig. 8-51)
   2. Inflammatory mass[108]
   3. Dermatological conditions
   4. Hematoma (Fig. 8-52)
   5. Secondary invasion from bone
   6. Bursal swelling (including iliopsoas bursa)
   7. Aneurysms
   8. Arteriovenous malformations or fistulae[12]
   9. Gardner's syndrome[91] (familial subcutaneous tumors, osteomas, and colonic polyps)
  10. Accessory muscle mass
  11. Endometrioma of limb[79]
  12. Ganglion
  13. Xanthomatosis of tendons[83] (can be associated with familial hypercholesterolemia)
  14. Hyperkeratosis and warts (Figs. 8-53, 8-54)
  15. Malignant teratoma
  16. Parosteal (nodular) fasciitis of the hand[68]

Cavernous hemangioma (see Figs. 8-45, 8-46) is not an uncommon soft-tissue tumor of the extremities, with predilections for sites distal to the elbow and knee. *Radiologically*, lobulated soft-tissue masses that may contain phleboliths are seen. The regional bone may be deformed and overgrown. If associated with enchondromatosis it is known as *Maffucci's syndrome. Giant-cell tumor of a tendon sheath*, or *fibroxanthoma*, is a common soft-tissue swelling seen most often in the hand, foot, wrist, or ankle. Erosion of an adjacent bone may occur.

The most common soft-tissue malignant neoplasms reported in AFIP material[65] are *liposarcomas*, which are most frequently encountered in the fifth decade. In the extremities, the most common type is the well-differentiated myxoid, which has a predilection for the medial thigh and popliteal area.

Lipoblastomatosis[56] is an unusual benign neoplastic condition of embryonal fat. It occurs most fre-

(Text continued on p. 661)

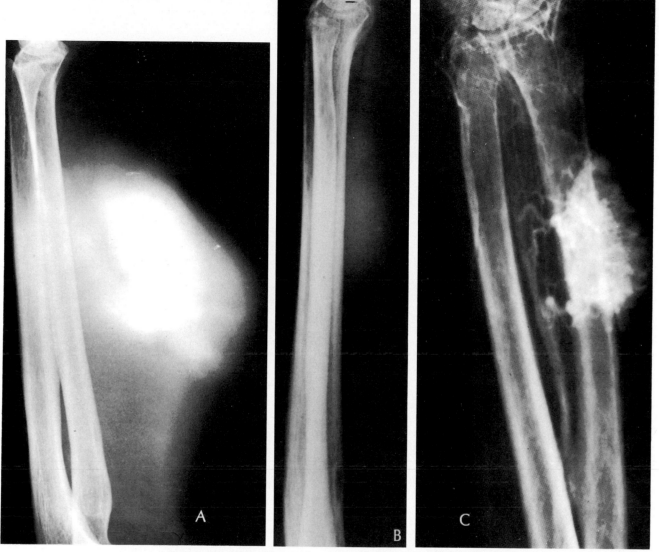

FIG. 8–33. Rhabdomyosarcoma. **A.** A large, lobulated soft-tissue mass without calcification may be seen. No bone involvement is present. **B.** Nine-month interval film following surgery. Soft-tissue mass has recurred at the distal aspect of the forearm. The bone is not invaded, but spotty osteoporosis is present. **C.** Arteriogram, taken on same day as **B**. There is persistence of contrast material in a large vascularized area corresponding to the limits of recurrent tumor.

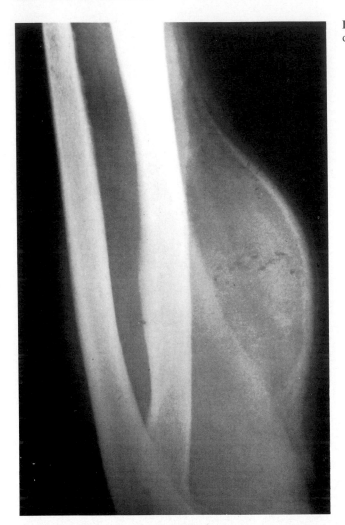

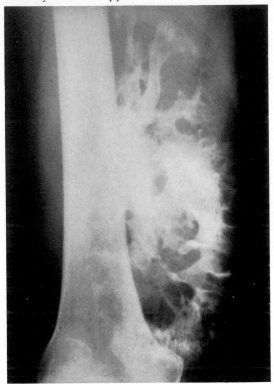

FIG. 8–34. Lipoma of the forearm. Note radiolucent ovoid mass between soft-tissue planes.

FIG. 8–35. Lipoma of the thigh, containing extensive ossification. The radiolucent character of the fatty tissue is apparent.

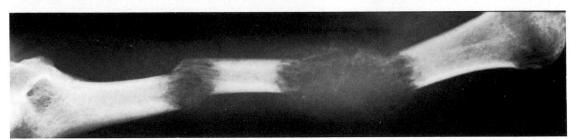

FIG. 8–36. Metastases to the humerus from a primary liposarcoma of the thigh. Several osteolytic areas may be seen. The large, proximal, osteolytic area has an expansile "blowout" appearance, and the large distal area shows a pathological fracture.

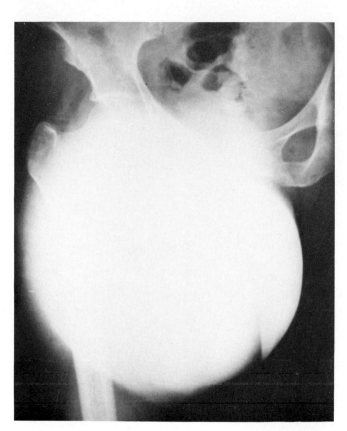

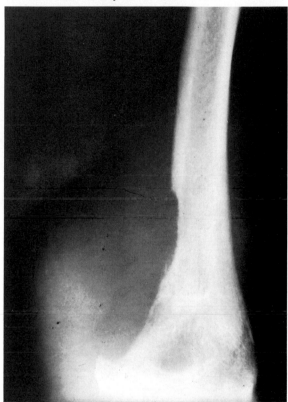

FIG. 8–37. Liposarcoma (thigh). A huge soft-tissue mass, which has not invaded the bone, is seen in the thigh. No fat density can be ascertained. The patient later developed extensive pulmonary metastases.

FIG. 8–38. Fibrosarcoma of the distal arm which has invaded the distal humerus and caused cortical destruction. No calcifications within the soft-tissue mass are apparent. The mass is not encapsulated or delimited. The cortex along the entire area of involvement is destroyed.

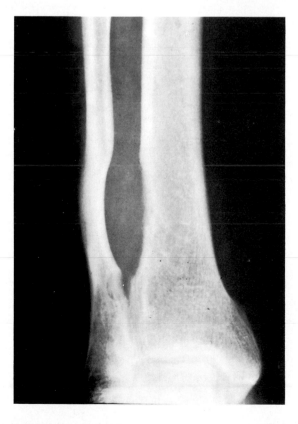

FIG. 8–39. Small fibrosarcoma of the distal leg. There is pressure deformity of the fibula and invasion of a portion of the distal tibial cortex, with cortical destruction.

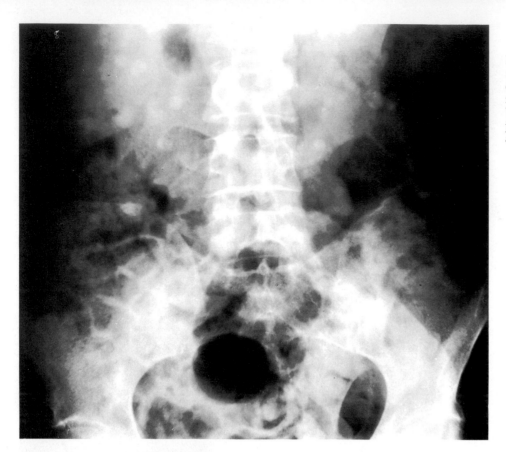

FIG. 8–40. Neurofibromatosis. Multiple small rounded densities of various sizes, representing skin neurofibromas, may be seen projected over the abdomen and abdominal wall.

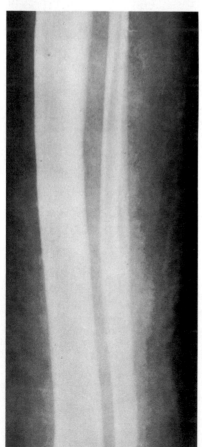

FIG. 8–41. Neurofibromatosis. There is marked soft-tissue enlargement due to plexiform neurofibroma. Mild tibial and fibular scoliosis is also present.

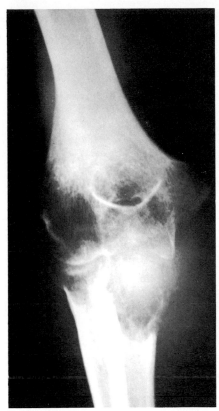

FIG. 8–42. Neurofibrosarcoma. Invasion and destruction of the proximal ulna is present. Lobulated soft-
tissue masses at the distal arm may
also be seen.

FIG. 8–43. Neurofibrosarcoma. Extensive destruction in the sacroiliac
region is present. Note several skin neurofibromas and a soft-tissue mass
in the pelvis.

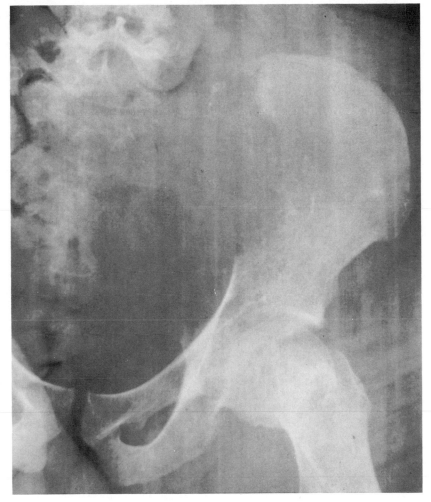

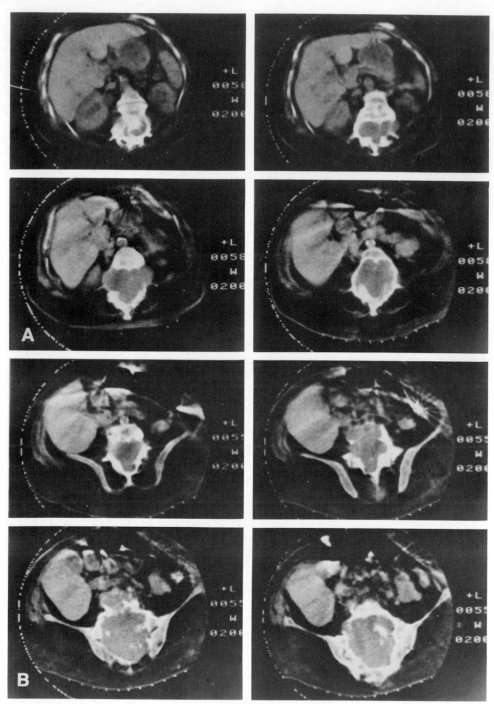

FIG. 8–44. A, B. CT scans of the lumbar spine. A large, long-segment expansile mass in the canal is noted, which on biopsy proved to be a ganglioneuroma.

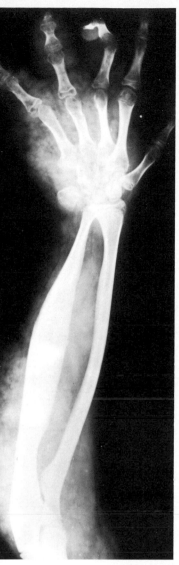
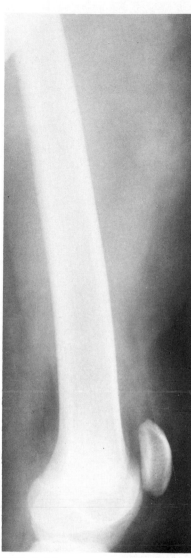

FIG. 8–45. Hemangioma (forearm and hand). Note soft-tissue swelling, with small irregular lobulations. The bones are deformed and the ulna has a fusiform contour. Several phleboliths are also present.

FIG. 8–46. Hemangioma of the thigh. Lateral view of the femur showing extensive lobulated soft-tissue masses.

FIG. 8–45   FIG. 8–46

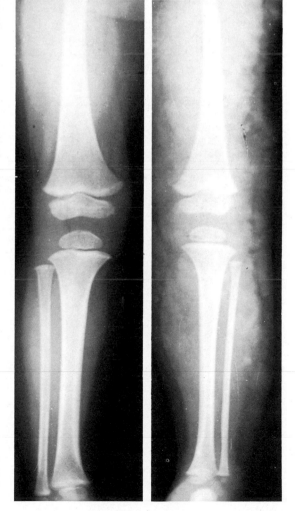

FIG. 8–47. Lymphangioma. Lobular soft-tissue masses and soft-tissue enlargement in the left leg may be noted. This has resulted in lack of bone development, both in length and in caliber. (Courtesy of Dr. Harvey White, Children's Hospital, Chicago, IL)

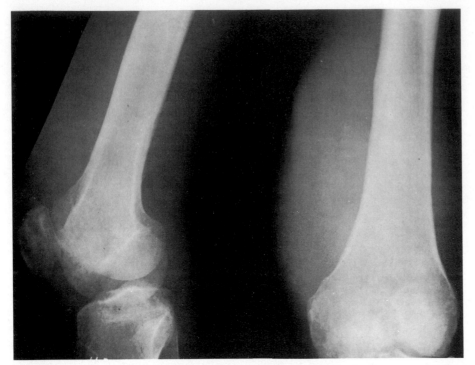

FIG. 8–48. Synovioma of the knee. Note large soft-tissue mass in the suprapatellar region, associated with spotty osteoporosis of the distal femur and patella. Several lobulations in the soft tissue can be seen posteriorly, and the cortex at the distal posterior femur is beginning to be eroded.

FIG. 8–49. Granular cell myoblastoma. A small, well-circumscribed, soft-tissue mass at the dorsum of the wrist may be seen. There is no invasion of soft tissues. The fascial planes adjacent to the mass are intact and there is no involvement of bone. Differentiation from other benign soft-tissue tumors is not possible radiologically.

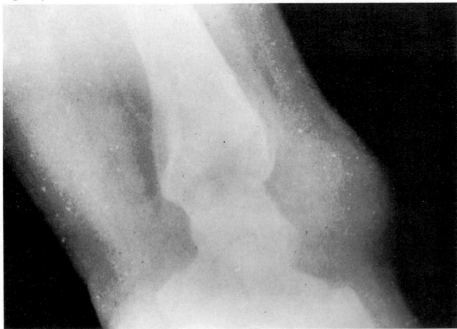

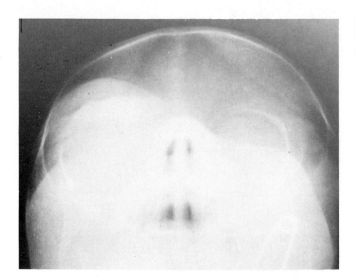

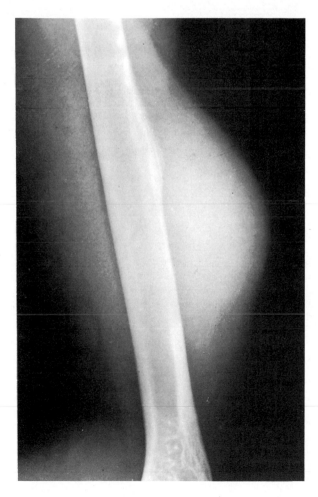

FIG. 8–50. Mesenchymoma (orbit). A lobulated, irregular soft-tissue mass overlying the left orbit is noted, with destruction of the orbital roof.

FIG. 8–51. Metastatic adenocarcinoma invading the tibia and causing the formation of a large, lobulated, soft-tissue mass.

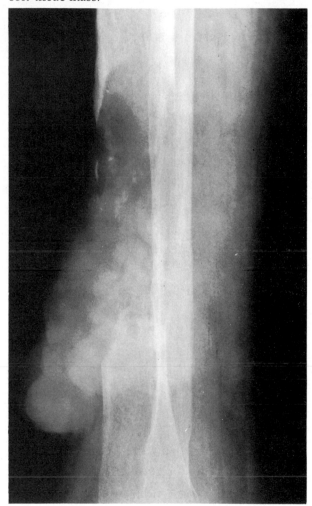

FIG. 8–52. Chronic hematoma, confirmed by two biopsies. Note smooth soft-tissue mass at the outer aspect of the arm and a small amount of laminated periosteal new bone formation. The laminations appear thick.

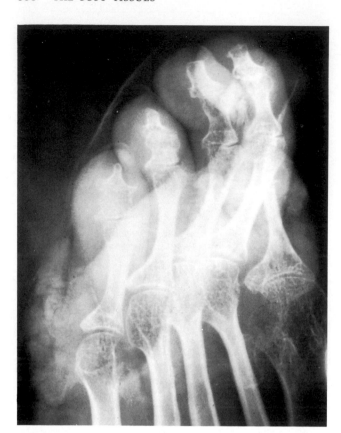

FIG. 8–53. Hyperkeratosis plantaris. Note irregular, lobulated soft-tissue masses, and resorption and thinning of the great toe. (From Greenfield GB, Rosado W, Rothbarth F: Benign proliferative skin lesions causing destructive and resorptive bone changes. Am J Roentgen 97:733–735, 1966)

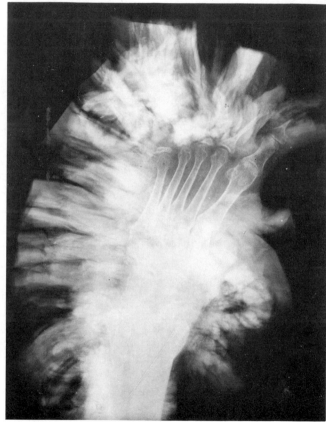

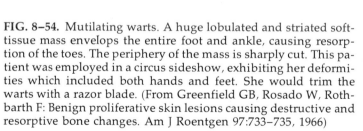

FIG. 8–54. Mutilating warts. A huge lobulated and striated soft-tissue mass envelops the entire foot and ankle, causing resorption of the toes. The periphery of the mass is sharply cut. This patient was employed in a circus sideshow, exhibiting her deformities which included both hands and feet. She would trim the warts with a razor blade. (From Greenfield GB, Rosado W, Rothbarth F: Benign proliferative skin lesions causing destructive and resorptive bone changes. Am J Roentgen 97:733–735, 1966)

quently in the first year of life, and should not be confused with myxoid liposarcoma. The latter is the most common soft-tissue sarcoma in adults, but rarely occurs in children. The lower extremity is most frequently involved. A soft-tissue mass with relative radiolucency is seen which may evoke a bone reaction.

Fibrosarcoma is probably the second most common soft-tissue sarcoma of the extremities. An ill-defined soft-tissue mass of water density without distinct margination is seen. Small calcific flecks may be present, and the adjacent bone may be invaded with a typical "saucerized" appearance (see Fig. 8–38). *Benign fibromas* occur and are given a variety of names, such as pedunculated fibroma and juvenile aponeurotic fibroma. *Parosteal nodular fasciitis* of the hand[68] is a very rare but distinct entity that represents a benign proliferation of spindle-cell stroma, containing reactive bone and occasionally cartilage. The age of reported incidence is 23 to 40 years. Painful soft-tissue swelling of the hand and fingers with periosteal new bone formation is seen. This condition is to be differentiated from a malignant neoplasm or an infectious process.

Another common type of soft-tissue malignancy is the *rhabdomyosarcomas*. One-half of these are the embryonal type that affect infants and young children. These tumors are usually found in the head, neck, and retroperitoneum. Only 5% were found in the extremities. The second subgroup is the alveolar type, which involves the extremities more frequently, and affects older children and young adults. The least common is the pleomorphic type, which involves skeletal muscle in adults.

Another tumor that occurs not infrequently is the *synovioma* or *synovial sarcoma*. Only 10% of these tumors are located primarily within a joint capsule. They can arise from a tendon sheath anywhere along a limb. There is a tendency toward calcification. The age incidence is between 18 and 35 years. In contrast, pigmented villonodular synovitis rarely, if ever, calcifies.

A group of tumors that has received recent attention are the *pseudosarcomas*. These are "quasineoplastic benign proliferations of connective tissue" which, because of their cellularity and frequently rapid growth, are readily mistaken for sarcoma (Enzinger).[14, 65] These entities represent reactive cellular proliferations of obscure etiology.

Aggressive fibromatosis[36] (musculoaponeurotic fibromatosis of the shoulder girdle, extra-abdominal desmoid) is a benign proliferation of fibrous tissue that, when located about the shoulder, exhibits a characteristic behavior. It is seen as a soft-tissue mass without calcification in the shoulder or upper portion of the back (Fig. 8–55). It is highly aggres-

FIG. 8–55. Aggressive fibromatosis. A large, lobulated soft-tissue mass is seen in the right shoulder region which has markedly displaced the scapula away from the chest wall.

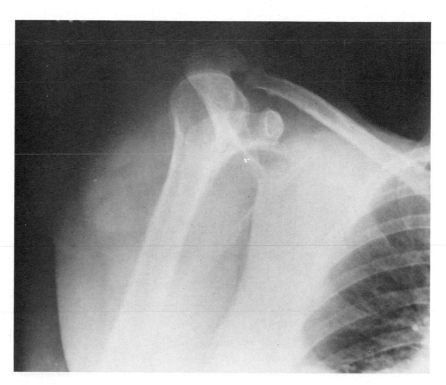

sive and tends to invade adjacent soft tissues. It has a high recurrence rate but typically does not metastasize. The mean age of occurrence is 23 years, and the tumor may be tender and painful.

Malignant fibrous histiocytoma[99] is an unusual tumor that may involve soft tissue or bone, and typically presents in the fifth and sixth decades of life. The tumor is thought to be of histiocytic origin with a wide variety of histologic patterns. It may be encapsulated. The patient typically presents with a soft-tissue mass in a limb. Such a mass may have been present for some time, but recently shows rapid increase in size and causes pain. *Radiologically*, an ill-defined soft-tissue mass with possible punctate calcifications is seen. Adjacent bone may be destroyed. Angiography shows increased vascularity.

In a review of 449 soft-tissue tumors from the M.D. Anderson Hospital and Tumor Institute (Martin RG et al),[65] the most common types found were:

TUMOR TYPE	NUMBER FOUND
Liposarcoma	107
Tumors of fibroblastic origin	96
Rhabdomyosarcoma	82
Unclassified sarcoma	59
Leiomyosarcoma	25
Synovial sarcoma	12

All malignant soft-tissue tumors may metastasize and invade bone. Rhabdomyosarcomas have a great tendency to do so. This gives an appearance of saucerization and possibly sclerosis.

In the young adult and middle age groups, fibrosarcoma and unclassified sarcoma are most common. In the older age group, liposarcoma, rhabdomyosarcoma, and leiomyosarcoma are more likely. The thigh is the most common site of malignant soft-tissue tumors.

The differential diagnosis of masses in special areas is summarized below.

DIFFERENTIAL DIAGNOSIS OF MASSES IN SPECIAL AREAS

I. An extrapleural mass associated with a lytic or destructive area in a rib can be due to:
1. Metastases (including carcinoma of prostate) (Fig. 8–56)
2. Multiple myeloma
3. Lymphoma
4. Tuberculosis (need not be calcified)
5. Aneurysmal bone cyst
6. Myelofibrosis with extramedullary hematopoiesis
7. Ewing's tumor

II. A paraspinal soft-tissue mass or paramediastinal stripe[77] can be due to:
1. Tuberculosis
2. Purulent spondylitis
3. Metastatic tumor (Figs. 8–57, 8–58)
4. Primary tumor of vertebra
5. Vertebra plana (eosinophilic granuloma)
6. Leukemia and lymphoma
7. Paget's disease (uncalcified osteoid)
8. Extramedullary hematopoiesis (Fig. 3–40)
9. Intraspinal tumors projecting through intervertebral spaces
10. Hematoma from trauma (should show progressive resolution)
11. Mediastinal effusion[106]
12. Osteoarthritis
13. Absent or occluded inferior vena cava with dilated azygous system[85]

LOCALIZED SOFT-TISSUE EDEMA

Localized edema can have an obstructive or inflammatory basis. *Radiologically*, there is an increase in thickness of the subcutaneous fat with prominence of the fibrous septa, causing a coarsened reticular pattern. The fascial planes are obliterated. In other cases, only soft-tissue prominence may be seen. *Obstructive edema* can be due to venous or lymphatic occlusion. Venous occlusion can be demonstrated by phlebography or cavography. Lymphedema may by primary or secondary. Lymphangiography is required for differentiation. *Primary lymphedema*[52] (Fig. 8–59) is due to a congenital lymphatic structural abnormality with no evidence of central obstruction. This condition can be divided into four groups:

1. Hypoplasia (fewer and larger lymphatic channels)
2. Varicose channels (frequently associated with dermal backflow)
3. Aplasia of lymphatics (rare)
4. Dermal backflow
5. Lymphaticoosseous communication[1]

The lymphangiogram may show sparse, dilated lymphatics with filled dermal and accessory lymphatic channels, and extravasation of contrast material into interstitial tissues, perineural spaces, and veins. Communication between hyperplastic superficial lymphatics and the epiphyseal portions of the bones of the lower extremity in primary lymphedema was demonstrated by lymphangiography in one patient.[1]

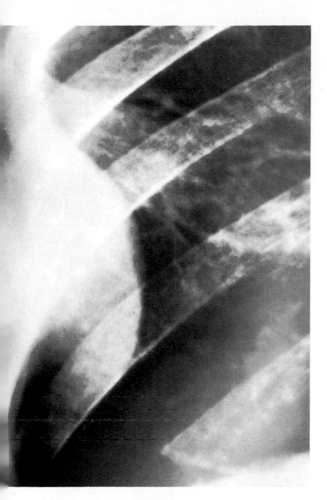

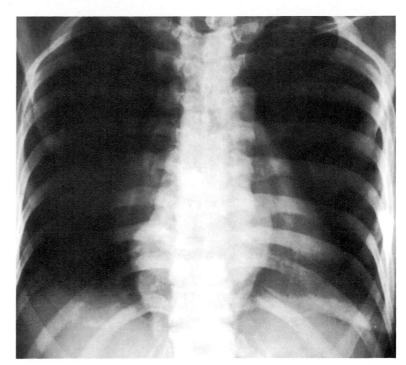

FIG. 8–56. Metastasis to a rib from carcinoma of the prostate, with an extrapleural sign. A soft-tissue mass may be noted with a smooth tapering margin. Associated rib destruction is seen.

FIG. 8–58. Large paraspinal soft-tissue mass from metastatic breast carcinoma. Note absence of the right breast shadow.

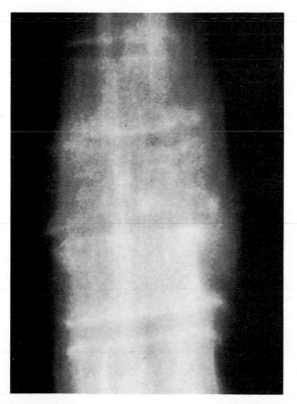

FIG. 8–57. Metastatic carcinoma of the lung to the vertebral column. There is destruction of a dorsal vertebral body with a paraspinal soft-tissue mass, well demonstrated by tomography.

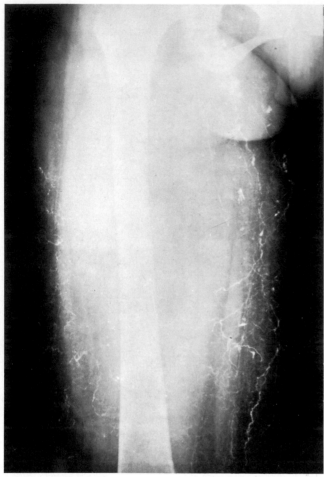

FIG. 8–59. Primary lymphedema—lymphangiogram. There is fill of dermal lymphatic channels without evidence of central lymphatic obstruction. Lymphatic varicosities may be seen. (From Love L, Kim SE: Clinical aspects of lymphangiography. Med Clin N Amer 51:227–248, 1967)

Secondary lymphedema (Fig. 8–60) results from lymphatic obstruction, which may be caused by:

1. Tumor
2. Inflammation
3. Radiation therapy
4. Postsurgical (particularly postmastectomy)
5. Trauma
6. Nodes
7. Filariasis

The lymphangiogram shows numerous filled lymphatic channels to the point of obstruction. Collateral lymphatics are visualized. *Inflammatory edema* may be primarily due to infectious, traumatic, thermal (Fig. 8–61), or neoplastic causes. It may also manifest as an accompanying soft-tissue inflammatory component to a disease such as benign cortical hyperostosis, vitamin A intoxication, Sudeck's atrophy, melorheostosis, thyroid acropachy, acromegaly, or neurofibromatosis.

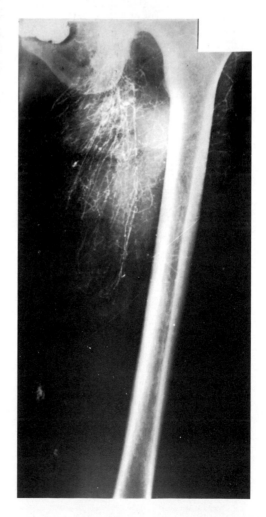

FIG. 8–60. Secondary lymphedema. There is central obstruction at the inguinal chain, with numerous filled lymphatics and collateral lymphatics. (From Love L, Kim SE: Clinical aspects of lymphangiography. Med Clin N Amer 51:227–248, 1967)

FIG. 8–61. Frostbite—edema of the fingers.

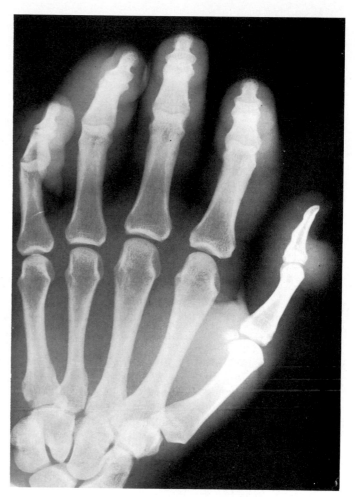

FIG. 8–62. Clubbing of the fingers. There is soft-tissue edema at the distal tufts of the fingers, which can result from a huge variety of causes. No bone changes are visible.

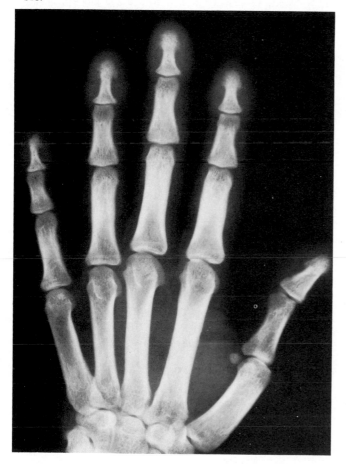

EDEMA IN SPECIAL AREAS OF DIAGNOSTIC SIGNIFICANCE

Clubbing of the fingers (Fig. 8–62) can be associated with a variety of intrathoracic and extrathoracic conditions. Clubbing, in general, is not to be confused with pulmonary hypertrophic osteoarthropathy,[37] which consists of a triad of clubbing, periosteal elevation, and painful joints in association with an intrathoracic lesion. Only one or two aspects of the triad may be present. Causes of clubbing of the fingers are summarized below.

CAUSES OF CLUBBING OF THE FINGERS

1. Acromegaly
2. Subacute Bacterial Endocarditis
3. Pulmonary Causes (Pulmonary Hypertrophic Osteoarthropathy)
   a) Brochogenic carcinoma
   b) Pulmonary metastases
   c) Lung abscess
   d) Empyema
   e) Tuberculosis
   f) Bronchiectasis
   g) Histoplasmosis
   h) Pulmonic cysts
   i) Pleural mesothelioma
   j) Benign tumors
   k) Pulmonary arteriovenous fistula
4. Alveolocapillary Block
   a) Interstitial pulmonary fibrosis
   b) Sarcoidosis
   c) Scleroderma
   d) Asbestosis
   e) Alveolar-cell carcinoma
5. Pulmonary Insufficiency
6. Common Cardiovascular Causes
   a) Patent ductus arteriosus
   b) Tetralogy of Fallot
   c) Pulmonic stenosis
   d) Ventricular septal defect
7. Diarrheal States
   a) Ulcerative colitis
   b) Tuberculous enteritis
   c) Sprue
   d) Amebic dysentery
   e) Bacillary dysentery
   f) Parasitic infestation
8. Hepatic Cirrhosis
9. Myxedema
10. Polycythemia
11. Chronic Urinary Tract Infections
12. Hyperparathyroidism
13. Pachydermoperiostosis
14. Thyroid Acropachy
15. Idiopathic

Thickening of the heel pads or the soft tissue inferior to the plantar aspect of the calcaneus can be seen in the following conditions:

1. Acromegaly (greater than 23 mm) (Fig. 5–110)
2. Obesity
3. Myxedema
4. Thyroid acropachy
5. Generalized edema
6. Genetic

SOFT-TISSUE DEFICIT

Diminution of the soft-tissue mass can occur in various conditions from atrophy or lack of development. It can be local or generalized, unilateral or bilateral. Among the causes are malnutrition, disuse atrophy, cachexia, neurological diseases, and muscular dystrophies.

The ratio of muscle tissue to fat is of diagnostic significance in infants, a reciprocal relationship existing in some diseases. Litt and Altman[60] have tabulated disorders of infancy altering the muscle ratio. A summary is presented below.

DISEASES AFFECTING MUSCLE-TO-FAT RATIO

I. Relative Increase of Subcutaneous Fat (Figs. 8–63, 8–64)
   1. Diminution of muscle
      a) Spinal atrophy, progressive (Werdnig–Hoffman)
      b) Amyotonia congenita (Oppenheim)
      c) Benign congenital hypotonia (Walton)
      d) Poliomyelitis, myelomeningocele, other neurological states
      e) Arthrogryposis multiplex congenita
      f) Disseminated lipogranulomatosis
   2. Increase in subcutaneous fat
      a) Cushing's syndrome

(Fat may occur in fascial spaces and between muscle fibers in some of the above diseases.)

II. Relative Diminution of Subcutaneous Fat
   1. Diminution of subcutaneous fat
      a) Malnutrition
      b) Diencephalic syndrome
      c) Total lipodystrophy[114]
      d) Hyperthyroidism
      e) Progeria
      f) Renal tubular acidosis
      g) Hurler's disease
      h) Morquio's disease
      i) Debilitating diseases
   2. Increase in Muscle Mass
      a) Congenital muscular hypertrophy (de Lange)
      b) Pseudohypertrophic stage of muscular dystrophy

(In addition to the above diseases, congenital absence of muscle groups may occur.)

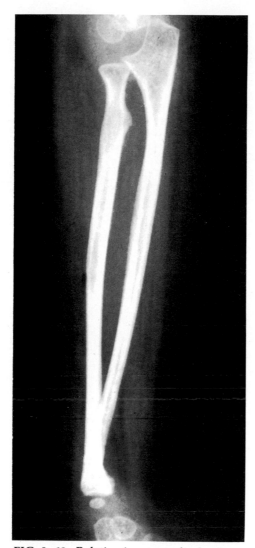

FIG. 8–63. Relative increase of subcutaneous fat infiltrating muscular planes. This picture can result from causes listed on page 666.

FIG. 8–64. Progressive muscular dystrophy (lower extremities). A large amount of subcutaneous fat is present with a small muscle mass and fat infiltrating muscular planes. Bilateral congenital hip dislocations, coxa valga, and marked overtubulation of the bones are noted.

CONTRACTURES

Congenital ring contractions of the extremities are due to focal tissue deficiencies caused by localized ischemia. There are deep circular grooves in the soft tissues, sometimes involving the bone (Fig. 8–65). These may proceed to complete amputations. Experimental evidence shows that these changes are secondary to ischemia from excessive contractions of the uterine muscles during the fifth and sixth weeks of pregnancy, and that this syndrome is not hereditary.[53] *Acquired ring contractions* of an extremity may be present, owing to a circular foreign object, such as a rubber band, that is neglected. This causes ulceration of the soft tissue and growth over the object. The bones may be involved. *Ainhum*[6,28] is a tropical disease, affecting chiefly males, wherein a deep constricting furrow around the base of the fifth toe occurs, leading to auto-amputation. Concentric bone erosion can be seen radiographically (Figs. 8–66, 8–67). The etiology is unknown. *Arthrogryposis multiplex congenita*[87]

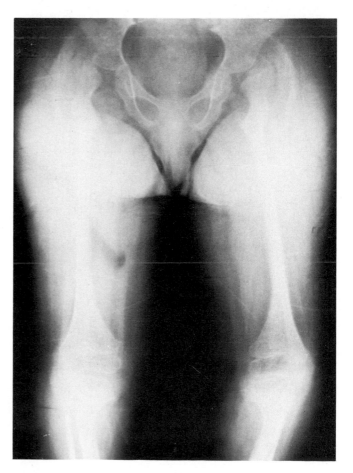

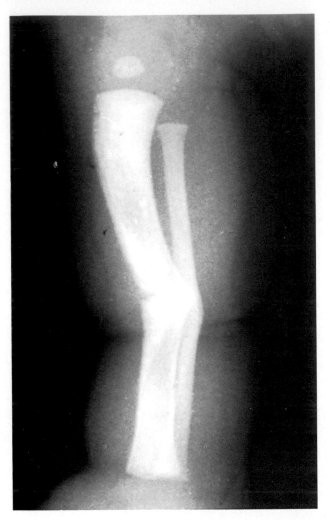

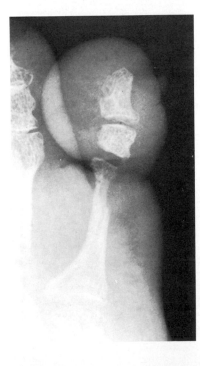

FIG. 8–65. Congenital ring contraction. A congenital soft-tissue stenotic band may be noted in the leg, with an associated pseudarthrosis in the midtibia. (Courtesy of Dr. Harvey White, Children's Memorial Hospital, Chicago, IL)

FIG. 8–66. Ainhum. Soft-tissue constriction at the midportion of the little toe. There is a gap in the bone and a pencillike deformity of the proximal phalanx.

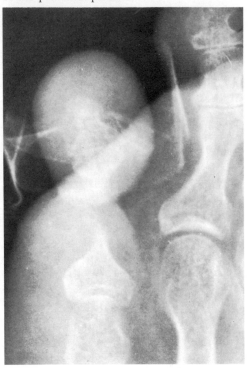

FIG. 8–67. Ainhum. Soft-tissue constriction at the midportion of the little toe, with thinning of the regional bone.

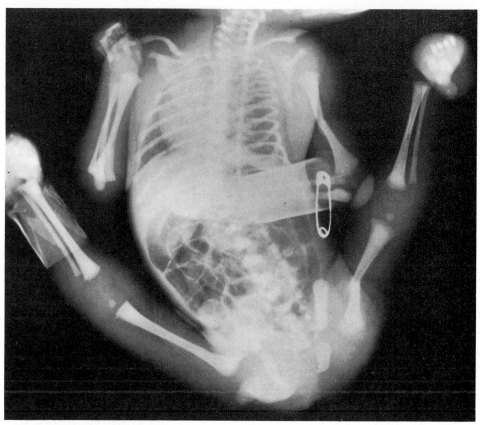

FIG. 8–68. Arthrogryposis multiplex congenita. Note contractures of all the extremities, and fractures of the left humerus and femur.

(amyoplasia) consists of a generalized failure of muscular development of the fetus resulting in widespread contractures and deformities (Fig. 8–68). The muscle bundles are small. There is an excess of fat, and the flexor aspects of the knees and elbows may be webbed. Bone changes include fractures, congenital amputations, carpal and tarsal fusions, clubfoot, hip dislocation, tibia recurvatum, hypoplasia of the mandible, and brachycephaly. When amyoplasia is associated with multiple bone dysplasia, labyrinthine deafness, regional losses of skin and hair pigmentation, and slate-blue irises, it is known as the *syndrome of Rocher–Sheldon*. *Dupuytren's contracture* is a contraction of the palmar fascia. Palmar induration is present and the fingers cannot be extended (Fig. 8–69). *Burns*, when sufficiently severe, result in contractures (Fig. 8–70). *Volkmann's ischemic contracture*[96] is usually seen in the forearm and sometimes in the leg. It is due to arterial insufficiency following injury or casting. There is a fibrosing myositis that results in flexion deformities (Fig. 8–71) *Camplodactyly* is a flexion contracture constantly involving the proximal interphalangeal joint of the little finger, and occasionally of the other fingers. The etiology is unknown, and it may be congenital or acquired. It is bilateral in the majority of cases. The palmar fascia is normal (Fig. 8–72). *Congenital contractural arachnodactyly*[9] is an autosomal, dominantly transmitted syndrome with multiple contractures and Marfanlike features of arachnodactyly and scoliosis. Normal intelligence and a characteristic ear shape are present.

(Text continued on p. 673)

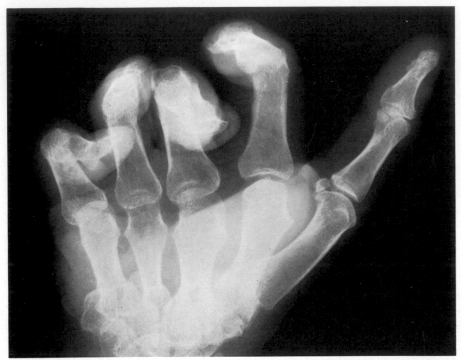

FIG. 8–69. Dupuytren's contracture. Note flexion
of the fingers.

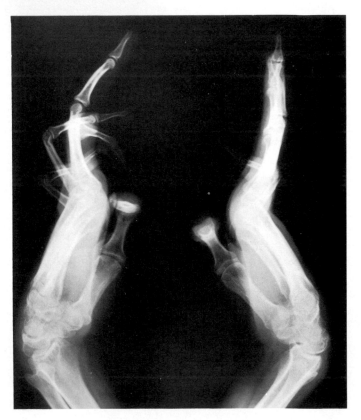

FIG. 8–70. Contractures resulting from burns. Note
flexion of the wrists and of several fingers, including
both thumbs.

FIG. 8–71. Volkmann's ischemic contracture. There is flexion of the fingers and dorsiflexion of the wrist following casting; this condition is caused by arterial insufficiency. Regional osteoporosis is also present.

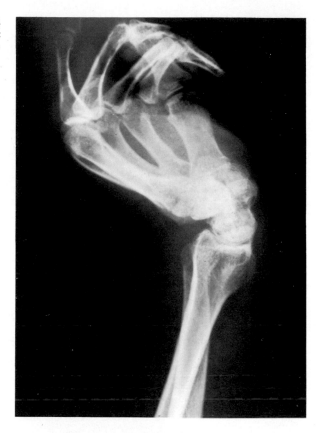

FIG. 8–72. Camptodactyly (hands)—male, age 14 years, with congenital flexion deformities and webbing. Involvement of third, fourth, and fifth digits. Flexion deformities at the proximal interphalangeal joints are seen, with shortening of the skin at the flexor aspect. No osteoporosis is present. (From Currarino G, Waldman I: Camptodactyly. Am J Roentgen 92:1312–1321, 1964)

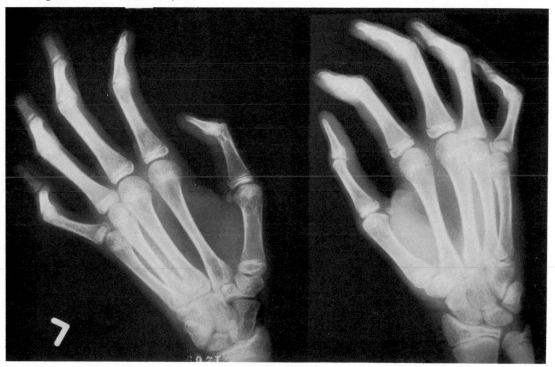

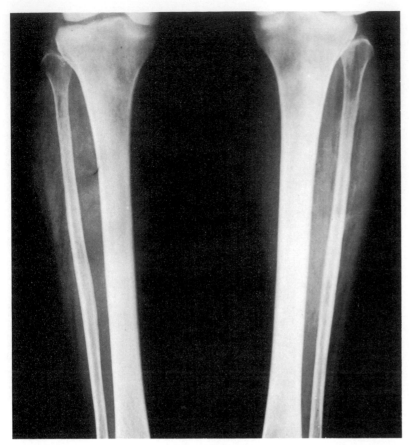

FIG. 8–73. Bilateral gas gangrene of the legs following an automobile accident. Gas is seen dissecting along subcutaneous tissues and muscle fibers.

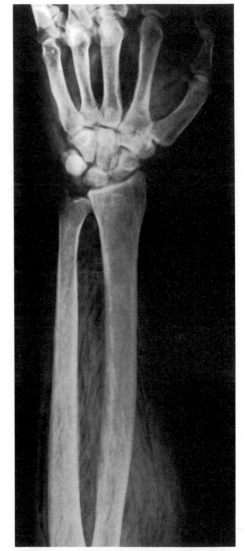

FIG. 8–74. Gas gangrene of the hand and forearm — advanced. There is extensive dissection of gas along muscle fibers of the forearm.

SOFT-TISSUE EMPHYSEMA

Gas in the soft tissue can be recognized radiographically by increased radiolucency. This can be caused by infiltration of air, gas phlegmon, or gas abscess. The gas can be subcutaneous or intramuscular. *Infiltration* or air may follow fractured ribs with lung injury, fractured air passages, tracheostomy, or thoracotomy. Air can infiltrate the thorax, neck, and arm with a subcutaneous or intramuscular distribution. Air can also be introduced into the soft tissues through open wounds or hypodermoclysis. In the absence of infection, serial films will show progressive resorption of air in the latter instances. *Gas phlegmon* or *gas gangrene* results from an infection of the tissues with various clostridia. Gas may appear soon after injury or may develop weeks after a penetrating wound. The distribution of gas may be superficial with diffuse subcutaneous gas bubbles showing a netlike structure. This type is said to have a better prognosis than the deep intramuscular type of gas gangrene, in which gas spreads along the muscle fibers (Fig. 8–73, 8–74). *Gas abscess* is a localized gas-forming infection of soft tissues without the malignant spread of gas gangrene. It can be differentiated from localized infiltration of air by the lack of gas resorption on serial films. Gas-forming infection in the feet of diabetics is common (Fig. 8–75). It has also been reported as a complication of chickenpox.

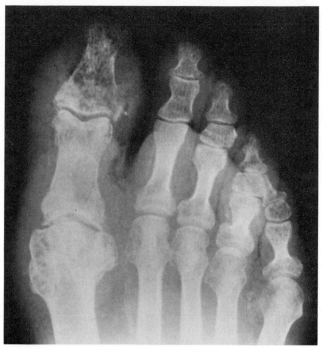

FIG. 8–75. Diabetic gangrene (left foot). Air in the soft tissues about the great toe is noted, as well as vascular calcification. Destruction of bone of the lateral base of the distal phalanx is also seen.

REFERENCES

1. Abe R: Lymphaticoosseous communication and primary lymphedema. Radiology 129:375–378, 1978

2. Aegerter E, Kirkpatrick J A: Orthopedic Diseases, 4th ed. Philadelphia, W B Saunders, 1975

3. Albright F, Reifenstein E C: The Parathyroid Glands and Metabolic Bone Disease: Selected Studies. Baltimore, Williams & Wilkins, 1948

4. Angervall L, Enzinger F M: Extraskeletal neoplasm resembling Ewing's sarcoma. Cancer 36:240–251, 1975

5. Aubrey D A, Andrews G S: Mammary osteogenic sarcoma. Brit J Radiol 58:472–474, 1971

6. Aukland G, Ball J, Griffiths D: Ainhum. J Bone Joint Surg 39–B:513–519, 1957

7. Ayella R J: Hemangiopericytoma. Radiology 97:611–612, 1970

8. Baldursson H, Evans E B, Dodge W F, Jackson W T: Tumoral calcinosis with hyperphosphatemia. A report of a family with incidence in 4 siblings. J Bone Joint Surg 51–A:913–925, 1969

9. Beals R K, Hecht F: Congenital contractural arachnodactyly. A hereditable disorder of connective tissue. J Bone Joint Surg 53–A:987–993, 1971

10. Berger P E, Heidelberger K P, Poznanski A K: Extravasation of calcium gluconate as a cause of soft-tissue calcification in infancy. Am J Roentgen 121:109–117, 1974

11. Blery M, Barre B: Maladie des calcifications tendineuses multiples. J Radiol Electrol 59:271–273, 1978

12. Bliznak J, Staple T W: Radiology of angiodysplasias of the limb. Radiology 110:35–44, 1974

13. Booker R J: Lipoblastic tumors of the hands and feet. Review of the literature and report of 33 cases. J Bone Joint Surg 47–A:727–740, 1965

14. Broder M S, Leonidas J C, Mittay H A: Pseudosarcomatous fasciitis: An unusual cause of soft-tissue calcification. Radiology 107:173–174, 1973

15. Budin J A, Feldman F: Soft-tissue calcifications in systemic lupus erythematosus. Am J Roentgen 124:358–364, 1975

16. Bundens W D, Brighton C T, Weitzman G: Primary ar-

ticular-cartilage calcifications with arthritis (pseudogout syndrome). J Bone Joint Surg 47–A:111–122, 1965

17. Burgener F A, Landman S: The radiological manifestations of fibroxanthosarcomas. Fortschr Roentgenstr 125:123–128, 1976

18. Caffey J, Silverman F N: Pediatric X-ray Diagnosis, 5th ed. Chicago, Year Book Publishers, 1967

19. Cavanagh R C: Tumors of the soft tissues of the extremities. Seminars Roentgen 8:73–89, 1973

20. Chaplin D M, Harrison M H M: Pseudomalignant osseous tumour of soft tissue. J Bone Joint Surg 54–B:334–340, 1972

21. Chinn D et al: Heterotopic bone formation in metastatic tumor from transitional-cell carcinoma of the urinary bladder. J Bone Joint Surg 58–A:881–883, 1976

22. Chung B S: Drug-induced myositis ossificans circumscripta. JAMA 226:469, 1973

23. Chung S M K, Janes J M: Diffuse pigmented villonodular synovitis of the hip joint. Review of the literature and report of 4 cases. J Bone Joint Surg 47–A:292–303, 1965

24. Condon R R, Allen R P: Congenital generalized fibromatosis. Radiology 76:444–448, 1961

25. Coventry M B, Harrison E G, Martin J F: Benign synovial tumors of the knee: A diagnostic problem. J Bone Joint Surg 48–A:1350–1358, 1966

26. Dillon E, Parkin G J S: The role of diagnostic radiology in the diagnosis and management of rhabdomyosarcoma in young persons. Clin Rad 29:53–59, 1978

27. Enzinger F M, Shiraki M: Musculoaponeurotic fibromatosis of the shoulder girdle (extraabdominal desmoid). Analysis of 30 cases followed up for 10 or more years. Cancer 20:1131–1140, 1967

28. Fetterman L E, Hardy R, Lehrer H: The clinicoroentgenological features of ainhum. Am J Roentgen 100:512–522, 1967

29. Fine G, Stout A P: Osteogenic sarcoma of the extraskeletal soft tissues. Cancer 9:1027–1043, 1956

30. Gay B B, Weens S H: Roentgenologic evaluation of disorders of muscle. Seminars Roentgen 8:25–36, 1973

31. Goldman A B: Myositis ossificans circumscripta: A benign lesion with a malignant differential diagnosis. Am J Roentgen 126:32–40, 1976

32. Gondos B: Roentgen manifestations in progressive systemic sclerosis (diffuse scleroderma). Am J Roentgen 84:235–247, 1960

33. Gonzalez–Crussi F, Enneking W F, Arean V M: Infiltrating angiolipoma. J Bone Joint Surg 48–A:1111–1124, 1966

34. Goodman A H, Briggs R C: Deep leiomyoma of an extremity. J Bone Joint Surg 47–A:529–532, 1965

35. Greenfield G B, Escamilla C H, Schorsch H A: The hand as an indicator of generalized disease. Am J Roentgen 99:736–745, 1967

36. Greenfield G B, Rubenstone A L, Lo M: Aggressive fibromatosis. Skel Rad 2:43–46, 1977

37. Greenfield G B, Schorsch H A, Shkolnik A: The various roentgen appearances of pulmonary hypertrophic osteoarthropathy. Am J Roentgen 101:927–931, 1967

38. Gunn D R, Young W B: Myositis ossificans as a complication of tetanus. J Bone Joint Surg 41–B:535–540, 1959

39. Hadley M, MacDonald A F: Epidermolysis bullosa. Brit J Radiol 33:646–649, 1960

40. Harwood–Nash D C F, Reilly B J: Calcification of the basal ganglia following radiation therapy. Am J Roentgen 108:392–395, 1970

41. Heilburn N, Kuhn W G: Erosive bone lesions and soft-tissue ossifications associated with spinal cord injuries (paraplegia). Radiology 48:570–593, 1947

42. Henry M J, Grimes H A, Lane J W: Intervertebral disk calcification in childhood. Radiology 89:81–84, 1967

43. Hug I, Guncaga J: Tumoral calcinosis with sedimentation sign. Brit J Radiol 47:734–736, 1974

44. Hutcheson J, Klatte E C, Kremp R: The angiographic appearance of myositis ossificans circumscripta. A case report. Radiology 102:57–58, 1972

45. Jaffe H L: Tumors and Tumorous Conditions of the Bones and Joints. Philadelphia, Lea & Febiger, 1958

46. James A E et al: Roentgen findings in pseudoxanthoma elasticum (P X E). Am J Roentgen 106:642–647, 1969

47. Jeffreys T E, Stiles P J: Pseudomalignant osseous tumor of soft tissue. J Bone Joint Surg 48–B:488–492, 1966

48. Jokl P, Federico J: Myositis ossificans traumatica association with hemophilia (Factor XI deficiency) in a football player. JAMA 237:2215–2216, 1977

49. Karasick D, O'Hara E A: Juvenile aponeurotic fibroma. Radiology 123:725–726, 1977

50. Karpas C M, Merendino V S: Uterine osteogenic sarcoma: Histochemical studies and report of a case. Obstet Gynec 24:629–633, 1964

51. Kauffman S L, Stout A P: Extraskeletal osteogenic sarcomas and chondrosarcomas in children. Cancer 16:432–439, 1963

52. Kinmonth J B, Taylor G W, Tracy G D, Marsh J D: Primary lymphedema: Clinical and lymphangiographic studies of series of 107 patients in which lower limbs were affected. Brit J Surg 45:1–10, 1957

53. Kino Y: Clinical and experimental studies of the congenital constriction band syndrome with an emphasis on its etiology. J Bone Joint Surg 57–A:636–643, 1975

54. Kolawole T M, Bohrer S P: Tumoral calcinosis with "fluid levels" in the tumoral masses. Am J Roentgen 120:461–465, 1974

55. Kuhn J P, Rosenstein B J, Oppenheimer E H: Metastatic calcification in cystic fibrosis. A report of 2 cases. Radiology 97:59–64, 1970

56. Lanploh J T et al: Lipoblastomatosis. A case report. J Bone Joint Surg 60–A:130–132, 1978

57. Leffert R D: Lipomas of the upper extremity. J Bone Joint Surg 54–A:1262–1266, 1972

58. Levine H A, Enrile F: Giant-cell tumor of patellar tendon coincident with Paget's disease. J Bone Joint Surg 53–A:335–340, 1971

59. Linscheid R L, Soule E H, Henderson E D: Pleomorphic rhabdomyosarcomata of the extremities and limb girdles. A clinicopathological study. J Bone Joint Surg 47–A:715–726, 1965

60. Litt R E, Altman D H: Significance of the muscle cylinder ratio in infancy. Am J Roentgen 100:80–87, 1967

61. Lorentzon R, Larsson S E, Boquist L: Extraosseous osteosarcoma. J Bone Joint Surg 61–B:205–208, 1979

62. Louis D S, Dick H M: Ossifying fibrolipoma of the median nerve. J Bone Joint Surg 55–A:1082–1084, 1973

63. Love L, Kim S E: Clinical aspects of lymphangiography. Med Clin N Amer 51:227–248, 1967

64. Mann T S: Acute calcific synovitis of the knee. J Bone Joint Surg 48–B:57–63, 1966

65. Martin R G et al: In Anderson M D: Hospital and Tumor Institute. Tumors of Bone and Soft Tissue. Chicago, Year Book Publishers, 1965

66. Maurer R M, Langford O L: Rothmund's syndrome: A cause of resorption of phalangeal tufts and dystrophic calcification. Radiology 89:706–708, 1967

67. McAlister W H, Koehler P R: Diseases of the adrenal. Radiol Clin N Amer 5:205–220, 1967

68. McCarthy E F et al: Parosteal (nodular) fasciitis of the hand. J Bone Joint Surg 58–A:714–716, 1976

69. McCarty D J, Haskin M E: Roentgenographic aspects of pseudogout. Am J Roentgen 90:1248–1257, 1963

70. McDonald P: Malignant sacrococcygeal teratoma: A report of 4 cases. Am J Roentgen 118:444–449, 1973

71. McKusick V A, Goodman R M: Pinnal calcification. JAMA 179:230–232, 1962

72. Melnick J C, Silverman F N: Intervertebral disc calcification in childhood. Radiology 80:399–408, 1963

73. Meschan I, Farrer–Meschan R M F: Roentgen Signs in Clinical Practice, vol 1. Philadelphia, W B Saunders, 1966

74. Mitra M, Sen A K, Deb H K: Myositis ossificans traumatica. A complication of tetanus. A report of a case and review of the literature. J Bone Joint Surg 58–A:885–886, 1977

75. Murphy N B: Ossifying lipoma. Brit J Radiol 47:97–98, 1974

76. Naidich T P, Siegelman S S: Paraarticular soft-tissue changes in systemic diseases. Seminars Roentgen 8:101–116, 1973

77. Norman A: Segmental bulge of the linear thoracic paraspinal shadow (paravertebral line). An early sign of disease of the thoracic spine. J Bone Joint Surg 44–A:352–358, 1962

78. Norman A, Dorfman H D: Juxtacortical circumscribed myositis ossificans: Evolution and radiographic features. Radiology 96:301–306, 1970

79. Novak E: Gynecological and Obstetrical Pathology with Clinical and Endocrine Relations, p 472. Philadelphia, W B Saunders, 1947

80. Ozonoff M B, Flynn F J: Roentgenologic features of dermatomyositis of childhood. Am J Roentgen 118:206–212, 1973

81. Palmer P E S: Tumoural calcinosis. Brit J Radiol 39:518–525, 1966

82. Parker M D, Irwin R S: Mycobacterium kansasii tendinitis and fasciitis. J Bone Joint Surg 57–A:557–559, 1975

83. Pastershank S P, Yip S, Sodhi H S: Cerebrotendinous xanthomatosis. J Canad Assn Rad 25:282–286, 1974

84. Paterson D C: Myositis ossificans circumscripta. J Bone Joint Surg 52–B:296–301, 1970

85. Petersen R W: Infrahepatic interruption of the inferior vena cava with azygous continuation (persistent right cardinal vein). Radiology 84:304–307, 1965

86. Pirkey E L, Hurt J: Roentgen evaluation of the soft tissues in orthopedics. Am J Roentgen 82:271–276, 1959

87. Poznanski A K, La Rowe P C: Radiographic manifestations of the arthrogryposis syndrome. Radiology 95:353–358, 1970

88. Reszel P A, Soule E H, Coventry M B: Liposarcoma of the extremities and limb girdles. A study of 222 cases. J Bone Joint Surg 48–A:229–244, 1966

89. Robbins L, Hanelin J: Soft-tissue roentgenography. In Golden's Diagnostic Roentgenology, vol 3, chap 17. Baltimore, Williams & Wilkins, 1964

90. Rosborough D: Ectopic bone formation associated with multiple congenital anomalies. J Bone Joint Surg 48–B:499–503, 1966

91. Ross P: Gardner's syndrome. Am J Roentgen 96:298–301, 1966

92. Rubin E H, Rubin M, Leiner G C, Escher D J W: Thoracic Diseases, Emphasizing Cardiopulmonary Relationships. Philadelphia, W B Saunders, 1961

93. Schanche A F, Bierman S M, Sopher R L, O'Loughlin B J: Disseminated lipogranulomatosis, early roentgen changes. Radiology 82:675–678, 1964

94. Schinz H R, Baensch W E, Friedl E, Uehlinger E: Roentgen Diagnostics. New York, Grune & Stratton, 1952

95. Schlenker J D, Clark D D, Weckesser E C: Calcinosis circumscripta of the hand in scleroderma. J Bone Joint Surg 55–A:1051–1056, 1973

96. Seddon H J: Voldmann's ischemia in the lower limb. J Bone Joint Surg 48–B:627–636, 1966

97. Shackelford G D, Barton L L, McAlister W H: Calcified subcutaneous fat necrosis in infancy. J Canad Assn Rad 26:203–207, 1976

98. Soule E H: Primary soft tissues of the extremities. Classification: Histogenesis and incidence. Instructional course lectures. The American Academy of Orthopedic Surgeons, 2:3–11, Ann Arbor, J W. Edwards, 1954

99. Spector D B, Miller J, Viloria J: Malignant fibrous histiocytoma. J Bone Joint Surg 61–A:190–193, 1979

100. Staple T W, Melson G L, Evens R G: Miscellaneous soft-tissue lesions of the extremities. Seminars Roentgen 8:117–127, 1973

101. Steel H H: Turtle-egg tumors. A late sequel of parenteral quinine. J Bone Joint Surg 46–A:134–136, 1964

102. Steinfeld J R, Schuit K E, Keats T E: Calcification in Cooper's ligament. Am J Roentgen 121:107–108, 1974

103. Stout A P: Pathology and classification of tumors of the soft tissues. Am J Roentgen 66:903–909, 1951

104. Symeonides P: Bursal chondromatosis. J Bone Joint Surg 48–B:371–373, 1966

105. Taveras J M, Wood E H: Diagnostic Neuroradiology. Baltimore, Williams & Wilkins, 1964

106. Trackler R T, Brinker R A: Widening of the left paravertebral

pleural line on supine chest roentgenograms in free pleural effusions. Am J Roentgen 96:1027–1034, 1966

107. Trapnell D H: Calcification of nerves in leprosy. Brit J Radiol 38:796–797, 1965

108. Tucker R E et al: Pyomyositis mimicking malignant tumor. Three case reports. J Bone Joint Surg 60–A:701–703, 1978

109. Twigg H L, Zvaifler N J, Nelson C W: Chondrocalcinosis. Radiology 82:655–659, 1964

110. Vix V A: Articular and fibrocartilage calcification in hyperparathyroidism: Associated hyperuricemia. Radiology 83:468–471, 1964

111. Voss H: Uber die Parostalen und Para-artikulären Knochenneubildungen bie Organischen Nervenkrankheiten. Fortschr Roentgenstr 55:423–441, 1937

112. Weinberger G, Levinsohn E M: Computed tomography in the evaluation of sarcomatous tumors of the thigh. Am J Roentgen 130:115–118, 1978

113. Weitzman G: Lipoma arborescens of knee. Report of a case. J Bone Joint Surg 47–A:1030–1034, 1965

114. Wesenberg R L, Gwinn J L, Barnes G R: The roentgenographic findings in total lipodystrophy. Am J Roentgen 103:154–164, 1968

115. Yaghmai I: Myositis ossificans: Diagnostic value of arteriography. Am J Roentgen 128:811–816, 1977

116. Yaghmai I, Mirbod P: Tumoral calcinosis. Am J Roentgen 111:573–578, 1971

117. Zadek I: Ossifying hematoma in the thigh. A case report. J Bone Joint Surg 51–A:386–390, 1969

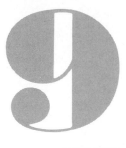

THE JOINTS

GENERAL CONSIDERATIONS

Joints are classified into three types: fibrous, cartilaginous, and synovial.

Fibrous joints are immovable, and include structures such as the cranial sutures. They are referred to as *synarthroses*.

Cartilaginous joints contain hyaline cartilage or fibrocartilage in the space between bone ends. A limited amount of motion is possible in the latter, and they are termed *amphiarthroses*. Examples are the intervertebral disks, the "joints" of Lushka in the cervical spine, and the symphysis pubis. The sacroiliac joint in its upper portion is amphiarthrodial, while the lower portion is synovial.

The majority of joints are *synovial*, or *diarthroses*. They are freely movable. The articular surfaces are covered with hyaline cartilage, and the joint is surrounded by a capsule and ligaments. The outer layer of the joint capsule is the stratum fibrosum, and the inner layer consists of vascularized connective tissue, the stratum synoviale or synovium. The synovium does not cover the articular cartilage. It merges with the periosteum covering the intracapsular portions of bone. The synovium secretes the highly viscous synovial fluid that lubricates the joints and nourishes the articular cartilage. The joints of the extremities, with few exceptions, are diarthrodial, as are the small apophyseal joints of the spine.

The significance of this classification lies in the fact that in those arthritides of generalized synovial involvement, only diarthrodial joints will be primarily affected. It should be noted that the spine has two systems, the amphiarthrodial intervertebral disks and the diarthrodial apophyseal articulations.

CLASSIFICATION OF ARTHRITIS

The classsification of arthritis and rheumatism adopted by the American Rheumatism Association in 1963, and modified to date,[218] is presented below.

CLASSIFICATION OF THE RHEUMATIC DISEASES*

I. *Polyarthritis of Unknown Etiology*

  A. Rheumatoid arthritis
  B. Juvenile rheumatoid arthritis (including Still's disease)
  C. Ankylosing spondylitis
  D. Psoriatic arthritis
  E. Reiter's syndrome
  F. Others

II. *"Connective Tissue" Disorders (Acquired)*

  A. Systemic lupus erythematosus
  B. Progressive systemic sclerosis (scleroderma)
  C. Polymyositis and dermatomyositis
  D. *Necrotizing arteritis and other forms of vasculitis*
    1. *Polyarteritis nodosa*
    2. *Hypersensitivity angiitis*
    3. *Wegener's granulomatosis*
    4. *Takayasu's (pulseless) disease*
    5. *Cogan's syndrome*
    6. *Giant-cell arteritis (including polymyalgia rheumatica)*
  E. Amyloidosis
  F. Others

III. *Rheumatic Fever*

IV. *Degenerative Joint Disease (Osteoarthritis, Osteoarthrosis)*

  A. Primary
  B. Secondary

V. *Nonarticular Rheumatism*

  A. Fibrositis
  B. Intervertebral disk and low back syndromes

* Adapted from the 1963 ARA Nomenclature and Classification of Arthritis and Rheumatism (tentative). Additions and modifications are italicized.

(Reprinted from: Primer on the Rheumatic Diseases, 7th ed. JAMA (Suppl) 224:662–812, 1973, by permission of The Arthritis Foundation, The Journal of the American Medical Association, and Gerald P. Rodnam, M.D., editor.)

C. Myositis and myalgia
D. Tendinitis and peritendinitis (bursitis)
E. Tenosynovitis
F. Fasciitis
G. Carpal–tunnel syndrome
H. Others

CLASSIFICATION OF THE RHEUMATIC DISEASES

VI. *Diseases with which Arthritis is Frequently Associated*

A. Sarcoidosis
B. Relapsing polychondritis
C. Schönlein–Henoch purpura
D. Ulcerative colitis
E. Regional enteritis
F. Whipple's disease
G. Sjögren's syndrome
H. Familial Mediterranean fever
I. Others

VII. *Associated with Known Infectious Agents*

A. Bacterial
1. Gonococcus
2. *Meningococcus*
3. Pneumococcus
4. *Streptococcus*
5. Staphylococcus
6. Salmonella
7. Brucella
8. Streptobacillus moniliformis (Haverhill fever)
9. Mycobacterium tuberculosis
10. Treponema pallidum (syphilis)
11. Treponema pertenue (yaws)
12. Others
(See also Rheumatic fever, III)
B. Rickettsial
C. Viral
1. *Rubella*
2. *Mumps*
3. *Viral hepatitis*
4. *Others*
D. Fungal
E. Parasitic

VIII. *Traumatic and/or Neurogenic Disorders*

A. Traumatic arthritis (the result of direct trauma)
B. Neuropathic arthropathy (Charcot joints)
1. Syphilis (tabes dorsalis)
2. Diabetes mellitus (diabetic neuropathy)
3. Syringomyelia
4. *Myelomeningocele*

5. *Congenital insensitivity to pain (including familial dysautonomia)*
6. Others
C. Shoulder-hand syndrome
D. Mechanical derangement of joints
E. Others

IX. *Associated with Known or Strongly Suspected Biochemical or Endocrine Abnormalites*

A. Gout
B. *Chondrocalcinosis articularis ("pseudogout")*
C. Alkaptonuria (ochronosis)
D. Hemophilia
E. Sickle-cell disease and other hemoglobinopathies
F. Agammaglobulinemia (hypogrammaglobulinemia)
G. Gaucher's disease
H. Hyperparathyroidism
I. Acromegaly
J. *Thyroid acropachy*
K. Hypothyroidism
L. Scurvy (hypovitaminosis C)
M. Hyperlipoproteinemia type II (xanthoma tuberosum and tendinosum)
N. *Fabry's disease (angiokeratoma corporis diffusum or glycolipid lipidosis)*
O. *Hemochromatosis*
P. Others

X. *Neoplasms*

A. Synovioma
B. Primary juxta-articular bone tumors
C. Metastatic malignant tumors
D. Leukemia
E. Multiple myeloma
F. Benign tumors of articular tissue
G. Others

XI. *Allergy and Drug Reactions*

A. Arthritis due to specific allergens (*e.g.,* serum sickness)
B. Arthritis due to drugs
C. Others

XII. *Inherited and Congenital Disorders*

A. Marfan syndrome
B. *Homocystinuria*
C. Ehlers–Danlos syndrome
D. *Osteogenesis imperfecta*
E. *Pseudoxanthoma elasticum*
F. *Cutis laxa*

G. *Mucopolysaccharidoses (including Hurler's syndrome)*
H. *Arthrogryposis multiplex congenita*
I. *Hypermobility syndromes*
J. *Myositis (or fibrodysplasia) ossificans progressiva*
K. *Tumoral calcinosis*
L. *Werner's syndrome*
M. Congenital dysplasia of the hip
N. Others

XIII. *Miscellaneous Disorders*

A. Pigmented villonodular synovitis and tenosynovitis
B. Behçet's syndrome
C. Erythema nodosum
D. *Relapsing panniculitis (Weber–Christian disease)*
E. Avascular necrosis of bone
F. Juvenile osteochondritis
G. Osteochondritis dissecans
H. Erythema multiforme (Stevens–Johnson syndrome)
I. Hypertrophic osteoarthropathy
J. Multicentric reticulohistiocytosis
K. *Disseminated lipogranulomatosis (Farber's disease)*
L. *Familial lipochrome pigmentary arthritis*
M. Tietze's syndrome
N. *Thrombotic thrombocytopenic purpura*
O. Others

ROENTGEN FEATURES OF JOINT DISEASE

A. Peripheral Joints
  1. The soft tissues
  2. Soft-tissue calcification and debris
  3. Joint effusion
  4. Loss of bone density
  5. The joint space
  6. Erosions and "cysts"
  7. Resorption of bone
  8. The ossification centers and small bones
  9. Subchondral sclerosis
  10. Osteophytes
  11. Periosteal new bone formation
  12. Malalignment
  13. Subluxation and dislocation
  14. Disorganization
  15. Ankylosis
  16. The distribution pattern
  17. The time and sequence of changes
B. Spinal
  18. The disk space
  19. The vertebral body
  20. The apophyseal joints
  21. The atlantoaxial articulation
  22. The paravertebral area

DISCUSSION OF ROENTGEN FEATURES OF JOINT DISEASE

The soft tissues may show swelling or atrophy. Swelling is to be differentiated from joint effusion in the hands. Clubbing of the terminal phalanges is seen in pulmonary hypertrophic osteoarthropathy, hyperparathyroidism, and pachydermoperiostosis. Subungual hyperkeratosis is present in psoriatic arthritis and Reiter's syndrome. Eccentric soft-tissue swellings are seen in gout due to tophi, and in thyroid acropachy. Soft-tissue masses due to nodules in rheumatoid arthritis, granulomatous diseases, amyloid, and xanthoma may be noted. Diffuse soft-tissue swelling of a finger may be seen in infectious arthritis, neurotrophic arthritis, Reiter's syndrome, juvenile rheumatoid arthritis, psoriatic arthritis, and metastatic tumor. Rheumatoid arthritis has a typical distribution of soft-tissue swelling about the proximal interphalangeal joints.

Soft-tissue atrophy may be present in chronic long-standing disease. It is seen in the terminal phalanges in scleroderma and with Raynaud's phenomenon. Atrophy of the thenar and hypothenar muscles, giving a concave rather than convex hypothenar border, may be seen with systemic lupus erythematosus as well as neurological diseases.

Soft-tissue calcifications may be metastatic calcifications, calcinosis, or dystrophic calcifications. They may be para-articular, or if in specialized structures, in vessels, tendons, joint capsule, articular cartilage, or fibrocartilage. Para-articular and capsular metastatic calcifications may be seen in chronic renal disease, especially with hemodialysis, hypo- and hyperparathyroidism, and chondrocalcinosis.

Calcinosis is often seen in scleroderma, and also in the CRST syndrome. Dystrophic calcification may be present in calcific tendinitis, as well as in gouty tophi, and in tumoral calcinosis. Vascular calcification occurs most frequently in diabetes mellitus, and also in chronic renal disease with hyperparathyroidism. Articular hyaline and fibrocartilage calcification are characteristic of chondrocalcinosis.

Soft-tissue debris, calcific or ossific, is typical of the hypertrophic type of neuropathic arthropathy.

Joint effusion is characteristic of synovitis or early arthritis. In the hands, effusions of the proximal interphalangeal and metacarpophalangeal joints are typical of rheumatoid arthritis. Knee effusions may be detected by fullness of the suprapatellar joint extension, seen on lateral view, and by curved radiolucent lines medial and lateral to the distal femoral shaft in the suprapatellar region, seen on anteroposterior roentgenographs.[89] Posterior displacement of the fabella would also indicate a joint effusion. Hip effusion in children may be detected by displacement and increased convexity of the surrounding fat planes owing to capsular distension.[170] There are two obturator signs. The first refers to displacement of the fat line between the obturator interpus muscle medially, and the intrapelvic contents. This is due to muscular edema which shares in the inflammatory process of the hip joint. The second obturator sign refers to asymmetry of the obturator foramina on the anteroposterior radiograph. Because it is painful for the child to extend the hip completely in the presence of effusion, an involuntary pelvic rotation results (Fig. 9–1).

When traction is applied to a normal hip joint, blood gases come out of solution owing to reduced pressure. This phenomenon is termed the *vacuum sign*. In the presence of joint effusion, the vacuum sign will not appear. If the amount of fluid increases, joint widening will occur. If further fluid accumulates, particularly in the hip and shoulder in children, dislocation will ensue. Another characteristic of effusion is haziness. Loss of the sharp, white, subchondral cortical line also occurs.

Loss of bone density associated with various arthritides, in the absence of other metabolic bone diseases, represents osteoporosis. In arthritis, synovial hyperemia leads to early periarticular osteoporosis in those conditions where pain or functional impairment is constantly present. Other conditions, such as Sudeck's atrophy, burns, regional migratory osteoporosis, and connective tissue diseases may give a similar picture. In chronic conditions, osteoporosis proceeds to a uniform bone atrophy. Senescent osteoarthritis is concomitant with osteoporosis of aging. Subchondral demineralization occurs in rapidly developing processes such as septic arthritis. Certain of the arthritides are often characterized by a relative lack of osteoporosis. These are gout, neurotrophic arthropathy, psoriatic arthritis, Reiter's syndrome, and pigmented villonodular synovitis.

The joint space may be widened or narrowed. The normal hip joint space is slightly over 4 mm.[67] Widening of the joint space in early stages is due to effusion, and may be seen in almost any of the arthritides. Acromegaly characteristically shows widening due to cartilage hypertrophy, and this finding combined with osteoarthritis is diagnostic. Widening in late stages may be due to interposed fibrous tissue or debris. This finding in the distal interphalangeal joints is typical of psoriatic arthritis. Bone resorption, as in neurotrophic disease, may also result in widening.

Joint space narrowing is due to cartilage destruction and is a universal phenomenon. Rheumatoid arthritis typically results in uniform joint space narrowing, while that in osteoarthritis is most marked in the weight-bearing areas. This is most apparent in the knee and the hip. In rheumatoid arthritis of the knee, all three joint compartments are uniformly narrowed. In osteoarthritis, usually the medial, but sometimes the lateral, joint compartment shows the greatest narrowing. In rheumatoid arthritis of the hip, uniform narrowing results in medial migration of the femoral head, while in osteoarthritis, the superior aspect is narrowed. This sometimes results in lateral drift of the head.

An objective measurement of this finding is the center-edge angle (C–E angle).[94] A vertical line is drawn from the central point of the femoral head, and another line from this point to the acetabular edge (Fig. 9–2). The normal range of this angle is between 20° and 40° with an average of 36°.[9,87]

Erosions occur in many of the arthritides. The absence of erosions in the hands is typical of Jaccoud's arthritis, Reiter's syndrome, and systemic lupus erythematosus. Rheumatoid arthritis results in three types of erosions, termed by Martel[148] as marginal, compressive, and superficial surface erosions. Initially there is a preerosive stage with cortical thinning and a dot-dash effect, best seen in the metacarpal heads. Marginal erosions progress from an ill-defined surface erosion to a circumscribed, well-defined radiolucency. They may be fuzzily marginated or "punched-out," but do not have a sclerotic margin in rheumatoid arthritis. Erosions are initially located near capsule or tendon attachments, as the cartilage protects subchondral bone. This is particularly true of juvenile rheumatoid arthritis.

After articular cartilage is destroyed, subchondral bone is eroded. In pyogenic arthritis, where cartilage is rapidly destroyed by proteolytic enzymes, early erosions in contact areas of articular cartilage occur.

In contrast to rheumatoid arthritis, erosions in gout tend to have a well-defined sclerotic margin. Erosions of bone remote from the articular surface also occur in gout. There is a characteristic overhanging margination in this disease with the axis of the margin directed away from the central axis of the bone.[144] Erosions in osteoarthritis also have well-defined margins.

Erosions seen *en face* appear as "cysts." "Cysts" may also form due to pressure of synovial fluid

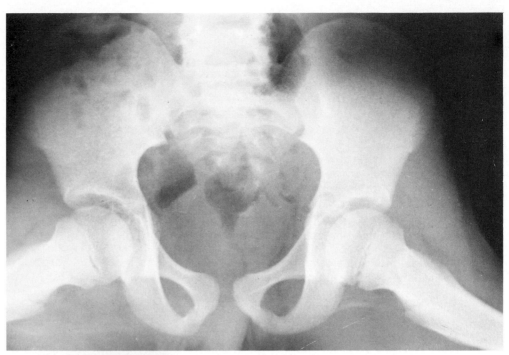

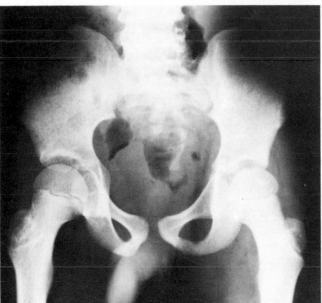

FIG. 9–1. Frog-leg and anteroposterior views of the pelvis showing both obturator signs. Asymmetry of the obturator foramina is noted. The obturator internus muscle is prominent on the left.

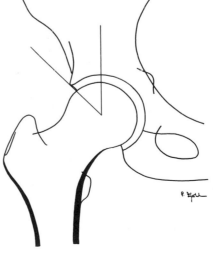

FIG. 9–2. Center-edge (C-E) angle. A vertical line is drawn from the central point of the femoral head, and another line from this point to the acetabular edge. (Drawing courtesy of Dr. P. Sirijintakarn)

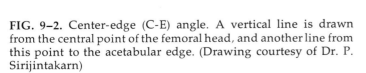

through defects in articular cartilage, and form ingrowth of granulation tissue into bone.

Resorption of bone in the vicinity of joints occurs in rheumatoid arthritis and psoriatic arthritis, and is characteristic of the atrophic type of neuropathic arthropathy. In the hands and feet, tapering of the convex member is usually seen, along with exaggeration of concavity of the opposite side to give a "pencil-in-cup" appearance. Both sides of the joint may be tapered, resulting in marked deformity. Resorption of an entire humeral head may occur. Resorption of the terminal phalangeal tufts occurs in a wide variety of conditions (see pp. 477–478).

The ossification centers and small bones show changes when the onset of arthritis is during the growth period. Juvenile rheumatoid arthritis, juvenile articular tuberculosis, and hemophilia may all cause changes in time of appearance and fusion of the epiphyseal ossification centers. A characteristic appearance is enlargement, irregularity of contour, osteoporosis, and coarsening of the trabecular pattern of the epiphyses. Shortening or lengthening of the extremity may occur.

Subchondral sclerosis or eburnation of subchondral bone is characteristic of osteoarthritis. Rheumatoid arthritis in the weight-bearing joints may develop a secondary subchondral sclerosis after cartilage destruction. Friction of opposed bone ends is followed by sclerosis.

Osteophytes in the peripheral joints, or marginal exostoses, are a characteristic feature of primary osteoarthritis. They overhang the periphery of articulating surfaces. They are continuous with the adjacent bone, and consist of trabeculae and fatty marrow, often covered partly by fibrocartilage or periosteum. They represent outgrowths of subchondral bone. Shifting and reduplication of the bone-cartilage border produce "flat exostoses" or irregularity of the contour of the articular surface. Reduplications result from new bone formation between the original calcified cartilage, and a newly formed zone above it. This is best seen in the femoral head.

Periosteal new bone formation may be seen in the inflammatory arthritides. Less than 5% of patients with adult rheumatoid arthritis show this finding. When seen in the hands, the periosteal new bone is sparse and thin, and occurs near involved joints. Juvenile rheumatoid arthritis typically shows thick periosteal new bone. Reiter's syndrome also characteristically exhibits thick and fluffy new bone formation. Periostitis associated with psoriatic arthritis is rare. The infective arthritides also show new bone in the areas of involvement. Ankylosing spon-

dylitis may be associated with irregular new bone formation at sites of muscle attachments, called "whiskering." Periosteal new bone formation in the hands may also be seen in pulmonary hypertrophic osteoarthropathy, thyroid acropachy, and pachydermoperiostosis. Fluffy periosteal new bone formation at the base of the distal phalanx of the great toe may be seen in Reiter's syndrome and psoriatic arthritis.

Malalignment refers to abnormalities of axial relationships of adjacent bones. They may manifest as deviation, flexion, or hyperextension. Deviation results when pathological changes in the tendons lead to muscular imbalance. A characteristic appearance is ulnar deviation of the fingers at the metacarpophalangeal joints. It is typically seen in rheumatoid arthritis, systemic lupus erythematosus, and Jaccoud's arthritis. In rheumatoid arthritis ulnar deviation is not easily reversible and is associated with erosions. In the latter two conditions the converse is true.

Characteristic deformities of flexion and hyperextension include the "boutonnière" deformity and the "swan-neck" deformity of the fingers. The former consists of flexion of the proximal interphalangeal joint and hyperextension of the distal. It may be associated with rheumatoid arthritis, systemic lupus erythematosus, and Jaccoud's arthritis. The latter deformity comprises hyperextension of the proximal interphalangeal joint and flexion of the distal joint.

Subluxation and dislocation may result from progress of deviation, from large effusions, or from destruction of the bone ends. Carpal malpositions may occur in rheumatoid arthritis. Telescoping of the fingers results in a *"main-en-lorgnette"* deformity. Large effusions of the shoulder or hip in infants result in dislocations.

Disorganization of a large joint is typical of neuropathic arthropathy. Fragmentation of bone ends, dislocation, and soft-tissue debris are seen. Arthritis mutilans refers to a destructive arthritis of the hands or feet, usually associated with a *"main-en-lorgnette"* deformity. It may result from rheumatoid arthritis, juvenile rheumatoid arthritis, psoriatic arthritis, leprosy, diabetes mellitus, or chronic infection.

Ankylosis may be fibrous or bony. Bony ankylosis assumes a different distribution and frequency pattern in the various arthritides. Interphalangeal bony ankylosis is more common in juvenile rheumatoid arthritis and in psoriatic arthritis. Carpal and tarsal bony ankylosis is more frequently seen in rheumatoid arthritis and juvenile rheumatoid arthritis. Bony ankylosis of the hip and knee is most frequently seen in juvenile rheumatoid arthritis, adult rheumatoid arthritis, and infectious arthritis. Bony ankylosis in osteoarthritis is rare.

The distribution pattern of joint lesions is a most valuable diagnostic indicator. Although individual lesions may appear similar, the sites of predilection of the various arthritides differ. For example, in the hands the distal interphalangeal joints are more often involved with osteoarthritis and psoriatic arthritis. Rheumatoid arthritis typically involves the proximal interphalangeal joints, metacarpophalangeal joints, and specific sites at the wrist. Reiter's syndrome characteristically predilects the lower extremities.

The time and sequence of changes and the characteristic evolution of the disease are important considerations, particularly with respect to correlation of radiologic and clinical findings. Certain diseases are apparent radiologically prior to typical clinical manifestations, while some do not show roentgen findings until late in their clinical course. Examples of the former are early rheumatoid arthritis, ankylosing spondylitis, and tuberculous arthritis. Examples of the latter are gout, hemophilia, and pyogenic arthritis.

The evolution of the roentgen picture is also of importance. For example, in pyogenic arthritis, destruction precedes osteoporosis, while in tuberculous arthritis the reverse is true.

The disk space may show changes of narrowing or calcification. Localized narrowing may be due to herniation of the nucleus pulposus, disk degeneration, infection, congenital anomaly, or atrophy accompanying fusion of the segmental apophyseal joints. Universal joint space narrowing is suggestive of ochronosis. The last condition also may cause generalized calcification of the intervertebral disks. Localized calcification of a disk may be idiopathic, posttraumatic, or infective.

The vertebral body may show the various changes of bone pathology described in previous chapters. A specific change of ankylosing spondylitis is "squaring" of the anterior margins due to bone resorption. Marginal osteophytes are typical of spondylosis. They are distinguished by their horizontal take-off, in contrast to syndesmophytes, which have a vertical orientation. The latter are most characteristic of ankylosing spondylitis. Posterior osteophytes may encroach upon the intervertebral foramina, causing neurological symptoms.

End-plate irregularities and erosions may also be seen, which are common to several afflictions. Exu-berant osteophyte formation is known as Forestier's disease.

The apophyseal joints may show narrowing and irregularity in both rheumatoid arthritis and ankylosing spondylitis. Subchondral sclerosis is seen in true osteoarthritis of the spine. Bony ankylosis is most commonly seen in ankylosing spondylitis and juvenile rheumatoid arthritis, but also may occur in psoriasis and rheumatoid arthritis. Ankylosing spondylitis typically involves the lower spine. Apophyseal fusion is often accompanied by atrophic narrowing of the corresponding intervertebral space. Congenital fusion may also occur.

The atlantoaxial articulation is a critical area, as quadriplegia or death may result from the subluxations which frequently occur in several arthritides. The most common causal disease is rheumatoid arthritis. Erosions and destruction of the odontoid process may also occur, as well as congenital hypoplasia or absence.

Radiography of the neck in flexion is often required to demonstrate atlantoaxial subluxation.

The paravertebral area may be the site of characteristic lesions. Coarse peripheral syndesmophytes may be seen in psoriatic arthritis or Reiter's syndrome. Arcuate paravertebral calcifications have also been described. A soft-tissue mass may occur in association with various processes, while a calcified paravertebral mass is typical of tuberculous spondylitis. Calcification of the interspinous ligament is seen in ankylosing spondylitis.

LABORATORY STUDIES[43, 160]

There are three laboratory studies particularly useful in the diagnosis of the inflammatory arthritides: the rheumatoid factor, antinuclear antibodies, and HLA.

Rheumatoid factor is an antibody in the serum capable of agglutinating various red blood cells or particles coated with gamma globulin. The current test uses latex particles so coated, and is positive if clumping is seen. The test is positive in about 90% of patients with classic rheumatoid arthritis. Severe disease correlates with classic rheumatoid arthritis and high titers of rheumatoid factor. The other collagen diseases—SLE, scleroderma, dermatomyositis, and polyarteritis nodosa—are also associated with the presence of rheumatoid factor. Various chronic infectious diseases and lymphoproliferative disorders, also have a positive rheumatoid factor, as does 4% of the normal population, with a low titer. The test is usually negative in the inflammatory arthritides with spinal involvement or psoriasis.

Antinuclear antibodies represent autoreactivity against nuclear constituents. Different antibodies react against different constituents. Antinative DNA is specific for SLE and is demonstrated in the LE cell test. Fluorescein tagging and radioisotope labeling are techniques now used for the autoantibodies. SLE and mixed connective tissue disease are nearly 100% positive. Scleroderma is positive in up to one-half of cases, as is Sjögren's syndrome. Rheumatoid arthritis is positive in 10% to 30% of patients. In the normal population antinuclear antibodies occur in up to 10% in a low titer. Other diseases, such as some liver disease, pulmonary fibrosis, burns, thyroiditis, myosthenia gravis, and Addison's disease also are associated with antinuclear antibodies.

HLA,[160] or *human leukocyte antigen*, represents the major human histocompatibility complex. It is a gentically determined system. Histocompatibility antigens determine "foreignness." HLA antigens are associated either positively or negatively with certain disease states. The chromosomal loci for the HLA genes have been assigned to the short arm of chromosome 6. According to WHO nomenclature, there are four major loci, designated HLA–A to HLA–D. There are several known alleles for each locus designated by an arabic numeral; *e.g.*, HLA–A2, HLA–B7, HLA–B8, and so forth. The loci A, B, and C carry alleles that code for antigens detectable by serologic methods. This system has been shown to be related to immune response capability and to some diseases associated with this response. One allele, HLA–B27, is associated with ankylosing spondylitis in about 90% of patients. It also has a high association with Reiter's syndrome. It is also present in about one-half of patients with psoriatic arthritis, particularly those with spondylitis.[229] Ten percent of the normal white population also carries the HLA–B27 antigen. The HLA–B8 antigen is also associated with a variety of disease states.

RHEUMATOID ARTHRITIS

Rheumatoid arthritis[64,102,218] is a common chronic disease characterized by nonsuppurative inflammation of the diarthrodial joints, frequently associated with a variety of extra-articular manifestions.

The average age of onset in adults is 40 years. Below that average, the ratio of females to males is 3:1, while above 40 years of age the sex incidence is approximately equal.

The clinical criteria for the diagnosis of rheumatoid arthritis have been developed by the American Rheumatism Association,[218] and are presented as follows.

The classification of progression of rheumatoid arthritis[218] is presented below.

CRITERIA FOR DIAGNOSIS AND CLASSIFICATION OF RHEUMATIC DISEASES

1. *Diagnostic Criteria for Rheumatoid Arthritis*

A. *Classical Rheumatoid Arthritis*

This diagnosis requires seven of the following criteria. In criteria one through five the joint signs or symptoms must be continuous for at least 6 weeks. (Any one of the features listed under "Exclusions" will exclude a patient from this and all other categories).

1. Morning stiffness
2. Pain on motion or tenderness in at least one joint (observed by a physician)
3. Swelling (soft-tissue thickening or fluid, not bony overgrowth alone) in at least one joint (observed by a physician)
4. Swelling (observed by a physician) of at least one other joint (any interval free of joint symptoms between the two joint involvements may not be more than 3 months)
5. Symmetrical joint swelling (observed by a physician) with simultaneous involvement of the same joint on both sides of the body (Bilateral involvement of proximal interphalangeal, metacarpophalangeal, or metatarsophalangeal joints is acceptable without absolute symmetry). Terminal phalangeal joint involvement will not satisfy this criterion.
6. Subcutaneous nodules (observed by a physician) over bony prominences, on extensor surfaces, or in juxta-articular regions
7. Roentgenographic changes typical of rheumatoid arthritis (which must include at least bony decalcification localized to or most marked adjacent to the involved joints and not just degenerative changes). Degenerative changes do not exclude patients from any group classified as rheumatoid arthritis.

(Reprinted from: Primer on the Rheumatic Diseases, 7th ed. JAMA (Suppl) 224:662–812, 1973, by permission of The Arthritis Foundation, The Journal of the American Medical Association, and Gerald P. Rodnan, M.D., editor)

8. Positive agglutination test—demonstration of the "rheumatoid factor" by any method which, in two laboratories, has been positive in not over 5% of normal controls—or positive streptococcal agglutination test. [The latter is now obsolete.]

9. Poor mucin precipitate from synovial fluid (with shreds and cloudy solution)

10. Characteristic histologic changes in synovium with three or more of the following: marked villous hypertrophy; proliferation of superficial synovial cells often with palisading; marked infiltration of chronic inflammatory cells (lymphocytes or plasma cells predominating) with tendency to form "lymphoid nodules"; deposition of compact fibrin either on surface or interstitially; foci of necrosis

11. Characteristic histologic changes in nodules showing granulomatous foci with central zones of cell necrosis, surrounded by a palisade of proliferated macrophages, and peripheral fibrosis and chronic inflammatory cell infiltration, predominantly perivascular

B. *Definite Rheumatoid Arthritis*
This diagnosis requires five of the above criteria. In criteria one through five the joint signs or symptoms must be continuous for at least 6 weeks.

C. *Probable Rheumatoid Arthritis*
This diagnosis requires three of the above criteria. In at least one of criteria one through five the joint signs or symptoms must be continuous for at least 6 weeks.

D. *Possible Rheumatoid Arthritis*
This diagnosis requires two of the following criteria and total duration of joint symptoms must be at least 3 weeks.
1. Morning stiffness
2. Tenderness or pain on motion (observed by a physician) with history of recurrence or peristence for 3 weeks
3. History or observation of joint swelling
4. Subcutaneous nodules (observed by a physician)
5. Elevated sedimentation rate or C-reactive protein
6. Iritis [of dubious value as a criterion except in the case of juvenile rheumatoid arthritis]

E. *Exclusions*
1. The typical rash of *systemic lupus erythematosus* (with butterfly distribution, follicle plugging, and areas of atrophy)
2. High concentration of *lupus erythematosus*

cells (four or more in two smears prepared from heparinized blood incubated not over 2 hours) [or other clearcut evidence of systemic lupus erythematosus]

3. Histologic evidence of *periarteritis nodosa* with segmental necrosis of arteries associated with nodular leukocytic infiltration extending perivascularly and tending to include many eosinophils

4. Weakness of neck, trunk, and pharyngeal muscles or persistent muscle swelling or *dermatomyositis*

5. Definite *scleroderma* (not limited to the fingers). [The latter is an arguable point.]

6. A clinical picture characteristic of *rheumatic fever* with migratory joint involvement and evidence of endocarditis, especially if accompanied by subcutaneous nodules or erythema marginatum or chorea. (An elevated antistreptolysin titer will not rule out the diagnosis of rheumatoid arthritis.)

7. A clinical picture characteristic of *gouty arthritis* with acute attacks of swelling, redness, and pain in one or more joints, especially if relieved by colchicine

8. Tophi

9. A clinical picture characteristic of acute *infectious arthritis* of bacterial or viral origin with: an acute focus of infection or in close association with a disease of known infectious origin, chills, fever, and an acute joint involvement, usually migratory initially (especially if there are organisms in the joint fluid or response to antibiotic therapy)

10. *Tubercle bacilli* in the joints or histological evidence of joint tuberculosis

11. A clinical picture characteristic of *Reiter's syndrome* with urethritis and conjunctivitis associated with acute joint involvement, usually migratory initially

12. A clinical picture characteristic of the *shoulder-hand syndrome* with unilateral involvement of shoulder and hand, with diffuse swelling of the hand followed by atrophy and contractures

13. A clinical picture characteristic of *hypertrophic osteoarthropathy* with clubbing of fingers and/or hypertrophic periostitis along the shafts of the long bones especially if an intrapulmonary lesion (or other appropriate underlying disorder) is present

14. A clinical picture characteristic of *neuroarthropathy* with condensation and destruc-

    tion of bones of involved joints and with as-
    sociated neurologic findings

15. *Homogentisic acid* in the urine, detectable
    grossly with alkalinization.
16. Histologic evidence of *sarcoid* or positive
    Kveim test
17. *Multiple myeloma* as evidenced by marked
    increase in plasma cells in the bone marrow,
    or Bence–Jones protein in the urine.
18. Characteristic skin lesions of *erythema nodo-
    sum*
19. *Leukemia* or *lymphoma* with characteristic
    cells in peripheral blood, bone marrow, or
    tissues
20. *Agammaglobulinemia*

It should be noted that these criteria were developed prior to the new classification of rheumatic
diseases adopted by the American Rheumatism Association in 1963, in which ankylosing spondylitis,
psoriatic arthritis, and arthritis associated with ulcerative colitis and regional enteritis are listed as
distinct from rheumatoid arthritis.

(Data from Ropes MW et al: 1958 Revision of diagnostic criteria for rheumatoid arthritis. Bull Rheum Dis 9:175–176, 1958;
Blumberg B et al: ARA nomenclature and classification of arthritis and rheumatism (tentative). Arthritis Rheum 7:93–97, 1965)

CRITERIA FOR DETERMINATION OF PROGRESSION
OF RHEUMATOID ARTHRITIS AND OF
FUNCTIONAL CAPACITY OF PATIENTS WITH THE
DISEASE

1. *Classification of Progression of Rheumatoid
Arthritis*[218]

Stage I, Early
    **1. No destructive changes on roentgeno-
        graphic examination
     2. Roentgenologic evidence of osteoporosis
        may be present.
Stage II, Moderate
    **1. Roentgenologic evidence of osteoporosis,

(Reprinted from: Primer on the Rheumatic Diseases, 7th ed.
JAMA (Suppl) 224:662–812, 1973, by permission of The Arthritis
Foundation, The Journal of the American Medical Association,
and Gerald P. Rodnan, M.D., editor)

    with or without slight subchondral bone de-
    struction; slight cartilage destruction may be
    present.
    **2. No joint deformities, although limitation of
        joint mobility may be present
     3. Adjacent muscle atrophy
     4. Extra-articular soft-tissue lesions, such as
        nodules and tenovaginitis, may be present.
Stage III, Severe
    **1. Roentgenologic evidence of cartilage and
        bone destruction, in addition to osteoporo-
        sis
    **2. Joint deformity, such as subluxation, ulnar
        deviation or hyperextension, without fi-
        brous or bony ankylosis
     3. Extensive muscle atrophy.
     4. Extra-articular soft-tissue lesions, such as
        nodules and tenovaginitis, may be present.
Stage IV, Terminal
    **1. Fibrous or bony ankylosis.
     2. Criteria of stage III

(The criteria prefaced by a double asterisk are
those which must be present to permit classification of a patient in any particular stage or grade.)

2. *Classification of Functional Capacity in
Rheumatoid Arthritis*

Class I—Complete functional capacity with ability to carry on all usual duties without handicaps.
Class II—Functional capacity adequate to conduct
normal activities despite handicap of discomfort
or limited mobility of one or more joints.
Class III—Functional capacity adequate to per-
form only few or none of the duties of usual occupa-
tion or of self care.
Class IV—Largely or wholly incapacitated with
patient bedridden or confined to wheelchair, permitting little or no self care.

(Data from Steinbrocker O, Traeger CH, Batterman RC: Therapeutic criteria in rheumatoid arthritis. JAMA, 140:659–662, 1949)

In the classification of rheumatic diseases
adopted by the American Rheumatism Association
in 1963, ankylosing spondylitis, psoriatic arthritis,
and arthritis associated with ulcerative colitis and
regional enteritis are listed as distinct from rheumatoid arthritis.[218]
Juvenile rheumatoid arthritis refers to rheumatoid
disease with an onset before the age of 16 years.
Females are more often affected than males. A number of features differ from those of adult disease,

including the occurrence of severe systemic disease and persistent monarticular or pauciarticular arthritis.

A peak in age incidence occurs between 2 and 5 years, and another peak between 9 and 12 years.

About 20% of children affected suffer from high spiking fevers, polyarthralgia, hepatosplenomegaly, lymphadenopathy, rash, pleuropericarditis, and possibly myocarditis. This condition is referred to as *Still's disease*. This picture has also been reported in adults.[31,61]

In the remaining patients, arthritis is present at the onset of illness. In 50% it is polyarticular; in 30% a single joint, most often the knee, is involved; and in the remainder it is pauciarticular. A serious systemic manifestation is iridocyclitis, which may lead to visual impairment. Rheumatoid factor is found in only 10% to 20% of children, and there may be high peripheral white-cell counts.

Felty's syndrome[223] refers to rheumatoid arthritis associated with splenomegaly and neutropenia. The patients are prone to recurrent infections.

Radiologically, rheumatoid arthritis involves the peripheral and axial skeleton. In the extremities, any synovial joint may show changes. There is, however, a predilection for the metacarpophalangeal joints and proximal interphalangeal joints of the hands and feet, the carpal joints as a group, and the distal radioulnar and radiocarpal joints. The acromioclavicular and sternoclavicular joints may be involved. The temporomandibular joints, knees, calcanei, ankles, hips, elbows, and shoulders may all be affected.

In the spine, there is a predilection for the cervical area, and only minimal changes are seen in the dorsolumbar spine. Sacroiliac involvement is uncommon.

It is this pattern of distribution that is important for radiological diagnosis, as well as the characteristic and predictable changes that occur at each site. The disease is usually symmetrical in later stages, but occasionally may be asymmetrical or monarticular. The latter form usually does not give rise to extensive destruction.

In the hands, the earliest changes include periarticular soft-tissue swelling due to joint effusion, hyperplastic synovitis, and periarticular edema (Figs. 9–3, 9–4). A technique has been described in which the hands are immersed in a 1:1 water-ethanol solution and xeroradiographed at low kv. This method shows the joint swelling in the preerosive stage to better advantage.[138, 139] It is spindle-shaped and most commonly seen in the proximal

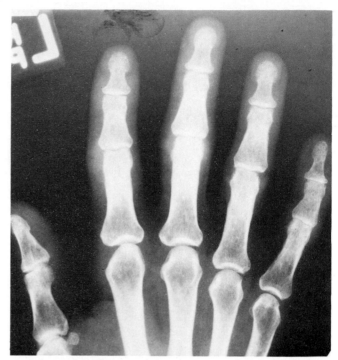

FIG. 9–3. Rheumatoid arthritis (hand)—early changes. Periarticular soft-tissue swellings of the proximal interphalangeal joints and the metacarpophalangeal joints are noted. A periarticular distribution of osteoporosis is also seen.

interphalangeal joints and the metacarpophalangeal joints.[143] Periarticular osteoporosis is another early finding, resulting from local hyperemia and disuse (Fig. 9–5). Widening of the joint space also occurs, but is difficult to demonstrate radiologically. This is seen only in early stages, when due to effusion. Preerosive cortical changes occur, best seen at the distal metacarpals. Initially, cortical thinning is seen, which progresses to a "skip" pattern or dot-dash type of deossification.

The pattern of erosions in the hand most frequently comprises the distal first three metacarpals and their corresponding proximal phalangeal bases, the base of the distal phalanx of the thumb, and the proximal interphalangeal joint of the middle finger.[148]

Anatomical and mechanical factors influence the sites of destruction and the progress of the disease, best ilustrated in the metacarpophalangeal joints.[151] (Fig. 9–6).

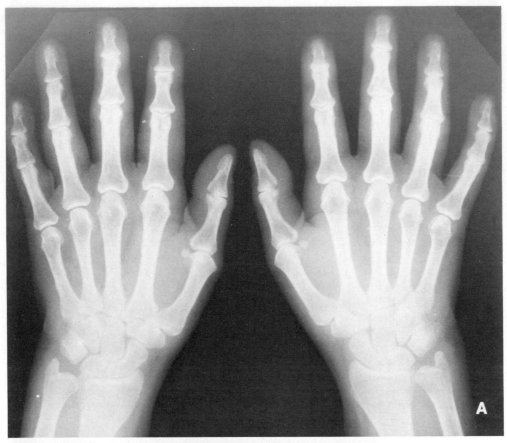

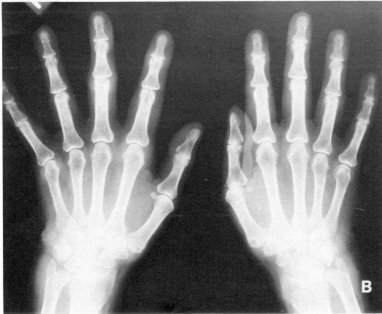

FIG. 9–4. Rheumatoid arthritis (hands and wrists). **A.** There is soft-tissue swelling bilaterally about the proximal interphalangeal joints as well as soft-tissue swelling of the wrists. **B.** Three-year interval film. Erosive changes have developed at both wrists, notably at the bases of the proximal first metacarpals, the trapezium, the radial aspects of the midnavicular, and the radial aspect of the midcapitate. Cyst formation is noted at the distal radii and ulnae. Only the most minimal erosions have developed at the proximal interphalangeal joints, although soft-tissue swelling persists.

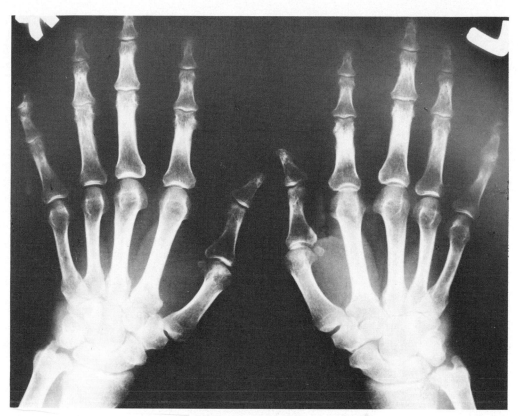

FIG. 9–5. Rheumatoid arthritis (hands)—early stage. A periarticular osteoporotic pattern is seen.

These articulations are the condyloid kind, formed by the reception of the larger, rounded metacarpal heads on the shallow cavities of the bases of the proximal phalanges. Each joint has a volar and 2 collateral ligaments. The volar ligaments are thick fibrocartilaginous structures, situated between the collateral ligaments to which they are connected. They are loosely united to the metacarpal heads but very firmly attached to the bases of the proximal phalanges.

The surface area of the articular cartilage on the metacarpal head is greater than that on the base of the proximal phalanx, leaving an area of articular cartilage always exposed at the former site. The synovium is attached around the margins of the articular catilage. On the metacarpals, it is reflected proximally along the neck, forming synovial pouches; greatest on the dorsal surface, and least on the volar surface. Thus a pouch with a double layer of synovium lies directly on cortical bone with no intervening articular cartilage. The relatively thin cortical bone at these sites is perforated by vascular foramina.

FIG. 9–6. Sagittal section of a metacarpophalangeal joint showing synovial pouches and articular cartilage relationships. (Drawing courtesy of Dr. P. Sirijintakarn)

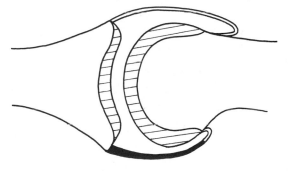

The synovium is the initial site of pathological changes in rheumatoid arthritis. The double layer of diseased tissue at the sites of the synovial pouches in contact with thin cortical bone, which is pierced by vascular foramina, gives rise to the initial erosive lesions. A possible mechanism is the invasion of diseased synovium along the nutrient vessels initiating destruction, with further pressure erosion leading to pseudocyst formation in areas of cortical bone adjacent to articular cartilage.

This mechanism explains the distribution of early bone changes, which are erosions at the margins of articular cartilage in the metacarpal heads. Up to 75% of patients may show erosions under the radial or ulnar collateral ligaments, while volar erosions are seen less frequently (Fig. 9–7). About one-quarter of patients at surgery may show a coalescence forming a collar of erosion around the metacarpal neck (Fig. 9–8). Erosions are less extensive at the base of the proximal phalanx, but may be present at the margins (Fig. 9–9), and may coalesce to form a ring. This is to be expected since no synovial pouches are present at this site.

The radiological patterns of erosions of the hand and wrist have been classified by Martel as marginal erosions, compressive erosions, superficial surface resorption, and pseudocyst formation.[148]

Marginal erosions arise through the above described mechanism, and are most evident radiologically at the radiovolar aspect of the metacarpal head. They also may be seen on the ulnar aspect. Conventional radiography does not demonstrate the dorsal aspects to good advantage. Norgaard[174] has suggested the utilization of the semisupinated position to show early changes, particularly erosions at the dorsoradial aspects of the proximal phalangeal bases (Figs. 9–10, 9–11).

Compressive erosions are due to the effect of muscular forces acting on osteoporotic bone, and their effect on the position of the joint. As the proximal phalanx undergoes volar subluxation and ulnar deviation, more articular cartilage on the dorsal and dorsoradial aspects lies in continual contact with diseased synovium.

The proliferating rheumatoid synovium releases

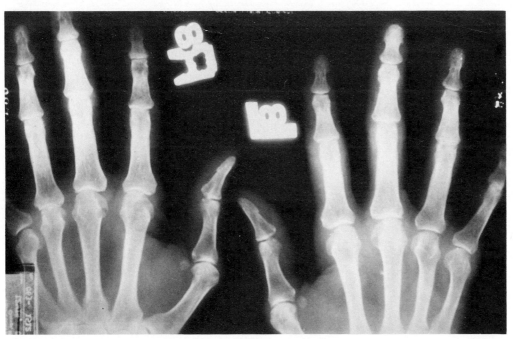

FIG. 9–7. Rheumatoid arthritis (hands)—early erosive stage. Marginal erosions of several metacarpal heads, minimal erosions of the bases of the proximal phalanges, and minimal erosions at the margins of several proximal interphalangeal joints are seen. Joint space narrowing in several areas is also noted.

lysosomal enzymes which degrade cartilage. The destroyed cartilage is replaced by pannus. Erosions of the proximal phalangeal bases as well as the metacarpal heads are greatest, therefore, at the dorsal aspects in the event of volar subluxation. Muscular forces may compress the bone ends into one another, causing bony invaginations, splaying, or irregular surfaces. This is a common occurrence.

Superficial surface resorption refers to a subtle erosion of the subperiosteal cortex along the shaft. It appears as a thinning of the cortex with fraying of the subperiosteal margin, somewhat reminiscent of hyperparathyroidism (Fig. 9–12). It may be accompanied by minimal periosteal new bone formation. The dorsal aspect of the first metacarpal and the proximal phalanx of the thumb are reported to be the most frequent sites.[148] It may be due to tenosynovitis.

Pseudocysts owe their appearance to marginal erosions seen *en face* and appear unconnected to the joint. They may attain large size, and may result from pressure erosion of the spongiosa following penetration of diseased tissue through the cortex.

The joint space becomes narrowed due to cartilage degeneration and destruction. Joint space narrowing without erosions may be present (Fig. 9–13).

The characteristic malalignment of the metacarpophalangeal joints is ulnar deviation of the phalanges (Fig. 9–14). Normally, the axes of the radials form a straight line. Deviation results in angulation of the axis. Subluxation refers to displacement of the articular surfaces (Figs. 9–15, 9–16), but the axes of the bones may or may not remain normal. Ulnar deviation and subluxation in rheumatoid arthritis are usually accompanied by erosions, and are irreversible. Reversible, nonerosive metacarpophalangeal malalignments suggest systemic lupus erythematosus or Jaccoud's arthritis.

Metacarpophalangeal bony ankylosis is not observed. Soft-tissue atrophy is common in later stages. In the proximal interphalangeal joints, the earliest sign may be a fusiform soft-tissue swelling. Joint space narrowing may be seen in early stages of the disease. Early joint space narrowing with an intact subchondral cortical margin is almost pathognomonic of rheumatoid arthritis.[56] Marginal erosions of the distal end of the proximal phalanx and the base of the middle phalanx occur, most commonly in the middle finger (Fig. 9–17). Compressive erosions, with "ball and socket" configurations or splaying of the bone ends, may occur in all proximal interphalangeal joints (Figs. 9–18, 9–19, 9–20).

(Text continued on p. 701)

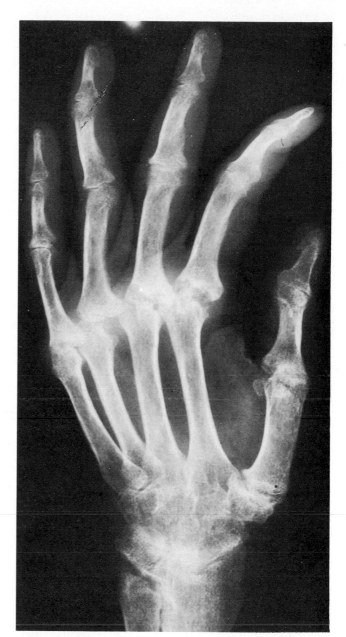

FIG. 9–8. Rheumatoid arthritis (hand)—advanced stage. Marked erosion of the metacarpal heads is seen involving all aspects at the second, third, and fifth metacarpals. Bony ankylosis at the wrist is noted, as well as a uniform osteoporosis.

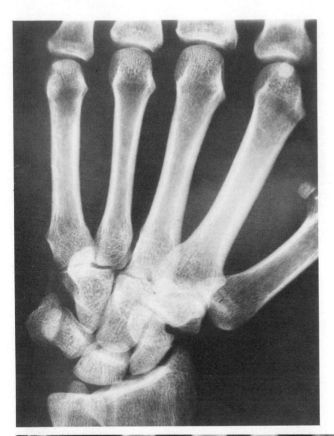

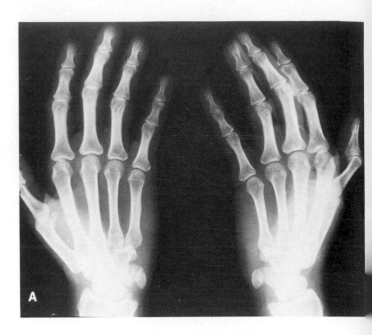

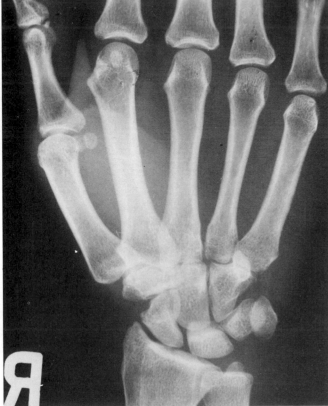

FIG. 9–9. Rheumatoid arthritis (both hands)—early stage. Minimal erosions at the margins of the bases of the proximal phalanges are seen. The distal metacarpals appear normal, and there is no narrowing of the joint spaces.

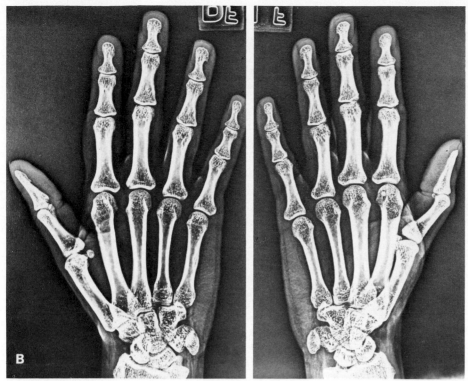

FIG. 9–10. Norgaard position (semisupination). **A.** Conventional radiograph. **B.** Xeroradiograph. This technique shows earlier changes at the bases of the proximal phalanges.

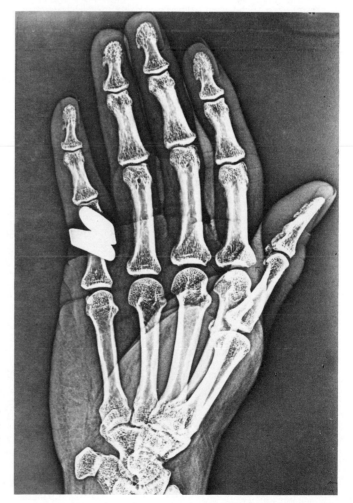

FIG. 9–11. Early rheumatoid arthritis (hand)—xeroradiograph in Norgaard position. Very minimal marginal erosive changes at the radial aspects of the bases of the proximal phalanges of the index and middle fingers are seen.

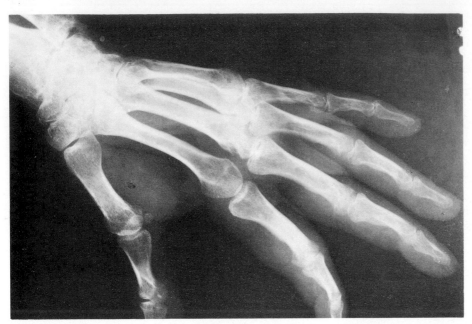

FIG. 9–12. Rheumatoid arthritis (hand and wrist). Erosions of the metacarpal heads of the middle, index, and little fingers are noted, as well as marked erosive changes in the carpus. Superficial surface resorption at the shaft of the first metacarpal is also seen.

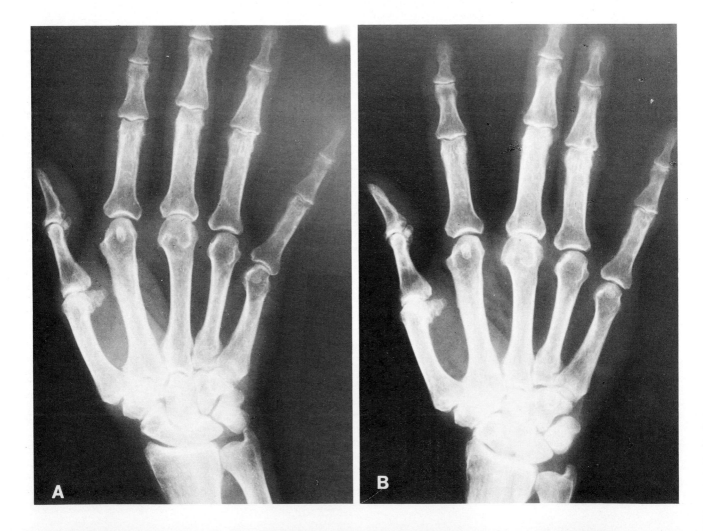

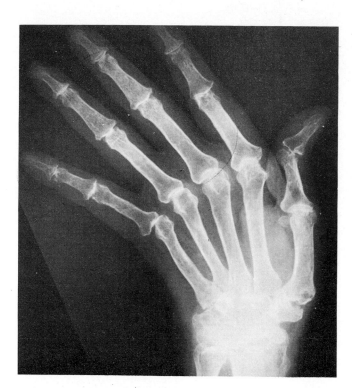

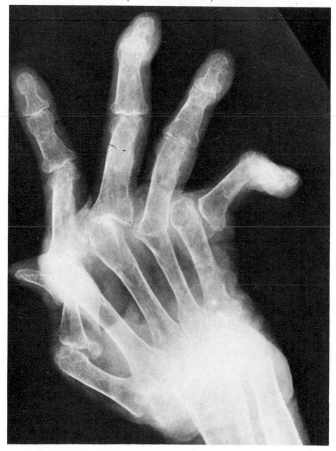

FIG. 9–14. Advanced rheumatoid arthritis (hand and wrist). Marked ulnar deviation at the metacarpophalangeal joints is noted, with hyperextension of the distal phalanx of the thumb. Joint space narrowing and erosions are also seen.

FIG. 9–15. Far-advanced rheumatoid arthritis (hand and wrist). Ulnar deviation and luxations at the metacarpophalangeal joints are noted, as well as dislocation at the carpus and at the interphalangeal joint of the thumb. Severe uniform osteoporosis is also present.

◀ FIG. 9–13. Rheumatoid arthritis (hand). A. Rheumatoid changes with narrowing of the third and fifth metacarpophalangeal joints and the third, fourth, and fifth proximal interphalangeal joints, with only minimal erosive changes. B. Same patient 3 years later. Joint space narrowing and soft-tissue swelling persist. Minimal erosive changes and pseudocyst formation have developed at the proximal interphalangeal joints of the ring and little fingers.

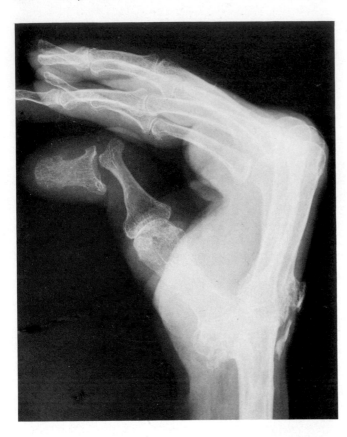

FIG. 9–16. Far-advanced rheumatoid arthritis (hand). Subluxations at the metacarpophalangeal joints associated with contracture of the hand, and dislocation at the interphalangeal joint of the thumb, are noted.

FIG. 9–17. Rheumatoid arthritis (hands) — early stage. Soft-tissue swelling at the proximal interphalangeal joints, associated with minimal marginal erosions, is noted. Similar changes at several distal interphalangeal joints are also seen. Joint space narrowing is also noted.

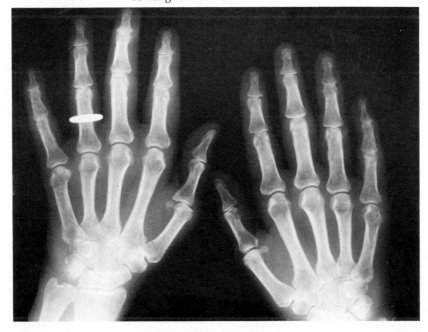

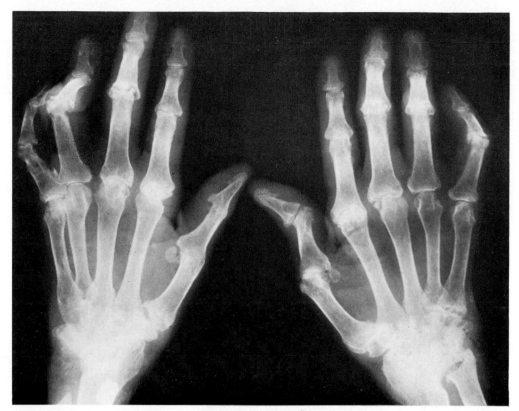

FIG. 9–18. Rheumatoid arthritis (hands and wrists). Compressive erosion at the proximal interphalangeal joints and several metacarpophalangeal joints, associated with pseudocyst formation, and soft-tissue swelling are noted. Marginal erosions and joint space narrowing are also seen. Severe carpal changes are noted with erosions, sclerosis, and partial fusion. A characteristic gouge defect at the ulnar aspect of the distal radius on the left is also seen.

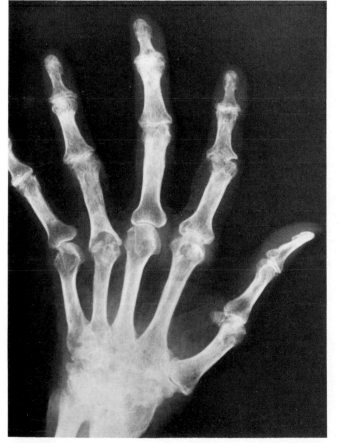

FIG. 9–19. Rheumatoid arthritis (hand). Compressive erosions are seen at the proximal interphalangeal joints, most pronounced in the index finger. A "ball and socket" compressive erosion is noted at the metacarpophalangeal joint of the ring finger. Carpal fusion is also noted.

699

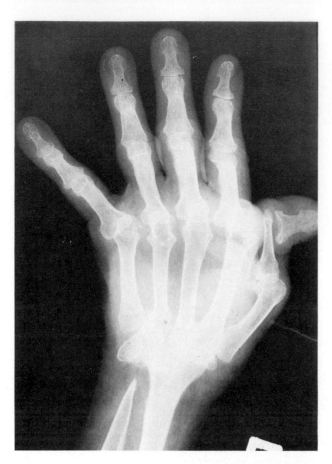

FIG. 9–20. Rheumatoid arthritis (hand and wrist)—advanced. Subluxation at the metacarpophalangeal joints is present. There is total dislocation at the interphalangeal joint of the thumb, with tapering of the distal aspect of the proximal phalanx and a cup-shaped deformity at the base of the distal phalanx. Tapering at the distal ulna is also seen.

FIG. 9–21. Rheumatoid arthritis (hands). Characteristic "boutonnière" deformities with flexion at the proximal interphalangeal joints and extension at the distal interphalangeal joints are noted at the index and middle fingers bilaterally.

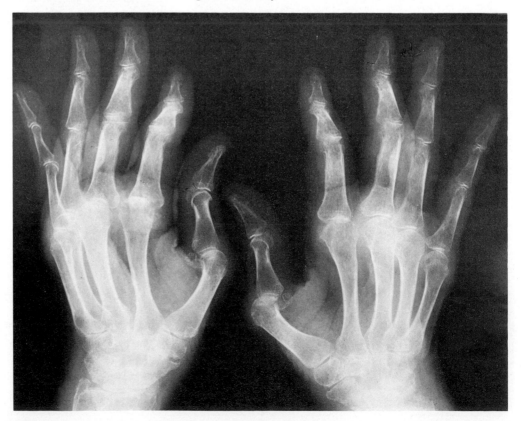

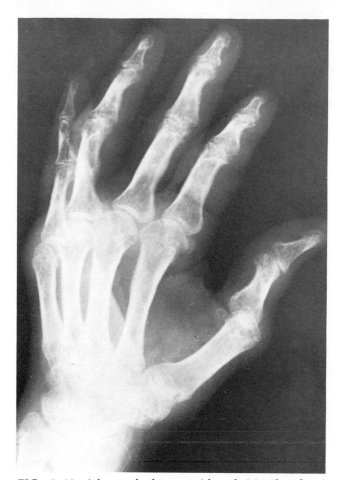

A characteristic deformity of the fingers, the "boutonnière" deformity (Fig. 9–21), occurs in rheumatoid arthritis. This may also be associated with systemic lupus erythematosus and Jaccoud's arthritis.[64] There is flexion deformity of the proximal interphalangeal joint and extension deformity of the distal interphalangeal joint, as though a "carnation were secured in a lapel." This is due to detachment of the extensor tendon from the middle phalanx, volar displacement, and resultant action as a flexor.

An opposite deformity may occur, referred to as a "swan-neck" deformity (Fig. 9–22). This is also seen in scleroderma, systemic lupus erythematosus, Jaccoud's arthritis, and psoriatic arthritis. The deformity occurs when the extensor tendon is shortened, resulting in hyperextension of the proximal interphalangeal joint, and compensatory flexion of the distal interphalangeal joint. In the thumb, the distal phalanx is often subluxed dorsally, with an associated flexion of the metacarpophalangeal joint.

Bony ankylosis of the interphalangeal joints may rarely occur (Fig. 9–23).

FIG. 9–22. Advanced rheumatoid arthritis (hand). A "swan-neck" deformity with hyperextension at the proximal interphalangeal joint and flexion at the distal interphalangeal joint is noted in the little finger. Marked osteoporosis is present as well as partial carpal fusion.

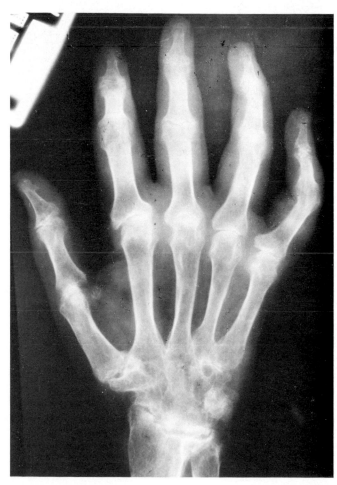

FIG. 9–23. Rheumatoid arthritis (hand). Bony ankylosis at the proximal interphalangeal joints of the index and little fingers, and partial ankylosis at the ring finger, have occurred. Compressive erosion at the proximal interphalangeal joints of the middle finger is seen, as well as joint space narrowing and marginal erosions at the metacarpophalangeal joints. Carpal fusion has also occurred.

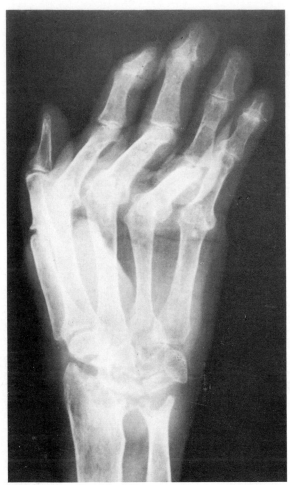

FIG. 9–24. Rheumatoid arthritis (hand)—far advanced. *"Main-en-lorgnette"* deformity with shortening of several proximal phalanges by compressive erosions and shortening by metacarpophalangeal dislocations. Severe erosions at the carpus and at the distal radius and ulna are noted.

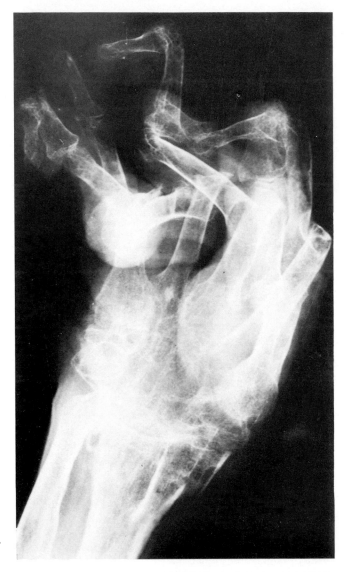

FIG. 9–25. Rheumatoid arthritis (hand and wrist)—severe arthritis mutilans.

FIG. 9–26. Rheumatoid arthritis (hand and wrist). Osteoporosis is noted, as well as mild marginal erosions along several metacarpophalangeal joints and at the ulnar styloid process. Periosteal new bone formation is noted along the radial aspects of the shafts of the proximal phalanges of the ring and little fingers. Minimal marginal erosions at several distal interphalangeal joints are also present.

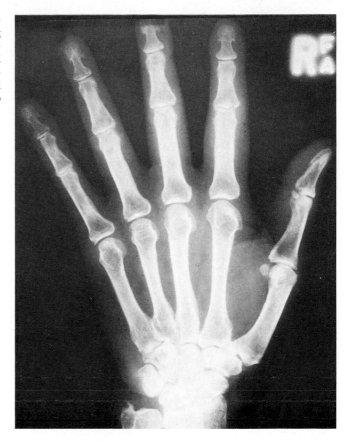

The distal interphalangeal joints are relatively spared in rheumatoid arthritis.

The disease may progress to extensive destruction of the bone ends, with "telescoping" of the fingers, the *"main-en-lorgnette"* or opera glass hand (Figs. 9–24, 9–25).

Periosteal new bone formation is sparse and thin. A thicker reaction is much more common in juvenile rheumatoid arthritis (Fig. 9–26). Secondary osteoarthrosis with subchondral sclerosis and marginal osteophyte formation may develop due to altered joint mechanics, but usually does not overshadow the features of rheumatoid arthritis[148] (Fig. 9–27).

In the wrist, soft-tissue swelling is an early change, most pronounced medial to the distal ulna and ulnar styloid process. The adjacent fat lines are obliterated. Osteoporosis may be seen early, often preceding erosions. All intracarpal joints are generally involved. Erosions at the wrist evolve by the same mechanism as in the hand (*i.e.*, between the articular cartilage and ligamentous attachments

(Fig. 9–28)). Frequent sites of erosion are the ulnar styloid, groove of the distal ulna (Fig. 9–29), radioulnar joint with "notching" of the distal radius, midscaphoid at its radial aspect, distal trapezium as well as proximal, midcapitate, and radial styloid, not on the radial aspect. The volar margins of the distal radius and ulna, and the triquetrum may show compressive erosions. A pattern of bone fragmentation involving the navicular, distal radius and ulna, and an elongated bony spicule overlying the radiocarpal joint, which is associated with carpal fusion, has been described by Resnick.[209] The carpal bones progress to definitive patterns of malposition.[42] Widening of the joint spaces of the distal radioulnar, the scaphoid-capitate, and the scaphoid-lunate joints is characteristic (Figs. 9–30, 9–31). Midcarpal angulation may also occur. Widening of the carpal spaces is not likely to occur in less than 2 to 3 years after onset.

Volar dislocation at the radiocarpal joint may ensue, as well as diastasis of the distal radioulnar joint with dorsal displacement of the distal ulna.

(*Text continued on p. 707*)

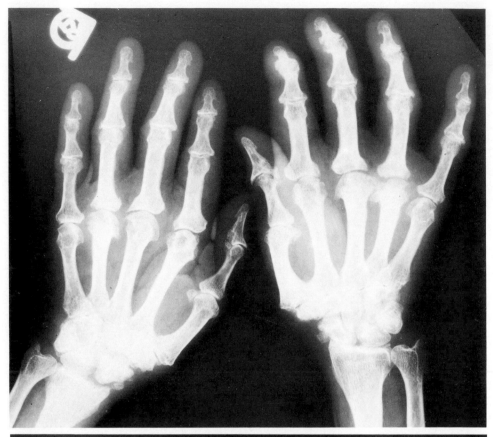

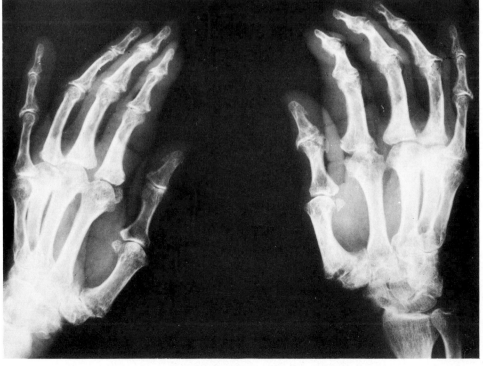

FIG. 9–27. Rheumatoid arthritis with secondary osteoarthritis (hands) — anteroposterior and oblique views. Joint space narrowing and erosions are seen, as well as pseudocyst formation. Hypertrophic lipping at multiple metacarpal heads and at the bases of the proximal and distal phalanges is noted.

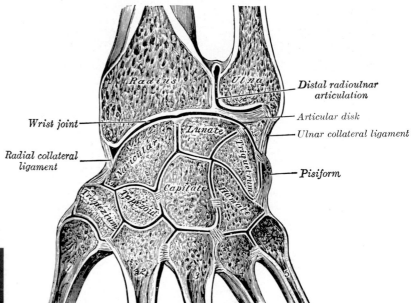

FIG. 9–28. Vertical section through the articulations at the wrist, showing the synovial cavities. (From Gray H: Anatomy of the Human Body, 29th ed. Philadelphia, Lea & Febiger, 1973)

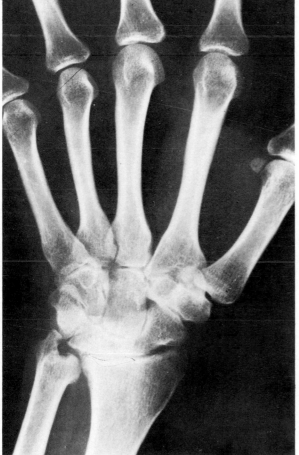

FIG. 9–29. Rheumatoid arthritis (wrist). Narrowing of the radiocarpal joint space is seen, as well as an erosion in the notch of the distal ulna.

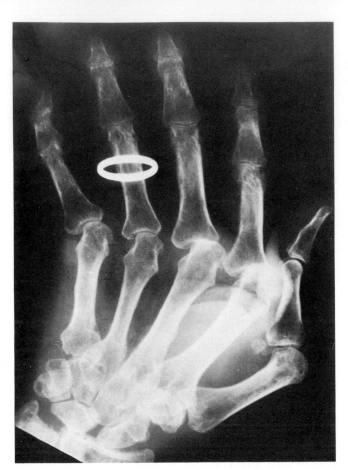

FIG. 9–30. Rheumatoid arthritis (wrist and hand). Scaphoid-lunate separation is present, as well as multiple erosions and pseudocyst formations. Subluxations at the metacarpophalangeal joints. with ulnar deviation and marginal erosions are also seen.

FIG. 9–31. Rheumatoid arthritis (wrist). Anteroposterior and lateral views. Subluxation of the lunate posteriorly is noted, with lunate-scaphoid separation. Erosions at the radial aspect of the lunate and the capitate are also seen, as well as erosion of the radial styloid process and the notch of the ulna.

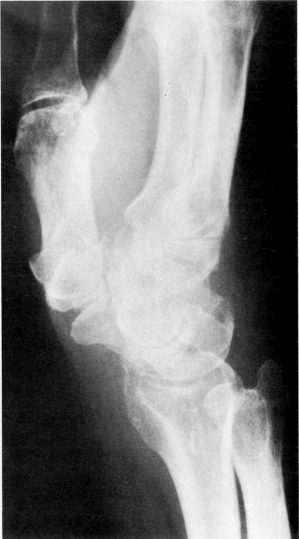

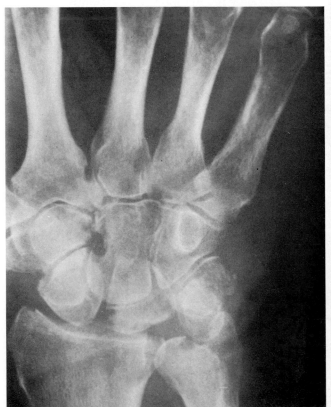

FIG. 9–32. Rheumatoid arthritis (hand and wrist)—far advanced arthritis mutilans. Fusion of the carpal bones, the carpal and metacarpal bones, and the joints between the bases of the metacarpals is seen.

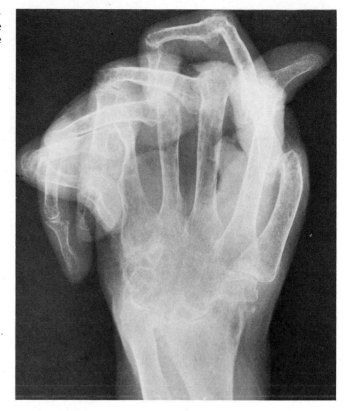

FIG. 9–33. Rheumatoid arthritis (foot). Metatarsal head erosions are noted, most marked at the third and fifth metatarsals. The configuration of the erosion at the fifth metatarsal head has been termed by Martel a "pocket erosion," producing a hooklike contour.

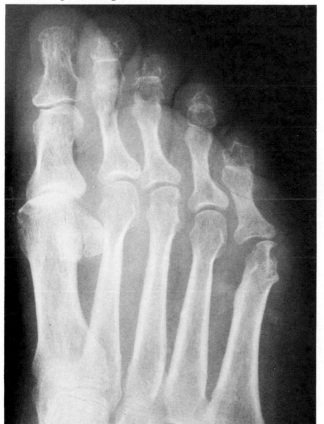

Deviation of the radiocarpal joint causing the scaphoid to lie in the hallow of the distal radius may also occur.

As the disease progresses, bony ankylosis is commonly seen in the intracarpal, carpometacarpal, and intermetacarpal joints (Fig. 9–32). Radioulnar ankylosis may rarely be seen.

The feet[194, 197] show changes analogous to those found in the hands. Metatarsophalangeal erosions are frequent (Fig. 9–33). The most common site being the medial-plantar aspect of the metatarsal head. The most frequent deformity is hallux valgus (Fig. 9–34). Fibular deviation of the toes at the metatarsophalangeal joints occurs, except for the little toe. Subluxations may occur.

Flexion deformities of the proximal and distal interphalangeal joints may occur, and may be associated with hyperextension deformities of the metatarsophalangeal joints (Fig. 9–35). The midfoot may show a planovalgus deformity (Fig. 9–36). Soft-tissue swelling may cause spreading of the metatarsal heads (Fig. 9–37).

(Text continued on p. 711)

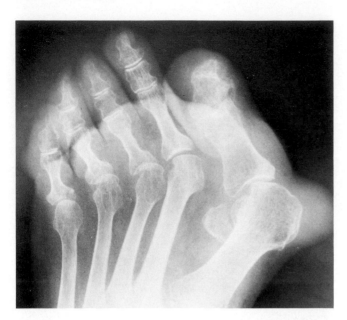

FIG. 9–34. Rheumatoid arthritis (foot). Marked hallux valgus deformity associated with soft-tissue swelling. Fibular deviation of the remaining toes is also noted at the metatarsophalangeal joints. Joint space narrowing and marginal erosions at the latter sites are also seen.

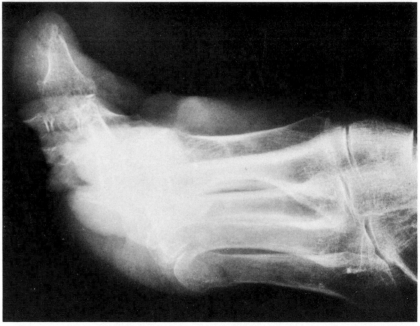

FIG. 9–35. Rheumatoid arthritis (foot). Hyperextension with subluxation at the metatarsophalangeal joints associated with flexion at the proximal interphalangeal joints, resulting in "cocked-up" toes.

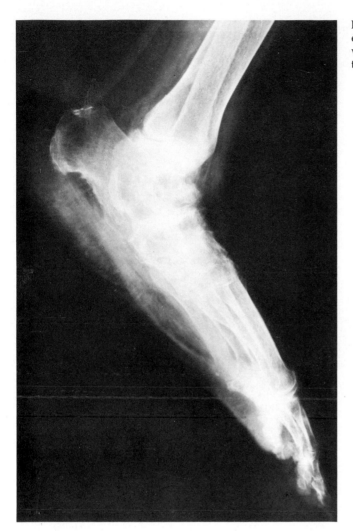

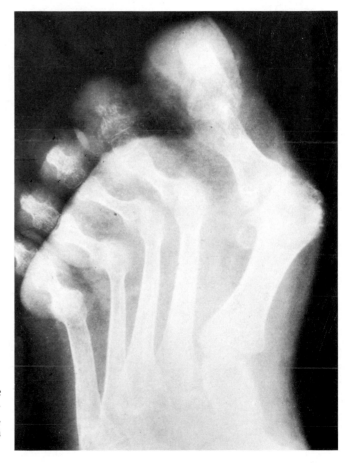

FIG. 9–36. Rheumatoid arthritis (foot). Pes planus and erosions at the inferior aspect of the calcaneus are seen, as well as slight irregularity at the posterior-superior aspect of the calcaneus.

FIG. 9–37. Rheumatoid arthritis (foot). Marked soft-tissue swelling is noted, which has caused spreading of the metatarsal heads and thickening of the toes. Hallux valgus is seen, as well as fibular deviation of the second, third, and fourth toes, and subluxation.

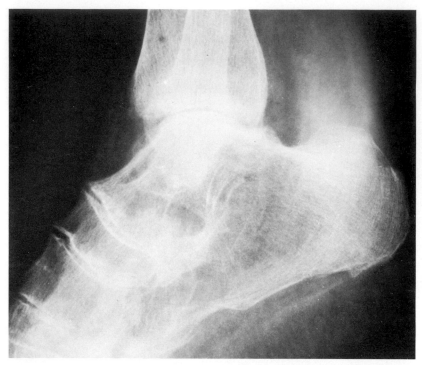

FIG. 9–38. Rheumatoid arthritis (calcaneus). Thickening of the Achilles tendon is seen, and an erosion at the posterior-superior aspect of the calcaneus is noted. Spur formation at the posterior and inferior aspects of the calcaneus is seen.

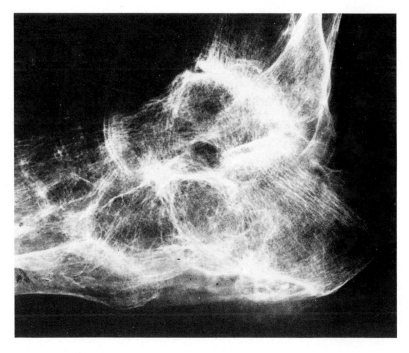

FIG. 9–39. Rheumatoid arthritis. Ankylosis at the ankle joint and tarsus has occurred. Severe osteoporosis is present. Periosteal new bone formation along the distal fibula is also noted.

The posterior aspect of the calcaneus at the site of the Achilles tendon, frequently shows changes.[204] A triangular radiolucency representing a fatty bursa between the Achilles tendon and the posterior superior aspect of the calcaneus is normally present. With rheumatoid involvement, the tendon becomes thickened and the lucency becomes obliterated. Erosion at this site occurs (Fig. 9–38). Erosion may also be seen at the calcaneal posterior plantar surface, and is often associated with a well-marginated bony spur. Late changes lead to bony ankylosis, frequently in the tarsals (Fig. 9–39).

In the elbow, soft-tissue changes are influenced by anatomic structure. Three fat pads are present between the synovial membrane and the capsule, two anterior and one posterior. These fill the fossae of the distal humerus. The posterior fat pad is the largest and is pressed deeply into the olecranon groove by the triceps tendon. The anterior fat pads superimpose on lateral view, and may be normally visible. In any condition leading to joint hemorrhage, effusion, or synovitis, the anterior fat pad may be displaced anteriorly and the posterior fat pad displaced so that it becomes visible. The differential of the elbow fat pad sign is given below.[164]

DIFFERENTIAL DIAGNOSIS OF POSITIVE ELBOW FAT PAD SIGN[164]

A. Hemarthrosis
   1. Trauma
   2. Hemophilia
B. Transudate
   1. Rheumatoid arthritis
   2. Other inflammatory arthritides
   3. Gout
   4. Pseudogout
   5. Osteoarthrosis
   6. Neuropathic
C. Exudate
   1. Infectious arthritis
D. Neoplasms
   1. Leukemia
   2. Metastases
   3. Synovial sarcoma
   4. Osteoid osteoma
E. Miscellaneous
   1. Pigmented villonodular synovitis
   2. Osteochondrosis dissecans
   3. Osteochondromatosis

In rheumatoid arthritis, this is a frequent occurrence (Fig. 9–40), and may precede bony changes, or may be displaced when there is only periarticular

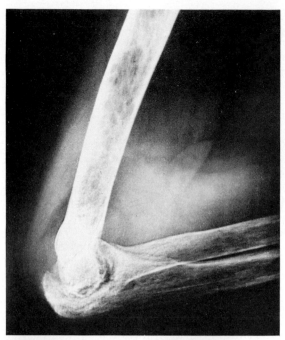

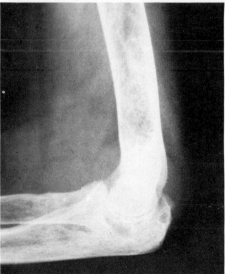

FIG. 9–40. Rheumatoid arthritis (elbow). Bilateral positive fat pad signs are seen, with displacement of both anterior and posterior fat pads away from the distal humerus. Erosive changes of rheumatoid arthritis and osteoporosis are also noted.

demineralization. A positive fat pad sign in the absence of trauma most probably indicates rheumatoid arthritis.[100]

A large bursa is situated posterior to the olecranon which does not communicate with the joint space. An associated bursitis is frequently present, and is seen as a soft-tissue mass. It may cause erosion of the posterior aspect of the olecranon process (Fig. 9–41).

The elbow is a common site for rheumatoid nodules, which occur in about 25% of patients. These are well-circumscribed, painless masses in the subcutaneous tissue, attaining a size of up to several centimeters. They may at times be subperiosteal. They are situated adjacent to the olecranon process and along the proximal extensor surface of the forearm. Nodules in similar locations may be seen in gout; however, they are not as discrete as rheumatoid nodules, and are more likely to produce bony erosions.

Osteoporosis occurs in the elbow in rheumatoid arthritis. A periarticular distribution is seen in early stages, and progresses to a uniform loss of density.

Cartilage destruction is uniform, and narrowing of the entire joint occurs (Fig. 9–42). Symmetrical involvement of both elbows is typical. Marginal erosions (Fig. 9–43) and irregularities develop, with disappearance of the articular cortex (Fig. 9–44).

Subchondral cysts or cystlike lesions, in large numbers and of large size, may be the prominent feature. Spontaneous fracture of the olecranon process due to erosions and cyst formation may occur,[193] usually through the midpoint of the trochlear notch. Extensive destruction and erosion may ensue, leading to subluxation (Fig. 9–45) and a picture of a nonspecific end-stage. Bony ankylosis rarely may occur (Fig. 9–46), although this is more common in juvenile rheumatoid arthritis.

Soft-tissue changes of rheumatoid arthritis in the knee include chronic intracapsular effusion. The fluid tends to accumulate in the suprapatellar pouch. On lateral view, this may be seen as fullness in the suprapatellar area with displacement of the fat lines away from the femur (Fig. 9–47). In the anteroposterior view, a curved radiolucent line lateral and/or medial to the distal femoral shaft in the suprapatellar area indicates this condition.[91] A more dramatic soft-tissue change may occur with massive distension of the popliteal bursae, where communication with the capsule frequently ex-

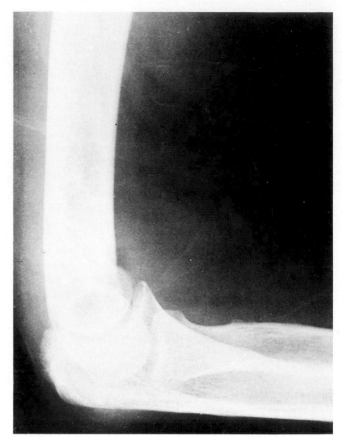

FIG. 9–41. Rheumatoid arthritis (elbow). Erosions at the posterior aspect of the olecranon process are seen.

ists.[178] A huge distended bursa may extend to the calf, and rarely the ankle. Synovial fluid may leak out into the surrounding tissues, causing severe pain (Fig. 9–48). Osteoporosis may develop, and progresses to a uniform pattern. The hallmark of rheumatoid arthritis in the knee is uniform joint space narrowing of all three compartments: the medial, lateral, and retropatellar (Fig. 9–49). This is in contrast to osteoarthritis, where the joint space is principally narrowed in the medial compartment. The uniformity of joint space narrowing suggests that the earliest change may be biochemical with atrophy of cartilage, and that surface erosion then follows.[37,158]

(Text continued on p. 718)

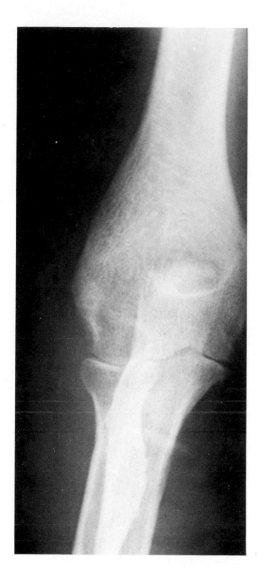

FIG. 9–42. Rheumatoid arthritis (elbow). Uniform narrowing of the joint space is noted, as well as periarticular osteoporosis.

FIG. 9–43. Rheumatoid arthritis (elbow). A large "pocket" erosion at the radial aspect of the distal humerus is noted, with associated soft-tissue swelling.

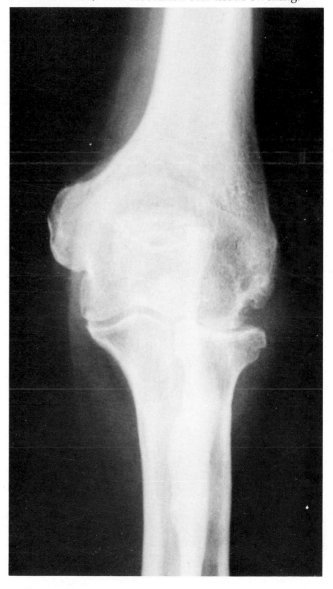

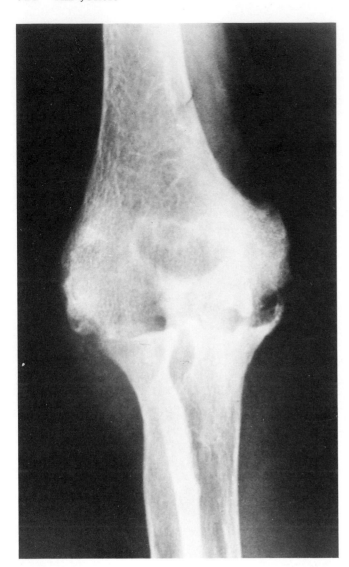

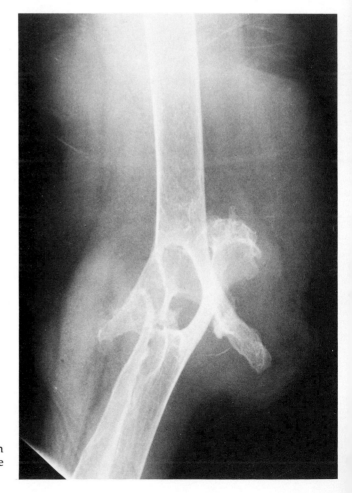

FIG. 9–44. Rheumatoid arthritis (elbow). Extensive erosions have led to disappearance of the articular cortex. Erosions at the humeral epicondyles are also present.

FIG. 9–45. Rheumatoid arthritis (elbow). Extensive destruction and subluxation are seen, associated with marked soft-tissue swelling. Severe osteoporosis is also present.

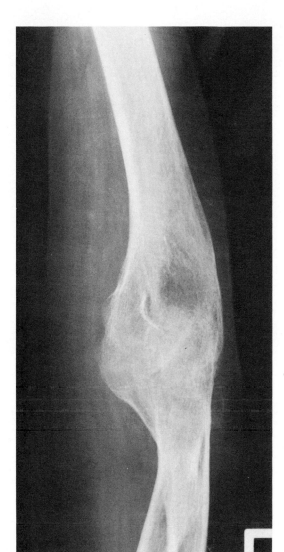

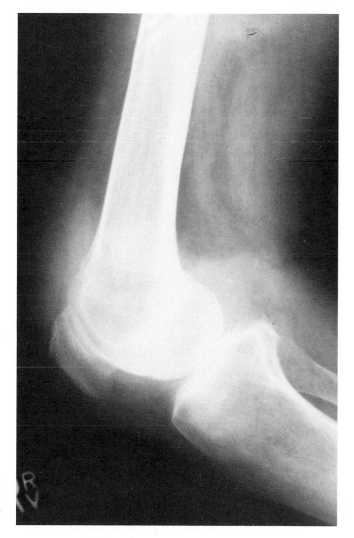

FIG. 9–46. Rheumatoid arthritis (elbow). There has been complete bony ankylosis of the elbow joint.

FIG. 9–47. Rheumatoid arthritis (knee). Effusion in the suprapatellar region is noted, with displacement of fat lines away from the femur. A Baker's cyst posteriorly is also present.

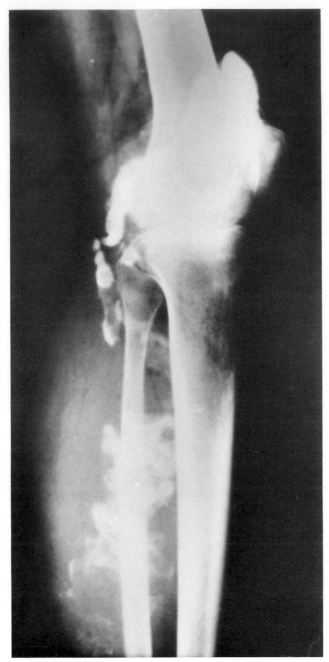

FIG. 9–48

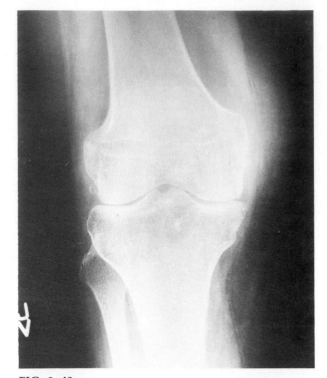

FIG. 9–49

FIG. 9–50

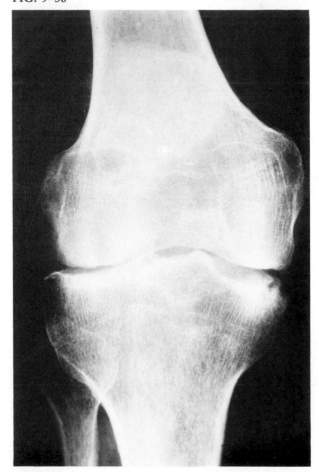

◀ **FIG. 9–48.** Rheumatoid arthritis (arthrogram)—giant ruptured bursa of the knee. Contrast material has dissected down the calf. (Courtesy of Dr. Dharmashi V. Bhate, VA Hosptial, Hines, IL)

◀ **FIG. 9–49.** Rheumatoid arthritis (knee). Uniform narrowing of the knee joint space is seen. Osteoporosis is also noted.

◀ **FIG. 9–50.** Rheumatoid arthritis (knee). Marginal erosions at the medial tibial margin and the lateral femoral margin are seen, associated with joint space narrowing.

FIG. 9–51. Rheumatoid arthritis (knee)—anteroposterior and lateral views. Advanced changes with destruction of the articular cortex at the medial and lateral aspects of the femorotibial joint are seen, with a compressive erosion of the entire tibial plateau. Erosion of the posterior distal femur from the posterior tibial lip is also seen, as well as narrowing of the patellofemoral joint. Severe osteoporosis is present. Vascular calcification may also be seen.

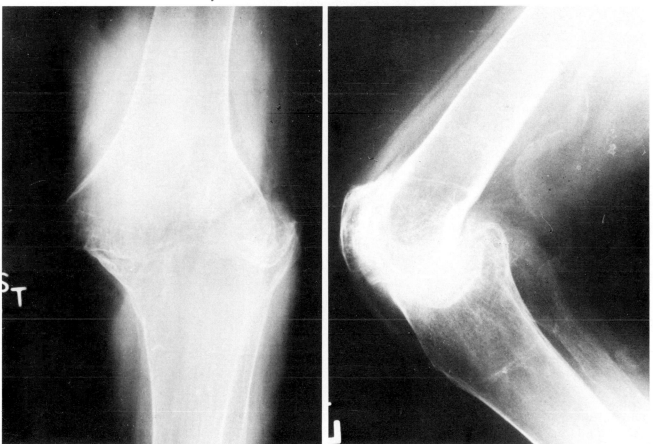

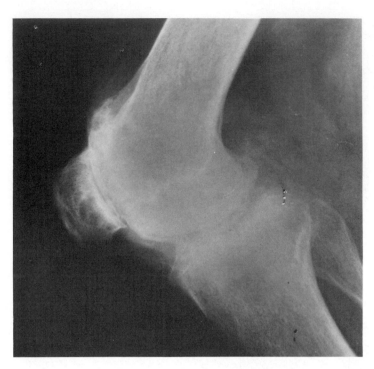

FIG. 9–52. Rheumatoid arthritis (knee). Pseudocysts are seen in the patella and at the femoral aspect of the patellofemoral joint. Secondary hypertrophic spurring in the suprapatellar region is also noted, as well as minimal posterior periosteal new bone formation.

FIG. 9–53. Rheumatoid arthritis (knee). There has been extreme narrowing of the knee joint space with cortical erosion, eburnation, and pseudocyst formation, as well as secondary hypertrophic changes.

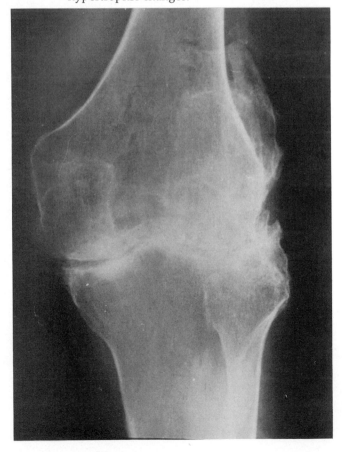

Erosions are less frequent in the knee than in the hands, but marginal erosions may develop (Fig. 9–50). Erosions of the central portion of the medial femoral condyle may occasionally be seen. The process may progress to destruction of major portions of the articular cortex (Fig. 9–51). Pseudocysts (geodes), which on occasion are quite large, may form in later stages[35] (Fig. 9–52). Secondary eburnation of the subarticular cortex may result (Figs. 9–53, 9–54). Sparse, thin periosteal new bone formation may at times be seen, particularly at the distal femoral metaphyses (Fig. 9–55). The intercondylar notch appears prominent in some cases (Fig. 9–56), but erosions may be exaggerated by radiographic projection of a semiflexed position.

The tibiofibular joint communicates with the knee joint in 10% of adults.[202] It may be involved in rheumatoid arthritis showing joint space narrowing and erosive changes.

In the shoulder, initiation of the rheumatoid process is rare. Ligamentous laxity permits upward displacement of the humeral head by muscle pull, with resultant erosion of the inferior distal aspect of the clavicle (Fig. 6–172). Erosion at the acromioclavicular joint also contributes to a characteristic tapered appearance, with an intact cortical margin (Fig. 9–57). This is in contrast to hyper-

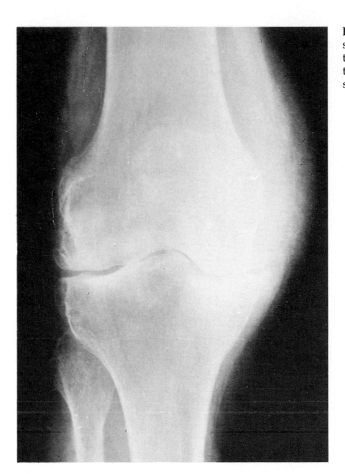

FIG. 9–54. Rheumatoid arthritis (knee). Uniform joint space narrowing has occurred. Secondary eburnation of the articular surface is seen, and also marginal spur formation. Ligamentous ossification to a minor degree laterally is seen, as well as soft-tissue swelling.

FIG. 9–55. Rheumatoid arthritis (knee). Minimal periosteal new bone formation at the distal femoral metaphyses is noted, as well as joint space narrowing and osteoporosis.

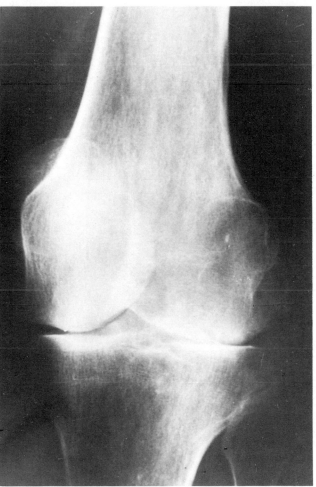

parathyroidism, where subperiosteal bone resorption renders irregularity to the cortex of the distal clavicle. Elongated erosion on the undersurface of the distal clavicle may be seen in rheumatoid arthritis related to inflammatory changes in the coracoclavicular ligament.[210]

The hallmark of rheumatoid arthritis in the humeral head is erosion. Initially, marginal erosions at the ends of the articular cartilage occur (Fig. 9–58). These are often seen above the greater tuberosity and at the inferior margin of articular cartilage. Large erosions may evolve as well as pseudocysts (Fig. 9–59). Sclerotic margins, as well as patches of bony sclerosis due to the healing process, may develop (Fig. 9–60). The above changes appear similar to those of osteoarthritis, hemophilia, and gout.

Erosion of the glenoid fossa (Fig. 9–61), and at the site of attachment of the coracoclavicular ligament (Fig. 9–62), may occasionally be seen.

(Text continued on p. 722)

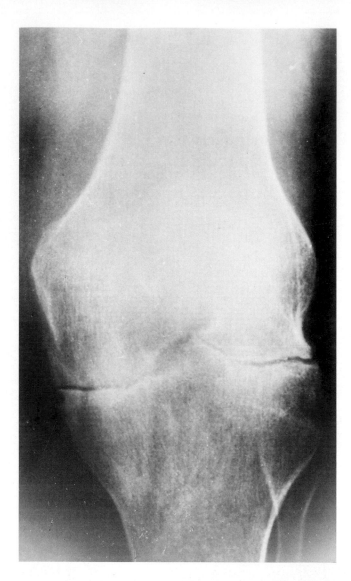

FIG. 9–56. Rheumatoid arthritis (knee). Marked joint space narrowing and erosion at the intercondylar notch at the femur are noted. Marginal erosion at the medial aspect of the tibia is also seen.

FIG. 9–57. Rheumatoid arthritis (shoulder). Erosion of the distal clavicle is noted at the acromioclavicular joint, leading to a tapered appearance.

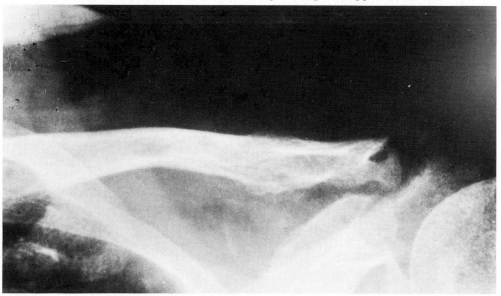

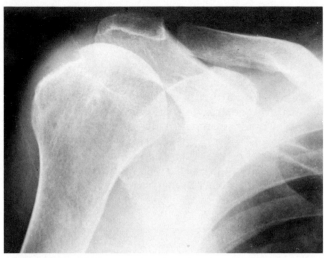

FIG. 9–58. Rheumatoid arthritis (shoulder). Erosion of the humeral head in the area above the greater tuberosity, at the margin of the articular cartilage, is seen.

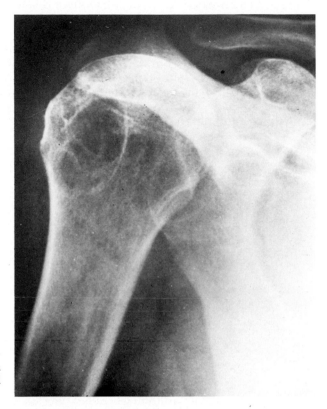

FIG. 9–59. Rheumatoid arthritis (shoulder). A large pseudo-cyst in the outer aspect of the humeral head is noted with a thin, sharp, sclerotic margin. A small erosion at the distal clavicle is also seen.

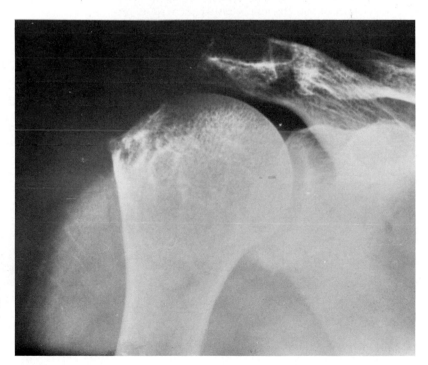

FIG. 9–60. Rheumatoid arthritis (shoulder). Erosions of the humeral head along the articular cartilage margin are seen, with sclerotic margins.

Severe resorptive changes occur at times in advanced disease. Pressure erosions of the humeral neck may result in a "hatchet-shaped" appearance (Fig. 9–63). Resorption of a portion or the entire humeral head may occur, with subsequent dislocation (Fig. 9–64).

Arthrograms of the shoulder in rheumatoid arthritis show nodular filling defects, irregularity of capsular attachments, bursal filling defects, and visualization of lymphatic channels. These may also show rotator cuff tear, biceps sheath dilatation, and frozen shoulder.[48] The latter is seen as a contracted joint space and obliterated axillary pouch. Arthrog-

raphy is the only means to distinguish between a rheumatoid flare-up and a rotator cuff tear, which is evidenced by the presence of contrast material in the subacromial bursa (Fig. 9–65).

The sternoclavicular joint is not infrequently involved, with widening and erosions.

Rheumatoid arthritis in the hips is characterized by uniform destruction of the articular cartilage, followed by erosions and superimposed degenerative changes.

This is in contrast to osteoarthritis, where narrowing occurs at the superior or weight-bearing aspect (Fig. 9–66). Narrowing of the medial portion of

FIG. 9–61. Rheumatoid arthritis (shoulder). Erosion of the glenoid fossa is noted.

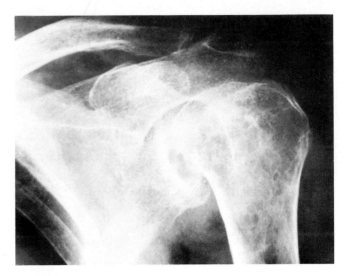

FIG. 9–62. Rheumatoid arthritis (shoulder). Erosion at the attachment of the coracoclavicular ligament at the inferior aspect of the clavicle is noted, as well as erosions of the humeral head.

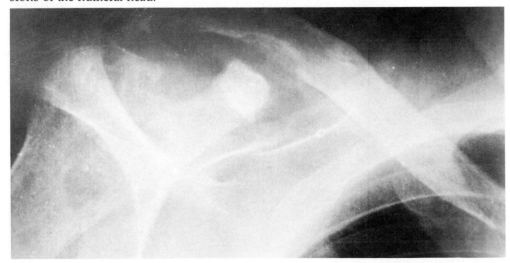

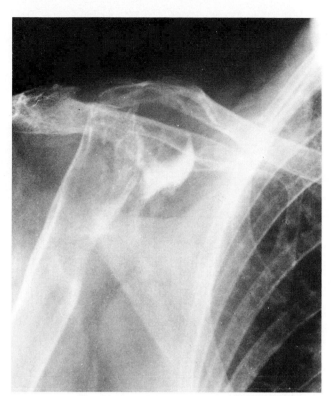

FIG. 9–63. Advanced rheumatoid arthritis (shoulder). Severe resorption of the humeral head and erosion at the humeral neck have resulted in a "hatchet-shaped" appearance. Erosion of the distal clavicle is also noted.

the joint space results in a medial drift of the femoral head.[6, 94] This medial drift leads to resorption and remodeling of the acetabulum to cause protrusion (Fig. 9–67). Erosions occur, and subchondral pseudocysts in both femoral head and acetabulum may be seen. Destruction and superimposed ischemic necrosis of the femoral head are late sequelae (Fig. 9–68). Concurrent progressive osteoporosis parallels the bone and joint changes. Erosions at the greater trochanter may rarely be seen (Fig. 9–69).

Rheumatoid arthritis, as well as osteoarthrosis, may give rise to large pelvic retroperitoneal or inguinal soft-tissue masses. This is due to massive enlargement of the iliopsoas bursa, which communicates with the hip joint.[10, 242] Hip joint involvement in this disease may rarely be monarticular, but is more frequently a component of polyarticular disease.

The extreme stage of rheumatoid arthritis in the extremities is "arthritis mutilans," with extensive destruction and disorganization of the joint with little remaining articular surface.

Spinal involvement in rheumatoid arthritis typically predilects the cervical region. The changes consist of subluxation,[29,44,190] erosions, intervertebral disk narrowing, osteoporosis, fusions, rarely granulomatous vertebral lesions,[76] and even a rheumatoid cyst has been reported.[134]

(Text continued on p. 727)

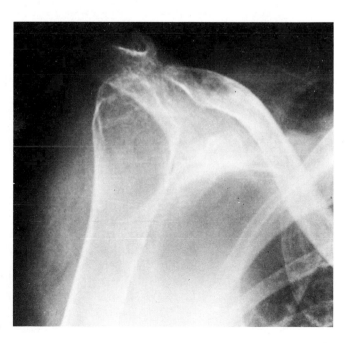

FIG. 9–64. Advanced rheumatoid arthritis (shoulder). Resorption of the humeral head has occurred, with subsequent dislocation.

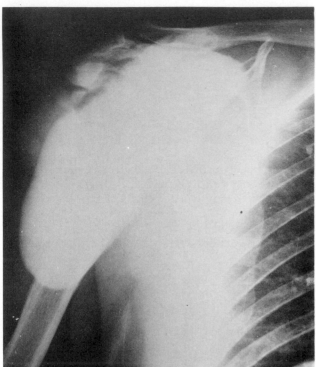

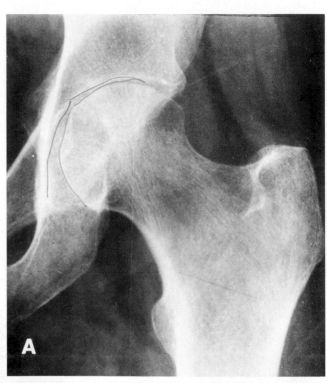

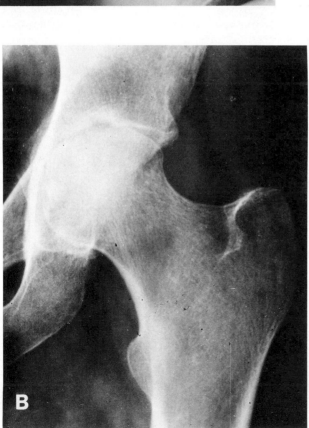

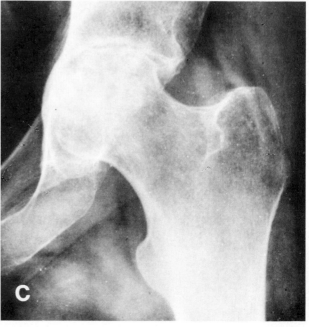

FIG. 9–65. Rheumatoid arthritis (arthrogram of shoulder). Contrast material fills a massively distended joint capsule. (Courtesy of Dr. Dharmashi V. Bhate, VA Hospital, Hines, IL)

FIG. 9–67. Rheumatoid arthritis (hip). Joint space narrowing and acetabular protrusion are noted on the left. Joint space narrowing is also seen on the right, to a lesser extent. Calcification in Cooper's ligament is incidentally seen. (From Steinfeld J R et al: Am J Roentgen 121:107–108, 1974)

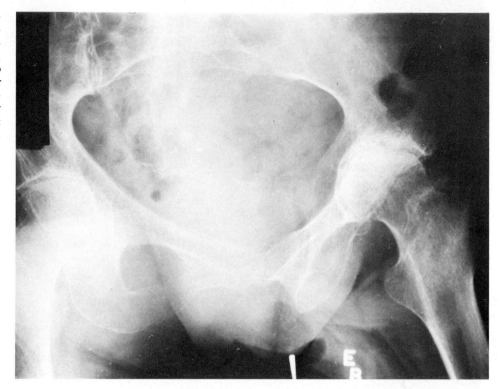

FIG. 9–68. Advanced rheumatoid arthritis (hip). Large erosions and pseudocysts at the medial aspect of the femoral head are noted. The overlying articular cortex has apparently collapsed partially.

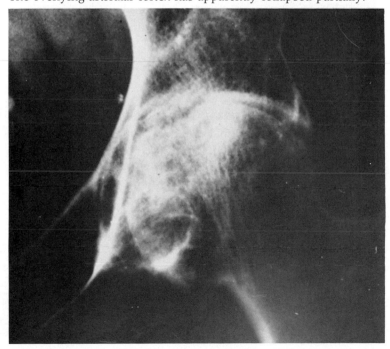

FIG. 9–66. A. Rheumatoid arthritis (hip). Uniform joint space narrowing is noted. **B.** Same patient, 1 year after **A**. Further progressive narrowing of the hip joint is noted, as well as subchondral erosions of both femoral head and acetabulum, and mild reactive sclerosis. **C.** Same patient as in **A** and **B**, 1½ years after **B**. Further progression of rheumatoid arthritis to minimal acetabular protrusion is seen.

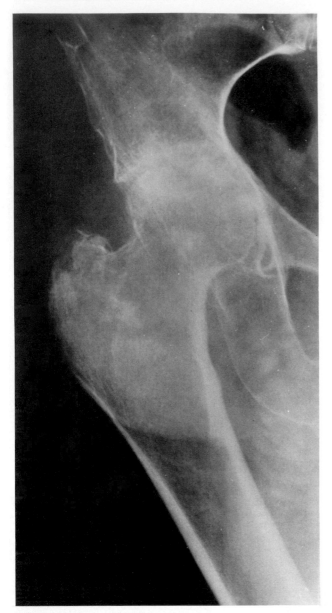

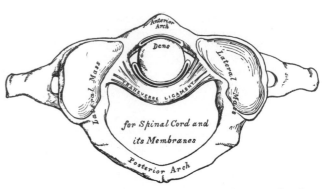

FIG. 9–70. Articulation between the dens and atlas. (From Gray H: Anatomy of the Human Body, 29th ed. Philadelphia, Lea & Febiger, 1973)

FIG. 9–71. Rheumatoid arthritis (atlantoaxial subluxation). There is widening of the joint space between the atlas and the odontoid process. (Courtesy of Dr. Harold Rosenbaum, University of Kentucky Medical Center, Lexington, KY)

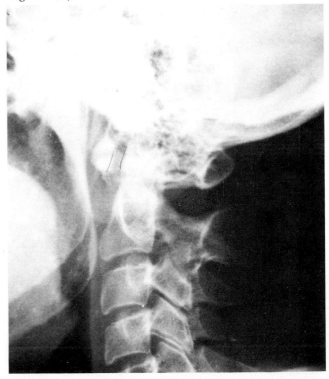

FIG. 9–69. Rheumatoid arthritis (hip). Uniform joint space narrowing is noted, as well as subchondral erosions. Erosion at the superior aspect of the greater trochanter is also noted.

The most frequent site of subluxation is at the atlantoaxial joint. The odontoid process is situated in close proximity to the anterior ring of the axis. The normal upper limit of separation in adults is 2.5 mm, while in children it may be as much as 4 mm. The odontoid process is secured firmly by the strong transverse check ligament that attaches to each side of the ring, preventing joint separation during flexion and extension of the neck (Figs. 9–70, 9–71). Two synovial joints are present, one anterior to the odontoid process, and one posteriorly between the transverse ligament and the odontoid process. Synovial inflammation leads to loosening of the ligamentous attachments and laxity of the transverse ligament, allowing atlantoaxial subluxation. This is most often associated with rheumatoid arthritis, but may also occur in ankylosing spondylitis, and in association with psoriasis. Severe neurological symptoms and even death may ensue due to compression of the spinal cord. Subluxation is best demonstrated in flexion views of the cervical spine, where a joint distance of greater than 2.5 mm confirms the diagnosis. The apparent joint space may be exaggerated by odontoid erosions. There may be circumferential erosion of the odontoid.[38] Rarely, the entire odontoid process may be amputated by erosions, or pathological fracture may occur.

Upward translocation of the odontoid in rheumatoid patients without platybasia has been recorded as a cause of urgent neurological syndromes and death.[191] The normal distance from the tip of the dens to McGregor's base line (posterior edge of hard palate to lower occipital curve) is 4.5 mm above the baseline. Several patients had distances of 10 mm and upward. Destruction and collapse of various parts of the occipito-atlanto-axial region lead to upward translocation.

Subluxations may also be present at other levels in the cervical spine, most commonly between C–4 and C–5. Occasionally multiple subluxations occur, showing a "stepladder" pattern. These subluxations are often accompanied by intervertebral disk space narrowing. Characteristically, no or very minimal osteophyte formation is seen in this condition. Occasionally secondary superimposed degenerative changes may lead to spur formation. Rheumatoid arthritis may be differentiated from spondylosis by the distribution of changes. Spondylosis usually begins in the intervertebral disk space between C–5 and C–6. If this is spared, inflammatory arthritis should be suspected.

Frequent sites of erosion include: the odontoid process, particularly at the posterior base; vertebral

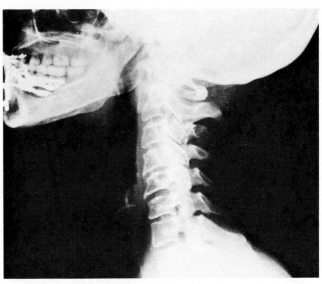

FIG. 9–72. Rheumatoid arthritis (cervical spine). Narrowing of the apophyseal joints in the middle and lower cervical region with fusion in the lower cervical region is noted. Only minimal intervertebral space narrowing is seen.

end-plates, where the lesions may resemble Schmorl's nodes in early stages; apophyseal joints; and the spinous processes, which may show tapering.

Ankylosis, if present, usually involves the apophyseal joints at one or a few levels (Fig. 9–72), but general ankylosis is rare in adults. The dorsal and lumbar spine show osteoporosis, perhaps augmented by steroid therapy. Rarely, rheumatoid nodules occur in the medulla of vertebral bodies, leading to collapse. A rheumatoid cyst, extending from a lumbar apophyseal joint into the epidural space and compressing the cauda equina, has been reported. Smooth erosion of the superior margins of the upper ribs occurs in rheumatoid arthritis as well as in other conditions (Fig. 6–180; see p. 481). The postulated mechanisms are pressure erosions from the scapula on osteoporotic bone, and resorption of bone at muscle attachments.

The sacroiliac joints occasionally exhibit minimal erosions in rheumatoid arthritis, with unilateral or a typical asymmetric distribution. Joint space narrowing without reactive sclerosis may also be seen, or rarely fusion of the joint. The temporomandibular joint is relatively often involved, as is, with a lesser frequency, the sternoclavicular joint.

A reported complication of rheumatoid arthritis

is necrotizing vasculitis with occlusion and resulting gangrene.[46]

Septic arthritis also occurs as a complication of rheumatoid arthritis.[71,196] Stress fractures of the long bones have been reported in this condition.[228] Unilateral changes of rheumatoid arthritis may be seen in patients with hemiplegia, since the immobilization paralysis prevents arthritic changes from advancing.[263]

Rheumatoid arthritis may present with an atypical appearance which may cause some confusion with gout.[192] The changes found are subarticular erosions with well-defined or sclerotic margins, erosions along the diaphysis, destruction of cartilage with hypertrophic bone formation simulating an overhanging margin, and localized soft-tissue swellings which could be mistaken for tophi. Localized, often large subcutaneous nodules about the joints of the hand and associated with only mild erosive changes have been described as a variant of the disease and termed *rheumatoid nodulosis*.[26]

JUVENILE RHEUMATOID ARTHRITIS

Juvenile rheumatoid arthritis[149] has radiologic manifestations that differ somewhat from those of the adult form of this disease. The distribution of involved joints differs, with a predilection for those joints undergoing most rapid growth. Monarticular disease is more common than in adults. Periosteal new bone formation is frequent, reflecting a greater growth potential. The growth potential modifies the evolution of the disease with premature appearance of epiphyseal ossification centers associated with ultimate smaller size, but early increase in size due to hyperemia.

A minority of patients are positive for IgM rheumatoid factor. These seropositive patients have early development of erosions at the metacarpal, interphalangeal, and metatarsal joints.[7] Progressive destruction occurs in untreated cases. Among seronegative patients three patterns of disease are seen: (1) systemic illness without early radiological changes (Still's disease); (2) Pauciarticular disease (few joints involved with frequent growth anomalies), and (3) generalized polyarthritis. Growth stimulation and early epiphyseal fusion result in either increase or decrease in length. Brachydactyly is common. Overconstriction of the diaphyses may occur (Figs. 9–73, 2–17). The articular cartilage is destroyed relatively late in the disease. There is a tendency toward ankylosis and dislocations of larger joints. Carpal and tarsal ankyloses are frequent. Erosions appear late. Radiolucent submetaphyseal bands are frequent and represent a nonspecific change. Compression fractures of the epiphyses may be seen.

The knee, ankle, and wrist are most frequently involved, with the hand, elbow, hip (Fig. 9–74), foot, shoulder, and cervical spine following, as reported by Martel *et al.*[149]

The knee shows soft-tissue swelling, overgrowth of the epiphyses, "squaring" of the inferior margin of the patella,[39] and overconstriction of the component shafts, as well as joint space narrowing. This appearance is identical to that seen in hemophilia, and even erosion of the femoral intercondylar notch may be present (Fig. 9–75). The hips may show acetabular protrusion, dislocation, or fusion (Fig. 9–76). Coxa valga, irregular and poorly formed femoral heads, and acetabular dysplasia may also occur, as well as iliac hypoplasia. Ischemic necrosis of the femoral heads, possibly caused by steroid therapy, may somtimes be seen.

Micrognathia is often present, with erosion of the mandibular condyle, and broad fossae.

In the spine, the cervical region is predilected as in adult disease. Subluxations, particularly atlantoaxial, are common (Fig. 9–77). There is a greater tendency to develop apophyseal joint ankylosis, which begins at the higher level and proceeds downward. Undergrowth of the vertebral bodies and intervertebral disks at the affected levels occurs, leading to block fusion. The spinous processes may show tapering. Mild sacroiliac arthritis may rarely occur. Vertebral end-plate destruction is rare. Compression fractures occur in the spine, possibly secondary to osteoporosis aggravated by steroid therapy. Dorsolumbar scoliosis may occur in advanced disease.[220]

In late stages, a generalized osteoporosis may be present. Bizarre deformities with subluxations due to growth disturbances and contractures are seen at times. Joint space narrowing leads to secondary osteoarthrosis. Periarticular calcification and digital arterial calcification have been reported.

ANKYLOSING SPONDYLITIS

Ankylosing spondylitis[19,179,218] is a chronic, progressive arthritis characterized by involvement of the sacroiliac joints, the spinal apophyseal joints, and the paravertebral soft tissues. The age of onset is usually in the latter second or early third decade of

FIG. 9–73. Juvenile rheumatoid arthritis (hands and wrists). Marked osteoporosis is present. Overconstriction of all of the diaphyses is noted. Enlargement and increased trabeculation of the carpal bones with some irregularity of contour is noted, as well as irregularity of the distal radial epiphysis and of the metacarpal heads. Shortening of the third and the fourth metacarpals and shortening of the ulna are noted. "Boutonnière" deformities of the fingers are seen, as well as compressive erosion of the base of the distal phalanges of the middle finger and thumb.

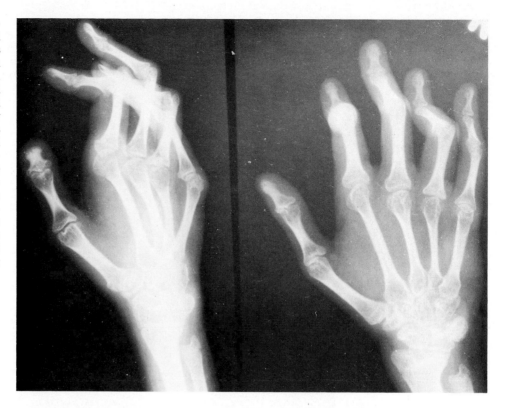

FIG. 9–74. Juvenile rheumatoid arthritis (hip); same patient as in Fig. 2–17. Osteoporosis of the right hip and resorptive changes of the right femoral head are seen.

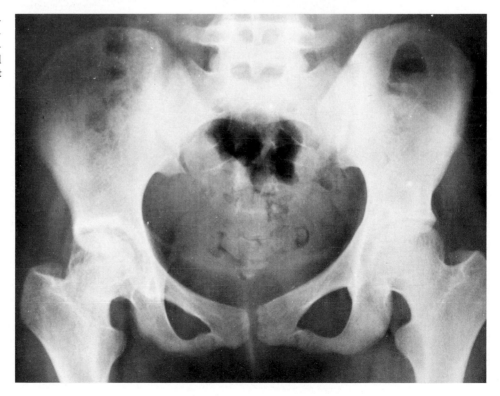

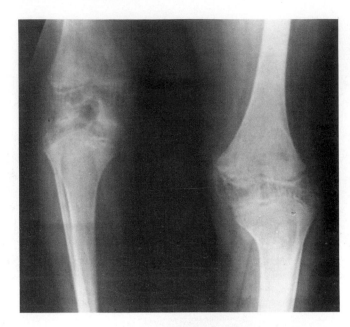

FIG. 9–75. Juvenile rheumatoid arthritis (knees). There has been shortening of the right lower extremity. Enlargement of the epiphyseal ossification centers is noted, with joint space narrowing. Erosion of the intercondylar notch on the right is also seen, as well as overconstriction. Surgical fusion of the left knee has been performed.

FIG. 9–76. Juvenile rheumatoid arthritis. Marked osteoporosis is present. There is bony ankylosis of the left hip. Enlargement of the right femoral head is seen. Erosive changes at both ischia and symphysis pubis are also noted. Fusion of both sacroiliac joints is seen.

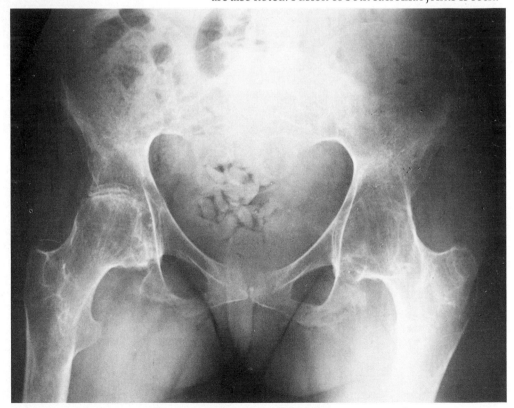

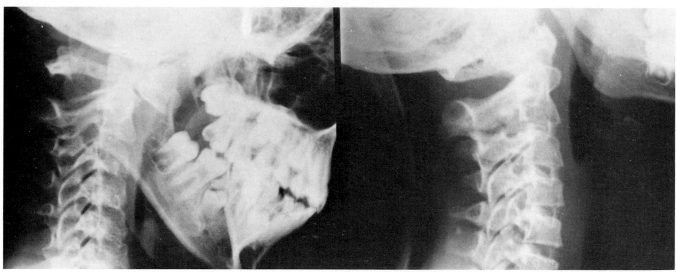

FIG. 9–77. Cervical spine in flexion and extension views. Extension view shows normal atlantoaxial relationships. Flexion view shows marked anterior atlantoaxial subluxation.

life, and approximately 90% of patients are males.

Clinically, the onset is usually insidious, with low back pain, sarcoiliac or hip pain, or less commonly pain with sciatic distribution. Iridocyclitis, which may precede arthritis, occurs in about 25% of patients. Aortic insufficiency and cardiac conduction disturbances develop in about 4% and 10% of cases, respectively. The clinical manifestations may be atypical in women, with an older age of onset, higher incidence of peripheral joint disease, and milder disease course. Almost all patients are positive for HLA–B27 antigen. The clinical criteria for this disease have been standardized (Rome Criteria) and are presented below.[199]

ROME CRITERIA FOR ANKYLOSING SPONDYLITIS[207]

1. Low back pain and stiffness of over 3 months' duration not relieved by rest
2. Pain and stiffness in the thoracic region
3. Limited motion in the lumbar spine
4. Limited chest expansion
5. A history of iritis or its sequelae
6. Radiographic evidence of bilateral sacroiliac changes characteristic of ankylosing spondylitis

The diagnosis is definite if four of the five clinical criteria are met, or if No. 6 and one other are fulfilled.

The blood rheumatoid factor is characteristically absent. The disease may arrest at any stage. In some patients, progressive spinal rigidity and kyphosis lead to extreme disability.

The sacroiliac joints are almost invariably affected. The hips are involved in about 50% of patients, and the shoulders and knees in about 30%. The knees often show only a transient inflammation. The other peripheral joints are involved less frequently.

Pathologically, the morphologic features of the proliferative chronic synovitis involving the diarthrodial joints are indistinguishable from those seen in rheumatoid arthritis.[218] There is a great tendency toward capsular fibrosis and bony ankylosis. In the paraspinal area, the formation of bony bridges between adjacent bodies, or syndesmophytes, is characteristic. These represent ossifications of the outer lamellae of the annulus fibrosus and the immediately adjacent paravertebral connective tissue. Amyloidosis has been reported at necropsy in a small percentage of patients.

Radiologically, the principal sites of involvement are the sacroiliac joints and the spine. Other sites include the hips, shoulders, knees, ankles, costovertebral and costotransverse joints, manubriosternal joint, symphysis pubis, rarely the temporomandibular joints,[199] and the os calcis. Involvement of the small joints of the hands and feet is unusual. Arthritis mutilans does not occur.

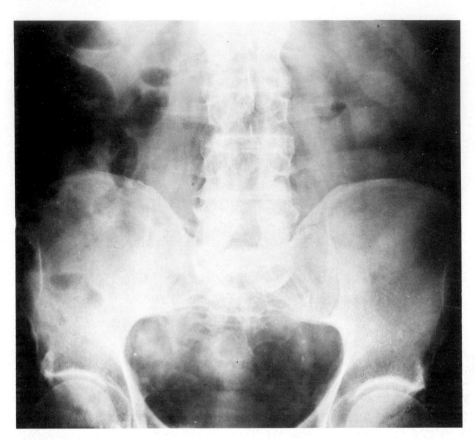

FIG. 9–78. Ankylosing spondylitis (lumbar spine and pelvis). Loss of definition of the sacroiliac joints is seen, with narrowing on the left. Osteoporosis is present. Syndesmophyte formation in the spine can be seen. A lower lumbar laminectomy has been performed for low back pain, a not infrequent occurrence prior to the establishment of the diagnosis. Osteophyte formation on the right at the L-4 to L-5 level is also seen.

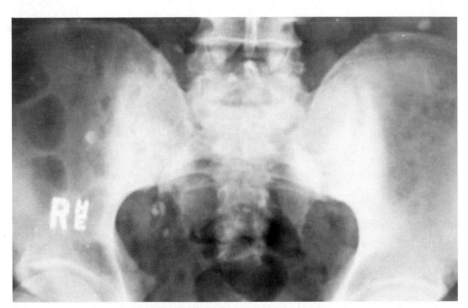

FIG. 9–79. Ankylosing spondylitis. Dense reactive sclerosis about both sacroiliac joints and erosions of the sacroiliac joints are noted.

FIG. 9–80. Ankylosing spondylitis (pelvis). Complete bony ankylosis of both sacroiliac joints has occurred. Syndesmophyte formation in the lower lumbar spine may be seen. Marked osteoporosis is present, as well as mild narrowing of the hip joint spaces.

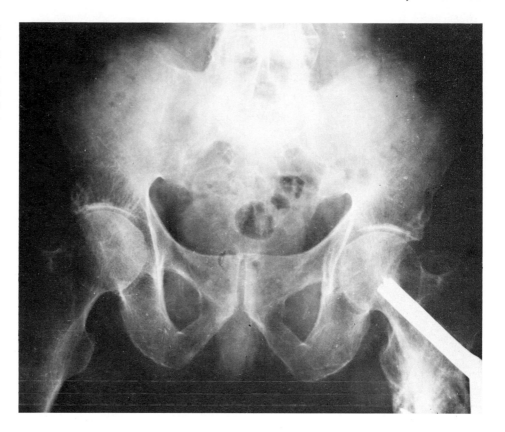

In the sacroiliac joints, the process is invariably bilateral, most often symmetrical, and present at the time the earliest lesions are seen in the spine.

The initial finding may be a loss of definition of the joint margins (Fig. 9–78). Osteoporosis or a dense reactive sclerosis may be present at this stage. Erosions may occur (Fig. 9–79). The iliac borders are affected before the sacral margins. The joint spaces become narrowed. Some patients progress to fibrous and bony ankylosis (Fig. 9–80), with regression of the dense reactive sclerosis. A thin, dense line may be the only residual of the joint, or complete disappearance may occur. Ossification of the amphiarthrodial upper third of the joint completes the end stage.

In the spine, the changes consist of arthritis of the apophyseal joints, osteitis of the vertebral bodies, syndesmophyte formation, disk degeneration, erosions, kyphosis, subluxations, ankylosis, osteoporosis, pathological fractures, and vertebral destructive lesions. The process begins in the lumbar region, with dorsolumbar and lumbosacral involvement.

The posterior diarthrodial joints of the dorsolumbar spine are involved with an inflammatory synovitis which results in haziness, erosions, and subchondral sclerosis. This process proceeds to massive ankylosis (Figs. 9–81, 9–82). The cervical spine is involved in later stages (Fig. 9–83).

Osteitis results in superficial erosions of the vertebral body margins, causing a loss of normal anterior concavity and giving a square appearance to the bodies (Fig. 9–84). This change may later regress, and only the superior margins may be affected. Bony bridges, or syndesmophytes, form between the vertebral bodies. These are seen laterally (Fig. 9–85) and anteriorly (Fig. 9–86), and can be differentiated from osteophytes by their vertical rather than horizontal orientation. Secondary degenerative spondylosis may result in osteophyte formation. The end result is a "bamboo spine" with universal syndesmophytosis (Fig. 9–87). Posterior interspinous ligament ossification fuses the spinous processes, and is seen on frontal projections as a solid midline linear vertical density (Fig. 9–88). Costovertebral ankylosis may also occur (Fig. 9–89).

Superficial erosions of the vertebral end-plates (Fig. 9–90) and erosions of the spinous processes

(*Text continued on p. 739*)

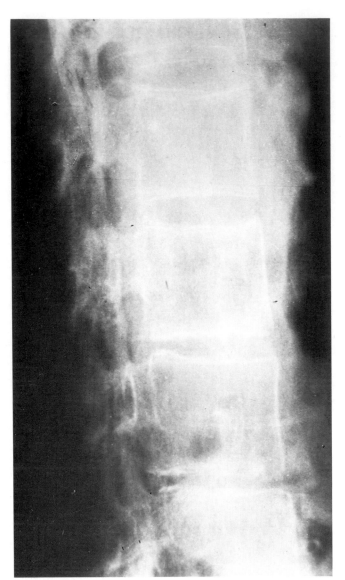

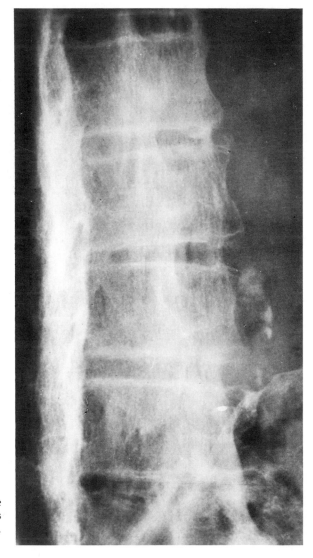

FIG. 9–81. Ankylosing spondylitis (lumbar spine). Massive ankylosis of the posterior diarthrodial joints is seen, associated with "squaring" of the anterior vertebral bodies and joint space narrowing in the lower lumbar area. Marked osteoporosis is also present.

FIG. 9–82. Ankylosing spondylitis (lumbar spine)—oblique view. Ossification of the outer fibers of the annulus fibrosus is seen, indicating this component in syndesmophyte formation. Fusion of the diarthrodial joints is noted.

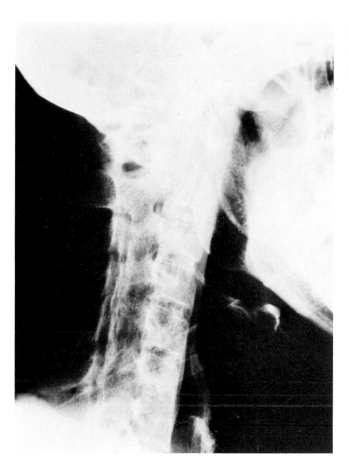

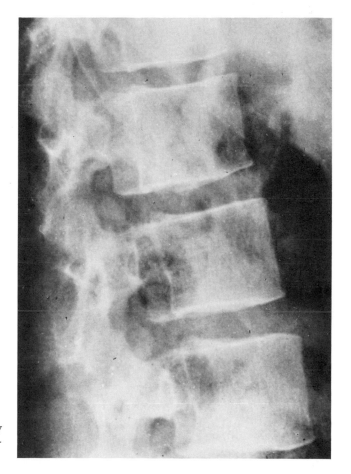

FIG. 9–83. Ankylosing spondylitis (cervical spine) — lateral view. Massive ankylosis of the diarthrodial joints is present, as well as osteoporosis, ''squaring'' of the vertebral bodies, and prevertebral calcification. The anteroposterior diameter of the lower cervical vertebral bodies is shortened.

FIG. 9–84. Ankylosing spondylitis (lumbar spine) — early change. The vertebral bodies have lost their normal anterior concavity, resulting in a square appearance.

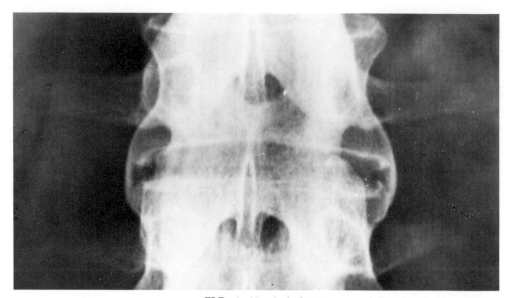

FIG. 9–85. Ankylosing spondylitis (spine) — syndesmophyte formation. Bony bridges between the margins of adjacent vertebrae are seen laterally.

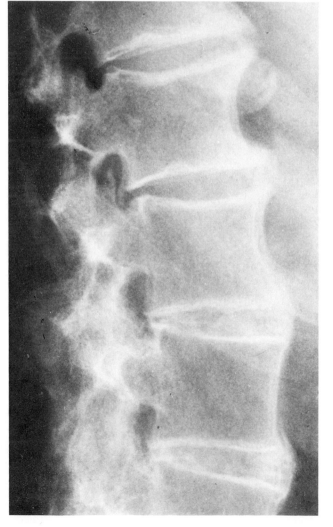

FIG. 9–86. Ankylosing spondylitis (lumbar spine). Anterior syndesmophyte formation in the midlumbar region is seen, and secondary osteophyte formation in the upper lumbar and dorsal lumbar region is noted. The vertical orientation of the syndesmophytes contrasts with the horizontal orientation of the osteophytes. Posterior fusion of the diarthrodial joints is noted, as well as osteoporosis.

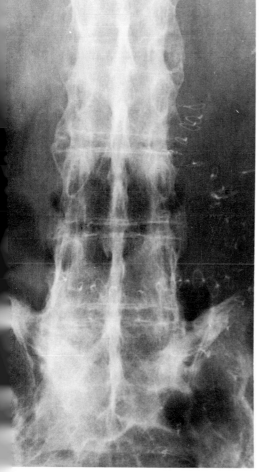

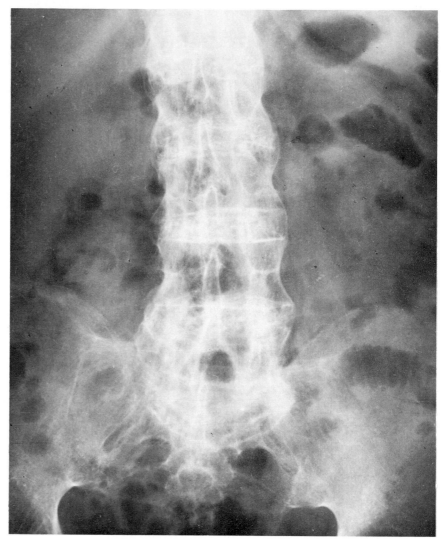

FIG. 9–87. Ankylosing spondylitis—universal syndesmophytosis resulting in a "bamboo spine." Osteoporosis is present, as well as bony ankylosis of both sacroiliac joints. The syndesmophytes originate from the corners of the vertebral bodies. Intervertebral disk calcifications are also present.

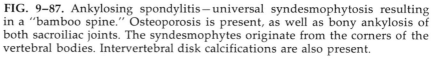

FIG. 9–88. Ankylosing spondylitis (lumbar spine). There has been ossification of the posterior interspinous ligament, which is seen as a solid midline linear vertical density. Syndesmophytosis and osteoporosis are also noted.

737

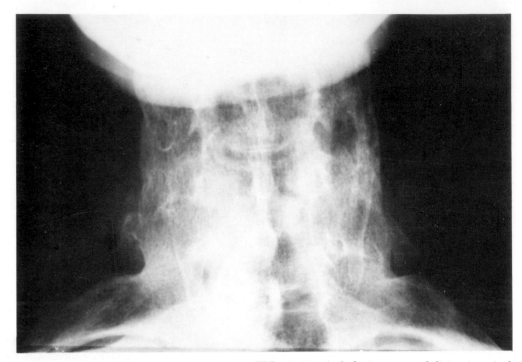

FIG. 9–89. Ankylosing spondylitis (cervical spine). There has been costovertebral ankylosis at the first ribs bilaterally, as well as bony ankylosis of the articular pyramids.

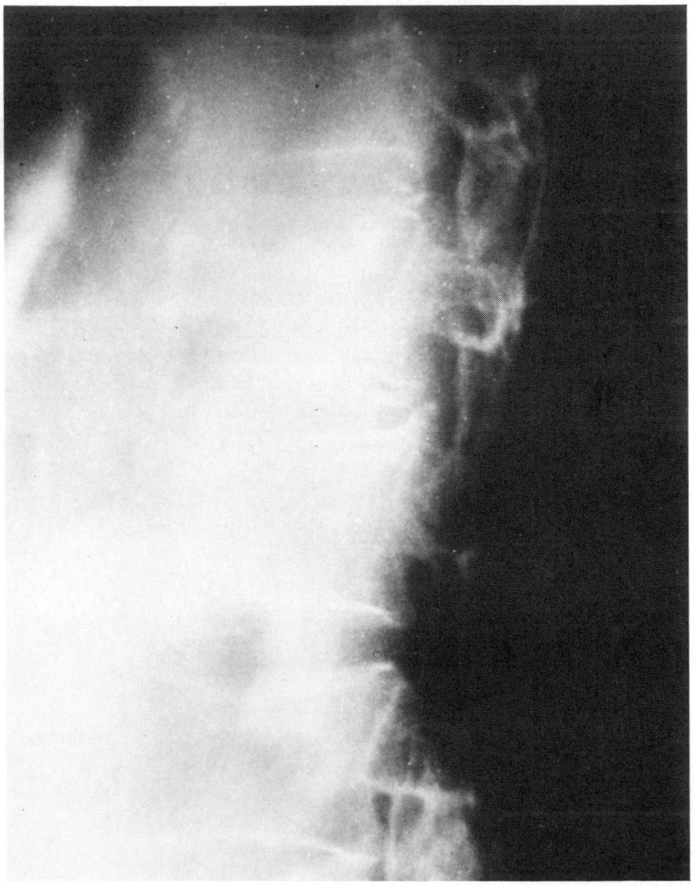

FIG. 9–90. Ankylosing spondylitis (lumbar spine). Erosion of the superior end-plate of the second lumbar vertebra has occurred. Marked osteoporosis is present, as well as bony ankylosis of the diarthrodial joints.

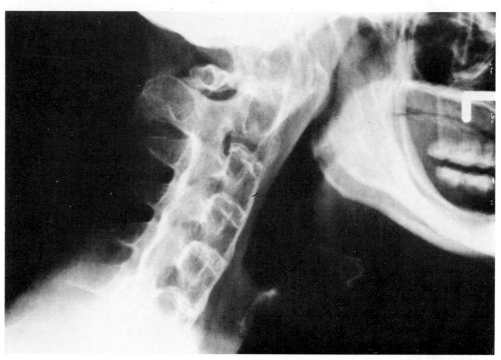

FIG. 9–91. Ankylosing spondylitis (cervical spine). Erosion of the spinous processes, giving a tapered appearance, is seen. Bony ankylosis of the diarthrodial joints, syndesmophytosis, and marked osteoporosis are present. Atlantoaxial subluxation, as evidenced by the forward position of the ring of C-1, is also present.

leading to tapering (Fig. 9–91) may occur. Bone resorption from the anterior surface of the lower cervical spine may be seen in late stages (Fig. 9–92).

Intervertebral disk narrowing accompanies posterior ankylosis. The spine becomes straightened and may develop extreme kyphosis (Fig. 9–93). Subluxations, rarely at the atlantoaxial joint, may occur as in rheumatoid arthritis with similar serious potential. The rigid osteoporotic spine is prone to fractures (Fig. 9–94). Fusion may occur in the subluxed position.

Destructive lesions in the vertebral bodies have been reported in this condition.[15,49,70,217] In the early stage they may be due to granulomas. Destructive changes involving an intervertebral disk and contiguous portions of vertebral bodies at the level of an unfused segment results from the focus of spinal motion at this site.[217] Similar findings result from fracture of the posterior elements.

The larger appendicular joints, particularly the hips and shoulders, are often involved with features similar to, yet differing from, those of rheumatoid arthritis. There is less osteoporosis and

more reactive sclerosis (Fig. 9–95). The end stage is bony ankylosis (Fig. 9–96), while in rheumatoid arthritis it is fibrous ankylosis with severe erosion of the articular bone ends. A bony spur at the superior aspect of the junction between the femoral head and neck is sometimes seen.

The os calcis may show erosions above the site of attachments of the Achilles tendon, as in rheumatoid arthritis and Reiter's syndrome. Reactive sclerosis sometimes occurs.

A distinctive appearance is seen at the sites of muscle attachments at points of stress. Irregular proliferative new bone formation giving a "whiskering" effect is seen, sometimes associated with reactive sclerosis. This is particularly common at the ischial tuberosities, iliac margins, and the calcaneus.

When the disease begins in adolescence, or earlier, it is referred to as *juvenile ankylosing spondylitis*.[7,119] It is predominantly seen in males. The mean age of onset is 10 to 12 years. Juvenile patients also have presence of HLA-B27 antigen, and the distribution of involved joints may be different.[216] The

(Text continued on p. 742)

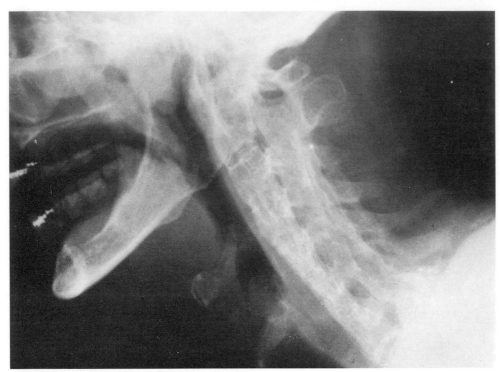

FIG. 9–92. Ankylosing spondylitis (cervical spine). Resorption of the vertebral bodies and ankylosis of the posterior joints are seen.

FIG. 9–93. Ankylosing spondylitis (dorsal spine). Moderate arcuate kyphosis is present, as well as squaring of the anterior vertebrae and prevertebral calcification. Calcification in the intervertebral disks is also seen, as is osteoporosis.

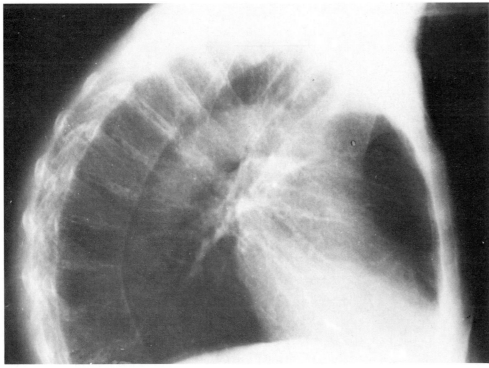

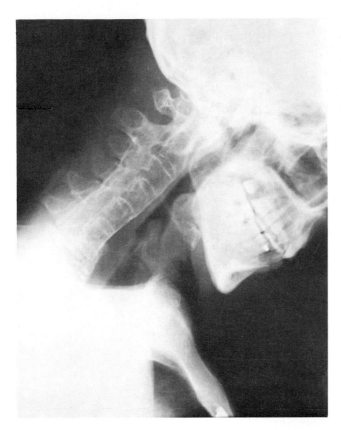

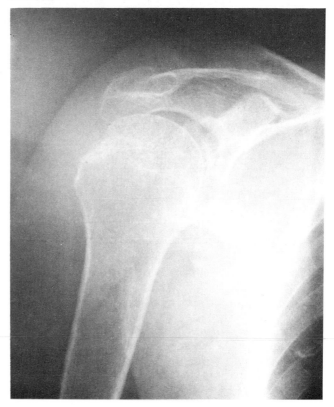

FIG. 9–94. Ankylosing spondylitis (cervical spine). A fracture at the level of C-6 and C-7 is seen, with a distinct break at the fused diarthrodial joints. Angulation is noted at the two fused blocks of bodies. Bone resorption from the anterior surface of the vertebral bodies has narrowed the anteroposterior diameter regionally. Partial ossification of the ligamentum nuchae is also noted.

FIG. 9–95. Ankylosing spondylitis (shoulder). Erosion at the region of the greater tuberosity is seen, with reactive sclerosis.

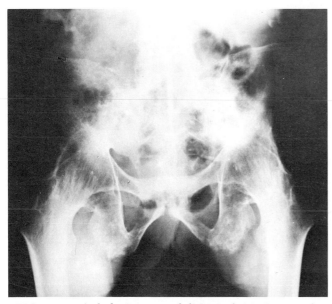

FIG. 9–96. Ankylosing spondylitis (pelvis). Bony ankylosis of both hips has occurred. Loss of bone density with coarsening of the trabecular pattern is seen. Partial ankylosis of the symphysis pubis is also noted, as well as ossification of the interspinous ligament of the lumbar spine. Marginal irregularity of both ischia, with a "whiskering" effect, is also present.

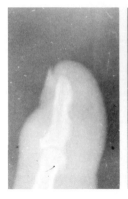
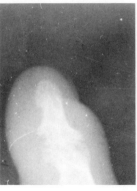
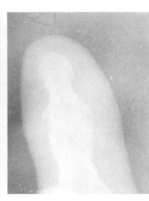

FIG. 9–97. Psoriatic arthritis (distal interphalangeal joints). Characteristic soft-tissue thickening is noted, as well as marginal erosions. (Courtesy of Dr. Antonio Pizarro, Hines VA Hospital, Hines, IL)

appendicular joints are more frequently involved, and may predominate throughout the course of the disease. There is a tendency toward arthritis of the hip, shoulder, elbow, wrist, knee, ankle, and foot. The metatarsophalangeal joints are the most frequently involved of the small joints.

Ankylosing spondylitis associated with primary hyperparathyroidism has been reported.[28, 108]

PSORIATIC ARTHRITIS

Psoriatic arthritis[14,116,208,244,261] represents a diverse spectrum of disease, which is a distinct clinical entity. Up to 7% of patients with psoriasis may be affected.

Three major groups are recognized. The most common are those patients with an asymmetric peripheral polyarthritis, including those with predominantly distal interphalangeal joint changes. There are those patients with arthritis mutilans, frequently complicated by *"main-en-lorgnette"* deformity and involvement of the sacroiliac joints. Finally there is a group with a pattern indistinguishable from that of rheumatoid arthritis. The joint changes may precede skin lesions, by a long interval in some patients. There is a close relationship between nail and joint involvement. A characteristic spondylitis also occurs in this condition.

Histologically, the synovitis is similar to that of rheumatoid arthritis. Rheumatoid factor and rheumatoid nodules are typically not present. The serum uric acid level is often elevated. It is probable that the incidence of rheumatoid arthritis in psoriatic patients is no greater than the coincidental coexistence of these two relatively common diseases.

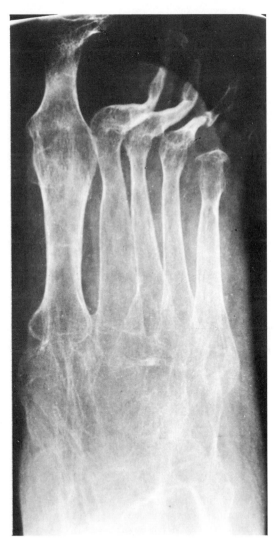

FIG. 9–98. Psoriatic arthritis (foot). Severe osteoporosis is noted, as well as bony ankylosis of the interphalangeal joints of the toes, the metatarsophalangeal joints, and the tarsus.

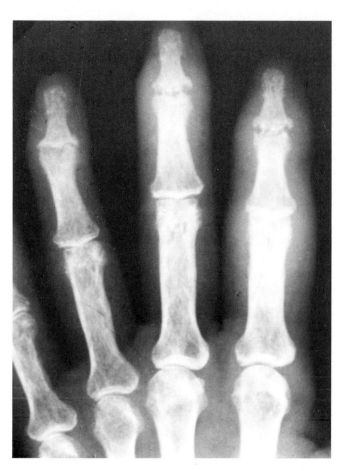

FIG. 9–99. Psoriatic arthritis (hand). Widening of the distal interphalangeal joints with marginal irregularity is noted. Soft-tissue swelling and osteoporosis are also present.

FIG. 9–100. Psoriatic arthritis (foot). Marginal erosions at the interphalangeal joint of the great toe are noted, as well as marginal new bone formation at the base of the distal phalanx. Erosions at the fifth metatarsal head are also noted, as is periosteal new bone formation along the shaft of the fifth metatarsal.

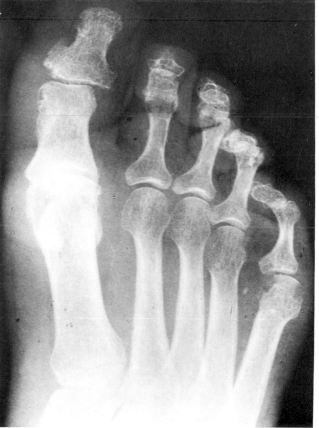

Radiologically, the specific signs of psoriatic arthritis have been elicited by Avila *et al*,[14] and are as follows:

1. Destructive arthritis involving predominantly the distal interphalangeal joints of the fingers and the interphalangeal joints of the toes. The appearance is that of rheumatoid arthritis, but the distribution pattern is different (Fig. 9–97)
2. Bony ankylosis of the interphalangeal joints of the hands and feet (Fig. 9–98)
3. Destruction of interphalangeal joints of the hands and feet, with abnormally wide joint spaces, and sharply demarcated adjacent bony surfaces. The only other condition with this finding is reticulohistiocytoma, a very rare disorder. This finding is therefore almost pathognomonic of psoriatic arthritis (Figs. 9–99, 6–177)
4. Destruction of the interphalangeal joint of the great toe, associated with irregular bony proliferation at the base of the distal phalanx (Fig. 9–100)
5. Resorption of the tufts of the distal phalanges of the hands and feet (Fig. 6–177)

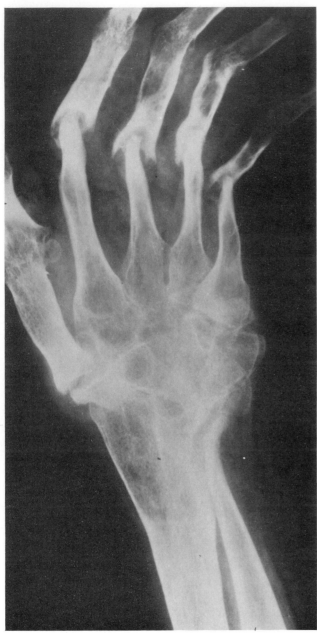

FIG. 9–101. Psoriatic arthritis (hand and wrist). Tapering of the distal metacarpals, two through five, associated with cupping of the bases of the proximal phalanges, is seen with tapering of the distal ulna. Fusions of the carpus and of the interphalangeal joints are also noted.

Symmetrical involvement of all of the distal interphalangeal joints is relatively infrequent.

Resorption of the terminal tufts may occur without arthritis in association with psoriasis, and also occurs in many other conditions (see pp. 477–478).

Advanced cases may proceed to a "pencil-in-cup" deformity, suggesting a neurotrophic component (Fig. 9–101).

Accessory signs in some patients include a lack of osteoporosis. This may be explained by the intermittent character of the arthritis, with no pain between exacerbations. There is also a characteristic lack of ulnar deviation. In addition, periosteal reaction of linear or fluffy type, near the joints and along the shafts, is occasionally seen.

Calcaneal erosions may also occur, with reactive bone sclerosis and fluffy periosteal new bone formation, as well as calcaneal spurs.

Resorption at the temporomandibular joints may also occur.

Some patients develop arthritis mutilans, with extreme resorption and erosion of the metacarpals and phalanges, shortening of the digits with "telescoping" of the fingers, and complete carpal fusion (Fig. 9–102). In the feet, the most destructive changes are at the metatarsophalangeal joints. Tapering of the bone ends and cuplike deformities are often associated.

The sacroiliac joints may show unilateral or bilateral involvement. The sequence of events is blurring of the subchondral margins, erosions (Fig. 9–103), narrowing of the joint space, and reactive sclerosis. The process may proceed to bony ankylosis.

In the spine, the characteristic finding is the presence of coarse, asymmetrical syndesmophytes, which skip areas of the spine (Fig. 9–104). They differ in appearance from those seen in ankylosing spondylitis in that they do not originate from the vertebral margins, but rather from the midvertebral body. They are also more superficially situated. The distribution of syndesmophytes is in the lumbar, dorsal, and initially lower cervical spine. In addition to syndesmophytes, paravertebral ossification is common. A fluffy arc of new bone is seen adjacent to, but separate from, the contiguous vertebral body. This is not seen in the cervical spine.

Another common finding in the cervical spine is atlantoaxial subluxation. Changes that rarely occur include "squaring" of vertebral bodies and apophyseal joint fusion.

FIG. 9–102. Psoriatic arthritis (hand and wrist)—arthritis mutilans. "Pencil-in-cup" deformities and dislocations of the metacarpophalangeal joints are seen, with "telescoping" of the fingers, causing a *"main-en-lorgnette"* deformity. Bony fusion at the interphalangeal joints and at the carpus is seen. Tapering of the distal ulna is also noted.

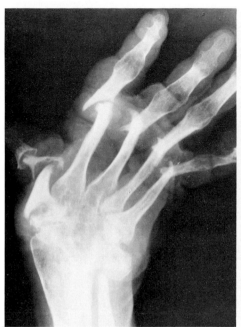
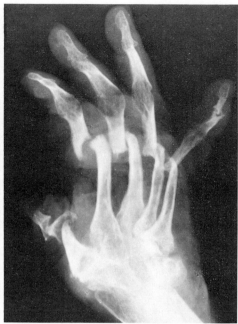

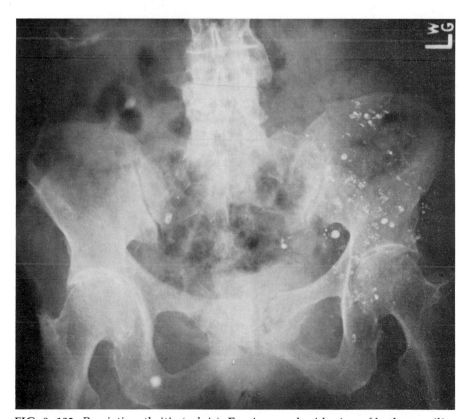

FIG. 9–103. Psoriatic arthritis (pelvis). Erosions and widening of both sacroiliac joints are seen, with mild marginal sclerosis. Coarse asymmetrical syndesmophytes in the lower lumbar spine are seen, as well as a paravertebral ossification at the right side.

Those patients with psoriatic arthritis showing changes radiologically indistinguishable from rheumatoid arthritis may be differentiated from those with coincident rheumatoid disease by lack of serum rheumatoid factor, rheumatoid nodules, and cardiopulmonary lesions.

REITER'S SYNDROME (REITER DISEASE)

Reiter's syndrome[145,235,257] is a condition of unproven etiology characterized by a triad of urethritis, arthritis, and conjunctivitis. Two additional consistent features are balanitis and a characteristic dermatitis, *keratodermia blennorrhagicum.* The symptoms are not always present simultaneously. The disease chiefly affects young adult males. It appears to have a venereal transmission, but Reiter's original case and cases seen in Europe followed severe diarrhea. The disease may be confused with psoriatic arthritis, as the skin lesions and roentgen features show some similarity. The course is usually self-limited, subsiding in 6 weeks to 6 months, but recurrences occur in up to 50% of patients.

Radiologically, the sacroiliac joints, heels, and toes are most frequently affected. The disease characteristically shows a predilection for arthritis of the lower extremities including the knee, ankle, metatarsophalangeal joints, proximal interphalangeal joints of the toes, and interphalangeal joint of the great toe (Fig. 9–105 *A*). The hip is only infrequently involved, as is the spine. In the upper extremities the proximal interphalangeal joints are most commonly affected, followed by the distal interphalangeal joints, which are uncommonly involved. Metacarpophalangeal involvement is rare (Fig. 9–105 *B*). The wrists and elbows may also be involved, but less frequently. Shoulder involvement is rare. There is some variation of reported involved sites in different series, possibly due to differing stages of the disease. The typical distribution pattern is asymmetrical.

The initial change is periarticular swelling. Joint space narrowing and destruction may follow, more commonly in the smaller than in the larger peripheral joints. The distribution is unifocal or multifocal, and panarthritis is rare. Periarticular osteoporosis is less frequently seen in Reiter's syndrome than in rheumatoid arthritis. Periosteal new bone formation in either a linear or fluffy pattern is frequently seen, particularly in the calcaneus, shafts of the metatarsals, distal tibia and fibula, and phalanges of the hands and feet.

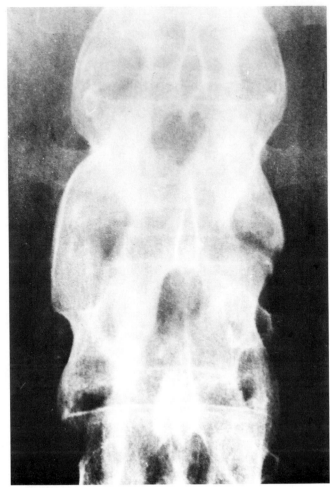

FIG. 9–104. Lumbar spine. Coarse asymmetrical syndesmophytes, which originate from the midaspect of the vertebral bodies rather than from the corners, are seen.

FIG. 9–105. Top. Reiter's syndrome (foot). Marginal destructive changes at the interphalangeal joints of the great toe are seen, associated with fluffy periosteal new bone formation at the proximal aspect of the distal phalanx. This finding is similar to what may be seen in psoriatic arthritis. (Courtesy of Dr. Antonio Pizarro). **Bottom.** Reiter's syndrome (hand and wrist). Periarticular osteoporosis, a boutonniere deformity of the little finger, and subluxation at the metacarpophalangeal joint of the index finger is seen, as well as a distal ulnar prosthesis. (Courtesy of Dr. Dharmashi V. Bhate, VA Hospital, Hines, IL)

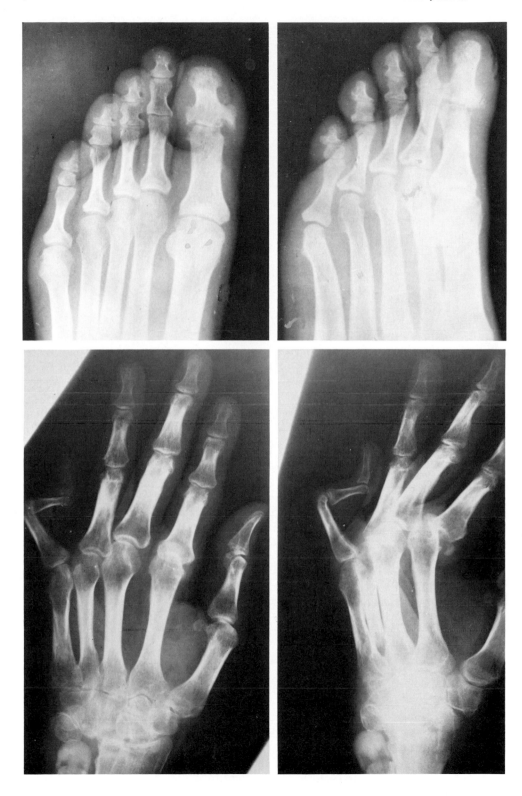

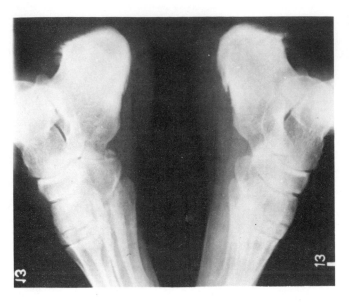

FIG. 9–106. Reiter's syndrome (both heels). Fluffy periosteal new bone formation along the posterior and inferior aspects of both calcanei is noted, associated with bone sclerosis. (Courtesy of Dr. Antonio Pizarro, Hines VA Hospital, Hines, IL)

In the feet, the disease may progress to a picture of arthritis mutilans, termed *Launois' deformity* in Reiter's syndrome. The calcaneus may show erosions and spur formation, as well as fluffy periosteal new bone formation and increase in density and size (Figs. 9–106, 9–107). The knee may show soft-tissue swelling, and less commonly uniform joint space narrowing. A Pellegrini-Stieda type of tendon calcification-ossification may occasionally be seen.

Sacroiliac joint involvement may be unilateral or bilateral, with joint space narrowing, erosions, and sclerosis. Joint obliteration is typically not seen.

The spine shows asymmetrical involvement with coarse, nonmarginal syndesmophytes in some patients, similar to that seen in psoriatic arthritis. The distribution is discontinuous, with skipped segments. Paravertebral ossification or calcification, not attached to the vertebrae, also occurs. A single case of Reiter disease with atlantoaxial subluxation has been reported.

POLYARTHRITIS ASSOCIATED WITH OTHER DISEASES

SYSTEMIC LUPUS ERYTHEMATOSUS[21,172,256]

Joint manifestations of this connective tissue disease include subluxations and malalignment, effusion, osteoporosis, and soft-tissue atrophy. Erosion, joint space narrowing, and destruction appear only minimally. Para-articular calcification may also be rarely seen. Ischemic necrosis, reported in the humeral and femoral heads, may be due to steroid therapy or possibly the primary disease process (Fig. 9–108). It has also been reported in the navicular and metacarpals. Atlantoaxial subluxation without erosions also may be present.

The hand shows characteristic findings. Soft-tissue atrophy is severe with concave rather than convex margins to the thenar and hypothenar borders (Fig. 9–109).

Osteoporosis is present with a periarticular or diffuse pattern. Joint swelling may be seen.

The characteristic finding is malalignment in the absence of erosions. A "bountonnière" or "swanneck" deformity may be present (see section on *Rheumatoid Arthritis*), as well as multiple subluxations. Subluxation of the interphalangeal joints of the thumbs is often seen (Fig. 9–110). Ease of reversibility of deformities is typical. Severe ulnar deviation may exist (Fig. 9–111), causing pressure erosion of adjacent bone ends. The deformities might be explained by neuromuscular weakness, wasting, and contractures, rather than bony erosion and destruction. Sclerosis of the terminal phalanges may also been seen. Resorption of the terminal phalanges may occur in patients with Raynaud's phenomenon.

JACCOUD'S ARTHRITIS[166, 250]

Jaccoud's arthritis represents an uncommon sequela resulting in deformity of the hands follow-

FIG. 9–107. Reiter's syndrome (calcaneus). Note resorption at the posterior aspect of the calcaneus, periostitis at the inferior aspect, and bone sclerosis. (Courtesy of Dr. Miriam Liberson, Chief Radiologist, West Side Veteran's Administration Hospital, Chicago, IL)

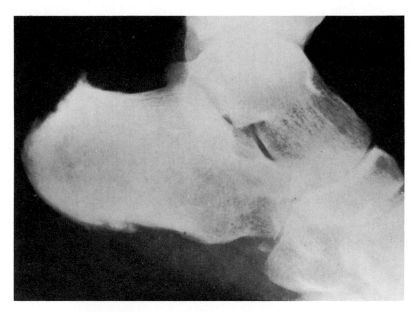

FIG. 9–108. Systemic lupus erythematosus (hand and wrist). Extensive carpal destruction secondary to ischemic necrosis is seen. Minimal periosteal new bone formation along the distal ulna is noted, but there is only minimal osteoporosis.

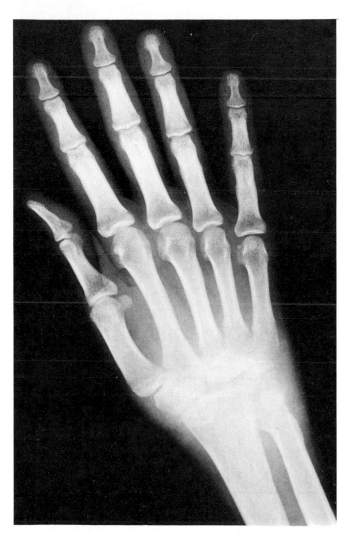

ing rheumatic fever. The patients develop a periarticular swelling of the small joints of the hands and feet, most frequently the metacarpophalangeal joints, and occasionally the proximal interphalangeal joints. This occurs during the subsiding stage of rheumatic fever. The disease progresses to deformity which may be due to periarticular fascial and tendon fibrosis rather than to synovitis.

Ulnar deviation at the metacarpophalangeal joints is seen, along with soft-tissue swelling, subluxation, and flexion deformity (Fig. 9–112). The ulnar deviation is easily reversible in early stages. Hyperextension at the interphalangeal joints may also be present. The bone is typically not involved. Erosions are said to follow in some cases.

ENTEROPATHIC ARTHRITIS[40, 163]

Approximately 10% or less of patients with ulcerative colitis and regional enteritis have associated arthritis. In approximately 25% of patients who develop spondylitis, the spondylitis precedes the

(Text continued on p. 753)

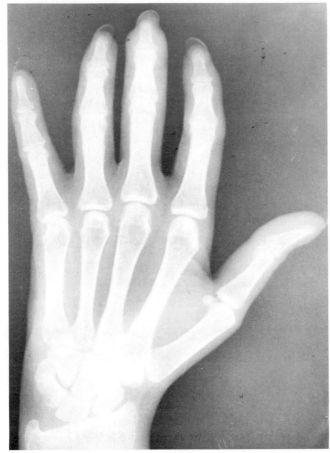

FIG. 9–109. Systemic lupus erythematosus (hand). Osteoporosis is noted, as well as soft-tissue atrophy with a concave margin at the hypothenar aspect. Joint space narrowing at the proximal interphalangeal joints and the metacarpophalangeal joints of the fifth finger is noted, with no erosive changes. Mild ulnar deviation is also present at the metacarpophalangeal joints.

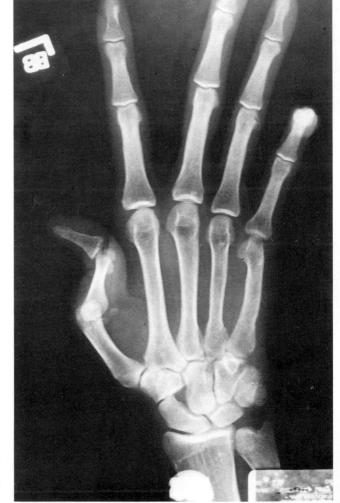

FIG. 9–110. Lupus erythematosus (hand). Subluxation at the interphalangeal joint of the thumb is seen, as well as moderate osteoporosis. Terminal phalangeal osteosclerosis of the index finger is also present.

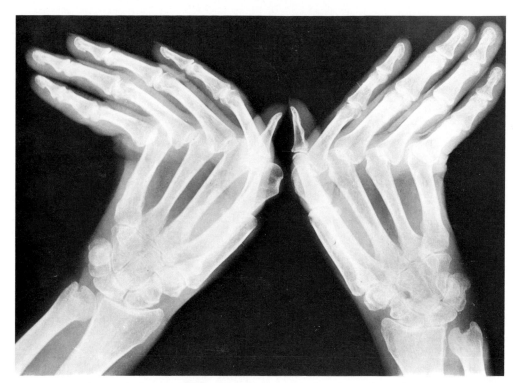

FIG. 9–111. Systemic lupus erythematosus (hands). Extreme ulnar deviation is seen with subluxations. No erosions at the metacarpophalangeal joints are seen. Minimal erosion at the left capitate is present, as well as mild erosions in the notch of the ulna.

FIG. 9–112. Jaccoud's arthritis (hands). Ulnar deviation at the metacarpophalangeal joints bilaterally is present, as well as mild osteoporosis. No erosions are seen.

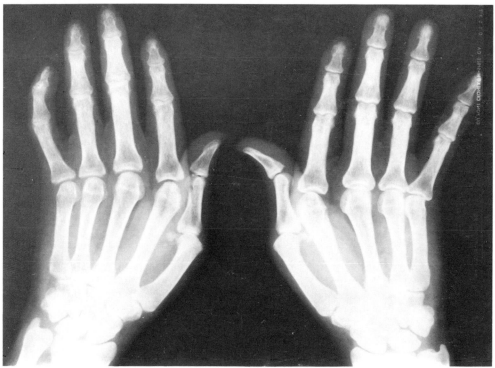

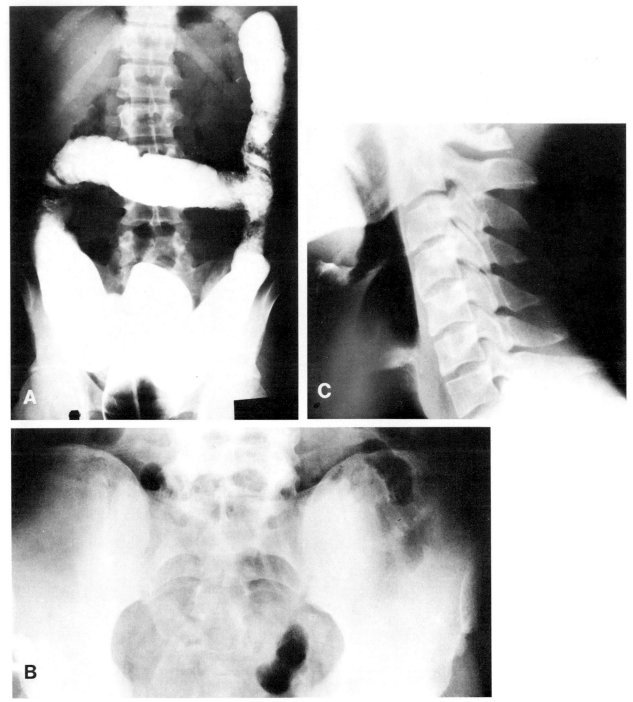

FIG. 9–113. Enteropathic arthritis — male, age 30 years, with ulcerative colitis. **A.** Film of the colon showing changes of ulcerative colitis. **B.** Bilateral sacroiliac joint involvement, with sclerosis and erosions. **C.** Cervical spine. Syndesmophyte formation between C-4 and C-5, and squaring of C-7, are noted.

appearance of the primary disease. The arthritis may develop simultaneously, but usually follows bowel disease. *Clinical features* include a migratory type of arthritis or arthralgia, symmetrically involving the peripheral joints, signs of ankylosing spondylitis, and erythema nodosum, and uveitis in some patients. Laboratory studies are not helpful.

Radiologically, soft-tissue swelling, peripherally most common in the knee and elbow, are seen. The hands, wrists, and feet may be involved. Periarticular osteoporosis occurs. Joint space narrowing and erosions follow, with less severity than in rheumatoid arthritis. Periostitis may also be present. The most common sites of involvement are the sacroiliac joints, which are typically symmetrically involved (Fig. 9–113). The most prominent finding is sclerosis; however, widening, erosions, and ankylosis may also occur. Spinal ankylosis with marginal syndesmophyte formation indistinguishable from that of ankylosing spondylitis has been reported in about 6% of patients with ulcerative colitis and regional enteritis.

The disease manifests itself either as a central or a peripheral type. The two types coexist only in a minority of patients. Migratory polyarthritis and monarticular arthritis have been reported in patients with antibiotic-associated colitis. Arthritis has also been reported associated with intestinal bypass procedure for morbid obesity.[222]

Whipple's disease, or *intestinal lipodystrophy,* is another enteric condition associated with arthritic changes. Nonspecific peripheral arthritic changes, as well as unilateral or bilateral sacroiliac fusion, may rarely be detected radiologically. Typical ankylosing spondylitis has not been reported in this condition.

SCLERODERMA[203,206,260]

In addition to terminal phalangeal resorption and soft-tissue calcification, erosive arthritis may rarely be seen in *scleroderma*. Pencil-in-cup deformities of the distal interphalangeal joints have been described, as well as joint space narrowing with bone resorption at the proximal interphalangeal joints (Fig. 9–114). Osteoporosis may be present. Selective involvement of the first carpometacarpal joint occurs with osseous erosions and radial subluxation

FIG. 9–114. Scleroderma (hands). Marked resorption of the terminal phalanges is present, associated with minimal calcifications in the left thumb. Severe bone resorption at several proximal interphalangeal joints is noted, as well as at the metacarpophalangeal joints. Subluxations at several proximal interphalangeal joints are also seen. Marked osteoporosis is present.

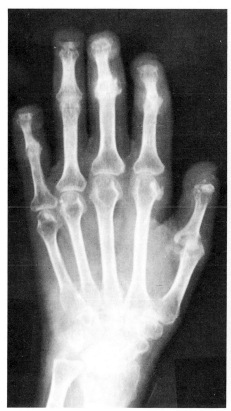 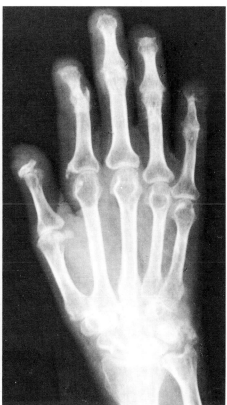

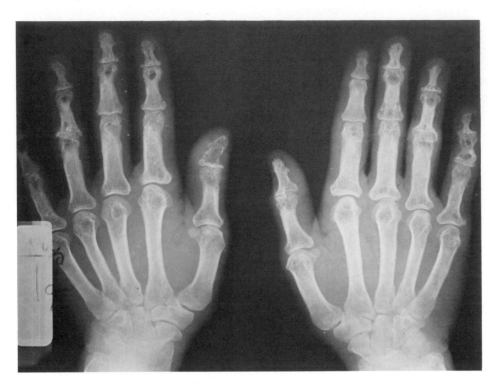

FIG. 9–115. Sarcoidosis (hands). Extensive destructive lesions of the phalanges are seen with punched-out areas, as well as an expansile lesion of the distal phalanx of the right thumb. (Courtesy of Dr. Dharmashi V. Bhate, VA Hospital, Hines, IL)

of the metacarpal base. Intra-articular calcification may occur in addition to periarticular calcification.

MIXED CONNECTIVE TISSUE DISEASE[175, 251]

Mixed connective tissue disease is a syndrome with an overlap of features of scleroderma, SLE, polymyositis, and rheumatoid arthritis. Patients possess an antinuclear antibody which reacts with a ribonuclease-sensitive extractable nuclear antigen. Radiographs of the hands show osteoporosis, both periarticular and diffuse. Periarticular soft-tissue swelling, narrowing of the joint spaces, and erosions may be seen. Subluxation and marked ulnar deviation of the phalanges also may occur, as well as resorption of the terminal tufts and soft-tissue atrophy.

SARCOIDOSIS

In addition to involvement of bone with granulation tissue, the hand may rarely show arthritic changes. Narrowing of the interphalangeal joint spaces with marginal spur formation may be seen (Fig. 9–115). Marginal erosive changes with slight ulnar deviation of the fingers may very rarely occur (Fig. 9–116). "Penciling" of phalanges has also been described.

FAMILIAL MEDITERRANEAN FEVER[25]

Familial Mediterranean fever is a disease of unknown etiology with recurrent episodes of fever and pleuroperitonitis. It occurs in the Eastern Mediterranean region and is associated with a high incidence of sacroiliac arthritis with erosions, sclerosis, and fusion. Monoarthritis, or migratory arthritis involving the knee, ankle, and hip may occur. Complete recovery is the rule.

Several generalized diseases may have a component of polyarthritis or arthralgia. There may be a transient arthritis, with little or no roentgen changes, or erosive changes may develop at times in some cases. Some of these diseases are listed below.

POLYARTHRITIS-ASSOCIATED DISEASES OTHER THAN THOSE DESCRIBED ABOVE[97]

1. Polyarteritis
2. Dermatomyositis (Fig. 9–117)
3. Sjögren's syndrome
4. Henoch–Schönlein purpura
5. Dysgammaglobulinemia
6. Amyloidosis[86]
7. Relapsing polychondritis

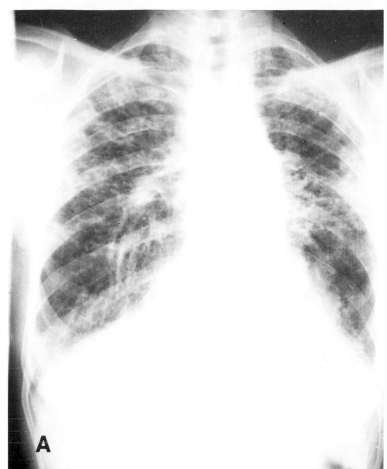

FIG. 9–116. Sarcoidosis—female, age 41 years. **A.** Posteroanterior chest film showing interstitial fibrotic changes of sarcoidosis. **B.** Right hand. Loss of bone density and accentuation of the bony trabecular pattern are noted. Ulnar deviation of the index and middle fingers is seen. Definitive marginal erosions, most pronounced at the base of the proximal phalanx of the index finger, but also at the distal aspect of the middle phalanx of the index finger and the distal aspect of the proximal phalanx of the middle finger, are seen.

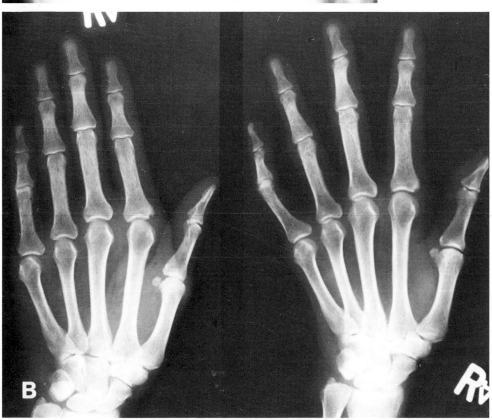

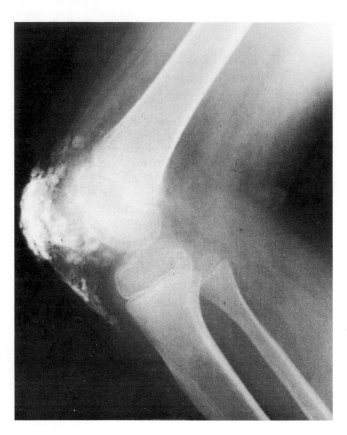

FIG. 9–117. Dermatomyositis (knee). Periarticular swelling and calcification are present.

TABLE 9–1. Types of Hemophilia.

Disorder	Deficient Factor	Inherittance Pattern
Hemophillia A (classic hemophilia)	VIII (AGH)	Sex-linked recessive
Hemophilia B (Christmas disease)	IX (PCT)	Sex-linked recessive
Factor XI deficiency (hemophilia C)	XI (PTA)	Autosomal dominant; incomplete penetrance
Factor X deficiency (Stuart disease)	X	Autosomal recessive
Factor VII deficiency	VII (stable)	Autosomal recessive
Factor V deficiency (parahemophilia)	V (labile)	Autosomal recessive
Hypothrombinemia	II (prothrombin)	Autosomal recessive
Afibrinogenemia	I (fibrinogen)	Autosomal recessive
Dysfibrinogenemia	Altered I	Autosomal recessive
FSF deficiency (Factor XIII deficiency)	XIII	Autosomal recessive
von Willebrand's disease (pseudohemophilia A)	VIII	Autosomal dominant
Thrombocytopenia	Platelets	Autosomal dominant and recessive

(Modified from Conn H. F., Conn R. B.: Current Diagnosis, Philadelphia, WB Saunders, 1974)

Primary amyloidosis[86] may result in infiltration of the synovium, capsule, and adjacent structures. Soft-tissue swelling occurs, as well as bone erosions. Subluxations have been reported. Nonarticular skeletal manifestations include destructive lesions, pathological fractures, and vertebral collapse.

HEMOPHILIA

Hemophilia[23, 243] causes an alteration of the normal textural appearance of bone, combined with growth disturbance and intra-articular, intraosseous, and subperiosteal hemorrhages. The normal clotting mechanism can be summarized in simplified form as follows:

1. Thromboplastin precursors + platelet factors form thromboplastin
2. Thromboplastin + Ca^{++} + factors V, VII, X allow prothrombin to form thrombin
3. Thrombin allows fibrinogen to form fibrin

The disease is caused by functional deficiency of a clotting factor. The various types are summarized in Table 9–1.[43]

Hemophilias A and B are sex-linked recessives and can occur only in males, transmitted by female carriers. They have identical radiological appearances.

Hemophilia C is a mendelian dominant, can affect both males and females, is less severe, and only rarely has bone and joint involvement. Severe hemarthrosis is unusual in hemorrhagic diseases other than hemophilia. The severity of hemophilia varies from patient to patient. Partial deficiencies may occur with milder bleeding tendencies. The functional plasma level of factor VIII or IX in the mild form may be 20% to 60%, in the moderate form 5% to 20%, and in the severe form 1% to 5%. The last may bleed spontaneously.

Clinically, in hemophilia A and B, the symptoms of hemorrhage begin in the first year of life and reach a peak of severity before puberty. The bleeding is always considered to be due to trauma. Subcutaneous, intramuscular, intra-articular and internal hemorrhages occur. Joint changes are almost always present on reaching adult life. A mild form of hemophilia with onset of symptoms at age 4 years or later exists; hemarthrosis is rare in this form.

The skeletal roentgen changes are caused by intra-articular hemorrhages, intraosseous hemorrhages, and subperiosteal hemorrhages.

Nonskeletal radiological changes include visceral, retroperitoneal, and intramural hemorrhages of the gastrointestinal tract.

The knees, elbows, and ankles are the joints most commonly involved with *intra-articular hemorrhages*. Because the affected joints tend to hemorrhage recurrently, the involvement of the various joints will not be uniform. Severe and permanent deformities result. Initially there is increased density of the periarticular soft tissue and distension of the joint space (Fig. 9–118), followed by chronic synovitis from repeated hemorrhage (Fig. 9–119). The increased density of soft tissue results from hemosiderin deposition. Limitation of motion causes disuse osteoporosis (Fig. 9–120). The thickened synovial membrane causes marginal erosion of the articular cartilage and subchondral bone erosion. The cartilage is destroyed and the joint space narrows. Secondary osteoarthritic changes develop. A multitude of subchondral cysts develop, both from a secondary degenerative process and from intraosseous hemorrhage. Although hemophilia may exist without subchondral cyst formation (Fig. 9–121), the large number and variations in size of these cysts are characteristic.

Hemorrhage may occur into the epiphyseal cartilage, causing slipped epiphyses, premature fusion, and deformity. Tibiotalar slant is common (Fig. 9–122).

Humerus varus is a common consequence. There may be enlargement, dysgenesis, or accelerated maturation of the epiphysis due to chronic hyperemia (Fig. 9–123). There may be marked osteoporosis with the trabeculae striated parallel to the bone. In the knee, widening of the intercondylar notch due to hemorrhage at the insertions of the cruciate ligaments is almost pathognomonic (Figs. 9–124, 9–125). Flattening of the inferior apex of the patella because of interference with growth may also occur if the onset in the joint originated at an early age (Fig. 9–126). This can also be seen in juvenile rheumatoid arthritis. Widening of the radial notch of the ulna has also been described.[185] Severe degenerative arthritis of the hip also develops in this condition.[73]

Intraosseous hemorrhages can cause lytic or cystic lesions in bone (Fig. 9–127). If the hemorrhage occurs in an epiphysis, a picture similar to that of aseptic necrosis may result.

Subperiosteal hemorrhages are relatively uncommon. There may be minimal periosteal reaction adjacent to an involved joint that can progress to cor-

(Text continued on p. 762)

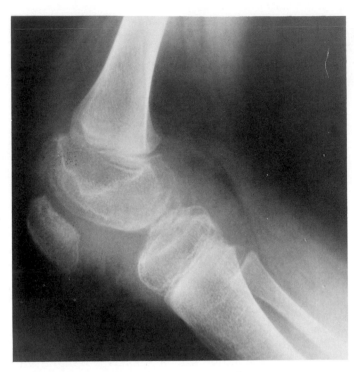

FIG. 9–118. Hemophilia (knee). Marked soft-tissue swelling of intracapsular effusion and hemorrhage are noted, with bulging of the pericapsular fat pad and fullness of the suprapatellar space. Enlargement and irregularity of the epiphyseal ossification centers are also seen.

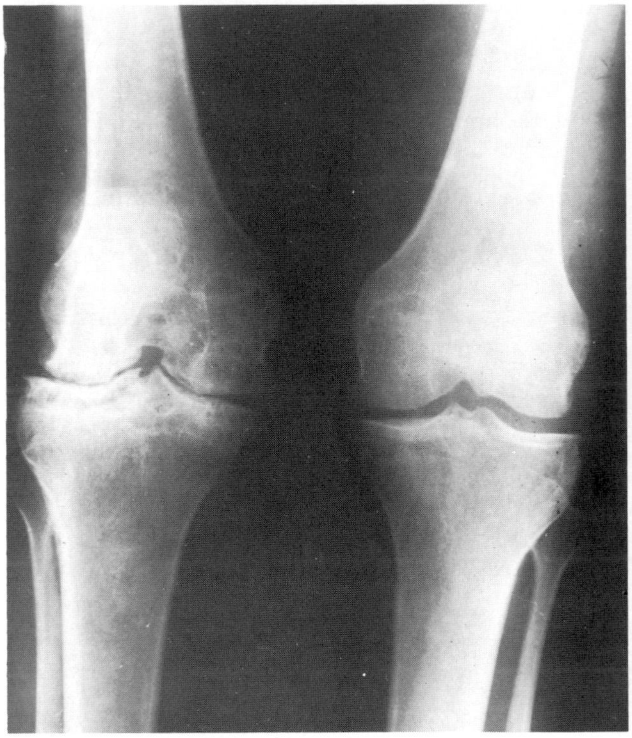

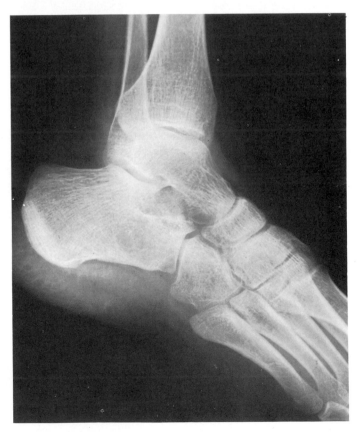

FIG. 9–119. Hemophilia (both knees). The changes in the right knee are more advanced than the changes in the left knee. Periarticular soft-tissue swelling, increased density, and minimal erosion at the lateral joint margins are the only significant findings in the left knee. The right knee reveals marked narrowing of the joint space, cyst formation, and widening of the intercondylar notch.

FIG. 9–120. Hemophilia—male, age 19 years. Osteoporosis is seen, with loss of bone density, accentuation of the trabecular pattern, and cortical thinning.

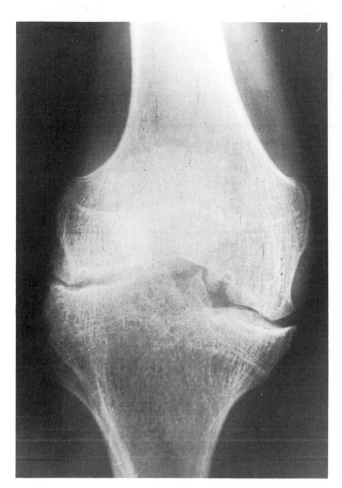

FIG. 9–121. Hemophilia (knee). Severe arthritic change without cyst formation. Note narrowing of the joint space, deformity of the medial tibial epiphysis, secondary to hemorrhage, and secondary osteoarthritic changes. There is no widening of the intercondylar notch.

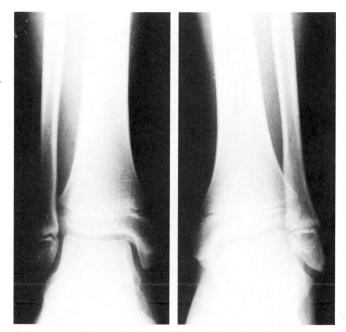

FIG. 9–122. Hemophilia (ankles). Tibiotalar slant on the left is noted.

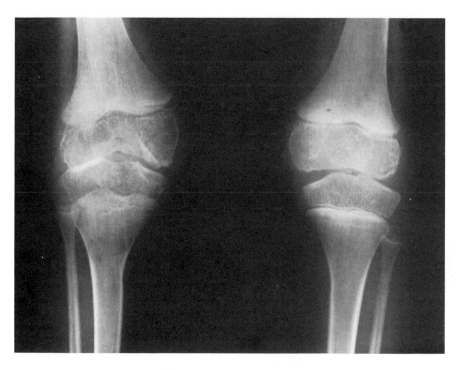

FIG. 9–123. Hemophilia (knees). Note enlargement of epiphyseal ossification centers bilaterally, more marked on the right due to chronic hyperemia. Arthritic changes are present bilaterally, also more severe on the right, where there is widening of the intercondylar notch.

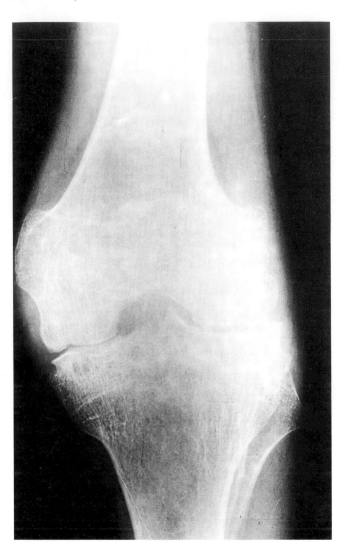

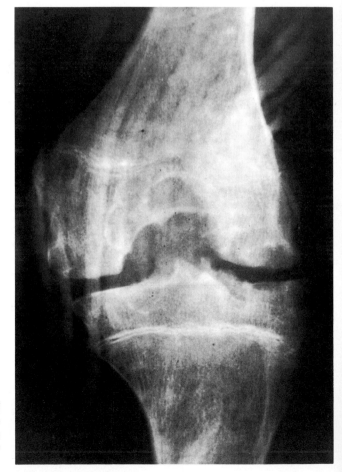

FIG. 9–124. Hemophilia (knee). Prominence of the inter-condylar notch is noted, as well as subchondral cyst forma-tion in the tibia. Narrowing of the joint space is also seen, as well as epiphyseal irregularity.

FIG. 9–125. Hemophilia (knee). There is marked widening of the intercondylar notch, a pathognomonic finding of hemophi-lic arthropathy, caused by hemorrhage at the insertions of the cruciate ligaments. Irregularities of the articular surfaces may also be noted.

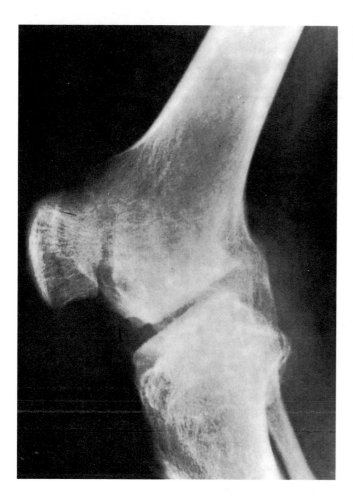

FIG. 9–126. Hemophilia (knee)—lateral view. Flattening of the inferior margin of the patella and advanced arthritic changes may be seen.

FIG. 9–127. Hemophilia (shoulder)—intraosseous hemorrhage. There is an area of radiolucency in the greater tuberosity and a smaller satellite area of radiolucency at its superior aspect. Loss of bone density and coarsening of the trabecular pattern may also be seen.

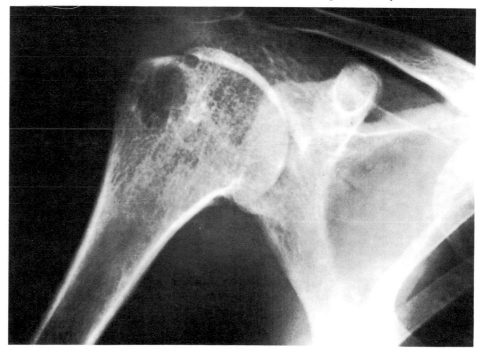

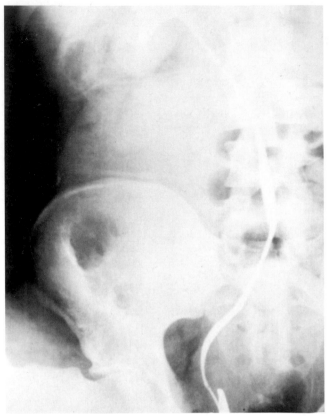

FIG. 9–128. Hemophilic pseudotumor (pelvis). A large soft-tissue mass is seen, associated with right iliac bone destruction and a small calcific or ossific rim. The ureter is displaced medially. (Courtesy of Dr. Harold Rosenbaum, Lexington, KY)

tical thickening. A large subperiosteal hematoma causes pressure erosion of the cortex. A Codman's triangle may be present. Bone spicules and calcification also may be seen. This is the hemophilic pseudotumor[23,62,81] most common in the femur and in the iliac bone. A large area of destruction with an associated soft-tissue mass in the iliac bone is sometimes present.

Ectopic bone formation in the pelvic region is a rare manifestation, resulting from hemorrhage with metaplasia and subsequent ossification (Fig. 9–128). Only the area of the iliacus and the adductor minimus muscles have been reported as sites of ectopic new bone formation. Chondrocalcinosis has been reported as associated with hemophilia.[105] Patients with synovial hemangiomas of the knee have been described as showing changes which simulate hemophilic arthropathy.[212] Adjacent phleboliths document the hemangiomas.

RETICULOHISTIOCYTOMA

Reticulohistiocytoma[24,77,146] *(lipoid dermatoarthritis)* is a rare, grave condition of unknown etiology in which cutaneous xanthomas are followed by arthritis and osseous erosive and resorptive changes leading to crippling deformities. The disease may resolve spontaneously. Blood chemistry values have been normal.

Radiologically, articular cartilage and subchondral bone destruction are present with marginal erosions, similar to those of rheumatoid arthritis. The distal interphalangeal joints of the hands and feet show early involvement. Involvement progresses to the phalanges, with severe resorption and telescoping of the digits. The distal clavicle may also show resorption (Fig. 9–129). Other joints may be involved, including the shoulders, elbows (Fig. 9–130), wrists (Fig. 9–131), hips (with destruction of the femoral heads and acetabular protrusion) (Fig. 9–132), knees, spine, and ribs. Resorption of the calcaneus may also occur (Fig. 9–133). The cervical spine may be involved with vertebral body and odontoid process destruction. Sacroiliac fusion and ischial erosion have also been described.

GOUT

Gout[88, 255] is a condition of hyperuricemia with crystal deposition and its resultant effects, which can be caused by a multiplicity of mechanisms. It may be due to an overproduction of uric acid or a failure of renal excretion of uric acid. If overproduction can be explained on the basis of excessive breakdown of nucleoproteins in diseases such as polycythemia, anemia, myelofibrosis, leukemia, lymphoma, multiple myeloma, psoriasis, glycogen storage disease,[239] hemoglobin E disease,[124] or is due to renal failure, the process is termed secondary gout (Figs. 9–134, 9–135). If overproduction of uric acid is caused by an inherited enzyme defect or has an unknown etiology, the process is referred to as *primary gout.* Several biochemically distinct forms are present in the category of primary gout. These include undefined specific defects, as well as the following enzyme defects: glucose-6-phosphatase, hypoxanthine-guanine phosphoribosyl transferase, glutamine-pp-ribose-p amidotransferase, and glutathione reductase. The symptomatology and roentgen appearance are similar in both primary and secondary forms.

(Text continued on p. 766)

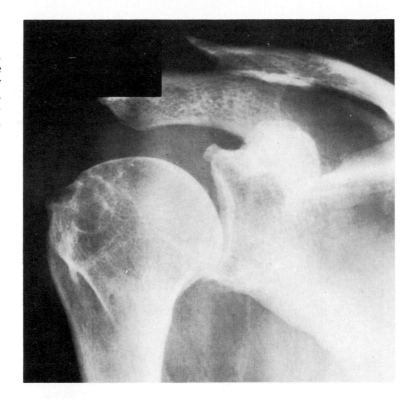

FIG. 9–129. Reticulohistiocytoma (shoulder). Note resorption of the distal clavicle. Cystlike changes in the region of the greater tuberosity of the humerus are present. (From Schwarz E, Fish A: Reticulohistiocytoma: A rare dermatologic disease with roentgen manifestations. Am J Roentgen 83:692–697, 1960)

FIG. 9–130. Reticulohistiocytoma (elbow). Cystic dissolutions of the articular surface and subchondral areas are seen. Soft-tissue mass can be noted at the medial aspect of the elbow joint.

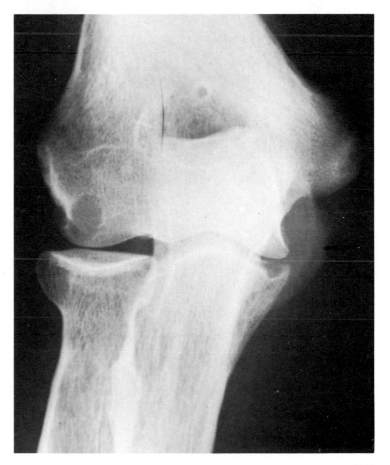

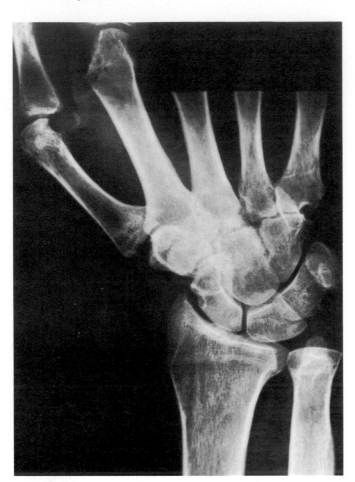

FIG. 9–131. Reticulohistiocytoma (wrist). Narrowing of the carpal-metacarpal joint spaces is present, with subchondral cystlike areas. Resorptive changes at the distal metacarpals and a smooth erosive defect at the distal ulna may be seen. This picture is not dissimilar to that of rheumatoid arthritis.

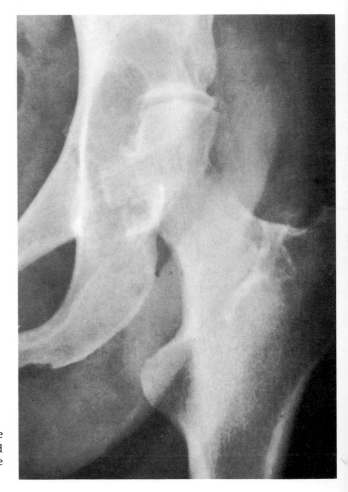

FIG. 9–132. Reticulohistiocytoma (hip). Marked resorptive changes of both the femoral head and the acetabulum, and resorption along the femoral neck and the greater trochanter are seen.

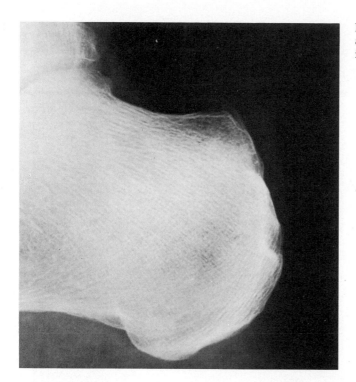

FIG. 9–133. Reticulohistiocytoma (calcaneus). Resorption at the posterior aspect of the calcaneus at the region of the insertion of the Achilles tendon is seen.

FIG. 9–134. Secondary gout (hands) associated with chronic renal disease. A tophus and destructive changes at the distal interphalangeal joint of the right ring finger are noted, as well as multiple marginal erosions and intraosseous cyst formation, particularly at the distal aspects of both first metacarpals. Joint space narrowing in several areas has also occurred.

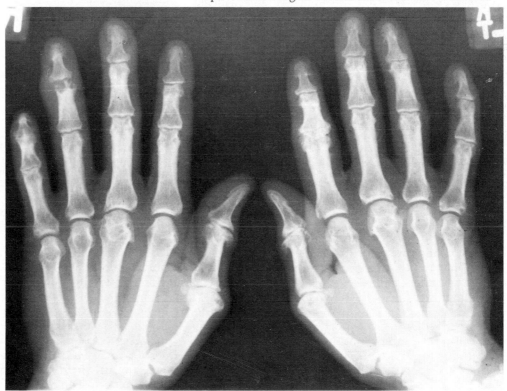

Pathogenesis: uric acid is a purine. All known uric acid in the body is derived from the oxidation of xanthine according to the following pathway:

Hypoxanthine
  Xanthine
    oxydase
Xanthine
  Xanthine
    oxydase
Uric Acid
  Uricase
Allantoin

Humans, in contrast to lower forms of life, lack hepatic uricase, which catalyzes the production of soluble allantoin from relatively insoluble uric acid. The major portion of uric acid must be excreted by way of the kidneys. In the event of overproduction, uric acid accumulates in the blood and is deposited as sodium urate in the tissues. One mechanism of primary gout is thought to be a partial deficiency of the enzyme phosphorylribosyltransferase, which restores guanine and hypoxanthine to guanylic and inosinic acids. There is no agreement regarding the presence or absence of a specific renal defect in the excretion of uric acid.

Gouty tophi are composed of sodium urate. They may be deposited in cartilage, collagen, and chondroid. The principal organs affected are the joints, kidneys, and heart.

In the joints, crystals are deposited in the synovia, and are carried by the synovial fluid to the articular surfaces. This causes an inflammatory reaction and granulation tissue, or pannus formation. The latter erodes cartilages and bone. Tophi, which range up to several centimeters in size, are deposited in cartilage, synovia, ligaments, bursa, and subcutaneous tissues. They cause extensive involvement of the joints and severe destruction of bone.

Clinically, primary gout is transmitted as an autosomal dominant with low penetrance in the female. Only 10% of cases are in females, in whom it occurs postmenopausally (Fig. 9–136). In males, symptomatology usually begins after the age of 40 years. Juvenile gout is a rare occurrence but not unknown. Middlemiss[154] reported one case in a boy with onset of symptoms at the age of 5½ years. Resnick et al[213] reported a series of patients with onset of gout in adolescence. Gout is less common in blacks.

Repeated attacks of acute arthritis usually occur, involving chiefly the first metatarsophalangeal joint

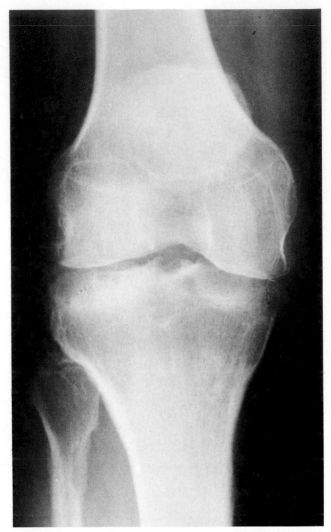

FIG. 9–135. Gout (knee) secondary to chronic renal failure. Destructive changes at the lateral tibial plateau have occurred; same patient as in Fig. 9–134.

(Fig. 9–137). Peripheral joint involvement is frequent, and central joint involvement is less common. The joint manifestations are effusion and acute inflammation, which subside after days or weeks. The attacks become progressively more frequent and severe, extend to multiple joints, and progress to extensive destructive changes. Uric acid stones, renal failure, and cardiac disease also occur. A serum uric acid level of 6 mg% or higher constitutes hyperuricemia.

A rare syndrome of hyperuricemia and mental retardation in children—the *Lesch–Nyhan syndrome*—

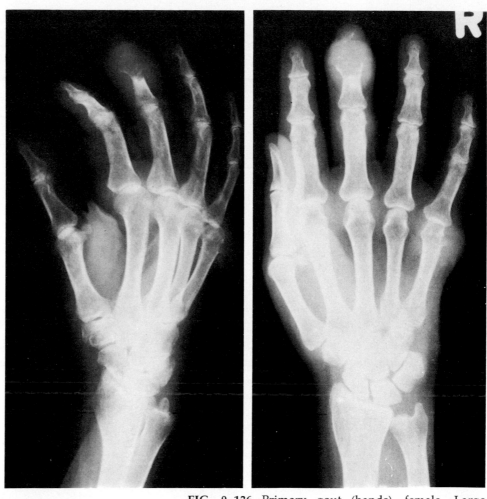

FIG. 9–136. Primary gout (hands)—female. Large tophi are seen at the distal middle finger, with extensive destruction of the distal phalanx and the distal portion of the middle phalanx, as well as at the fifth metacarpophalangeal joint, where joint space narrowing and marginal erosion have occurred.

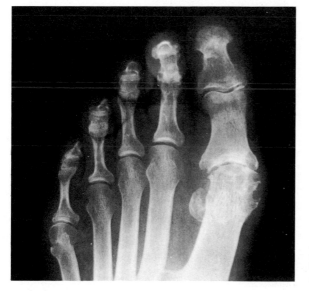

FIG. 9–137. Gout in its typical location in the first metatarsophalangeal joint. Joint space narrowing and marginal erosion are present.

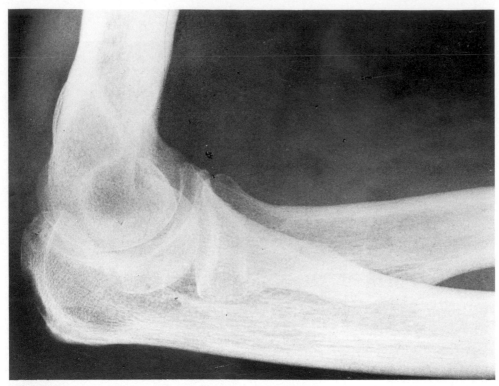

FIG. 9–138. Gout (elbow). A tophus posterior to the olecranon process is noted, which has caused erosion.

Nat Cooper
level

FIG. 9–139. Gout (elbow). A large tophus at the elbow is noted, which has stimulated the formation of an olecranon spur. A small amount of calcification within the tophus can be discerned.

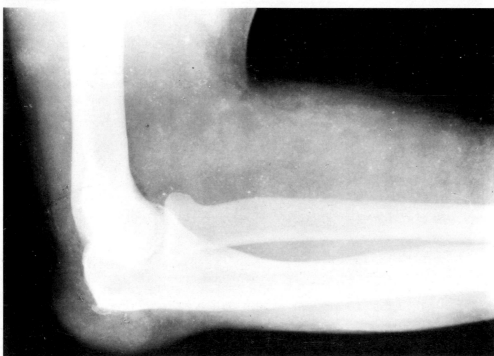

is due to total deficiency of the enzyme hypoxanthine-guanine phosphorylribosyltransferase. This defect is transmitted by a recessive gene on the X chromosome, and hence occurs in male children. There is a characteristic pattern of mental retardation and abnormal aggressive behavior with self-mutilation by biting of the fingers and lips, chorioathetosis, hyperuricemia, and uric acid nephrolithiasis.

Radiologically, the earliest changes in gout are joint effusions and swellings. A tophus is not uncommonly seen posterior to the olecranon process, where erosion or spur formation may occur (Figs. 9–138, 9–139). Destructive changes occur late in the course of the disease. The pannus of granulation tissue causes uniform narrowing of the joint, and subchondral and marginal erosions. These lesions have been described as cystlike or "punched-out"; they have little surrounding reactive sclerosis and are associated with little regional osteoporosis (Fig. 9–140). A typical location is at the metatarsophalangeal joints of the first toes (Fig. 9–141), but all small joints may be involved. Periosteal reaction may also be present. A feature distinguishing gout from the other arthritides is the presence of destructive lesions in bone that are remote from the articular surface (Fig. 9–142). Many of the lesions are expansile with overhanging margins which are displaced away from the axis of the bone.[144] Secondary calcification within tophi or degenerated

tissue may occur, particularly if vitamin D is administered (Fig. 9–143). Severe bony destructive lesions ensue (Fig. 9–144) which are not related to the amount of urate in the soft tissues. Bony ankylosis may occur. Changes in the sacroiliac joints[5] include sclerosis and marginal irregularity, focal osteoporosis, and "cysts" with sclerotic margins. Obliteration of the joint space has been described. Rarely, the spine may be involved.[262] Narrowing of the intervertebral space and end-plate erosion, as well as erosion of the odontoid process and subluxation of the first cervical vertebra, have been reported.

Ischemic necrosis of the femoral heads may also occur as well as medullary bone infarcts.[225]

A finding that has been emphasized by Steinbach is the presence, in a high percentage of gout patients, of calcification in articular cartilage and the menisci of the knee. This "chondrocalcinosis" is to be regarded as a secondary manifestation of gout. It is also seen in the pseudogout syndrome and other conditions (see p. 791).

Terminal phalangeal resorption also may occur, as well as flexion deformities (Fig. 9–145). In the rare cases of juvenile gout, growth disturbances of the long bones due to epiphyseal injury have been described. Rupture of the quadriceps tendons with downward displacement of the patellae has been reported.[132] A synovial popliteal cyst may develop,

(Text continued on p. 773)

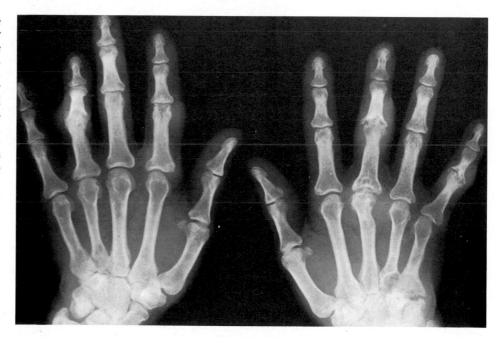

FIG. 9–140. Gout (hands). Note widely distributed periarticular swellings. There is joint space narrowing, marginal erosions, and subchondral erosions of several interphalangeal joints. Bony ankylosis of the right proximal fourth interphalangeal joint has occurred, with flexion deformity. Osteolytic lesions at the left proximal fourth and fifth metacarpals may be noted. The lesions have little surrounding reactive sclerosis. Significant regional osteoporosis is not present.

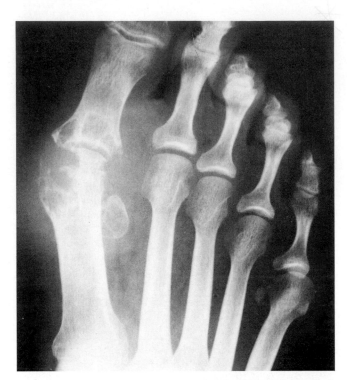

FIG. 9–141. Far-advanced gout (first metatarsophalangeal joint). Soft-tissue swelling is seen, as well as marked destruction of the distal first metatarsal. Displacement and a cystlike lesion in the sesamoid bone are also noted. Cystlike lesions at the base of the proximal phalanx and marginal erosions are seen. This is the only lesion in the foot.

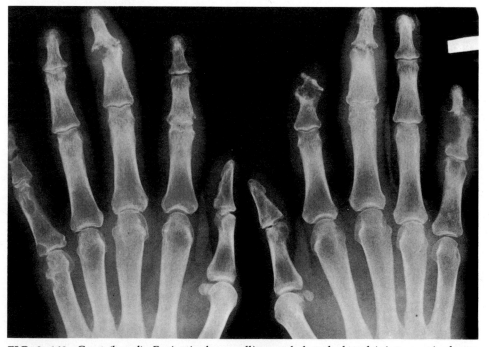

FIG. 9–142. Gout (hand). Periarticular swelling, subchondral and joint marginal erosions may be noted. Destructive changes of bone have taken place at a distance from the joint: destroyed medial aspect of the middle phalanx of the left fifth finger; and cystlike or "punched-out" lesion in the proximal phalanx of the right fifth finger, approximately 1 cm distant from the joint surface. Severe resorption of the terminal phalanx of the left index finger has occurred.

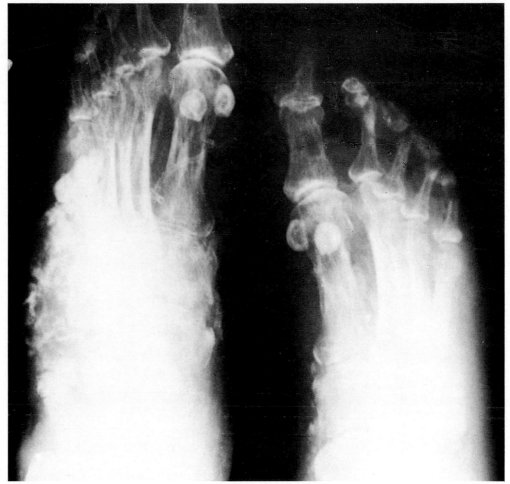

FIG. 9–143. Gout (feet). The patient has had vitamin D administration, with subsequent marked soft-tissue and vascular calcification.

FIG. 9–144. Gout. Severe destructive changes in the tarsus are seen. Destructive changes at the second metatarsophalangeal joint are also noted, as well as fusion at the first metatarsophalangeal joint. Secondary hypertrophic changes have occurred.

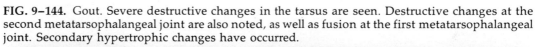

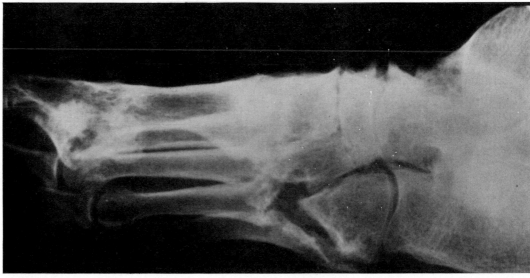

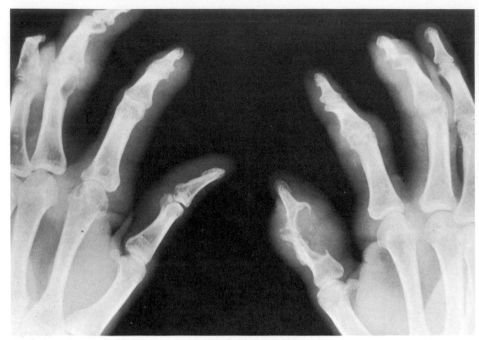

FIG. 9–145. Gout (hand). Resorption at the terminal phalanx of the right fourth finger is present, as well as flexion deformities, periarticular swellings and bone and joint destruction. A large, smoothly marginated destructive lesion in the left thumb is prominent, with overhanging margins.

FIG. 9–146. Osteoarthritis (hands). Heberden's nodes are seen at the distal interphalangeal joints resulting from spur formation and subluxation of the distal phalanges.

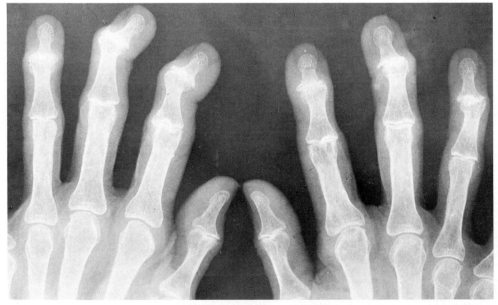

similar to those seen in rheumatoid arthritis.[181] It may dissect and simulate deep vein thrombosis.[131] Chronic synovitis rather than tophus deposition may rarely predominate in the picture of presentation of gout. Rheumatoid arthritis is then simulated with joint space narrowing and popliteal cysts.[247] The coexistence of gout and rheumatoid arthritis in the same patient is extremely rare, with only four documented cases reported in the literature.[230] Severe deformities of the hands with telescoping of the digits may occur during allopurinol treatment owing to rapid resorption of osseous tophi which are not replaced by bone matrix.[80]

A roentgen appearance of the hands with erosions similar to those of gout has been described in lymphoma cutis.[33]

OSTEOARTHRITIS (OSTEOARTHROSIS, DEGENERATIVE JOINT DISEASE, HYPERTROPHIC ARTHRITIS)

Osteoarthritis[64,82,96,102,195,211,241,246,252] is a noninflammatory progressive disorder of movable joints. It is characterized by deterioration of articular cartilage and new bone formation at the joint margins and in the subchondral regions. It is by far the most common form of arthritis. It is estimated that 40 million Americans have osteoarthritic changes in the hands and feet, and that 175,000 Americans over 65 years of age are incapacitated by osteoarthritis of the hip.

Clinically, the disease may be classified as primary or secondary. *Primary osteoarthritis* occurs with intrinsic degeneration of articular cartilage as the initial change. This form of osteoarthritis chiefly affects women. It is painful and at times inflammatory and degenerative. Erosive changes are present in small joints, chiefly the distal interphalangeal joints of the fingers and the first carpometacarpal joints. Bony protuberances at the dorsal margins of the distal interphalangeal joints are common, and are referred to as Heberden's nodes (Fig. 9–146). A mucoid cyst or subluxation at this site may be associated.

Less frequently, similar nodes are seen in the proximal interphalangeal joints, referred to as Bouchard's nodes (Fig. 9–147). A genetic predisposition to Heberden's nodes has been suggested.

Osteoarthritis, particularly involving weight-bearing joints and the spine, may result from senescent changes in cartilage. Other predisposing factors, such as obesity, Wilson's disease, acromegaly

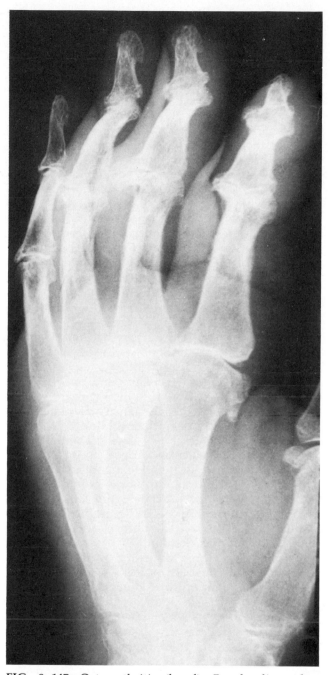

FIG. 9–147. Osteoarthritis (hand)—Bouchard's nodes. Marked spur formation at the proximal interphalangeal joints is noted.

(Fig. 9–148), disordered proprioceptive sense, and alcaptonuria, as well as local structural abnormality, stress abnormality, trauma, burns, inflammation, and hemorrhage, contribute to the development of osteoarthritis. Joint space narrowing may also result from disuse atrophy of cartilage. When a cause can be defined, the disease is termed *secondary osteoarthritis*.

Osteoarthritis is usually slowly progressive, with changes measured in terms of years. Rarely, an inflammatory synovitis and joint effusion may be associated. In other instances, subchondral erosion may proceed more rapidly in a joint with painful soft-tissue swelling. The latter condition is termed *erosive osteoarthritis*. The major clinical complaints are pain, stiffness after rest, aching in bad weather, crepitation, limitation of motion, and possibly malalignment in the osteoarthritic joint. The joints of major clinical concern are those of the hip and the knee.

Pathologic changes include fraying and fibrillation of degenerating cartilage, with depletion of chondrocytes and of protein-polysaccharides. Theories of pathogenesis include changes in enzymes, chondrocyte function, and nutrition.

The cartilage becomes yellow and opaque, with focal areas of malacia and roughening of the surface in early degenerative change. The surface later frays and fibrillates, with deep cracks. Minute fragments of cartilage may induce an acute synovitis. In the final stages, the articular surface becomes totally denuded of cartilage. Remodeling of subchondral bone results in eburnation. Bony spurs, following cartilage hyperplasia, at times very large, form at the site of joint margins and attachments of ligaments and tendons. Osteoporosis and local pressure inhibit spur formation.

Radiologically, the changes of primary and secondary osteoarthritis are basically similar. The typical pattern is nonuniform joint space narrowing, subchondral sclerosis, spur formation, subarticular cysts or pseudocysts which may precede or be concurrent with the other changes, and lack of periarticular osteoporosis. Microfractures and focal areas of ischemic necrosis may develop, as well as alignment abnormalities. Periosteal new bone formation is sparse except in certain characteristic areas. Synovial membrane may be stimulated to form new bone. Subchondral radiolucencies may be due to an ingrowth of granulation tissue through defects in articular cartilage, pressure atrophy from fluid forced through these defects by intra-articular pressure, or subchondral metaplasia.[125] A subchondral pseudocyst may collapse resulting in flattening and irregularity of a segment of the articular surface.

"Loose bodies" may become detached and fall free in the joint. The end stage in certain areas may rarely be bony ankylosis.

Primary osteoarthritis is widespread and involves small and large joints. Changes in the spine are difficult to categorize. Secondary osteoarthritis affects those joints subject to abnormality or insult. Articular changes of senescence rarely give rise to severe clinical complaints, but when they do, they can be considered a form of primary osteoarthritis. Studies suggest that the changes in degenerative cartilage are not merely a further progression of the aging process, but may reflect an abnormality specific for osteoarthritis.

The large joints most frequently involved with primary osteoarthritis are those of the hip and the knee. The femoral head migrates in the acetabulum, usually superior but also superomedial.[195] It may migrate in other directions with lesser frequency. Osteophyte formation at the patellar insertion of the quadriceps tendon can result in severe vertical ridging at the anterior superior surface of the patella.[82] Involvement of the shoulder girdle is much less common (Fig. 9–149, 9–150), except for the acromioclavicular joint. Tibiotalar joint involvement is not seen.

In the hands, all joints may be involved; however, there is a predilection for the distal interphalangeal joints (Fig. 9–151) and the first carpometacarpal joint (Fig. 9–152). The proximal interphalangeal joints may also be involved, and less frequently the metacarpophalangeal joints.[150] The basic changes are joint space narrowing, subchondral sclerosis, and marginal spur formation. Marginal erosions are not seen. Malalignment at the interphalangeal joints due to uneven joint space narrowing may occur.

Rarely, bony ankylosis of the interphalangeal joints may be seen.[240] Subchondral cysts occur, some of which may collapse. These features would have to be differentiated from those of rheumatoid arthritis.

One or more of the metacarpophalangeal joints not uncommonly show uniform narrowing (Fig. 9–153). Marginal erosions are not present. Osteophytosis may be present as well as small, discrete subchondral radiolucencies, usually 1 to 3 mm in diameter. Flexion deformities, volar subluxations, and ulnar deviation are not seen. The uniform narrowing may be on the basis of disuse atrophy of cartilage. These changes have to be differentiated again from those of rheumatoid arthritis, and from the more severe findings in hemochromatosis and pseudogout in this region.

(*Text continued on p. 779*)

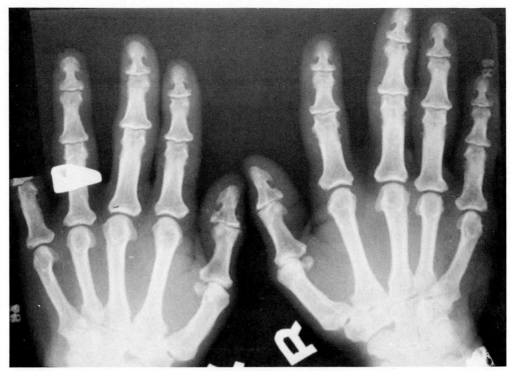

FIG. 9–148. Acromegaly with osteoarthritis (hands). Joint space widening is present with mild marginal spur formation, particularly at the bases of the proximal phalanges. Pseudocyst formation at several sites is also seen. The typical "spadelike" configuration of the terminal tufts is noted.

FIG. 9–149. Osteoarthritis (shoulder). Marked spur formation at the inferior aspect of the glenoid, as well as of the medial aspect of the humeral head, is noted.

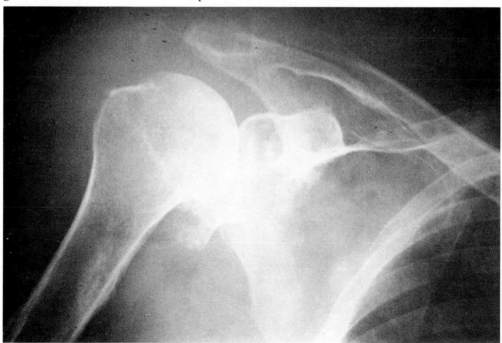

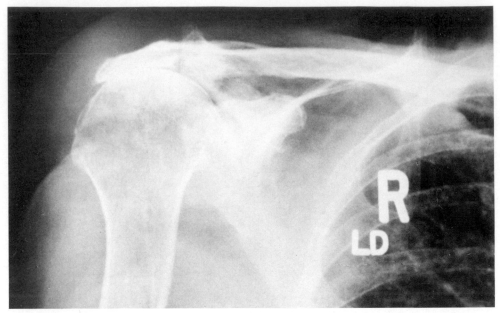

FIG. 9–150. Osteoarthritis (shoulder) secondary to rotator-cuff injury. Upward elevation of the humeral head, due to unopposed pull of the deltoid muscle is seen, with erosion of the inferior aspect of the acromial process, and spur formation most marked at the medial aspect of the humeral head. Acromioclavicular arthritic changes are also present.

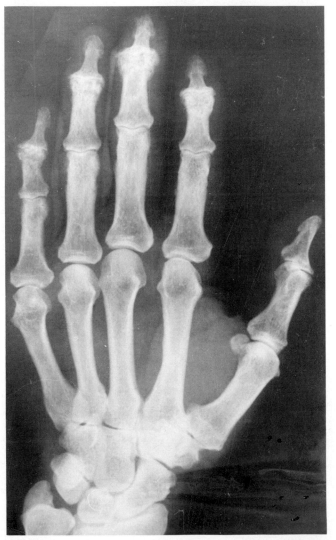

FIG. 9–151. Osteoarthritis (hand). Typical distribution of involvement of the distal interphalangeal joints, showing joint space narrowing and spur formation as well as subchondral cysts. The other joints of the hand are not significantly involved.

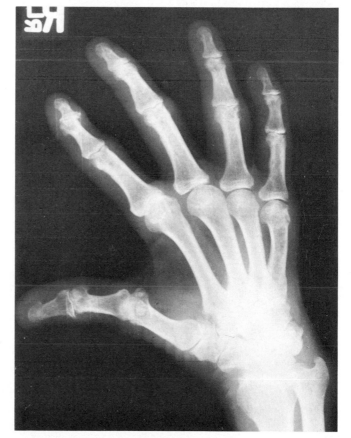

FIG. 9–152. Osteoarthritis (hand and wrist). Involvement of only the first carpometacarpal joint is seen, with joint space narrowing and marginal spur formation. This is a typical location for initial or early change.

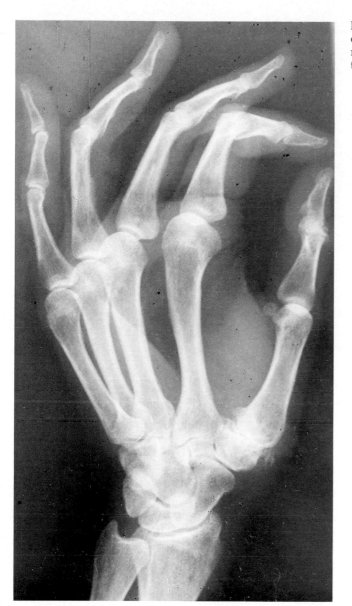

FIG. 9–153. Osteoarthritis (hand). Uniform narrowing of the metacarpophalangeal joint space of the index finger is noted, with maximum involvement of this finger with osteoarthritis at the distal interphalangeal joint. Joint space narrowing, marginal osteophyte formation, and subluxation are seen, forming a typical Heberden's node. A disuse factor may contribute to the narrowing.

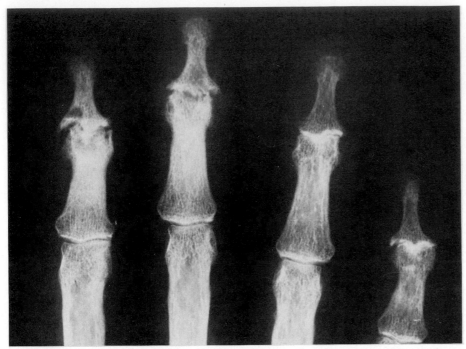

FIG. 9–154. Erosive osteoarthritis (hand). Irregular destruction of the subchondral cortex at the distal interphalangeal joint of the index finger, and to a lesser extent of the middle finger, is seen.

FIG. 9–155. Former ballerina, age 57 years, who now suffers from severe osteoarthritis of the hips. Note flattening of both femoral heads, cyst formation, and sclerosis, upward subluxation, and erosion of the roofs of both acetabula with spur formation.

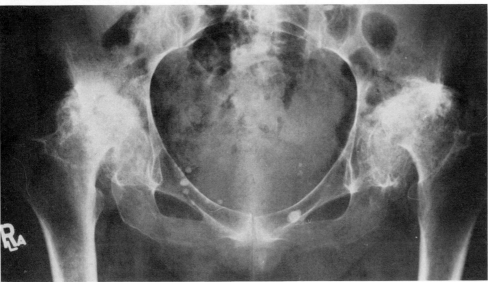

Erosive osteoarthritis[114, 245] is an inflammatory form of osteoarthritis generally limited to the hands, and affecting predominantly post-menopausal women. The interphalangeal joints and the trapeziometacarpal joint are chiefly involved. *Clinically*, a symmetrical synovitis of the interphalangeal joints of the hand, the wrist, and the knees[252] is seen. Joint space narrowing occurs. Severe irregular destruction of the subchondral cortex may be associated with marked soft-tissue swelling (Fig. 9–154). Osteophyte formation and sclerosis follow. The wrist may be involved at its radial aspect, the first carpometacarpal, and the trapezioscaphoid joints.[83] Severe shortening of the fingers may proceed to a *"main-en-lorgnette"* deformity.

Diffuse involvement of the intracarpal joints, and radiocarpal and distal radioulnar joint involvement are not seen in primary osteoarthritis.

In the feet, the most common site of involvement is the first metatarsophalangeal joints. The first tarsometatarsal and talonavicular joints are not uncommonly involved.

In the hips,[103, 152] the etiology may be primary[167] or secondary to a wide variety of disturbances, some of which are summarized below. Involvement is often unilateral.

ETIOLOGY OF SECONDARY OSTEOARTHRITIS OF THE HIP

1. Athletic activity in adolescence[168, 226] (Fig. 9–155)
2. Slipped capital femoral epiphysis
3. Congenital dislocation of the hip
4. Fracture
5. Idiopathic coxa vara
6. Obesity
7. Legg–Perthes' disease
8. Ischemic necrosis of the femoral head
9. Acromegaly[22]
10. Acetabular dysplasia
11. Multiple epiphyseal dysplasia
12. Disorders of cartilage (*e.g.*, ochronosis)
13. Endocrine disturbances
14. Previous infective arthritis
15. Previous rheumatoid arthritis
16. Disturbances of stress forces

Severe degenerative arthritis in old age is referred to as *malum coxae senilis.*

Narrowing of the joint space is seen, with the greatest narrowing at the superior, weight-bearing surface.[94] There is usually no medial migration of the femoral head as is seen in rheumatoid arthritis. Subchondral sclerosis and well-marginated cystlike radiolucencies are present. A large "cyst" may be connected to the joint cavity by a narrow "bottleneck" opening. A cyst may collapse, resulting in deformity of the articular surface. Further characteristic deformities develop, including: flattening of the femoral head; varus angulation and "flat exostosis" formation at the superior margin of the junction between the femoral head and neck; a double contour of the medial aspect of the femoral head; medial spur formation; and buttressing of the medial femoral neck. Osteophytosis of the acetabular margins is also frequent (Fig. 9–156). The acetabulum may become shallow, and subluxation of the femoral head may occur (Fig. 9–157).

Bursal extension into the pelvis, presenting as an intrapelvic mass, has been described in osteoarthritis as well as rheumatoid arthritis.[10]

Arteriographic studies show hyperemia of the involved joint.[169] Venous engorgement and increased intraosseous pressure have also been demonstrated.[12]

In the event of paraplegia or polio, uniform narrowing of the hip joint may be seen.

The knee has three compartments; the lateral and medial femorotibial, and the retropatellar. Narrowing of the knee joint space in osteoarthritis[142] does not involve all three to a uniform extent. In primary osteoarthritis, the weight-bearing portion with greatest stress, usually the medial compartment, shows initial and greatest narrowing (Fig. 9–158). A varus or valgus deformity may develop with subsequent subluxation. Marked spur formation at the joint margins, and of the intercondyloid eminences, may develop, as well as at the margins of the patella (Fig. 9–159). Subchondral sclerosis and "cyst" formation also is characteristic (Fig. 9–160). A Baker's cyst and superior distension of the joint space may be present (Fig. 9–161). A frequently associated finding in advanced disease is chondrocalcinosis involving the hyaline articular cartilage as well as the menisci.

Chondromalacia patellae[177] is a related condition occurring in younger individuals. A softening of cartilage, chiefly at the posterior surface of the patella, occurs. Hypertrophic spurs at the patellar margins in a young individual should raise suspicion of this possibility. It is thought to be related to trauma.

In the spine, two distinct articular systems are affected: the apophyseal joints, which are diarthrodial, and the intervertebral articulations, which are amphiarthrodial. Changes in the former are comparable to changes in the peripheral joints and are termed *spinal osteoarthritis*. Degenerative changes in the latter are termed *spondylosis*, or *spondylosis*

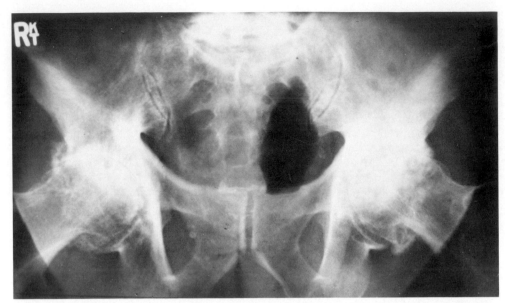

FIG. 9–156. Osteoarthritis (both hips). On the right there has been narrowing of the joint space in the superior portion of the hip joint. Marginal sclerosis and subchondral cysts are seen. A prominent spur at the junction of the femoral head and neck is noted, as well as spur formation inferiorly at the femoral head. On the left there has been destruction at the superior aspect of the joint space. The joint space persists medially, where a double contour to the medial aspect of the femoral head is seen, which terminates in an inferior spur. A "bump" is seen at the superior junction between the femoral head and neck. Cortical thickening at the medial aspects of the femoral necks is also seen, as well as osteophyte formation at the acetabular margins.

FIG. 9–157. Osteoarthritis (both hips) with flattening of the femoral heads and outward displacement. The C-E (center-edge) angle has become decreased.

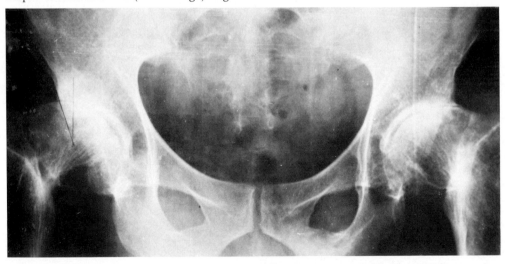

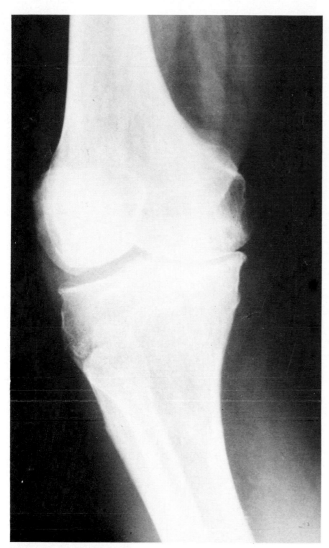

FIG. 9–158. Osteoarthritis (knee). Narrowing of the medial compartment of the knee joint space with resultant varus deformity is noted. Subchondral cyst formation at the medial femoral condyle and mild marginal spur formation are also seen.

deformans. The levels of the two changes usually correlate, although they may be independent of one another. Narrowing of an intervertebral disk may result in secondary apophyseal osteoarthritis.

Spondylosis deformans is regarded by Jaffe[102] as being in the "category of secondary osteoarthritis, since the condition follows in the wake of avulsion of fibers of the annulus fibrosus of the intervertebral disk from the site of anchorage of these fibers in the marginal ridge of the vertebral body." This is initiated by disk degeneration.

It is usually located in the lower cervical, lower thoracic and lower lumbar segments, as well as the lumbosacral region. Exostotic protuberances from the anterior and lateral borders and less frequently posterior borders of the vertebral margins, termed *osteophytes*, are seen. They blend with the vertebral bodies, with a continuous cortex. Their departure is in a horizontal direction, although later they may curve and fuse with one another (Fig. 9–162). Osteophytes are to be differentiated from syndesmophytes, which have a vertical direction and occur in inflammatory disease of the spine. Another type of osteophyte has been described, called the *traction spur.*[137] It also is horizontally directed but arises about 2 mm away from the vertebral margin at the site of attachment of the outermost fibers of the annulus. It is said to denote segmental instability (Fig. 9–163).

Spondylosis of the cervical spine is most likely to cause severe symptoms because of the relatively

(Text continued on p. 784)

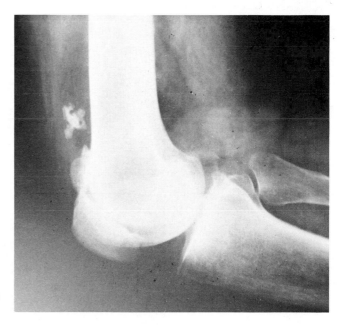

FIG. 9–159. Osteoarthritis (knee). Narrowing of the patellofemoral joint space with marginal spur formation is noted, as well as a calcification in the suprapatellar region.

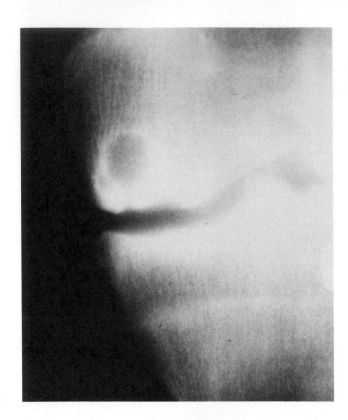

FIG. 9–160. Osteoarthritis (knee). Tomogram of subchondral cyst, showing narrow channel of communication to articular surface where erosion has occurred.

FIG. 9–161. Degenerative osteoarthritis (knee joint) — oblique and lateral views of arthrogram. Contrast material fills a pronounced superior extension of the knee joint space, as well as a Baker's cyst posteriorly.

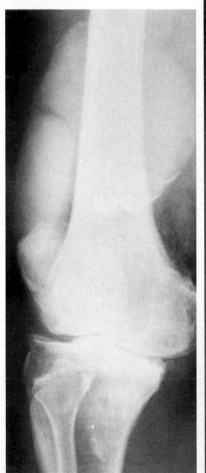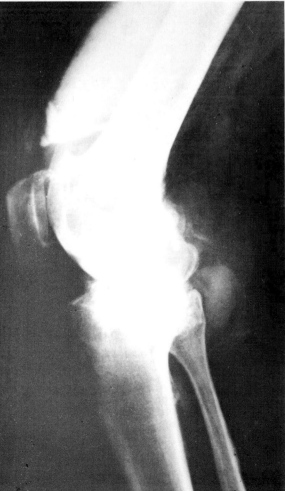

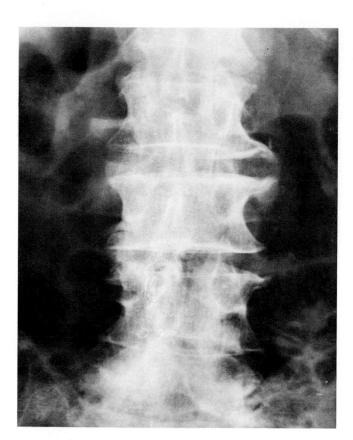

FIG. 9–162. Spondylosis (lumbar spine) with osteophyte formation. Note the horizontal take-off of the marginal osteophytes.

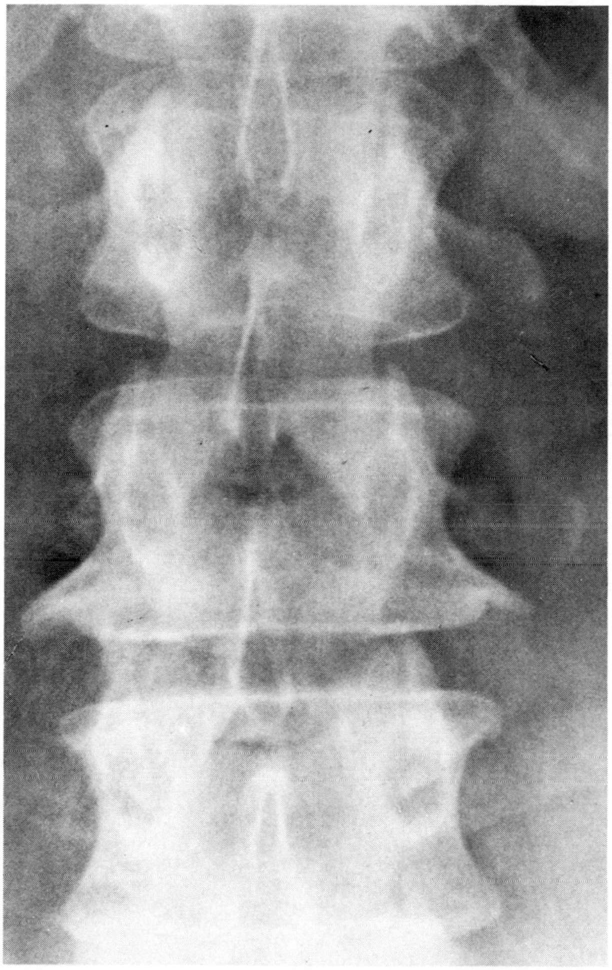

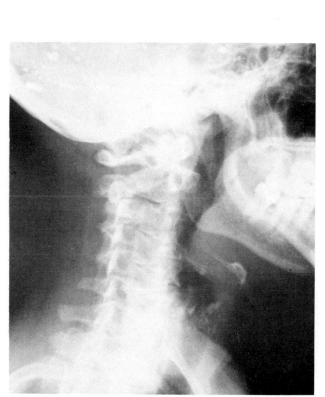

FIG. 9–163. Lumbar spine—traction spur. Horizontally directed spurs, about 3 mm superior to the vertebral margins of L-2, are seen.

FIG. 9–164. Spondylosis (cervical spine)—oblique view. Encroachment of hypertrophic spurs into the intervertebral foramina is seen.

narrow cervical canal and intervertebral foramina. Posterior osteophytes may form a ridge that compresses the cervical cord. Spurs on the lateral lips of the uncovertebral "joints" of Lushka may narrow or encroach upon the intervertebral foramina, resulting in neurological symptomatology (Fig. 9–164). These spurs have a radiolucent cartilage cap, so that their true size is not radiographically indicated. Subluxations may also occur. Disk degeneration may be evident as narrowing of the intervertebral space, or as a radiolucency in the space, termed the *vacuum sign*. There is a tendency for the C–5 and C–6 levels to be initially involved (Fig. 9–165) Osteophytes may regress after spinal stabilization procedures.

Exuberant anterior and lateral osteophytes, very large and superficially located, that are irregular and may fuse together, are termed *ankylosing hyperostosis*[153] or *Forestier's disease* (Figs. 9–166, 9–167) Peripheral joint manifestations may sometimes be associated with this condition. It is now termed *diffuse idiopathic skeletal hyperostosis*.[214, 248] It affects middle-aged and elderly patients. Hyperostosis at ligamentous attachments in the pelvis, symphysis pubis, calcaneus, tarsals, patella, olecranon, humerus, and hands may be seen. Hyperostosis of the attachments of the interosseous membranes of the forearm and leg also occur, as well as pelvic "whiskering." When the cervical spine is involved, dysphagia due to anterior displacement of the esophagus results. The apophyseal joints are not fused, and the intervertebral spaces need not be narrowed. Ossification of the posterior longitudinal ligament has also been reported.[200]

Osteoarthritis commonly occurs in the sacroiliac joints showing subchondral bone sclerosis.

Schmorl's nodes, or herniation of the nucleus pulposus into the vertebral bodies, is not an uncommon occurrence. Central or marginal herniation may be seen (Fig. 9–168)

Wilson's disease[4, 159] has as its skeletal manifestations osteoarthritis, osteochondrosis dissecans, marginal bone fragmentation, and cystic changes in areas of tendon and ligament insertions. Schmorl's nodes, bone fragmentation, and subchondral changes are seen in the spine. Renal failure leads to rickets, osteomalacia, pseudofractures, pathological fractures, loss of bone density, and para-articular calcifications.

Kashin–Beck disease[233] refers to a degenerative osteoarthritis of the joints of the spine and extremities. It almost always occurs in children. It is slowly progressive, and may result in shortening of extremities and reduction of height. Extraskeletal ab-

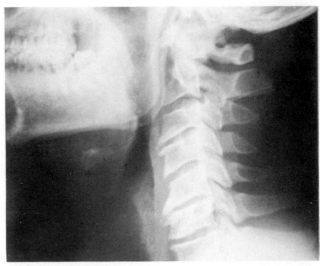

FIG. 9–165. Spondylosis (cervical spine). Straightening of the cervical spine and spur formation, most marked at the levels of C-5 and C-6, are seen. Apparent detachment of bony spurs at the inferior margins of C-3 and C-5 do not represent fractures, but rather intercalary bone formation.

FIG. 9–166. Ankylosing hyperostosis or Forestier's disease. Large exuberant irregular osteophytes seen anteriorly in the cervical spine: some of them are separated by a radiolucency from the anterior vertebral margins. The spurs approximate the tracheal air shadow. Dysphagia was present.

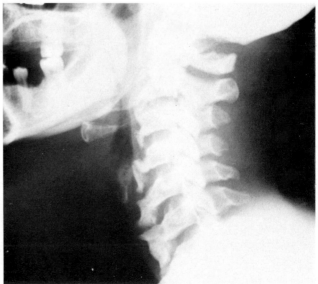

FIG. 9–167. Ankylosing hyperostosis or Forestier's disease. Marked superficial anterior osteophytes, which are partially separated from the anterior vertebral margins by a radiolucent line at the bodies of C-4 and C-5 are seen. These have fused together at the fourth, fifth, and sixth segments. Unattached ossicles at the tips of the spinous processes of C-6 and C-7 are also seen.

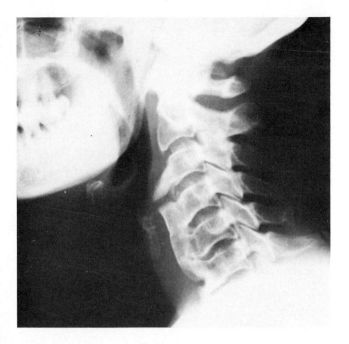

FIG. 9–168. Schmorl's nodes. Central herniations of the nucleus pulposus into several vertebral bodies, as well as marginal herniation of C-4 with an apparent detached fragment, are noted.

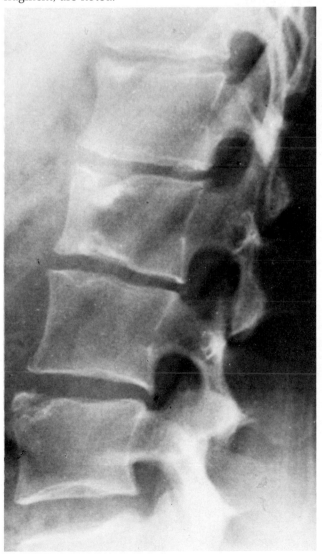

normalities also occur. It is due to excess intake of iron and is endemic in parts of Asia.

Narrowing of the hip joint space also occurs as a complication of slipped capital femoral epiphysis. It is then termed *acute chondrolysis*. The hip joint space may partially reconstitute Idiopathic chondrolysis also occurs. It has been reported following burns.

Vibration syndrome refers to severe degenerative arthritis of the wrist with ischemic necrosis of the carpal bones and marked subchondral cyst formation. It is due to chronic repeated trauma such as seen in air-hammer drillers (Fig. 9–169)

SPINAL STENOSIS[60, 118]

Narrowing or stenosis of the spinal canal is an important structural change which is recently gaining attention. Clinically significant changes may occur in the cervical or lumbar areas. Congenital or developmental spinal stenosis may occur in such conditions such as achondroplasia. However, the majority of cases are acquired. The stenosis may be localized, and in the lumbar spine it is more likely to occur in the lower-most two lumbar segments. In considering spinal stenosis, the anatomical regions of interest are the sagittal diameter or central canal, the lateral recesses and the intervertebral foramina, or the lateral canals. Degenerative lesions leading to

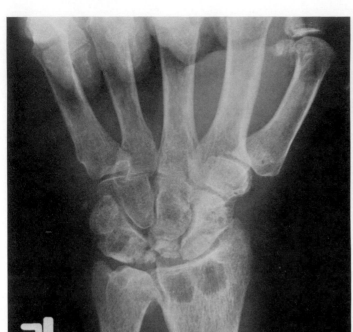

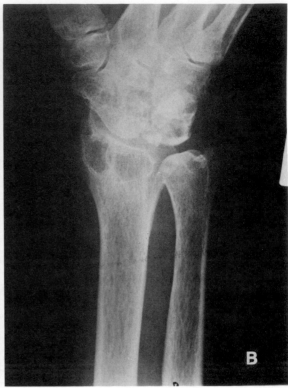

TABLE 9–1. Degenerative Lesions in the Lumbar Spine

Recurrent Rotational Strains (Compression Injury)		
POSTERIOR JOINTS ◄————Three-Joint Complex————► INTERVERTEBRAL DISC		
Synovial Reaction		Circumferential Tears
Cartilage Destruction	HERNIATION◄Radial Tears	
Osteophyte Formation		Internal Disruption
Capsular Laxity ————————► Instability ◄———————— Loss Disc Height		
Subluxation ————► LATERAL NERVE ENTRAPMENT◄Disc Resorption		
Enlargement Articular Processes (and Laminae) ————► ONE LEVEL ◄———— Osteophytes at Back of Vertebral Bodies CENTRAL STENOSIS		
Effect of Recurrent Strains at Levels Above and Below the Original Lesion		
Multilevel Degenerative Lesions		
MULTILEVEL SPINAL STENOSIS		

(Data from Kirkaldy–Willis WH, University Hospital, Saskatoon)

FIG. 9–169. Vibration syndrome—anteroposterior and oblique views of the wrist. Ischemic necrosis of the lunate with fragmentation has occurred, as well as sclerosis of the navicular, and cyst formation in the carpal bones and distal radius and ulna. A small bone fragment is seen medially at the carpus.

stenosis have been described as a function of the three-joint complex (intervertebral disc and two small joints) by Kirkaldy–Willis. A flow chart of the pathogenesis is presented in Table 9–1. Central canal stenosis may result from hypertrophic spur formation posteriorly, spondylolisthesis, intervertebral disc protrusion or herniation, or other diseases such as Paget's disease. A lateral recess stenosis usually results from hypertrophic changes of the inferior articular facets. Lateral canal stenosis may develop from hypertrophic spur formation or narrowing of the intervertebral spaces with subsequent diminution of height of the lateral canal. Plain roentgenographic examination with oblique views, tomography, computed tomography (Fig. 9–170), and myelography are the radiological examinations that demonstrate this condition.

NEUROTROPHIC ARTHROPATHY

Neurotrophic arthropathy, or *Charcot's joint,*[64, 97] is an extreme progression of degenerative osteoarthritis following a loss of proprioceptive or pain sensation. The normal protective reactions are not invoked. Relaxation of supporting structures leads to joint instability. Trauma, acute or cumulative, results in degenerative changes, subchondral frac-

tures, and total joint disorganization. The etiology and joint predilection of neurotrophic arthropathy are summarized below.

The neurotrophic joint may paradoxically be painful due to capsular distension and soft-tissue trauma.

Radiologically, the two classical forms are atrophic arthropathy and hypertrophic arthropathy. Differing opinions exist on whether or not one can change into the other (Fig. 6–140). Atrophic arthropathy is encountered more often in the upper extremities, while hypertrophic arthropathy is seen more often in the lower extremities. The spine only shows hypertrophic changes. The underlying disease does not determine which form predominates.

Atrophic arthropathy is seen as resorption of the bone ends. Osteoporosis is present, and destruction may proceed to dislocation. No osteophytes, sclerosis, fragmentation, or soft-tissue debris is present Tapering of the distal aspect of the bone (Fig. 6–185), with a "mortar and pestle" or "pencil-in-cup" deformity, are seen. There is a pointing of the convex member, and a hollowing or broadening of the concave member of a small joint. Joint effusion usually precedes destructive changes.

Hypertrophic arthropathy also is initiated by effusion. The progress is usually slow, but may on

ETIOLOGY OF NEUROPATHIC ARTHROPATHY AND JOINTS INVOLVED[97]

Disease	*Joints Most Frequently Involved*
Lues (tabes dorsalis) (Fig. 9–171)	Knee, hip, ankle, lower spine
Syringomyelia (Fig. 9–172)	Shoulder, elbow, cervical spine
Diabetes mellitus[34,41,84] (Fig. 9–173)	Tarsal, tarsometatarsal, metatarsophalangeal
Congenital insensitivity to pain[52,236] (Fig. 9–174)	Ankle, tarsal, knee
Intra-articular steroid injection[18]	Hip, knee
Meningomyelocele (Fig. 9–175)	Ankle, tarsal
Postrenal transplant[2]	Hip, knee, shoulder
Acrodystrophic neuropathy[17]	Knee, ankle, metatarsophalangeal
Amyloid neuropathy[182]	Ankle, tarsal
Spina bifida	Depends on level
Spinal trauma	Depends on level
Brain injury	Other areas may be affected.
Leprosy	
Neurological diseases[27]	
Prolonged analgesic use	

(Text continued on p. 791)

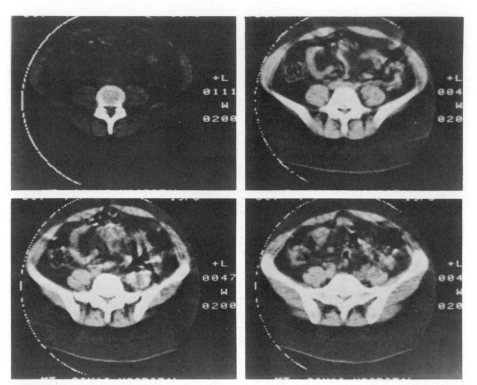

FIG. 9–170. Spinal stenosis (lumbo-sacral spine)—computed tomography. Hypertrophy of the inferior articular facets resulting in narrowing of the lateral recesses of the fifth lumbar vertebra, as well as narrowing of the sagittal diameter of the first sacral segment, is seen.

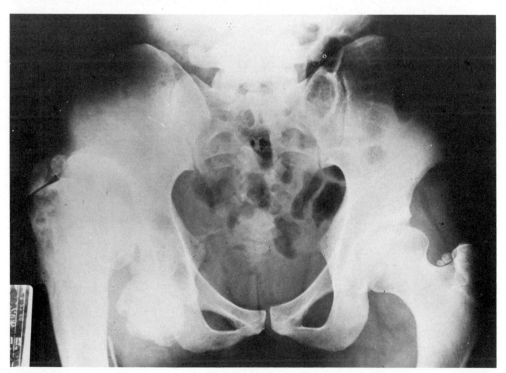

FIG. 9–171. Luetic Charcot's joints. Hypertrophy of the left femoral head is seen, with well-organized ossific deposits in the area superior to the femoral head and inferior to the acetabulum. Acetabular erosion is present. Charcot changes in the lower spine may also be seen.

FIG. 9–172. Syringomyelia (elbow), bony sclerosis, destruction, widening of the ulnar notch, soft-tissue debris, and bone formation are noted.

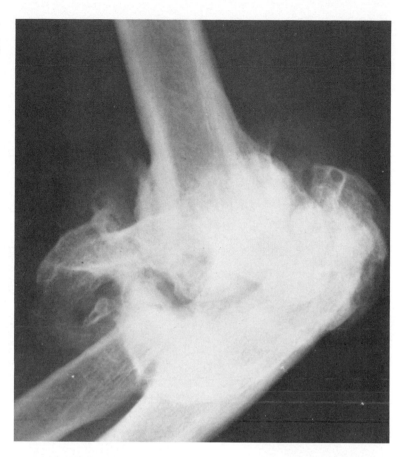

FIG. 9–173. Diabetes mellitus (tarsus). Marked disorganization and sclerosis of the tarsus are noted with involvement of the proximal metatarsals.

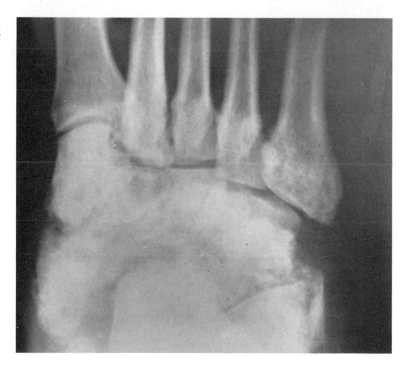

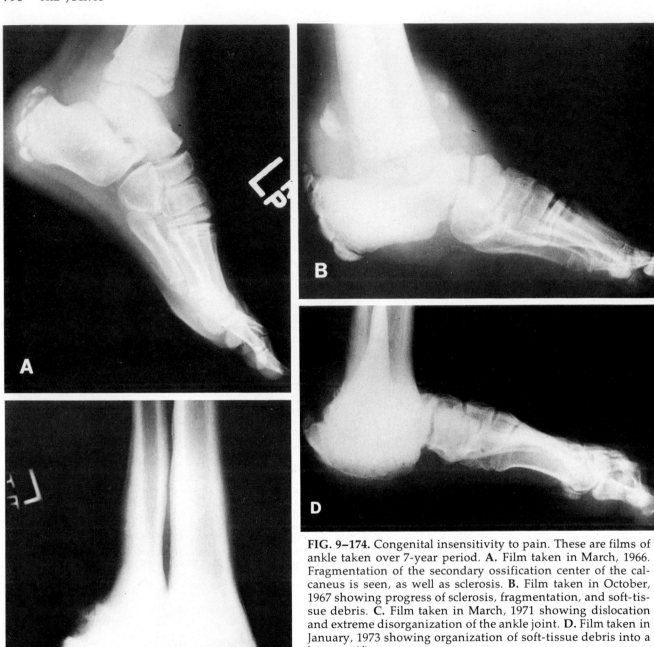

FIG. 9–174. Congenital insensitivity to pain. These are films of ankle taken over 7-year period. **A.** Film taken in March, 1966. Fragmentation of the secondary ossification center of the calcaneus is seen, as well as sclerosis. **B.** Film taken in October, 1967 showing progress of sclerosis, fragmentation, and soft-tissue debris. **C.** Film taken in March, 1971 showing dislocation and extreme disorganization of the ankle joint. **D.** Film taken in January, 1973 showing organization of soft-tissue debris into a large ossific mass.

FIG. 9–175. Meningomyelocele (tarsal bones). There has been disorganization of the left bases of the third and fourth metatarsals, with erosion of the fifth metatarsal. Similar changes to a lesser extent are noted on the right. A picture of osteoporosis is present, and there is no reactive sclerosis. Soft-tissue swelling is seen.

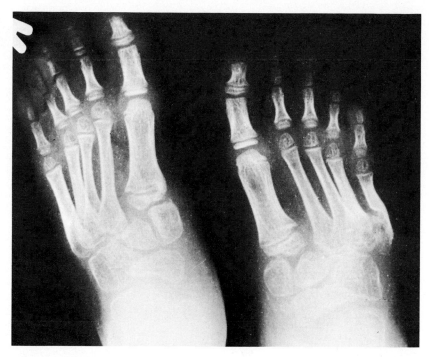

rare occasions be rapid. The joint space becomes narrowed. Marked bony sclerosis occurs (Fig. 9–176). Osteoporosis does not occur in this form, even with advanced changes. Fractures and fragmentation of the articular surfaces follow (Fig. 9–177). A large amount of bony soft-tissue debris forms, and later fuses together into a large, dense, well-organized bony mass with an integral cortex. This mass may fuse with the bone. The bone fragments may break out of the periarticular space and dissect along muscle planes.[65] Some may be resorbed.[93] Periosteal new bone formation may occur. Subluxation and dislocation proceed to destruction, malalignment of articular surfaces, and finally to total disorganization of the joint, appearing as if it were pounded by a sledgehammer (Fig. 9–178). Lisfranc's fracture-dislocation at the tarsometatarsal joints has also been described, particularly in patients with diabetes.[72] In children neuropathic injuries to the lower extremities may be seen as long bone fractures, epiphyseal separation, Charcot joints, and soft-tissue ulceration.[227]

In the spine, narrowing of the involved intervertebral disk spaces with very marked osteophyte formation is seen (Fig. 9–179). This can occur at multiple levels with "skip" areas in between. Sclerosis and fragmentation of the involved vertebral bodies occurs (Fig. 6–142). Paraspinal soft-tissue masses containing ossific debris are present. The lumbar and dorsal segments are most frequently affected.

CHONDROCALCINOSIS

Chondrocalcinosis[97] refers to the presence of calcification in articular hyaline cartilage or fibrocartilage. The calcium may be in the form of calcium pyrophosphate, calcium hydroxyapatite, or calcium orthophosphate. Chondrocalcinosis may be associated with several different conditions, summarized below.

CONDITIONS ASSOCIATED WITH CHONDROCALCINOSIS

1. Pseudogout
2. Hyperparathyroidism[50]
3. Degenerative arthritis
4. Ochronosis
5. Gout
6. Hemochromatosis
7. Wilson's disease
8. Acromegaly
9. Hypophosphatasia

One or several joints may be involved.

(Text continued on p. 795)

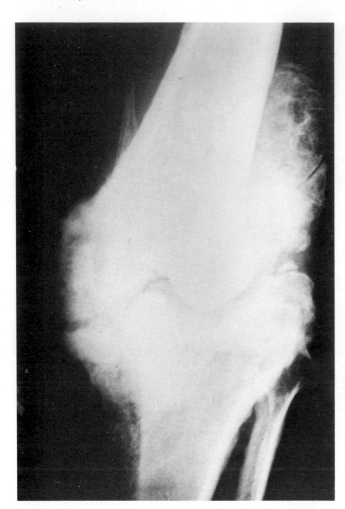

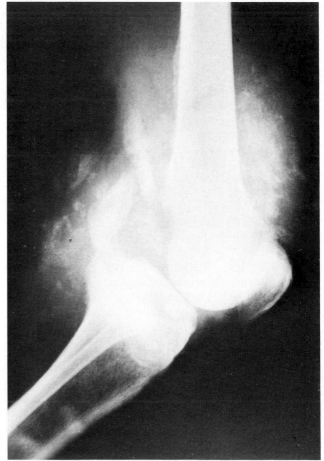

FIG. 9–176. Hypertrophic Charcot's joint (knee). Extremely dense sclerosis is seen, as well as dislocation, disorganization, and soft-tissue debris which has organized into an ossific mass.

FIG. 9–177. Charcot's joint (knee). Fractures and fragmentation of the articular surface are seen, as well as fine, disorganized soft-tissue debris. Considerable soft-tissue swelling is also noted.

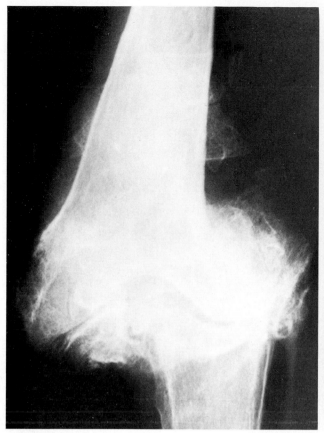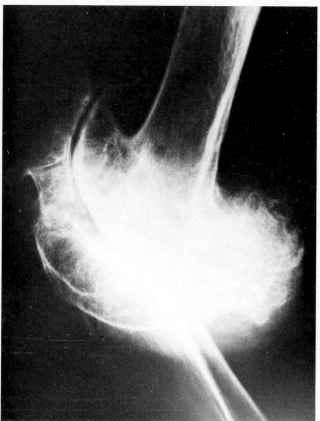

FIG. 9–178. Charcot's joint (knee)—anteroposterior and lateral views. There has been total disorganization of the knee joint.

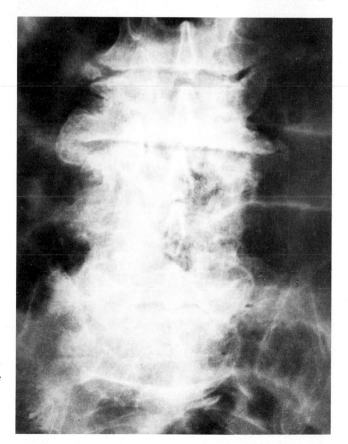

FIG. 9–179. Charot's spine. Marked narrowing of the intervertebral disk spaces and very exaggerated osteophyte formation associated with severe bone sclerosis are seen.

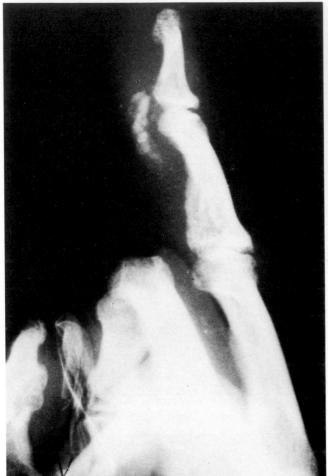

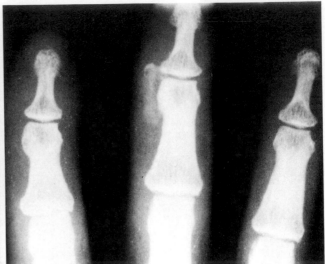

FIG. 9–180. Pseudogout syndrome. Periarticular soft-tissue calcification at the distal interphalangeal joint is seen.

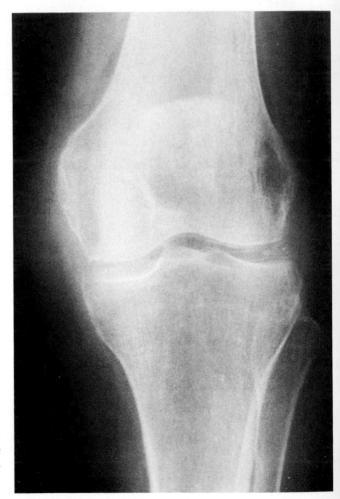

FIG. 9–181. Pseudogout syndrome (knee). Hyaline articular cartilage calcification and calcification of the fibrocartilage of the menisci are seen. The hyaline cartilage calcification is seen as a fine line that parallels the articular surface. The meniscal calcification is seen as a punctate linear pattern.

PSEUDOGOUT SYNDROME (CALCIUM PYROPHOSPHATE DIHYDRATE DEPOSITION DISEASE (CPPC))

Pseudogout[97,205] is a crystal-induced acute or chronic combination of synovitis and arthritis. The characteristic crystal in the synovial fluid is calcium pyrophosphate dihydrate, which can best be identified under polarized light microscopy. The crystals show weak positive birefringence. Chronic effusions have both extra- and intracellular crystals. The crystals are rhombic or rod-shaped.

Clinically, severe attacks of acute joint pain and inflammation may occur, with an average duration of about 2 weeks. The knee is most frequently involved. Mild attacks and chronic low-grade inflammation may also be present. Several associated diseases have been described, most frequently diabetes mellitus, hypertension, atherosclerosis, azotemia, and hyperuricemia. The mean age of onset of symptoms is 57 years.

This syndrome represents a metabolic disturbance consisting of excessive production or impaired degradation of pyrophosphate. A low concentration of pyrophosphate is normally present in plasma. Pyrophosphatase rapidly transforms pyrophosphate to orthophosphate. Inhibition of the activity of this enzyme, as, for example, in hemochromatosis, leads to crystal deposition.

Radiologically, the disease is characterized by the presence of calcification in intra-articular fibrocartilage, hyaline cartilage, articular capsule, and para-articular soft tissues (Fig. 9–180).

Fibrocartilage shows a characteristic punctate and linear pattern of calcification. Hyaline articular cartilage appears as a delicate radiopaque line paralleling the articular cortex. The knees (Fig. 9–181), wrists (Fig. 9–182), hips (Fig. 9–183), symphysis pubis (Fig. 9–184), and intervertebral disk (Fig. 9–185) are most commonly involved, and any joint may be affected.

A distinctive type of osteoarthritis has been described as being associated with this condition, showing a predilection for the metacarpophalangeal joints, as well as those of the elbows, wrists, ankles, and knees.[13, 147] It may also be seen in the radiocarpal compartment of the wrist and the patellofemoral compartment of the knee.

Flattening of the metacarpal heads, with sclerosis and "cyst" formation, as well as narrowing of the joint space, may be seen. Marginal spur formation also may occur. Subchondral cysts, particularly in the knee, may attain large size. An identical picture in the metacarpophalangeal joints may be present in hemochromatosis. The process may progress to extensive collapse and fragmentation of subchondral bone resulting in joint disintegration, with multiple intra-articular loose bodies. This is seen most often in the knees, hips, talocalcaneal joints, glenohumeral joints, and cervical spine. Cervical spine involvement may be severe with intervertebral disk calcification, and vertebral body and intervertebral space destruction. Atlantoaxial subluxation, anterior osseous fragmentation, and apophyseal joint changes may also occur.

Pseudogout, with typical symptoms and crystals in the joint, may occur without radiologically demonstrable calcifications, and joint calcifications may be asymptomatic.

Intervertebral disk calcification is seen in the annulus fibrosis. Calcification may also be present in tendons and bursae, and in the pinna of the ear. Calcification of capsule, synovium tendons, intra-articular ligaments, and soft tissues occurs. The most frequent areas to show calcifications are the knee, symphysis pubis, and wrist.

HYDROXYAPATITE DEPOSITION DISEASE

Hydroxyapatite deposition disease (HADD) is another crystal-induced arthropathy, along with gout and pseudogout. It is a common cause of periarticular disease, such as in the rotator cuff tendon or the trochanteric bursa. Hydroxyapatite crystals may also be deposited intra-articularly. This may be either primary or secondary. The picture may range from monoarticular periarthritis to polyarticular disease, and may progress to joint erosions and joint destruction. There may be simultaneous HADD and CPPD in the same joint.

Radiologically, amorphous calcifications about or within joints or bursae may be seen, with a wide spectrum of appearance.

Conditions associated with secondary HADD include collagen vascular disease, renal failure, and osteoarthritis.

HEMOCHROMATOSIS[104,221,249,254]

Hemochromatosis is a chronic disease in which excess iron is deposited in parenchymal tissues. This leads to fibrosis and functional insufficiency of those organs that are severely involved. The disease may be inherited (idiopathic) or acquired.[233] Idiopathic disease may be due to a deficiency of hepatic xanthine oxidase.

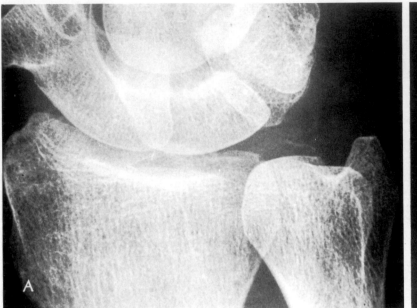

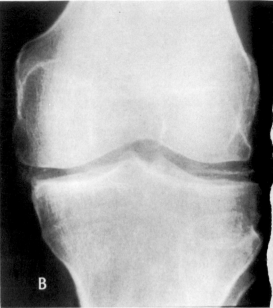

FIG. 9–182. Pseudogout syndrome. **A.** An exceptionally fine linear streak of calcification may be seen at the distal ulna. **B.** Knee—same patient. Calcific deposits in the articular cartilage and in the menisci are present.

FIG. 9–183. Pseudogout syndrome (hip). Note hyaline cartilage calcification paralleling articular cortex of the femoral head.

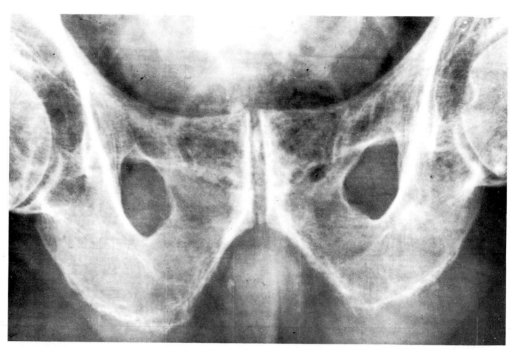

FIG. 9–184. Chondrocalcinosis. A vertical calcification in the symphysis pubis is seen.

Twenty to 50% of patients show bone and joint changes that are roentgenologically detectable.

Clinically, with respect to the arthropathy, the most frequent sites of involvement are the metacarpophalangeal joints and the interphalangeal joints. The wrists, elbows, shoulders, hips, and knees are less frequently involved. There is a history of chronic painful arthritis which varies in severity. Joint movement may be limited. Acute episodes of inflammatory synovitis may be superimposed on a chronic picture. These attacks may occur in joints with or without chondrocalcinosis. The serum alkaline phosphatase may be elevated, but this finding is thought to be due to hepatic damage. The serum calcium and phosphorus values are normal. The peak age incidence is 55 to 65 years, and males are more frequently affected than females.

Radiologically, the findings are osteoporosis, chondrocalcinosis, and a distinctive arthropathy.

The osteoporosis may have a component resulting from androgen deficiency, although generalized

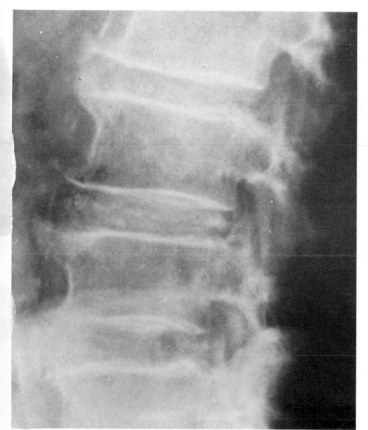

FIG. 9–185. Pseudogout syndrome. Calcification of the intervertebral discs is noted, as well as marginal hypertrophic lipping. (Courtesy of Dr. Dharmashi V. Bhate, VA Hospital, Hines, IL)

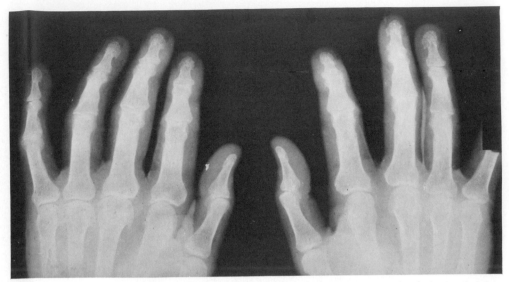

FIG. 9–186. Hemochromatosis (hand). Narrowing of the metacarpal phalangeal joint spaces most marked at the index and middle fingers, bilaterally, is noted with marginal spur formation. A peculiar flattening of the metacarpal heads is present.

FIG. 9–187. Hemochromatosis (hand). Marked degenerative arthritis is present at several distal and proximal interphalangeal joints. There is a peculiar enlargement of the heads of the metacarpals with cyst formation and subluxations at several metacarpal-phalangeal joints. (Courtesy of Dr. Dharmashi V. Bhate, VA Hospital, Hines, IL)

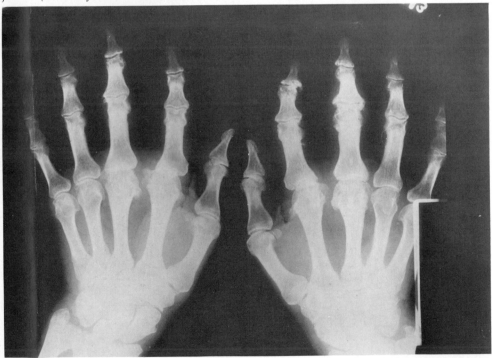

osteoporosis is slight. Disuse osteoporosis in involved areas is frequent. The pattern of periarticular osteoporosis, frequently seen in rheumatoid arthritis, is not usually present. Loss of density, thinning of the cortex, and sparse fine bony trabeculae may be seen.

Chondrocalcinosis, due to deposition of calcium pyrophosphate dihydrate in hyaline cartilage and fibrocartilage, is a frequent finding in this condition. Calcification in hyaline cartilage is said to be more marked in patients with hemochromatosis than in patients with idiopathic chondrocalcinosis. Fibrocartilage calcification in the menisci of the knees, the triangular ligaments of the wrists, and the pubic symphysis is seen. Hyaline cartilage calcification in the shoulder, elbow, hip, knee, and ankle may also be present. Pseudosyndesmophyte formation and calcification in the longitudinal ligaments of the lumbar spine[32] and in the soft tissues about the heel, has been reported. The calcification in articular cartilage is seen as a thin radiopacity paralleling the articular surface. Synovial iron deposition about the knee has also been described.

Arthritic changes are most frequently seen in the second and third metacarpophalangeal joints. The other metacarpophalangeal joints are less frequently involved.

The main features are joint space narrowing, subarticular cysts and erosions, osteophytosis, irregularity and sclerosis of the articular surface subluxations, and a peculiar flattening and widening of the metacarpal heads (Figs. 9–186, 9–187).

The initial lesion is probably the subarticular cyst, 1 to 3 mm in diameter, appearing in a metacarpal head. These cysts are bounded by a sclerotic rim. Small marginal osteophytes may develop with or without joint space narrowing. The width of the joint space may be reduced, not necessarily in a uniform manner, and subluxation may result. Widening of a metacarpophalangeal joint space may rarely occur. Cysts may also be present in the carpal bones, in the head of the ulna, and in the ulnar styloid. Erosion may occur at the last site. Cysts in the shafts of the phalanges and metacarpals may also be seen. Changes in the hips and shoulders (Fig. 9–188), in addition to chondrocalcinosis, may rarely suggest ischemic necrosis of bone.

A possible mechanism that has been suggested is that the synovial deposition of iron inhibits pyrophosphatase activity, and allows the deposition of calcium pyrophosphate in cartilage.

In the differential diagnosis, idiopathic pseudogout and rheumatoid arthritis are the entities that warrant the most serious consideration.

Radiologically, pseudogout would be most difficult to differentiate from hemochromatosis, since an identical metacarpophalangeal arthritis may be seen in this condition, as well as cartilage calcification. Clinical differentiation would have to be made.

Rheumatoid arthritis may be clinically excluded by serologic studies. In addition, the characteristic periarticular osteoporosis, marginal erosions, ulnar deviation and soft-tissue swelling are not present in hemochromatotic osteoarthropathy.

FIG. 9–188. Hemochromatosis (shoulder). Narrowing of the glenohumeral joint, bony sclerosis, and a large inferior spur at the humeral head is noted. (Courtesy of Dr. Dharmashi V. Bhate, VA Hospital, Hines, IL)

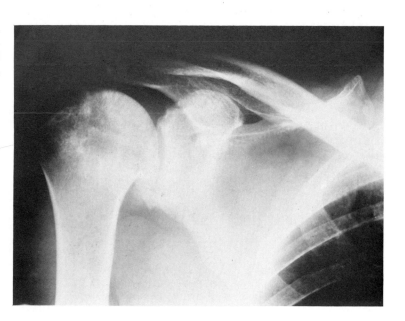

Ochronosis is an inborn error of metabolism in which pigmentation of connective tissue occurs in patients with alkaptonuria. Only some alkaptonurics develop ochronotic arthropathy. Alkaptonuria is asymptomatic unless pigment is deposited in cartilage and other connective tissues. Pigmentation and spondylosis develop in the majority of patients past 30 years of age.

The disease is caused by complete deficiency of the enzyme homogentisic acid oxidase, which converts homogentisic acid to maleylacetoacetic acid, in the metabolic pathways of phenylalanine and tyrosine. In some patients with this defect, an "ochre" or dark yellow pigment is deposited in cartilage and other connective tissue, causing pigmentation, degeneration, and calcification. The pigment is believed to be a polymer derived from homogentisic acid. The urine turns dark on standing, or when alkalinized, owing to oxidation of homogentistic acid.

This is a rare disease. The peak incidence of ochronotic arthropathy is in the fifth decade. The sex ratio is 2:1 males to females.

Ochronotic spondylosis is more common that peripheral arthropathy.

Radiologically, in the spine the lumbar region is said to be initially affected, followed by the dorsal and cervical areas. Narrowing of the intervertebral spaces occurs, associated with calcification due to deposition of hydroxyapatite. Dense laminated calcification is seen in the disk, with relative sparing of the centralmost portions (Fig. 9–189). Marginal osteophytes, as well as osteoporosis of vertebral bodies, develops (Fig. 9–190). Calcification of the interspinous ligament has also been described. The vacuum phenomenon in the intervertebral disks at multiple sites is not an uncommon occurrence. Kyphosis and scoliosis may occur. The apophyseal joints are not involved, and a "bamboo" spine is not seen.

In the peripheral joints, a degenerative type of arthritis occurs, although this is less frequently seen than spondylosis. The most commonly involved joints are those of the shoulders (Fig. 9–191), hips, and knees. Synovial effusion precedes a picture of

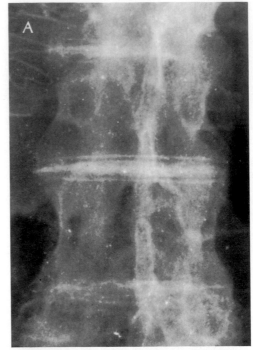

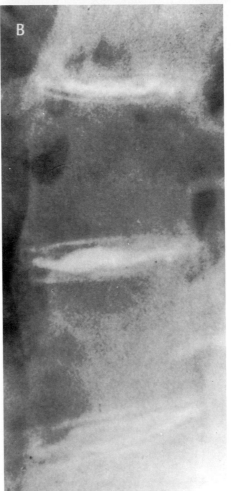

FIG. 9–189. Ochronosis (lumbar spine). **A.** Narrowing of the intervertebral spaces and dense intervertebral calcifications. **B.** Lateral view, showing generalized intervertebral calcifications with a laminated structure.

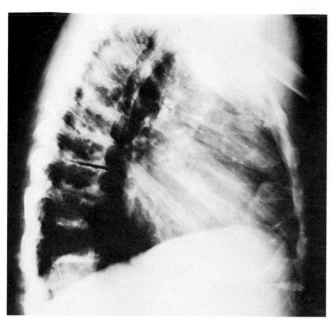

FIG. 9–190. Ochronosis (dorsal spine). Marked disk-space narrowing, calcification, and secondary osteophyte formation are noted.

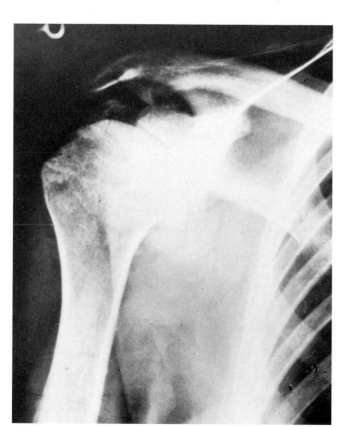

FIG. 9–191. Ochronosis (shoulder). Severe degenerative arthritis with joint space narrowing, marginal sclerosis, and marked spur formation at the inferior aspect of both humeral head and glenoid is noted. This is the same patient as in previous figure.

osteoarthritis. In the knee, calcification of the menisci may be present. Joint space narrowing, marginal osteophytes, and subchondral sclerosis are seen. Calcified loose bodies may also occur, as well as ligamentous ossifications. Rupture of the Achilles tendon has been reported. There may be flattening of the femoral and humeral heads.

The small joints of the hands and feet are not involved.

INFECTIOUS ARTHRITIS

BACTERIAL ARTHRITIS[113]

Bacterial arthritis results from invasion of the synovial membrane and joint cavity by any of a large variety of microorganisms. The more common organisms that cause acute pyogenic arthritis are listed below.

MICROORGANISMS CAUSING ACUTE PYOGENIC ARTHRITIS[97]

More Common:

Staphylococcus aureus
Streptococcus pyogenes*
Diplococcus pneumoniae
Neisseria gonorrhoeae

Less Common:

Hemophilus influenzae* [253]
Pseudomonas aeruginosa
Klebsiella aerobacter
Coliform organisms
Salmonellae
Brucella
Proteus[90]
Pseudomonas pseudomalii
Clostridium welchii[113]
Clostridium bifermentans[171]
Serratia marcescens[219]
Corynebacterium pyogenes[173]

* More common in children

FIG. 9–192. Septic arthritis (hand). Patient on steroid therapy. Periarticular osteoporosis is present, as well as soft-tissue swelling at the proximal interphalangeal joint of the middle and little fingers. Periosteal new bone formation along the proximal shaft of the proximal phalanx of the middle finger is also seen.

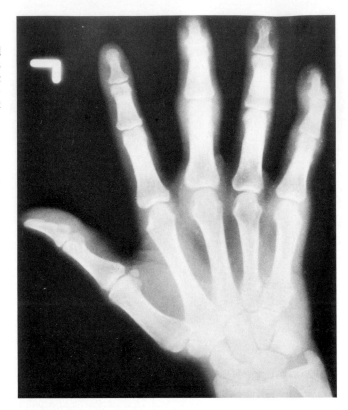

FIG. 9–193. Patient who lacerated his knuckle while striking a blow to the mouth of an adversary. **A.** Initial film showing soft-tissue air about the metacarpophalangeal joint. The bony structure appears intact. **B.** Oblique view taken after short interval showing cortical destruction of the metacarpal head, as well as joint space narrowing.

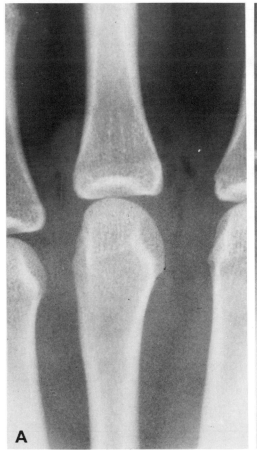

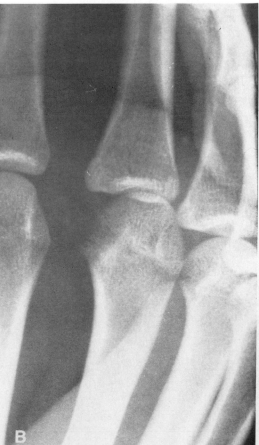

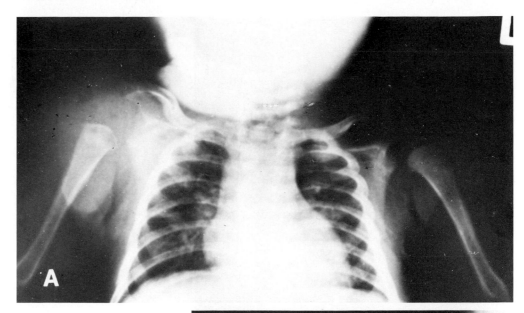

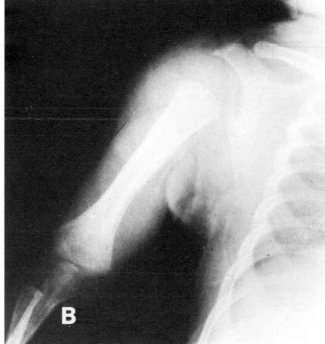

The organisms may gain entry by the hematogenous route, by extension from osteomyelitis, needling or trauma, or secondary to joint surgery. An increased incidence of septic arthritis occurs in patients with rheumatoid arthritis and with hypogammaglobulinemia, and in the elderly, the chronically ill, cancer patients, those on immunosuppressive drugs, those with sickle-cell anemia, and those with neurotrophic arthritis. Ten to 20% of staphylococcal and 75% to 85% of gonococcal infections involve two or more joints.

There has been a sharp rise in incidence of osteomyelitis in recent years, particularly spondylitis, as a complication of intravenous drug abuse.[115] Pseudomonas and Klebsiella are common causative organisms. Young adults are most frequently involved. The intervertebral spaces of the spine are most frequently affected, as well as the sacroiliac joints, symphysis pubis, sternoclavicular joints, radial styloid, and knee.

Clinically, in pyogenic arthritis, severe acute inflammation with pain, tenderness, swelling, and redness, as well as constitutional symptoms with high fever, usually occur. Some cases, however, may present with minimal inflammatory signs.

Radiologically, the basic changes in pyogenic arthritis are soft-tissue swelling (Figs. 9–192, 9–193 *A, B*, 9–194), followed by rapid destruction of cartilage and bone (Fig. 9–195). Sequestration and periosteal new bone formation follow if osteomyelitis is present. Destructive changes precede osteoporosis, the opposite of what happens in tuberculous arthritis. Osteoporosis develops rapidly when joint destruction is present. The bony changes usually be-

FIG. 9–194. Septic arthritis (shoulder)—male infant, age 2 months. **A.** Initial film showing marked soft-tissue swelling, air in the soft tissues, and a destructive metaphyseal focus. **B.** One-month interval film. There has been reduction in the amount of soft-tissue swelling. A sclerotic margin around the destructive focus is noted, and periosteal new bone formation along the humeral shaft is seen.

803

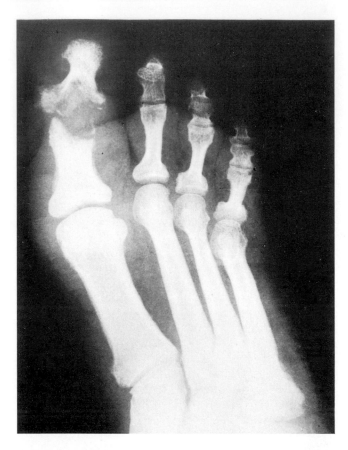

FIG. 9–195. Septic arthritis (foot). Diabetic patient with previous amputation of little toe and metatarsal. There is marked destruction at the interphalangeal joint of the great toe. Periosteal new bone formation along the shaft of the proximal phalanx and along the first metatarsal shaft is also seen. The destructive change has preceded osteoporosis.

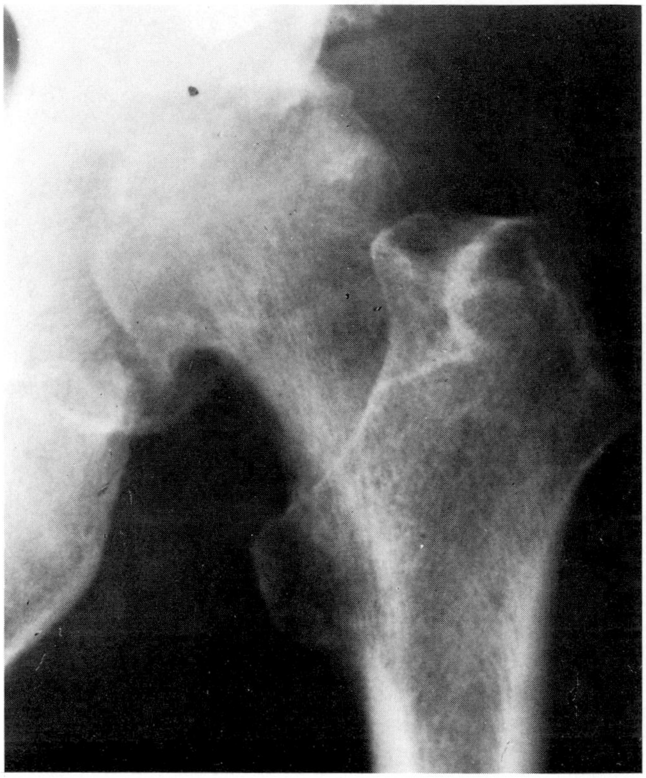

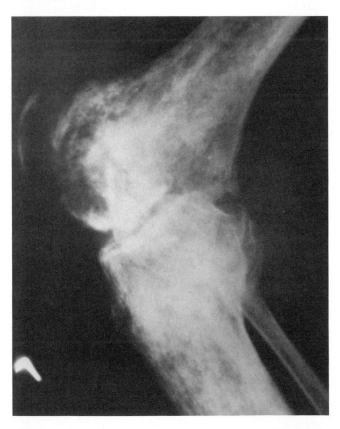

FIG. 9–196. Septic arthritis (hip)—male, age 63 years. Marked subchondral destruction of both femoral head and acetabulum has occurred. Considerable osteoporosis is present. Lateral displacement of the femoral head may also be seen.

FIG. 9–197. Hemoglobin SC disease with salmonella arthritis and osteomyelitis (knee). Joint space narrowing has occurred and considerable subchondral destruction is present.

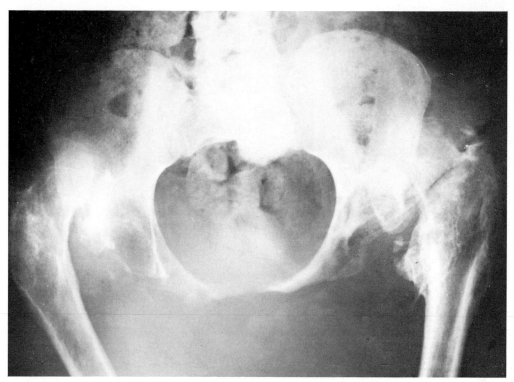

FIG. 9–198. Paraplegia with decubitus ulcer and septic arthritis of both hips, with extensive destruction and dislocations bilaterally.

come evident 8 to 10 days following the onset of symptoms.

Cartilage destruction at areas of contact with opposing articular surfaces results in early joint narrowing and subchondral destruction of bone, causing loss of the entire cortical outline (Figs. 9–196, 9–197, 9–198). This is in contrast to tuberculous arthritis, where marginal bone destruction is initially seen. Reactive sclerosis follows. Healing may result in an irregular articular surface or bony ankylosis (Fig. 9–199).

Large joints, such as those of the knee and the hip, are more often affected than the small joints. In infants, pathological dislocations of the hip and shoulder are common due to extreme distention of the capsule (Fig. 9–200). The apparent dislocation of a hip in an infant prior to ossification of the epiphyseal center may actually be due to a pathological epiphyseal separation caused by osteomyelitis. An arthrogram would demonstrate the condition.[75, 112]

In the shoulder, initial plain films may be normal in septic arthritis. Subsequent examinations may show osteoporosis and joint space narrowing, sub-luxations of the humeral head, and erosions. Rotator cuff tears not uncommonly occur[8] and can be demonstrated by arthrography. In the knee, the patella becomes displaced away from the femur, concurrent with distention of the suprapatellar bursa.

In the spine,[84] the intervertebral spaces are involved early in inflammatory processes, in contrast to vertebral body involvement in metastatic disease.

Initially, prevertebral edema is followed by joint space narrowing. Destruction of the vertebral endplates follows. Collapse of the bodies may occur (Fig. 9–201). Healing changes are evidenced by sclerosis, osteophyte formation, and bony fusion.

Severe and prolonged pyogenic arthritis may result in the presence of dystrophic periarticular calcifications.[234]

Sympathetic joint effusion refers to transudative fluid in a joint adjacent to a site of inflammation. It usually presents as an acute arthritis. It has been described in septic arthritis, but is more commonly seen in other conditions summarized on page 808.[16]

(Text continued on p. 808)

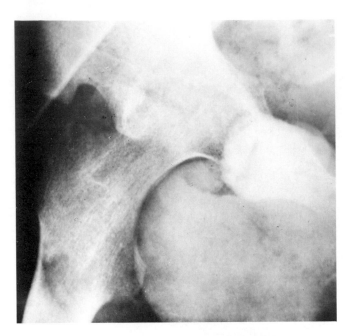

FIG. 9–199. Septic arthritic (hip) resulting from decubitus ulcer in a paraplegic. Healing changes with total joint space narrowing and partial bony ankylosis are observed.

FIG. 9–200. Septic arthritic (left shoulder) — female infant, age 10 months. A. Initial film showing soft-tissue swelling and metaphyseal destruction. B. One-month interval film showing dislocation of the left shoulder.

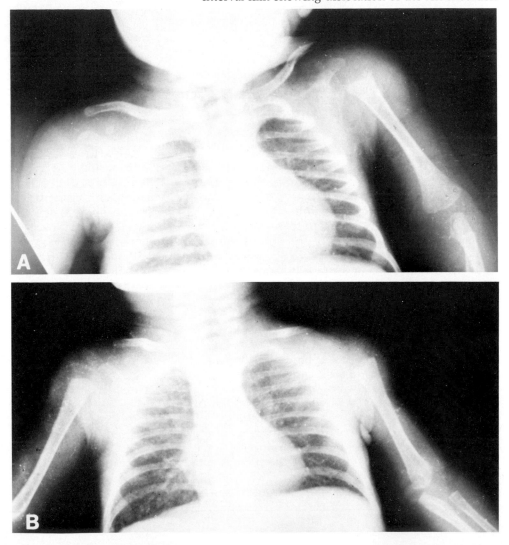

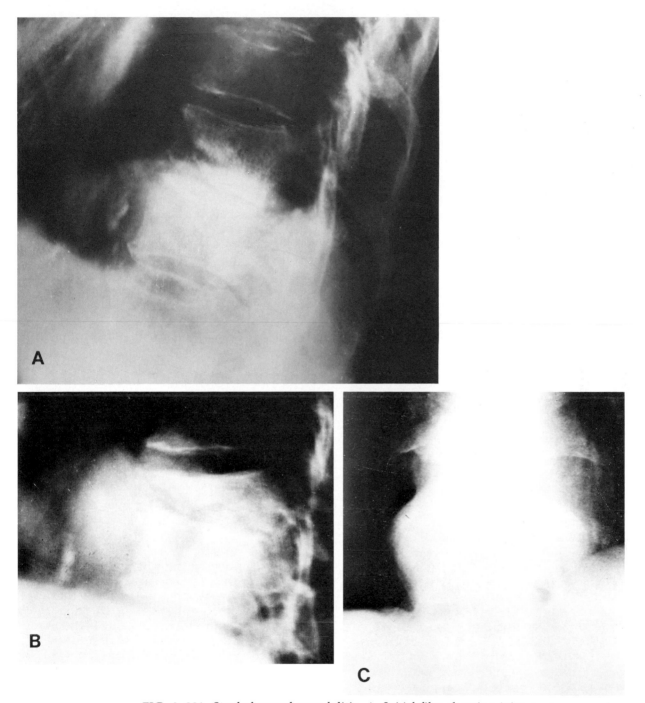

FIG. 9–201. Staphylococcal spondylitis. **A.** Initial film showing joint space narrowing and destructive focus at the anterior aspect of the vertebral body. **B.** Seven-month interval film. There has been collapse of the involved vertebral body with destruction of the vertebral plate. **C.** Anteroposterior view showing marked paravertebral soft-tissue masses.

Sarcoidosis
Erythema nodosum
Calcific periarthritis
Gout
SLE
Pulmonary hypertrophic osteoarthropathy
Dialysis arthritis
Septic arthritis

An occult carcinoma of the colon has been reported as presenting with pyogenic arthritis.[136]

TUBERCULOUS ARTHRITIS[20,64,78]

Tuberculous arthritis and spondylitis occur in only 1% of patients with tuberculosis. Of those with skeletal involvement, 50% have spinal disease, 30% have hip or knee disease, and 20% have inflammation of other joints. The initial symptoms are mild, and progress of the process is very slow. It is most often monarticular.

The disease may affect the joint by hematogenous spread, or from direct extension from a focus in bone. About 50% of patients with skeletal tuberculosis do not show active pulmonary disease.

In the peripheral joints, a caseating granulomatous synovitis occurs. Proteolytic enzymes are lacking, resulting in relatively late cartilaginous destruction.

Mycobacterium tuberculosis of the human type is the causative agent in the majority of cases. The bovine strain and atypical mycobacteria may affect some patients.

Radiologically, a characteristic triad of osteoporosis, joint space narrowing, and marginal erosions has long been considered to be the hallmark of this disease (Fig. 9–202). The osteoporosis is severe (Fig. 9–203), and may be present distal to the involved joint in an extremity. This stage causes a hazy appearance of the joint structures. The osteoporosis develops slowly, and occurs prior to destructive changes. This is in contrast to what is seen in pyogenic arthritis. In children, localized hyperemia may result in premature appearance and enlargement of the epiphyseal ossification centers (Fig. 9–204). The appearance is somewhat similar to that of juvenile rheumatoid arthritis or hemophilia.

Articular cartilage in contact with its opposing member is involved relatively late in direct primary synovial tuberculosis. The articular cartilage is first destroyed at its periphery, where there is little or no contact or pressure (Fig. 9–205). In the knee, the

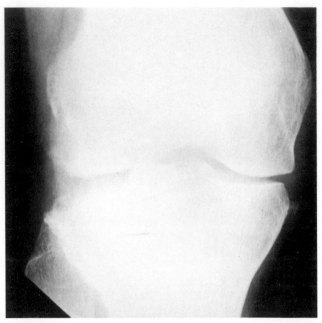

FIG. 9–202. Tuberculosis of the knee with characteristic triad of osteoporosis, joint space narrowing, and marginal erosions.

noncontact central areas are also eroded early (Fig. 9–206). Joint space narrowing thus occurs late in tuberculous arthritis, in contrast to the early narrowing in purulent arthritis.

In joints such as that of the shoulder, the initial destruction is typically widespread because of a small surface contact area of articular cartilage. The appearance in the humeral head, called *caries sicca*, is of multiple large erosive and destructive lesions (Fig. 9–207).

Late in the disease, the articular cartilage is destroyed and joint space narrowing occurs. The subchondral bone then becomes involved. Destructive foci tend to lie directly opposite each other. Cortical irregularity and sequestrations occur, along with some sclerosis. Sequestra in opposing bones in contact, called "kissing sequestra," may be seen (Fig. 9–208). In the sacroiliac joints, marked destruction with widening of the joint may occur (Fig. 9–209). Little or no periosteal or bone reaction occurs.

Healing occurs with increase in bone density, and may be accompanied by extensive soft-tissue calcification. There may be fibrous ankylosis, in which case the articular cortex appears irregular, or total bony ankylosis may ensue.

Spinal involvement is discussed under *tuberculous osteomyelitis* (see Chap. 6).

Secondary pyogenic infection may complicate the picture.

(Text continued on p. 812)

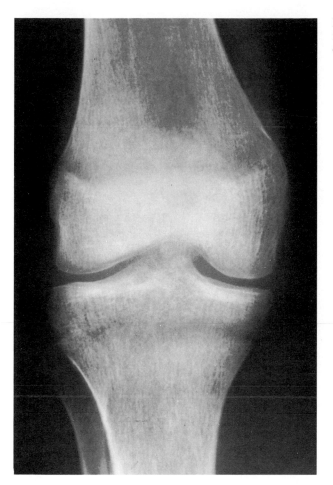

FIG. 9–203. Tuberculosis (knee). Marked local osteoporosis is present with a metaphyseal radiolucent band and subchondral osteoporosis.

FIG. 9–204. Tuberculosis of the left knee in a child. Severe osteoporosis is noted, as well as irregularity of the epiphyseal ossification centers. Destruction of the articular cortex of bone at the lateral aspect of the knee joint is also seen.

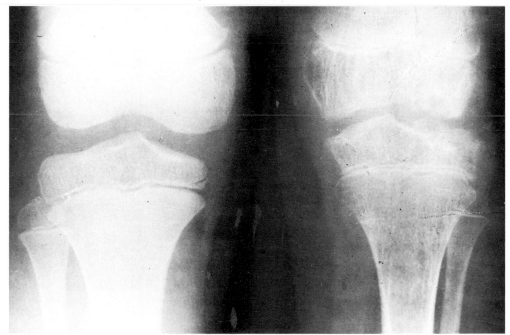

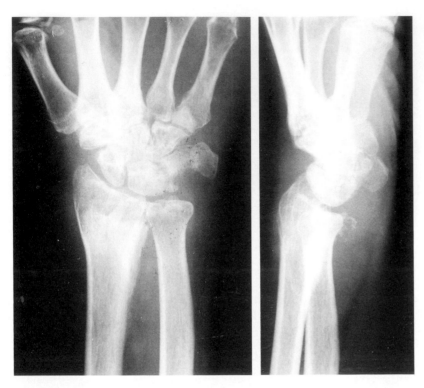

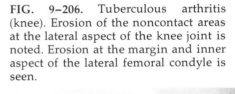

FIG. 9–205. Tuberculous arthritis (wrist). Osteoporosis, erosions, and destruction are seen. Extensive destruction at the noncontact area of the triangular bone is noted.

FIG. 9–206. Tuberculous arthritis (knee). Erosion of the noncontact areas at the lateral aspect of the knee joint is noted. Erosion at the margin and inner aspect of the lateral femoral condyle is seen.

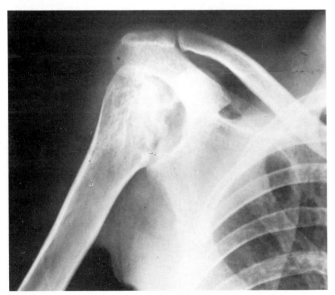

FIG. 9–207. Tuberculous arthritis of the soulder in its typical form. Marked destruction of the humeral head is noted. This is the picture of "caries sicca."

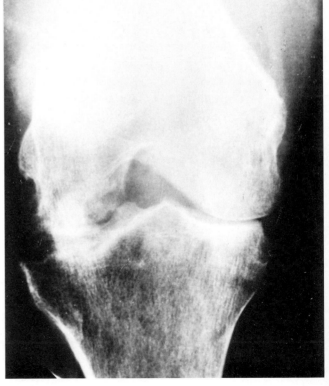

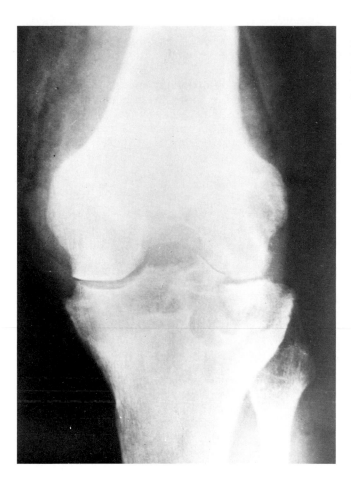

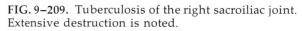

FIG. 9–208. Advanced tuberculosis of the knee. Involvement chiefly of the lateral aspect of the joint space is seen, with extensive cortical destruction, and destruction of the noncontact areas in the midportion of the knee joint as well. Two opposing small dense areas laterally, the so-called "kissing sequestra," are noted.

FIG. 9–209. Tuberculosis of the right sacroiliac joint. Extensive destruction is noted.

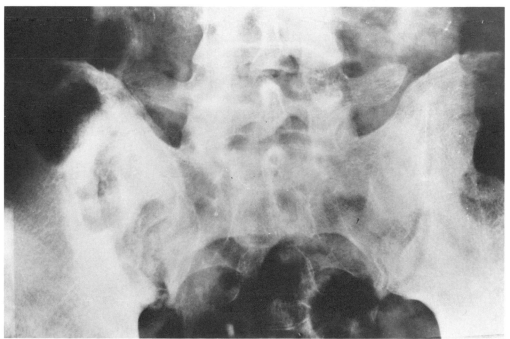

FUNGAL ARTHRITIS

Fungal arthritis may rarely be encountered, showing a varied radiological picture. Coccidioidomycosis, histoplasmosis, blastomycosis,[133] cryptococcosis, and sporotrichosis occur, in approximately that order of frequency. Coccidioidomycosis has been reported as presenting in the spine with a picture similar to Pott's disease.[258] Laboratory studies are necessary for diagnosis. Acute guinea-worm synovitis of the knee joint has been reported.[238] Yaws osteitis has been reported as resulting in concentric bone atrophy and *"doigt-en-lorgnette"* deformity.[110] Aspergillis terreus,[232] usually encountered as a complication of neoplastic disease, has been reported as involving the spine in an immunocompetent patient.

VIRAL SYNOVITIS AND ARTHRITIS

These result in acute transient polyarthritis with little tendency toward chronicity (Fig. 9–210). The most common cause is rubella. Polyarthritis involving the small joints of the hands is very frequent in some epidemics. The duration of the arthritis averages 9 days. Mumps, variola, and serum hepatitis are some of the other virus diseases associated with transient arthritis.

LYME ARTHRITIS[53]

Lyme arthritis is a syndrome characterized by a skin rash, severe systemic manifestations, and nondeforming oligoarthritis. The cause is unknown, but an infectious agent, possibly a virus, is thought to be transmitted by ticks. It has been reported in New England, New York, and Wisconsin. Migratory arthritis involving the knees, shoulders, and elbows occurs. This may be followed by recurrent episodes of oligoarthritis separated by periods of complete remission. No persistent synovitis or permanent joint deformities were seen.

TUMORS OF JOINTS

SYNOVIOMA

Synovioma or *synovial sacroma*[99] is a highly malignant fibroblastic neoplasm. The age incidence is between 18 and 35 years. It is usually located near a joint, with only 10% of lesions primarily within the joint capsule. The lower extremities are most often involved, especially the knees. It can also arise from a tendon sheath anywhere along a limb. The buttocks, back, neck, chest, hands, feet, abdominal wall, and orbits are other reported sites.

Radiologically, a soft-tissue mass is seen, which may be lobulated or quite large (Figs. 9–211, 8–48). There is a tendency toward calcification, which may be the only definitive finding. The regional bone may show osteoporosis or invasion (Fig. 9–212). Irregular destructive changes of bone or of the involved joint may be seen (Fig. 9–213).

OSTEOID OSTEOMA

Osteoid Osteoma may produce effects on an adjacent joint. An intracapsular osteoid osteoma, particularly in the hip, may produce osteoporosis and synovitis. Similar changes may rarely result in an osteoid osteoma more remote from a joint (see Chap. 7).

PIGMENTED VILLONODULAR SYNOVITIS AND VILLONODULAR TENOSYNOVITIS[47,107,117]

Pigmented villonodular synovitis and villonodular tenosynovitis are chronic, proliferative, inflammatory reactions occurring in the synovia of the joints, bursae, and tendons. They have previously been called giant-cell tumors and xanthomas. Young adults are most commonly affected, with a history of intermittent pain and swelling of a joint. *Radiologically*, joint swellings with lobular soft-tissue masses are seen. They may extend beyond the capsule, or rarely be entirely extracapsular. These do not calcify but may appear dense, owing to hemosiderin deposits. The disease is usually monarticular. *Endosteal villonodular synovitis* is a term defined by Aegerter[1] to indicate erosion or invasion of bone in this condition, which may affect subchondral or articular marginal areas (Figs. 9–214, 9–215). Cystlike defects of varying sizes may be present, with sharp and sclerotic margins. Some cases may progress to joint destruction. The usual absence of joint space narrowing and regional osteoporosis serves to differentiate this condition from rheumatoid arthritis or tuberculosis. Lack of calcification aids in differentiation from synovioma.

The lesions are usually monarticular; however, biarticular involvement has been reported.[45,58,69] Temporomandibular joint lesions have also been reported.[126]

(*Text continued on p. 815*)

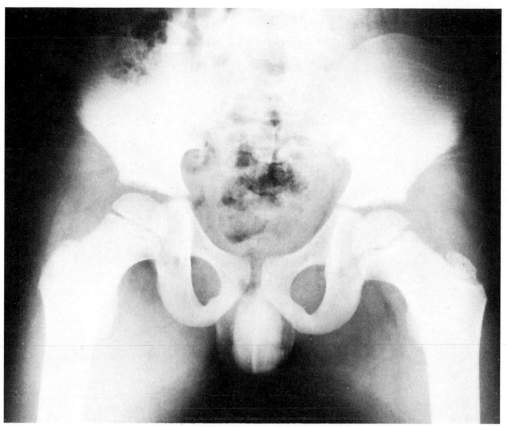

FIG. 9–210. Synovitis of the right hip in a child. Capsular distention is seen by displacement of the fat lines of the right hip. Soft-tissue swelling is also present.

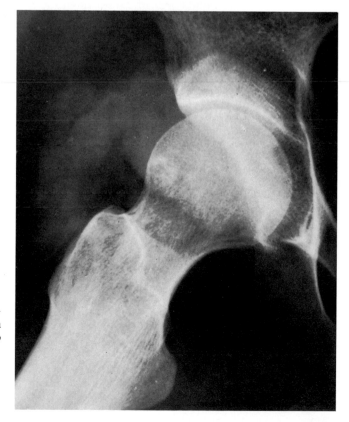

FIG. 9–211. Recurrent synovioma of the hip joint. Lobulated irregular soft-tissue masses may be seen. There is a minimal amount of calcification at the outer aspect, and no evidence of bone invasion.

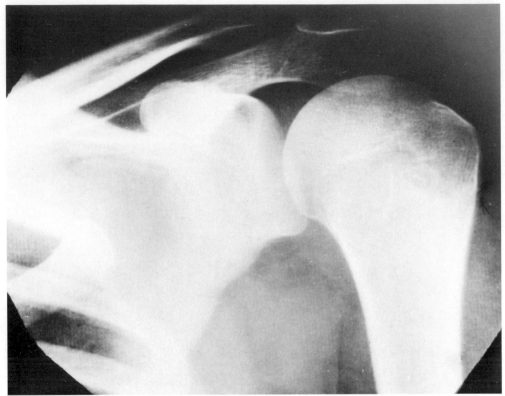

FIG. 9–212. Synovioma of the shoulder joint—female, age 19 years. Osteoporosis of the humerus and a destructive area in the region of the greater tuberosity are noted.

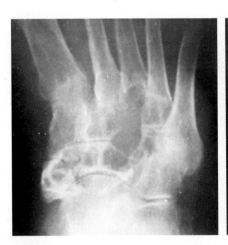 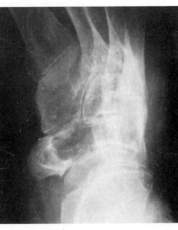

FIG. 9–213. Synovioma of the tarsus. Extensive tarsal destruction and destruction of the metatarsal bases are seen. (Courtesy of Dr. Antonio Pizarro, Hines VA Hospital, Hines, IL)

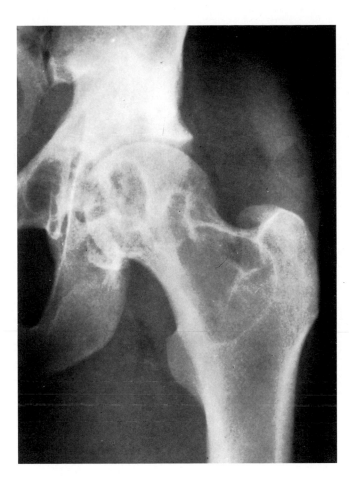

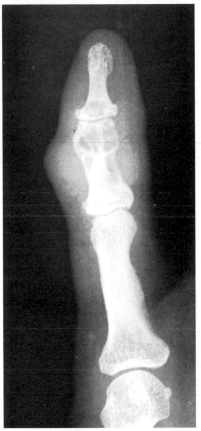

FIG. 9–214. Pigmented villonodular synovitis (hip)—endosteal type. Note multiple large and small erosions of the femoral head and neck in the acetabular region. The joint space is maintained. Bulging of the soft-tissue fascial planes at the superior aspect of the hip joint may be seen.

FIG. 9–215. Pigmented villonodular tenosynovitis (finger). Note soft-tissue swelling in the middle phalanx of the fifth finger, associated with multiple bone erosions.

SYNOVIAL OSTEOCHONDROMATOSIS OR CHONDROMATOSIS[155, 186]

Synovial osteochondromatosis or *chondromatosis* as defined by Jaffe[101] is the condition in which foci of cartilage develop in synovial membrane through metaplasia. Cartilage becomes detached, enters the joint cavity, and increases in amount as it is nourished by synovial fluid. The cartilage eventually becomes calcified and ossified. The disease is usually monarticular, occurring in young adults or the middle-aged. Males are more frequently affected than females.

Radiologically, the most frequent areas of involvement are the knee joints, the hip, elbow, and shoulder. Hip involvement has been reported as presenting with an intrapelvic mass.[57] Bursae may be involved, as well as periarticular tendons.[135] Involvement of the ankle,[98] knee,[55] and temporomandibular joint has also been reported.[3, 237]

The characteristic finding is multiple small calcified or ossified densities within the joint capsule

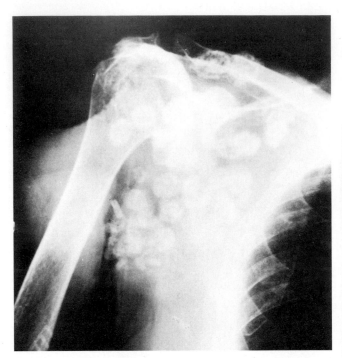

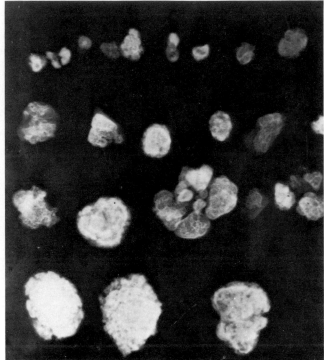

FIG. 9–216. Synovial osteochondromatosis (shoulder). Posttraumatic or degenerative type. Multiple calcific densities of varying sizes within a distended shoulder joint capsule are seen. The calcifications have a dense periphery.

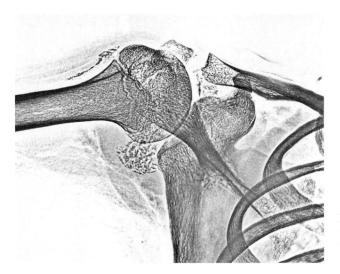

FIG. 9–217. Radiograph of specimen osteochondromas showing configuration and variation in size. Posttraumatic or degenerative type.

FIG. 9–218. Synovial osteochondromatosis (shoulder), idiopathic type (not biopsied)—xeroradiograph of asymptomatic female, age 13 years. Multiple small intracapsular calcifications are noted.

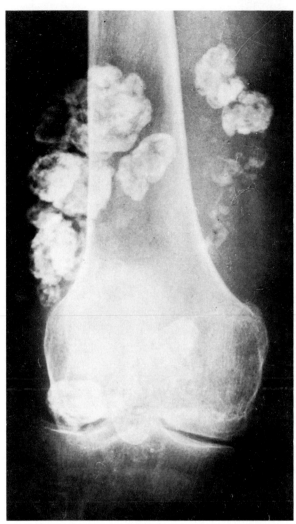

FIG. 9–219. Knee. Large-sized synovial osteochondromas associated with degenerative disease of the knee are seen.

(Figs. 9–216, 9–217, 9–218). Osteoporosis is usually absent. Joint space narrowing and osteophyte formation may be seen at times.

Multiple larger or fewer intra-articular calcifications and ossifications are more likely to result from trauma, neuropathic arthropathy, or osteochondrosis dissecans (Fig. 9–219). The lesions of osteochondromatosis tend to increase in size after incomplete synovectomy.

INTRACAPSULAR CHONDROMA[162]

Intracapsular chondroma or para-articular chondroma represents extrasynovial chondrometaplasia in the fibrous capsule or connective tissue of a joint. This is a rare condition, and is in contrast to the synovial origin of synovial chondromatosis. It usually affects the knee, where a solitary density is seen, typically inferior to the patella. It may attain a size as large as 5 cm.

SYNOVIAL CHONDROSARCOMA[54, 156]

Synovial chondrosarcoma is a very rare tumor that may arise *de novo* or develop in a joint that harbors synovial osteochondromatosis. A large mass with invasion of bone may be seen. If synovial chondromatosis is present, the calcifications may be displaced away from the joint.

SYNOVIAL HEMANGIOMA[63, 127]

Synovial hemangioma is a rare condition that most often involves the knee. Other joints have been reported as being affected, including the elbow and temporomandibular joint. Adolescents and young adults are most susceptible. The involved joint is enlarged, with some limitation of motion, and is somewhat painful. Joint aspiration may yield hemorrhagically discolored fluid. The adjacent soft tissues or bone may also show concomitant angiomas. Muscle atrophy may be present. There are two types, circumscribed and diffuse.

Radiologically, the picture is often normal. Nearby soft-tissue phleboliths may be seen, as well as a soft-tissue density in the region of the joint. Muscle atrophy and discrepancy in limb length, accelerated maturation of the epiphyses, and destructive regional bone changes may all be present. Osteoporosis, osteoarthritis, periosteal bone formation, and ankylosis have been described. Changes similar to those in hemophilia have also been described.

Arthrography may demonstrate a lobulated synovial mass, while arteriography may show a network of tortuous, irregular small vessels.

LIPOMA

Lipoma, or a true primary benign fatty neoplasm of the synovium, is a rare condition encountered almost exclusively in the knee joint. Partial ossification of a lipoma has been reported. Fatty tumors secondary to, or associated with, other conditions also may occur. *Lipoma arborescens*[30] is a polypoid, fatty, synovial proliferation most often associated with degenerative joint disease. Soft-tissue swelling is noted radiologically which need not be radiolucent. Arthrography may demonstrate a lobulated

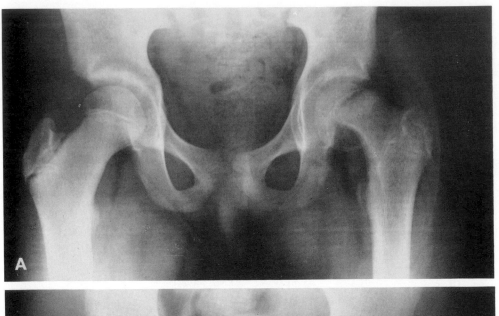

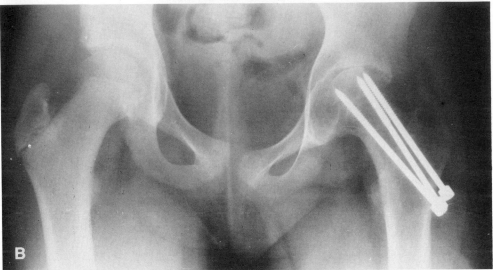

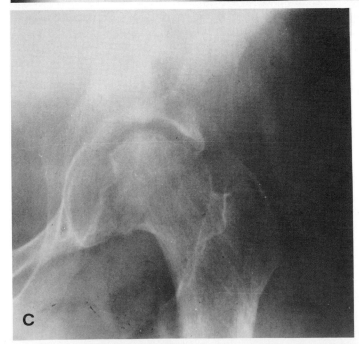

FIG. 9–220. Slipped capital femoral epiphysis that has developed acute chondrolysis. **A.** Anteroposterior view showing posterior and medial displacement of the femoral capital epiphyseal ossification center. The joint space is normal. **B.** Film taken after pinning; the patient complained of severe pain in the hip joint. Marked narrowing of the superior aspect of the joint space is noted. **C.** Film of the hip taken after removal of pins. The hip joint space has partially reconstituted. Irregularity of the femoral head and the acetabulum is noted.

radiolucent defect. *Hoffa's disease* represents a post-traumatic inflammatory hypertrophy of the sub-synovial fat present in the region of the patellar ligament.

Radiolucent masses have been reported as being seen on plain films in the elbow and subdeltoid bursa in chronic rheumatoid arthritis.[259] Pedunculated lesions of mature fat covered by synovium have been noted at surgery.

MISCELLANEOUS

Osteolysis with detritic synovitis is a new syndrome described by Resnick *et al*[201] and reported in a 71-year-old woman. Severe destructive mutilating arthropathy of the hands with distal phalangeal deformity and resorption, as well as resorption along the shafts of the metacarpals and phalanges, resorption of the distal clavicles, and involvement of the central skeleton and long bones is seen. Synovial ulceration and necrosis occurs.

Primary biliary cirrhosis is reported as showing distinctive changes in the hands.[176] Erosive arthritis with marginal erosions about the interphalangeal joints and to a lesser extent the metacarpophalangeal joints is seen. Loss of bone density is present. Intraosseous lytic defects are also described, as is chondrocalcinosis. Acroosteolysis and subperiosteal bone resorption may also be seen, the latter probably due to secondary hyperparathyroidism.

Acute chondrolysis may develop following treatment for slipped capital femoral epiphysis. Rapid and painful narrowing of the joint space occurs. The joint space may reconstitute (Fig. 9–220 *A-C*). The etiology is speculative. This condition has also been described following burns.[183]

DIFFERENTIAL DIAGNOSIS OF SEVERAL ROENTGEN FEATURES RELATED TO THE ARTHRITIDES

1. *Osteoporosis of the wrist* (Fig. 9–221)
   Rheumatoid arthritis
   Tuberculous arthritis
   Regional migratory osteoporosis
   Sudeck's atrophy
   Burns
2. *Arthritis with relative lack of osteoporosis*
   Gout
   Neurotrophic arthritis
   Early septic arthritis

(*Text continued on p. 822*)

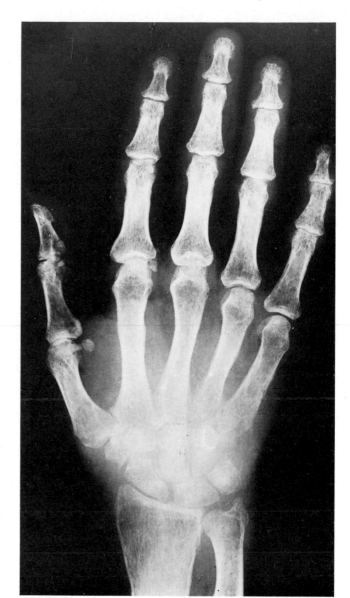

FIG. 9–221. Osteoporosis of the wrist.

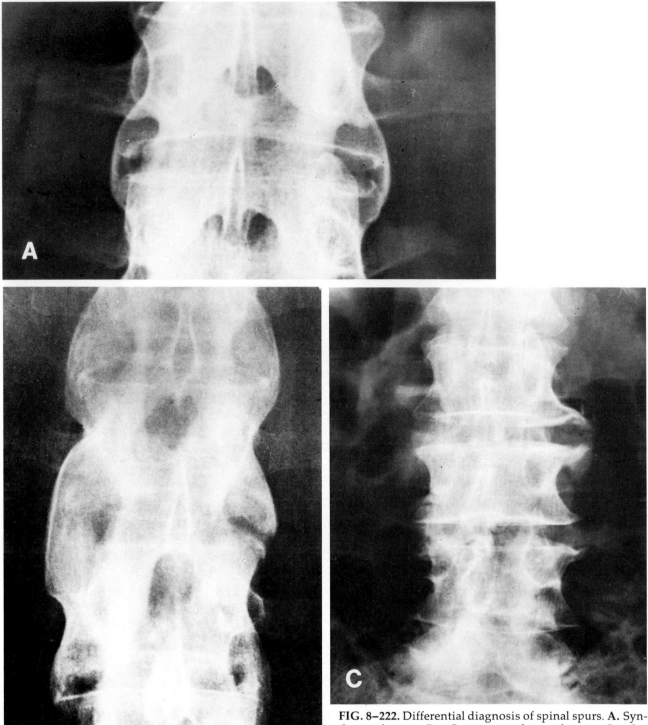

FIG. 8–222. Differential diagnosis of spinal spurs. **A.** Syndesmophytes. **B.** Coarse syndesmophytes. **C.** Osteophytes. **D.** Traction spur. **E.** Forestier's disease. **F.** Charcot's spine.

(Continued)

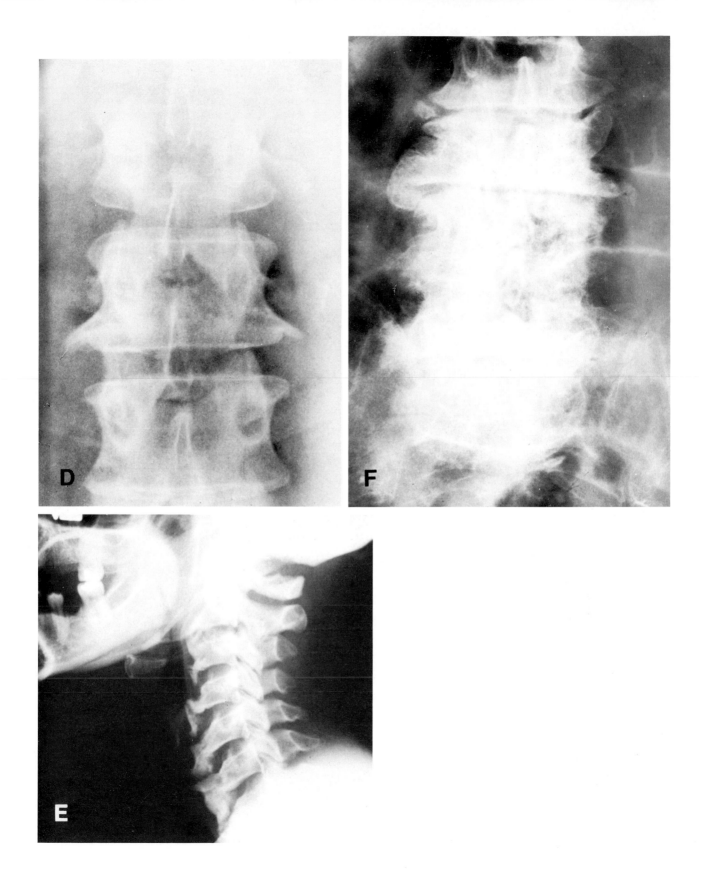

Pigmented villonodular synovitis
Psoriatic arthritis
Reiter's syndrome
Sarcoidosis
3. *"Boutonnière" and "swan-neck" deformities*
Rheumatoid arthritis
Juvenile rheumatoid arthritis
Systemic lupus erythematosus
Psoriatic arthritis
Jaccoud's arthritis
Camptodactyly
4. *Easily correctable ulnar deviation*
Systemic lupus erythematosus
Jaccoud's arthritis
5. *Thicker periosteal new bone formation*
Reiter's syndrome
Psoriatic arthritis
Juvenile rheumatoid arthritis
Infectious arthritis
6. *Uniform swelling of a digit*
Infectious arthritis
Psoriatic arthritis
Reiter's syndrome
Neurotrophic arthritis
7. *Arthritis mutilans*
Rheumatoid arthritis
Juvenile rheumatoid arthritis
Psoriatic arthritis
Leprosy
Diabetes mellitus
Chronic infection
Lipoid dermatoarthritis
8. *Relative absence of erosions in hands*
Systemic lupus erythematosus
Jaccoud's arthritis
Reiter's syndrome
9. *Enlarged or irregular epiphyseal ossification centers*
Juvenile rheumatoid arthritis
Hemophilia
Juvenile tuberculous arthritis
10. *"Cystic" lesions in humeral head*
Rheumatoid arthritis
Lipoid dermatoarthritis
Gout
Hemophilia
Ankylosing spondylitis
Osteoarthritis (rare)
11. *Atlantoaxial subluxation*
Rheumatoid arthritis
Juvenile rheumatoid arthritis
Psoriatic arthritis

Mongoloidism
Congenital hypoplasia or absence of the dens
Ankylosing spondylitis (rare)
Systemic lupus erythematosus
Morquio's syndrome
12. *Sacroiliac fusion*
Ankylosing spondylitis (almost always symmetrical)
Juvenile rheumatoid arthritis
Reiter's syndrome (may be asymmetrical)
Psoriatic arthritis (may be asymmetrical)
Enteropathic arthritis
Polyvinyl chloride intoxication
Relapsing polychondritis
Gaucher's disease
Paraplegia
Rheumatoid arthritis (rare and asymmetrical)
13. *Asymmetrical sacroiliac destruction*
Tuberculosis
Pyogenic arthritis
Gout
14. *Migration of femoral head*
Rheumatoid arthritis—inward
Paget's arthritis—inward
Osteoarthritis—outward
15. *Erosion of intercondylar notch of knee*
Hemophilia
Juvenile rheumatoid arthritis
Tuberculous arthritis
16. *Tibiotalar slant*
Hemophilia
Juvenile rheumatoid arthritis
Multiple epiphyseal dysplasia
17. *Calcaneal erosions*
Rheumatoid arthritis
Ankylosing spondylitis
Reiter's syndrome
Psoriatic arthritis
Lipoid dermatoarthritis
Hyperparathyroidism
18. *Premature degenerative joint disease*
Chondromalacia patellae
Ochronosis
Wilson's disease
Hemochromatosis
Neuropathic arthropathy
Kashin–Beck disease
19. *Spinal spurs*
See illustration (Fig. 9–222)
20. *Some changes in the hand*
See short atlas of hand radiographs (Fig. 9–223)

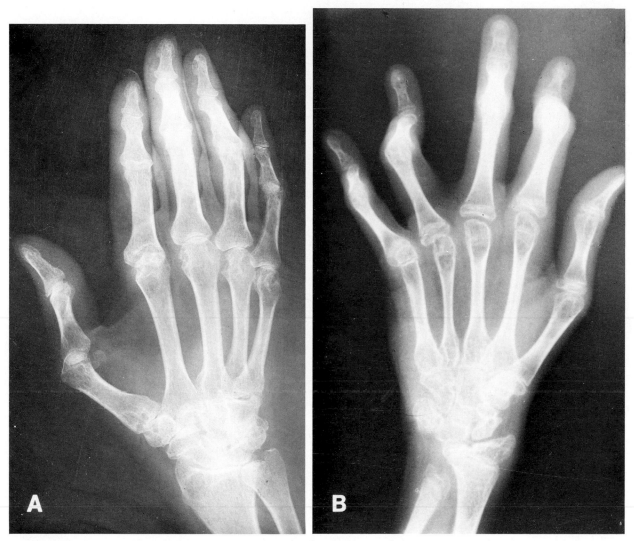

FIG. 9–223. A short atlas of hand radiographs. **A.** Rheumatoid arthritis. **B.** Juvenile rheumatoid arthritis. **C.** Psoriatic arthritis. **D.** Systemic lupus erythematosus. **E.** Gout. **F.** Enchondromatosis. **G.** Metastases. **H.** Sarcoidosis. **I.** Osteoarthritis. **J.** Hemochromatosis. **K.** Leprosy. **L.** Pigmented villonodular synovitis. **M.** Burns. **N.** Infectious arthritis. **O.** Acromegaly. **P.** Macrodactyly. **Q.** "Freiberg's" of hand. **R.** Pulmonary hypertrophic osteoarthropathy. **S.** Terminal phalangeal osteosclerosis. **T.** Scleroderma. **U.** Thyroid acropachy. **V.** Hemangiomatosis. **W.** Calcinosis universalis. **X.** Paget's disease.

(Continued)

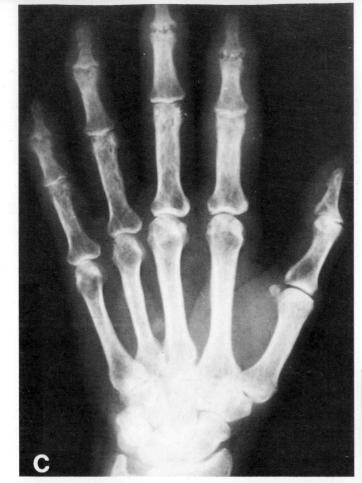

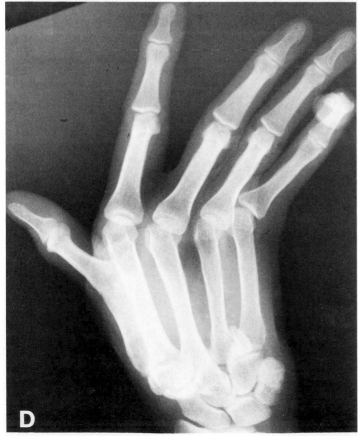

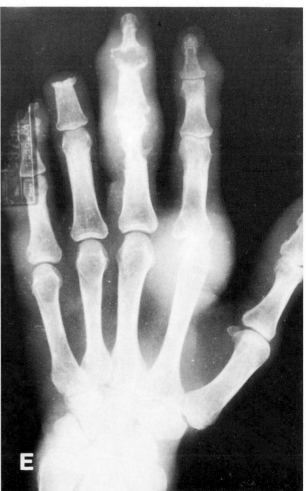

(Continued)

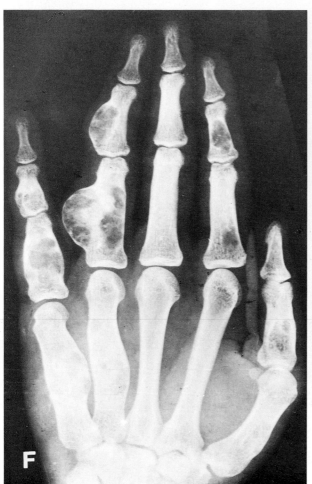

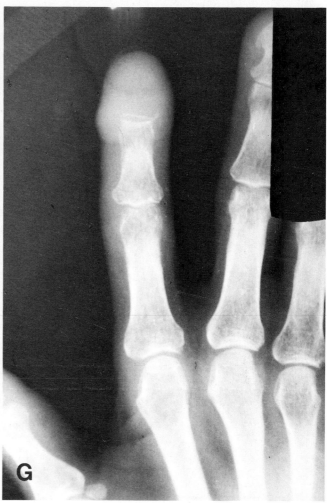

(Continued)

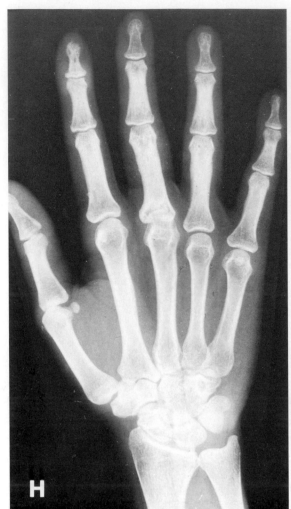
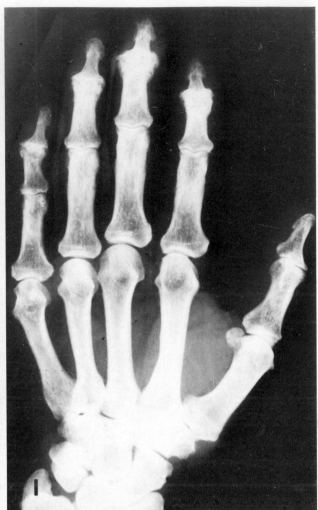

(Continued)

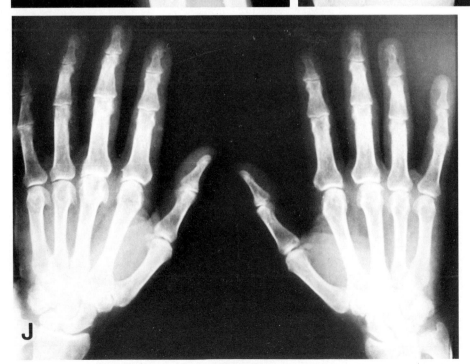

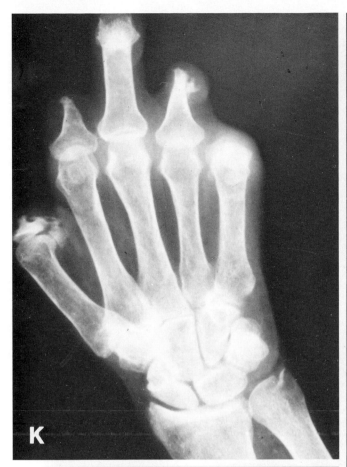

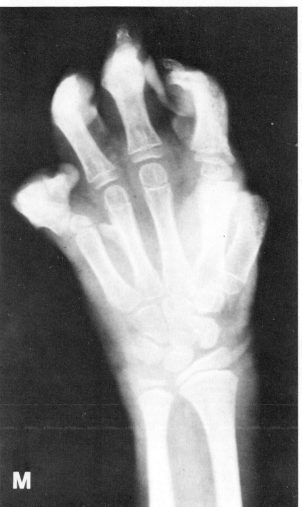

(Continued)

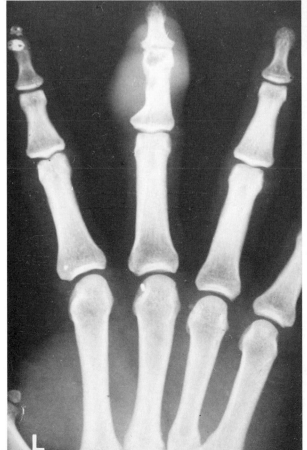

827

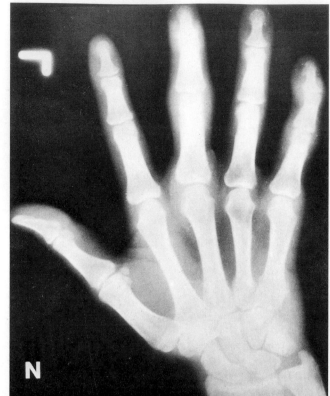

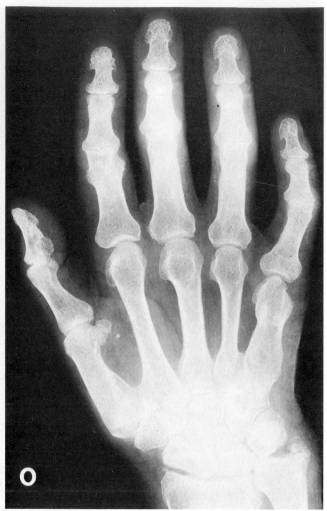

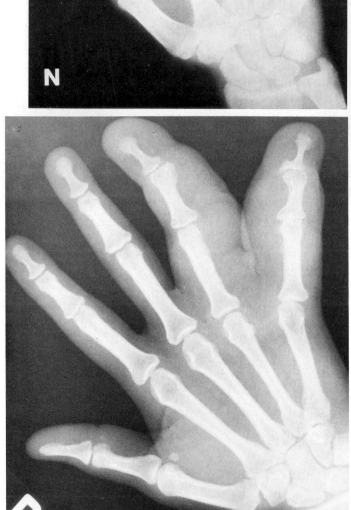

(Continued)

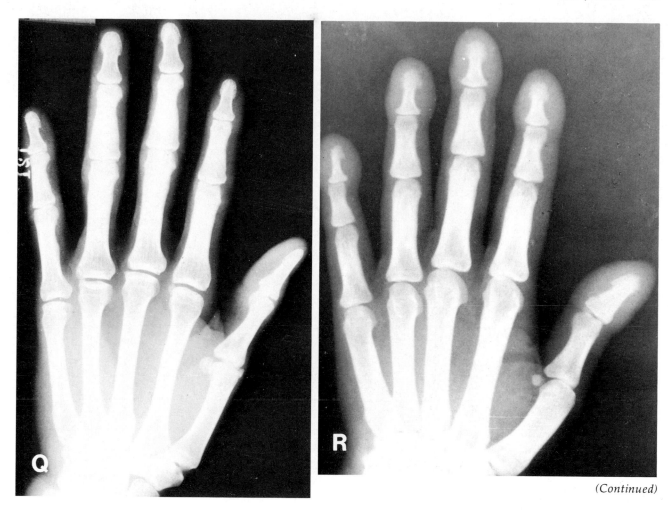

(Continued)

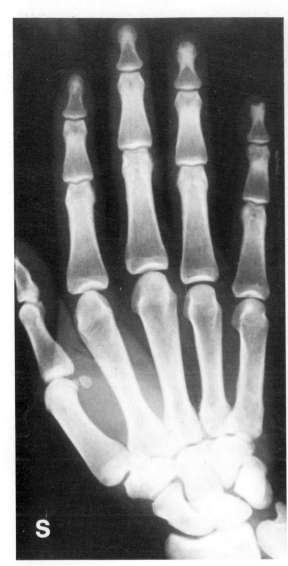

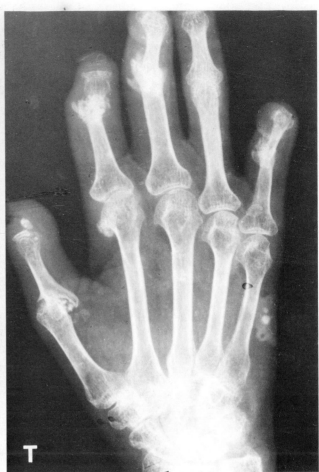

(Continued)

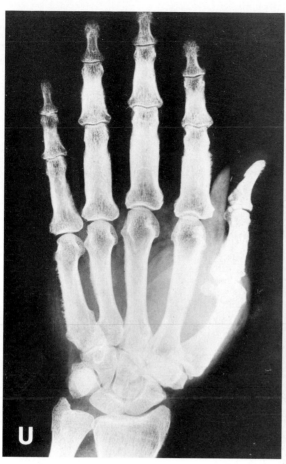

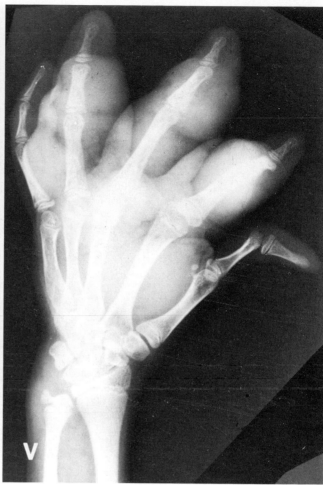

(Continued)

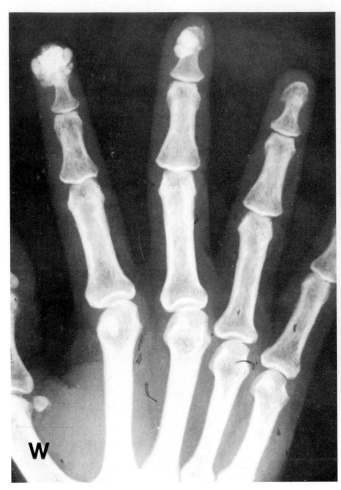

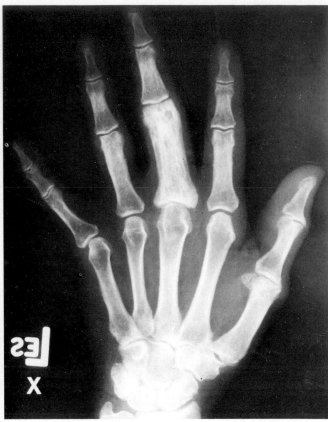

REFERENCES

1. Aegerter E, Kirkpatrick J A: Orthopedic Diseases, 4th ed. Philadelphia, W B Saunders, 1975

2. Aichroth P, Branfoot A C, Huskisson E C, Loughride L W: Destructive joint changes following kidney transplantation. J Bone Joint Surg 53–B:488–494, 1971

3. Akhtar M et al: Synovial chondromatosis of the temporomandibular joint. Report of a case. J Bone Joint Surg 59–A:266–267, 1977

4. Aksoy M, Camli N, Dincol K, Erdem S, Akgun T: Osseous changes in Wilson's disease. A radiologic study of 9 patients. Radiology 102:505–510, 1972

5. Alarcon–Segovia D, Cetina J A, Diaz–Jovanen E: Sacroiliac joints in primary gout: Clinical and roentgenographic study of 143 patients. Am J Roentgen 118:438–443, 1973

6. Anderson J, Stewart A M: The significance of the magnitude of the medial hip joint space. Brit J Radiol 43:238–239, 1970

7. Ansell B M, Kent P A: Radiological changes in juvenile chronic polyarthritis. Skel Rad 1:129–144, 1977

8. Armbuster T G: Extra-articular manifestations of septic arthritis of the glenohumeral joint. Am J Roentgen 129:667–672, 1977

9. Armbuster T G et al: The adult hip: An anatomic study. Part I: The bony landmarks. Radiology 128:1–10, 1978

10. Armstrong P, Saxton H: Iliopsoas bursa. Brit J Radiol 45:493–495, 1972

11. Arnold W D, Hilgartner M W: Hemophilic arthropathy. J Bone Joint Surg 59–A:287–305, 1977

12. Arnoldi C C, Linderholm H, Mussbichler H: Venous engorgement and intraosseous hypertension in osteoarthritis of the hip. J Bone Joint Surg 54–B:409–421, 1972

13. Atkins C J, McIvor J, Smith P M: Chondrocalcinosis and arthropathy: Studies in haemochromatosis and in idiopathic chondrocalcinosis. Quart J Med 39:71–82, 1970

14. Avila R, Pugh D G, Slocumb C H, Winkelmann R K: Psoriatic arthritis. A roentgenologic study. Radiology 75:691–701, 1960

15. Bachynski J E: An expanding lesion of the intervertebral disc in a case of ankylosing spondylitis. J Canad Assn Radiol 21:110–112, 1970

16. Baker S B, Robinson D R: Sympathetic joint effusion in septic arthritis. JAMA 240:1989, 1979

17. Banna M, Foster J B: Roentgenologic features of acrodystrophic neuropathy. Am J Roentgen 115:186–190, 1972

18. Bentley G, Goodfellow J W: Disorganization of the knees following intra-articular hydrocortisone injections. J Bone Joint Surg 51–B:498–502, 1969

19. Beren D L: Roentgen features of ankylosing spondylitis. Clin Orthop 74:20–33, 1971

20. Berney S, Goldstein M, Bishko F: Clinical and diagnostic features of tuberculous arthritis. Am J Med 53:36–42, 1972

21. Bleifeld C J, Inglis A E: The hand in systemic lupus erythematosus. J Bone Joint Surg 56–A:1207–1215, 1974

22. Bluestone R, Bywaters E G L, Hartog M, Holt P J L: Acromegalic arthropathy. Ann Rheum Dis 30:243–258, 1972

22a. Bonavita J A, Dalinka M K, Schumacher H R Jr: Hydroxyapatite deposition disease. Radiology 134:621–625, 1980

23. Brant E E, Jordan H H: Radiologic aspects of hemophilic pseudotumors in bone. Am J Roentgen 115:525–539, 1972

24. Brodey P A: Multicentric reticulohistiocytosis: A rare cause of destructive polyarthritis. Radiology 114:327–328, 1975

25. Brodey P A, Wolff S M: Radiographic changes in the sacroiliac joints in familial Mediterranean fever. Radiology 114:331–333, 1975

26. Brower A C: Rheumatoid nodulosis: Another cause of juxtaarticular nodules. Radiology 125:669–670, 1977

27. Bruckner F E, Kendall B E: Neuroarthropathy in Charcot–Marie–Tooth disease. Ann Rheum Dis 28:577–583, 1969

28. Bunch T W, Hunder G G: Ankylosing spondylitis and primary hyperparathyroidism. JAMA 225:1108–1109, 1973

29. Bunton R W, Grennan D M, Palmer D G: Lateral subluxation of the atlas in rheumatoid arthritis. Brit J Radiol 51:963–967, 1978

30. Burgan D W: Lipoma aborescens of the knee. Another cause of filling defects on a knee arthrogram. Radiology 101:583–584, 1971

31. Bywaters E G L: Still's disease in the adult. Ann Rheum Dis 30:138–148, 1971

32. Bywaters E G L, Hamilton E B D, Williams R: The spine in idiopathic haemochromatosis. Ann Rheum Dis 30:453–465, 1971

33. Campbell J B, Reeder M M, Sewell J: Lymphoma cutis with osseous involvement. Radiology 103:99–100, 1972

34. Campbell W L, Feldman F: Bone and soft-tissue abnormalities of the upper extremity in diabetes mellitus. Am J Roentgen 124:7–16, 1975

35. Carter A R, Liyanage S P: Large subarticular cysts (geodes) adjacent to the knee joint in rheumatoid arthritis. Clin Rad 26:353–538, 1975

36. Cecil R L, Loeb R F: A Textbook of Medicine, 13th ed. Philadelphia, W B Saunders, 1971

37. Chaplin D M: The pattern of bone and cartilage damage in the rheumatoid knee. J Bone Joint Surg 53–B:711–717, 1971

38. Chevrot A, Correas G, Pallardy G: Atteinte cervicale de la polyarthrite rhumatoide. J Radiol Electrol 59:545–550, 1978

39. Chlosta E M, Kuhns L R, Holt J F: The "patellar ratio" in hemophilia and juvenile rheumatoid arthritis. Radiology 116:137–138, 1975

40. Clark R L, Muhletaler C A, Margulies S I: Colitic arthritis. Clinical and radiographic manifestations. Radiology 101:585–594, 1971

41. Clouse M E, Gramm H F, Legg M, Flood T: Diabetic osteoarthropathy: Clinical and roentgenographic observations in 90 cases. Am J Roentgen 121:22–34, 1974

42. Collins L C, Lidsky L D, Sharp J T, Moreland J: Malposition of carpal bones in rheumatoid arthritis. Radiology 103:95–98, 1972

43. Conn H F, Conn R B: Current Diagnosis. Philadelphia, W B Saunders, 1974

44. Crellin R Q, Maccabe J J, Hamilton E B D: Severe subluxation of the cervical spine in rheumatoid arthritis. J Bone Joint Surg 52–B:244–251, 1970

45. Crosby E B, Inglis A, Bullough P G: Multiple joint involvement with pigmented villonodular synovitis. Radiology 122:671–672, 1977

46. Cummings J K, Taleisnik J: Peripheral gangrene as a complication of rheumatoid arthritis. Report of a case and review of the literature. J Bone Joint Surg 53–A:1001–1006, 1971

47. Davis S, Lawton G, Lowy M: Pigmented villonodular synovitis: Bone involvement of the fingers. Clin Rad 26:357–361, 1975

48. DeSmet A A, Ting Y M, Weiss J J: Shoulder arthrography in rheumatoid arthritis. Radiology 116:601–605, 1975

49. Dihlmann W, Delling G: Discovertebral destructive lesions (so-called Anderson lesions) associated with ankylosing spondylitis. Skel Rad 3:10–16, 1978

50. Dodds W J, Steinback H L: Primary hyperparathyroidism and articular cartilage calcification. Am J Roentgen 104:884–892, 1968

51. Dodds W J, Steinbach H L: Triangular cartilage calcification in the wrists: Its incidence in elderly patients. Am J Roentgen 105:850–852, 1969

52. Drummond R P, Rose G K: A 21-year review of a case of congenital indifference to pain. J Bone Joint Surg 57–B:241–243, 1975

53. Dryer R F, Goellner P G, Carney A S: Lyme arthritis in Wisconsin. JAMA 241:498–499, 1979

54. Dunn E J, McGauran M H, Nelson P, Greer R B: Synovial chondrosarcoma. Report of a case. J Bone Joint Surg 56–A:811–813, 1974

55. Dunn W A, Whisler J H: Synovial chondromatosis of the knee with associated extracapsular chondromas. J Bone Joint Surg 55–A:1747–1748, 1973

56. Edeiken J, Hodes P J: Roentgen Diagnosis of Diseases of Bone, 2nd ed. Baltimore, Williams & Wilkins, 1973

57. Eisenberg K S, Johnston J O: Synovial chondromatosis of the hip joint presenting as an intrapelvic mass. A case report. J Bone Joint Surg 54–A:176–178, 1972

58. Eisenberg R L, Hedgecock M U: Bilateral pigmented villonodular synovitis of the hip. Brit J Radiol 51:916, 1978

59. El-Khoury G Y, Mickelson M R: Chondrolysis following slipped capital femoral epiphysis. Radiology 123:327–330, 1977

60. Epstein B S, Epstein J A, Jones M D: Lumbar spinal stenosis. Radiol Clin N Amer 15:227–239, 1977

61. Fabricant M S, Chandor S B, Friou G J: Still disease in adults. A cause of prolonged undiagnosed fever. JAMA 225:273–276, 1973

62. Forbes C D et al: Bilateral pseudotumors of the pelvis in a patient with Christmas disease: With notes on localization by radioactive scanning and ultrasonography. Am J Roentgen 121:173–176, 1974

63. Forrest J, Staple T W: Synovial hemangioma of the knee. Demonstration by arthrography and arteriography. Am J Roentgen 112:512–516, 1971

64. Forrester D M, Brown J C, Nesson J W: The Radiology of Joint Disease, 2nd ed. Philadelphia, W B Saunders, 1978

65. Forrester D M, Magre G: Migrating bone shards in dissecting Charcot joints. Am J Roentgen 130:133–136, 1978

66. Frank P, Gleeson J A: Destructive vertebral lesions in ankylosing spondylitis. Brit J Radiol 48:755–758, 1975

67. Fredensborg N, Nilsson B E: The joint space in normal hip radiographs, Radiology 126:325–326, 1978

68. Friedman A C, Naidich T P: The fabella sign: Fabella displacement in synovial effusion and popliteal fossa masses. Radiology 127:113–121, 1978

69. Gehweiler J A, Wilson J W: Diffuse biarticular pigmented villonodular synovitis. Radiology 93:845–852, 1969

70. Gelman M I, Umber J S: Fractures of the thoracolumbar spine in ankylosing spondylitis. Am J Roentgen 130:485–491, 1978

71. Gelman M I, Ward J R: Septic arthritis: A complication of rheumatoid arthritis. Radiology 122:17–23, 1977

72. Giesecke S B, Dalinka M K, Kyle G C: Lisfrancs fracture-dislocation: A manifestation of peripheral neuropathy. Am J Roentgen 131:139–141, 1978

73. Gilchrist G S, Hajedory A B, Stauffer R N: Severe degenerative joint disease, mild and moderately severe hemophilia. JAMA 238:2383–2385, 1977

74. Giustra P E, Furman R S, Roberts L, Killoran P J: Synovial osteochondromatosis involving the elbow. Am J Roentgen 127:347–348, 1976

75. Glassberg G B, Ozonoff M B: Arthrographic findings in septic arthritis of the hip in infants. Radiology 128:151–155, 1978

76. Glay A, Rona G: Nodular rheumatoid vertebral lesions versus ankylosing spondylitis. Am J Roentgen 94:631–638, 1965

77. Gold R H, Metzger A L, Mirra J N, Weinberger H J, Killegrew K: Multicentric reticulohystiocytosis (lipoid dermatoarthritis): An erosive polyarthritis with distinctive clinical, roentgenographic, and pathological features. Am J Roentgen 124:610–624, 1975

78. Goldblatt M, Cremin B J: Osteoarticular tuberculosis: Its presentation in coloured races. Clin Radiol 29:669–677, 1978

79. Goldman A B, Schneider R, Martel W: Acute chondrolysis complicating slipped capital femoral epiphysis. Am J Roentgen 130:945–950, 1978

80. Gottlieb N L, Gray R G: Allopurinol-associated hand and foot deformities in chronic tophaceous gout. JAMA 238:1663–1664, 1977

81. Grauthoff H et al: Haemophilic pseudotumours and iliac haematomas: Radiological and clinical findings. Fortschr Roentgenstr 129:614–620, 1978

82. Greenspan A, Norman A, Tchans F K: Tooth sign in patellar degenerative disease. J Bone Joint Surg 59–A:483–485, 1977

83. Greenway G: Carpal involvement in inflammatory (erosive) osteoarthritis. J Canad Assn Rad 30:95–98, 1979

84. Griffiths H E D, Jones D M: Pyogenic infection of the spine. J Bone Joint Surg 53–B:383–391, 1971

85. Griffiths H J, Rossini A A: A case of lipoatrophic diabetes. Radiology 114:329–330, 1975

86. Grossman R E, Hensley G T: Bone lesions in primary amyloidosis. Am J Roentgen 101:872–875, 1967

87. Guerra J et al: The adult hip: An anatomic study. Part II: The soft-tissue landmarks. Radiology 128:11–20, 1978

88. Gutman A B: Views on the pathogenesis and management of primary gout – 1971. J Bone Joint Surg 54–A:357–372, 1972

89. Hall F M: Radiographic diagnosis and accuracy in knee joint effusions. Radiology 115:49–54, 1975

90. Hardin J G: Occult chronic septic arthritis due to proteus mirabilis. JAMA 240:1889–1890, 1978

91. Harris R D, Hecht H L: Suprapatellar effusions. A new diagnostic sign. Radiology 97:1–4, 1970

92. Harrison M O, Freiberger R H, Ranawat C S: Arthrography of the rheumatoid wrist joint. Am J Roentgen 112:480–486, 1971

93. Harrison R B: Charcot's joint: Two new observations. Am J Roentgen 128:807–809, 1977

94. Hermodsson I: Roentgen appearances of arthritis of the hip. Acta Radiol 12:865–881, 1972

95. Hirsch J H, Killien F C, Troupin R H: The arthropathy of hemochromatosis. Radiology 118:591–596, 1976

96. Hoaglund F T: Osteoarthritis. Orthop Clin N Amer 2:3–18, 1971

97. Hollander J L, McCarty D J: Arthritis and Allied Conditions, 8th ed. Philadelphia, Lea & Febriger, 1972

98. Holm C L: Primary synovial chondromatosis of the ankle. J Bone Joint Surg 58–A:878–880, 1970

99. Horowitz A L, Resnick I, Watson R C: The roentgen features of synovial sarcomas. Clin Rad 24:481–484, 1973

100. Jackman R J, Pugh D G: The positive elbow fat pad sign in rheumatoid arthritis. Am J Roentgen 108:812–818, 1970

101. Jaffe H L: Tumors and Tumorous Conditions of the Bones and Joints. Philadelphia, Lea & Febiger, 1958

102. Jaffe H L: Metabolic, Degenerative, and Inflammatory Diseases of Bones and Joints. Philadelphia, Lea & Febiger, 1972

103. Jeffery A K: Osteogenesis in the osteoarthritic femoral head. J Bone Joint Surg 55–B:262–272, 1973

104. Jensen P S: Hemochromatosis: A disease often silent but not invisible. Am J Roentgen 126:343–351, 1976

105. Jensen P S, Putman C E: Chondrocalcinosis and haemophilia. Clin Rad 28:401–405, 1977

106. Jensen P S, Putman C E: Current concepts with respect to chondrocalcinosis and the pseudogout syndrome. Am J Roentgen 123:531–539, 1975

107. Jergesen H E, Mankin J H, Schiller A L: Diffuse pigmented villonodular synovitis of the knee mimicking primary bone neoplasm. A report of 2 cases. J Bone Joint Surg 60–A:825–829, 1978

108. Jimenea C V, Frame B, Chaykin L B, Sigler J W: Spondylitis of hypoparathyroidism. Clin Orthrop 74:84–89, 1971

109. Johnson C, Kersley G D, Airth G R: Rib lesions in rheumatoid disease. Brit J Radiol 43:269–270, 1970

110. Jones B S: Doigt-en-lorgnette and concentric bone atrophy associated with healed yaws osteitis. J Bone Joint Surg 54–B:341–345, 1972

111. Kanefield D G et al: Destructive lesions of the spine in rheumatoid ankylosing spondylitis. J Bone Joint Surg 51–A:1369–1375, 1969

112. Kaye J J, Winchester P H, Freiberger R H: "Neonatal septic dislocation" of the hip: True dislocation or pathological epiphyseal separation. Radiology 114:671–674, 1975

113. Kelly P J, Martin W J, Coventry M B: Bacterial (suppurative) arthritis in the adult. J Bone Joint Surg 52–A:1595–1602, 1970

114. Kidd K L, Peter J B: Erosive osteoarthritis. Radiology 86:640–647, 1966

115. Kido D, Bryan D, Halpern M: Hematogenous osteomyelitis in drug addicts. Am J Roentgen 118:356–363, 1973

116. Killebrew K, Gold R H, Sholkoff S D: Psoriatic spondylitis. Radiology 108:9–16, 1973

117. Kindblom L G, Gunterberg G: Pigmented villonodular synovitis involving bone. A case report. J Bone Joint Surg 60–A:830–832, 1978

118. Kirkaldy–Willis W H: Lecture series. University Hospital, Saskatchewan, Canada

119. Kleinman P et al: Juvenile ankylosing spondylitis. Radiology 125:775–780, 1977

120. Korn J A, Gilbert M S, Siffert R S, Jacobson J H: Clostridium welchii arthritis. A case report. J Bone Joint Surg 57–A:555–557, 1975

121. Kraft E, Spyropoulos E, Finby N: Neurogenic disorders of the foot in diabetes mellitus. Am J Roentgen 124:17–24, 1975

122. Kreel L, Urguhart W: Two unusual radiologic features in rheumatoid arthritis. Brit J Radiol 36:715–719, 1963

123. Lachman R S, Yamauchi T, Klein J: Neonatal systemic candidiasis and arthritis. Radiology 105:631–632, 1972

124. Lambeth J T, Burns–Cox C J, MacLean R: Sacroiliac gout associated with hemoglobin E and hypersplenism. Radiology 95:413–415, 1970

125. Landells J W: The bone cysts of osteoarthritis. J Bone Joint Surg 35–B:643–649, 1953

126. Lapayouker M S, Miller W T, Levy W M, Harwick R D: Pigmented villonodular synovitis of the temporomandibular joint. Radiology 108:313–316, 1973

127. Larsen I J, Landry R M: Hemangioma of the synovial membrane. J Bone Joint Surg 51–A:1210–1212, 1969

128. Laskar F J, Sargison K D: Ochronotic arthropathy. A review with 4 case reports. J Bone Joint Surg 52–B:653–666, 1970

129. Latchaw R E, Meyer G W: Reiter disease with atlantoaxial subluxation. Radiology 126:303–304, 1978

130. Levitin P M, Gough W W, Davis J S: HLA-B27 antigen in women with ankylosing spondylitis. JAMA 235:2621–2622, 1976

131. Levitin P M, Keats T E: Dissecting synovial cyst of the popliteal space in gout. Am J Roentgen 124:32–33, 1975

132. Levy M, Seelenfreund M, Maur P, Fried A, Lurie M: Bilateral spontaneous and simultaneous rupture of the quadriceps tendon in gout. J Bone Joint Surg 53–B:510–513, 1971

133. Liggett A S, Silberman Z: Blastomycosis of the knee joint. A case report. J Bone Joint Surg 52–A:1445–1449, 1970

134. Linquist P R, McDonnell D E: Rheumatoid cyst causing extradural compression. J Bone Joint Surg 52–A:1235–1240, 1970

135. Lynn M D, Lee J: Periarticular tenosynovial chondrometaplasia. Report of a case at the wrist. J Bone Joint Surg 54–A:650–652, 1972

136. Lyon L J, Nevins M A: Carcinoma of the colon presenting as pyogenic arthritis. JAMA 241:2060, 1979

137. Macnab I: The traction spur. An indicator of segmental instability. J Bone Joint Surg 53–A:663–670, 1971

138. Mäkëla P, Haaslanti J O: Immersion technique in soft-tissue radiography of the hands. Acta Rad (Diagn) 19:89–96, 1978

139. Mäkëla P, Virtama P: "The Preerosive" radiologic signs of rheumatoid arthritis in soft-tissue radiography of the hands. Skel Rad 2:213–220, 1978

140. Mankin H J, Dorfman H, Lippiello L, Zarins A: Biochemical and metabolic abnormalities in articular cartilage from osteoarthritic human hips. II. Correlation of morphology with biochemical and metabolic data. J Bone Joint Surg 53–A:523–537, 1971

141. Mankin H J, Lippiello L: Biochemical and metabolic abnormalities in articular cartilage from osteoarthritic human hips. J Bone Joint Surg 52–A:424–434, 1970

142. Marmor L: Osteoarthritis of the knee. JAMA 218:213–215, 1971

143. Martel W: The pattern of rheumatoid arthritis in the hand and wrist. Radiol Clin N Amer 2:221–234, 1964

144. Martel W: The overhanging margin of bone. A roentgenologic manifestation of gout. Radiology 91:755–756, 1968

145. Martel W et al: Radiologic features of Reiter disease. Radiology 132:1–10, 1979

146. Martel W, Abell M R, Duff I F: Cervical spine involvement in lipoid-dermato-arthritis. Radiology 77:613–617, 1961

147. Martel W, Champion C K, Thompson G R, Carter T L: A roentgenologically distinctive arthropathy in some patients with the pseudogout syndrome. Am J Roentgen 109:587–605, 1970

148. Martel W, Hayes J T, Duff I F: The pattern of bone erosion in the hand and wrist in rheumatoid arthritis. Radiology 84:204–214, 1965

149. Martel W, Holt J F, Cassidy J T: Roentgenologic manifestations of juvenile rheumatoid arthritis. Am J Roentgen 88:400–423, 1962

150. Martel W, Snarr J W, Horn J R: The metacarpophalangeal joints in interphalangeal osteoarthritis. Radiology 108:1–7, 1973

151. McMaster M: The natural history of the rheumatoid metacarpo-phalangeal joint. J Bone Joint Surg 54–B:687–697, 1972

152. Meachim G, Hardinge K, Williams D R: Methods for correlating pathological and radiological findings in osteoarthrosis of the hip. Brit J Radiol 45:670–676, 1972

153. Meeks L W, Renshaw T S: Vertebral osteophytosis and dysphagia. Two case reports of the syndrome recently termed ankylosing hyperostosis. J Bone Joint Surg 55–A:197–201, 1973

154. Middlemiss J H, Raper A B: Skeletal changes in the hemoglobinopathies. J Bone Joint Surg 48–B:693–702, 1966

155. Milgram J W: Synovial osteochondromatosis: A histopathological study of 30 cases. J Bone Joint Surg 59–A:792–801, 1977

156. Milgram J W, Addison R G: Synovial osteochondromatosis of the knee. Chondromatous recurrence with possible chondrosarcomatous degeneration. J Bone Joint Surg 58–B:264–266, 1976

157. Miller J L, Soltani K, Tourtellotte C D: Psoriatic acroosteolysis without arthritis. A case study. J Bone Joint Surg 53–A:371–374, 1971

158. Mills K: Pathology of the knee joint in rheumatoid arthritis. J Bone Joint Surg 52–B:746–756, 1970

159. Mindelzun R, Elkin M, Scheinberg I H, Sternlieb I: Skeletal changes in Wilson's disease. Radiology 94:127–132, 1970

160. Moore S B: H L A. Mayo Clin Proc 54:385–393, 1979

161. Moseley J E: Bone Changes in Hematological Disorders. New York, Grune & Stratton, 1963

162. Mosher J F, Kettlekamp O B, Crawford J C: Intracapsular or paraarticular chondroma. A report of 3 cases. J Bone Joint Surg 48–A:1561–1569, 1966

163. Mueller C E, Seeger J F, Martel W: Ankylosing spondylitis and regional enteritis. Radiology 112:579–581, 1974

164. Murphy W A, Siegel M J: Elbow fat pads with new signs and extended differential diagnosis. Radiology 124:659–665, 1977

165. Murphy W A, Siegel M J, Gilula L A: Arthrography in the diagnosis of unexplained chronic hip pain with regional osteopenia. Am J Roentgen 129:283–287, 1977

166. Murphy W A, Staple T W: Jaccoud's arthropathy reviewed. Am J Roentgen 118:300–307, 1973

167. Murray R O: The aetiology of primary osteoarthritis of the hip. Brit J Radiol 38:810–824, 1965

168. Murray R O, Duncan C: Athletic activity in adolescence as an etiological factor in degenerative hip disease. J Bone Joint Surg 53–B:406–419, 1971

169. Müssbichler H: Arteriographic findings in patients with degenerative osteoarthritis of the hip. Radiology 107:21–27, 1973

170. Neuhauser E B D, Wittenborg M H: Synovitis of the hips in infancy and childhood. Radiol Clin N Amer 1:13–16, 1963

171. Nolan B, Leers W D, Schatzker J: Septic arthritis of the knee due to clostridium bifermentans. Report of a case. J Bone Joint Surg 54–A:1275–1278, 1972

172. Noonan C D, Odone D T, Engelman E P, Splitter S D: Roentgen manifestations of joint disease in systemic lupus erythematosus. Radiology 80:837–843, 1963

173. Norenberg D D: Corynebacterium pyogenes septic arthritis with plasma-cell synovial infiltrate and monoclonal gammopathy. Arch Int Med 138:810–811, 1978

174. Norgaard F: Earliest roentgen changes in polyarthritis of the rheumatoid type. Continued investigations. Radiology 92:299–303, 1969

175. O'Connell D J, Bennett R M: Mixed connective tissue disease: Clinical and radiological aspects of 20 cases. Brit J Radiol 50:620–625, 1977

176. O'Connell D J, Marx W J: Hand changes in primary biliary cirrhosis. Radiogy 129:31–35, 1978

177. Outerbridge R E: The etiology of chondromalacia patellae. J Bone Joint Surg 43–B:752–757, 1961

178. Pastershank S P, Mitchell D M: Knee joint bursal abnormalities in rheumatoid arthritis. J Canad Assn Rad 28:199–203, 1977

179. Patton J T: Differential diagnosis of inflammatory spondylitis. Skel Rad 1:77–85, 1976

180. Pearson K D, Wells S A, Keiser H R: Familial medullary carcinoma of the thyroid, adrenal pheochromocytoma, and parathyroid hyperplasia. Radiology 107:249–255, 1973

181. Peavy P W, Franco D J: Gout: Presentation as a popliteal cyst. Radiology 111:103–104, 1974

182. Peitzman S J et al: Charcot arthropathy secondary to amyloid neuropathy. JAMA 235:1345–1347, 1976

183. Pellici P M, Wilson P D: Chondrolysis of the hips associated with severe burns. J Bone Joint Surg 61–A:592–596, 1979

184. Perovic M N, Kopits S E, Thompson R C: Radiological evaluation of the spinal cord in congenital atlantoaxial dislocation. Radiology 109:713–716, 1973

185. Perri G: Widening of the radial notch of the ulna: A new articular change in haemophilia. Clin Rad 29:61–62, 1978

186. Prager R J, Mall J C: Arthrographic diagnosis of synovial chondromatosis. Am J Roentgen 127:344–346, 1976

187. Preger L et al: Roentgenographic skeletal changes in the glycogen storage diseases. Am J Roentgen 107:840–847, 1969

188. Price C H G, Goldie W: Paget's sarcoma of bone. A study of

80 cases from the Bristol and Leeds bone tumour registries. J Bone Joint Surg 51–B:205–224, 1969

189. Pudlowski R M, Gilula L A, Kyriakos M: Intraarticular lipoma with osseous metaplasia: Radiographic-pathologic correlation. Am J Roentgen 132:471–473, 1979

190. Rana N A, Nancock D O, Taylor A R, Hill A G S: Atlantoaxial subluxation in rheumatoid arthritis. J Bone Joint Surg 55–B:458–470, 1973

191. Rana N A, Hancock D O, Taylor A R, Hill A GS: Upward translocation of the dens in rheumatoid arthritis. J Bone Joint Surg 55–B:471–477, 1973

192. Rappaport A S, Sosman J L, Weissman B N: Lesions resembling gout in patients with rheumatoid arthritis. Am J Roentgen 126:41–45, 1976

193. Rappaport A S, Sosman J L, Weissman B N: Spontaneous fractures of the olecranon process in rheumatoid arthritis. Radiology 119:83–84, 1976

194. Resnick D: Roentgen features of the rheumatoid mid and hind foot. J Canad Assn Rad 27:99–107, 1976

195. Resnick D: Patterns of migration of the femoral head in osteoarthritis of the hip: Roentgenographic-pathologic correlation and comparison with rheumatoid arthritis. Am J Roentgen 124:62–74, 1975

196. Resnick D: Pyarthrosis complicating rheumatoid arthritis. Radiology 114:581–586, 1975

197. Resnick D: The interphalangeal joint of the great toe in rheumatoid arthritis. J Canad Assn Rad 26:255–262, 1975

198. Resnick D: Patterns of peripheral joint disease in ankylosing spondylitis. Radiology 110:523–532, 1974

199. Resnick D: Temporomandibular joint involvement in ankylosing spondylitis: Comparison with rheumatoid arthritis and psoriasis. Radiology 112:587–591, 1974

200. Resnick D et al: Association of diffuse idiopathic skeletal hyperostosis (DISH) and calcification and ossification of the posterior longitudinal ligament. Am J Roentgen 131:1049–1053, 1978

201. Resnick D et al: Osteolysis with detritic synovitis. A new syndrome. Arch Intern Med 138:1003–1005, 1978

202. Resnick D et al: Proximal tibiofibular joint: Anatomic pathologic-radiographic correlation. Am J Roentgen 131:133–138, 1978

203. Resnick D et al: Selective involvement of the first carpometacarpal joint in scleroderma. Am J Roentgen 131:283–286, 1978

204. Resnick D et al: Calcaneal abnormalities in articular disorders. Radiology 125:355–366, 1977

205. Resnick D et al: Clinical, radiographic, and pathologic abnormalities in calcium pyrophosphate dihydrate deposition disease (CPPD): Pseudogout. Radiology 122:1–15, 1977

206. Resnick D et al: Intra-articular calcification in scleroderma. Radiology 124:685–688, 1977

207. Resnick D et al: Clinical and radiographic abnormalities in ankylosing spondylitis. A comparison of men and women. Radiology 119:293–297, 1976

208. Resnick D, Broderick T W: Bony proliferation of terminal

toe phalanges in psoriasis: The "ivory" phalanx. J Canad Assn Rad 28:187–189, 1977

209. Resnick D, Gmelich J T: Bone fragmentation in the rheumatoid wrist. Radiographic and pathologic consideration. Radiology 114:315–321, 1975

210. Resnick D, Niwayama G: Resorption of the undersurface of the distal clavicle in rheumatoid arthritis. Radiology 120:75–77, 1976

211. Resnick D, Niwayama G, Goergen T G: Comparison of radiographic abnormalities of the sacroiliac joint in degenerative disease and ankylosing spondylitis. Am J Roentgen 128:189–196, 1977

212. Resnick D, Oliphant M: Hemophilialike arthropathy of the knee associated with cutaneous and synovial hemangiomas. Report of 3 cases and review. Radiology 114:323–326, 1975

213. Resnick D, Reinke R T, Taketa R M: Early-onset gouty arthritis. Radiology 114:67–73, 1975

214. Resnick D, Shaul S R, Robins J M: Diffuse idiopathic skeletal hyperostosis (DISH): Forrestier's disease with extraspinal manifestations. Radiology 115:513–524, 1975

215. Resnick D, Utsinger P D: The wrist arthropathy of "pseudogout" occurring with and without chondrocalcinosis. Radiology 113:633–641, 1974

216. Riley M J, Ansell B M, Bywaters E G L: Radiologic manifestations of ankylosing spondylitis according to age at onset. Ann Rheum Dis 30:138–148, 1971

217. Rivelis M, Freiberger R H: Vertebral destruction at unfused segments in late ankylosing spondylitis. Radiology 93:251–256, 1969

218. Rodnan G P (ed): Primer on the Rheumatic Diseases, 7th ed. JAMA (Suppl) 224:662–812, 1973

219. Rogala E J, Cruess R L: Multiple pyogenic arthritis due to serratia marcescens following renal homotransplantation. Report of a case. J Bone Joint Surg 54–A:1283–1287, 1972

220. Rombouts J J, Rombouts–Lindemans C: Scoliosis in juvenile rheumatoid arthritis. J Bone Joint Surg 56–B:478–483, 1974

221. Ross P, Wood B: Osteoarthropathy in idiopathic hemochromatosis. Am J Roentgen 109:575–580, 1970

222. Rothschild B M, Masi A T, June P L: Arthritis associated with ampicillin colitis. Arch Intern Med 137:1605–1607, 1977

223. Sandusky W R, Rudolf L E, Leavell B S: Splenectomy for control of neutropenia in Felty's syndrome. Ann Surg 167:744–751, 1968

224. Sarmiento A, Elkins R W: Giant intra-articular osteochondroma of the knee. A case report. J Bone Joint Surg 57–A:560–561, 1975

225. Schabel S I et al: Bone infarction in gout. Skel Rad 3:42–47, 1978

226. Schneider H J, King A Y, Bronson J L, Miller E H: Stress injuries and developmental change of lower extremities in ballet dancers. Radiology 113:627–632, 1974

227. Schneider R, Goldman A B, Bohne W H O: Neuropathic in-

juries to the lower extremities in children. Radiology 128:713–718, 1978

228. Schneider R, Kaye J J: Insufficiency and stress fractures of the long bones occurring in patients with rheumatoid arthritis. Radiology 116:595–599, 1975

229. Schumacher T M et al: HLA-B27 associated arthropathies. Radiology 126:289–297, 1978

230. Schwartzberg M et al: Rheumatoid arthritis and chronic gouty arthropathy. JAMA 240:2658–2659, 1978

231. Schwarz G S, Berenyi M R, Siegel M W: Atrophic arthropathy and diabetic neuritis. Am J Roentgen 106:523–529, 1969

232. Seligsohn R, Rippon J W, Lerner S A: Aspergillus terreus osteomyelitis. Arch Intern Med 137:918–920, 1977

233. Sella E J, Goodman A H: Arthropathy secondary to transfusion hemochromatosis. J Bone Joint Surg 55–A:1077–1081, 1973

234. Shawker T H, Dennis J M: Periarticular calcifications in pyogenic arthritis. Am J Roentgen 113:650–654, 1971

235. Sholkoff S D, Glickman M G, Steinbach H L: Roentgenology of Reiter's syndrome. Radiology 97:497–503, 1970

236. Siegelman S S, Heimann W G, Manin M C: Congenital indifference to pain. Am J Roentgen 97:242–250, 1966

237. Silver C M, Simon S D, Litchman H M, Dyckman J: Synovial chondromatosis of the temporomandibular joint. A case report. J Bone Joint Surg 53–A:777–780, 1971

238. Sivaramappa M, Reddy C R R M, Devi C S, Reddy A C, Reddy P K, Murthy D R: Acute guinea-worm synovitis of the knee joint. J Bone Joint Surg 51–A:1324–1330, 1969

239. Smith E E, Kurlander G J, Powell R C: Two rare causes of secondary gouty arthritis. Am J Roentgen 100:550–553, 1967

240. Smukler N M, Edeiken J, Guiliano V J: Ankylosis in osteoarthritis of the finger joints. Radiology 100:525–530, 1971

241. Solomon L: Patterns of osteoarthritis of the hip. J Bone Joint Surg 58–B:176–183, 1976

242. Staple T W: Arthrographic demonstration of iliopsoas bursa extension of the hip joint. Radiology 102:515–516, 1972

243. Steel W M, Duthie R B, O'Connor B T: Haemophilic cysts. J Bone Joint Surg 51–B:614–626, 1969

244. Sundaram M, Patton J T: Paravertebral ossification in psoriasis and Reiter's disease. Brit J Radiol 48:628–633, 1975

245. Swezey R L, Alexander S J: Erosive osteoarthritis and the main-en-lorgnette deformity (opera glass hand). Arch Intern Med 128:269–272, 1971

246. Thomas R H, Resnick D, Alazraki N P, Daniel D, Greenfield R: Compartmental evaluation of osteoarthritis of the knee. A comparative study of available diagnostic modalities. Radiology 116:585–594, 1975

247. Trentham D E, Masi A T: Chronic synovitis in gout simulating rheumatoid arthritis. JAMA 235:1358–1360, 1976

248. Tsukamoto Y, Onitsuka H, Lee K: Radiologic aspects of diffuse idiopathic skeletal hyperostosis in the spine. Am J Roentgen 129:913–918, 1977

249. Twersky J: Joint changes in idiopathic hemochromatosis. Am J Roentgen 124:139–144, 1975

250. Twigg H L, Smith B F: Jaccoud's arthritis. Radiology 80:417–421, 1963

251. Udoff E J, Genant H K, Kozin F, Ginsburg M: Mixed connective tissue disease. The spectrum of radiographic manifestations. Radiology 124:613–618, 1977

252. Utsinger P D et al: Roentgenologic, immunologic, and therapeutic study of erosive (inflammatory) osteoarthritis. Arch Intern Med 138:693–697, 1978

253. Wale J J, Hunt D D: Acute hematogenous pyarthrosis caused by hemophilus influenzae. J Bone Joint Surg 50–A:1657–1662, 1968

254. Wardle E N, Patton J T: Bone and joint changes in haemochromatosis. Ann Rheum Dis 28:15–23, 1969

255. Watt I, Middlemiss H: The radiology of gout. Clin Radiol 26:27–36, 1975

256. Weissman B N, Rappaport A S, Sossman J L, Schur P H: Radiographic findings in the hands in patients with systemic lupus erythematosus. Radiology 126:313–317, 1978

257. Weldon W V, Scalettar R: Roentgen changes in Reiter's syndrome. Am J Roentgen 86:344–350, 1961

258. Wesselius L J, Brooks R J, Gall E P: Vertebral coccidioidomycosis presenting as Pott's disease. JAMA 238:1397–1398, 1977

259. Weston W J: The intrasynovial fatty masses in chronic rheumatoid arthritis. Brit J Radiol 46:213–216, 1973

260. Wild W, Beetham W P: Erosive arthropathy in systemic scleroderma. JAMA 232:511–512, 1975

261. Wright V: Psoriatic arthritis: Comparative radiographic study of rheumatoid arthritis and arthritis associated with psoriasis. Ann Rheum Dis 20:123–132, 1961

262. Vinstein A L, Cockerill E M: Involvement of the spine in gout. A case report. Radiology 103:311–312, 1972

263. Yaghmai I, Rooholamini S M, Faunce H F: Unilateral rheumatoid arthritis. Protective effect of neurologic deficits. Am J Roentgen 128:299–301, 1977

INDEX